Retinal Disorders

Genetic Approaches to Diagnosis and Treatment

SECOND EDITION

A subject collection from *Cold Spring Harbor Perspectives in Medicine*

OTHER SUBJECT COLLECTIONS FROM *COLD SPRING HARBOR PERSPECTIVES IN MEDICINE*

Combining Human Genetics and Causal Inference to Understand Human Disease and Development
Lung Cancer: Disease Biology and Its Potential for Clinical Translation
Influenza: The Cutting Edge
Leukemia and Lymphoma: Molecular and Therapeutic Insights
Addiction, Second Edition
Hepatitis C Virus: The Story of a Scientific and Therapeutic Revolution
The PTEN Family
Metastasis: Mechanism to Therapy
Genetic Counseling: Clinical Practice and Ethical Considerations
Bioelectronic Medicine
Function and Dysfunction of the Cochlea: From Mechanisms to Potential Therapies
Next-Generation Sequencing in Medicine
Prostate Cancer
RAS and Cancer in the 21st Century
Enteric Hepatitis Viruses
Bone: A Regulator of Physiology
Multiple Sclerosis
Cancer Evolution

SUBJECT COLLECTIONS FROM *COLD SPRING HARBOR PERSPECTIVES IN BIOLOGY*

Synthetic Biology and Greenhouse Gases
Wound Healing: From Bench to Bedside
The Endoplasmic Reticulum, Second Edition
Sex Differences in Brain and Behavior
Regeneration
The Nucleus, Second Edition
Auxin Signaling: From Synthesis to Systems Biology, Second Edition
Stem Cells: From Biological Principles to Regenerative Medicine
Heart Development and Disease
Cell Survival and Cell Death, Second Edition
Calcium Signaling, Second Edition
Engineering Plants for Agriculture
Protein Homeostasis, Second Edition
Translation Mechanisms and Control
Cytokines
Circadian Rhythms
Immune Memory and Vaccines: Great Debates
Cell–Cell Junctions, Second Edition
Prion Biology

Retinal Disorders

Genetic Approaches to Diagnosis and Treatment

SECOND EDITION

A subject collection from *Cold Spring Harbor Perspectives in Medicine*

EDITED BY

Eyal Banin
*Hadassah-Hebrew University
Medical Center*

Jean Bennett
University of Pennsylvania

Jacque L. Duncan
*University of California,
San Francisco*

Botond Roska
*Institute of Molecular and
Clinical Ophthalmology Basel*

José-Alain Sahel
University of Pittsburgh

COLD SPRING HARBOR LABORATORY PRESS
Cold Spring Harbor, New York • www.cshlpress.org

Retinal Disorders: Genetic Approaches to Diagnosis and Treatment, Second Edition
A subject collection from *Cold Spring Harbor Perspectives in Medicine*
Articles online at www.perspectivesinmedicine.org

Executive Editor	Richard Sever
Project Supervisor	Barbara Acosta
Permissions Administrator	Carol Brown
Production Editor	Diane Schubach
Production Manager/Cover Designer	Denise Weiss
Publisher	John Inglis

Front cover artwork: The vision of a person affected by inherited retinal diseases can be improved by various genetic modifications including gene augmentation therapy, the use of SiRNA, gene editing, and more. Even in cases in which photoreceptors have largely degenerated leading to blindness, optogenetic therapy that renders the inner retina light sensitive can improve vision. (Illustration by Veronique Juvin, SciArtWork.)

Library of Congress Cataloging-in-Publication Data

Names: Banin, Eyal, editor. | Bennett, Jean, editor. | Duncan, Jacque L., editor. | Roska, Botond, editor. | Sahel, José-Alain, editor.
Title: Retinal disorders : genetic approaches to diagnosis and treatment / edited by Eyal Banin, Jean Bennett, Jacque L. Duncan, Botond Roska and Jose-Alain Sahel.
Other titles: Cold Spring Harbor Perspectives in Medicine.
Description: Second edition. | Cold Spring Harbor, New York : Cold Spring Harbor Laboratory Press, [2024] | A subject collection from Cold Spring Harbor Perspectives in Medicine. | Includes bibliographical references and index. | Summary: "The retina is a layer of neural tissue that lines the inner eye and captures visual stimuli. This volume provides an update on retinal diseases, describing the genetic and pathophysiological basis of the diseases and advances in strategies to treat them"-- Provided by publisher.
Identifiers: LCCN 2023032500 (print) | LCCN 2023032501 (ebook) | ISBN 9781621824626 (cloth) | ISBN 9781621824633 (epub)
Subjects: MESH: Retinal Diseases--genetics | Eye Diseases, Hereditary--therapy | Genetic Therapy--methods | Collected Work
Classification: LCC RE551 (print) | LCC RE551 (ebook) | NLM WW 5 | DDC 617.7/35042--dc23/eng/20231002
LC record available at https://lccn.loc.gov/2023032500
LC ebook record available at https://lccn.loc.gov/2023032501

10 9 8 7 6 5 4 3 2 1

All World Wide Web addresses are accurate to the best of our knowledge at the time of printing.

For a complete catalog of all Cold Spring Harbor Laboratory Press publications, visit our website at www.cshlpress.org.

Contents

Preface, ix

INTRODUCTION

The Extraordinary Phenotypic and Genetic Variability of Retinal and Macular Degenerations:
The Relevance to Therapeutic Developments, 1
Isabelle Audo, Marco Nassisi, Christina Zeitz, and José-Alain Sahel

GENETICS AND PATHOPHYSIOLOGY OF INHERITED RETINAL DEGENERATIONS

History of Finding Genes and Mutations Causing Inherited Retinal Diseases, 11
Stephen P. Daiger, Lori S. Sullivan, Elizabeth L. Cadena, and Sara J. Bowne

Comparison of Worldwide Disease Prevalence and Genetic Prevalence of Inherited
Retinal Diseases and Variant Interpretation Considerations, 23
Mor Hanany, Sapir Shalom, Tamar Ben-Yosef, and Dror Sharon

Rodent Models of Retinal Degeneration: From Purified Cells in Culture to
Living Animals, 35
*Valérie Fradot, Sébastien Augustin, Valérie Fontaine, Katia Marazova, Xavier Guillonneau,
José A. Sahel, and Serge Picaud*

Retinal Degeneration Animal Models in Bardet–Biedl Syndrome and
Related Ciliopathies, 51
Clarisse Delvallée and Hélène Dollfus

Canine and Feline Models of Inherited Retinal Diseases, 71
Simon M. Petersen-Jones and András M. Komáromy

Pig Models in Retinal Research and Retinal Disease, 91
Maureen A. McCall

Toward Retinal Organoids in High-Throughput, 109
Stefan Erich Spirig and Magdalena Renner

GENE-BASED THERAPIES

Overview of Retinal Gene Therapy: Current Status and Future Challenges, 125
Jean Bennett

Contents

Lessons Learned from the Development of the First FDA-Approved Gene
Therapy Drug, Voretigene Neparvovec-rzyl, 135
Jean Bennett and Albert M. Maguire

Trial by "Firsts": Clinical Trial Design and Regulatory Considerations in the Development
and Approval of the First AAV Gene Therapy Product in the United States, 151
Kathleen Z. Reape and Katherine A. High

Developing New Vectors for Retinal Gene Therapy, 163
Emilia A. Zin, Bilge E. Ozturk, Deniz Dalkara, and Leah C. Byrne

Immunology of Retinitis Pigmentosa and Gene Therapy-Associated Uveitis, 179
Paul Yang, Debarshi Mustafi, and Kathryn L. Pepple

Choroideremia: Toward Regulatory Approval of Retinal Gene Therapy, 201
Imran H. Yusuf and Robert E. MacLaren

RPGR-Related Retinopathy: Clinical Features, Molecular Genetics, and Gene
Replacement Therapy, 221
Shaima Awadh Hashem, Michalis Georgiou, Robin R. Ali, and Michel Michaelides

Gene Therapy for Rhodopsin Mutations, 231
Alfred S. Lewin and W. Clay Smith

X-Linked Retinoschisis, 247
Cristy A. Ku, Lisa W. Wei, and Paul A. Sieving

From Bench to Bedside—Delivering Gene Therapy for Leber Hereditary Optic
Neuropathy, 259
Benson S. Chen and Patrick Yu-Wai-Man

A Systematic Review of Optogenetic Vision Restoration: History, Challenges,
and New Inventions from Bench to Bedside, 283
Antonia Stefanov and John G. Flannery

Optogenetic Vision Restoration, 299
Volker Busskamp, Botond Roska, and José-Alain Sahel

Therapeutic Gene Editing in Inherited Retinal Disorders, 309
Jinjie Ling, Laura A. Jenny, Ashley Zhou, and Stephen H. Tsang

Alternative RNA Splicing in the Retina: Insights and Perspectives, 325
Casey J. Keuthan, Sadik Karma, and Donald J. Zack

NEUROPROTECTION

Pathomechanisms of Inherited Retinal Degeneration and Perspectives for Neuroprotection, 343
*Arianna Tolone, Merve Sen, Yiyi Chen, Marius Ueffing, Blanca Arango-Gonzalez,
and François Paquet-Durand*

Neurotrophic Factors in the Treatment of Inherited Retinal Diseases, 357
Laure Blouin, José-Alain Sahel, and Daniel C. Chung

Restoration of Rod-Derived Metabolic and Redox Signaling to Prevent Blindness, 365
Emmanuelle Clérin, Najate Aït-Ali, José-Alain Sahel, and Thierry Léveillard

Gene Therapies for Retinitis Pigmentosa that Target Glucose Metabolism, 381
Yunlu Xue and Constance L. Cepko

VISUAL PROSTHESIS

Electronic Retinal Prostheses, 389
Daniel Palanker

CELL-BASED THERAPIES

iPSC-RPE in Retinal Degeneration: Recent Advancements and Future Perspectives, 409
Tadao Maeda and Masayo Takahashi

Considerations for Developing an Autologous Induced Pluripotent Stem Cell (iPSC)-Derived
Retinal Pigment Epithelium (RPE) Replacement Therapy, 429
Devika Bose, Davide Ortolan, Mitra Farnoodian, Ruchi Sharma, and Kapil Bharti

Photoreceptor Cell Replacement Using Pluripotent Stem Cells: Current Knowledge
and Remaining Questions, 447
Christelle Monville, Olivier Goureau, and Karim Ben M'Barek

Cell-Based Therapies: Strategies for Regeneration, 461
Marina Pavlou and Thomas A. Reh

PLANNING FOR CLINICAL TRIALS AND IDENTIFYING OUTCOME
MEASURES IN IRDs

The Importance of Natural History Studies in Inherited Retinal Diseases, 477
Allison Ayala, Janet Cheetham, Todd Durham, and Maureen Maguire

Adaptive Optics Imaging of Inherited Retinal Disease, 493
Jacque L. Duncan and Joseph Carroll

Contents

Beyond the NEI-VFQ: Recent Experience in the Development and Utilization
of Patient-Reported Outcomes for Inherited Retinal Diseases, 507
Todd Durham, Judit Banhazi, Francesco Patalano, and Thiran Jayasundera

Mobility Testing and Other Performance-Based Assessments of Functional Vision
in Patients with Inherited Retinal Disease, 539
Daniel Chung, Colas Authié, and Laure Blouin

Current Status of Clinical Trials Design and Outcomes in Retinal Gene Therapy, 547
Boris Rosin, Eyal Banin, and José-Alain Sahel

Index, 557

Preface

Almost ten years ago, I felt honored to be invited to write a chapter for the previous edition of "Retinal Disorders" for Cold Spring Harbor Laboratory Press, edited by Richard Masland, Eric Pierce, and Joan Miller. When asked about the next edition, the late Richard Masland had suggested my name. While I was saddened by his recent passing, I felt honored and pleased to invite the leaders in the field to join me in preparing this new edition. My co-editors and I agreed that, given the accelerated path to a better understanding and management of these conditions, the time was ripe for revisiting entirely the biology, pathogenesis, and therapies of these blinding conditions.

Indeed, as the chapter written by Steve Daiger et al. emphasizes, understanding of the underlying genetic mechanisms has progressed significantly (Hanany et al.). Several chapters demonstrate the heterogeneity and complexity at both the genotypic and phenotypic levels of retinal degenerations (Audo et al.; Hanany et al.). Elusive genetic abnormalities remain to be elucidated but all are confident that it is just a matter of time given the power of the constantly maturing technologies.

This would, some years ago, have been considered as extremely promising in terms of preparing for gene-based therapies. However, recent years have demonstrated both the power of gene therapy and the multiple challenges in developing successfully cures or palliative approaches for more than one genetic defect (Bennett). Indeed, the approval of Luxturna by both the FDA and the EMA, following two decades of systematic work led by one of our co-editors, has illustrated the power of gene therapy, its impact on daily lives, and the ability to design clinical trials with relevant outcome measures, after successful discussions with the regulatory agencies (Bennett and Maguire; Reape and High). However, more than half a decade later, no other gene therapy or gene-based approach has yet met with a similar success, despite promising preliminary data (Chen and Yu-Wai-Man; Ku et al.; Lewin and Smith; Awadh Hashem et al.; Yusuf and MacLaren).

This volume tries to help in preparing for an even brighter future, capitalizing upon lessons learned from animal and in vitro models (Delvallée and Dollfus; Fradot et al.; McCall; Petersen-Jones and Komáromy; Spirig and Renner) and current trials, and the impressive progress of imaging (Blouin et al.; Chung et al.; Duncan and Carroll; Durham et al.); phenotypic characterization (Audo et al.); natural history studies (Ayala et al.); novel gene therapy technologies, for example, novel vectors (Zin et al.), gene editing (Ling et al.), optogenetics (Busskamp et al.; Stefanov and Flannery), and RNA technologies (Keuthan et al.); control of inflammation (Yang et al.); as well as cell-based therapies (Bose et al.; Maeda and Takahashi; Monville et al.; Pavlou and Reh); and prosthetics (Palanker). The latter, as well as neuroprotective approaches, offer opportunities to propose gene-independent approaches (Busskamp et al.; Clérin et al.; Stefanov and Flannery; Tolone et al.; Xue and Cepko). These are not curative but have the ability to delay significantly the evolution toward severe visual impairment.

Such progress will rely on the refinement of outcome measure methodologies, including real-life assessment of functional vision, on the design of trials based on a better understanding of the natural history of each condition, and the extension of this knowledge to even more rare diseases. Hopefully, as advocated by many, and understood by the leaders of initiatives like Bespoke, a more straightforward and predictable regulatory pathway will emerge for most, if not all, relying on progress in manufacturing, safety assessment, and understanding by all of the complexity of such rare conditions. Whereas no compromise on scientific rigor and safety should be contemplated, should we leave multiple patients and families in wait for the ideal therapy to meet all the gold standard requirements? Progressing toward severe visual impairment is not a safe path either, and a constructive, data-driven dialogue between academics, industry, and regulatory bodies should lead to creative approaches enabling the development and approval of breakthrough therapies.

The chapters in this volume describe progress but also uncertainties and attempts to overcome these limitations to navigate the narrow path toward hope, safely (Rosin et al.). We are enthusiastic about the promises of the multiple diagnostic, methodological, and therapeutic progress described here and the likelihood that most of these chapters will be outdated soon, as more therapies reach the approval stage. Future editions will undoubtedly include emerging methodologies for clinical trials as well as a better inclusion of patients' voices, including in the assessment of therapeutic benefit.

We are grateful to the editor, the editorial team, especially our project supervisor Barbara Acosta, and the readership of Cold Spring Harbor Laboratory Press for this opportunity to share our enthusiasm and questions.

JOSÉ-ALAIN SAHEL
EYAL BANIN
JEAN BENNETT
JACQUE DUNCAN
BOTOND ROSKA

The Extraordinary Phenotypic and Genetic Variability of Retinal and Macular Degenerations: The Relevance to Therapeutic Developments

Isabelle Audo,[1,2] Marco Nassisi,[1,3,4] Christina Zeitz,[1] and José-Alain Sahel[1,2,5]

[1]Sorbonne Université, INSERM, CNRS, Institut de la Vision, Paris 75012, France

[2]Centre Hospitalier National d'Ophtalmologie des Quinze-Vingts, National Rare Disease Center REFERET and INSERM-DGOS CIC 1423, Paris F-75012, France

[3]Department of Clinical Sciences and Community Health, University of Milan, Milan 20122, Italy

[4]Ophthalmology Unit, Fondazione IRCCS Ca' Granda Ospedale Maggiore Policlinico di Milano, Milan 20122, Italy

[5]Department of Ophthalmology, University of Pittsburgh Medical School, Pittsburgh, Pennsylvania 15213, USA

Correspondence: isabelle.audo@inserm.fr

Inherited retinal diseases (IRDs) are a clinically and genetically heterogeneous group of rare conditions leading to various degrees of visual handicap and to progressive blindness in more severe cases. Besides visual rehabilitation, educational, and socio-professional support, there are currently limited therapeutic options, but the approval of the first gene therapy product for *RPE65*-related IRDs raised hope for therapeutic innovations. Such developments are facing obstacles intrinsic to the disease and the affected tissue including the extreme phenotypic and genetic variability of IRDs and the fine tuning of visual processing through the complex architecture of the postmitotic neural retina. A precise phenotypic characterization is required prior to genetic testing, which now relies on high-throughput sequencing. Their challenges will be discussed within this article as well as their implications in clinical trial design.

Inherited retinal diseases (IRDs) are a large group of rare genetic conditions with a prevalence of about 1/3000 subjects worldwide (Bessant et al. 2001) that may be isolated or part of a syndromic disorder. IRDs may affect the entire retina such as in the most common one, rod-cone dystrophies (RCDs) also known as retinitis pigmentosa (RP), or only the macular region (i.e., macular dystrophies) with various degrees of visual handicap up to progressive blindness.

Besides visual rehabilitation, educational, and socio-professional support, there are currently limited therapeutic options for IRDs (Sahel et al. 2015). Nevertheless, the approval of the first gene therapy product for the treatment of *RPE65*-related IRDs after successful phases 1/2 (Maguire et al. 2008) and 3 (Russell et al. 2017) and ongoing clinical trials (Sahel et al. 2015) raised hope for therapeutic innovations. Such developments are facing obstacles intrinsic to the disease and the affected tissue including the extreme phenotypic and genetic variability of IRDs and the fine tuning of visual processing through the complex architecture of the postmitotic neural retina. We will be discussing some of these issues within this article.

PHENOTYPIC VARIABILITY OF IRDs MIRRORED BY AN EXTREME GENETIC HETEROGENEITY

IRDs are characterized by an extreme phenotypic variability, which is difficult to accurately capture within a clinical classification, an attempt being presented in Table 1. IRDs range from congenital, usually stationary disorders to early-, juvenile-, or adult-onset degenerative disorders. Each of these disorders will have a variable impact and degree of severity on visual function. Some dystrophies will progressively affect the entire retina usually leading to blindness, whereas disorders affecting only the central part, the macula, will be associated with a severe impact on visual acuity but with preserved peripheral vision. Most of these disorders primarily affect photoreceptor cells, namely, rod photoreceptors responsible for dim light vision, and cone photoreceptors associated with daylight, color, and precise vision (Lamb 2022). The primary site of dysfunction can also be the retinal pigment epithelium (RPE), which, among other functions, provides metabolic support essential to photoreceptor functioning and survival (Caceres and Rodriguez-Boulan 2020). The respective prevalence of each of these entities is not always precisely known but, by far, RCD (RP) is the most prevalent one, affecting about 1/4000 individuals worldwide, representing up to 70% of IRDs (Bocquet et al. 2013). This entity itself is associated with some phenotypic variability in the age at onset, the disease course, and the potential association with additional alterations as part of syndromic diseases. Usher syndrome, associated with variable degrees of deafness and vestibular dysfunction, is the most common syndromic form of RCD (Delmaghani and El-Amraoui 2022) followed by Bardet–Biedl syndrome, a ciliopathy that associates variable degrees of cognitive difficulties, obesity, hexadactilia, and kidney disease (Mockel et al. 2011). The

management and support of patients affected with these syndromic disorders is therefore not only challenged by the visual handicap but also by the other systemic alterations, which require a multidisciplinary management. Of note, despite the clinical heterogeneity of RCD/RP, symptoms and ophthalmic alterations may be consistent within this clinical heterogeneity with night blindness often being the first symptom followed by progressive peripheral visual field constriction and eventually the loss of central vision late in the disease leading to blindness in most severe cases. Clinical examination will typically reveal visual field constriction, generalized rod-cone dysfunction on the full-field electroretinogram (ff-ERG) and cardinal signs on fundus examination including a waxy pallor of the optic disc, narrowed retinal vessels, and pigmentary changes in the retinal periphery (Fig. 1). Macular dystrophies will manifest differently starting with decrease in visual acuity, color vision disturbances, and some pathognomonic macular alterations on fundus examination or fundus autofluorescence imaging (Fig. 2). With a more severe visual outcome, cone and cone-rod dystrophies have overlapping visual symptoms at onset in addition to photophobia. ff-ERG is instrumental for the differential diagnosis and visual prognosis (i.e., macular dystrophies have normal retinal function on ff-ERG while cone and cone-rod dystrophies show variable degrees of generalized cone and rod dysfunction) (Cornish et al. 2021).

The clinical heterogeneity of IRDs is mirrored by the genetic heterogeneity. Indeed, since the initial discovery of mutations in *RHO* underlying autosomal-dominant RCD as the first gene defect identified underlying IRDs (Dryja et al. 1990a,b), more than 250 genes have been associated with some forms of IRDs (web.sph.uth .edu/RetNet/home.htm). These genes encode proteins of various expression profiles and functions, some being specific to photoreceptors (e.g., involved in the phototransduction cascade) or the RPE (e.g., involved in the visual cycle), whereas others are associated with a more ubiquitous expression profile such as splicing factors (e.g., *PRPF31*, *PRPF8*, *PRPF3*) or proteins involved in the primary cilium maintenance, mutations in the latter potentially leading to syn-

Table 1. Attempt for a simplified clinical classification showing the phenotypic variability of inherited retinal diseases

Phenotypic variability	Cellular alterations	Diagnosis	Mode of inheritance	Prevalence	References
Stationary	Rod dysfunction	Riggs-type CSNB	AD, AR	Unknown	Zeitz et al. 2015
	Post-phototransduction dysfunction	Schubert–Bornschein-type CSNB	AR, XL	Unknown	Zeitz et al. 2015
	Cone dysfunction	Achromatopsia	AR	1/50,000	Aboshiha et al. 2016
		BCM	XL	1/100,000	De Silva et al. 2021
Degenerative	Generalized progressive rod then cone dysfunction and affiliated disorders	RCD, isolated	AR	1/4000	Verbakel et al. 2018
		RCD-type LCA/EORD	AR	1/100,000	Hanein et al. 2004
		Syndromic (e.g., Usher syndrome, BBS)	AR	1/20,000	Boughman et al. 1983; Mockel et al. 2011
		ESCS/Goldman–Favre syndrome	AR	<1/1,000,000	Yzer et al. 2013
	Chorioretinopathies	CHM	XL	1/100,000	Zeitz et al. 2021
		Bietti chorioretinal dystrophy	AR	Unknown	García-García et al. 2019
		Gyrate atrophy	AR	Unknown	Sergouniotis et al. 2012
	Generalized progressive cone +/– rod dysfunction	CD and CRD, isolated	AR, AD, XL	1/100,000	Gill et al. 2019
		CRD-type LCA/EORD	AR	1/100,000	Hanein et al. 2004
		Syndromic cone and cone-rod dystrophies (e.g., SCA7, BBS)	AD, AR	<1/1,000,000	Gill et al. 2019
	Inner retina	XL-retinoschisis	XL	1/100,000	Molday et al. 2012
	Macular dystrophies	Stargardt disease	AR	1/10,000	Rahman et al. 2020)
		Best disease	AD	1/10,000	Boon et al. 2009
		Pattern dystrophy including maternally inherited diabetes and deafness	AD, mitochondrial	Unknown	Rahman et al. 2020
		North Carolina macular dystrophy	AD	<1/1,000,000	Rahman et al. 2020
		Doyne Honeycomb retinal dystrophy	AD	<1/1,000,000	Rahman et al. 2020
		Sorsby fundus dystrophy	AD	<1/1,000,000	Rahman et al. 2020

(AD) Autosomal-dominant, (AR) autosomal-recessive, (XL) X-linked, (CSNB) congenital stationary night blindness, (BCM) blue cone monochromacy, (SCA7) spinocerebellar ataxia type 7, (BBS) Bardet–Biedl syndrome, (ESCS) enhanced S-cone syndrome, (CHM) choroideremia, (LCA) Leber congenital amaurosis, (EORD) early-onset retinal dystrophies, (RCD) rod-cone dystrophies, (CRD) cone-rod dystrophy.

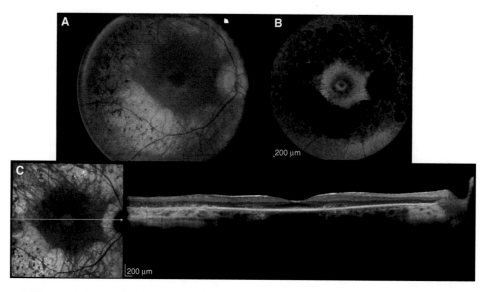

Figure 1. Characteristic retinal alterations of rod-cone dystrophy, also known as retinitis pigmentosa, in a 50-yr-old man with biallelic *USH2A* variants (allele 1: c.1036A > C, p.(Asn346His); allele 2: c.2276G > T, p.(Cys759Phe) (right eye). (*A*) Fundus photograph showing a pale optic disc, narrowed retinal vessels, chorioretinal atrophy, and pigmentary changes in the mid-periphery with perifoveal changes. (*B*) Short-wavelength fundus autofluorescence showing peripheral loss of autofluorescence. (*C*) Spectral domain optical coherence tomography showing outer retinal alteration outside the foveal region.

dromic disease defined as ciliopathies (Bujakow-ska et al. 2017).

The genetic complexity goes even further since distinct mutations within the same gene can lead to distinct phenotypes or inheritance (Fig. 3), while a similar phenotype can be associated with distinct genotypes. For instance, an RP phenotype may be associated with genetic variants in more than 70 distinct genes (web .sph.uth.edu/RetNet/home.htm) while some of these genes may be associated with several distinct IRDs depending on the genetic variants. Similarly, maculopathies with flecks are more commonly associated with *ABC44* variants following an autosomal-recessive inheritance, but similar phenotypes may also be associated with variants in *PRPH2* or less commonly in *ELOVL4*, both gene defects following an autosomal-dominance inheritance.

Biallelic variants in the ATP-binding cassette, subfamily A, member 4 (*ABCA4*, OMIM* 601691) are underlying Stargardt disease (OMIM#248200), the most common form of macular dystrophy, but may also lead to cone,

cone-rod dystrophy (CORD3, OMIM#604116), and possibly RP (RP19, OMIM#601718) with some degree of phenotype/genotype correlation, genetic variants leading to a more severe ABCA4 dysfunction being associated with more severe phenotypes (Cremers et al. 2020). Similarly, monoallelic *BEST1* (OMIM*607854) variants were initially associated with the second-most-common macular dystrophy, autosomal-dominant Best vitelliform macular dystrophy (OMIM# 153700) (Petrukhin et al. 1998), whereas monoallelic-specific splice site variants were found underlying autosomal-dominant vitreoretinochoroidopathy (ADVIRC, OMIM#19 3220) (Burgess et al. 2009) and biallelic changes in autosomal-recessive bestrophynopathy (ARB, OMIM# 611809) (Burgess et al. 2008). *RPGR* (OMIM*312610) variants are the most common cause of X-linked RCD (RP3, OMIM#300029) (Meindl et al. 1996) but also X-linked CRD (OMIM#304020) (Yang et al. 2002; Nassisi et al. 2022), both having distinct impact on visual function. Even more relevant for patients' management and counseling, certain genes may be asso-

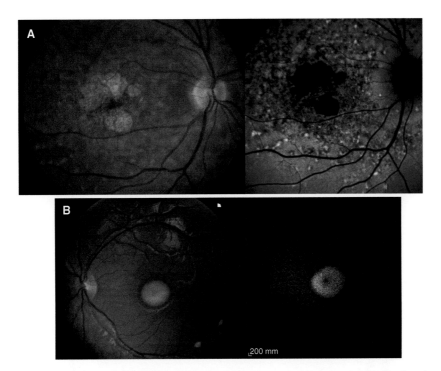

Figure 2. Characteristic retinal alterations for the two most common macular dystrophies on fundus photographs and short-wavelength fundus autofluorescence: (*A*) Stargardt macular dystrophy, and (*B*) Best vitelliform dystrophy (*BEST 1* heterozygous variant: c.889C > T, p.(Pro297Ser)).

ciated with either isolated retinal disorders or syndromic diseases (e.g., biallelic *USH2A* variants leading either to autosomal-recessive RCD or Usher type 2 [Eudy et al. 1998; Bernal et al. 2003]; *CLN3* variants can lead to a severe and eventually lethal syndromic neurological disorder—Batten disease—or to an isolated retinal dystrophy [Smirnov et al. 2021]). Finally, even within the same gene defect, there is a high inter- and intrafamilial variability, variable expression, and incomplete penetrance (Farrar et al. 2017).

A precise delineation of phenotype/genotype correlation is therefore essential for a better understanding of IRD, an improved patients' management, but also to support therapeutic research.

MASSIVE PARALLEL SEQUENCING APPLIED TO IRDs

The past two decades have seen tremendous technological developments in the field of massive parallel sequencing accelerating gene discovery and delivering high-throughput analytic tools particularly suited to encompass the genetic heterogeneity of IRDs. Indeed, nearly 300 genes have been associated with specific forms of IRDs (web .sph.uth.edu/RetNet/sum-dis.htm#D-graph, last accessed March 13, 2023). Targeted next-generation sequencing (NGS) has indeed passed from a research setting (Audo et al. 2012) to diagnostic laboratories with a genetic resolution rate reaching about 70% (Shah et al. 2020; Britten-Jones et al. 2023). In addition, whole-exome sequencing (WES) and further whole-genome sequencing (WGS) have also entered the diagnostic area and provide a more comprehensive genetic analysis. In addition to providing a better coverage of coding regions, the latter covers also noncoding intronic and regulatory regions and allows a more precise analysis of DNA structural alterations such as copy number variations and other large genomic changes or repeat expansions (Dolzhenko et al. 2017; Chen et al. 2019). This massive

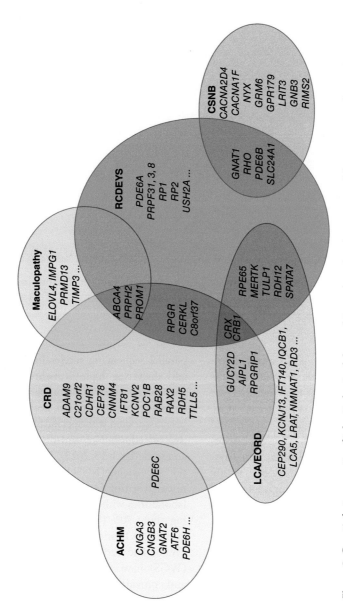

Figure 3. Genetic heterogeneity of inherited retinal dystrophies and overlapping genotype/phenotype correlation. (ACHM) Achromatopsia, (CRD) cone-rod dystrophy, (CSNB) congenital stationary night blindness, (LCA/EORD) Leber congenital amaurosis/early-onset retinal degeneration, (RCD) rod-cone dystrophy, also known as RP.

parallel sequencing however generates a significant volume of data to be stored and analyzed through relevant bioinformatic algorithms, which became more efficient along with the development of the techniques and the reduction of their cost. In this context, a detailed phenotypic characterization and a precise phenotype/genotype delineation has become increasingly essential to pinpoint the genetic cause among the numerous genetic variants obtained with high-throughput sequencing. The issue of unsolicited or incidental genetic findings, which should be discussed with the patient prior to genetic testing, can be resolved by performing phenotype-based in silico panels on a predefined list of genes associated with the disease of interest. This option reduces the number of variants to analyze and limits the interpretation to genomic regions within the strict expertise of the interpreting biologist. A variant interpretation has been refined with the American College of Medical Genetics and Genomics guidelines (Richards et al. 2015). Nevertheless, variants of unknown significance remain a real issue when it comes to accurate genetic counseling and access to therapies or selection for clinical trials (Hoffman-Andrews 2017). To improve variant classification, a precise phenotypic characterization may help in addition to variant segregation within a given family, which should be sought systematically. The implementation of functional tests, such as mini-gene assays to validate putative RNA mis-splicing, for instance, cilia-based assays, or biochemical tests (Sangermano et al. 2018; Yang et al. 2019; Westin et al. 2021; Lange et al. 2022), when relevant, are essential to refine variant classification. But these require an additional technology that is not always present in a diagnostic setting. Finally, an incentive should be given to report any new variant in available databases, such as the Leiden Open Variation Database (databases.lovd.nl/shared/genes) or ClinVar (www.ncbi.nlm.nih.gov/clinvar/), a requirement for certain genetic journals prior to publication (e.g., *Human Mutation*), which should be made mandatory for any diagnostic genetic laboratory. Indeed, an exhaustive reporting of all identified variants would help further develop the genetic landscape of IRD, which still needs to be completed. In this respect, a recent meta-analysis of targeted NGS panels applied to IRDs revealed a genetic diagnostic yield between 52% and 74% (Britten-Jones et al. 2023). More recently applied, WGS constitutes an unprecedented powerful tool to solve additional cases, although recent studies suggest that this added improvement may be limited (Wen et al. 2023) with only 2.1% additional cases for which WGS identified structural variants that were missed by NGS or WES (Wen et al. 2023). Expanding IRD cohorts analyzed through WGS, with improved bioinformatic pipelines and variant classification, will help better address the impact of WGS to resolve genetically unsolved cases. Newer technologies such as long-read sequencing may bring further insight in providing a better genome mapping of structural variants and highly repetitive regions as well as providing important phase information (Amarasinghe et al. 2020).

Finally, there are so far very few studies addressing the role of epigenetics in IRDs, which could account, to some extent, for the intrafamilial phenotypic variability or for some of the genetically unresolved cases (Dvoriantchikova et al. 2022). Further studies would be needed to establish the role of epigenetics in the clinical and genetic heterogeneity of IRDs, with a major obstacle residing in the lack of direct access to the diseased tissue.

A better understanding of the genetic landscape of IRDs, along with the development of deep phenotyping and relevant phenotype/genotype correlation, is essential to support the development of therapeutic trials.

NEED FOR A BETTER PHENOTYPIC DELINEATION AND OUTCOME MEASURE TO FACILITATE CLINICAL TRIALS

The past decades have seen an increased number of clinical trials in IRDs, which led to the approval of the first gene-augmentation therapy for *RPE65*-related IRDs (Russell et al. 2017). This active translational research is challenged by the phenotypic and genetic heterogeneity of IRDs. In this context, a panel of experts in the field recently established the priorities needed to accelerate therapeutic research facing these challenges (Thompson et al. 2015, 2020). The first priority was identified as "the use of natural history studies to guide clinical trial design" (Thompson et al. 2015). These natural history studies will have to face the intrinsic phenotypic variability of IRDs, even within a single genotype, by including a significant number of patients to reach statistical power. They will provide relevant information on disease progression and determine biomarkers and clinical end points better suited to document disease severity and progression, while potentially identifying a relevant window of intervention, which will be essential for trial design.

The selection of relevant outcomes and end points for clinical trials may directly affect the success of innovative therapeutic strategies. While for other acute diseases (e.g., exudative neovascular age-related macular degeneration, uveitis) (Schmetterer et al. 2023) improvement of visual acuity is generally considered the most important clinical outcome, for IRDs it may not be the most relevant criteria. In most cases, a reasonable objective of a therapy in IRDs would be delaying disease progression and stabilizing visual acuity over time, improving it being elusive when associated with photoreceptor degeneration. Indeed, the phase 2/3 studies for X-linked RP (NCT03116113) and for choroideremia (NCT03496012) did not meet the primary outcome of a 15-letter gain in visual acuity from baseline, an outcome accepted by the FDA, whereas other end points, such as no change in visual acuity or visual field from baseline, may have been relevant for the disease and the patients. A close dialogue with regulatory agencies prior to clinical trial design to better discuss the specificity of IRDs, in light of the phenotypic and genetic heterogeneity, along with natural history data may help to better define outcome measures and end points in IRDs. The development of standardized testing guidelines would take into account (1) the different definition of "therapeutic efficacy" for specific types of IRDs and interventions; (2) the correlation of each surrogate outcome with accepted clinically meaningful outcomes for assessing efficacy; and (3) the reproducibility and reliability of the outcome measures evaluated (Thompson et al. 2020). Furthermore, the current advancing use of artificial intelligence and machine learning is leading to the opportunity of standardizing outcome measures across multiple trial sites and may take into account genetic heterogeneity (Sumaroka et al. 2019, 2020). Nevertheless, while highly standardized clinical tests are important for the evaluation of potential treatments, the development of new clinical outcomes that reflect the needs of patients (e.g., patient-reported outcomes and performance-based tests) would be highly relevant (Thompson et al. 2020).

CONCLUDING REMARKS

IRDs are characterized by a significant phenotypic and genetic heterogeneity. The advent of genomic testing along with deep phenotyping offers a unique opportunity to better delineate phenotype/genotype correlations and subsequently support improved management of IRD patients, but also to provide more accurate biomarkers for successful clinical trials.

ACKNOWLEDGMENTS

IHU FOReSIGHT (ANR-18-IAHU-0001) supported by French state funds managed by the Agence Nationale de la Recherche within the Investissements d'Avenir program.

REFERENCES

Aboshiha J, Dubis AM, Carroll J, Hardcastle AJ, Michaelides M. 2016. The cone dysfunction syndromes. *Br J Ophthalmol* **100:** 115–121. doi:10.1136/bjophthalmol-2014-306505

Amarasinghe SL, Su S, Dong X, Zappia L, Ritchie ME, Gouil Q. 2020. Opportunities and challenges in long-read sequencing data analysis. *Genome Biol* **21:** 30. doi:10.1186/s13059-020-1935-5

Audo I, Bujakowska KM, Léveillard T, Mohand-Saïd S, Lancelot ME, Germain A, Antonio A, Michiels C, Saraiva JP, Letexier M, et al. 2012. Development and application of a next-generation-sequencing (NGS) approach to detect known and novel gene defects underlying retinal diseases. *Orphanet J Rare Dis* **7:** 8. doi:10.1186/1750-1172-7-8

Bernal S, Ayuso C, Antinolo G, Gimenez A, Borrego S, Trujillo MJ, Marcos I, Calaf M, Del Rio E, Baiget M. 2003. Mutations in USH2A in Spanish patients with autosomal recessive retinitis pigmentosa: high prevalence and phenotypic variation. *J Med Genet* **40:** e8. doi:10.1136/jmg.40.1.e8

Bessant DA, Ali RR, Bhattacharya SS. 2001. Molecular genetics and prospects for therapy of the inherited retinal dystrophies. *Curr Opin Genet Dev* **11:** 307–316. doi:10.1016/S0959-437X(00)00195-7

Bocquet B, Lacroux A, Surget MO, Baudoin C, Marquette V, Manes G, Hebrard M, Sénéchal A, Delettre C, Roux AF, et al. 2013. Relative frequencies of inherited retinal dystro-

Cite this article as *Cold Spring Harb Perspect Med* doi: 10.1101/cshperspect.a041652

phies and optic neuropathies in Southern France: assessment of 21-year data management. *Ophthalmic Epidemiol* **20**: 13–25. doi:10.3109/09286586.2012.737890

Boon CJ, Klevering BJ, Leroy BP, Hoyng CB, Keunen JE, den Hollander AI. 2009. The spectrum of ocular phenotypes caused by mutations in the BEST1 gene. *Prog Retin Eye Res* **28**: 187–205. doi:10.1016/j.preteyeres.2009.04.002

Boughman JA, Vernon M, Shaver KA. 1983. Usher syndrome: definition and estimate of prevalence from two high-risk populations. *J Chronic Dis* **36**: 595–603. doi:10.1016/0021-9681(83)90147-9

Britten-Jones AC, Gocuk SA, Goh KL, Huq A, Edwards TL, Ayton LN. 2023. The diagnostic yield of next generation sequencing in inherited retinal diseases: a systematic review and meta-analysis. *Am J Ophthalmol* **249**: 57–73. doi:10.1016/j.ajo.2022.12.027

Bujakowska KM, Liu Q, Pierce EA. 2017. Photoreceptor cilia and retinal ciliopathies. *Cold Spring Harb Perspect Biol* **9**: a028274. doi:10.1101/cshperspect.a028274

Burgess R, Millar ID, Leroy BP, Urquhart JE, Fearon IM, De Baere E, Brown PD, Robson AG, Wright GA, Kestelyn P, et al. 2008. Biallelic mutation of BEST1 causes a distinct retinopathy in humans. *Am J Hum Genet* **82**: 19–31. doi:10.1016/j.ajhg.2007.08.004

Burgess R, MacLaren RE, Davidson AE, Urquhart JE, Holder GE, Robson AG, Moore AT, Keefe RO, Black GC, Manson FD. 2009. ADVIRC is caused by distinct mutations in BEST1 that alter pre-mRNA splicing. *J Med Genet* **46**: 620–625. doi:10.1136/jmg.2008.059881

Caceres PS, Rodriguez-Boulan E. 2020. Retinal pigment epithelium polarity in health and blinding diseases. *Curr Opin Cell Biol* **62**: 37–45. doi:10.1016/j.ceb.2019.08.001

Chen S, Krusche P, Dolzhenko E, Sherman RM, Petrovski R, Schlesinger F, Kirsche M, Bentley DR, Schatz MC, Sedlazeck FJ, et al. 2019. Paragraph: a graph-based structural variant genotyper for short-read sequence data. *Genome Biol* **20**: 291. doi:10.1186/s13059-019-1909-7

Cornish EE, Vaze A, Jamieson RV, Grigg JR. 2021. The electroretinogram in the genomics era: outer retinal disorders. *Eye (Lond)* **35**: 2406–2418. doi:10.1038/s41433-021-01659-y

Cremers FPM, Lee W, Collin RWJ, Allikmets R. 2020. Clinical spectrum, genetic complexity and therapeutic approaches for retinal disease caused by ABCA4 mutations. *Prog Retin Eye Res* **79**: 100861. doi:10.1016/j.preteyeres.2020.100861

Delmaghani S, El-Amraoui A. 2022. The genetic and phenotypic landscapes of Usher syndrome: from disease mechanisms to a new classification. *Hum Genet* **141**: 709–735. doi:10.1007/s00439-022-02448-7

De Silva SR, Arno G, Robson AG, Fakin A, Pontikos N, Mohamed MD, Bird AC, Moore AT, Michaelides M, Webster AR, et al. 2021. The X-linked retinopathies: physiological insights, pathogenic mechanisms, phenotypic features and novel therapies. *Prog Retin Eye Res* **82**: 100898. doi:10.1016/j.preteyeres.2020.100898

Dolzhenko E, van Vugt J, Shaw RJ, Bekritsky MA, van Blitterswijk M, Narzisi G, Ajay SS, Rajan V, Lajoie BR, Johnson NH, et al. 2017. Detection of long repeat expansions from PCR-free whole-genome sequence data. *Genome Res* **27**: 1895–1903. doi:10.1101/gr.225672.117

Dryja TP, McGee TL, Hahn LB, Cowley GS, Olsson JE, Reichel E, Sandberg MA, Berson EL. 1990a. Mutations within the rhodopsin gene in patients with autosomal

dominant retinitis pigmentosa. *N Engl J Med* **323**: 1302–1307. doi:10.1056/NEJM199011083231903

Dryja TP, McGee TL, Reichel E, Hahn LB, Cowley GS, Yandell DW, Sandberg MA, Berson EL. 1990b. A point mutation of the rhodopsin gene in one form of retinitis pigmentosa. *Nature* **343**: 364–366. doi:10.1038/343364a0

Dvoriantchikova G, Lypka KR, Ivanov D. 2022. The potential role of epigenetic mechanisms in the development of retinitis pigmentosa and related photoreceptor dystrophies. *Front Genet* **13**: 827274. doi:10.3389/fgene.2022.827274

Eudy JD, Weston MD, Yao S, Hoover DM, Rehm HL, Ma-Edmonds M, Yan D, Ahmad I, Cheng JJ, Ayuso C, et al. 1998. Mutation of a gene encoding a protein with extracellular matrix motifs in Usher syndrome type IIa. *Science* **280**: 1753–1757. doi:10.1126/science.280.5370.1753

Farrar GJ, Carrigan M, Dockery A, Millington-Ward S, Palfi A, Chadderton N, Humphries M, Kiang AS, Kenna PF, Humphries P. 2017. Toward an elucidation of the molecular genetics of inherited retinal degenerations. *Hum Mol Genet* **26**: R2–R11.

García-García GP, Martínez-Rubio M, Moya-Moya MA, Pérez-Santonja JJ, Escribano J. 2019. Current perspectives in Bietti crystalline dystrophy. *Clin Ophthalmol* **13**: 1379–1399. doi:10.2147/OPTH.S185744

Gill JS, Georgiou M, Kalitzeos A, Moore AT, Michaelides M. 2019. Progressive cone and cone-rod dystrophies: clinical features, molecular genetics and prospects for therapy. *Br J Ophthalmol* **103**: 711–720. doi:10.1136/bjophthalmol-2018-313278

Hanein S, Perrault I, Gerber S, Tanguy G, Barbet F, Ducroq D, Calvas P, Dollfus H, Hamel C, Lopponen T, et al. 2004. Leber congenital amaurosis: comprehensive survey of the genetic heterogeneity, refinement of the clinical definition, and genotype-phenotype correlations as a strategy for molecular diagnosis. *Hum Mutat* **23**: 306–317. doi:10.1002/humu.20010

Hoffman-Andrews L. 2017. The known unknown: the challenges of genetic variants of uncertain significance in clinical practice. *J Law Biosci* **4**: 648–657. doi:10.1093/jlb/lsx038

Lamb TD. 2022. Photoreceptor physiology and evolution: cellular and molecular basis of rod and cone phototransduction. *J Physiol* **600**: 4585–4601. doi:10.1113/JP282058

Lange KI, Best S, Tsiropoulou S, Berry I, Johnson CA, Blacque OE. 2022. Interpreting ciliopathy-associated missense variants of uncertain significance (VUS) in *Caenorhabditis elegans*. *Hum Mol Genet* **31**: 1574–1587. doi:10.1093/hmg/ddab344

Maguire AM, Simonelli F, Pierce EA, Pugh EN, Mingozzi F, Bennicelli J, Banfi S, Marshall KA, Testa F, Surace EM, et al. 2008. Safety and efficacy of gene transfer for Leber's congenital amaurosis. *N Engl J Med* **358**: 2240–2248. doi:10.1056/NEJMoa0802315

Meindl A, Dry K, Herrmann K, Manson F, Ciccodicola A, Edgar A, Carvalho MR, Achatz H, Hellebrand H, Lennon A, et al. 1996. A gene (RPGR) with homology to the RCC1 guanine nucleotide exchange factor is mutated in X-linked retinitis pigmentosa (RP3). *Nat Genet* **13**: 35–42. doi:10.1038/ng0596-35

Mockel A, Perdomo Y, Stutzmann F, Letsch J, Marion V, Dollfus H. 2011. Retinal dystrophy in Bardet-Biedl syndrome and related syndromic ciliopathies. *Prog Retin Eye Res* **30**: 258–274. doi:10.1016/j.preteyeres.2011.03.001

Molday RS, Kellner U, Weber BH. 2012. X-linked juvenile retinoschisis: clinical diagnosis, genetic analysis, and molecular mechanisms. *Prog Retin Eye Res* **31**: 195–212. doi:10.1016/j.preteyeres.2011.12.002

Nassisi M, De Bartolo G, Mohand-Said S, Condroyer C, Antonio A, Lancelot ME, Bujakowska K, Smirnov V, Pugliese T, Neidhardt J, et al. 2022. Retrospective natural history study of *RPGR*-related cone- and cone-rod dystrophies while expanding the mutation spectrum of the disease. *Int J Mol Sci* **23**: 7189. doi:10.3390/ijms23137189

Petrukhin K, Koisti MJ, Bakall B, Li W, Xie G, Marknell T, Sandgren O, Forsman K, Holmgren G, Andreasson S, et al. 1998. Identification of the gene responsible for Best macular dystrophy. *Nat Genet* **19**: 241–247. doi:10.1038/915

Rahman N, Georgiou M, Khan KN, Michaelides M. 2020. Macular dystrophies: clinical and imaging features, molecular genetics and therapeutic options. *Br J Ophthalmol* **104**: 451–460. doi:10.1136/bjophthalmol-2019-315086

Richards S, Aziz N, Bale S, Bick D, Das S, Gastier-Foster J, Grody WW, Hegde M, Lyon E, Spector E, et al. 2015. Standards and guidelines for the interpretation of sequence variants: a joint consensus recommendation of the American College of Medical Genetics and Genomics and the Association for Molecular Pathology. *Genet Med* **17**: 405–424. doi:10.1038/gim.2015.30

Russell S, Bennett J, Wellman JA, Chung DC, Yu ZF, Tillman A, Wittes J, Pappas J, Elci O, McCague S, et al. 2017. Efficacy and safety of voretigene neparvovec (AAV2-hRPE65v2) in patients with RPE65-mediated inherited retinal dystrophy: a randomised, controlled, open-label, phase 3 trial. *Lancet* **390**: 849–860. doi:10.1016/S0140-6736(17)31868-8

Sahel JA, Marazova K, Audo I. 2015. Clinical characteristics and current therapies for inherited retinal degenerations. *Cold Spring Harb Perspect Med* **5**: a017111. doi:10.1101/cshperspect.a017111

Sangermano R, Khan M, Cornelis SS, Richelle V, Albert S, Garanto A, Elmelik D, Qamar R, Lugtenberg D, van den Born LI, et al. 2018. *ABCA4* midigenes reveal the full splice spectrum of all reported noncanonical splice site variants in Stargardt disease. *Genome Res* **28**: 100–110. doi:10.1101/gr.226621.117

Schmetterer L, Scholl H, Garhöfer G, Janeschitz-Kriegl L, Corvi F, Sadda SR, Medeiros FA. 2023. Endpoints for clinical trials in ophthalmology. *Prog Retin Eye Res* doi:10.1016/j.preteyeres.2022.101160

Sergouniotis PI, Davidson AE, Lenassi E, Devery SR, Moore AT, Webster AR. 2012. Retinal structure, function, and molecular pathologic features in gyrate atrophy. *Ophthalmology* **119**: 596–605. doi:10.1016/j.ophtha.2011.09.017

Shah M, Shanks M, Packham E, Williams J, Haysmoore J, MacLaren RE, Németh AH, Clouston P, Downes SM. 2020. Next generation sequencing using phenotype-based panels for genetic testing in inherited retinal diseases. *Ophthalmic Genet* **41**: 331–337. doi:10.1080/13816810.2020.1778736

Smirnov VM, Nassisi M, Solis Hernandez C, Méjécase C, El Shamieh S, Condroyer C, Antonio A, Meunier I, Andrieu C, Defoort-Dhellemmes S, et al. 2021. Retinal phenotype of patients with isolated retinal degeneration due to *CLN3* pathogenic variants in a French retinitis pigmentosa cohort. *JAMA Opthalmol* **139**: 278–291. doi:10.1001/jamaophthalmol.2020.6089

Sumaroka A, Garafalo AV, Semenov EP, Sheplock R, Krishnan AK, Roman AJ, Jacobson SG, Cideciyan AV. 2019. Treatment potential for macular cone vision in Leber congenital amaurosis due to *CEP290* or *NPHP5* mutations: predictions from artificial intelligence. *Invest Ophthalmol Vis Sci* **60**: 2551–2562. doi:10.1167/iovs.19-27156

Sumaroka A, Cideciyan AV, Sheplock R, Wu V, Kohl S, Wissinger B, Jacobson SG. 2020. Foveal therapy in blue cone monochromacy: predictions of visual potential from artificial intelligence. *Front Neurosci* **14**: 800. doi:10.3389/fnins.2020.00800

Thompson DA, Ali RR, Banin E, Branham KE, Flannery JG, Gamm DM, Hauswirth WW, Heckenlively JR, Iannaccone A, Jayasundera KT, et al. 2015. Advancing therapeutic strategies for inherited retinal degeneration: recommendations from the Monaciano Symposium. *Invest Ophthalmol Vis Sci* **56**: 918–931. doi:10.1167/iovs.14-16049

Thompson DA, Iannaccone A, Ali RR, Arshavsky VY, Audo I, Bainbridge JWB, Besirli CG, Birch DG, Branham KE, Cideciyan AV, et al. 2020. Advancing clinical trials for inherited retinal diseases: recommendations from the Second Monaciano Symposium. *Transl Vis Sci Technol* **9**: 2. doi:10.1167/tvst.9.7.2

Verbakel SK, van Huet RAC, Boon CJF, den Hollander AI, Collin RWJ, Klaver CCW, Hoyng CB, Roepman R, Klevering BJ. 2018. Non-syndromic retinitis pigmentosa. *Prog Retin Eye Res* **66**: 157–186. doi:10.1016/j.preteyeres.2018.03.005

Wen S, Wang M, Qian X, Li Y, Wang K, Choi J, Pennesi ME, Yang P, Marra M, Koenekoop RK, et al. 2023. Systematic assessment of the contribution of structural variants to inherited retinal diseases. *Hum Mol Genet* doi:10.1093/hmg/ddad032

Westin IM, Jonsson F, Österman L, Holmberg M, Burstedt M, Golovleva I. 2021. EYS mutations and implementation of minigene assay for variant classification in EYS-associated retinitis pigmentosa in northern Sweden. *Sci Rep* **11**: 7696. doi:10.1038/s41598-021-87224-9

Yang Z, Peachey NS, Moshfeghi DM, Thirumalaichary S, Chorich L, Shugart YY, Fan K, Zhang K. 2002. Mutations in the RPGR gene cause X-linked cone dystrophy. *Hum Mol Genet* **11**: 605–611. doi:10.1093/hmg/11.5.605

Yang U, Gentleman S, Gai X, Gorin MB, Borchert MS, Lee TC, Villanueva A, Koenekoop R, Maguire AM, Bennett J, et al. 2019. Utility of in vitro mutagenesis of RPE65 protein for verification of mutational pathogenicity before gene therapy. *JAMA Ophthalmol* **137**: 1381–1388. doi:10.1001/jamaophthalmol.2019.3914

Yzer S, Barbazetto I, Allikmets R, van Schooneveld MJ, Bergen A, Tsang SH, Jacobson SG, Yannuzzi LA. 2013. Expanded clinical spectrum of enhanced S-cone syndrome. *JAMA Ophthalmol* **131**: 1324–1330. doi:10.1001/jamaophthalmol.2013.4349

Zeitz C, Robson AG, Audo I. 2015. Congenital stationary night blindness: an analysis and update of genotype–phenotype correlations and pathogenic mechanisms. *Prog Retin Eye Res* **45**: 58–110. doi:10.1016/j.preteyeres.2014.09.001

Zeitz C, Nassisi M, Laurent-Coriat C, Andrieu C, Boyard F, Condroyer C, Démontant V, Antonio A, Lancelot ME, Frederiksen H, et al. 2021. *CHM* mutation spectrum and disease: an update at the time of human therapeutic trials. *Hum Mutat* **42**: 323–341. doi:10.1002/humu.24174

History of Finding Genes and Mutations Causing Inherited Retinal Diseases

Stephen P. Daiger, Lori S. Sullivan, Elizabeth L. Cadena, and Sara J. Bowne

School of Public Health, University of Texas Health Science Center, Houston, Texas 77030-3900, USA

Correspondence: Stephen.P.Daiger@uth.tmc.edu

This is a brief history of the work by many investigators throughout the world to find genes and mutations causing inherited retinal diseases (IRDs). It largely covers 40 years, from the late-1980s through today. Perhaps the best reason to study history is to better understand the present. The "present" for IRDs is exceptionally complex. Mutations in hundreds of genes are known to cause IRDs; tens of thousands of disease-causing mutations have been reported; clinical consequences are highly variable, even within the same family; and genetic testing, counseling, and clinical care are highly advanced but technically challenging. The aim of this review is to account for how we have come to know and understand, at least partly, this complexity.

In reporting progress in gene discovery for inherited retinal diseases (IRDs), it is important to keep in mind the ultimate goal of the research. The goal was, and is, to find the underlying cause of inherited retinal disease in each affected individual (those who wish to participate in the research) and to use this information to provide clinical benefits to patients and their families. A secondary, although integral, goal is to use this information to better understand the pathophysiology of ocular diseases and the biology of normal vision to improve health and welfare in general. We should be judged on how well we are meeting these goals, not just on advances in gene discovery per se. Other works have touched on these goals and show that, indeed, great progress has been made, although perhaps not as fast as we might wish.

HISTORICAL CHANGES IN TERMS AND CONCEPTS

There are several terms and concepts that have evolved over the years, but which, realistically, are still in flux.

First, there is the question as to whether IRDs are "dystrophies," "degenerations," or simply "diseases." Dystrophy implies an abnormality present early in development; degeneration implies a progressive disorder. But some IRDs only affect the retina later in life and some conditions are congenital but not progressive. "Disease" has the advantage of being neutral, but still implies a substantial burden on the patient, which is certainly true of IRDs.

Second, IRD-causing genes may be referred to by the disease name, the gene name, the protein name, the disease symbol, the gene symbol, or the protein symbol. Further, the names and symbols have changed through the years. For example, the locus, gene, and protein on the short arm of chromosome 1 causing Leber congenital amaurosis (LCA) has alternatively been called LCA2, RP20, *RPE65*, retinal pigment epithelium-specific 65 kD protein, and retinoid isomerohydrolase RPE65 (RPE65 database; www.ncbi.nlm.nih.gov/gene/6121). Each IRD gene has its own naming history. As a rule, be aware of alternate names and symbols, and state clearly to which you refer.

Third, IRDs are assumed to be monogenic, Mendelian diseases. That is, it is expected that in a given affected individual, and usually in affected first-degree relatives, only one specific gene is involved, although the gene may be autosomal or X-linked, and the mode of inheritance either dominant or recessive. It is also assumed that there are no common phenocopies, that is, diseases that are not monogenic but mimic the symptoms of an IRD. We already know exceptions to these rules. For example, some forms of retinitis pigmentosa (RP) are caused by a mutation in *PRPH2* plus a mutation in *ROM1* (i.e., digenic disease; Dryja et al. 1997). Symptoms of early-onset age-related macular degeneration may overlap with Stargardt disease (Cremers et al. 2020). And, most strikingly, mutations in some genes can be either dominant-acting or recessive (Sullivan et al. 2014, 2017).

Fortunately, these are relatively rare cases and the assumption of monogenic disease without phenocopies is generally valid. However, it is important to not lose sight of these possibilities. Also, it remains to be seen whether these assumptions hold for the 20%, at least, of IRD patients and families whose genetic cause cannot be determined yet.

Finally, perhaps the most important conceptual change over the past 40 years is recognition that these are not unrelated disorders, with unique, nonoverlapping names (e.g., RP, LCA, Stargardt disease). In fact, although there are many different IRD-causing genes, and many possible clinical consequences, these blinding diseases overlap in symptoms, causes, and shared disease pathways, and probably in ways not yet understood. Fundamentally, there is no one-for-one mapping be-

tween the disease name and the underlying causative gene. For this reason, it has been suggested that, after clinical evaluation and genetic testing, the "name" for the condition in an affected individual should be the mode of inheritance, the disease gene, and clinical type (e.g., "dominant rhodopsin [RHO] retinitis pigmentosa"). How best to name the condition in a way of most value to the patient and family but of sufficient accuracy for technical use is an ongoing discussion.

RESEARCH SUPPORT

Although not limited to genetics alone, it is important to acknowledge the remarkable, absolutely essential financial support for IRD research provided by foundations and agencies for decades. For example, the Foundation Fighting Blindness (FFB), originally called the National Retinitis Pigmentosa Foundation, has funded nearly $1 billion U.S. dollars of research on IRDs since its founding in 1971 (www.fightingblindness.org/about/mission-and-history). Many additional national and international organizations, all working together, have provided comparable support. These include Retina International, established in parallel with the FFB in the 1970s, and FFB chapters and allied organizations in most U.S. states and several countries (www.fightingblindness.org). Further, the National Eye Institute (NEI) of the U.S. National Institutes of Health (NIH) has had a specific, strategic focus on IRDs since the 1980s. This has directed several billion U.S. dollars to IRD research in both NIH extramural and intramural programs (National Eye Institute, www.nei.nih.gov/sites/default/files/2022-04/NEI%20FY%202023%20CJ%20Chapter_508_Final.pdf). Comparable funding has been awarded by government programs in Europe and Asia. This is a very incomplete list; it is just a reminder that no progress would have been made, or will be made in the future, if not for the incredibly generous support by individual donors, dedicated foundations, and committed governments.

1850–1980: EARLY RESEARCH

Any history of genetics should include a reminder of the enormous advances in understanding human inheritance in the past 150 years. There have been a series of scientific revolutions: Darwinian evolution, Mendel's rules of inheritance, Garrod's inborn errors of metabolism, chromosomal biology, and the structure of DNA leading to the "Central Dogma," culminating (for now) in the Human Genome Project (HGP) (Cohn et al. 2023). All of these findings and concepts are directly relevant to inherited eye diseases and part of the shared language spoken by experts in this field. This review assumes these as background, but it is important to remember that this is not universally shared, common knowledge, hence the need for, among other clinical specialists, genetic counselors to work with IRD patients and families.

Among the earliest descriptions of RP, and recognition of RP as an inherited disease, were publications by Donders (1855, 1857) and von Graefe (1858) in German.

There followed a series of papers in the early 1900s demonstrating the Mendelian nature of RP. In 1981, Heckenlively described 20 RP cases, clearly demonstrating either dominant, recessive, or X-linked inheritance (Heckenlively et al. 1981). Other forms of inherited retinal disease were reported in turn, and by 1985 it was clearly established that RP, LCA, and other inherited retinopathies were Mendelian in nature and amenable to detection by genetic techniques then in development (Marmor et al. 1983; Heckenlively 1988).

1980–1990: CHROMOSOMAL ASSIGNMENT

Arguably, the first useful technique for finding IRD genes was linkage mapping (Ott 1991). After many DNA-based, polymorphic genetic markers were discovered (e.g., restriction-fragment length polymorphisms [RPFLs]) (Lander and Botstein 1986), it became possible to assign disease-causing genes to specific chromosomal regions. The linkage regions were (and are) large relative to actual genes, that is, millions of DNA base pairs (BPs) versus thousands but, still, mapping firmly localized the disease genes. Among the early successes were mapping retinoblastoma to chromosome 13q14.2 (Sparkes et al. 1983), X-linked RP to Xp11.23 (Bhattacharya et al. 1984),

and autosomal-dominant RP (adRP) to 3q22.1 (McWilliam et al. 1989). However, these early successes did not lead directly to the causative genes and they only began to hint at the underlying genetic heterogeneity of IRDs. Nonetheless, by the year 2000, more than 100 IRD genes had been localized by linkage mapping (RetNet; web.sph.uth.edu/RetNet).

1990–2000: EARLY BENEFITS OF THE HUMAN GENOME PROJECT

The official start of the HGP was in 1990 (Lander et al. 2001; Venter et al. 2001). One of the revolutionary aspects of funding for the HGP was that sequence data had to be released to the public very quickly, even within 24 h of sequencing. For geneticists working on IRDs, this meant that, drop-by-drop, sequence data were released that might overlap with one of the mapped genes.

For those of us doing linkage mapping, it was a ritual to come into work each morning and look at GenBank, the go-to sequence database, to see if data covering our favorite region had been released overnight. If so, we immediately began sequencing patient DNAs to see if we could find the actual, underlying disease-causing gene and mutation or mutations. In general, this was called positional cloning or reverse genetics: for a monogenic disease, independent of any hypothesis as to the cause, use linkage mapping to localize the gene, then sequence the region and find the likely DNA damage. Often, once the gene was found, the essential next step was to try to understand why this gene was the cause of retinal disease, that is, to generate an actual hypothesis.

From 1900 to 2000, roughly 75 IRD genes were identified by positional cloning (RetNet, web.sph.uth.edu/RetNet), all dependent on sequence data from the HGP. This was the beginning of recognition that these are exceptionally heterogeneous disorders. One ironic consequence of finding genes based on overnight data was that many new IRD genes were reported nearly simultaneously by groups working independently. For example, the *RPE65* gene causing recessive LCA (Gu et al. 1997; Marlhens et al. 1997) and *RP1* gene causing adRP (Pierce et al. 1999; Sullivan et al. 1999) were each discovered, independently, by more than one group. Although this was, and is, daunting for researchers, it is hugely beneficial to patients.

In response to the rapid identification of novel IRD genes during this period, the RetNet database was initiated in 1996 (RetNet, web.sph.uth.edu/RetNet). RetNet, the Retinal Information Network, is a currated list of IRD genes, including the disease (or diseases) known to be caused by mutations in the gene, primary references, and other information. Web pages are updated as new genes are reported. The number of IRD genes known at various times in the past can be ascertained from archived RetNet pages. Finally, skipping ahead to the next decade, one profound outcome of identification of a myriad of IRD-causing genes was recognition of broad biochemical and pathological pathways underlying many of these diseases (Wright et al. 2010). A concomitant development was recognition that many of the IRDs with distinctively different clinical names actually overlap in causative genes and shared pathways (Berger et al. 2010). This is the justification for referring to all of the named, inherited retinal diseases as a single category, "IRDs."

2000–2010: THE MODERN ERA OF HUMAN GENETICS

The HGP transformed biology across the board, of course, not just for inherited diseases. In addition to the sequence data—by now encompassing millions of humans and tens of thousands of other species—the HGP introduced a steady stream of new, more powerful sequencing techniques and analytical methods (Heather and Chain 2016). Manual Sanger sequencing was replaced by automated, fluorescent Sanger sequencing; then Sanger sequencing was displaced by short-read, high-throughput, next-generation sequencing (NGS). Single-molecule, long-read sequencing, for example using Oxford Nanopore technology or PacBio sequencing, is the follow-on from NGS (Mastrorosa et al. 2023). Most recently, a combination of methods was used to produce the first, intact, telomere-to-telomere, human DNA sequence (Nurk et al. 2022).

These extraordinary technology advances were accompanied by equally exceptional computational advances. Many extremely powerful analytic methods for sequence analysis were developed in parallel. Extremely large DNA sequence databases were compiled, and powerful visualization methods, for example, the UCSC and Enterez genome browsers (Sayers et al. 2021; Nassar et al. 2023), were released. Most of the analytical and database resources were, and are, publicly available. In combination, informaticists refer to this as the "analytic pipeline," connecting raw sequence data with final conclusions regarding disease-causing genes and mutations, and, ultimately, clinical care.

These developments revolutionized finding genes and mutations causing IRDs. Far beyond this, though, to geneticists living through this period, the HGP was among the greatest scientific achievements in human history, with yet unimaginable benefits and risks.

All of these developments contributed to very rapid progress in finding the causes of IRDs. During this period, at least 80 new IRD genes were reported and the number of known disease-causing mutations increased to more than 1000 (Stenson et al. 2020; RetNet, web.sph.uth.edu/RetNet). This was the first clear recognition that, first, IRDs are genetically heterogeneous; second, in a population of patients, each disease gene will have many different pathogenic variants (allelic heterogeneity); and, third, testing just a few genes in an affected person will have low yield. To illustrate this last point, by 2007 it was known that mutations in more than 20 genes could be the cause of adRP (Daiger et al. 2007).

2010 TO PRESENT: BECOMING A MATURE CLINICAL SCIENCE

Major Trends

It is reasonable to describe the period from 2010 to the present as the consolidation and maturation of IRD genetics as a clinical science (but perhaps naive since there is much yet to do). During this period:

- the number of known IRD genes and mutations increased substantially;

- new genetic technologies were applied to IRD testing; and large-scale population screening was undertaken;

- genetic data became widely available through international databases; and

- genetic testing became an essential component of diagnostics, natural history studies, and clinical trials; and testing standards and guidelines were developed and promulgated.

Three broad developments define this period. First, as knowledge of IRD genetics increased profoundly, and genetic testing methods improved in parallel, it became possible to find the underlying disease-causing gene and mutation or mutations in the majority of IRD patients and families. Roughly speaking, it is now possible to determine the disease-causing genotype in 60%–70% of IRD cases based on certified testing in a commercial or academic laboratory, and in an additional 15% of cases based on research testing (Duncan et al. 2018; Thompson et al. 2020).

Second, noncommercial and commercial services have made substantial contributions to genetic testing, not just to advance knowledge of the field but, principally, as a prerequisite to developing and administering gene-specific and mutation-specific therapies.

Third, with each passing year, the subject of IRD genetics has become more complicated, novel mutation types have been discovered, and more exceptions to "textbook" genetics have been discovered. In retrospect, this last is the natural outcome of in-depth understanding of a complex area of human biology, but it presents a distinct challenge in communicating genetic findings to patients and families.

By 2010, roughly 150 IRD genes had been identified; currently more than 350 are known (RetNet, web.sph.uth.edu/RetNet).

Definition of an IRD Gene

There is a trivial debate regarding the definition of an "IRD gene"—although it has substantial clinical implications. Most of the first IRD genes discovered cause "simple" forms of retinal disease, either nonsyndromic such as RP or neurosensory such as Usher syndrome (Zahid 2018). As more genes were found, though, it became clear that many cases of inherited retinal degeneration were accompanied by additional symptoms (e.g., developmental abnormalities, neurologic disorders, and/or kidney disease). Further, some fall into the class of "ciliopathies," affecting ciliated processes throughout the body. Generically, the latter are syndromic and/or systemic disorders (Bujakowska et al. 2017; Chen et al. 2019). Whether these are all "true" IRDs is basically irrelevant; they are part of any reasonable count of IRD genes since they affect the retina and the earliest symptoms are often seen by ophthalmologists. However, the fact that so many IRD genes are syndromic or systemic, that is, pleiotropic in a genetic sense, has major implications for diagnosis, prognosis, and treatment.

Population-Based Genetic Screening

Reasonable estimates are that more than 300,000 Americans are affected with one or another form of IRD and millions worldwide (Daiger et al. 2007). As the number of known IRD genes grew, there was an obvious need to optimize genetic testing and to screen as many affected people as possible. Diagnostic testing was originally limited to certified academic laboratories, but a number of commercial testing facilities now dominate the field. Testing was restricted to genes associated with the patient's diagnosis (e.g., genes causing recessive LCA). This proved problematic, though. Since different mutations in the same gene may cause distinctly different diseases, limiting testing to the "typical" disease associated with a gene excludes other possibilities. Two alternative approaches are whole exome sequencing or whole genome sequencing. Both have advantages and disadvantages. Currently, most IRD testing is based on panel testing of all known IRD genes, specifically, exome sequencing augmented with noncoding sequences known to harbor IRD mutations and optimized for sequencing-refractory regions of the genome (Consugar et al. 2015). This is an evolving area of genetic testing, in general, likely to change significantly in coming years.

The need to know the full spectrum of disease-causing genes and mutations, and the hope of placing patients into gene-specific clinical trials, spurred development of several large IRD screening projects. One of the earliest, eyeGENE, the National Ophthalmic Disease Genotyping and Phenotyping Network, was established in 2008 by the National Eye Institute of the NIH (Goetz et al. 2012). Currently, more than 6400 eyeGENE patient samples have been tested for mutations in IRD genes using a variety of methods. In 2014, the Foundation Fighting Blindness, Columbia, MD, began My Retina Tracker to register IRD patients on a voluntary basis, and offer genetic testing if requested (Fisher et al. 2016; Zhao et al. 2021). To date, more than 20,000 individuals are registered and 10,000 have completed genetic testing.

A similar service, ID Your IRD, is offered by Invitae Corporation and Spark Therapeutics (McClard et al. 2022). Similar IRD screening services exist in Europe, Asia, and elsewhere; and several large-scale, focused screening projects have been conducted, for example, the Irish Target 5000 project (Stephenson et al. 2021). This list is necessarily very incomplete, and does not do justice to the many academic, regional, national, and international IRD screening projects. Suffice it to say, genetic screening of IRD patients and families has been a hugely successful worldwide enterprise, and the number of genotype-known patients is greater than 100,000.

Mutation Databases

The success in finding IRD genes (and many other disease genes, of course), and the ever-increasing number of reported IRD mutations, motivated development of comprehensive, gene-specific mutation databases. An early example is the Human Gene Mutation Database (HGMD), which became publicly available in 1996 (Cooper and Krawczak 1996). More recently, Leiden Open Variation Databases (LOVD), proposed in 2006 by Leiden University, The Netherlands, have served as templates for a number of mutation databases (Fokkema et al. 2005). Mutations in thousands of genes are now registered in one or more LOVD, covering all, or nearly all, known IRD genes (Cremers et al. 2014).

Determining Pathogenicity

One of the most pressing problems in genetic testing is distinguishing pathogenic from nonpatho-genic variants. This is a multifaceted problem. First, sequencing strategy, such as sequencing coverage and depth, affects which rare variants are detected and whether other, potentially pathogenic variants are missed. Second, different analytical methods may give different conclusions regarding pathogenicity or are uninformative. Third, confirming segregation of a potentially pathogenic variant in a family is informative but may not be feasible. Similarly, published reports of the variant found in other IRD patients is supportive of pathogenicity, but absence of a published variant is uninformative. Further, it is helpful to look for the variant in large databases, such as gnomAD (Gudmundsson et al. 2022), since if the variant is not extremely rare it is probably not pathogenic. However, if the patient is from a population that is underrepresented in the database this can be misleading. Finally, and fundamentally, pathogenicity must be confirmed by functional testing, including, for example, computer modeling of protein folding (Buel and Walters 2022), and animal, cellular, and organoid models (Ludwig and Gamm 2021; Moshiri 2021).

There has been exceptional progress in all of these areas for all human DNA variants, not just IRD mutations. Still, a significant fraction of possible IRD mutations is classified as "variants of uncertain significance (VUSs)," to the frustration of patients, clinicians, and counselors alike.

Of the many developments in evaluating pathogenicity of rare human DNA variants, two are particularly relevant to the present state of IRD genetics. The first is "standards and guidelines for the interpretation of sequence variants" proposed by the American College of Medical Genetics and Genomics (ACMG) in 2015 (Richards et al. 2015). The ACMG guidelines propose several lines of evidence and suggest specific variant categories: pathogenic, likely pathogenic, uncertain significance, likely benign, and benign. With a number of refinements since then, these have become the de facto requirements for rating potential disease-causing variants, including IRD mutations.

The second development was a response to the need for validation of disease-causing genes and mutations for gene-based therapies. This is applicable to all inherited diseases but especially to IRDs since the first FDA-approved gene therapy drug, Luxturna, effectively set the stage for future approvals (Russell et al. 2017). Discussions with the FDA, and reasonable expectations, suggest that pathogenicity of potential disease-causing mutations should be confirmed prior to initiation of therapy (Duncan et al. 2018; Thompson et al. 2020). To address this need, the NIH National Human Genome Research Institute (NHGRI), has established the ClinGen program to set standards for confirming that mutations in specific genes are the cause of specific inherited diseases, and has designated ClinVar as the authoritative database for validated, pathogenic variants (Rehm et al. 2015). ClinGen committees specific to inherited retinal diseases include the Leber Congenital Amaurosis/early-onset Retinal Dystrophy Variant Curation Expert Panel (LCA/eoRD), Optic Nerve Atrophy Variant Curation Expert Panel, and the X-linked Inherited Retinal Disease Variant Curation Expert Panel (Lee et al. 2021).

Finally, standards for genetic testing of patients with inherited eye diseases, including retinal diseases, have been proposed by the America Academy of Ophthalmology (Stone 2003; Stone et al. 2014 [AAO Task Force on Genetic Testing; www.aao.org/education/clinical-statement/recommendations-genetic-testing-of-inherited-eye-d]).

IRD Genetics Expands Understanding of Human Genetics

In addition to a profound improvement in finding genes and mutations causing IRDs, genetic testing for these disorders has revealed novel, or at least underappreciated, concepts in human genetics broadly. Examples include:

- Novel mutations in genes first identified as causing autosomal-recessive IRDs may cause dominant disease and vice versa. For a dominant disease, it is not surprising that compound heterozygous or homozygous mutations may cause more complex diseases or may not be viable. However, in some cases, two IRD mutations in a "dominant" IRD gene may also cause retinal disease, and retinal disease alone, albeit

usually a more severe form than the dominant phenotype. Examples include rare, homozygous mutations in two genes, *RP1* and *HK1*, both known to cause adRP (Sullivan et al. 1999, 2014; Kabir et al. 2016). Conversely, some mutations in genes commonly associated with recessive retinal disease (e.g., *SAG*), may be dominant-acting (Sullivan et al. 2017). That this occurs is not surprising since functional consequences of different mutations in the same gene may range from extremely mild to severe, but it reinforces that there is no simple mapping from an IRD gene to the clinical phenotype.

- Although many IRD mutations are rare, and limited to one or a few families, some have achieved appreciable frequency as a result of founder effect. For rare inherited diseases, a single mutation seen in unrelated patients may arise because of recurrent mutations (e.g., a mutation "hotspot") or from a single ancestral source (e.g., as a founder mutation) (Jobling et al. 2004). That is, a recessive mutation may attain appreciable frequency by drift alone, and a dominant mutation may segregate in families over many generations if the disease is of late onset or has limited effect on reproduction. "Common" IRD mutations are predominately founder mutations, whereas recurrent mutations are uncommon. The most striking example is the RHO Pro23His mutation, which causes adRP. This is a frequent cause of adRP in the United States but rare elsewhere: It is a founder mutation that arose in a single European ancestor several hundreds of years ago (Dryja et al. 1990). Another example is the SAG Cys147Phe mutation, which is a common cause of adRP in Hispanic families in the Southwest United States but rare otherwise (Sullivan et al. 2017). Finally, a recessive example is the intronic CEP290 2991 + 1655A → G mutation, which is a common cause of LCA—as high as 21% of cases—in Canada and Europe, but rare elsewhere (den Hollander et al. 2006).

- Mutations in the same gene may cause distinctly different phenotypes, even within the same family. It is a truism that there is considerable clinical variation within and between IRD families, especially in age of onset and rate of progression (Heckenlively 1988). However, in many cases, clinical variability is even more striking. First, some mutations causing dominant disease may skip generations, that is, are nonpenetrant, for example in *PRPF31* (Rivolta et al. 2006; Venturini et al. 2012). Second, for example, mutations in the *USH2A* gene cause recessive Usher syndrome, other *USH2A* mutations cause RP, and still others cause variable forms of disease even among individuals with the same genotype within the same family (Koenekoop et al. 2023). Third—another example—*RPGR* mutations may cause X-linked RP in males, or cone-rod dystrophy, or both within a family (De Silva et al. 2021); and female carriers may be unaffected or have symptomatic RP, again, varying within families (Fahim and Daiger 2016; Fahim et al. 2020). Fundamentally, exceptional clinical variability is a hallmark of IRD-causing genes. Again, there is no one-for-one relationship between genes and clinical phenotype. However, this raises the possibility that factors modifying clinical expression, once understood, will reveal novel therapeutic targets.

- Large families with multiple affected individuals over several generations may have more than one disease-causing gene segregating independently. It is reasonable to hypothesize that every affected member of a multigeneration IRD family has the same underlying disease genotype; indeed, this is the rational for linkage mapping. However, there are now several published instances of more than one disease genotype segregating independently in a family (Jones et al. 2017). Note that this is distinct from mutations in different genes that, working together, cause IRD in a single person (i.e., digenic disease). This is further confirmation that as IRD screening encompasses more patients and families, many "non-textbook" possibilities are to be expected.

- Although highly diverse, IRD genes fall into broad biochemical and functional categories, revealing novel biological pathways. Over all, perhaps the most underappreciated aspect of the impact of finding IRD genes is the numerous contributions to understanding the basic biology of vision. Although the functions of IRD genes are highly diverse, many fall into broad categories such as phototransduction, the visual cycle, or photoreceptor structure (Berger et al. 2010; Wright et al. 2010). Finding new genes in these pathways adds to our understanding of vision. However, other genes are surprises, suggesting previously unsuspected retinal biology. The most striking example is a set of genes coding for splice-complex proteins, *PRPF3*, *PRPF4*, *PRPF6*, *PRPF8*, *PRPF31*, and *SNRNP200* (Yang et al. 2021). Although the splice complex is an essential component of all nucleated eukaryotic cells, specific mutations in each of these genes cause adRP with no other apparent findings. Why this is so is not known, but it clearly hints at a component of mRNA splicing unique to the retina. A final example is the broad class of ciliopathies, inherited diseases that affect cilia, including the connecting cilium in photoreceptors (Bujakowska et al. 2017; Chen et al. 2019). Many of the earliest examples of this class of disease were identified as the cause of one or another form of IRD, although it is now known that many other human diseases are the result of ciliary dysfunction.

These few examples just skim the surface of the deep biological insights that finding genes and mutations causing IRDs have revealed over the past 40 years.

PRESENT AND NEAR FUTURE

How well have we met the explicit goal of IRD genetics, that is, to assist in finding treatments and cures for these diseases? A fair appraisal: We have accomplished a great deal but there is more to do. We have a much better understanding of genes and mutations causing IRDs, and there are extensive commercial and noncommercial services for testing. Genetic testing is now a routine part of clinical care for IRD patients in many communities. Testing is effective, that is, provides positive results, in from 60% to 80% of patients, depending on the tests available and patient demographics. Genetic test results are now integral to the many clinical trials and natural history studies currently underway. This is success, indisputably.

But substantial problems and issues remain. First, we need to find the remaining "elusive" genes and mutations causing IRDs, that is, to solve the 20%–40% of unsolved cases. This includes determining pathogenicity of VUSs. To address this, the near future will provide advanced sequencing methods, improved computational pipelines, rapid functional assays, and other tools. Second, we need a better understanding of factors that contribute to variation in clinical expression, including environmental factors, lifestyle choices, and biological modifiers. These studies are long term but made possible by access to genotype-known patients, if they wish, through programs such as My Retina Tracker and the Irish Target 5000 Project.

Third, there is a critical gap in understanding the relationship between genotype and phenotype: the pathway between an IRD mutation at conception and the clinical consequences is essentially unknown for any form of IRD. Solving this will require advances in molecular, biochemical, cellular, and histological research, among other disciplines. As challenging as this may be, in the long term, this information will be critical for developing safe and effective therapies. Further, IRDs are the ideal candidates for these studies, and are certain to improve our understanding of the basic biology of all diseases, as they have already for decades.

Finally, it is time to address equity, fairness, and access to care. For all complex medical problems, but especially for IRD patients, there is a need for expert clinical evaluation, knowledgeable counseling, appropriate testing, effective follow-up, and many other resources. Additionally, initial treatments are, and will be, expensive, requiring specialized facilities. For some patients and families these resources are immediately available, but not for most. Solutions are not at all obvious or easy, but must be considered.

But what a wonderful opportunity! Decades of research on inherited retinal diseases have brought us to the point where preventing the loss of vision, and restoring vision, are not only possible but are in our immediate future. Now we need to figure out how to make this available to the widest number of people possible, as soon as possible.

REFERENCES

Berger W, Kloeckener-Gruissem B, Neidhardt J. 2010. The molecular basis of human retinal and vitreoretinal diseases. *Prog Retin Eye Res* **29:** 335–375. doi:10.1016/j.preteyeres.2010.03.004

Bhattacharya SS, Wright AF, Clayton JF, Price WH, Phillips CI, McKeown CM, Jay M, Bird AC, Pearson PL, Southern EM, et al. 1984. Close genetic linkage between X-linked retinitis pigmentosa and a restriction fragment length polymorphism identified by recombinant DNA probe L1.28. *Nature* **309:** 253–255. doi:10.1038/309253a0

Buel GR, Walters KJ. 2022. Can AlphaFold2 predict the impact of missense mutations on structure? *Nat Struct Mol Biol* **29:** 1–2. doi:10.1038/s41594-021-00714-2

Bujakowska KM, Liu Q, Pierce EA. 2017. Photoreceptor cilia and retinal ciliopathies. *Cold Spring Harb Perspect Biol* **9:** a028274. doi:10.1101/cshperspect.a028274

Chen HY, Welby E, Li T, Swaroop A. 2019. Retinal disease in ciliopathies: recent advances with a focus on stem cell-based therapies. *Transl Sci Rare Dis* **4:** 97–115.

Cohn R, Scherer S, Hamosh A. 2023. *Thompson & Thompson genetics and genomics in medicine.* Elsevier, New York.

Consugar MB, Navarro-Gomez D, Place EM, Bujakowska KM, Sousa ME, Fonseca-Kelly ZD, Taub DG, Janessian M, Wang DY, Au ED, et al. 2015. Panel-based genetic diagnostic testing for inherited eye diseases is highly accurate and reproducible, and more sensitive for variant detection, than exome sequencing. *Genet Med* **17:** 253–261. doi:10.1038/gim.2014.172

Cooper DN, Krawczak M. 1996. Human gene mutation database. *Hum Genet* **98:** 629. doi:10.1007/s004390050272

Cremers FP, den Dunnen JT, Ajmal M, Hussain A, Preising MN, Daiger SP, Qamar R. 2014. Comprehensive registration of DNA sequence variants associated with inherited retinal diseases in Leiden open variation databases. *Hum Mutat* **35:** 147–148. doi:10.1002/humu.22458

Cremers FPM, Lee W, Collin RWJ, Allikmets R. 2020. Clinical spectrum, genetic complexity and therapeutic approaches for retinal disease caused by ABCA4 mutations. *Prog Retin Eye Res* **79:** 100861. doi:10.1016/j.preteyeres.2020.100861

Daiger SP, Bowne SJ, Sullivan LS. 2007. Perspective on genes and mutations causing retinitis pigmentosa. *Arch Ophthalmol* **125:** 151–158. doi:10.1001/archopht.125.2.151

den Hollander AI, Koenekoop RK, Yzer S, Lopez I, Arends ML, Voesenek KE, Zonneveld MN, Strom TM, Meitinger T, Brunner HG, et al. 2006. Mutations in the CEP290 (NPHP6) gene are a frequent cause of Leber congenital amaurosis. *Am J Hum Genet* **79:** 556–561. doi:10.1086/507318

De Silva SR, Arno G, Robson AG, Fakin A, Pontikos N, Mohamed MD, Bird AC, Moore AT, Michaelides M, Webster AR, et al. 2021. The X-linked retinopathies: physiological insights, pathogenic mechanisms, phenotypic features and novel therapies. *Prog Retin Eye Res* **82:** 100898. doi:10.1016/j.preteyeres.2020.100898

Donders F. 1855. Torpeur de la retine congenital e hereditarie [Contributions to the pathological anatomy of the eye]. *Ann Ocul (Paris)* **34:** 270–273.

Donders F. 1857. Beitrage zur pathologischen anatomie des auges. *Graefes Arch Clin Exp Ophthalmol*: **l**: 106–118; 103: 139–165.

Dryja TP, McGee TL, Reichel E, Hahn LB, Cowley GS, Yandell DW, Sandberg MA, Berson EL. 1990. A point mutation of the rhodopsin gene in one form of retinitis pigmentosa. *Nature* **343**: 364–366. doi:10.1038/343364a0

Dryja TP, Hahn LB, Kajiwara K, Berson EL. 1997. Dominant and digenic mutations in the peripherin/RDS and ROM1 genes in retinitis pigmentosa. *Invest Ophthalmol Vis Sci* **38**: 1972–1982.

Duncan JL, Pierce EA, Laster AM, Daiger SP, Birch DG, Ash JD, Iannaccone A, Flannery JG, Sahel JA, Zack DJ, et al. 2018. Inherited retinal degenerations: current landscape and knowledge gaps. *Transl Vis Sci Technol* **7**: 6. doi:10.1167/tvst.7.4.6

Fahim AT, Daiger SP. 2016. The role of X-chromosome inactivation in retinal development and disease. *Adv Exp Med Biol* **854**: 325–331. doi:10.1007/978-3-319-17121-0_43

Fahim AT, Sullivan LS, Bowne SJ, Jones KD, Wheaton DKH, Khan NW, Heckenlively JR, Jayasundera KT, Branham KH, Andrews CA, et al. 2020. X-chromosome inactivation is a biomarker of clinical severity in female carriers of RPGR-associated X-linked retinitis pigmentosa. *Ophthalmol Retina* **4**: 510–520. doi:10.1016/j.oret.2019.11.010

Fisher JK, Bromley RL, Mansfield BC. 2016. My Retina Tracker: an on-line international registry for people affected with inherited orphan retinal degenerative diseases and their genetic relatives—a new resource. *Adv Exp Med Biol* **854**: 245–251. doi:10.1007/978-3-319-17121-0_33

Fokkema IF, den Dunnen JT, Taschner PE. 2005. LOVD: easy creation of a locus-specific sequence variation database using an "LSDB-in-a-box" approach. *Hum Mutat* **26**: 63–68. doi:10.1002/humu.20201

Goetz KE, Reeves MJ, Tumminia SJ, Brooks BP. 2012. eyeGENE(R): a novel approach to combine clinical testing and researching genetic ocular disease. *Curr Opin Ophthalmol* **23**: 355–363. doi:10.1097/ICU.0b013e32835715c9

Gu SM, Thompson DA, Srikumari CR, Lorenz B, Finckh U, Nicoletti A, Murthy KR, Rathmann M, Kumaramanickavel G, Denton MJ, et al. 1997. Mutations in RPE65 cause autosomal recessive childhood-onset severe retinal dystrophy. *Nat Genet* **17**: 194–197. doi:10.1038/ng1097-194

Gudmundsson S, Singer-Berk M, Watts NA, Phu W, Goodrich JK, Solomonson M; Genome Aggregation Database Consortium; Rehm HL, MacArthur DG, O'Donnell-Luria A. 2022. Variant interpretation using population databases: lessons from gnomAD. *Hum Mutat* **43**: 1012–1030. doi:10.1002/humu.24309

Heather JM, Chain B. 2016. The sequence of sequencers: the history of sequencing DNA. *Genomics* **107**: 1–8. doi:10.1016/j.ygeno.2015.11.003

Heckenlively JR. 1988. *Retinitis pigmentosa*. J.B. Lippincott, Philadelphia.

Heckenlively JR, Martin DA, Rosales TO. 1981. Telangiectasia and optic atrophy in cone-rod degenerations. *Arch Ophthalmol* **99**: 1983–1991. doi:10.1001/archopht.1981.03930020859009

Jobling MA, Hurles M, Tyler-Smith C. 2004. *Human evolutionary genetics: origins, peoples & disease*. Garland Science, New York.

Jones KD, Wheaton DK, Bowne SJ, Sullivan LS, Birch DG, Chen R, Daiger SP. 2017. Next-generation sequencing to solve complex inherited retinal dystrophy: a case series of multiple genes contributing to disease in extended families. *Mol Vis* **23**: 470–481.

Kabir F, Ullah I, Ali S, Gottsch AD, Naeem MA, Assir MZ, Khan SN, Akram J, Riazuddin S, Ayyagari R, et al. 2016. Loss of function mutations in RP1 are responsible for retinitis pigmentosa in consanguineous familial cases. *Mol Vis* **22**: 610–625.

Koenekoop R, Arriaga M, Trzupek KM, Lentz J. 2023. Usher syndrome type II. In *GeneReviews [Internet]*. University of Washington, Seattle.

Lander ES, Botstein D. 1986. Mapping complex genetic traits in humans: new methods using a complete RFLP linkage map. *Cold Spring Harb Symp Quant Biol* **51** (Pt 1): 49–62. doi:10.1101/SQB.1986.051.01.007

Lander ES, Linton LM, Birren B, Nusbaum C, Zody MC, Baldwin J, Devon K, Dewar K, Doyle M, FitzHugh W, et al. 2001. Initial sequencing and analysis of the human genome. *Nature* **409**: 860–921. doi:10.1038/35057062

Lee K, Place E, Ayyagari R, Chen R, Goetz K, Hufnagel RB, Reis L, Roosing S, Souzeau E, Yu-Wai-Man P, et al. 2021. Establishing standardized criteria to improve the interpretation of genetic testing for ocular disorders. *Invest Ophthalmol Vis Sci* **62**: 1566.

Ludwig AL, Gamm DM. 2021. Outer retinal cell replacement: putting the pieces together. *Transl Vis Sci Technol* **10**: 15. doi:10.1167/tvst.10.10.15

Marlhens F, Bareil C, Griffoin JM, Zrenner E, Amalric P, Eliaou C, Liu SY, Harris E, Redmond TM, Arnaud B, et al. 1997. Mutations in RPE65 cause Leber's congenital amaurosis. *Nat Genet* **17**: 139–141. doi:10.1038/ng1097-139

Marmor MF, Aguirre G, Arden G, Berson E, Birch DG, Boughman JA, Carr R, Chatrian GE, Del Monte M, Dowling J, et al. 1983. Retinitis pigmentosa: a symposium on terminology and methods of examination. *Ophthalmology* **90**: 126–131. doi:10.1016/S0161-6420(83)34587-5

Mastrorosa FK, Miller DE, Eichler EE. 2023. Applications of long-read sequencing to Mendelian genetics. *Genome Med* **15**: 42. doi:10.1186/s13073-023-01194-3

McClard CK, Pollalis D, Jamshidi F, Kingsley R, Lee SY. 2022. Utility of no-charge panel genetic testing for inherited retinal diseases in a real-world clinical setting. *J Vitreoretin Dis* **6**: 351–357. doi:10.1177/24741264221100936

McWilliam P, Farrar GJ, Kenna P, Bradley DG, Humphries MM, Sharp EM, McConnell DJ, Lawler M, Sheils D, Ryan C, et al. 1989. Autosomal dominant retinitis pigmentosa (ADRP): localization of an ADRP gene to the long arm of chromosome 3. *Genomics* **5**: 619–622. doi:10.1016/0888-7543(89)90031-1

Moshiri A. 2021. Animals models of inherited retinal disease. *Int Ophthalmol Clin* **61**: 113–130. doi:10.1097/IIO.0000000000000368

Nassar LR, Barber GP, Benet-Pagès A, Casper J, Clawson H, Diekhans M, Fischer C, Gonzalez JN, Hinrichs AS, Lee BT, et al. 2023. The UCSC genome browser database: 2023 update. *Nucleic Acids Res* **51**: D1188–D1195. doi:10.1093/nar/gkac1072

Nurk S, Koren S, Rhie A, Rautiainen M, Bzikadze AV, Mikheenko A, Vollger MR, Altemose N, Uralsky L,

Gershman A, et al. 2022. The complete sequence of a human genome. *Science* 376: 44–53. doi:10.1126/science.abj6987

Ott J. 1991. *Analysis of human genetic linkage.* The Johns Hopkins University Press, Baltimore.

Pierce EA, Quinn T, Meehan T, McGee TL, Berson EL, Dryja TP. 1999. Mutations in a gene encoding a new oxygen-regulated photoreceptor protein cause dominant retinitis pigmentosa. *Nat Genet* 22: 248–254. doi:10.1038/10305

Rehm HL, Berg JS, Brooks LD, Bustamante CD, Evans JP, Landrum MJ, Ledbetter DH, Maglott DR, Martin CL, Nussbaum RL, et al. 2015. ClinGen—the clinical genome resource. *N Engl J Med* 372: 2235–2242. doi:10.1056/NEJMsr1406261

Richards S, Aziz N, Bale S, Bick D, Das S, Gastier-Foster J, Grody WW, Hegde M, Lyon E, Spector E, et al. 2015. Standards and guidelines for the interpretation of sequence variants: a joint consensus recommendation of the American College of Medical Genetics and Genomics and the Association for Molecular Pathology. *Genet Med* 17: 405–424. doi:10.1038/gim.2015.30

Rivolta C, McGee TL, Frio TR, Jensen RV, Berson EL, Dryja TP. 2006. Variation in retinitis pigmentosa-11 (*PRPF31* or *RP11*) gene expression between symptomatic and asymptomatic patients with dominant *RP11* mutations. *Hum Mutat* 27: 644–653. doi:10.1002/humu.20325

Russell S, Bennett J, Wellman JA, Chung DC, Yu ZF, Tillman A, Wittes J, Pappas J, Elci O, McCague S, et al. 2017. Efficacy and safety of voretigene neparvovec (AAV2-hRPE65v2) in patients with RPE65-mediated inherited retinal dystrophy: a randomised, controlled, open-label, phase 3 trial. *Lancet* 390: 849–860. doi:10.1016/S0140-6736(17)31868-8

Sayers EW, Beck J, Bolton EE, Bourexis D, Brister JR, Canese K, Comeau DC, Funk K, Kim S, Klimke W, et al. 2021. Database resources of the national center for biotechnology information. *Nucleic Acids Res* 49: D10–D17. doi:10.1093/nar/gkaa892

Sparkes RS, Murphree AL, Lingua RW, Sparkes MC, Field LL, Funderburk SJ, Benedict WF. 1983. Gene for hereditary retinoblastoma assigned to human chromosome 13 by linkage to esterase D. *Science* 219: 971–973. doi:10.1126/science.6823558

Stenson PD, Mort M, Ball EV, Chapman M, Evans K, Azevedo L, Hayden M, Heywood S, Millar DS, Phillips AD, et al. 2020. The Human Gene Mutation Database (HGMD): optimizing its use in a clinical diagnostic or research setting. *Hum Genet* 139: 1197–1207. doi:10.1007/s00439-020-02199-3

Stephenson KAJ, Zhu J, Wynne N, Dockery A, Cairns RM, Duignan E, Whelan L, Malone CP, Dempsey H, Collins K, et al. 2021. Target 5000: a standardized all-Ireland pathway for the diagnosis and management of inherited retinal degenerations. *Orphanet J Rare Dis* 16: 200. doi:10.1186/s13023-021-01841-1

Stone EM. 2003. Finding and interpreting genetic variations that are important to ophthalmologists. *Trans Am Ophthalmol Soc* 101: 437–484.

Stone EM, Aldave AJ, Drack AV, MacCumber MW, Sheffield VC, Traboulsi E, Weleber RG; AAO Task Force on Genetic Testing. 2014. *Recommendations for genetic testing of inherited eye diseases.* American Academy of Ophthalmology, San Francisco.

Sullivan LS, Heckenlively JR, Bowne SJ, Zuo J, Hide WA, Gal A, Denton M, Inglehearn CF, Blanton SH, Daiger SP. 1999. Mutations in a novel retina-specific gene cause autosomal dominant retinitis pigmentosa. *Nat Genet* 22: 255–259. doi:10.1038/10314

Sullivan LS, Koboldt DC, Bowne SJ, Lang S, Blanton SH, Cadena E, Avery CE, Lewis RA, Webb-Jones K, Wheaton DH, et al. 2014. A dominant mutation in hexokinase 1 (HK1) causes retinitis pigmentosa. *Invest Ophthalmol Vis Sci* 55: 7147–7158. doi:10.1167/iovs.14-15419

Sullivan LS, Bowne SJ, Koboldt DC, Cadena EL, Heckenlively JR, Branham KE, Wheaton DH, Jones KD, Ruiz RS, Pennesi ME, et al. 2017. A novel dominant mutation in *SAG*, the arrestin-1 gene, is a common cause of retinitis pigmentosa in Hispanic families in the Southwestern United States. *Invest Ophthalmol Vis Sci* 58: 2774–2784. doi:10.1167/iovs.16-21341

Thompson DA, Iannaccone A, Ali RR, Arshavsky VY, Audo I, Bainbridge JWB, Besirli CG, Birch DG, Branham KE, Cideciyan AV, et al. 2020. Advancing clinical trials for inherited retinal diseases: recommendations from the Second Monaciano Symposium. *Transl Vis Sci Technol* 9: 2. doi:10.1167/tvst.9.7.2

Venter JC, Adams MD, Myers EW, Li PW, Mural RJ, Sutton GG, Smith HO, Yandell M, Evans CA, Holt RA, et al. 2001. The sequence of the human genome. *Science* 291: 1304–1351. doi:10.1126/science.1058040

Venturini G, Rose AM, Shah AZ, Bhattacharya SS, Rivolta C. 2012. CNOT3 is a modifier of PRPF31 mutations in retinitis pigmentosa with incomplete penetrance. *PLoS Genet* 8: e1003040. doi:10.1371/journal.pgen.1003040

von Graefe A. 1858. Exceptionnelles verhalten des gesichtsfeldes bei pigmernentartung der netzhaut [Exceptional behavior of the visual field in pigmentary degeneration of the retina]. *Graefes Arch Clin Exp Ophthalmol* 4: 250–253.

Wright AF, Chakarova CF, Abd El-Aziz MM, Bhattacharya SS. 2010. Photoreceptor degeneration: genetic and mechanistic dissection of a complex trait. *Nat Rev Genet* 11: 273–284. doi:10.1038/nrg2717

Yang C, Georgiou M, Atkinson R, Collin J, Al-Aama J, Nagaraja-Grellscheid S, Johnson C, Ali R, Armstrong L, Mozaffari-Jovin S, et al. 2021. Pre-mRNA processing factors and retinitis pigmentosa: RNA splicing and beyond. *Front Cell Dev Biol* 9: 700276. doi:10.3389/fcell.2021.700276

Zahid S. 2018. *Retinal dystrophy gene atlas.* Springer, Cham, Switzerland.

Zhao PY, Branham K, Schlegel D, Fahim AT, Jayasundera KT. 2021. Association of no-cost genetic testing program implementation and patient characteristics with access to genetic testing for inherited retinal degenerations. *JAMA Ophthalmol* 139: 449–455. doi:10.1001/jamaophthalmol.2021.0004

Comparison of Worldwide Disease Prevalence and Genetic Prevalence of Inherited Retinal Diseases and Variant Interpretation Considerations

Mor Hanany,[1] Sapir Shalom,[1,2] Tamar Ben-Yosef,[3] and Dror Sharon[1]

[1]Department of Ophthalmology, Hadassah Medical Center, Faculty of Medicine, The Hebrew University of Jerusalem, Jerusalem 91120001, Israel

[2]Department of Military Medicine and "Tzameret," Faculty of Medicine, Hebrew University of Jerusalem and Medical Corps, Israel Defense Forces, Jerusalem 9112102, Israel

[3]Ruth & Bruce Rappaport Faculty of Medicine, Technion-Israel Institute of Technology, Haifa 3200003, Israel

Correspondence: dror.sharon1@mail.huji.ac.il

One of the considerations in planning the development of novel therapeutic modalities is disease prevalence that is usually defined by studying large national/regional populations. Such studies are rare and might suffer from inaccuracies and challenging clinical characterization in heterogeneous diseases, such as inherited retinal diseases (IRDs). Here we collected reported disease prevalence information on various IRDs in different populations. The most common IRD, retinitis pigmentosa, has an average disease prevalence of ~1:4500 individuals, Stargardt disease ~1:17,000, Usher syndrome ~1:25,000, Leber congenital amaurosis ~1:42,000, and all IRDs ~1:3450. We compared these values to genetic prevalence (GP) calculated based on allele frequency of autosomal-recessive IRD mutations. Although most values did correlate, some differences were observed that can be explained by discordant, presumably null mutations that are likely to be either nonpathogenic or hypomorphic. Our analysis highlights the importance of performing additional disease prevalence studies and to couple them with population-dependent allele frequency data.

A major feature in the characterization of a genetic disease is to determine its prevalence in various worldwide populations, a process that requires comprehensive national or regional health information and should be performed on a large population size to obtain accurate data on rare diseases (de la Paz et al. 2010). Disease prevalence is defined as the proportion of affected individuals in a specific population, and can be presented as "point prevalence" representing data collected at a specified point in time or as "period prevalence" representing data collected during a specified period of time. Disease prevalence is different from disease incidence, which is a measure of the number of new cases of a disease in a specific population during a specified time period. Disease prevalence is usually considered as a minimal value since it is reasonable to assume that not all patients are included in such analyses. One of the major motivations in obtaining accurate disease prevalence information is related to the development of therapeutic modalities. Gene-based therapy is currently being developed for specific genes and one of the major factors in deciding which genes to target is the predicted number of affected individuals due to mutations in these genes.

Unfortunately, performing such analyses is not possible in many parts of the globe, either due to lack of available information or to incomplete or inaccurate clinical information. As part of the characterization of inherited retinal diseases (IRDs), disease prevalence of specific phenotypes (such as retinitis pigmentosa [RP]) or multiple IRD phenotypes have been reported, mainly limited to the European and North American populations. For the current study, we collected information regarding the prevalence of clinically identified IRDs (Table 1; Fig. 1) and compared it to genetic carrier data obtained from large genomic databases (Table 2), included in our recent report (Hanany et al. 2020).

DISEASE PREVALENCE VERSUS GENETIC PREVALENCE OF IRDS

Among all IRDs, the prevalence of RP, the most prevalent IRD form, was studied most extensively and is usually cited in the scientific literature as ranging between 1 in 3000 and 1 in 5000 individuals (Pagon 1988; Sharon et al. 2020), with a predicted total of about 1.5 million expected affected individuals worldwide (Pagon 1988). Our literature survey (Table 1; Fig. 1) yielded 14 studies (eight from Europe and the United Kingdom, three from Asia, two from the United States, and one from Israel), in which a population size >100,000 was studied. While in some studies only nonsyndromic RP cases were included, others either reported all RP cases (including both syndromic and nonsyndromic cases) or did not provide information regarding inclusion/exclusion criteria. In some studies, the analysis was done on a specific age interval, as shown in Table 1. Despite these discrepancies, we included all

large-scale RP studies in Table 1. The prevalence of RP (not limited to specific age groups) ranges from 1 in 2086 in the vicinity of Jerusalem (Sharon and Banin 2015) to 1 in 9017 in South Korea (Na et al. 2017). The latter study represents an excellent example of a comprehensive population-based retrospective cohort study, which is nationwide (and therefore including over 50 million residents of South Korea) in which over 5000 RP patients were identified (Table 1). This study was made possible thanks to the Rare Intractable Disease (RID) program that is integrated into the Korean National Health Insurance (NHI) system and is run by the government, allowing registration of patients using predefined criteria, therefore ensuring diagnostic accuracy. Such large cohort studies are expected to yield more accurate results. Interestingly, a relatively low disease prevalence value was obtained in this study (~1 in 9000 at all ages and ~1 in 6000 for individuals over the age of 40 yr). The variability in disease prevalence among different studies (up to 4.3-fold) might stem from different population structures (e.g., endogamous versus nonendogamous populations leading to high versus low rates of consanguineous unions). Based on these studies, we calculated the minimal (nonsyndromic) and maximal (all RP cases) average prevalence of RP as 1 in 4660 and 1 in 4499, respectively (Table 1). It should be noted that in some of the studies, data are available for both the whole population and for individuals over a certain age (usually 40–50 yr). Since some IRD phenotypes (including forms of RP) have a relatively late disease onset, the higher values obtained in the more aged group might better reflect disease prevalence.

In addition to these studies, a large study was also performed in Spain (Perea-Romero et al. 2021); however, as the authors noted, it might only include patients from specific parts of the country and, therefore, we decided not to include it in the above calculated average. The prevalence obtained in this study was relatively low (1 in 27,436 for nonsyndromic RP and 1 in 13,121 for all RP cases). It also should be noted that some studies reported RP prevalence by performing a cross-sectional cohort analysis in which a few thousand individuals participated

Table 1. Prevalence of clinically identified IRDs compared to genetic carrier data obtained from large genomic databases

City/state/country	Prevalence[a]	References	Studied ages	Size of studied population	No. of reported affected Individuals
The prevalence of RP in large-scale studies					
South Korea	1:9017#	Na et al. 2017	All	>50,000,000	5692
	1:6000#		>40		
Denmark	1:6134	Haim 2002	All	5,129,254	837
	(1:3948*)				
Northern France	1:4225	Puech et al. 1991	All	4,000,000	931
Norway (south-east region)	1:6127*	Holtan et al. 2020	All	2,977,723	486
Virginia, USA	1:3700*	Boughman et al. 1980	All	2,479,000	670
Slovenia	1:7934	Peterlin et al. 1992	All	1,999,477	252
Maine, USA	1:5193	Bunker et al. 1984	All	1,124,660	236
	(1:4756*)				
Birmingham, UK	1:4869*	Bundey and Crews 1984	All	~1,000,000	214
	1:3195*		45–64		
Jerusalem, Israel	1:2086	Sharon and Banin 2015	All	945,000	453
Norway	1:4440	Grøndahl 1987	All	815,000	101
Switzerland	1:6931*	Ammann et al. 1965	All	700,000	101
Iceland	1:5800	Thorsteinsson et al. 2021	All	364,000	63
China	1:4000#	You et al. 2013	55–85	279,715	71
China	1:3784#	Hu 1987	All	196,777	52
Average	1:4660				
	1:4499[a*]				
The prevalence of Stargardt disease in large-scale studies					
The Netherlands	1:22,680	Runhart et al. 2021	All	17,282,163	762
Northern France	1:8627	Puech et al. 1991	All	4,000,000	431
Norway (south-east region)	1:53,173	Holtan et al. 2020	All	2,977,723	56
Iceland	1:17,000	Thorsteinsson et al. 2021	All	364,000	21
Average	1:16,832				
The prevalence of Usher syndrome in large-scale studies					
Louisiana, USA	1:22,727	Boughman et al. 1983	All	~4,000,000	143
Northern France	1:68,886	Puech et al. 1991	All	4,000,000	57
Eastern Spain	1:23,810	Espinós et al. 1998	All	3,875,234	89
Norway (south-east region)	1:40,000	Holtan et al. 2020	All	2,977,723	39
Denmark	1:20,000	Rosenberg et al. 1997	20–49	2,335,971	118
Birmingham, UK	1:16,085	Hope et al. 1997	>15	788,146	49
	1:10,574		30–49		
Heidelberg, Germany	1:16,129	Spandau and Rohrschneider 2002	All	517,000	424
Norway	1:27,778	Grøndahl 1987	All	815,000	28

Continued

Table 1. *Continued*

City/state/country	Prevalence[a]	References	Studied ages	Size of studied population	No. of reported affected Individuals
Iceland	1:40,444	Thorsteinsson et al. 2021	All	364,000	9
Average	1:24,971				
The prevalence of Leber congenital amaurosis (LCA) in large-scale studies					
Northern France	1:60,485	Puech et al. 1991	All	4,000,000	65
Norway (south-east region)	1: 66,172	Holtan et al. 2020	All	2,977,723	45
Denmark	1:25,063	Bertelsen et al. 2013	0–17	1,204,235	48
Average	1:41,932				
The prevalence of all IRDs in large-scale studies					
Northern France	1:2409	Puech et al. 1991	All	4,000,000	1660
Norway (south-east region)	1: 4347	Holtan et al. 2020	All	2,977,723	685
	1: 3856		16–66		514
Denmark	1:7692	Bertelsen et al. 2013	0–17	1,204,235	153
Iceland	1:2600	Thorsteinsson et al. 2021	All	364,000	140
Average	1:3449				

[a]Most data are provided for nonsyndromic RP cases only; however, in a few studies marked with *, syndromic cases were also included. These studies were not included in the average calculation. In some cases, marked with #, the authors did not indicate whether syndromic cases were included in the study.

and were clinically evaluated. Such studies suffer from a few drawbacks, including the enrichment of individuals with visual defects in the cohort (individuals with reduced vision might be more interested in providing information on their visual condition compared to individuals with normal vision), the relatively low number of studied individuals, and, more importantly, a low number of identified affected individuals in the study (usually less than 10). These studies are therefore prone to large variability and a tendency for overestimating disease prevalence. For example, three studies in which less than 10,000 individuals participated in India and Singapore concluded that 1 in 930 individuals (Sen et al. 2008), 1 in 750 individuals ages 31–70 yr (Nangia et al. 2012), and 1 in 1660 individuals ages 40–80 yr (Teo et al. 2021) are likely to be affected with RP, extrapolating to a total of 1.4 million expected affected individual in India alone (Nangia et al. 2012). A similar study in China identified four individuals with RP out of 4027 individuals, leading to a prevalence calculation of about 1 in 1000 and a total of 1.3 million expected affected individuals (Xu et al. 2006).

This is in contrast to large-scale prevalence studies indicating a total of 1.5 million affected individuals worldwide. Since the number of RP patients characterized in these studies is low, these estimates might not reflect the real prevalence in these populations.

Since other IRD phenotypes are less frequent than RP, assessing their prevalence is even more challenging and therefore only a few such studies were reported (Fig. 1). We provide here information on large-scale studies performed aiming to estimate the prevalence of Stargardt disease (STGD), Usher syndrome (USH), Leber congenital amaurosis (LCA), achromatopsia (ACHM), congenital stationary night blindness (CSNB), and all IRDs combined (Table 1).

STGD is a macular degeneration phenotype mainly caused by biallelic mutations in the *ABCA4* gene. The prevalence of the "classic" form of STGD is expected to be much lower than the calculated prevalence of *ABCA4* mutations, since mutations in this gene can cause various phenotypes (indeed including juvenile maculopathy, but also cone-rod degeneration [CRD], rarely RP) and even late-onset STGD

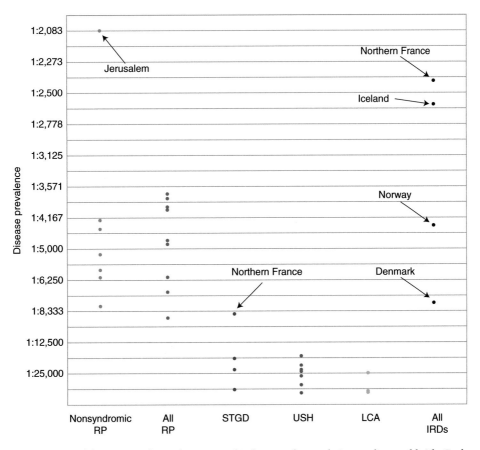

Figure 1. Summary of disease prevalence data reported in large-scale population studies worldwide. Each point represents a prevalence result obtained in a single study for each indicated phenotype. Black arrows point to highlighted studies with an indication of the city/country in which the study was performed. More accurate information can be found in Table 1. (RP) Retinitis pigmentosa, (STGD) Stargardt disease, (USH) Usher syndrome, (LCA) Leber congenital amaurosis, (IRDs) inherited retinal diseases.

often diagnosed as "early AMD" (Runhart et al. 2019; Cremers et al. 2020). Thus, the prevalence of STGD is mentioned in the scientific literature mainly as very rough estimations or speculations ranging from 1 in 1000 individuals (Riveiro-Alvarez et al. 2009) to 1 in 10,000 individuals (Michaelides et al. 2003; Tsang and Sharma 2018b) with no concrete period prevalence values. Endemiological analysis of STGD in the United Kingdom aiming to study its incidence in a 1-yr interval reported 81 new cases with a calculated disease incidence of 1 in 787,401 individuals (Spiteri Cornish et al. 2017). The prevalence of STGD was estimated in four large-scale studies in North Europe only (Table 1) with an average of 1 in 16,832 individuals and

large variability (1 in 8627 in Northern France vs. 1 in 53,173 in Norway). The largest reported study was performed in the Netherlands covering a population of over 17 million individuals (Runhart et al. 2021). This nationwide retrospective cohort study was based on the collaborative RD5000 disease registry that allows ongoing systematic collection, analysis, and interpretation of health data and diagnostic trends (van Huet et al. 2014). Establishing similar databases in other countries will enhance the ability of the scientific community to obtain more accurate large-scale disease prevalence and incidence data for STGD as well as additional IRDs.

USH is a heterogeneous syndrome causing RP and sensorineural hearing loss, which might

Table 2. A comparison of genetic prevalence (GP) and disease prevalence

Disease	GP	GP ratio	Number of expected affected	Percentage out of IRD GP	Disease prevalence (see Table 1)
Nonsyndromic RP	1.5×10^{-4}	1:6563	1,158,063	23.69%	1:4499–1:4660
STGD	1.5×10^{-4}	1:6578	1,155,328	23.64%	1:16,832
STGD late onset	8.2×10^{-5}	1:12,173	624,317	12.77%	–
USH	5.0×10^{-5}	1:19,891	382,084	7.82%	1:24,971
ACHM	1.8×10^{-5}	1:54,795	138,699	2.84%	–
CSNB	2.4×10^{-5}	1:41,543	182,943	3.74%	–
LCA	4.3×10^{-5}	1:23,109	328,876	6.73%	1:41,932
All IRDs	7.3×10^{-4}	1:1367	5,558,970	100.00%	1:3449

(RP) Retinitis pigmentosa, (STGD) Stargardt disease, (USH) Usher syndrome, (ACHM) achromatopsia, (CSNB) congenital stationary night blindness, (LCA) Leber congenital amaurosis, (IRDs) inherited retinal diseases.

be congenital (USH type 1) or appear later in life. The prevalence of USH was estimated in nine large-scale studies (Table 1) performed in Europe (seven studies), the United Kingdom (one study), and the United States (one study), with an average of 1 in 24,971 affected individuals showing relatively small variability between studies. Additional studies on USH (Tazetdinov et al. 2008; Kimberling et al. 2010; Yoshimura et al. 2021) used estimations and extrapolations to predict the disease prevalence and were not included in the average calculation presented here.

LCA is considered the most severe nonsyndromic IRD due to early-onset, mostly congenital, retinal degeneration. The prevalence of LCA was evaluated in three large-scale studies performed in North Europe (Table 1) with an average prevalence of 1 in 41,932 affected individuals. In other studies, prevalence estimations ranged from 1 in 33,000 to 1 in 81,000 (Allikmets 2004; Koenekoop 2004; Stone 2007; Tsang and Sharma 2018a).

For other IRDs, only isolated studies were performed. For example, the prevalence of ACHM, a congenital cone dysfunction phenotype, was reported as high as 4%–10% in the Pingelapese (Brody et al. 1970) in a small population of 285 individuals due to a single founder mutation in *CNGB3* and as 1 in 12,500 in the Jerusalem area (Zelinger et al. 2015) in a population of about one million residents that has a relatively high rate of consanguinity. These two studies do not represent other populations and

therefore there are currently no prevalence studies of ACHM in large populations worldwide. The prevalence of ACHM has been roughly estimated as ranging from 1 in 30,000 to 1 in 50,000 individuals (Alexander et al. 2007; Roosing et al. 2014; Mayer et al. 2017; Weisschuh et al. 2018; Hlavatá et al. 2019) with no concrete evidence.

Similarly, the prevalence of CSNB, a congenital night blindness disease, was studied in only two non-representative large-scale studies in Israel, reaching a prevalence of 1 in 6210 individuals in the vicinity of Jerusalem (AlTalbishi et al. 2019) and 1 in 10,661 among individuals ages 16–20 (Rosner et al. 1993). On the other hand, based on the population frequency of a single *TRPM1* founder mutation in Ashkenazi Jews (ASH) (Alu insertion in exon 10), an estimate of 1 in 4025 homozygous individuals in this population were predicted by allele frequency calculations (Hirsch et al. 2019).

Only four large-scale studies reported the prevalence of all IRDs, all of which were conducted on the North European population (Table 1; Fig. 1) with an average of 1 in 3449 individuals. Another large-scale study in Spain did not cover the whole population, reaching a relatively low prevalence of 1 in 7673 individuals (Perea-Romero et al. 2021).

We have previously reported a worldwide carrier frequency (CF) and genetic prevalence (GP) analysis of autosomal-recessive (AR) IRD mutations and diseases in a way allowing GP calculation for each IRD phenotype in various

Cite this article as *Cold Spring Harb Perspect Med* doi: 10.1101/cshperspect.a041277

worldwide populations separately as well as a combined worldwide value. It would therefore be interesting to know whether the overall GP data are in correlation with disease prevalence for various IRDs. However, before performing such comparisons, a few limitations should be pointed out: (1) While GP is based on AR mutations only, disease prevalence includes all possible inheritance patterns (and mainly autosomal-dominant and X-linked in addition to AR) and is therefore expected to yield higher values. (2) By calculating GP, only mutations in genes that were already reported to cause disease when mutated are included in the analysis, while in disease prevalence calculations, all affected individuals, regardless of the causative gene, are included. For example, recent studies showed that using IRD gene panels and whole exome sequencing (WES), the cause of disease was identified in only 50%–75% of samples. Again, this is likely to yield a higher disease prevalence value compared to GP. (3) While GP calculates the number of individuals harboring a pathogenic IRD genotype (including those who have not yet manifested the disease at a level that led them to be clinically diagnosed), disease prevalence considers only affected, identified individuals. Therefore, the first two arguments will result in a higher value for disease prevalence compared to GP, while the third argument will result in a higher GP value in noncongenital phenotypes. Table 2 depicts the calculated GP value for each studied phenotype versus the appropriate disease prevalence when available. Nonsyndromic RP is a heterogeneous disease for which ~70%–80% of causative genes have been identified, with an average age of onset of 25 yr. Therefore, one would expect a higher disease prevalence compared to GP, and indeed GP (1 in 6563 individuals) shows a lower value compared to disease prevalence (a range of 1 in 4499 to 1 in 4660 individuals).

On the other hand, STGD is caused by biallelic *ABCA4* mutations in the vast majority of cases with an earlier age of onset compared to RP. Although these features are likely to result in a similar value of GP and disease prevalence, GP (1 in 6578) is consistently higher than disease prevalence (1 in 16,832) in such calculations, not including late-

onset STGD. This difference can be explained by three *ABCA4* features, which are rarely seen in other IRD genes: first, recent studies showed that *ABCA4* mutations tend to be located in *cis* (Lee et al. 2021), therefore causing a higher GP value, since in *cis* mutations are counted twice in the allele frequency analysis. In addition, at least 16 *ABCA4* variants are considered hypomorphic and are likely to be pathogenic only when paired in *trans* with a null or severe pathogenic variant. Although the GP calculation does take such pairing of hypomorphic-null pairs into account, other known *ABCA4* variants might also be hypomorphic, but not yet identified as such, therefore elevating GP values. And third, a recent study (Runhart et al. 2020) reported imbalance of disease prevalence between males and females, therefore affecting the measured disease prevalence of STGD, since in the GP calculations no difference was assumed between males and females. On the other hand, recently a group of variants was found to be associated with late-onset STGD, and therefore disease prevalence will tend to be relatively low (since individuals with a genotype that should lead to this phenotype do not show symptoms until a relatively late age), indeed as is the case. The genetic analysis of *ABCA4* is extensively studied by various research groups (Zernant et al. 2017; Cremers et al. 2020) and therefore additional information might be accumulated in the coming years that might resolve this discrepancy.

The remaining studied phenotypes (USH, ACHM, CSNB, and LCA) are exclusively or mainly AR and congenital, therefore similar values are expected for GP and disease prevalence, indeed as is the case for USH. For LCA, however, disease prevalence is low compared to GP, which might be explained by the observation that mutations in autosomal-recessive LCA (arLCA) genes can cause other phenotypes (e.g., RP and CRD) (den Hollander et al. 2008). No representative reliable disease prevalence data are available for ACHM and CSNB, and GP is currently the only available measurement (ACHM—1 in 54,795 and CSNB—1 in 41,543 individuals). Similarly, GP for all IRD cases is calculated as 1 in 1367 individuals, which is higher than the reported disease prevalence (1 in 3449), probably due to the inclusion of phenotypes with relatively late disease onset.

In summary, estimations of disease prevalence that are based on large populations and are therefore likely to be reliable are rare and usually limited to specific populations. Thus, our ability to determine disease prevalence is limited, with the exception of RP, which has been studied in multiple geographical regions. Under this constraint indirect estimations of disease prevalence, such as GP and CF, which are performed on large genomic databases (e.g., gnomAD), provide important support for studies based on identification of prevalent clinical phenotypes, and, in less studied phenotypes such as CSNB and ACHM, they may provide the major resource for estimating disease frequencies. One should of course be aware of the above-listed differences between these two methods, and use the information in an appropriate way. Yet another reason for the differences between GP and disease prevalence data might be the inclusion of either hypomorphic or even nonpathogenic variants in the GP analysis, as discussed in the next section. In addition, while disease prevalence data usually include all inheritance types, GP data analyses largely and practically only reflect AR mutations. Dominant mutations are likely to be excluded or are extremely rare in public genetic databases due to exclusion criteria and therefore their frequency is unlikely to correlate with disease prevalence. Similarly, X-linked mutations are expected to affect all hemizygous males and some heterozygous females, and therefore their frequency in public databases is also expected to be lower than their actual contribution to disease prevalence.

DISCORDANCE BETWEEN EXPECTED AND OBSERVED PREVALENCE OF SPECIFIC IRD-RELATED VARIANTS

One of the possible explanations for different estimations of disease prevalence compared to GP might be the inclusion of sequence variants that are suspected or even reported as being pathogenic, but are either hypomorphic (causing disease only when combined with a severe mutation) or actually nonpathogenic. The vast majority of pathogenic recessive mutations are considered fully penetrant. However, recent studies on large cohorts of patients indicated

that 26 missense variants in *ABCA4* are hypomorphic and cause disease only in *trans* with a severe mutation (Zernant et al. 2018; Bauwens et al. 2019; Cremers et al. 2020). Since large sets of both patients and controls of the same ethnicity need to be analyzed, such hypomorphic alleles are difficult to identify.

Aiming to examine whether such variants exist, we studied a population for which reliable genetic data of controls as well as IRD patients exit: the ASH population. Based on the Israeli Central Bureau of Statistics data from 2019, 4.36 million individuals out of the ~7.2 million Jewish Israeli citizens are of full ASH origin. Over the last 20 yr, we recruited over 5000 Israeli patients with IRDs, who are predicted to represent ~50% of all IRD cases in the country (Sharon et al. 2020). This allows measuring the frequency of each causative variant (and mainly the most common ones) in this cohort. Similarly, the gnomAD v2.1 database includes next-generation-sequencing data of 5185 ASH individuals (5040 WES and 145 whole genome sequencing). Allele frequency was calculated from gnomAD data, and the number of expected affected individuals was calculated based on the Hardy–Weinberg equilibrium. For large deletions that cause IRDs in the ASH population, no gnomAD entries are available, and we therefore used data previously published on large sets of ASH controls to calculate GP (Stone et al. 2011; Chiang et al. 2018; Hirsch et al. 2019). For the current study, we performed chi-square analysis of the observed versus the expected number of individuals who are homozygous for each variant (Fig. 2) in 187 genes reported to cause an AR-IRD. The observed value was obtained for each IRD variant by summing the number of ASH individuals who are affected with IRDs and are homozygous for a causative IRD variant. Since our cohort is expected to include about 50% of all IRD cases in Israel, the number of expected affected individuals was corrected accordingly.

Interestingly, four apparent null variants (two in *CDH23*, one in *PCDH15*, and one in *TMEM216*) showed very high allele frequency (AF) of over 1% in ASH samples while none of them has been identified in IRD patients, and we

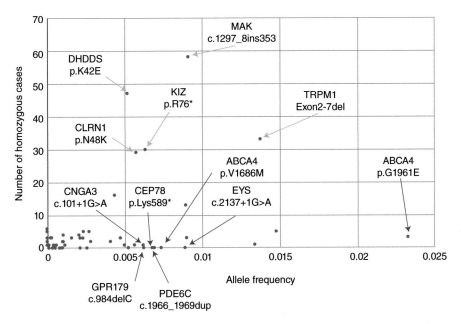

Figure 2. Graph representing allele frequency (AF) on the *x*-axis versus the observed number of homozygous cases in the studied cohort on the *y*-axis. Green arrows point to well-established reported founder mutations that show no significant difference between expected and observed data, while red arrows point to nonconcordant sequence variants showing a relatively high AF with no or a very low number of observed homozygous cases, indicating that these variants are either nonpathogenic or hypormorphic.

therefore concluded that these variants do not cause IRDs and they were excluded from subsequent analyses. All four variants affect regions in which multiple annotations at the RNA and protein levels are possible (*CDH23* variants c.101_105delAGGCG and c.101_105dupAGGCG are part of the 5′ untranslated region in most transcripts, *PCDH15* variant c.106 + 2T > C and *TMEM216* variant c.432-2_432-1insA are located next to alternative exons) and are likely to represent variants that should not be considered null and therefore are not part of the analysis.

Excluding hypomorphic variants, the most frequent ASH mutations in gnomAD were the following: *ABCA4*-p.Gly1961Glu (621 expected homozygotes in the Israeli population), *TRPM1*-chr15:31355203-31391647del (413 expected homozygotes), *CACNA2D4*-chr12:1,948,911-1,984,652 (313 expected homozygotes), and *WFS1*-c.1672C > T (256 expected homozygotes).

Aiming to identify variants that show a significant difference between the expected and observed number of homozygotes, we calculated

chi-square values for each variant and identified outliers. The analysis (Fig. 2) revealed well-established mutations that show no significant difference between the number of expected and observed homozygotes (Fig. 2, green arrows), including mutations in *MAK*, *DHDDS*, *TRPM1*, *KIZ*, and *CLRN1*. On the other hand, differences between the expected and observed number of homozygotes were obtained for various variants (Fig. 2, red arrows), some of which were reported in the literature as pathogenic. The *ABCA4*-p.G1961E variant, for example, has an expected value of 621 homozygotes; however, only three homozygotes were observed in our cohort. Although homozygosity for this variant has been previously reported as causing bull's eye maculopathy (Cella et al. 2009), recent allele frequency calculations (Hanany et al. 2018), as well as data on *cis*-acting modifiers (Lee et al. 2021), indicate that not all p.G1961E alleles are pathogenic and in some populations (e.g., the African and the Israeli populations) it is likely to assume that most p.G1961E variants are nonpathogenic, as also indicated in the current analysis (Fig. 2).

Our analysis also highlighted another nonconcordant *ABCA4* variant, p.V1686M, which might indicate that this variant should be considered as hypomorphic.

In addition, two of the nonconcordant variants are suspected canonical splice-site mutations in *EYS* (c.2137 + 1G > A in intron 13) and *CNGA3* (c.101 + 1G > A in intron 2), which have relatively high allele frequencies (Fig. 2), indicating that these are not fully penetrant pathogenic alleles. Both exons are not known to undergo alternative splicing and therefore there might be a nearby weak in-frame splice-site that can compensate for the mutation and produce a lower level of fully functional protein or normal level of partially functional protein. This hypothesis needs to be evaluated experimentally.

CONCLUDING REMARKS

One of the considerations in planning the development of novel therapeutic modalities is disease prevalence, which is usually defined by studying large national or regional populations. Such studies are rare and might suffer from inaccuracies and challenging clinical characterization in heterogeneous diseases, such as IRDs. Our effort of collecting data on large disease prevalence studies worldwide revealed a small number of such studies, most of which are limited to North Europe and North America. It is therefore highly important both to increase the number of IRD disease prevalence studies worldwide and to expand studies to areas or populations that currently have no or very little information regarding disease prevalence (Africa, South America, the Middle East, Asia, East Europe, etc.). In parallel to expanding such phenotype-based prevalence studies, GP studies can support the findings of more prevalent diseases and serve to assess the expected prevalence of phenotypes that are rare. In this context, expanding genetic databases (such as gnomAD), both in the number of participants and the studied populations, will assist in determining the set of pathogenic variants for many genetic diseases and the identification of hypomorphic mutations as well as mutations that were mistakenly labeled as pathogenic. Such combined improvement will allow not only to improve genetic analysis but also to identify the most appropriate genes and mutations that should be at higher priority for development of gene-based therapies as well as the populations in which such therapies would be highly relevant.

ACKNOWLEDGMENTS

The study was supported by the Israel Science Foundation (grant No. 1778/20) and the Foundation Fighting Blindness (BR-GE-0518-0734).

REFERENCES

Alexander JJ, Umino Y, Everhart D, Chang B, Min SH, Li Q, Timmers AM, Hawes NL, Pang JJ, Barlow RB, et al. 2007. Restoration of cone vision in a mouse model of achromatopsia. *Nat Med* 13: 685–687. doi:10.1038/nm1596

Allikmets R. 2004. Leber congenital amaurosis: a genetic paradigm. *Ophthalmic Genet* 25: 67–79. doi:10.1080/13816810490514261

AlTalbishi A, Zelinger L, Zeitz C, Hendler K, Namburi P, Audo I, Sheffer R, Yahalom C, Khateb S, Banin E, et al. 2019. TRPM1 mutations are the most common cause of autosomal recessive congenital stationary night blindness (CSNB) in the Palestinian and Israeli populations. *Sci Rep* 9: 12047. doi:10.1038/s41598-019-46811-7

Ammann F, Klein D, Franceschetti A. 1965. Genetic and epidemiological investigations on pigmentary degeneration of the retina and allied disorders in Switzerland. *J Neurol Sci* 2: 183–196. doi:10.1016/0022-510X(65)90079-1

Bauwens M, Garanto A, Sangermano R, Naessens S, Weisschuh N, De Zaeytijd J, Khan M, Sadler F, Balikova I, Van Cauwenbergh C, et al. 2019. ABCA4-associated disease as a model for missing heritability in autosomal recessive disorders: novel noncoding splice, *cis*-regulatory, structural, and recurrent hypomorphic variants. *Genet Med* 21: 1761–1771. doi:10.1038/s41436-018-0420-y

Bertelsen M, Jensen H, Larsen M, Lorenz B, Preising MN, Rosenberg T. 2013. Prevalence and diagnostic spectrum of generalized retinal dystrophy in Danish children. *Ophthalmic Epidemiol* 20: 164–169. doi:10.3109/09286586.2013.776692

Boughman JA, Conneally PM, Nance WE. 1980. Population genetic studies of retinitis pigmentosa. *Am J Hum Genet* 32: 223–235.

Boughman JA, Vernon M, Shaver KA. 1983. Usher syndrome: definition and estimate of prevalence from two high-risk populations. *J Chronic Dis* 36: 595–603. doi:10.1016/0021-9681(83)90147-9

Brody JA, Hussels I, Brink E, Torres J. 1970. Hereditary blindness among Pingelapese people of Eastern Caroline Islands. *Lancet* 295: 1253–1257. doi:10.1016/S0140-6736(70)91740-X

Bundey S, Crews SJ. 1984. A study of retinitis pigmentosa in the city of Birmingham. II: Clinical and genetic heterogeneity. *J Med Genet* **21:** 421–428. doi:10.1136/jmg.21.6.421

Bunker CH, Berson EL, Bromley WC, Hayes RP, Roderick TH. 1984. Prevalence of retinitis pigmentosa in Maine. *Am J Ophthalmol* **97:** 357–365. doi:10.1016/0002-9394(84)90636-6

Cella W, Greenstein VC, Zernant-Rajang J, Smith TR, Barile G, Allikmets R, Tsang SH. 2009. G1961e mutant allele in the Stargardt disease gene ABCA4 causes bull's eye maculopathy. *Exp Eye Res* **89:** 16–24. doi:10.1016/j.exer.2009.02.001

Chiang JPW, Luo H, Duan J, Ekstein J, Hirsch Y. 2018. Founder Ashkenazi Jewish mutations of large deletion in the inherited retinal dystrophy genes. *Ophthalmic Genet* **39:** 135–136. doi:10.1080/13816810.2017.1318928

Cremers FPM, Lee W, Collin RWJ, Allikmets R. 2020. Clinical spectrum, genetic complexity and therapeutic approaches for retinal disease caused by ABCA4 mutations. *Prog Retin Eye Res* **79:** 100861. doi:10.1016/j.preteyeres.2020.100861

de la Paz MP, Villaverde-Hueso A, Alonso V, János S, Zurriaga Ó, Pollán M, Abaitua-Borda I. 2010. Rare diseases epidemiology research. In *Rare diseases epidemiology* (ed. De La Paz M, Groft SC), pp. 17–39. Springer, Dordrecht, Netherlands

den Hollander AI, Roepman R, Koenekoop RK, Cremers FP. 2008. Leber congenital amaurosis: genes, proteins and disease mechanisms. *Prog Retin Eye Res* **27:** 391–419. doi:10.1016/j.preteyeres.2008.05.003

Espinós C, Millán JM, Beneyto M, Nájera C. 1998. Epidemiology of Usher syndrome in Valencia and Spain. *Community Genet* **1:** 223–228.

Grøndahl J. 1987. Estimation of prognosis and prevalence of retinitis pigmentosa and Usher syndrome in Norway. *Clin Genet* **31:** 255–264. doi:10.1111/j.1399-0004.1987.tb02804.x

Haim M. 2002. The epidemiology of retinitis pigmentosa in Denmark. *Acta Ophthalmol Scand Suppl* **80:** 1–34. doi:10.1046/j.1395-3907.2002.00001.x

Hanany M, Allon G, Kimchi A, Blumenfeld A, Newman H, Pras E, Wormser O, Birk OS, Gradstein L, Banin E, et al. 2018. Carrier frequency analysis of mutations causing autosomal-recessive-inherited retinal diseases in the Israeli population. *Eur J Hum Genet* **26:** 1159–1166. doi:10.1038/s41431-018-0152-0

Hanany M, Rivolta C, Sharon D. 2020. Worldwide carrier frequency and genetic prevalence of autosomal recessive inherited retinal diseases. *Proc Natl Acad Sci* **117:** 2710–2716. doi:10.1073/pnas.1913179117

Hirsch Y, Zeevi DA, Lam BL, Scher SY, Bringer R, Cherki B, Cohen CC, Muallem H, Chiang J, Pei W, et al. 2019. A founder deletion in the TRPM1 gene associated with congenital stationary night blindness and myopia is highly prevalent in Ashkenazi Jews. *Hum Genome Var* **6:** 45. doi:10.1038/s41439-019-0076-4

Hlavatá L, Ďuďáková Ľ, Moravíková J, Zobanová A, Kousal B, Lišková P. 2019. Molecular genetic cause of achromatopsia in two patients of Czech origin. *Cesk Slov Oftalmol* **75:** 272–276.

Holtan JP, Selmer KK, Heimdal KR, Bragadóttir R. 2020. Inherited retinal disease in Norway—a characterization

of current clinical and genetic knowledge. *Acta Ophthalmol* **98:** 286–295. doi:10.1111/aos.14218

Hope CI, Bundey S, Proops D, Fielder AR. 1997. Usher syndrome in the city of Birmingham—prevalence and clinical classification. *Br J Ophthalmol* **81:** 46–53. doi:10.1136/bjo.81.1.46

Hu DN. 1987. Prevalence and mode of inheritance of major genetic eye diseases in China. *J Med Genet* **24:** 584–588. doi:10.1136/jmg.24.10.584

Kimberling WJ, Hildebrand MS, Shearer AE, Jensen ML, Halder JA, Trzupek K, Cohn ES, Weleber RG, Stone EM, Smith RJH. 2010. Frequency of Usher syndrome in two pediatric populations: implications for genetic screening of deaf and hard of hearing children. *Genet Med* **12:** 512–516. doi:10.1097/GIM.0b013e3181e5afb8

Koenekoop RK. 2004. An overview of Leber congenital amaurosis: a model to understand human retinal development. *Surv Ophthalmol* **49:** 379–398. doi:10.1016/j.survophthal.2004.04.003

Lee W, Zernant J, Nagasaki T, Molday LL, Su PY, Fishman GA, Tsang SH, Molday RS, Allikmets R. 2021. Cis-acting modifiers in the ABCA4 locus contribute to the penetrance of the major disease-causing variant in Stargardt disease. *Hum Mol Genet* **30:** 1293–1304. doi:10.1093/hmg/ddab122

Mayer AK, Van Cauwenbergh C, Rother C, Baumann B, Reuter P, De Baere E, Wissinger B, Kohl S; ACHM Study Group. 2017. CNGB3 mutation spectrum including copy number variations in 552 achromatopsia patients. *Hum Mutat* **38:** 1579–1591. doi:10.1002/humu.23311

Michaelides M, Hunt DM, Moore AT. 2003. The genetics of inherited macular dystrophies. *J Med Genet* **40:** 641–650. doi:10.1136/jmg.40.9.641

Na K-H, Kim HJ, Kim KH, Han S, Kim P, Hann HJ, Ahn HS. 2017. Prevalence, age at diagnosis, mortality, and cause of death in retinitis pigmentosa in Korea—a nationwide population-based study. *Am J Ophthalmol* **176:** 157–165. doi:10.1016/j.ajo.2017.01.014

Nangia V, Jonas JB, Khare A, Sinha A. 2012. Prevalence of retinitis pigmentosa in India: the Central India Eye And Medical Study. *Acta Ophthalmol* **90:** e649–e650. doi:10.1111/j.1755-3768.2012.02396.x

Pagon RA. 1988. Retinitis pigmentosa. *Surv Ophthalmol* **33:** 137–177. doi:10.1016/0039-6257(88)90085-9

Perea-Romero I, Gordo G, Iancu IF, Del Pozo-Valero M, Almoguera B, Blanco-Kelly F, Carreño E, Jimenez-Rolando B, Lopez-Rodriguez R, Lorda-Sanchez I, et al. 2021. Genetic landscape of 6089 inherited retinal dystrophies affected cases in Spain and their therapeutic and extended epidemiological implications. *Sci Rep* **11:** 1526. doi:10.1038/s41598-021-81093-y

Peterlin B, Canki-Klain N, Morela V, Stirn B, Rainer S, Cerar V. 1992. Prevalence of retinitis pigmentosa in Slovenia. *Clin Genet* **42:** 122–123. doi:10.1111/j.1399-0004.1992.tb03222.x

Puech B, Kostrubiec B, Hache JC, François P. 1991. Epidemiology and prevalence of hereditary retinal dystrophies in the northern France. *J Fr Ophtalmol* **14:** 153–164.

Riveiro-Alvarez R, Aguirre-Lamban J, Lopez-Martinez MA, Trujillo-Tiebas MJ, Cantalapiedra D, Vallespin E, Avila-Fernandez A, Ramos C, Ayuso C. 2009. Frequency of ABCA4 mutations in 278 Spanish controls: an insight into the prevalence of autosomal recessive Stargardt disease. *Br J Ophthalmol* **93:** 1359–1364. doi:10.1136/bjo.2008.148155

Roosing S, Thiadens AA, Hoyng CB, Klaver CC, den Hollander AI, Cremers FP. 2014. Causes and consequences of inherited cone disorders. *Prog Retin Eye Res* **42:** 1–26. doi:10.1016/j.preteyeres.2014.05.001

Rosenberg T, Haim M, Hauch AM, Parving A. 1997. The prevalence of Usher syndrome and other retinal dystrophy-hearing impairment associations. *Clin Genet* **51:** 314–321. doi:10.1111/j.1399-0004.1997.tb02480.x

Rosner M, Hefetz L, Abraham FA. 1993. The prevalence of retinitis pigmentosa and congenital stationary night blindness in Israel. *Am J Ophthalmol* **116:** 373–374. doi:10.1016/S0002-9394(14)71358-3

Runhart EH, Valkenburg D, Cornelis SS, Khan M, Sangermano R, Albert S, Bax NM, Astuti GDN, Gilissen C, Pott JWR, et al. 2019. Late-onset Stargardt disease due to mild, deep-intronic ABCA4 alleles. *Investig Ophthalmol Vis Sci* **60:** 4249–4256. doi:10.1167/iovs.19-27524

Runhart EH, Khan M, Cornelis SS, Roosing S, Del Pozo-Valero M, Lamey TM, Liskova P, Roberts L, Stöhr H, Klaver CCW, et al. 2020. Association of sex with frequent and mild ABCA4 alleles in Stargardt disease. *JAMA Ophthalmol* **138:** 1035–1042. doi:10.1001/jamaophthalmol.2020.2990

Runhart EH, Dhooge P, Meester-Smoor M, Pas J, Pott JWR, van Leeuwen R, Kroes HY, Bergen AA, de Jong-Hesse Y, Thiadens AA, et al. 2021. Stargardt disease: monitoring incidence and diagnostic trends in the Netherlands using a nationwide disease registry. *Acta Ophthalmol* **100:** 395–402. doi:10.1111/aos.14996

Sen P, Bhargava A, George R, Ramesh SV, Hemamalini A, Prema R, Kumaramanickavel G, Vijaya L. 2008. Prevalence of retinitis pigmentosa in south Indian population aged above 40 years. *Ophthalmic Epidemiol* **15:** 279–281. doi:10.1080/09286580802105814

Sharon D, Banin E. 2015. Nonsyndromic retinitis pigmentosa is highly prevalent in the Jerusalem region with a high frequency of founder mutations. *Mol Vis* **21:** 783–792.

Sharon D, Ben-Yosef T, Goldenberg-Cohen N, Pras E, Gradstein L, Soudry S, Mezer E, Zur D, Abbasi AH, Zeitz C, et al. 2020. A nationwide genetic analysis of inherited retinal diseases in Israel as assessed by the Israeli inherited retinal disease consortium (IIRDC). *Hum Mutat* **41:** 140–149. doi:10.1002/humu.23903

Spandau UHM, Rohrschneider K. 2002. Prevalence and geographical distribution of Usher syndrome in Germany. *Graefe's Arch Clin Exp Ophthalmol* **240:** 495–498. doi:10.1007/s00417-002-0485-8

Spiteri Cornish K, Ho J, Downes S, Scott NW, Bainbridge J, Lois N. 2017. The epidemiology of Stargardt disease in the United Kingdom. *Ophthalmol Retin* **1:** 508–513. doi:10.1016/j.oret.2017.03.001

Stone EM. 2007. Leber congenital amaurosis—a model for efficient genetic testing of heterogeneous disorders: LXIV Edward Jackson memorial lecture. *Am J Ophthalmol* **144:** 791–811.e6. doi:10.1016/j.ajo.2007.08.022

Stone EM, Luo X, Héon E, Lam BL, Weleber RG, Halder JA, Affatigato LM, Goldberg JB, Sumaroka A, Schwartz SB, et al. 2011. Autosomal recessive retinitis pigmentosa caused

by mutations in the MAK gene. *Invest Ophthalmol Vis Sci* **52:** 9665–9673. doi:10.1167/iovs.11-8527

Tazetdinov AM, Dzhemileva LU, Khusnutdinova EK. 2008. Molecular genetics of Usher syndrome. *Genetika* **44:** 725–733.

Teo CL, Cheung N, Poh S, Thakur S, Rim TH, Cheng CY, Tham YC. 2021. Prevalence of retinitis pigmentosa in Singapore: the Singapore epidemiology of eye diseases study. *Acta Ophthalmol* **99:** e134–e135. doi:10.1111/aos.14483

Thorsteinsson DA, Stefansdottir V, Eysteinsson T, Thorisdottir S, Jonsson JJ. 2021. Molecular genetics of inherited retinal degenerations in Icelandic patients. *Clin Genet* **100:** 156–167. doi:10.1111/cge.13967

Tsang SH, Sharma T. 2018a. Leber congenital amaurosis. *Adv Exp Med Biol* **1085:** 131–137. doi:10.1007/978-3-319-95046-4_26

Tsang SH, Sharma T. 2018b. Stargardt disease. *Adv Exp Med Biol* **1085:** 139–151. doi:10.1007/978-3-319-95046-4_27

van Huet RAC, Oomen CJ, Plomp AS, van Genderen MM, Klevering BJ, Schlingemann RO, Klaver CCW, van den Born LI, Cremers FPM; RD5000 Study Group. 2014. The RD5000 database: facilitating clinical, genetic, and therapeutic studies on inherited retinal diseases. *Invest Ophthalmol Vis Sci* **55:** 7355–7360. doi:10.1167/iovs.14-15317

Weisschuh N, Stingl K, Audo I, Biskup S, Bocquet B, Branham K, Burstedt MS, De Baere E, De Vries MJ, Golovleva I, et al. 2018. Mutations in the gene PDE6C encoding the catalytic subunit of the cone photoreceptor phosphodiesterase in patients with achromatopsia. *Hum Mutat* **39:** 1366–1371. doi:10.1002/humu.23606

Xu L, Hu L, Ma K, Li J, Jonas JB. 2006. Prevalence of retinitis pigmentosa in urban and rural adult Chinese: the Beijing Eye Study. *Eur J Ophthalmol* **16:** 865–866. doi:10.1177/112067210601600614

Yoshimura H, Nishio SY, Isaka Y, Kurokawa T, Usami SI; Interactable Hearing Disorder Consortium. 2021. A nationwide epidemiologic, clinical, genetic study of Usher syndrome in Japan. *Acta Otolaryngol* **141:** 841–846. doi:10.1080/00016489.2021.1966500

You QS, Xu L, Wang YX, Liang QF, Cui TT, Yang XH, Wang S, Yang H, Jonas JB. 2013. Prevalence of retinitis pigmentosa in North China: the Beijing Eye Public Health Care Project. *Acta Ophthalmol* **91:** e499–e500. doi:10.1111/aos.12163

Zelinger L, Cideciyan AV, Kohl S, Schwartz SB, Rosenmann A, Eli D, Sumaroka A, Roman AJ, Luo X, Brown C, et al. 2015. Genetics and disease expression in the CNGA3 form of achromatopsia: steps on the path to gene therapy. *Ophthalmology* **122:** 997–1007. doi:10.1016/j.ophtha.2014.11.025

Zernant J, Lee W, Collison FT, Fishman GA, Sergeev YV, Schuerch K, Sparrow JR, Tsang SH, Allikmets R. 2017. Frequent hypomorphic alleles account for a significant fraction of ABCA4 disease and distinguish it from age-related macular degeneration. *J Med Genet* **54:** 404–412. doi:10.1136/jmedgenet-2017-104540

Zernant J, Lee W, Nagasaki T, Collison FT, Fishman GA, Bertelsen M, Rosenberg T, Gouras P, Tsang SH, Allikmets R. 2018. Extremely hypomorphic and severe deep intronic variants in the ABCA4 locus result in varying Stargardt disease phenotypes. *Cold Spring Harb Mol Case Stud* **4:** a002733. doi:10.1101/mcs.a002733

Rodent Models of Retinal Degeneration: From Purified Cells in Culture to Living Animals

Valérie Fradot,[1] Sébastien Augustin,[1] Valérie Fontaine,[1] Katia Marazova,[1] Xavier Guillonneau,[1] José A. Sahel,[1,2] and Serge Picaud[1]

[1]Sorbonne Université, INSERM, CNRS, Institut de la Vision, Paris F-75012, France

[2]Department of Ophthalmology, The University of Pittsburgh School of Medicine, Pittsburgh, Pennsylvania 15213, USA

Correspondence: serge.picaud@inserm.fr

Rodent models of retinal degeneration are essential for the development of therapeutic strategies. In addition to living animal models, we here also discuss models based on rodent cell cultures, such as purified retinal ganglion cells and retinal explants. These ex vivo models extend the possibilities for investigating pathological mechanisms and assessing the neuroprotective effect of pharmacological agents by eliminating questions on drug pharmacokinetics and bioavailability. The number of living rodent models has greatly increased with the possibilities to achieve transgenic modifications in animals for knocking in and out genes and mutations. The Cre-*lox* system has further enabled investigators to target specific genes or mutations in specific cells at specific stages. However, chemically or physically induced models can provide alternatives to such targeted gene modifications. The increased diversity of rodent models has widened our possibility to address most ocular pathologies for providing initial proof of concept of innovative therapeutic strategies.

The ultimate goal of vision research is to understand the underlying mechanisms of vision as well as visual pathologies, prevent vision loss, and restore sight in blind patients. Inherited retinal degenerations that lead to blindness are as yet mostly untreatable, apart from one approved gene augmentation therapy for retinal disease associated with mutations in the *RPE65* gene. Additional examples of highly prevalent retinal degenerative diseases that are currently an unmet need include the nonneovascular (dry) form of age-related macular degeneration as well as the loss of retinal ganglion cells (RGCs) in glaucoma that often occurs despite available treatments. The need for novel treatments is urged by the high number of blind patients worldwide rising above 30 million (Bourne et al. 2017; GBD 2019 Blindness and Vision Impairment Collaborators et al. 2021) with an expected doubling of blind and tripling of visually impaired patients, respectively, due mostly to population aging at the 2050 horizon (Bourne et al. 2017).

To develop treatments for the prevention of retinal diseases, there is a clear need to develop models that will allow better understanding of normal processes of vision as well as pathological mechanisms leading to blindness or severe visual impairment. In addition to naturally occurring rodent animal models of retinal diseases, the recent development of transgenic animals has transformed the analysis of normal and pathological mechanisms of vision. Transgenic animals have not only provided living models of retinal diseases, they also allowed the production of animals containing the green fluorescent protein (GFP) in different cell types. Via fluorescent-activated cell sorting (FACS), this permits generation of purified cell cultures as well as analysis of gene expression patterns in specific cell types. In addition to the culture of purified rodent retinal cells, culture of the whole retina has also provided interesting models to assess molecular mechanisms in a fully wired structure with the ease to apply various pharmacological agents in the medium, either toxic or therapeutic. Recently, the development of retinal organoids from stem cells or induced pluripotent stem cells (iPSCs) from control or patient cells further expands the potential of these in vitro approaches to develop therapeutic strategies (Reichman et al. 2014, 2017). These in vitro models of retinal diseases also carry an additional benefit in that they adhere to the 3R objectives of reduction, refinement, and replacement of animal experimentation.

We therefore propose here to review different rodent models, ranging from single cell types in culture to living animals, as tools for the development of novel therapeutic strategies for retinal degenerative diseases.

RODENT MONOLAYER CELL CULTURES

In vitro culture of rodent retinal cells was obtained with different cell types, from retinal pigment epithelium (RPE) cells to retinal neurons including photoreceptors and retinal ganglion cells (Hicks and Courtois 1990, 1992; Malecaze et al. 1993; Heidinger et al. 1998). Several methods are available to separate retinal pigmented epithelium cells from the retina and obtain a pure preparation for seeding in culture dishes (Hicks et al. 1990). These cells can divide until confluence, reconstituting in a layer similar to that seen in vivo. However, for large studies on

retinal pigment epithelium such as light toxicity, we recently preferred porcine eyes available in large quantities to obtain more cells (Arnault et al. 2013; Fontaine et al. 2016, 2021; Marie et al. 2018). This method is also relevant for primates, including human eyes under condition of a reduced postmortem delay. Using freshly removed macaque eyes, we were able to apply trypsin in the eyecup and harvest RPE cells that survived for several weeks. With opportunity to get human donor eyes, we established that a postmortem delay of <10 h is the key for success of the purification protocol. Glial cells were also prepared and cultured from overnight incubated rat eyes following mere retinal dissociation (Hicks and Courtois 1990; Heidinger et al. 1998) or from dissociated porcine retina on a density gradient (Guidry 1996).

Rat retinal ganglion cells were also purified by a technique named "immunopanning" using Thy1 antibody (Barres et al. 1988) to then assess the effect of different trophic factors on their survival in vitro (Meyer-Franke et al. 1995). This approach was also used to investigate axonal growth and myelinization (Watkins et al. 2008). Although these postnatal day 5 (P5) retinal ganglion cells required a combination of brain-derived neurotrophic factor (BDNF), ciliary neurotrophic factor (CNTF), and components like forskolin to survive (Watkins et al. 2008), we found that adult rat retinal ganglion cells prepared in the same manner did not require these factors although conditioning media from Müller cells or mesenchymal cells were neuroprotective (Fuchs et al. 2005; Roubeix et al. 2015). We also demonstrated that these retinal ganglion cells were sensitive to tumor necrosis factor α (TNF-α) through nuclear factor κ-light-chain enhancer of activated B cells (NF-κB) activation (Fuchs et al. 2005). Furthermore, we showed that vascular endothelial growth factor (VEGF) is an autocrine/paracrine trophic factor for these adult retinal ganglion cells in culture (Froger et al. 2020). Taurine was also found to support their survival in vitro (Froger et al. 2012).

Photoreceptor cells were also purified from the rodent retina by cutting the tissue in its thickness at the level of the outer plexiform layer to then investigate photoreceptor sensitivity to fac-

 Cite this article as *Cold Spring Harb Perspect Med* doi: 10.1101/cshperspect.a041311

tors such as fibroblast growth factor (FGF) (Fontaine et al. 1998). However, these isolated photoreceptors, mainly rods, did not survive for very long in culture beyond P10. Adult porcine photoreceptors purified similarly were found to survive on a glial feeder layer for weeks (Picaud et al. 1998). For the analysis of cone survival, other species such as chick and pig have been used to test survival medium and factors, because of the very low number of mouse cone photoreceptors (Léveillard et al. 2004; Balse et al. 2005). Porcine cones were purified by lectin panning (Balse et al. 2005) with a survival effect promoted by a glial conditioned medium (Balse et al. 2005). Such purified cone photoreceptor cells enabled us to identify blue violet light as the most toxic to cone cells even at intensities that the retina is exposed to during the summertime in France (Marie et al. 2020).

RETINAL EXPLANTS

To preserve the retinal architecture with original synaptic connections, the whole retina was kept in culture with great success at the water/air interface first on small rafts and then on insert wells (Caffé et al. 1993; Soderpalm et al. 1994; Pinzón-Duarte et al. 2000; Vallazza-Deschamps et al. 2005), allowing us to assess retinal cell development while controlling the extracellular medium (Caffé et al. 1993; Soderpalm et al. 1994; Pinzón-Duarte et al. 2000). These explant cultures offer the advantage of very precisely controlling the extracellular medium for application of toxic molecules for modeling neuronal degeneration or to assess the efficacy of pharmacological agents for neuroprotection (Vallazza-Deschamps et al. 2005; Froger et al. 2013). Depending on the cell of interest, the retinal pigment epithelium can be kept in contact with the retina for investigating photoreceptor survival (Vallazza-Deschamps et al. 2005), whereas assessing retinal ganglion cell survival does not require its presence (Froger et al. 2012). For instance, phosphodiesterase blockers were applied to model photoreceptor degeneration (Vallazza-Deschamps et al. 2005), whereas retinal ganglion cell loss was induced by application of a glutamate receptor agonist, MK801 (Froger et al. 2013). Retinas from various animal models of photoreceptor

degeneration (e.g., rd1, P23H rhodopsin) were also used in such studies to screen for neuroprotective molecules because these explants bypass all problems of molecule bioavailability that may exist in vivo via application directly in the culture medium (Vallazza-Deschamps et al. 2005; Sen et al. 2021a,b). Reverse magnetofection was even applied to deliver small interfering RNA (siRNA) in rodent retinal explant (Bassetto et al. 2021). These ex vivo retinal explant cultures can thus provide an interesting modality to limit in vivo animal experimentation while demonstrating efficacy of a drug, such as in neuroprotection. Since these early studies in rodents, retinal explants were further developed with other species like the bovine retina (Peynshaert et al. 2017) or even with postmortem human retina (Busskamp et al. 2010; Fradot et al. 2011) to investigate retinal gene delivery.

LIVING ANIMALS

Retinal function and structure including effects of degenerative processes as well as various treatments can be documented in living rodents using a wide range of noninvasive technologies that are also applied in humans. These include monitoring visual behavior and assessing acuity through the optomotor response (Abdeljalil et al. 2005), quantifying rod and cone–derived retinal function by electroretinography (Orhan et al. 2015), and documenting retinal structure by fundus color and autofluorescence imaging (Paques et al. 2007), optical coherence tomography (OCT) (Orhan et al. 2015), and scanning laser ophthalmoscopy (Paques et al. 2005). Isolating the retina allows recording the ex vivo activity in retinal ganglion cells using a multielectrode array to further characterize the functional change in the diseased tissue. Waves of activity were thus observed in the degenerating retina with features highly reminiscent to those described during development (Stasheff 2008; Kolomiets et al. 2010). Then, histopathology provides access to cell counting in both sections or retinal flat mounts (Clérin et al. 2011) while investigating the degree of reactive gliosis with increased expression of the glial fibrillary acidic protein in Müller cells at or around the lesion area (Picaud et al. 1993) or the migration and transformation of microglial cells from stellate cells to an amoeboid morphology (Gaucher et al. 2007).

Increased Intraocular Pressure

Increase of intraocular pressure (IOP) is a main risk factor in the development of glaucoma, and animal models of glaucoma can be created by increasing the IOP in the eye through different strategies. Thus, the disease was modeled by transiently increasing the intraocular pressure for a limited period (1 h) in the anterior chamber (Mohand-Said et al. 1997). In addition, increase of IOP can be induced by cauterization of episcleral veins (Froger et al. 2012). A similar result was obtained by laser photocoagulation of episcleral and limbal veins (Salinas-Navarro et al. 2010). Injection of polystyrene or magnetic beads in the anterior chamber was also used to block the mouse trabecular meshwork, thereby raising the IOP (Cone et al. 2010; Mao et al. 2013). In clinical practice, many different topical treatments that lower IOP have proved efficient in attenuating disease progression toward blindness. However, unfortunately, even when controlling the pressure, some patients still experience retinal ganglion cell loss and additional effective treatments for this highly prevalent disease are sorely needed.

Light Damage

Light damage models are widely used to investigate intracellular mechanisms that lead to photoreceptor cell death, a common feature in retinitis pigmentosa and age-related macular degeneration. Photochemical damage to the retina occurs after short or prolonged exposures of mild or intense light in mice and rats. The "white light damage" model targets photoreceptors, whereas the "blue light damage" model (excitation peak 440 nm) induces primarily RPE cell photosensitization. These models have been shown to have a major impact on photoreceptor and RPE function, inducing photochemical damage and leading to cell death (Wu et al. 2005). It is also possible to couple transgenic models sharing cellular features of AMD with light damage. Thus, transgenic

$Abca4^{-/-}$ or $Abca4^{-/-}Rdh8^{-/-}$ mice that accumulate RPE lipofuscin at increased levels are more susceptible to retinal light damage than wild-type mice (Maeda et al. 2008, 2009; Wu et al. 2014; Fontaine et al. 2016).

Laser-Induced Subretinal Inflammation

Laser treatments were applied to generate choroidal neovascularization (CNV) as a model of the neovascular ("wet") form of age-related macular degeneration (Combadière et al. 2007). This model allowed analysis of different treatment modalities including anti-VEGF treatments and studying the role of inflammation in CNV formation. It involves the induction of CNV using laser photocoagulation that penetrates the Bruchs membrane, which mimics the pathological processes seen in diseases such as age-related macular degeneration (AMD) (Grossniklaus et al. 2010). Subretinal inflammation is induced in pigmented mice with a laser mounted on a slit lamp. The injury induces a neutrophil and macrophage (macrophage/microglial cell) infiltration that can be quantified using Ly-6G and IBA-1 immunostainings on retinal and choroidal flat mounts or by FACS analysis at different time points after laser injury. Ly-6G$^+$ neutrophils are significantly recruited to the injury site, reaching their maximum at 10 h and being cleared at day 3. IBA-1$^+$ macrophages are recruited at day 3, reach a maximum at day 4, and diminish thereafter. Agonists and antagonists can be administered at different time points after laser injury by intravitreal injection (Camelo et al. 2012; Levy et al. 2015) or systemic treatment (Lavalette et al. 2011). Even sizeable molecules (such as antibodies) penetrate the post–laser injury retina and can affect subretinal inflammation. Choroidal neovascularization is evaluated by angiography or by OCT in vivo and by immunostained flat mounts postmortem. Although the trigger to induce neovascularization is very different from the human disease, mechanisms of downstream subretinal inflammation and neo-angiogenesis are likely similar. For instance, aflibercept, which blocks murine as well as human VEGF, inhibits CNV in this model similar to its effect in humans (Ma et al. 2016).

Oxygen-Induced Retinopathy

Ischemic retinopathies, including retinopathy of prematurity (ROP), vein occlusion, and diabetic retinopathy (DR) are all characterized by primary retinal ischemia. If left untreated, they can progress to neuronal dysfunction and proliferative forms of retinopathies causing rapid and irreversible vision loss. Unlike humans, adult rodents do not develop a proliferative response to experimental ischemic situations even following laser-induced vein occlusion or diabetes induction. To address the mechanisms of proliferative retinopathies, Smith et al. described a model of oxygen-induced retinopathy in newborn mice (Smith et al. 1994). The treatment relies on exposing neonatal mice to alternating periods of high and low oxygen levels. This results in retinal vascular abnormalities resembling those observed in human retinopathy of prematurity and diabetic retinopathy. As a consequence, it has since become a widely used model for studying the pathophysiology and potential treatments of ischemic retinopathies.

In addition to the vascular abnormalities observed in human retinopathy of prematurity, persistent rod photoreceptor dysfunction is observed in adulthood despite the clinical resolution of vascular abnormalities (Fulton et al. 2009). A similar observation is made in the mouse and rat oxygen-induced retinopathy models (Liu et al. 2005; Vessey et al. 2011). This long-term loss of rod photoreceptor function, while cone function remains intact, has been attributed to differential metabolic adaptation of rods and cones to ischemic stress (Fulton et al. 2009). Overall, while the oxygen-induced retinopathy model is widely used to study pathological retinal neovascularization, it also allows for the investigation of rod photoreceptor responses to acute ischemia as well as long-term modifications of rod photoreceptor activity.

Pharmacological Models

Different pharmacological treatments were shown to induce retinal degeneration. For instance, treatments limiting taurine transport by introducing β-alanine or guanidinoethane sulfonate in the diet were first reported to induce photoreceptor degeneration (Pasantes-Morales et al. 1983). More recently, similar treatments were shown to preferentially affect cone photoreceptors and retinal ganglion cells (Gaucher et al. 2012; García-Ayuso et al. 2019). This more precise description of the damaging effect of taurine deficiency resulted from the investigation of the retinal toxicity of vigabatrin, an antiepileptic drug still prescribed in infantile spams, which was shown to induce taurine deficiency in rodents and patients (Jammoul et al. 2009). It was first reported to generate a destruction of the outer nuclear layer in albino animals (Butler et al. 1987), and we showed that the earlier cone and retinal ganglion cell degeneration is related to taurine deficiency associated with phototoxicity (Duboc et al. 2004; Jammoul et al. 2009, 2010).

In glaucoma, the loss of retinal ganglion cells was often attributed to glutamate excitotoxicity (Lipton 2003). Supporting this hypothesis, memantine, an N-methyl-D-aspartate (NMDA) receptor antagonist, was found to be neuroprotective in different animal models of glaucoma (Wolde-Mussie et al. 2002). As a consequence, glaucomatous conditions are often modeled by intraocular injection of a glutamate NMDA receptor agonist (Torero Ibad et al. 2011). However, memantine was not found to be efficient in the treatment of glaucomatous patients (Danesh-Meyer and Levin 2009).

Pharmacological treatments with streptozotocin or alloxan were also applied to induce diabetes in rodents (Barber et al. 1998; Park et al. 2003; Martin et al. 2004; Gaucher et al. 2007). These treatments allowed to demonstrate neuronal apoptosis or a microglial reaction in the treated animals. The neurodegenerative process in these animal models was very variable from photoreceptors to retinal ganglion cells. These models also showed some alterations of the vascular system occurring with time (Song et al. 2004), but in general they do not develop diabetic retinopathy similar to that which can be observed in human diabetic patients.

Naturally Occurring Models

Many mice display spontaneous phenotypes of retinal degeneration in the photoreceptor layer, and they were named numerically in the order that they were identified: rd1, rd2, rd10, etc. (Chang et al. 2002). The rd1 mouse (*Pde6b^{rd1}*, also known as the rd mouse) was described in 1924 by Keeler as "leading to absence of the visual cells (rods), the external nuclear layer, and the external molecular layer" (Keeler 1924). Subsequently, it was found that the phenotype results from a spontaneous recessive mutation in the β-subunit of the rod-phosphodiesterase (PDE) gene *Pde6b^{rd1}* (Bowes et al. 1990). The model is associated with massive death of rods in the first weeks of postnatal life, followed by the death of cones, thus mimicking an early-onset severe retinal degeneration as in patients affected by retinitis pigmentosa, who can in some cases have a mutation in the homolog human gene (Farber 1995). rd10 mice carry a different recessive mutation in the same rod-*PDE* gene, leading to a similar but somewhat milder degeneration profile with slower rod loss (between P20 and P25) and slower secondary cone degeneration (Chang et al. 2002). The rd1 mouse was used in the laboratory of Jean Bennett to demonstrate the therapeutic potential of subretinal injection of a recombinant replication-defective adenovirus that contained the murine eDNA for wild-type β *PDE*, Ad.CMV β *PDE* (Bennett et al. 1996).

Other naturally occurring mouse models of retinal degeneration include the rds (retinal degeneration slow) mouse, because of a mutation in the *Prph* gene (rd2). The retinal phenotype of *Prph2 Rd2/Rd2* mouse consists of complete failure to develop photoreceptor outer segments and apoptotic loss of photoreceptor cells. This model allowed for demonstration of successful reversal of the retinal degeneration by gene augmentation therapy using a recombinant adeno-associated virus (AAV) vector encoding a *Prph2* transgene, showing stable generation of normal outer segments (Ali et al. 2000). The RD3 protein was reported to negatively modulate the activity of guanylate cyclase (Chen et al. 2022). The rd5 or tubby mouse (tub) displays not only retinal degeneration but also maturity-onset obesity, insulin resistance, and hearing deficits (Noben-Trauth et al. 1996). The rd6 phenotype is due to a mutation in the membrane-type frizzled-related protein (MFRP), which is normally expressed in the retinal pigment epithelium and ciliary body (Fogerty and Besharse 2011). The retinal degeneration 7 (rd7) is related to a mutation in the transcription factor *Nr2e3*, the mutation of which results in the production of photoreceptors with a hybrid rod and cone cell type responsible for enhanced S-cone syndrome phenotype (Corbo and Cepko 2005). The rd8 mutation in the *CrB1* gene is often discovered in different lines of C57BL/6N or embryonic stem cells such that it can generate confusing retinal phenotypes in transgenic animals and should be actively screened for (Mattapallil et al. 2012). The rd9 mouse carries a base-pair duplication in the purine reach domain (ORF) of the retinitis pigmentosa GTPase regulator (*RPGR*) thereby providing an appropriate model of X-linked retinitis pigmentosa (Thompson et al. 2012). The rd11 model is caused by mutation in the lysophosphatidylcholine acyltransferase-1 (*LPCAT1*) gene coding for a phospholipid biosynthesis/remodeling enzyme (Friedman et al. 2010). The rd12 mouse, which represent a model for Leber congenital amaurosis (Redmond and Hamel 2000), was used to demonstrate efficacy of gene therapy when reintroducing the correct gene sequence of *RPE65* (Pang et al. 2005). Similarly, the rd16 mouse, which represents a model for *CEP290*-elicited ciliogenesis defect, was used to assess a possible therapeutic intervention (Mookherjee et al. 2018).

Apart from these mouse models, a very common animal model in many research laboratories is the Royal College of Surgeon (RCS) rat, which shows an accumulation of debris below the retina. The retinal degeneration in this model is caused by a recessive mutation in the *Mertk* gene (D'Cruz et al. 2000; Nandrot et al. 2000), which is expressed in RPE cells, and plays an important role in phagocytosis of photoreceptor outer segments as part of their natural turnover (Vollrath et al. 2001). The failure of phagocytosis leads to accumulation of debris under the retina, leading to secondary degeneration of the photoreceptors. As such, it is often considered as a model of age-related macular degeneration, because photoreceptor loss follows upon primary dysfunction of the RPE. However, it is actually an inherited retinal disorder, and, in humans, mutations in the *Mertk* gene cause an early and severe form of retinitis pigmentosa or Leber congenital amaurosis. Gene augmentation therapy was shown to attenuate the course of disease in the RCS rat (Vollrath et al. 2001). Later, washout of the debris by subretinal surgery was also shown to prolong the survival of photoreceptors in this model (Lorach et al. 2018).

Finally, the *DBA2/2J* mouse serves as a common model for glaucoma because pigment dispersion in the anterior chamber and trabecular meshwork induces a major increase in intraocular pressure. Despite the high variability of this model, it was used to demonstrate efficacy of different molecules for the prevention of glaucoma such as memantine, timolol, or taurine (Schuettauf et al. 2002; Froger et al. 2012).

Electroporation for Gene Transfer

The Institute de la Vision in Paris has been a pioneer in the preclinical and clinical development of gene therapy for a severe pathology, Leber's hereditary optic neuropathy (LHON) (Carelli et al. 2023). To study the pathological background of this blinding disease, an animal model was created through the introduction of the human *ND4* gene harboring the *G11778A* mutation (responsible for 60% of LHON cases in humans) to rat eyes by in vivo electroporation (Ellouze et al. 2008). The treatment induced morphological and functional characteristics of human LHON with degeneration of retinal ganglion cells, a deleterious effect that was also confirmed in primary cell culture. Importantly, retinal ganglion cell loss was clearly associated with a decline in visual performance. Subsequent electroporation with wild-type *ND4* prevented both retinal ganglion cell loss and the impairment of visual function, providing proof of principle that optimized allotopic expression can be an effective treatment for LHON, thus opening the way to clinical studies on other devastating mitochondrial disorders. Following these discoveries, we have created the biotech company GenSight Biologics, which initiated the GS010 gene therapy clinical trial for *G11778A*-associated LHON (NCT02652780, NCT03406104). The study confirmed the clinical benefit of LUMEVOQ (lena-

dogene nolparvovec) for retinal ganglion cell preservation and bilateral improvement in visual acuity after unilateral injection in patients with LHON (Newman et al. 2021). Long-term follow-up demonstrated that this gene therapy is well tolerated in the short as well as long term (currently for a minimum of 5 years) (Vignal et al. 2018; Vignal-Clermont et al. 2021; Carelli et al. 2023; Newman et al. 2023).

Induced Genetic Models

To increase the frequency of mutagenesis in mouse colonies, *N*-ethyl-*N*-nitrosourea-induced (ENU) mutagenesis was applied and then followed by screening for mouse models of diseases. This approach was applied with great success to generate animals with clear eye phenotypes including retinal degeneration (Thaung et al. 2002). However, recent advances in molecular genetic techniques now allow to manipulate the genome with high precision and provide the ability to generate specific models of retinal diseases, especially models of rare diseases. These include gene knockouts but also knockin models in which specific mutations can be introduced into specific genes. The number of these transgenic animal models has increased exponentially in recent years, and therefore they cannot be fully reviewed here. A major example is the P23H rat and mouse, which reproduce a highly prevalent human mutation in the rhodopsin gene (Machida et al. 2000; Chrysostomou et al. 2009; Kolomiets et al. 2010; Orhan et al. 2015). This animal model was used to assess different therapeutic strategies such as the effect of the rod-derived cone viability factor RdCVF on cone survival (Yang et al. 2009). Similarly, the *Abca4-KO* mouse model has been largely utilized to understand the etiology of Stargardt disease or age-related macular degeneration (Weng et al. 1999). For the large *ABCA4* gene, which exceeds the loading capacity of AAV vectors, a lipid nanoparticle-based approach has demonstrated effectiveness for in vivo delivery in $Abca4^{-/-}$ mice (Sun et al. 2020, 2022). Development of therapies for Usher syndrome type 1 (USH1)—a major cause of combined inherited deafness–blindness in humans—has been hampered because mouse models only develop deafness but no retinal degeneration, as is the case in both harmonin ($Ush1c^{-/-}$) or sans ($Ush1g^{-/-}$) knockout mice (Trouillet et al. 2018). In fact, cone degeneration was observed only when transferring the transgene in an albino background (Trouillet et al. 2018), thereby suggesting a role for light and oxidative stress in the degenerative process of Usher retinal disease. This result was consistent with a previous study showing vulnerability of photoreceptors in the shaker 1 mouse ($Ush1b$ mutant) to moderate light exposure (Peng et al. 2011).

The etiology of age-related macular degeneration is multifactorial and associated with various genetic and environmental factors. The need to develop effective treatments for AMD has led to the generation of multiple rodent models by expressing genetic mutations commonly associated with the disease (Pennesi et al. 2012; Ratnapriya and Chew 2013; Fletcher et al. 2014; Veleri et al. 2015). Although there is no model that fully recapitulates all of the features of human AMD (particularly in view of the fact that rodents and indeed most species except primates and certain types of birds do not possess a macular structure), these models have helped in the discovery of pathophysiological mechanisms underlying AMD, such as inflammation and immune dysregulation, chronic oxidative damage, and alterations in lipid and carbohydrate metabolism, among others (Calippe et al. 2017; Beguier et al. 2020). Polymorphisms in the gene for complement factor H (CFH) B, C2, C3, and C9 have been associated with either conferring protection or susceptibility to the development and progression of AMD. The $Cfh^{-/-}$ mouse was used to study some aspects of the complement factor pathway in the pathogenesis of AMD, but one should bear in mind that the genetic variants associated with AMD do not lead to down-regulation of CFH. These mice also display systemic consumption of C3, deposition of C3a in the glomerular basement membrane and glomerulonephritis, contrary to the increase of C3 and C3a observed in AMD. In the retina, they develop mild loss of photoreceptors, reduced rod function, and increased deposition of complement in the photoreceptor layer (Coffey et al. 2007). Decreased visual acuity and reduction in rod-driven

ERG a- and b-wave responses were found at two years of age, together with thinning of the Bruch's membrane (Coffey et al. 2007), which is not typical of AMD. Transgenic *CFH Y402H* mice ($Cfh^{-/-}$ mice expressing the human AMD-related polymorphism CFH 402H under control of the human ApoE promoter) show a large number of drusen-like deposits at the age of 1 yr, increased number of microglial cells and macrophages in the subretinal space, thickening of Bruch's membrane, and basement membrane deposition of C3d as compared to wild-type mice (Ufret-Vincenty et al. 2010). However, they did not show photoreceptor atrophy even under a high-fat diet but they showed clear differences from mice expressing the "wild-type" CFH 402Y protein (Landowski et al. 2019). Transgenic mice overexpressing C3 show several features of AMD such as proliferation and migration of endothelial cells within the retina, disruption of the RPE with migration of pigmented cells into the retina, complement deposition, and atrophy of the photoreceptor outer segments. However, the C3-overexpressing animals demonstrate increased incidence of retinal detachments that is not consistent with AMD (reviewed in Pennesi et al. 2012). These *cfh* mouse models of AMD developed by Bowes Rickman and collaborators have enabled the unveiling of novel mechanisms contributing to AMD pathophysiology, including correlation between CFH levels and retinal integrity (Ding et al. 2015) and a link between the complement system and lipid pathways (Ding et al. 2015; Toomey et al. 2015; Landowski et al. 2019; Landowski and Bowes Rickman 2022). Importantly, they serve as tools for validation of potential therapeutic targets in AMD (for review, see Kelly et al. 2020; Landowski and Bowes Rickman 2022).

Our research in the field of AMD showed that under physiological conditions, the subretinal space is immunosuppressive and devoid of mononuclear phagocytes, a family of cells that includes monocytes and infiltrating and resident macrophages (reviewed in Guillonneau et al. 2017). A common feature of early and advanced dry and neovascular forms of AMD is the activation of macrophages in the inner retina and the chronic accumulation of subretinal mononuclear phagocytes. We showed that the homeostatic elimination of mononuclear phagocytes that infiltrate the photoreceptor cell layer depends on thrombospondin 1 (TSP1)-mediated activation of their CD47 receptor. Accordingly, $Thbs1^{-/-}$ and $Cd47^{-/-}$ mice develop age-related subretinal mononuclear phagocyte accumulation similar to AMD patients. Importantly, we demonstrated that both major genetic AMD risk factors, the CFH H402 variant and 10q26 risk haplotype, inhibit TSP1-mediated CD47 activation and MP elimination, promoting chronic pathogenic inflammation (Calippe et al. 2017; Beguier et al. 2020). Our findings described a comprehensive mechanism of how these two prominent AMD-risk haplotypes, the variant of complement factor H and a minor haplotype of the chromosome 10q26, account for most of the genetic risk for AMD and promote AMD pathogenesis. This work provides a rationale for therapeutic restoration of immune privilege in the subretinal space to induce the resolution of subretinal chronic inflammation that promotes photoreceptor destruction and blindness in AMD. In agreement with these results, several mouse models targeting inflammatory mediators and apolipoproteins have been generated and reported to partially replicate AMD features, including subretinal drusen-like accumulations, thickening of Bruch's membrane, an increase in autofluorescence and lipofuscin granules, and photoreceptor degeneration (Combadière et al. 2007). However, the Rd8 mutation of the $Crb1$ gene present in many mouse strains appears sufficient to generate most of these ocular phenotypes (Mattapallil et al. 2012). Unless explicitly excluding the rd8 mutation, it is therefore impossible to conclude which genetic alteration truly provokes AMD-like features. Alternatively, different models of oxidative damage leading to inflammation have been developed based on the particular susceptibility of the retina to oxidative injury associated with its high metabolic demand, high concentration of oxidizable polyunsaturated fatty acids, and presence of photosensitive molecules (such as rhodopsin or lipofuscin). Among them, ceruloplasmin/hephaestin$^{-/-}$ mice, $Sod1^{-/-}$ mice, $Sod2^{-/-}$ and $Sod2$ knockdown mice, and OXYS rat are commonly used models, allowing us to

evaluate the role of oxidative stress in the pathogenesis of AMD (Fletcher et al. 2014). Exposure to cigarette smoke, hydroquinone, high fat diet, and blue light also produced many AMD-like features (see light damage model above).

Myopia can also have a genetic origin (Tedja et al. 2018) such that many mutated mouse models were found to develop or to have increased susceptibility to develop myopia under application of different optical devices (Zeitz et al. 2023). For instance, mutations causing complete congenital stationary night blindness (cCSNB) in patients and animal models were often found to induce myopia (Zeitz et al. 2023). Thus, a substantial increase of the myopic shift was reported in $Gpr179^{-/-}$ mice compared to wild-type littermates following a 3-wk-long lens-induced myopia protocol (Wilmet et al. 2022). The adult $Gpr179^{-/-}$ mice have a significant decrease in both retinal dopamine and 3,4-dihydroxyphenylacetic acid, in agreement with previous observations that an alteration of the dopaminergic system correlated with an increased susceptibility to lens-induced myopia (Schwahn et al. 2000; Feldkaemper and Schaeffel 2013; Landis et al. 2020).

Cre-*lox* Gene Targeting

The Cre-*lox* system is a genetic tool permitting efficient and accurate control over the location and timing of gene expression and generation of mouse strains in which a transgene is either inducible or expressed only in certain tissues (Sauer and Henderson 1990; Lakso et al. 1992). Pioneering work by Botond Roska's group described approximately 100 mouse lines with either defined strata or, more specifically, retinal cell types marked with GFP allowing stratification-based screening for characterizing neuronal circuitry (Siegert et al. 2009). This strategy not only allowed us to sort specific cell types for genetic analysis but also to optically target cells for recording and functional characterization. For the anatomical analysis of the circuit, the approach can be combined with the Brainbow technology (Livet et al. 2007). This transgenic system allows for stochastic expression of multiple fluorescent protein genes through Cre-*lox* recombination (Livet et al. 2007; Dumas et al. 2015, 2022).

This strategy to selectively ablate gene expression in a specific cell type was applied to demonstrate expression of the nucleoredoxin-like-1 (*Nxnl1*) gene in cone photoreceptors (Mei et al. 2016). Indeed, when using a transgenic line expressing Cre recombinase under the control of a cone opsin promoter, cones of these mice were dysfunctional and degenerated by 8 mo of age. Similarly, silencing the expression of RdCVFL in cone-enriched culture resulted in reduced cell viability. These experiments indicated that the *Nxnl1* gene protects cones by two distinct pathways, by RdCVFL produced by cones themselves and by RdCVF released from rods (Léveillard et al. 2004; Aït-Ali et al. 2015). These results have provided the rationale for a future therapy combining both RdCVF and RdCVFL expression by gene therapy.

CONCLUDING REMARKS

Demonstrating "proof of principle" in one or more animal models opens the road to moving a candidate therapy toward human clinical trials. Considering that today the potential to translate novel therapies for retinal diseases to the clinic increases, there is a strong need for relevant animal models that can provide information about the natural history of the disease and its pathogenic pathways and genetic background. Among mammals, large animal models, particularly nonhuman primates that have a macula, can most faithfully reproduce the human conditions for assessing treatment efficacy and safety (Picaud et al. 2019). Furthermore, cell sizes, cell types, eye sizes, eye architectures, and immune responses often differ between species and especially between rodents and primates. Gene isoforms and redundancy may also easily differ in the different species. All these differences justify the need to assess the safety and efficiency of therapeutic strategies in primates prior to clinical trials for increasing their final success rate, as exemplified by the preclinical testing of retinal prostheses (Prévot et al. 2020), optogenetic therapy (Gauvain et al. 2021; Sahel et al. 2021), or cell therapy (Ben M'Barek et al. 2020). Developing an AMD model in nonhuman primates would be critical for the development of an efficient therapeutic treatment for dry AMD because not one of the multiple rodent models fully recapitulates the features of the human disease. However, nonhuman primates are difficult to manage and manipulate genetically and are expensive to maintain.

The limited number of spontaneously arising large animal models of retinal degeneration and ethical concerns are additional points to consider. This is why rodents, particularly mice, are most widely used for modeling of human disease and have helped to reveal the roles of oxidative damage, inflammation, immune dysregulation, and lipid metabolism in the development of AMD. The adaptation of human clinical eye examination technologies for assessment of retinal function and structure also in rodent eyes helped to enhance translational investigations of novel therapeutic approaches in relevant models. Today, the principle of the 3Rs—replacement (avoid/replace the use of animals), reduction (minimize the number of animals used), and refinement (minimize animal suffering and improve welfare)—is widely considered. Wherever possible at an early stage of translational research, a significant reduction in animal studies is achieved by alternative cellular and organotypic methods of in vitro, in vivo, and in silico mathematical models for disease modeling and outcome prediction.

ACKNOWLEDGMENTS

This work was supported by the French state funds managed by the Agence Nationale de la Recherche (ANR) within Programme Investissements d'Avenir: Laboratoire d'Excellence (LABEX) LIFESENSES (ANR-10-LABX-0065) and Institut Hospitalo-Universitaire FOReSIGHT (ANR-18-IAHU-0001), by Optic 2000, the City of Paris and Région Ile de France, by the National Institutes of Health (NIH) CORE Grant P30 EY08098 to the Department of Ophthalmology, the Eye and Ear Foundation of Pittsburgh, and from an unrestricted grant from Research to Prevent Blindness, New York, NY.

REFERENCES

Abdeljalil J, Hamid M, Abdel-mouttalib O, Stéphane R, Raymond R, Johan A, José S, Pierre C, Serge P. 2005. The optomotor response: a robust first-line visual screening method for mice. *Vision Res* 45: 1439–1446. doi:10.1016/j.visres.2004.12.015

Aït-Ali N, Fridlich R, Millet-Puel G, Clérin E, Delalande F, Jaillard C, Blond F, Perrocheau L, Reichman S, Byrne LC, et al. 2015. Rod-derived cone viability factor promotes cone survival by stimulating aerobic glycolysis. *Cell* 161: 817–832. doi:10.1016/j.cell.2015.03.023

Ali RR, Sarra GM, Stephens C, Alwis MD, Bainbridge JW, Munro PM, Fauser S, Reichel MB, Kinnon C, Hunt DM, et al. 2000. Restoration of photoreceptor ultrastructure and function in retinal degeneration slow mice by gene therapy. *Nat Genet* 25: 306–310. doi:10.1038/77068

Arnault E, Barrau C, Nanteau C, Gondouin P, Bigot K, Viénot F, Gutman E, Fontaine V, Villette T, Cohen-Tannoudji C, et al. 2013. Phototoxic action spectrum on a retinal pigment epithelium model of age-related macular degeneration exposed to sunlight normalized conditions. *PLoS ONE* 8: e71398. doi:10.1371/journal.pone.0071398

Balse E, Tessier LH, Fuchs C, Forster V, Sahel JA, Picaud S. 2005. Purification of mammalian cone photoreceptors by lectin panning and the enhancement of their survival in glia-conditioned medium. *Invest Ophthalmol Vis Sci* 46: 367–374. doi:10.1167/iovs.04-0695

Barber AJ, Lieth E, Khin SA, Antonetti DA, Buchanan AG, Gardner TW. 1998. Neural apoptosis in the retina during experimental and human diabetes. Early onset and effect of insulin. *J Clin Invest* 102: 783–791. doi:10.1172/JCI2425

Barres BA, Silverstein BE, Corey DP, Chun LL. 1988. Immunological, morphological, and electrophysiological variation among retinal ganglion cells purified by panning. *Neuron* 1: 791–803. doi:10.1016/0896-6273(88)90127-4

Bassetto M, Sen M, Poulhes F, Arango-Gonzalez B, Bonvin E, Sapet C, Ueffing M, Zelphati O. 2021. New method for efficient siRNA delivery in retina explants: reverse magnetofection. *Bioconjug Chem* 32: 1078–1093. doi:10.1021/acs.bioconjchem.1c00132

Beguier F, Housset M, Roubeix C, Augustin S, Zagar Y, Nous C, Mathis T, Eandi C, Benchaboune M, Drame-Maigné A, et al. 2020. The 10q26 risk haplotype of age-related macular degeneration aggravates subretinal inflammation by impairing monocyte elimination. *Immunity* 53: 429–441.e8. doi:10.1016/j.immuni.2020.07.021

Ben M'Barek K, Bertin S, Brazhnikova E, Jaillard C, Habeler W, Plancheron A, Fovet CM, Demilly J, Jarraya M, Bejanariu A, et al. 2020. Clinical-grade production and safe delivery of human ESC derived RPE sheets in primates and rodents. *Biomaterials* 230: 119603. doi:10.1016/j.biomaterials.2019.119603

Bennett J, Tanabe T, Sun D, Zeng Y, Kjeldbye H, Gouras P, Maguire AM. 1996. Photoreceptor cell rescue in retinal degeneration (rd) mice by in vivo gene therapy. *Nat Med* 2: 649–654. doi:10.1038/nm0696-649

GBD 2019 Blindness and Vision Impairment Collaborators; Vision Loss Expert Group of the Global Burden of Disease Study; et al. 2021. Causes of blindness and vision impairment in 2020 and trends over 30 years, and prevalence of avoidable blindness in relation to VISION 2020: the right to sight: an analysis for the global burden of disease study. *Lancet Glob Health* 9: e144–e160. doi:10.1016/S2214-109X(20)30489-7

Bourne RRA, Flaxman SR, Braithwaite T, Cicinelli MV, Das A, Jonas JB, Keeffe J, Kempen JH, Leasher J, Limburg H, et al. 2017. Magnitude, temporal trends, and projections of the global prevalence of blindness and distance and near vision impairment: a systematic review and meta-analysis. *Lancet Glob Health* 5: e888–e897. doi:10.1016/S2214-109X(17)30293-0

Bowes C, Li T, Danciger M, Baxter LC, Applebury ML, Farber DB. 1990. Retinal degeneration in the rd mouse is caused by a defect in the β subunit of rod cGMP-phosphodiesterase. *Nature* 347: 677–680. doi:10.1038/347677a0

Busskamp V, Duebel J, Balya D, Fradot M, Viney TJ, Siegert S, Groner AC, Cabuy E, Forster V, Seeliger M, et al. 2010. Genetic reactivation of cone photoreceptors restores visual responses in retinitis pigmentosa. *Science* 329: 413–417. doi:10.1126/science.1190897

Butler WH, Ford GP, Newberne JW. 1987. A study of the effects of vigabatrin on the central nervous system and retina of Sprague Dawley and Lister–Hooded rats. *Toxicol Pathol* 15: 143–148. doi:10.1177/019262338701500203

Caffé AR, Söderpalm A, van Veen T. 1993. Photoreceptor-specific protein expression of mouse retina in organ culture and retardation of rd degeneration in vitro by a combination of basic fibroblast and nerve growth factors. *Curr Eye Res* 12: 719–726. doi:10.3109/02713689308995767

Calippe B, Augustin S, Beguier F, Charles-Messance H, Poupel L, Conart JB, Hu SJ, Lavalette S, Fauvet A, Rayes J, et al. 2017. Complement factor H inhibits CD47-mediated resolution of inflammation. *Immunity* 46: 261–272. doi:10.1016/j.immuni.2017.01.006

Camelo S, Raoul W, Lavalette S, Calippe B, Cristofaro B, Levy O, Houssier M, Sulpice E, Jonet L, Klein C, et al. 2012. Delta-like 4 inhibits choroidal neovascularization despite opposing effects on vascular endothelium and macrophages. *Angiogenesis* 15: 609–622. doi:10.1007/s10456-012-9290-0

Carelli V, Newman NJ, Yu-Wai-Man P, Biousse V, Moster ML, Subramanian PS, Vignal-Clermont C, Wang AG, Donahue SP, Leroy BP, et al. 2023. Indirect comparison of lenadogene nolparvovec gene therapy versus natural history in patients with Leber hereditary optic neuropathy carrying the m.11778G > A MT-ND4 mutation. *Ophthalmol Ther* 12: 401–429. doi:10.1007/s40123-022-00611-x

Chang B, Hawes NL, Hurd RE, Davisson MT, Nusinowitz S, Heckenlively JR. 2002. Retinal degeneration mutants in the mouse. *Vision Res* 42: 517–525. doi:10.1016/S0042-6989(01)00146-8

Chen Y, Bräuer AU, Koch KW. 2022. Retinal degeneration protein 3 controls membrane guanylate cyclase activities in brain tissue. *Front Mol Neurosci* 15: 1076430. doi:10.3389/fnmol.2022.1076430

Chrysostomou V, Stone J, Valter K. 2009. Life history of cones in the rhodopsin-mutant P23H-3 rat: evidence of long-term survival. *Invest Ophthalmol Vis Sci* 50: 2407–2416. doi:10.1167/iovs.08-3003

Clérin E, Wicker N, Mohand-Saïd S, Poch O, Sahel JA, Léveillard T. 2011. e-conome: an automated tissue counting platform of cone photoreceptors for rodent models of retinitis pigmentosa. *BMC Ophthalmol* **11**: 38. doi:10 .1186/1471-2415-11-38

Coffey PJ, Gias C, McDermott CJ, Lundh P, Pickering MC, Sethi C, Bird A, Fitzke FW, Maass A, Chen LL, et al. 2007. Complement factor H deficiency in aged mice causes retinal abnormalities and visual dysfunction. *Proc Natl Acad Sci* **104**: 16651–16656. doi:10.1073/pnas.0705079104

Combadière C, Feumi C, Raoul W, Keller N, Rodéro M, Pézard A, Lavalette S, Houssier M, Jonet L, Picard E, et al. 2007. CX3CR1-dependent subretinal microglia cell accumulation is associated with cardinal features of age-related macular degeneration. *J Clin Invest* **117**: 2920–2928. doi:10.1172/JCI31692

Cone FE, Gelman SE, Son JL, Pease ME, Quigley HA. 2010. Differential susceptibility to experimental glaucoma among 3 mouse strains using bead and viscoelastic injection. *Exp Eye Res* **91**: 415–424. doi:10.1016/j.exer.2010.06 .018

Corbo JC, Cepko CL. 2005. A hybrid photoreceptor expressing both rod and cone genes in a mouse model of enhanced S-cone syndrome. *PLoS Genet* **1**: e11. doi:10.1371/ journal.pgen.0010011

Danesh-Meyer HV, Levin LA. 2009. Neuroprotection: extrapolating from neurologic diseases to the eye. *Am J Ophthalmol* **148**: 186–191.e182. doi:10.1016/j.ajo.2009 .03.029

D'Cruz PM, Yasumura D, Weir J, Matthes MT, Abderrahim H, LaVail MM, Vollrath D. 2000. Mutation of the receptor tyrosine kinase gene *Mertk* in the retinal dystrophic RCS rat. *Hum Mol Genet* **9**: 645–651. doi:10.1093/hmg/9.4.645

Ding JD, Kelly U, Landowski M, Toomey CB, Groelle M, Miller C, Smith SG, Klingeborn M, Singhapricha T, Jiang H, et al. 2015. Expression of human complement factor H prevents age-related macular degeneration–like retina damage and kidney abnormalities in aged Cfh knockout mice. *Am J Pathol* **185**: 29–42. doi:10.1016/j.ajpath.2014 .08.026

Duboc A, Hanoteau N, Simonutti M, Rudolf G, Nehlig A, Sahel JA, Picaud S. 2004. Vigabatrin, the GABA-transaminase inhibitor, damages cone photoreceptors in rats. *Ann Neurol* **55**: 695–705. doi:10.1002/ana.20081

Dumas L, Heitz-Marchaland C, Fouquet S, Suter U, Livet J, Moreau-Fauvarque C, Chédotal A. 2015. Multicolor analysis of oligodendrocyte morphology, interactions, and development with Brainbow. *Glia* **63**: 699–717. doi:10 .1002/glia.22779

Dumas L, Clavreul S, Michon F, Loulier K. 2022. Multicolor strategies for investigating clonal expansion and tissue plasticity. *Cell Mol Life Sci* **79**: 141. doi:10.1007/s00018-021-04077-1

Ellouze S, Augustin S, Bouaita A, Bonnet C, Simonutti M, Forster V, Picaud S, Sahel JA, Corral-Debrinski M. 2008. Optimized allotopic expression of the human mitochondrial ND4 prevents blindness in a rat model of mitochondrial dysfunction. *Am J Hum Genet* **83**: 373–387. doi:10 .1016/j.ajhg.2008.08.013

Farber DB. 1995. From mice to men: the cyclic GMP phosphodiesterase gene in vision and disease. The Proctor Lecture. *Invest Ophthalmol Vis Sci* **36**: 263–275.

Feldkaemper M, Schaeffel F. 2013. An updated view on the role of dopamine in myopia. *Exp Eye Res* **114**: 106–119. doi:10.1016/j.exer.2013.02.007

Fletcher EL, Jobling AI, Greferath U, Mills SA, Waugh M, Ho T, de Iongh RU, Phipps JA, Vessey KA. 2014. Studying age-related macular degeneration using animal models. *Optom Vis Sci* **91**: 878–886. doi:10.1097/OPX .0000000000000322

Fogerty J, Besharse JC. 2011. 174delG mutation in mouse MFRP causes photoreceptor degeneration and RPE atrophy. *Invest Ophthalmol Vis Sci* **52**: 7256–7266. doi:10 .1167/iovs.11-8112

Fontaine V, Kinkl N, Sahel J, Dreyfus H, Hicks D. 1998. Survival of purified rat photoreceptors in vitro is stimulated directly by fibroblast growth factor-2. *J Neurosci* **18**: 9662–9672. doi:10.1523/JNEUROSCI.18-23-09662.1998

Fontaine V, Monteiro E, Brazhnikova E, Lesage L, Balducci C, Guibout L, Feraille L, Elena PP, Sahel JA, Veillet S, et al. 2016. Norbixin protects retinal pigmented epithelium cells and photoreceptors against A2E-mediated phototoxicity in vitro and in vivo. *PLoS ONE* **11**: e0167793. doi:10.1371/journal.pone.0167793

Fontaine V, Fournié M, Monteiro E, Boumedine T, Balducci C, Guibout L, Latil M, Sahel JA, Veillet S, Dilda PJ, et al. 2021. A2E-induced inflammation and angiogenesis in RPE cells in vitro are modulated by PPAR-α, -β/δ, -γ, and RXR antagonists and by norbixin. *Aging (Albany NY)* **13**: 22040–22058. doi:10.18632/aging.203558

Fradot M, Busskamp V, Forster V, Cronin T, Léveillard T, Bennett J, Sahel JA, Roska B, Picaud S. 2011. Gene therapy in ophthalmology: validation on cultured retinal cells and explants from postmortem human eyes. *Hum Gene Ther* **22**: 587–593. doi:10.1089/hum.2010.157

Friedman JS, Chang B, Krauth DS, Lopez I, Waseem NH, Hurd RE, Feathers KL, Branham KE, Shaw M, Thomas GE, et al. 2010. Loss of lysophosphatidylcholine acyltransferase 1 leads to photoreceptor degeneration in rd11 mice. *Proc Natl Acad Sci* **107**: 15523–15528. doi:10 .1073/pnas.1002897107

Froger N, Cadetti L, Lorach H, Martins J, Bemelmans AP, Dubus E, Degardin J, Pain D, Forster V, Chicaud L, et al. 2012. Taurine provides neuroprotection against retinal ganglion cell degeneration. *PLoS ONE* **7**: e42017. doi:10 .1371/journal.pone.0042017

Froger N, Jammoul F, Gaucher D, Cadetti L, Lorach H, Degardin J, Pain D, Dubus E, Forster V, Ivkovic I, et al. 2013. Taurine is a crucial factor to preserve retinal ganglion cell survival. *Adv Exp Med Biol* **775**: 69–83. doi:10 .1007/978-1-4614-6130-2_6

Froger N, Matonti F, Roubeix C, Forster V, Ivkovic I, Brunel N, Baudouin C, Sahel JA, Picaud S. 2020. VEGF is an autocrine/paracrine neuroprotective factor for injured retinal ganglion neurons. *Sci Rep* **10**: 12409. doi:10 .1038/s41598-020-68488-z

Fuchs C, Forster V, Balse E, Sahel JA, Picaud S, Tessier LH. 2005. Retinal-cell-conditioned medium prevents TNF-α-induced apoptosis of purified ganglion cells. *Invest Ophthalmol Vis Sci* **46**: 2983–2991. doi:10.1167/iovs.04-1177

Fulton AB, Hansen RM, Moskowitz A, Akula JD. 2009. The neurovascular retina in retinopathy of prematurity. *Prog Retin Eye Res* **28**: 452–482. doi:10.1016/j.preteyeres.2009 .06.003

García-Ayuso D, Di Pierdomenico J, Valiente-Soriano FJ, Martínez-Vacas A, Agudo-Barriuso M, Vidal-Sanz M, Picaud S, Villegas-Pérez MP. 2019. β-alanine supplementation induces taurine depletion and causes alterations of the retinal nerve fiber layer and axonal transport by retinal ganglion cells. *Exp Eye Res* **188**: 107781. doi:10.1016/j.exer.2019.107781

Gaucher D, Chiappore JA, Pâques M, Simonutti M, Boitard C, Sahel JA, Massin P, Picaud S. 2007. Microglial changes occur without neural cell death in diabetic retinopathy. *Vision Res* **47**: 612–623. doi:10.1016/j.visres.2006.11.017

Gaucher D, Arnault E, Husson Z, Froger N, Dubus E, Gondouin P, Dhérbecourt D, Degardin J, Simonutti M, Fouquet S, et al. 2012. Taurine deficiency damages retinal neurones: cone photoreceptors and retinal ganglion cells. *Amino Acids* **43**: 1979–1993. doi:10.1007/s00726-012-1273-3

Gauvain G, Akolkar H, Chaffiol A, Arcizet F, Khoei MA, Desrosiers M, Jaillard C, Caplette R, Marre O, Bertin S, et al. 2021. Optogenetic therapy: high spatiotemporal resolution and pattern discrimination compatible with vision restoration in non-human primates. *Commun Biol* **4**: 125. doi:10.1038/s42003-020-01594-w

Grossniklaus HE, Kang SJ, Berglin L. 2010. Animal models of choroidal and retinal neovascularization. *Prog Retin Eye Res* **29**: 500–519. doi:10.1016/j.preteyeres.2010.05.003

Guidry C. 1996. Isolation and characterization of porcine Müller cells. Myofibroblastic dedifferentiation in culture. *Invest Ophthalmol Vis Sci* **37**: 740–752.

Guillonneau X, Eandi CM, Paques M, Sahel JA, Sapieha P, Sennlaub F. 2017. On phagocytes and macular degeneration. *Prog Retin Eye Res* **61**: 98–128. doi:10.1016/j.preteyeres.2017.06.002

Heidinger V, Dreyfus H, Sahel J, Christen Y, Hicks D. 1998. Excitotoxic damage of retinal glial cells depends upon normal neuron-glial interactions. *Glia* **23**: 146–155. doi:10.1002/(SICI)1098-1136(199806)23:2<146::AID-GLIA6>3.0.CO;2-4

Hicks D, Courtois Y. 1990. The growth and behaviour of rat retinal Müller cells in vitro. 1: An improved method for isolation and culture. *Exp Eye Res* **51**: 119–129. doi:10.1016/0014-4835(90)90063-Z

Hicks D, Courtois Y. 1992. Fibroblast growth factor stimulates photoreceptor differentiation in vitro. *J Neurosci* **12**: 2022–2033. doi:10.1523/JNEUROSCI.12-06-02022.1992

Jammoul F, Wang Q, Nabbout R, Coriat C, Duboc A, Simonutti M, Dubus E, Craft CM, Ye W, Collins SD, et al. 2009. Taurine deficiency is a cause of vigabatrin-induced retinal phototoxicity. *Ann Neurol* **65**: 98–107. doi:10.1002/ana.21526

Jammoul F, Dégardin J, Pain D, Gondouin P, Simonutti M, Dubus E, Caplette R, Fouquet S, Craft CM, Sahel JA, et al. 2010. Taurine deficiency damages photoreceptors and retinal ganglion cells in vigabatrin-treated neonatal rats. *Mol Cell Neurosci* **43**: 414–421. doi:10.1016/j.mcn.2010.01.008

Keeler CE. 1924. The inheritance of a retinal abnormality in white mice. *Proc Natl Acad Sci* **10**: 329–333. doi:10.1073/pnas.10.7.329

Kelly UL, Grigsby D, Cady MA, Landowski M, Skiba NP, Liu J, Remaley AT, Klingeborn M, Bowes Rickman C. 2020.

High-density lipoproteins are a potential therapeutic target for age-related macular degeneration. *J Biol Chem* **295**: 13601–13616. doi:10.1074/jbc.RA119.012305

Kolomiets B, Dubus E, Simonutti M, Rosolen S, Sahel JA, Picaud S. 2010. Late histological and functional changes in the P23H rat retina after photoreceptor loss. *Neurobiol Dis* **38**: 47–58. doi:10.1016/j.nbd.2009.12.025

Lakso M, Sauer B, Mosinger B, Lee EJ, Manning RW, Yu SH, Mulder KL, Westphal H. 1992. Targeted oncogene activation by site-specific recombination in transgenic mice. *Proc Natl Acad Sci* **89**: 6232–6236. doi:10.1073/pnas.89.14.6232

Landis EG, Chrenek MA, Chakraborty R, Strickland R, Bergen M, Yang V, Iuvone PM, Pardue MT. 2020. Increased endogenous dopamine prevents myopia in mice. *Exp Eye Res* **193**: 107956. doi:10.1016/j.exer.2020.107956

Landowski M, Bowes Rickman C. 2022. Targeting lipid metabolism for the treatment of age-related macular degeneration: insights from preclinical mouse models. *J Ocul Pharmacol Ther* **38**: 3–32. doi:10.1089/jop.2021.0067

Landowski M, Kelly U, Klingeborn M, Groelle M, Ding JD, Grigsby D, Bowes Rickman C. 2019. Human complement factor H Y402H polymorphism causes an age-related macular degeneration phenotype and lipoprotein dysregulation in mice. *Proc Natl Acad Sci* **116**: 3703–3711. doi:10.1073/pnas.1814014116

Lavalette S, Raoul W, Houssier M, Camelo S, Levy O, Calippe B, Jonet L, Behar-Cohen F, Chemtob S, Guillonneau X, et al. 2011. Interleukin-1β inhibition prevents choroidal neovascularization and does not exacerbate photoreceptor degeneration. *Am J Pathol* **178**: 2416–2423. doi:10.1016/j.ajpath.2011.01.013

Léveillard T, Mohand-Saïd S, Lorentz O, Hicks D, Fintz AC, Clérin E, Simonutti M, Forster V, Cavusoglu N, Chalmel F, et al. 2004. Identification and characterization of rod-derived cone viability factor. *Nat Genet* **36**: 755–759. doi:10.1038/ng1386

Levy O, Calippe B, Lavalette S, Hu SJ, Raoul W, Dominguez E, Housset M, Paques M, Sahel JA, Bemelmans AP, et al. 2015. Apolipoprotein E promotes subretinal mononuclear phagocyte survival and chronic inflammation in age-related macular degeneration. *EMBO Mol Med* **7**: 211–226. doi:10.15252/emmm.201404524

Lipton SA. 2003. Possible role for memantine in protecting retinal ganglion cells from glaucomatous damage. *Surv Ophthalmol* **48**: S38–S46. doi:10.1016/S0039-6257(03)00008-0

Liu K, Akula JD, Falk C, Hansen RM, Fulton AB. 2005. The retinal vasculature and function of the neural retina in a rat model of retinopathy of prematurity. *Invest Ophthalmol Vis Sci* **47**: 2639–2647. doi:10.1167/iovs.06-0016

Livet J, Weissman TA, Kang H, Draft RW, Lu J, Bennis RA, Sanes JR, Lichtman JW. 2007. Transgenic strategies for combinatorial expression of fluorescent proteins in the nervous system. *Nature* **450**: 56–62. doi:10.1038/nature06293

Lorach H, Kang S, Dalal R, Bhuckory MB, Quan Y, Palanker D. 2018. Long-term rescue of photoreceptors in a rodent model of retinitis pigmentosa associated with MERTK mutation. *Sci Rep* **8**: 11312. doi:10.1038/s41598-018-29631-z

Ma J, Sun Y, López FJ, Adamson P, Kurali E, Lashkari K. 2016. Blockage of PI3K/mTOR pathways inhibits laser-induced choroidal neovascularization and improves outcomes relative to VEGF-A suppression alone. *Invest Ophthalmol Vis Sci* **57**: 3138–3144. doi:10.1167/iovs.15-18795

Machida S, Kondo M, Jamison JA, Khan NW, Kononen LT, Sugawara T, Bush RA, Sieving PA. 2000. P23h rhodopsin transgenic rat: correlation of retinal function with histopathology. *Invest Ophthalmol Vis Sci* **41**: 3200–3209.

Maeda A, Maeda T, Golczak M, Palczewski K. 2008. Retinopathy in mice induced by disrupted all-trans-retinal clearance. *J Biol Chem* **283**: 26684–26693. doi:10.1074/jbc.M804505200

Maeda A, Maeda T, Golczak M, Chou S, Desai A, Hoppel CL, Matsuyama S, Palczewski K. 2009. Involvement of all-trans-retinal in acute light-induced retinopathy of mice. *J Biol Chem* **284**: 15173–15183. doi:10.1074/jbc.M900322200

Malecaze F, Mascarelli F, Bugra K, Fuhrmann G, Courtois Y, Hicks D. 1993. Fibroblast growth factor receptor deficiency in dystrophic retinal pigmented epithelium. *J Cell Physiol* **154**: 631–642. doi:10.1002/jcp.1041540323

Mao W, Liu Y, Wordinger RJ, Clark AF. 2013. A magnetic bead-based method for mouse trabecular meshwork cell isolation. *Invest Ophthalmol Vis Sci* **54**: 3600–3606. doi:10.1167/iovs.13-12033

Marie M, Bigot K, Angebault C, Barrau C, Gondouin P, Pagan D, Fouquet S, Villette T, Sahel JA, Lenaers G, et al. 2018. Light action spectrum on oxidative stress and mitochondrial damage in A2E-loaded retinal pigment epithelium cells. *Cell Death Dis* **9**: 287. doi:10.1038/s41419-018-0331-5

Marie M, Forster V, Fouquet S, Berto P, Barrau C, Ehrismann C, Sahel JA, Tessier G, Picaud S. 2020. Phototoxic damage to cone photoreceptors can be independent of the visual pigment: the porphyrin hypothesis. *Cell Death Dis* **11**: 711. doi:10.1038/s41419-020-02918-8

Martin PM, Roon P, Van Ells TK, Ganapathy V, Smith SB. 2004. Death of retinal neurons in streptozotocin-induced diabetic mice. *Invest Ophthalmol Vis Sci* **45**: 3330–3336. doi:10.1167/iovs.04-0247

Mattapallil MJ, Wawrousek EF, Chan CC, Zhao H, Roychoudhury J, Ferguson TA, Caspi RR. 2012. The Rd8 mutation of the *Crb1* gene is present in vendor lines of C57BL/6N mice and embryonic stem cells, and confounds ocular induced mutant phenotypes. *Invest Ophthalmol Vis Sci* **53**: 2921–2927. doi:10.1167/iovs.12-9662

Mei X, Chaffiol A, Kole C, Yang Y, Millet-Puel G, Clerin E, Aït-Ali N, Bennett J, Dalkara D, Sahel JA, et al. 2016. The thioredoxin encoded by the rod-derived cone viability factor gene protects cone photoreceptors against oxidative stress. *Antioxid Redox Signal* **24**: 909–923. doi:10.1089/ars.2015.6509

Meyer-Franke A, Kaplan MR, Pfrieger FW, Barres BA. 1995. Characterization of the signaling interactions that promote the survival and growth of developing retinal ganglion cells in culture. *Neuron* **15**: 805–819. doi:10.1016/0896-6273(95)90172-8

Mohand-Said S, Weber M, Hicks D, Dreyfus H, Sahel JA. 1997. Intravitreal injection of ganglioside GM1 after ischemia reduces retinal damage in rats. *Stroke* **28**: 617–621; discussion 622. doi:10.1161/01.STR.28.3.617

Mookherjee S, Chen HY, Isgrig K, Yu W, Hiriyanna S, Levron R, Li T, Colosi P, Chien W, Swaroop A, et al. 2018. A CEP290 C-terminal domain complements the mutant CEP290 of Rd16 mice in trans and rescues retinal degeneration. *Cell Rep* **25**: 611–623 e616. doi:10.1016/j.celrep.2018.09.043

Nandrot E, Dufour EM, Provost AC, Péquignot MO, Bonnel S, Gogat K, Marchant D, Rouillac C, Sépulchre de Condé B, Bihoreau MT, et al. 2000. Homozygous deletion in the coding sequence of the *c-mer* gene in RCS rats unravels general mechanisms of physiological cell adhesion and apoptosis. *Neurobiol Dis* **7**: 586–599. doi:10.1006/nbdi.2000.0328

Newman NJ, Yu-Wai-Man P, Carelli V, Moster ML, Biousse V, Vignal-Clermont C, Sergott RC, Klopstock T, Sadun AA, Barboni P, et al. 2021. Efficacy and safety of intravitreal gene therapy for Leber hereditary optic neuropathy treated within 6 months of disease onset. *Ophthalmology* **128**: 649–660. doi:10.1016/j.ophtha.2020.12.012

Newman NJ, Yu-Wai-Man P, Subramanian PS, Moster ML, Wang AG, Donahue SP, Leroy BP, Carelli V, Biousse V, Vignal-Clermont C, et al. 2023. Randomized trial of bilateral gene therapy injection for m.11778G > A MT-ND4 Leber optic neuropathy. *Brain* **146**: 1328–1341. doi:10.1093/brain/awac421

Noben-Trauth K, Naggert JK, North MA, Nishina PM. 1996. A candidate gene for the mouse mutation tubby. *Nature* **380**: 534–538. doi:10.1038/380534a0

Orhan E, Dalkara D, Neuillé M, Lechauve C, Michiels C, Picaud S, Léveillard T, Sahel JA, Naash MI, Lavail MM, et al. 2015. Genotypic and phenotypic characterization of P23H line 1 rat model. *PLoS ONE* **10**: e0127319. doi:10.1371/journal.pone.0127319

Pang JJ, Chang B, Kumar A, Nusinowitz S, Noorwez SM, Li J, Rani A, Foster TC, Chiodo VA, Doyle T, et al. 2005. Gene therapy restores vision-dependent behavior as well as retinal structure and function in a mouse model of RPE65 Leber congenital amaurosis. *Mol Ther* **13**: 565–572. doi:10.1016/j.ymthe.2005.09.001

Paques M, Simonutti M, Roux MJ, Picaud S, Levavasseur E, Bellman C, Sahel JA. 2005. High resolution fundus imaging by confocal scanning laser ophthalmoscopy in the mouse. *Vision Res* **46**: 1336–1345. doi:10.1016/j.visres.2005.09.037

Paques M, Guyomard JL, Simonutti M, Roux MJ, Picaud S, Legargasson JF, Sahel JA. 2007. Panretinal, high-resolution color photography of the mouse fundus. *Invest Ophthalmol Vis Sci* **48**: 2769–2774. doi:10.1167/iovs.06-1099

Park SH, Park JW, Park SJ, Kim KY, Chung JW, Chun MH, Oh SJ. 2003. Apoptotic death of photoreceptors in the streptozotocin-induced diabetic rat retina. *Diabetologia* **46**: 1260–1268. doi:10.1007/s00125-003-1177-6

Pasantes-Morales H, Quesada O, Cárabez A, Huxtable RJ. 1983. Effects of the taurine transport antagonist, guanidinoethane sulfonate, and β-alanine on the morphology of rat retina. *J Neurosci Res* **9**: 135–143. doi:10.1002/jnr.490090205

Peng YW, Zallocchi M, Wang WM, Delimont D, Cosgrove D. 2011. Moderate light-induced degeneration of rod photoreceptors with delayed transducin translocation in shaker1 mice. *Invest Ophthalmol Vis Sci* **52**: 6421–6427. doi:10.1167/iovs.10-6557

Cite this article as *Cold Spring Harb Perspect Med* doi: 10.1101/cshperspect.a041311

Pennesi ME, Neuringer M, Courtney RJ. 2012. Animal models of age related macular degeneration. *Mol Aspects Med* **33:** 487–509. doi:10.1016/j.mam.2012.06.003

Peynshaert K, Devoldere J, Forster V, Picaud S, Vanhove C, De Smedt SC, Remaut K. 2017. Toward smart design of retinal drug carriers: a novel bovine retinal explant model to study the barrier role of the vitreoretinal interface. *Drug Deliv* **24:** 1384–1394. doi:10.1080/10717544.2017.1375578

Picaud S, Peichl L, Franceschini N. 1993. Dye-induced photolesion in the mammalian retina: glial and neuronal reactions. *J Neurosci Res* **35:** 629–642. doi:10.1002/jnr.490350606

Picaud S, Pattnaik B, Hicks D, Forster V, Fontaine V, Sahel J, Dreyfus H. 1998. GABAA and GABAC receptors in adult porcine cones: evidence from a photoreceptor-glia coculture model. *J Physiol* **513:** 33–42. doi:10.1111/j.1469-7793.1998.033by.x

Picaud S, Dalkara D, Marazova K, Goureau O, Roska B, Sahel JA. 2019. The primate model for understanding and restoring vision. *Proc Natl Acad Sci* **116:** 26280–26287. doi:10.1073/pnas.1902292116

Pinzón-Duarte G, Kohler K, Arango-González B, Guenther E. 2000. Cell differentiation, synaptogenesis, and influence of the retinal pigment epithelium in a rat neonatal organotypic retina culture. *Vision Res* **40:** 3455–3465. doi:10.1016/S0042-6989(00)00185-1

Prévot PH, Gehere K, Arcizet F, Akolkar H, Khoei MA, Blaize K, Oubari O, Daye P, Lanoë M, Valet M, et al. 2020. Behavioural responses to a photovoltaic subretinal prosthesis implanted in non-human primates. *Nat Biomed Eng* **4:** 172–180. doi:10.1038/s41551-019-0484-2

Ratnapriya R, Chew EY. 2013. Age-related macular degeneration-clinical review and genetics update. *Clin Genet* **84:** 160–166. doi:10.1111/cge.12206

Redmond TM, Hamel CP. 2000. Genetic analysis of RPE65: from human disease to mouse model. *Methods Enzymol* **316:** 705–724. doi:10.1016/S0076-6879(00)16758-8

Reichman S, Terray A, Slembrouck A, Nanteau C, Orieux G, Habeler W, Nandrot EF, Sahel JA, Monville C, Goureau O. 2014. From confluent human iPS cells to self-forming neural retina and retinal pigmented epithelium. *Proc Natl Acad Sci* **111:** 8518–8523. doi:10.1073/pnas.1324212111

Reichman S, Slembrouck A, Gagliardi G, Chaffiol A, Terray A, Nanteau C, Potey A, Belle M, Rabesandratana O, Duebel J, et al. 2017. Generation of storable retinal organoids and retinal pigmented epithelium from adherent human iPS cells in xeno-free and feeder-free conditions. *Stem Cells* **35:** 1176–1188. doi:10.1002/stem.2586

Roubeix C, Godefroy D, Mias C, Sapienza A, Riancho L, Degardin J, Fradot V, Ivkovic I, Picaud S, Sennlaub F, et al. 2015. Intraocular pressure reduction and neuroprotection conferred by bone marrow-derived mesenchymal stem cells in an animal model of glaucoma. *Stem Cell Res Ther* **6:** 177. doi:10.1186/s13287-015-0168-0

Sahel JA, Boulanger-Scemama E, Pagot C, Arleo A, Galluppi F, Martel JN, Esposti SD, Delaux A, de Saint Aubert JB, de Montleau C, et al. 2021. Partial recovery of visual function in a blind patient after optogenetic therapy. *Nat Med* **27:** 1223–1229. doi:10.1038/s41591-021-01351-4

Salinas-Navarro M, Alarcón-Martínez L, Valiente-Soriano FJ, Jiménez-López M, Mayor-Torroglosa S, Avilés-Tri-gueros M, Villegas-Pérez MP, Vidal-Sanz M. 2010. Ocular hypertension impairs optic nerve axonal transport leading to progressive retinal ganglion cell degeneration. *Exp Eye Res* **90:** 168–183. doi:10.1016/j.exer.2009.10.003

Sauer B, Henderson N. 1990. Targeted insertion of exogenous DNA into the eukaryotic genome by the Cre recombinase. *New Biol* **2:** 441–449.

Schuettauf F, Quinto K, Naskar R, Zurakowski D. 2002. Effects of anti-glaucoma medications on ganglion cell survival: the DBA/2J mouse model. *Vision Res* **42:** 2333–2337. doi:10.1016/S0042-6989(02)00188-8

Schwahn HN, Kaymak H, Schaeffel F. 2000. Effects of atropine on refractive development, dopamine release, and slow retinal potentials in the chick. *Vis Neurosci* **17:** 165–176. doi:10.1017/S0952523800171184

Sen M, Al-Amin M, Kicková E, Sadeghi A, Puranen J, Urtti A, Caliceti P, Salmaso S, Arango-Gonzalez B, Ueffing M. 2021a. Retinal neuroprotection by controlled release of a VCP inhibitor from self-assembled nanoparticles. *J Control Release* **339:** 307–320. doi:10.1016/j.jconrel.2021.09.039

Sen M, Kutsyr O, Cao B, Bolz S, Arango-Gonzalez B, Ueffing M. 2021b. Pharmacological inhibition of the VCP/proteasome axis rescues photoreceptor degeneration in RHO (P23H) rat retinal explants. *Biomolecules* **11:** 1528. doi:10.3390/biom11101528

Siegert S, Scherf BG, Del Punta K, Didkovsky N, Heintz N, Roska B. 2009. Genetic address book for retinal cell types. *Nat Neurosci* **12:** 1197–1204. doi:10.1038/nn.2370

Smith LE, Wesolowski E, McLellan A, Kostyk SK, D'Amato R, Sullivan R, D'Amore PA. 1994. Oxygen-induced retinopathy in the mouse. *Invest Ophthalmol Vis Sci* **35:** 101–111.

Soderpalm A, Szel A, Caffe AR, van Veen T. 1994. Selective development of one cone photoreceptor type in retinal organ culture. *Invest Ophthalmol Vis Sci* **35:** 3910–3921.

Song E, Dong Y, Han LN, Sui DM, Xu Q, Wang XR, Wu JX. 2004. Diabetic retinopathy: VEGF, bFGF and retinal vascular pathology. *Chin Med J (Engl)* **117:** 247–251.

Stasheff SF. 2008. Emergence of sustained spontaneous hyperactivity and temporary preservation of OFF responses in ganglion cells of the retinal degeneration (rd1) mouse. *J Neurophysiol* **99:** 1408–1421. doi:10.1152/jn.00144.2007

Sun D, Schur RM, Sears AE, Gao SQ, Vaidya A, Sun W, Maeda A, Kern T, Palczewski K, Lu ZR. 2020. Non-viral gene therapy for Stargardt disease with ECO/pRHO-ABCA4 self-assembled nanoparticles. *Mol Ther* **28:** 293–303. doi:10.1016/j.ymthe.2019.09.010

Sun D, Sun W, Gao SQ, Lehrer J, Naderi A, Wei C, Lee S, Schilb AL, Scheidt J, Hall RC, et al. 2022. Effective gene therapy of Stargardt disease with PEG-ECO/pGRK1-ABCA4-S/MAR nanoparticles. *Mol Ther Nucleic Acids* **29:** 823–835. doi:10.1016/j.omtn.2022.08.026

Tedja MS, Wojciechowski R, Hysi PG, Eriksson N, Furlotte NA, Verhoeven VJM, Iglesias AI, Meester-Smoor MA, Tompson SW, Fan Q, et al. 2018. Genome-wide association meta-analysis highlights light-induced signaling as a driver for refractive error. *Nat Genet* **50:** 834–848. doi:10.1038/s41588-018-0127-7

Thaung C, West K, Clark BJ, McKie L, Morgan JE, Arnold K, Nolan PM, Peters J, Hunter AJ, Brown SD, et al. 2002. Novel ENU-induced eye mutations in the mouse: models for human eye disease. *Hum Mol Genet* **11**: 755–767. doi:10.1093/hmg/11.7.755

Thompson DA, Khan NW, Othman MI, Chang B, Jia L, Grahek G, Wu Z, Hiriyanna S, Nellissery J, Li T, et al. 2012. Rd9 is a naturally occurring mouse model of a common form of retinitis pigmentosa caused by mutations in RPGR-ORF15. *PLoS ONE* **7**: e35865. doi:10.1371/journal.pone.0035865

Toomey CB, Kelly U, Saban DR, Bowes Rickman C. 2015. Regulation of age-related macular degeneration-like pathology by complement factor H. *Proc Natl Acad Sci* **112**: E3040–E3049. doi:10.1073/pnas.1424391112

Torero Ibad R, Rheey J, Mrejen S, Forster V, Picaud S, Prochiantz A, Moya KL. 2011. Otx2 promotes the survival of damaged adult retinal ganglion cells and protects against excitotoxic loss of visual acuity in vivo. *J Neurosci* **31**: 5495–5503. doi:10.1523/JNEUROSCI.0187-11.2011

Trouillet A, Dubus E, Degardin J, Estivalet A, Ivkovic I, Godefroy D, Garcia-Ayuso D, Simonutti M, Sahly I, Sahel JA, et al. 2018. Cone degeneration is triggered by the absence of USH1 proteins but prevented by antioxidant treatments. *Sci Rep* **8**: 1968. doi:10.1038/s41598-018-20171-0

Ufret-Vincenty RL, Aredo B, Liu X, McMahon A, Chen PW, Sun H, Niederkorn JY, Kedzierski W. 2010. Transgenic mice expressing variants of complement factor H develop AMD-like retinal findings. *Invest Ophthalmol Vis Sci* **51**: 5878–5887. doi:10.1167/iovs.09-4457

Vallazza-Deschamps G, Cia D, Gong J, Jellali A, Duboc A, Forster V, Sahel JA, Tessier LH, Picaud S. 2005. Excessive activation of cyclic nucleotide-gated channels contributes to neuronal degeneration of photoreceptors. *Eur J Neurosci* **22**: 1013–1022. doi:10.1111/j.1460-9568.2005.04306.x

Veleri S, Lazar CH, Chang B, Sieving PA, Banin E, Swaroop A. 2015. Biology and therapy of inherited retinal degenerative disease: insights from mouse models. *Dis Model Mech* **8**: 109–129. doi:10.1242/dmm.017913

Vessey KA, Wilkinson-Berka JL, Fletcher EL. 2011. Characterization of retinal function and glial cell response in a mouse model of oxygen-induced retinopathy. *J Comp Neurol* **519**: 506–527. doi:10.1002/cne.22530

Vignal C, Uretsky S, Fitoussi S, Galy A, Blouin L, Girmens JF, Bidot S, Thomasson N, Bouquet C, Valero S, et al. 2018. Safety of rAAV2/2-ND4 gene therapy for Leber hereditary optic neuropathy. *Ophthalmology* **125**: 945–947. doi:10.1016/j.ophtha.2017.12.036

Vignal-Clermont C, Girmens JF, Audo I, Said SM, Errera MH, Plaine L, O'Shaughnessy D, Taiel M, Sahel JA. 2021. Safety of intravitreal gene therapy for treatment of subjects with Leber hereditary optic neuropathy due to mutations in the mitochondrial *ND4* gene: the REVEAL study. *BioDrugs* **35**: 201–214. doi:10.1007/s40259-021-00468-9

Vollrath D, Feng W, Duncan JL, Yasumura D, D'Cruz PM, Chappelow A, Matthes MT, Kay MA, LaVail MM. 2001. Correction of the retinal dystrophy phenotype of the RCS rat by viral gene transfer of Mertk. *Proc Natl Acad Sci* **98**: 12584–12589. doi:10.1073/pnas.221364198

Watkins TA, Emery B, Mulinyawe S, Barres BA. 2008. Distinct stages of myelination regulated by γ-secretase and astrocytes in a rapidly myelinating CNS coculture system. *Neuron* **60**: 555–569. doi:10.1016/j.neuron.2008.09.011

Weng J, Mata NL, Azarian SM, Tzekov RT, Birch DG, Travis GH. 1999. Insights into the function of Rim protein in photoreceptors and etiology of Stargardt's disease from the phenotype in *abcr* knockout mice. *Cell* **98**: 13–23. doi:10.1016/S0092-8674(00)80602-9

Wilmet B, Callebert J, Duvoisin R, Goulet R, Tourain C, Michiels C, Frederiksen H, Schaeffel F, Marre O, Sahel JA, et al. 2022. Mice lacking Gpr179 with complete congenital stationary night blindness are a good model for myopia. *Int J Mol Sci* **24**: 219. doi:10.3390/ijms24010219

WoldeMussie E, Yoles E, Schwartz M, Ruiz G, Wheeler LA. 2002. Neuroprotective effect of memantine in different retinal injury models in rats. *J Glaucoma* **11**: 474–480. doi:10.1097/00061198-200212000-00003

Wu J, Seregard S, Algvere PV. 2005. Photochemical damage of the retina. *Surv Ophthalmol* **51**: 461–481. doi:10.1016/j.survophthal.2006.06.009

Wu L, Ueda K, Nagasaki T, Sparrow JR. 2014. Light damage in *Abca4* and *Rpe65^{rd12}* mice. *Invest Ophthalmol Vis Sci* **55**: 1910–1918. doi:10.1167/iovs.14-13867

Yang Y, Mohand-Said S, Danan A, Simonutti M, Fontaine V, Clerin E, Picaud S, Léveillard T, Sahel JA. 2009. Functional cone rescue by RdCVF protein in a dominant model of retinitis pigmentosa. *Mol Ther* **17**: 787–795. doi:10.1038/mt.2009.28

Zeitz C, Roger JE, Audo I, Michiels C, Sánchez-Farias N, Varin J, Frederiksen H, Wilmet B, Callebert J, Gimenez ML, et al. 2023. Shedding light on myopia by studying complete congenital stationary night blindness. *Prog Retin Eye Res* **93**: 101155. doi:10.1016/j.preteyeres.2022.101155

Retinal Degeneration Animal Models in Bardet–Biedl Syndrome and Related Ciliopathies

Clarisse Delvallée and Hélène Dollfus

Laboratoire de Génétique Médicale UMRS1112, Centre de Recherche Biomédicale de Strasbourg, CRBS, Institut de Génétique Médicale d'Alsace, IGMA, Strasbourg 67000, France

Correspondence: dollfus@unistra.fr

Retinal degeneration due to photoreceptor ciliary-related proteins dysfunction accounts for more than 25% of all inherited retinal dystrophies. The cilium, being an evolutionarily conserved and ubiquitous organelle implied in many cellular functions, can be investigated by way of many models from invertebrate models to nonhuman primates, all these models have massively contributed to the pathogenesis understanding of human ciliopathies. Taking the Bardet–Biedl syndrome (BBS) as an emblematic example as well as other related syndromic ciliopathies, the contribution of a wide range of models has enabled to characterize the role of the BBS proteins in the archetypical cilium but also at the level of the connecting cilium of the photoreceptors. There are more than 24 BBS genes encoding for proteins that form different complexes such as the BBSome and the chaperone proteins complex. But how they lead to retinal degeneration remains a matter of debate with the possible accumulation of proteins in the inner segment and/or accumulation of unwanted proteins in the outer segment that cannot return in the inner segment machinery. Many BBS proteins (but not the chaperonins for instance) can be modeled in primitive organisms such as *Paramecium*, *Chlamydomonas reinardtii*, *Trypanosoma brucei*, and *Caenorhabditis elegans*. These models have enabled clarifying the role of a subset of BBS proteins in the primary cilium as well as their relations with other modules such as the intraflagellar transport (IFT) module, the nephronophthisis (NPHP) module, or the Meckel–Gruber syndrome (MKS)/Joubert syndrome (JBTS) module mostly involved with the transition zone of the primary cilia. Assessing the role of the primary cilia structure of the connecting cilium of the photoreceptor cells has been very much studied by way of zebrafish modeling (*Danio rerio*) as well as by a plethora of mouse models. More recently, large animal models have been described for three BBS genes and one nonhuman primate model in rhesus macaque for *BBS7*. In completion to animal models, human cell models can now be used notably thanks to gene editing and the use of induced pluripotent stem cells (iPSCs). All these models are not only important for pathogenesis understanding but also very useful for studying therapeutic avenues, their pros and cons, especially for gene replacement therapy as well as pharmacological triggers.

Inherited retinal dystrophy (IRD) is at this time the most common cause of blindness in Europe in children and working-age adults, represented by a vast group of rare diseases with currently very limited effective cure/therapy available in clinical practice. IRD is a constellation of highly heterogeneous genetic diseases resulting in progressive loss of retinal cells (mostly photoreceptor [PR] cells and the retinal pigment epithelium [RPE] cells) leading to visual impairment and blindness affecting one in 3000 people (Bessant et al. 2001). Research in this field has reached many successes, notably with next-generation sequencing approaches demonstrating noncoding gene variations and enhancing novel gene identifications with now >300 IRD genes identified (RetNet: sph.uth.edu/retnet, last updated June 9, 2022). However, IRDs remains an immense challenge for therapy development because of the vastness of genetic and phenotypic variability remaining to be understood (Thompson et al. 2015). The pathogenic landscape is extremely complex ranging from functional visual cycle impairment, PR metabolism, or structure alterations to transcription/RNA splicing defect as well as ciliary defects, all leading to the degeneration of PR as a common result of those highly heterogeneous initial biological cellular triggers (Berger et al. 2010; Thompson et al. 2015). Most importantly, >25% of all IRDs are ciliopathy-related retinal degeneration (RD) (syndromic or nonsyndromic) linked to a dysfunction of the highly modified primary cilium structure of the PR (Wright et al. 2010; Estrada-Cuzcano et al. 2012a) of which 25% are syndromic associated with additional extraocular manifestations. More than 100 ciliary genes are associated with IRDs (Chen et al. 2019).

This review will focus on an emblematic syndromic ciliopathy, namely, Bardet–Biedl syndrome (BBS) (as well as illustrative other related ciliopathies) to showcase how various in vivo models used to study ciliary proteins can contribute to understanding the pathogenesis of IRDs and be used as tools for genomic validation or for exploring therapeutic avenues.

PHENOTYPE AND GENOTYPE OF BARDET–BIEDL SYNDROME (BBS): AN EMBLEMATIC CILIOPATHY

BBS and other related ciliopathies have been described more than a century ago on clinical grounds as an inherited disease with multiple organ manifestations and were recognized to be linked to primary cilium dysfunctions since

the early 2000s (Fliegauf et al. 2007; Chandra et al. 2022).

Cilia are highly conserved and ubiquitously expressed organelles consisting of an axoneme, a basal body, a transition zone, and a ciliary tip. The primary nonmotile cilium is a protrusion of the plasma membrane supported by a microtubule cytoskeleton present on the surface of almost all cells of the vertebrate body at some point of development and cellular functions. The primary cilium "9 + 0," as opposed to the "9 + 2" defining motile cilium, is unique at the cell surface and represents a major player in cell signaling (especially with the Sonic Hedgehog [SHH] or Wnt pathways) and cell communication with an enrichment of receptors such as G protein–coupled receptors at the level of the ciliary membrane (Goetz and Anderson 2010). The basal body is considered as a docking platform for proteins getting to the cilium and is surrounded by the transition zone that regulates the ciliary function and traffic. Intraflagellar transport (IFT) is bidirectional: anterograde regulated by kinesins and retrograde regulated by dyneins (Fig. 1).

Ciliopathies are defined by conditions due to pathogenic genetic variations in genes encoding ciliary-related proteins leading to isolated organ dysfunction (i.e., isolated retinal phenotype such as retinitis pigmentosa, isolated nephronophthisis [NPHP], a condition defined as a chronic tubulo-interstitial nephritis leading to kidney failure) or syndromic presentations shown by BBS and other syndromes. All belong to a continuously completed clinical spectrum encompassing well-known entities such as Joubert syndrome (JBTS), Senior–Loken syndrome (SLSN), oro-facial-digital (OFD) syndrome, and the lethal Meckel–Gruber syndrome (MKS), to mention the main ones (Hildebrandt et al. 2011; Reiter and Leroux 2017).

One of the ciliopathy clinical classical targets is the retina, mainly by affecting PR cells (although other retinal cells have also ciliated compounds) resulting in RD (Chandra et al. 2022). The vertebrate PRs are highly polarized and specialized neurons with the outer segment (OS) as a specific compartment where the photoreaction and phototransduction occurs at the levels of stacked discs aligned in the axoneme. The PR's

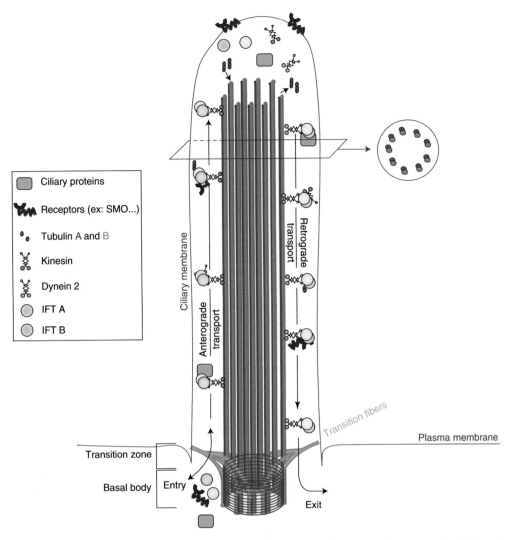

Figure 1. Schematic representation of a primary cilium. The transversal section at the axoneme level shows the 9 + 0 structure of the microtubule cytoskeleton composed of tubulin A and B. The basal body corresponds to a derived centriole that serves as a platform for the formation of the cilium. The transition zone is a specialized region that regulates the protein entry inside and outside the cilium. Ciliary proteins and signaling receptors are transported between the base and the apex of the cilium by the intraflagellar transport (IFT) proteins that interact with the molecular motors (kinesin and dynein). (Figure adapted from Delvallée 2020, p. 6, with permission from the author.)

modified cilium, namely, the connecting cilium (CC) and associated periciliary complex (PCC), is located at the junction of the inner segment (IS) and OS and is equivalent to the transition zone of primary cilia and play the role of a ciliary gate (Chen et al. 2021). The IS contains the Golgi, rough endoplasmic reticulum (ER), mitochondria, and microtubules.

Intense trafficking occurs at the CC with more than 1000 rhodopsin molecules transiting per second (Besharse 1986). Abnormal protein trafficking caused by defective IFT of proteins between the two segments of the PRs induces a proapoptotic reaction. The precise molecular triggers and mechanisms leading to PR death remains to be clearly identified but are based on the alteration of protein transport via the transition zone and in connection with all actors of the ciliary system. Various models have enlightened the pathogenesis of the PR degeneration in ciliopathies and are described in this review.

More than 1500 ciliary proteins (van Dam et al. 2019) are known to be involved in cilia formation, resorption, protein transports, and signaling cascades transduction, and ~700 ciliary genes have been identified as important in health or disease noticeably by way of the SYSCILIA consortium (Vasquez et al. 2021). Various proteins are necessary to the ciliary function and can be grouped according to modules matching groups of syndromic ciliopathies (Fig. 2). For example, IFT modules are composed of proteins interacting with two molecular motors (kinesin and dynein) to transport protein cargos inside/outside the cilium. Dyneins are acting in interaction with IFT proteins called "IFT A" involved in the retrograde transport (IFT139, 121, 143, 144, 122, 140), and kinesins are acting in interaction with IFT proteins, called "IFT B" in the antero-

grade transport (IFT54, 80, 20, 172, 38, 57, 52, 88, 46, 70, 56, 25, 27, 74, 81, 22) (Nakayama and Katoh 2018). Others modules related to diseases are localized at the cilia diffusion barrier, the transition zone, to select the protein cargo that enter in the cilium: the BBSome complex module (BBS1, 2, 4, 5, 7, 8, 9, 18), the MKS/JBTS module (AHI, B9D1, B9D2, CC2D2A, MKS1, TCTN1, TCTN2, TCTN3, TMEM17, TMEM67, TMEM 107, TMEM216, TMEM231), and the NPHP module (ATXN10, CEP290, INVS, NEK8, NPHP1, NPHP3, NPHP4, NPHP5, NPHP8, RPGRIP1L) (Gupta et al. 2021). Transport into and out of cilia is carefully regulated by IFT machinery and the BBSome. The BBSome functions as an adaptor to IFT complexes and recruits cargo for ciliary export via retrograde transport. The BBSome recruiting cargo needs the assistance of the small GTPase, ARL6/BBS3. The BBsome has a stepwise assembling process (with the top = BBS2 and BBS7, the base = BBS5, BBS8, and BBS9, and the joining proteins base-top = BBS1, BBS4, and BBS18). The BBS chaperonin com-

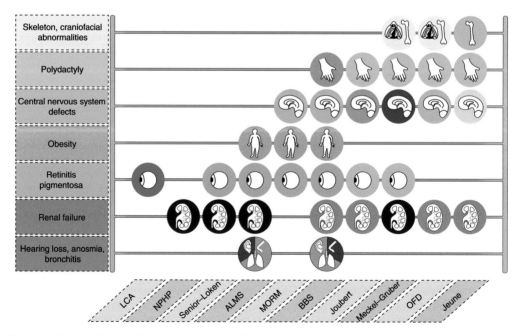

Figure 2. Abacus of ciliopathies. Representation of the major clinical features depending on the considered ciliopathy. (LCA) Leber's congenital amaurosis, (NPHP) nephronophthisis, (ALMS) Alström syndrome, (MORM) mental retardation, obesity, retinal dystrophy, and micropenis, (BBS) Bardet–Biedl syndrome, (OFD) oro-facial-digital. (Figure adapted from Delvallée 2020, p. 30, with permission from the author.)

plex, composed of three protein BBS (BBS6, BBS10, BBS12), is important for the formation of the BBSome (Álvarez-Satta et al. 2017). It has recently been shown that partially assembled BBSome is tolerated in PR as opposed to other cells where complete BBSome is required (Hsu et al. 2021).

Bardet–Biedl syndrome (BBS; OMIM: 209900) is an autosomal-recessive ciliopathy characterized by RD, associated with early-onset truncal obesity, postaxial polydactyly, renal dysfunction/failure, learning disabilities, and hypogonadism, among other rarer manifestations (Tobin and Beales 2007; Zaghloul and Katsanis 2009; Forsythe and Beales 2013). More than 24 BBS (BBS1–BBS24) genes have been identified. To date, a molecular diagnosis is achieved in clinical settings in ~80% of cases. The two most frequently mutated genes are BBS1 (~19%) and BBS10 (~12%). 75% of BBS1 patients are carriers of a recurrent mutation M390R (Mykytyn et al. 2002; Beales et al. 2003). Other BBS genes are less frequently mutated (3%–6% for BBS4 or BBS6, for instance) or even much rarer, such as BBS17/LZTLF1 or BBS18/BBIP1, only reported in a very low number of patients (Fig. 3A). Overall, reported pathogenic variants are very diverse with nonsense and missense variants, but rare intragenic deletions have been reported as well as other more complex variants such as a recurrent retrotransposon variant in BBS1 (Tavares et al. 2018; Delvallée et al. 2021). BBS is also emblematic as a model of genetic interaction with the concept of oligenism (Katsanis et al. 2001) and epistatic interactions for secondary variant models (Kousi et al. 2020). Eight BBS proteins (BBS1, BBS2, BBS4, BBS5, BBS7, BBS8, BBS9, BBS18) form a complex named BBsome, recently modeled with near atomic structure (Klink et al. 2020; Yang et al. 2020), whereas the other BBS proteins facilitate BBSome formation and general function for ciliary activities. The chaperonin complex, composed of BBS6, BBS10, and BBS12, is vertebrate specific and a key player for the formation of the BBSome (Álvarez-Satta et al. 2017) accounting for 30% of the mutational load (Fig. 3B).

In BBS, the RD is highly penetrant and typically of early onset in patients mostly described as a rod-cone degeneration or global PR degeneration leading to major visual impairment before the age of 10. In rare cases, the retinal phenotype may display dramatic clinical variability such as only or mainly cones affected, leading to alterations in central vision (with relative rod sparing and peripheral visual field preservation that can occur much latter with a cone-rod degeneration) compared to classical BBS cases (Scheidecker et al. 2015; Mauring et al. 2020). In addition, very delayed age-of-onset and/or very mild RD with preservation of functioning PRs for a very significant period have also been described by our group (Scheidecker et al. 2015) and others especially for BBS1 (Azari et al. 2006). Phenotype–genotype correlations for RD due to variants in BBS genes have been described by suggesting a slower degeneration for patients with BBS1 gene defects compared to patients with BBS10 gene defects for instance (Grudzinska Pechhacker et al. 2021). Nonsyndromic IRD have been associated with variants in BBS1, BBS2, BBS3/ARL6, BBS5, BBS8/TTC8, BBS14/CEP290, and BBS21/C8orf37 (Pretorius et al. 2011; Estrada-Cuzcano et al. 2012b; Murphy et al. 2015; Shevach et al. 2015; Fadaie et al. 2022). For example, the IVS1-2A>G mutation in the splice acceptor site of BBS8 exon 2A abolished the expression of the BBS8 PR-specific isoform that thus explained the limited retinal phenotype (Murphy et al. 2015). Structural studies have shown that the variants responsible for the nonsyndromic RD affect solvent-exposed residues compared to buried residues in full-spectrum BBS phenotype cases (Chou et al. 2019). This emphasizes the extreme sensitivity to PR due to a high transport rate unable to cope even with a slight alteration of BBSome (Datta et al. 2015; Hsu et al. 2017).

RD is also observed as highly penetrant in other syndromic ciliopathies such as the closely clinically related to BBS Alström syndrome (ALMS), due to gene alteration in one gene ALMS1, an ultrarare syndrome, and also characterized by constant early-onset severe RD (but with mostly prominent central involvement), obesity, and kidney dysfunction, but differing by the absence of polydactyly and the occurrence of insulin resistance, deafness, and cardiomyopathy. In other syndromic ciliopathies, RD can

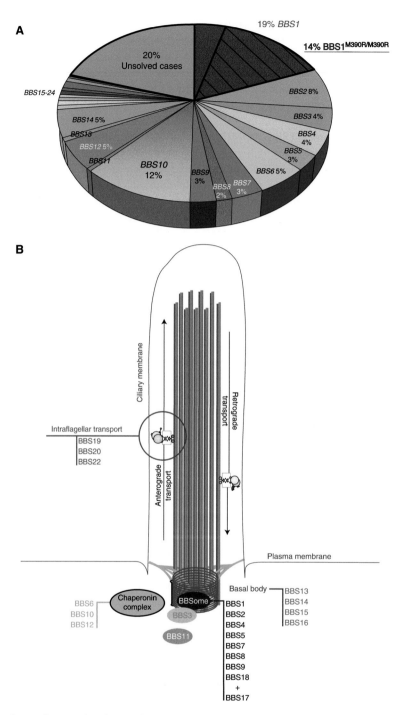

Figure 3. Incidence of genes related to Bardet–Biedl syndrome (BBS) and localization of corresponding proteins in a generic primary cilium. (*A*) Diagram representing the proportion of patient carriers of mutation in each BBS gene among the 80% of patients with a solved genetic diagnosis. *BBS1* and *BBS10* are the two major BBS contributors. (Panel *A* created from data in Forsyth and Gunay-Aygun 1993; updated July 23, 2020.) (*B*) Schematic representation showing the location of 22 out of the 24 BBS proteins (identified to date) in various zones of a primary cilium. (Panel *B* adapted from Delvallée 2020, pp. 16–17, with permission from the author.)

occur but not systematically; the main related ciliary syndromes with possible RD are briefly described hereafter.

JBTS (OMIM: 213300) is a rare autosomal-recessive ciliopathy characterized by central nervous system manifestations of developmental delay, neonatal breathing difficulties, apraxia, ataxia with hypoplasia of the cerebellar vermis, and occasional polydactyly (Bachmann-Gagescu et al. 2020). A subset of JBTS patients (30%) also develop RD mostly in the following genes: *AHI1*, *TMEM67*, *TCTN2*, *CEP290*, and *CC2D2A* (the last two can also cause isolated RD). 40 genes (*JBTS1–40*) have been reported and are all involved in ciliogenesis or ciliary function (Bachmann-Gagescu et al. 2015).

NPHP (OMIM: 256100) is another autosomal-recessive ciliopathy considered as the most common genetic cause of renal failure in childhood and characterized by a progressive tubule interstitial nephritis with medullary cysts leading to end-stage renal disease before 30 years. To date, >26 genes coding for ciliary proteins been identified with the NPHP phenotypes (*ANKS6*, *CC2D2A*, *CEP164*, *CEP290*, *CEP41*, *CEP83*, *DCDC2*, *FAN1*, *GLIS2*, *IFT172*, *INVS*, *IQCB1*, *MAPKBP1*, *NEK8*, *NPHP1*, *NPHP3*, *NPHP4*, *OFD1*, *PKHD1*, *RPGRIP1L*, *SDCCAG8*, *TCTN1*, *TMEM138*, *TMEM216*, *TMEM237*, *TMEM67*, *TRAF3IP1*, *TTC21B*, *WDR19*, *WDR35*, *XPNP EP3*, *ZNF423*). The most frequent variant is an *NPHP1* deletion (Snoek et al. 2018; Gupta et al. 2021) occasionally associated with RD. Indeed, 10% to 20% of the NPHP patients have extra features that can define specific syndromic entities. The Senior–Loken syndrome (OMIM: 266900, 606995, 606996, 609254, 610189, 613615, 614845, 616307, 616629) is characterized by NPHP and RD degeneration with a major gene being *NPHP5/IQCB1* coding for a centrosomal and transition zone protein that interacts with CEP290 to regulate the BBsome integrity and trafficking to the membrane (Barbelanne et al. 2015). *NPHP1*, *CFAP31*, *NPHP4*, *CEP290*, *SDCCAG8*, *WDR19*, *TRAF3IP1*, and *INVS* have also been associated with Senior–Loken syndrome. The Mainzer–Saldino syndrome (OMIM: 266920, 615630) is defined mainly by NPHP, RD, and cone-shaped epiphysis, and

have been associated with mutations in *IFT140*, *IFT172*, and *WDR19*.

The OFD is X-linked-dominant with facial, oral cavity, and digits malformations due to pathogenic variants in the *OFD1* gene coding for centrosomal/basal body OFD1 protein and controlling ciliogenesis but has been also implied in various ciliopathies including JBTS and RD (Webb et al. 2012; Wang et al. 2017; Chen et al. 2018; Morleo et Franco 2020).

GENERAL OVERVIEW OF CILIOPATHY MODELS: FROM PARAMECIA TO MONKEYS

In vitro cell models with immortalized cell lines or patient cells (mainly fibroblasts cultures from skin biopsies) have very much contributed to characterize ciliary proteins and complexes (see specific section) for all these syndromes. In vivo models are playing a crucial role in deciphering and understanding the pathogenesis, the variability of the natural history of ciliopathies. Moreover, they can be key players in early and now late stages of preclinical investigations.

In vivo modeling in the field of ciliary biogenesis and function has taken advantage of the very high level of conservation of a large number of ciliary proteins. BBSome and BBS3/ARL6 are present in most organisms pointing to a major role in the cilia evolution (however, the chaperonin module is vertebrate specific and seems to be acquired during evolution). Overall nonvertebrate and vertebrate models have proven to be of high value in deciphering the role of BBS proteins and other ciliopathies.

Nonvertebrate Models

Unicellular eukaryotic organisms have contributed extensively to the fundamental understanding of ciliary biogenesis and function including for BBS.

For instance, *Paramecium tetraurelia* is a unicellular and multiciliated sensory organism that can model numerous ciliopathies (Valentine and Van Houten 2021) such as, for example, OFD1 alteration-inducing anomalies at the level of the common docking of the basal body with an identical observation in human beings carrying mutations in OFD1 (Bengueddach et al. 2017). In *Paramecium*, KO of BBS genes cause prolonged backward swimming due to loss of K^+ and TRP/PKD2 ionic channels. RNAi experiments on *BBS7* and *BBS9* cause cilia loss or reduction of length (Valentine et al. 2012).

Historically, the example of the biflagellate alga *Chlamydomonas Reinardtii* in which the *Ift88* mutant showed no flagella is famous because it enabled the link with the *Ift88^{orpk}* mouse model that disclosed polycystic kidney (and also RD). This was a starting point to understand the role of cilia in human diseases (Pazour et al. 2000). *C. reinardtii* represents an invaluable source of functional and validation information for ciliopathy genes (Sánchez-Bellver et al. 2021). Especially for IFT, which is a conserved bidirectional mechanism in eukaryotic motile and nonmotile cilia, ensuring the molecular turnover of ciliary-related proteins contributing to the understanding of the identical PR ciliary gate actors (Khanna 2015). For example, the BBSome interactions with IFT proteins has been demonstrated for export of signaling proteins from the flagella (Lechtreck et al. 2009), suggesting that the BBSome is an adaptor to the IFT machinery. In addition, the exit of signaling proteins to the IS has also been demonstrated with BBS3 (ARL6/GTPase) for the signaling protein phospholipase D via the BBsome, suggesting regulatory mechanism for ciliary signaling protein removal out of cilia (Liu et al. 2021). The same stands for other BBS genes (Fauser et al. 2022) like *LZTFL1* for which *C. reinardtii* helped to model the BBSome recruitment at the basal body and its reassembly at the basal tip (Sun et al. 2021).

Trypanosoma brucei (the agent for sleeping sickness) has flagella important for virulence. KO of *BBS1*, *BBS4*, *BBS5*, *BBS6*, and *BBS9* does not show structural anomalies but presents a loss of virulence due to abnormal surface proteins modifying host–parasite interactions supporting a model, whereby the BBSome function is implied in postendocytic sorting of select surface proteins (Langousis et al. 2016).

Caenorhabditis elegans is characterized by sensory (nonmotile) cilia of the cephalic neurons. *Bbs C. elegans* mutants have shorter cilia and other dysfunctions implying functional sensory de-

fects. *Bbs* mutants have abnormal IFT A/B interactions; this model also contributed to dissect mechanisms such as showing that BBSome associated with the Bbs3 ARL6/small GTPase connects the complex to the ciliary via interactions with Bbs1 at the membrane (Hao et al. 2011) or that *Bbs8* mutants have defective endocytosis trafficking (Kaplan et al. 2012).

Drosophila melanogaster have a specific BBSome compared to the mammalian one. Their comparison is an interesting example of how evolutionary observations on conservation (or nonconservation) of subsets of proteins can help to disentangle the roles of each BBSome component in its assembly. *D. melanogaster* lacks BBS2 and BBS7 (but expresses ARL6/BBS3), whereas mouse models *Bbs2$^{-/-}$* and *Bbs7$^{-/-}$* are described as less severe on the PR phenotype than others raising the hypothesis of alleviated phenotypes linked to more "recent" BBS proteins (Chou et al. 2019; Chandra et al. 2022).

Vertebrate Models

Understanding ciliary defects leading to nonocular manifestations and RD requires modeling (including for PR) in vertebrates where all BBS genes are conserved. In vertebrates, ciliogenesis occurs once the progenitor has escaped the cell cycle and differentiates (Sánchez-Bellver et al. 2021). Most ciliary proteins have been shown to be located in the various compartments of the PR cells (basal body, periciliary membrane, CC, axoneme, OS, IS). In the PR, BBS proteins mostly locate at the basal body, noticeably the BBSome, and some are also found at the CC (i.e., BBS1, BBS8, BBS9) (Sánchez-Bellver et al. 2021).

Zebrafish Models for RD Studies in BBS and Related Ciliopathies

Zebrafish present many advantages with rapid development, high fecundity, transparent embryos, and a high level of human orthologs (82% of OMIM genes) including for ciliary proteins. Developing externally, embryos carry cilia in almost all cell types with similarities with human anatomy (Song et al. 2016). Zebrafish models could be obtained by a large-scale mutagenesis screen,

Cite this article as *Cold Spring Harb Perspect Med* doi: 10.1101/cshperspect.a041303

Talen, CRISPR/Cas9 editing, or Morpholino KO. Different techniques for a same gene may induce discrepancies in the results. As an example, CEP290 morphants can disclose phenotypes not reproduced with editing approaches (Song et al. 2016). Zebrafish have been extensively used to model ciliopathies for gene validation as well as for studying modifiers and genetic interactions (Tayeh et al. 2008; Davis et al. 2014).

The zebrafish retina is well laminated. An eye shape occurs at 11.5 hours postfertilization (hpf), a characteristic subcellular structure appears at 48 hpf, the presence of an internal connecting cilia and basal body with an IS is observed at 50 hpf, an OS is seen at 54 hpf, and the first visual response is detected at 70 hpf (Shi et al. 2017). Zebrafish is an ideal model to study IRDs, their retina is cone rich and this model has the ability to regenerate damaged neural cells including retina after injury by way of Müller cells (Perkins 2022).

Bbs protein-deficient zebrafish models display aberrant localization of rhodopsin to the IS, OS disorganization, and progressive PR degeneration (Perkins 2022). Morpholino suppression of *bbs2*, *bbs4*, *bbs5*, *bbs6*, *bbs7*, or *bbs*8 show shortening of the motile cilia in the Kupffer's vesicle with left–right patterning defects associated with reduction of retrograde transport of melanosomes of the skin (Yen et al. 2006). KO of bbs genes results in expansion of the sonic hedgehog expression resulting in fin bud abnormal patterning reminiscent of the patient polydactyly (Tayeh et al. 2008).

CRISPR/Cas9 editing targeting exon 4 of *bbs2* morphant showed impaired optokinetic response at day 5–6 days postfertilization (dpf). Transmission electron microscopy (TEM) discloses shorter cone OS in larval fish, whereas in the adult fish mislocalization of rhodopsin was observed mostly in cones leading to degeneration (Song et al. 2020). Accumulation of Stx3 (SNARE protein syntaxine-3) in the OS is in line with the OS featured as a "sink" for membrane proteins (Seo and Datta 2017) pointing to the role of BBSome in the protein exit of the OS via ciliary cargo. The rather slow degeneration process for *bbs* genes, compared to other ciliary genes, was observed and compared to similar differences in mice and human. Interest-

ingly, the PR regeneration (by way of multipotent neurogenic precursors) appeared in *bbs2* morphants after light damage (but not spontaneously without a trigger) (Song et al. 2020).

A CRISPR/Cas9 *bbs1* mutant has been generated and despite normal lamination and morphology, mutants showed impaired vision at 5 dpf with decreased electroretinogram (ERG) response on the B-wave. At 10 dpf, OS disorganization appeared with twisted and titled discs followed by an increase of the cone apoptosis. Alteration of lipid homeostasis of the OS was present and is in line with the role of BBSome as mediating retrograde transport to remove non-OS resident proteins (Masek et al. 2022).

Zebrafish have also been used to study the NPHP, SLSN, JBTS, and MKS modules. For instance, cc2d2a$^{-/-}$ zebrafish PR disclosed cilium-specific vesicle fusion defects resulting in opsin accumulation, a phenotype that could be opposed to the corresponding KO mice model, which presents mostly ciliogenesis defects (Naharros et al. 2017). *Ahi* zebrafish mutants show a JBTS phenotype with disrupted cone OS with unaltered axonemal structures, important vesiculation at the CC with massive OS disorganization with rhodopsin mislocalization (Lessieur et al. 2019).

Mouse Models for RD in BBS and Related Ciliopathies

More than 230 mouse models are known to recapitulate IRDs (Collin et al. 2020). They are spontaneous models (naturally occurring) or induced ones obtained by chemical induction (ENU) or genetically modified mostly by genetic engineering approaches (>70%). Ciliary function and trafficking defects represent, by far, the largest group of mice models described to date for RDs (Collin et al. 2020). Overall, key ciliary structures or processes that can be studied in mouse models are the following: ciliogenesis, OS morphogenesis, and PR homeostasis.

BBS protein expression increases after birth with a peak at postnatal day P15–16 when PRs terminate differentiation and disclose still low retinal function (Hsu et al. 2017). Compared to most ciliary mouse models, the disruption of the BBSome complex (observed for *Bbs1*, *Bbs2*,

Arl6/Bbs3, Bbs4, Bbs7, Ttc8/Bbs8, and *Bbip1/Bbs18*) and associated chaperones/regulators (*Bbs10, Bbs12,* and *Lztfl1/Bbs17*) lead to a quite moderate RD. Indeed, eye phenotype of Bbs knockout (KO) PR degeneration compared to other ciliary genes overall shows slower delay and lack of ciliogenesis defects suggesting functional redundancy among BBSome components. On the contrary, other genes (non-BBS) implied in the ciliary gate function of the connecting ciliary transition zone cause much more rapid RD (i.e., *Nphp1, Nphp4, Ahi1, Iqcb1, Tmeme67, Cep290,* and *Ift88*) with most PR eliminated by 3 to 4 weeks of age.

However, very high levels of variability occur by comparing different Bbs KO such as, for instance, slow degeneration in *Bbs5* KO mice compared to *Bbs8* KO models, even if *Bbs3* KO is the most severe. $Bbs4^{-/-}$, $Bbs8^{-/-}$, and $Bbs1^{M390R/M390R}$ mice have OS morphogenesis defects at an age preceding PR degeneration at P15–P16. Hsu et al. (2017) have shown that, with a similar genetic background, the rate of RD was different with the most severe being $Bbs3^{-/-}$ followed by $Bbs4^{-/-}$ and $Bbs8^{-/-}$ and with the slowest being $Bbs2^{-/-}$ and $Bbs7^{-/-}$. For *Bbs4* KO, the PR degeneration occurs after maturation with 90% of loss after 7 mo of age. In the $Bbs8^{-/-}$ model, RPE delayed maturation was observed before the PR maturation defects (Hsu et al. 2017) as also observed for RPE cells derived from iPSCs (induced pluripotent stem cells) in ciliopathy patients (May-Simera et al. 2018). Cones and rods are independently affected in BBS mouse models (Dilan et al. 2018).

$Bbs10^{-/-}$, $Bbs1^{M390R/M390R}$, and *CEP290*-mediated LCA mouse models exhibit perinatal RD with rhodopsin mislocalization in the PR and has been shown to induce an ER stress in the IS (Brun et al. 2019). Arrestin mislocalization in IS and OS has been observed in $Bbs5^{-/-}$ mice as Bbs5 is directly involved in arrestin translocation (Smith et al. 2013).

Ciliopathy mouse models (including Bbs) disclose various ciliopathy manifestations including obesity, renal defects, and RD, among others and have been observed in a plethora of Bbs mouse models since 2004: *Bbs1* (Kulaga et al. 2004), $Bbs1^{M390R}$ knockin mouse (Davis et al. 2007), *Bbs1* (Nishimura et al. 2004), *Bbs3* (Zhang et al. 2011), and *Bbs4* (Mykytyn et al. 2004; Eichers et al. 2006). For a summary of the ocular and extraocular manifestations occurring in Bbs mouse models reported to date, details can be found in Table 1. $Bbs^{-/-}$ mutant mice and $Bbs1^{M390R/M390R}$ recapitulate the phenotype of BBS including obesity, blindness, and sperm flagella shortening, but polydactyly and obvious kidney cysts are not observed.

An *Lztlf1* null mouse mutant has shown RD with mislocalization and accumulation of non-OS proteins in the OS and also loss of compartmentalization (as opposed to a defect of import) pointing to the BBsome as a gatekeeper (Datta et al. 2015).

Overall, Bbsome mouse models have enabled better understanding of the PR degeneration features. Bbsome is required for the protein trafficking in the primary cilia OS well known as a specific compartment that requires high directional IS to OS flux for OS renewal. The OS is considered as a "sink" for membrane protein that retrieved proteins that are in the OS to the IS such as Stx3. Aberrant accumulation of Stx3 in the OS has been observed in $Bbs8^{-/-}$, $Bbs4^{-/-}$, and $Bbs1^{M90R/M390R}$ mice during OS formation but also after (Hsu et al. 2017; Dilan et al. 2018). The mouse models $Bbs8^{gt/gt}$; Flp$^+$ with a restoration of Bbs8 expression at P15 (corresponding to a 1-year-old human being) is able to rescue the PR degeneration. Evaluating future therapeutic windows is still a challenge. Comparing various Bbs KO mice differences in rates of RD and visual function differences were observed for *Bbs5, Bbs6,* and *Bbs8* KOs (Kretschmer et al. 2019). $Bbs8^{-/-}$ mouse showed the fastest PR degeneration (blind at 6 mo of age) with loss of cone function at P25, whereas $Bbs5^{-/-}$ (also a Bbsome component) showed very little degeneration (relatively normal responses by 10 mo of age). $Bbs6^{-/-}$ mice (a chaperonin protein) showed a moderate rate of degeneration involving cones and rods. Redundancy and compensation on the one hand and nonoverlapping functions on the other hand are keys in understanding the phenotypic differences that remain to be fully understood.

Bbsome mouse models have been investigated to understand tissue-/cell-specific recruitment and regulation by which subcomplexes

Cite this article as *Cold Spring Harb Perspect Med* doi: 10.1101/cshperspect.a041303

Table 1. Phenotypes of Bbs mouse models reported since 2004

Bbs gene	Number of mouse strains	Type of gene defect	Embryonic lethality	Mutagenesis	Retinopathy[a]			Obesity	Renal defects	Polydactyly	Male infertility	Neuronal defect	References
					Retinal layer thickness	ERG response decrease	Rhodopsin mislocalization						
Bbs1	2	1 KO, 1 KI (M390R)	−(2/2)	HR	+(2/2)	+(2/2)	+(2/2)	+(2/2)	−(2/2)	−(2/2)	+(2/2)	+(1/2) NA (1/2)	Kulaga et al. 2004; Davis et al. 2007
Bbs2	1	KO	−	HR	+	+	+	+	+	−	+	NA	Nishimura et al. 2004
Bbs3/Arl6	2	2 KO	−(2/2)	HR	−(2/2)	NA (2/2)	NA (2/2)	−(2/2)	+(2/2)	NA (2/2)	+(2/2)	+(2/2)	Pretorius et al. 2011; Zhang et al. 2011
Bbs4	5	4 KO, 1 hypomorph	−(5/5)	HR	+(3/5) NA (2/5)	+(2/5) NA (3/5)	+(1/5) NA (4/5)	+(3/5) −(2/5)	NA (5/5)	−(1/5) NA (4/5)	+(3/5) NA (2/5)	+(1/5) NA (4/5)	Kulaga et al. 2004; Mykytyn et al. 2004; Eichers et al. 2006; Simons et al. 2011; Tsyklauri et al. 2021
Bbs5	4	3 KO, 1 conditional	−(4/4)	HR	+(2/4) NA (2/4)	+(2/4) NA (2/4)	+(1/4) NA (3/4)	+(1/4) −(1/4) NA (2/4)	+(2/4) NA (2/4)	NA 4/4	+(1/4) −(1/4) NA (2/4)	+(1/4) NA (3/4)	Kretschmer et al. 2019; Bales et al. 2020; Bentley-Ford et al. 2021
Bbs6/Mkks	2	2 KO	−(2/2)	HR	+(2/2)	+(1/2) NA (1/2)	+(2/2)	+(1/2) NA (1/2)	NA (2/2)	−(1/2) NA (1/2)	−(1/2) NA (1/2)	NA (2/2)	Fath et al. 2005; Ross et al. 2005; Kretschmer et al. 2019
Bbs7	1	KO	−	HR	+	NA	NA	+	−	−	+	+	Zhang et al. 2013
Bbs8/Ttc8	5	2 KO, 1 retina-specific KO, 2 conditional	−(5/5)	HR	+(5/5)	+(5/5)	+(1/5) NA (4/5)	+(1/5) NA (4/5)	+(1/5) NA (4/5)	− NA (5/5)	+ NA	+ NA	Tadenev et al. 2011; Hsu et al. 2017; Dilan et al. 2018; Kretschmer et al. 2019
Bbs10	1	KO	−	HR	+	+	+	+	−	NA	NA	NA	Cognard et al. 2015; Brun et al. 2019
Bbs12	1	KO	−	HR	+	+	NA	+	−	NA	NA	NA	Marion et al. 2012; Mockel et al. 2012
Bbs16/Sdccag8	3	2 hypomorph, 1 KO	−(2/3 died after birth)	HR	+(1/3) NA (2/3)	+(1/3) NA (2/3)	NA (3/3)	NA (3/3)	+(1/3) NA (2/3)	+(3/3)	NA (3/3)	+(2/3) NA (1/3)	Airik et al. 2014; Insolera et al. 2014; Weihbrecht et al. 2018
Bbs17/Lztfl1	2	2 KO	−(2/2)	HR	+(2/2)	+(1/2) NA (1/2)	+(1/2) −(1/2)	+(2/2)	−(2/2)	NA (2/2)	NA (2/2)	+(1/2) NA (1/2)	Datta et al. 2015; Jiang et al. 2016
Bbs18/Bbip1	1	1	−(pre-weaning lethality)	CRISPR/Cas9	NA	NA	NA	NA	NA	NA	NA	NA	Tsyklauri et al. 2021

Continued

Table 1. *Continued*

Bbs gene	Number of mouse strains	Type of gene defect	Embryonic lethality	Mutagenesis	Retinopathy[a] Retinal layer thickness	ERG response decrease	Rhodopsin mislocalization	Obesity	Renal defects	Polydactyly	Male infertility	Neuronal defect	References
Bbs19/ Ift27	2	1 KO, 1 germ cell–specific KO	−(1/2 died after birth)	HR	NA 2/2	NA 2/2	NA 2/2	NA 2/2	NA 2/2	+(1/2) NA (1/2)	−(1/2) NA (1/2)	+(1/2) NA (1/2)	Eguether et al. 2014; Zhang et al. 2017
Bbs20/ Ift172	5	3 KO, 1 developing limb-specific KO, 1 rod-specific KO	−(2/5) +(3/5)	1 ENU, 4 HR	+(1/5) NA (4/5)	+(1/5) NA (4/5)	+(1/5) NA (4/5)	NA (5/5)	NA (5/5)	+(2/5) NA (3/5)	NA (5/5)	+(2/5) NA (3/5)	Huangfu et al. 2003; Gorivodsky et al. 2009; Howard et al. 2010; Gupta et al. 2018
Bbs21/ C8orf37	3	3 KO	−	CRISPR/Cas9	+(1/3) NA (2/3)	+(3/3)	−(1/3) NA (2/3)	−(3/3)	−(3/3)	−(3/3)	−(3/3)	NA (3/3)	Sharif et al. 2018
Bbs22/ Ift74	1	1 germ cell–specific KO	−	HR	NA	NA	NA	NA	NA	NA	−	NA	Shi et al. 2019

Each line corresponds to a Bbs gene. Each column mentions the name of the gene, the total number of mouse model lineages, the targeted gene defect, the possible embryonic lethality, and the creation method, respectively. The other columns report the number of models disclosing a given phenotype as compared to the total number of models (e.g., 2/4). (HR) Homologous recombination, (KO) knockout model, (KI) knockin model, (ENU) ethylnitrosourea induced, (+) phenotype present, (−) phenotype absent, (NA) data not available.

[a]The retinopathy phenotype encompasses "retinal layer thickness, ERG response decrease, and rhodopsin mislocalization."

remain efficient in PR compared to other generic cell carriers of a primary cilia. A Bbsome subcomplex containing Bbs1, Bbs5, Bbs8, and Bbs9 can enter the PR cilia in absence of Bbs2 or Bbs7, whereas another Bbsome subcomplex containing Bbs1, Bbs2, Bbs5, Bbs7, and Bbs9 in the absence of Bbs8 is unable to enter the cilia in PR (independent of the presence of Bbs3/Arl6). This result is not generalizable to the primary cilia of other cell types showing that the ciliary protein selection by the BBSome is tissue specific (Hsu et al. 2021). Using Bbs mouse models including conditional $Bbs8^{\text{floxed/floxed}}$, showed that the lack of Bbsome function also negatively impacts retinal synaptogenesis with horizontal cells defects (Hsu et al. 2020).

By investigating other ciliopathy genes, interactions with Bbs genes have been shown. For instance, a study based on double-mutant mice of an allele of the MKS complex protein Mks1 and the Bbsome protein Bbs4 highlights interactions between the Mks transition zone complex and the Bbsome-mediating traffic of specific transmembrane receptors to the cilium. Moreover, the genetic interaction of Mks1 with components of IFT machinery suggests that the transition zone complex facilitates IFT to promote cilium assembly and structure (Goetz et al. 2017). $Nphp5^{-/-}$ mice PR do not fully develop; there is no OS at 1 mo and mislocalization of Bbs2 and Bbs8 inducing a dysfunctional Bbsome. As a point of interest, the $Nphp5^{-/-}$ mice as the $Nphp1^{-/-}$, $Nphp4^{-/-}$, and $Nphp6^{-/-}$ models only develop a retinal phenotype, whereas no kidney involvement was observed (Barbelanne et al. 2015; Ronquillo et al. 2016).

Large Animal Models: Dog Models

Canine progressive retinal atrophy (PRA) is the equivalent of IRDs in humans and linked to PR cell death with vast genetic heterogeneity. Whole exome and whole genome sequencing progress has facilitated gene identification (Bunel et al. 2019). To date, three natural dog models have been reported for BBS:BBS2 (Hitti-Malin et al. 2021), BBS4 (Chew et al. 2017), and BBS8/TTC8 (Downs et al. 2014; Mäkeläinen et al. 2020).

In the Golden Retriever dog, PRA has been found to be due to 1-bp deletion in *BBS8/TTC8* equivalent to human *BBS8* (Downs et al. 2014). Obesity, renal anomalies, sperm defects, and olfactory defect have been reported more recently (Mäkeläinen et al. 2020).

In the Hungarian Puli dog, a nonsense single-nucleotide variant (SNV) in *BBS4* causes a syndromic PRA (Chew et al. 2017), with phenotypes comparable to a $Bbs4^{-/-}$ mice model (Mykytyn et al. 2004) with spermatozoa flagella defects and obesity.

PRA occurs naturally in the Shetland sheepdog and is due to an SNV in exon 11 of *BBS2*. The RD was diagnosed quite late (6 yr) and was associated with excess weight and a voracious appetite as well some kidney issues and dysmorphic features (upturned nose, abnormal coat, dental anomalies) (Hitti-Malin et al. 2021).

These large animal models are highly valuable for pathogenesis investigations and for therapy approaches, on preclinical grounds, to study how to alleviate symptoms, especially at the level of visual impairment.

Nonhuman Primate Models

Nonhuman primate models are invaluable large animal models with a high value when it comes to preclinical testing of various therapeutic approaches but only very few have been identified as naturally occurring models (Neff 2020). Two siblings in a lineage of Rhesus macaques were found to have RD and kidney failure. Their genome sequencing revealed a frameshift variant in *BBS7*. A third younger case (3.5 yr) showed less advanced disease with RD confirmed by ERG with markedly reduced A- and B-waves (Peterson et al. 2019). In vivo imaging of the two older macaques showed severe macular degeneration with absence of PR layers. The histological investigations (at 4 and 6 yr) showed mainly broad loss of PR and inner retinal layers. No polydactyly or obesity was observed in contrast to *BBS7* patients who, however, disclose the same type of cone-rod RD also identical to the mouse model (Aleman et al. 2021).

Human Cell Models

To fully address the question of modeling, we cite here progress made with patient cells. Modeling of ciliopathies with patient-derived cellular models is surging due to recent technical advances permitting generation of 2D and 3D cellular models. Most commonly, the cells are derived from patient fibroblasts, but other cell sources exist as, for instance, urinary cells (URECS) (Ajzenberg et al. 2015; Ziegler et al. 2022). CRISPR/Cas9 editing is a very useful tool to generate or correct variants. These cellular models, derived from the patients themselves, are enabling better pathogenesis understanding, therapy generation (molecule screening), testing of various approaches, and, finally, can open up the path to regenerative medicine (Pollara et al. 2022). As far as BBS is concerned, fibroblast-derived iPSC for *BBS1*, *BBS10*, and *BBS2* have been generated. *BBS10* and *BBS1* iPSC showed neural crest cell expression profile defects (Barrell et al. 2019), deregulation of neurodevelopmental genes (Barabino et al. 2020), and neuronal function (Wang et al. 2021). With the same assays, the importance of BBS in ciliogenesis and hedgehog signaling for *BBS1*, *BBS10*, and BBS5 was disclosed (Hey et al. 2021). *BBS2* iPSC models have been used to test translational readthrough approaches (Eintracht et al. 2021).

MODELS AND THERAPY APPROACHES

Bbs mouse models have been used to address preclinical assays for various therapeutic approaches to alleviate the RD. Undoubtedly, other approaches, in addition to those cited herein (gene replacement and pharmacological therapies), can be considered such as gene editing or AOs (antisense oligonucleotides). They have already been used in other ciliary-related RD (Kim and Kim 2019); herein we cite only the ones relevant to BBS.

For gene-replacement therapy, AAV2/5-*Bbs1* subretinal gene therapy was applied to the $Bbs1^{M390R/M390R}$ mouse model showing improved ERG as well as improved rhodopsin localization. However, AAV-*Bbs1* applied to WT mice showed retinal toxicity (Seo et al. 2013). In another study, $Bbs4^{-/-}$ mice were crossed with transgenic mice carrying Bbs4 tagged with a lap tag under the control of a β-actin promoter. Rescue of various phenotypic traits such as obesity, male fertility, and RD were thus observed (Chamling et al. 2013). Subretinal injection of AAV5-*Bbs4* in $Bbs4^{-/-}$ mice rescued the rhodopsin mislocalization and ERG response (Simons et al. 2011).

Pharmacological treatment has also been investigated in Bbs mouse models (Duong Phu et al. 2021). In $Bbs12^{-/-}$, pharmacological modulation of retinal unfolded protein response by administering a combination of valproic acid, Guanabenz, and a specific caspase-12 inhibitor achieved efficient PR protection (Mockel et al. 2012). Tauroursodeoxycholic acid (TUDCA) was shown to improve vision in $Bbs1^{M390R/M390R}$ with subcutaneous injections (Drack et al. 2012). More recently, a $Bbs2^{-/-}$ mouse model disclosed monosialodihexosylganglioside accumulating in cilia, indicating impairment of glycosphingolipid (GSL) metabolism in BBS. On this basis, glucosylceramide synthase inhibitor Genz-667161 with per os administration showed global improvement with obesity, liver function, olfaction, and RD by increasing the thickness of the outer nuclear layer (Husson et al. 2020).

CONCLUSIONS

BBS in vivo models have indisputably contributed to better understanding of the pathogenesis underlying PR degeneration (and other tissues). Various models such as *Chlamydomonas reinhardtii*, zebrafish, mouse model studies, and edited cells can converge toward an explanation of the triggers underlying defects in BBSome in the PR with the OS "sink" concept in which membrane proteins are unable to return back to the IS and/or the accumulation of proteins in the IS. The overall integration of the ciliopathy models will enable understanding of variability, phenotype–genotype correlations, and, most importantly, to unveil robust therapeutic approaches still lacking to prevent visual loss in patients.

REFERENCES

Airik R, Slaats GG, Guo Z, Weiss AC, Khan N, Ghosh A, Hurd TW, Bekker-Jensen S, Schrøder JM, Elledge SJ, et al.

2014. Renal-retinal ciliopathy gene *Sdccag8* regulates DNA damage response signaling. *J Am Soc Nephrol* **25**: 2573–2583. doi:10.1681/ASN.2013050565

Ajzenberg H, Slaats GG, Stokman MF, Arts HH, Logister I, Kroes HY, Renkema KY, van Haelst MM, Terhal PA, van Rooij IA, et al. 2015. Non-invasive sources of cells with primary cilia from pediatric and adult patients. *Cilia* **4**: 8. doi:10.1186/s13630-015-0017-x

Aleman TS, O'Neil EC, O'Connor K, Jiang YY, Aleman IA, Bennett J, Morgan JIW, Toussaint BW. 2021. Bardet–Biedl syndrome-7 (*BBS7*) shows treatment potential and a cone-rod dystrophy phenotype that recapitulates the non-human primate model. *Ophthalmic Genet* **42**: 252–265. doi:10.1080/13816810.2021.1888132

Álvarez-Satta M, Castro-Sánchez S, Valverde D. 2017. Bardet–Biedl syndrome as a chaperonopathy: dissecting the major role of chaperonin-like BBS proteins (BBS6-BBS10-BBS12). *Front Mol Biosci* **4**: 55. doi:10.3389/fmolb.2017.00055

Azari AA, Aleman TS, Cideciyan AV, Schwartz SB, Windsor EAM, Sumaroka A, Cheung AY, Steinberg JD, Roman AJ, Stone EM, et al. 2006. Retinal disease expression in Bardet–Biedl syndrome-1 (*BBS1*) is a spectrum from maculopathy to retina-wide degeneration. *Invest Ophthalmol Vis Sci* **47**: 5004–5010. doi:10.1167/iovs.06-0517

Bachmann-Gagescu R, Dempsey JC, Phelps IG, O'Roak BJ, Knutzen DM, Rue TC, Ishak GE, Isabella CR, Gorden N, Adkins J, et al. 2015. Joubert syndrome: a model for untangling recessive disorders with extreme genetic heterogeneity. *J Med Genet* **52**: 514–522. doi:10.1136/jmedgenet-2015-103087

Bachmann-Gagescu R, Dempsey JC, Bulgheroni S, Chen ML, D'Arrigo S, Glass IA, Heller T, Héon E, Hildebrandt F, Joshi N, et al. 2020. Healthcare recommendations for Joubert syndrome. *Am J Med Genet A* **182**: 229–249. doi:10.1002/ajmg.a.61399

Bales KL, Bentley MR, Croyle MJ, Kesterson RA, Yoder BK, Gross AK. 2020. BBSome component BBS5 is required for cone photoreceptor protein trafficking and outer segment maintenance. *Invest Ophthalmol Vis Sci* **61**: 17. doi:10.1167/iovs.61.10.17

Barabino A, Flamier A, Hanna R, Héon E, Freedman BS, Bernier G. 2020. Deregulation of neuro-developmental genes and primary cilium cytoskeleton anomalies in iPSC retinal sheets from human syndromic ciliopathies. *Stem Cell Reports* **14**: 357–373. doi:10.1016/j.stemcr.2020.02.005

Barbelanne M, Hossain D, Chan DP, Peränen J, Tsang WY. 2015. Nephrocystin proteins NPHP5 and Cep290 regulate BBSome integrity, ciliary trafficking and cargo delivery. *Hum Mol Genet* **24**: 2185–2200. doi:10.1093/hmg/ddu738

Barrell WB, Griffin JN, Harvey JL, Danovi D, Beales P, Grigoriadis AE, Liu KJ. 2019. Induction of neural crest stem cells from Bardet–Biedl syndrome patient derived hiPSCs. *Front Mol Neurosci* **12**: 139. doi:10.3389/fnmol.2019.00139

Beales PL, Badano JL, Ross AJ, Ansley SJ, Hoskins BE, Kirsten B, Mein CA, Froguel P, Scambler PJ, Lewis RA, et al. 2003. Genetic interaction of BBS1 mutations with alleles at other BBS loci can result in non-Mendelian Bar-

det–Biedl syndrome. *Am J Hum Genet* **72**: 1187–1199. doi:10.1086/375178

Bengueddach H, Lemullois M, Aubusson-Fleury A, Koll F. 2017. Basal body positioning and anchoring in the multiciliated cell *Paramecium tetraurelia*: roles of OFD1 and VFL3. *Cilia* **6**: 6. doi:10.1186/s13630-017-0050-z

Bentley-Ford MR, Engle SE, Clearman KR, Haycraft CJ, Andersen RS, Croyle MJ, Rains AB, Berbari NF, Yoder BK. 2021. A mouse model of BBS identifies developmental and homeostatic effects of BBS5 mutation and identifies novel pituitary abnormalities. *Hum Molec Genet* **30**: 234–246. doi:10.1093/hmg/ddab039

Berger W, Kloeckener-Gruissem B, Neidhardt J. 2010. The molecular basis of human retinal and vitreoretinal diseases. *Prog Retin Eye Res* **29**: 335–375. doi:10.1016/j.preteyeres.2010.03.004

Besharse JC. 1986. Photosensitive membrane turnover: differentiated membrane domains and cell-cell interaction. In *The retina: a model for cell biological studies* (ed. Adler R, Farber D), pp. 297–352. Academic Press, Orlando, FL. doi:10.1016/B978-0-12-044275-1.50014-4

Bessant DAR, Ali RR, Bhattacharya SS. 2001. Molecular genetics and prospects for therapy of the inherited retinal dystrophies. *Curr Opin Genet Dev* **11**: 307–316. doi:10.1016/S0959-437X(00)00195-7

Brun A, Yu X, Obringer C, Ajoy D, Haser E, Stoetzel C, Roux MJ, Messaddeq N, Dollfus H, Marion V. 2019. In vivo phenotypic and molecular characterization of retinal degeneration in mouse models of three ciliopathies. *Exp Eye Res* **186**: 107721. doi:10.1016/j.exer.2019.107721

Bunel M, Chaudieu G, Hamel C, Lagoutte L, Manes G, Botherel N, Brabet P, Pilorge P, André C, Quignon P. 2019. Natural models for retinitis pigmentosa: progressive retinal atrophy in dog breeds. *Hum Genet* **138**: 441–453. doi:10.1007/s00439-019-01999-6

Chamling X, Seo S, Bugge K, Searby C, Guo DF, Drack AV, Rahmouni K, Sheffield VC. 2013. Ectopic expression of human BBS4 can rescue Bardet–Biedl syndrome phenotypes in Bbs4 null mice. *PLoS ONE* **8**: e59101. doi:10.1371/journal.pone.0059101

Chandra B, Tung ML, Hsu Y, Scheetz T, Sheffield VC. 2022. Retinal ciliopathies through the lens of Bardet–Biedl syndrome: past, present and future. *Prog Retin Eye Res* **89**: 101035. doi:10.1016/j.preteyeres.2021.101035

Chen X, Sheng X, Liu Y, Li Z, Sun X, Jiang C, Qi R, Yuan S, Wang X, Zhou G, et al. 2018. Distinct mutations with different inheritance mode caused similar retinal dystrophies in one family: a demonstration of the importance of genetic annotations in complicated pedigrees. *J Transl Med* **16**: 145. doi:10.1186/s12967-018-1522-7

Chen HY, Welby E, Li T, Swaroop A. 2019. Retinal disease in ciliopathies: recent advances with a focus on stem cell-based therapies. *Transl Sci Rare Dis* **4**: 97–115. doi:10.3233/TRD-190038

Chen HY, Kelley RA, Li T, Swaroop A. 2021. Primary cilia biogenesis and associated retinal ciliopathies. *Semin Cell Dev Biol* **110**: 70–88. doi:10.1016/j.semcdb.2020.07.013

Chew T, Haase B, Bathgate R, Willet CE, Kaukonen MK, Mascord LJ, Lohi HT, Wade CM. 2017. A coding variant in the gene Bardet–Biedl syndrome 4 (BBS4) is associated with a novel form of canine progressive retinal atrophy. *G3 (Bethesda)* **7**: 2327–2335. doi:10.1534/g3.117.043109

Chou HT, Apelt L, Farrell DP, White SR, Woodsmith J, Svetlov V, Goldstein JS, Nager AR, Li Z, Muller J, et al. 2019. The molecular architecture of native BBSome obtained by an integrated structural approach. *Structure* 27: 1384–1394.e4. doi:10.1016/j.str.2019.06.006

Cognard N, Scerbo MJ, Obringer C, Yu X, Costa F, Haser E, Le D, Stoetzel C, Roux MJ, Moulin B, et al. 2015. Comparing the Bbs10 complete knockout phenotype with a specific renal epithelial knockout one highlights the link between renal defects and systemic inactivation in mice. *Cilia* 4: 10. doi:10.1186/s13630-015-0019-8

Collin GB, Gogna N, Chang B, Damkham N, Pinkney J, Hyde LF, Stone L, Naggert JK, Nishina PM, Krebs MP. 2020. Mouse models of inherited retinal degeneration with photoreceptor cell loss. *Cells* 9: E931. doi:10.3390/cells9040931

Datta P, Allamargot C, Hudson JS, Andersen EK, Bhattarai S, Drack AV, Sheffield VC, Seo S. 2015. Accumulation of non-outer segment proteins in the outer segment underlies photoreceptor degeneration in Bardet–Biedl syndrome. *Proc Natl Acad Sci* 112: E4400–E4409. doi:10.1073/pnas.1510111112

Davis RE, Swiderski RE, Rahmouni K, Nishimura DY, Mullins RF, Agassandian K, Philp AR, Searby CC, Andrews MP, Thompson S, et al. 2007. A knockin mouse model of the Bardet–Biedl syndrome 1 M390R mutation has cilia defects, ventriculomegaly, retinopathy, and obesity. *Proc Natl Acad Sci* 104: 19422–19427. doi:10.1073/pnas.0708571104

Davis EE, Frangakis S, Katsanis N. 2014. Interpreting human genetic variation with in vivo zebrafish assays. *Biochim Biophys Acta* 1842: 1960–1970. doi:10.1016/j.bbadis.2014.05.024

Delvallée C. 2020. "Du génome humain au modèle murin: compréhension des ciliopathies." These de doctorat, Strasbourg, France. http://www.theses.fr/2020STRAJ039

Delvallée C, Nicaise S, Antin M, Leuvrey AS, Nourisson E, Leitch CC, Kellaris G, Stoetzel C, Geoffroy V, Scheidecker S, et al. 2021. A *BBS1* SVA F retrotransposon insertion is a frequent cause of Bardet–Biedl syndrome. *Clin Genet* 99: 318–324. doi:10.1111/cge.13878

Dilan TL, Singh RK, Saravanan T, Moye A, Goldberg AFX, Stoilov P, Ramamurthy V. 2018. Bardet–Biedl syndrome-8 (BBS8) protein is crucial for the development of outer segments in photoreceptor neurons. *Hum Mol Genet* 27: 283–294. doi:10.1093/hmg/ddx399

Downs LM, Wallin-Håkansson B, Bergström T, Mellersh CS. 2014. A novel mutation in TTC8 is associated with progressive retinal atrophy in the golden retriever. *Canine Genet Epidemiol* 1: 4. doi:10.1186/2052-6687-1-4

Drack AV, Dumitrescu AV, Bhattarai S, Gratie D, Stone EM, Mullins R, Sheffield VC. 2012. TUDCA slows retinal degeneration in two different mouse models of retinitis pigmentosa and prevents obesity in Bardet–Biedl syndrome type 1 mice. *Invest Ophthalmol Vis Sci* 53: 100–106. doi:10.1167/iovs.11-8544

Duong Phu M, Bross S, Burkhalter MD, Philipp M. 2021. Limitations and opportunities in the pharmacotherapy of ciliopathies. *Pharmacol Ther* 225: 107841. doi:10.1016/j.pharmthera.2021.107841

Eichers ER, Abd-El-Barr MM, Paylor R, Lewis RA, Bi W, Lin X, Meehan TP, Stockton DW, Wu SM, Lindsay E, et al. 2006. Phenotypic characterization of Bbs4 null mice reveals age-dependent penetrance and variable expressivity. *Hum Genet* 120: 211–226. doi:10.1007/s00439-006-0197-y

Eintracht J, Forsythe E, May-Simera H, Moosajee M. 2021. Translational readthrough of ciliopathy genes BBS2 and ALMS1 restores protein, ciliogenesis and function in patient fibroblasts. *EBioMedicine* 70: 103515. doi:10.1016/j.ebiom.2021.103515

Eguether T, San Agustin JT, Keady BT, Jonassen JA, Liang Y, Francis R, Tobita K, Johnson CA, Abdelhamed ZA, Lo CW, et al. 2014. IFT27 links the BBSome to IFT for maintenance of the ciliary signaling compartment. *Dev Cell* 31: 279–290. doi:10.1016/j.devcel.2014.09.011

Estrada-Cuzcano A, Neveling K, Kohl S, Banin E, Rotenstreich Y, Sharon D, Falik-Zaccai TC, Hipp S, Roepman R, Wissinger B, et al. 2012a. Mutations in C8orf37, encoding a ciliary protein, are associated with autosomal-recessive retinal dystrophies with early macular involvement. *Am J Hum Genet* 90: 102–109. doi:10.1016/j.ajhg.2011.11.015

Estrada-Cuzcano A, Roepman R, Cremers FPM, den Hollander AI, Mans DA. 2012b. Non-syndromic retinal ciliopathies: translating gene discovery into therapy. *Hum Mol Genet* 21: R111–R124. doi:10.1093/hmg/dds298

Fadaie Z, Whelan L, Dockery A, Li CHZ, van den Born LI, Hoyng CB, Gilissen C, Corominas J, Rowlands C, et al. 2022. BBS1 branchpoint variant is associated with non-syndromic retinitis pigmentosa. *J Med Genet* 59: 438–444. doi:10.1136/jmedgenet-2020-107626

Fath MA, Mullins RF, Searby C, Nishimura DY, Wei J, Rahmouni K, Davis RE, Tayeh MK, Andrews M, Yang B, et al. 2005. Mkks-null mice have a phenotype resembling Bardet–Biedl syndrome. *Hum Mol Genet* 14: 1109–1118. doi:10.1093/hmg/ddi123

Fauser F, Vilarrasa-Blasi J, Onishi M, Ramundo S, Patena W, Millican M, Osaki J, Philp C, Nemeth M, Salomé PA, et al. 2022. Systematic characterization of gene function in the photosynthetic alga *Chlamydomonas reinhardtii*. *Nat Genet* 54: 705–714. doi:10.1038/s41588-022-01052-9

Fliegauf M, Benzing T, Omran H. 2007. When cilia go bad: cilia defects and ciliopathies. *Nat Rev Mol Cell Biol* 8: 880–893. doi:10.1038/nrm2278

Forsyth R, Gunay-Aygun M. 1993. Bardet–Biedl syndrome overview. In *GeneReviews [Internet]* (ed. Adam MP, Everman DB, Mirzaa GM, et al.). University of Washington, Seattle. https://www.ncbi.nlm.nih.gov/books/NBK1363

Forsythe E, Beales PL. 2013. Bardet–Biedl syndrome. *Eur J Hum Genet* 21: 8–13. doi:10.1038/ejhg.2012.115

Goetz SC, Anderson KV. 2010. The primary cilium: a signalling centre during vertebrate development. *Nat Rev Genet* 11: 331–344. doi:10.1038/nrg2774

Goetz SC, Bangs F, Barrington CL, Katsanis N, Anderson KV. 2017. The Meckel syndrome–associated protein MKS1 functionally interacts with components of the BBSome and IFT complexes to mediate ciliary trafficking and hedgehog signaling. *PLoS ONE* 12: e0173399. doi:10.1371/journal.pone.0173399

Gorivodsky M, Mukhopadhyay M, Wilsch-Braeuninger M, Phillips M, Teufel A, Kim C, Malik N, Huttner W, Westphal H. 2009. Intraflagellar transport protein 172 is essential for primary cilia formation and plays a vital role in

Cite this article as *Cold Spring Harb Perspect Med* doi: 10.1101/cshperspect.a041303

patterning the mammalian brain. *Dev Biol* **325:** 24–32. doi:10.1016/j.ydbio.2008.09.019

Grudzinska Pechhacker MK, Jacobson SG, Drack AV, Scipio MD, Strubbe I, Pfeifer W, Duncan JL, Dollfus H, Goetz N, Muller J, et al. 2021. Comparative natural history of visual function from patients with biallelic variants in *BBS1* and *BBS10*. *Invest Ophthalmol Vis Sci* **62:** 26. doi:10.1167/iovs .62.15.26

Gupta PR, Pendse N, Greenwald SH, Leon M, Liu Q, Pierce EA, Bujakowska KM. 2018. Ift172 conditional knock-out mice exhibit rapid retinal degeneration and protein trafficking defects. *Hum Mol Genet* **27:** 2012–2024. doi:10.1093/hmg/ddy109

Gupta S, Ozimek-Kulik JE, Phillips JK. 2021. Nephronophthisis-pathobiology and molecular pathogenesis of a rare kidney genetic disease. *Genes (Basel)* **12:** 1762. doi:10 .3390/genes12111762

Hao L, Thein M, Brust-Mascher I, Civelekoglu-Scholey G, Lu Y, Acar S, Prevo B, Shaham S, Scholey JM. 2011. Intraflagellar transport delivers tubulin isotypes to sensory cilium middle and distal segments. *Nat Cell Biol* **13:** 790–798. doi:10.1038/ncb2268

Hey CAB, Larsen LJ, Tümer Z, Brøndum-Nielsen K, Grønskov K, Hjortshøj TD, Møller LB. 2021. BBS proteins affect ciliogenesis and are essential for Hedgehog signaling, but not for formation of iPSC-derived RPE-65 expressing RPE-like cells. *Int J Mol Sci* **22:** 1345. doi:10.3390/ijms22031345

Hildebrandt F, Benzing T, Katsanis N. 2011. Ciliopathies. *N Engl J Med* **364:** 1533–1543. doi:10.1056/NEJMra 1010172

Hitti-Malin RJ, Burmeister LM, Lingaas F, Kaukonen M, Pettinen I, Lohi H, Sargan D, Mellersh CS. 2021. A missense variant in the Bardet–Biedl syndrome 2 gene (BBS2) leads to a novel syndromic retinal degeneration in the Shetland sheepdog. *Genes (Basel)* **12:** 1771. doi:10 .3390/genes12111771

Howard PW, Howard TL, Maurer RA. 2010. Generation of mice with a conditional allele for Ift172. *Transgenic Res* **19:** 121–126. doi:10.1007/s11248-009-9292-x

Huangfu D, Liu A, Rakeman AS, Murcia NS, Niswander L, Anderson KV. 2003. Hedgehog signalling in the mouse requires intraflagellar transport proteins. *Nature* **426:** 83–87. doi:10.1038/nature02061.

Hsu Y, Garrison JE, Kim G, Schmitz AR, Searby CC, Zhang Q, Datta P, Nishimura DY, Seo S, Sheffield VC. 2017. BBSome function is required for both the morphogenesis and maintenance of the photoreceptor outer segment. *PLoS Genet* **13:** e1007057. doi:10.1371/journal.pgen .1007057

Hsu Y, Garrison JE, Seo S, Sheffield VC. 2020. The absence of BBSome function decreases synaptogenesis and causes ectopic synapse formation in the retina. *Sci Rep* **10:** 8321. doi:10.1038/s41598-020-65233-4

Hsu Y, Seo S, Sheffield VC. 2021. Photoreceptor cilia, in contrast to primary cilia, grant entry to a partially assembled BBSome. *Hum Mol Genet* **30:** 87–102. doi:10.1093/ hmg/ddaa284

Husson H, Bukanov NO, Moreno S, Smith MM, Richards B, Zhu C, Picariello T, Park H, Wang B, Natoli TA, et al. 2020. Correction of cilia structure and function alleviates multi-organ pathology in Bardet–Biedl syndrome mice.

Hum Mol Genet **29:** 2508–2522. doi:10.1093/hmg/ ddaa138

Insolera R, Shao W, Airik R, Hildebrandt F, Shi S. 2014. SDCCAG8 regulates pericentriolar material recruitment and neuronal migration in the developing cortex. *Neuron* **83:** 805–822. doi:10.1016/j.neuron.2014.06.029

Jiang J, Promchan K, Jiang H, Awasthi P, Marshall H, Harned A, Natarajan V. 2016. Depletion of BBS protein LZTFL1 affects growth and causes retinal degeneration in mice. *J Genet Genomics* **43:** 381–391. doi:10.1016/j. jgg.2015.11.006

Kaplan OI, Doroquez DB, Cevik S, Bowie RV, Clarke L, Sanders AAWM, Kida K, Rappoport JZ, Sengupta P, Blacque OE. 2012. Endocytosis genes facilitate protein and membrane transport in *C. elegans* sensory cilia. *Curr Biol* **22:** 451–460. doi:10.1016/j.cub.2012.01.060

Katsanis N, Ansley SJ, Badano JL, Eichers ER, Lewis RA, Hoskins BE, Scambler PJ, Davidson WS, Beales PL, Lupski JR. 2001. Triallelic inheritance in Bardet–Biedl syndrome, a Mendelian recessive disorder. *Science* **293:** 2256–2259. doi:10.1126/science.1063525

Khanna H. 2015. Photoreceptor sensory cilium: traversing the ciliary gate. *Cells* **4:** 674–686. doi:10.3390/ cells4040674

Kim YJ, Kim J. 2019. Therapeutic perspectives for structural and functional abnormalities of cilia. *Cell Mol Life Sci* **76:** 3695–3709. doi:10.1007/s00018-019-03158-6

Klink BU, Gatsogiannis C, Hofnagel O, Wittinghofer A, Raunser S. 2020. Structure of the human BBSome core complex. *eLife* **9:** e53910. doi:10.7554/eLife.53910

Kousi M, Söylemez O, Ozanturk A, Mourtzi N, Akle S, Jungreis I, Muller J, Cassa CA, Brand H, Mokry JA, et al. 2020. Evidence for secondary-variant genetic burden and non-random distribution across biological modules in a recessive ciliopathy. *Nat Genet* **52:** 1145–1150. doi:10 .1038/s41588-020-0707-1

Kretschmer V, Patnaik SR, Kretschmer F, Chawda MM, Hernandez-Hernandez V, May-Simera HL. 2019. Progressive characterization of visual phenotype in Bardet–Biedl syndrome mutant mice. *Invest Ophthalmol Vis Sci* **60:** 1132–1143. doi:10.1167/iovs.18-25210

Kulaga HM, Leitch CC, Eichers ER, Badano JL, Lesemann A, Hoskins BE, Lupski JR, Beales PL, Reed RR, Katsanis N. 2004. Loss of BBS proteins causes anosmia in humans and defects in olfactory cilia structure and function in the mouse. *Nat Genet* **36:** 994–998. doi:10.1038/ng1418

Langousis G, Shimogawa MM, Saada EA, Vashisht AA, Spreafico R, Nager AR, Barshop WD, Nachury MV, Wohlschlegel JA, Hill KL. 2016. Loss of the BBSome perturbs endocytic trafficking and disrupts virulence of *Trypanosoma brucei*. *Proc Natl Acad Sci* **113:** 632–637. doi:10 .1073/pnas.1518079113

Lechtreck KF, Johnson EC, Sakai T, Cochran D, Ballif BA, Rush J, Pazour GJ, Ikebe M, Witman GB. 2009. The *Chlamydomonas reinhardtii* BBSome is an IFT cargo required for export of specific signaling proteins from flagella. *J Cell Biol* **187:** 1117–1132. doi:10.1083/jcb.200909183

Lessieur EM, Song P, Nivar GC, Piccillo EM, Fogerty J, Rozic R, Perkins BD. 2019. Ciliary genes arl13b, ahi1 and cc2d2a differentially modify expression of visual acuity phenotypes but do not enhance retinal degeneration due to mutation of cep290 in zebrafish. *PLoS ONE* **14:** e0213960. doi:10.1371/journal.pone.0213960

Liu YX, Xue B, Sun WY, Wingfield JL, Sun J, Wu M, Lechtreck KF, Wu Z, Fan ZC. 2021. Bardet–Biedl syndrome 3 protein promotes ciliary exit of the signaling protein phospholipase D via the BBSome. *eLife* **10:** e59119. doi:10.7554/eLife.59119

Mäkeläinen S, Hellsand M, van der Heiden AD, Andersson E, Thorsson E, Holst BS, Häggström J, Ljungvall I, Mellersh C, Hallböök F, et al. 2020. Deletion in the Bardet–Biedl syndrome gene TTC8 results in a syndromic retinal degeneration in dogs. *Genes (Basel)* **11:** 1090. doi:10.3390/genes11091090

Marion V, Mockel A, De Melo C, Obringer C, Claussmann A, Simon A, Messaddeq N, Durand M, Dupuis L, Loeffler J, et al. 2012. BBS-induced ciliary defect enhances adipogenesis, causing paradoxical higher-insulin sensitivity, glucose usage, and decreased inflammatory response. *Cell Metab* **16:** 363–377. doi:10.1016/j.cmet.2012.08.005

Masek M, Etard C, Hofmann C, Hülsmeier AJ, Zang J, Takamiya M, Gesemann M, Neuhauss SC, Hornemann T, Strähle U, et al. 2022. Loss of the Bardet–Biedl protein Bbs1 alters photoreceptor outer segment protein and lipid composition. *Nat Commun* **13:** 1282. doi:10.1038/s41467-022-28982-6

Mauring L, Porter LF, Pelletier V, Riehm A, Leuvrey AS, Gouronc A, Studer F, Stoetzel C, Dollfus H, Muller J. 2020. Atypical retinal phenotype in a patient with Alström syndrome and biallelic novel pathogenic variants in ALMS1, including a de novo variation. *Front Genet* **11:** 938. doi:10.3389/fgene.2020.00938

May-Simera HL, Wan Q, Jha BS, Hartford J, Khristov V, Dejene R, Chang J, Patnaik S, Lu Q, Banerjee P, et al. 2018. Primary cilium-mediated retinal pigment epithelium maturation is disrupted in ciliopathy patient cells. *Cell Rep* **22:** 189–205. doi:10.1016/j.celrep.2017.12.038

Mockel A, Obringer C, Hakvoort TBM, Seeliger M, Lamers WH, Stoetzel C, Dollfus H, Marion V. 2012. Pharmacological modulation of the retinal unfolded protein response in Bardet–Biedl syndrome reduces apoptosis and preserves light detection ability. *J Biol Chem* **287:** 37483–37494. doi:10.1074/jbc.M112.386821

Morleo M, Franco B. 2020. OFD type I syndrome: lessons learned from a rare ciliopathy. *Biochem Soc Trans* **48:** 1929–1939. doi:10.1042/BST20191029

Murphy D, Singh R, Kolandaivelu S, Ramamurthy V, Stoilov P. 2015. Alternative splicing shapes the phenotype of a mutation in BBS8 to cause nonsyndromic retinitis pigmentosa. *Mol Cell Biol* **35:** 1860–1870. doi:10.1128/MCB.00040-15

Mykytyn K, Nishimura DY, Searby CC, Shastri M, Yen H, Beck JS, Braun T, Streb LM, Cornier AS, Cox GF, et al. 2002. Identification of the gene (BBS1) most commonly involved in Bardet–Biedl syndrome, a complex human obesity syndrome. *Nat Genet* **31:** 435–438. doi:10.1038/ng935

Mykytyn K, Mullins RF, Andrews M, Chiang AP, Swiderski RE, Yang B, Braun T, Casavant T, Stone EM, Sheffield VC. 2004. Bardet–Biedl syndrome type 4 (BBS4)-null mice implicate Bbs4 in flagella formation but not global cilia assembly. *Proc Natl Acad Sci* **101:** 8664–8669. doi:10.1073/pnas.0402354101

Naharros IO, Gesemann M, Mateos JM, Barmettler G, Forbes A, Ziegler U, Neuhauss SCF, Bachmann-Gagescu R. 2017. Loss-of-function of the ciliopathy protein Cc2d2a disorganizes the vesicle fusion machinery at the periciliary membrane and indirectly affects Rab8-trafficking in zebrafish photoreceptors. *PLOS Genet* **13:** e1007150. doi:10.1371/journal.pgen.1007150

Nakayama K, Katoh Y. 2018. Ciliary protein trafficking mediated by IFT and BBSome complexes with the aid of kinesin-2 and dynein-2 motors. *J Biochem* **163:** 155–164. doi:10.1093/jb/mvx087

Neff EP. 2020. A natural macaque model of Bardet–Biedl appears in Oregon. *Lab Anim (NY)* **49:** 17–17. doi:10.1038/s41684-019-0449-9

Nishimura DY, Fath M, Mullins RF, Searby C, Andrews M, Davis R, Andorf JL, Mykytyn K, Swiderski RE, Yang B, et al. 2004. Bbs2-null mice have neurosensory deficits, a defect in social dominance, and retinopathy associated with mislocalization of rhodopsin. *Proc Natl Acad Sci* **101:** 16588–16593. doi:10.1073/pnas.0405496101

Pazour GJ, Dickert BL, Vucica Y, Seeley ES, Rosenbaum JL, Witman GB, Cole DG. 2000. Chlamydomonas IFT88 and its mouse homologue, polycystic kidney disease gene tg737, are required for assembly of cilia and flagella. *J Cell Biol* **151:** 709–718. doi:10.1083/jcb.151.3.709

Perkins BD. 2022. Zebrafish models of inherited retinal dystrophies. *J Transll Genet Genom* **6:** 95–110. doi:10.20517/jtgg.2021.47

Peterson SM, McGill TJ, Puthussery T, Stoddard J, Renner L, Lewis AD, Colgin LMA, Gayet J, Wang X, Prongay K, et al. 2019. Bardet–Biedl syndrome in rhesus macaques: a non-human primate model of retinitis pigmentosa. *Exp Eye Res* **189:** 107825. doi:10.1016/j.exer.2019.107825

Pollara L, Sottile V, Valente EM. 2022. Patient-derived cellular models of primary ciliopathies. *J Med Genet* **59:** 517–527. doi:10.1136/jmedgenet-2021-108315

Pretorius PR, Aldahmesh MA, Alkuraya FS, Sheffield VC, Slusarski DC. 2011. Functional analysis of BBS3 A89V that results in non-syndromic retinal degeneration. *Hum Mol Genet* **20:** 1625–1632. doi:10.1093/hmg/ddr039

Reiter JF, Leroux MR. 2017. Genes and molecular pathways underpinning ciliopathies. *Nat Rev Mol Cell Biol* **18:** 533–547. doi:10.1038/nrm.2017.60

Ronquillo CC, Hanke-Gogokhia C, Revelo MP, Frederick JM, Jiang L, Baehr W. 2016. Ciliopathy-associated IQCB1/NPHP5 protein is required for mouse photoreceptor outer segment formation. *FASEB J* **30:** 3400–3412. doi:10.1096/fj.201600511R

Ross AJ, May-Simera H, Eichers ER, Kai M, Hill J, Jagger DJ, Leitch CC, Chapple JP, Munro PM, Fisher S, et al. 2005. Disruption of Bardet–Biedl syndrome ciliary proteins perturbs planar cell polarity in vertebrates. *Nat Genet* **37:** 1135. doi:10.1038/ng1644

Sánchez-Bellver L, Toulis V, Marfany G. 2021. On the wrong track: alterations of ciliary transport in inherited retinal dystrophies. *Front Cell Dev Biol* **9:** 623734. doi:10.3389/fcell.2021.623734

Scheidecker S, Hull S, Perdomo Y, Studer F, Pelletier V, Muller J, Stoetzel C, Schaefer E, Defoort-Dhellemmes S, Drumare I, et al. 2015. Predominantly cone-system dysfunction as rare form of retinal degeneration in patients with molecularly confirmed Bardet–Biedl syndrome. *Am*

Cite this article as *Cold Spring Harb Perspect Med* doi: 10.1101/cshperspect.a041303

J Ophthalmol 160: 364–372.e1. doi:10.1016/j.ajo.2015.05 .007

Seo S, Datta P. 2017. Photoreceptor outer segment as a sink for membrane proteins: hypothesis and implications in retinal ciliopathies. *Hum Mol Genet* 26: R75–R82. doi:10 .1093/hmg/ddx163

Seo S, Mullins RF, Dumitrescu AV, Bhattarai S, Gratie D, Wang K, Stone EM, Sheffield V, Drack AV. 2013. Subretinal gene therapy of mice with Bardet–Biedl syndrome type 1. *Invest Ophthalmol Vis Sci* 54: 6118–6132. doi:10 .1167/iovs.13-11673

Sharif AS, Yu D, Loertscher S, Austin R, Nguyen K, Mathur PD, Clark AM, Zou J, Lobanova ES, Arshavsky VY, et al. 2018. C8ORF37 is required for photoreceptor outer segment disc morphogenesis by maintaining outer segment membrane protein homeostasis. *J Neurosci* 38: 3160–3176. doi:10.1523/JNEUROSCI.2964-17.2018

Shevach E, Ali M, Mizrahi-Meissonnier L, McKibbin M, El-Asrag M, Watson CM, Inglehearn CF, Ben-Yosef T, Blumenfeld A, Jalas C, et al. 2015. Association between missense mutations in the *BBS2* gene and nonsyndromic retinitis pigmentosa. *JAMA Ophthalmol* 133: 312–318. doi:10.1001/jamaophthalmol.2014.5251

Shi Y, Su Y, Lipschutz JH, Lobo GP. 2017. Zebrafish as models to study ciliopathies of the eye and kidney. *Clin Nephrol Res* 1: 6–9.

Shi L, Zhou T, Huang Q, Zhang S, Li W, Zhang L, Hess RA, Pazour GJ, Zhang Z. 2019. Intraflagellar transport protein 74 is essential for spermatogenesis and male fertility in mice. *Biol Reprod* 101: 188–199. doi:10.1093/biolre/ ioz071

Simons DL, Boye SL, Hauswirth WW, Wu SM. 2011. Gene therapy prevents photoreceptor death and preserves retinal function in a Bardet–Biedl syndrome mouse model. *Proc Natl Acad Sci* 108: 6276–6281. doi:10.1073/pnas .1019222108

Smith TS, Spitzbarth B, Li J, Dugger DR, Stern-Schneider G, Sehn E, Bolch SN, McDowell JH, Tipton J, Wolfrum U, et al. 2013. Light-dependent phosphorylation of Bardet–Biedl syndrome 5 in photoreceptor cells modulates its interaction with arrestin1. *Cell Mol Life Sci* 70: 4603–4616. doi:10.1007/s00018-013-1403-4

Snoek R, van Setten J, Keating BJ, Israni AK, Jacobson PA, Oetting WS, Matas AJ, Mannon RB, Zhang Z, Zhang W, et al. 2018. NPHP1 (nephrocystin-1) gene deletions cause adult-onset ESRD. *J Am Soc Nephrol* 29: 1772–1779. doi:10.1681/ASN.2017111200

Song D, Zhang X, Jia S, Yelick P, Zhao C. 2016. Zebrafish as a model for human ciliopathies. *J Genet Genomics* 43: 107–120. doi:10.1016/j.jgg.2016.02.001

Song P, Fogerty J, Cianciolo LT, Stupay R, Perkins BD. 2020. Cone photoreceptor degeneration and neuroinflammation in the zebrafish Bardet–Biedl syndrome 2 (bbs2) mutant does not lead to retinal regeneration. *Front Cell Dev Biol* 8: 578528. doi:10.3389/fcell.2020.578528

Sun WY, Xue B, Liu YX, Zhang RK, Li RC, Xin W, Wu M, Fan ZC. 2021. *Chlamydomonas* LZTFL1 mediates phototaxis via controlling BBSome recruitment to the basal body and its reassembly at the ciliary tip. *Proc Natl Acad Sci* 118: e2101590118. doi:10.1073/pnas.210 1590118

Tadenev ALD, Kulaga HM, May-Simera HL, Kelley MW, Katsanis N, Reed RR. 2011. Loss of Bardet-Biedl syndrome protein-8 (BBS8) perturbs olfactory function, protein localization, and axon targeting. *Proc Natl Acad Sci* 108: 10320–10325. doi:10.1073/pnas.1016531108

Tavares E, Tang CY, Vig A, Li S, Billingsley G, Sung W, Vincent A, Thiruvahindrapuram B, Héon E. 2018. Retrotransposon insertion as a novel mutational event in Bardet–Biedl syndrome. *Mol Genet Genomic Med* 7: e00521. doi:10.1002/mgg3.521

Tayeh MK, Yen HJ, Beck JS, Searby CC, Westfall TA, Griesbach H, Sheffield VC, Slusarski DC. 2008. Genetic interaction between Bardet–Biedl syndrome genes and implications for limb patterning. *Hum Mol Genet* 17: 1956–1967. doi:10.1093/hmg/ddn093

Thompson DA, Ali RR, Banin E, Branham KE, Flannery JG, Gamm DM, Hauswirth WW, Heckenlively JR, Iannaccone A, Jayasundera KT, et al. 2015. Advancing therapeutic strategies for inherited retinal degeneration: recommendations from the Monaciano symposium. *Invest Ophthalmol Vis Sci* 56: 918–931. doi:10.1167/iovs.14-16049

Tobin JL, Beales PL. 2007. Bardet–Biedl syndrome: beyond the cilium. *Pediatr Nephrol* 22: 926–936. doi:10.1007/ s00467-007-0435-0

Tsyklauri O, Niederlova V, Forsythe E, Prasai A, Drobek A, Kasparek P, Sparks K, Trachtulec Z, Prochazka J, Sedlacek R, et al. 2021. Bardet–Biedl syndrome ciliopathy is linked to altered hematopoiesis and dysregulated self-tolerance. *EMBO Rep* 22: e50785. doi:10.15252/embr.202050785

Valentine M, Van Houten J. 2021. Using paramecium as a model for ciliopathies. *Genes (Basel)* 12: 1493. doi:10 .3390/genes12101493

Valentine MS, Rajendran A, Yano J, Weeraratne SD, Beisson J, Cohen J, Koll F, Van Houten J. 2012. Paramecium BBS genes are key to presence of channels in Cilia. *Cilia* 1: 16. doi:10.1186/2046-2530-1-16

Van Dam TJP, Kennedy J, van der Lee R, de Vrieze E, Wunderlich KA, Rix S, Dougherty GW, Lambacher NJ, Li C, Jensen VL, et al. 2019. Ciliacarta: an integrated and validated compendium of ciliary genes. *PLoS ONE* 14: e0216705. doi:10.1371/journal.pone.0216705

Vasquez SSV, van Dam J, Wheway G. 2021. An updated SYSCILIA gold standard (SCGSv2) of known ciliary genes, revealing the vast progress that has been made in the cilia research field. *Mol Biol Cell* 32: br13. doi:10.1091/ mbc.E21-05-0226

Wang X, Zheng C, Liu W, Yang H. 2017. Retinitis pigmentosa and bilateral idiopathic demyelinating optic neuritis in a 6-year-old boy with OFD1 gene mutation. *Case Rep Ophthalmol Med* 2017: 5310924. doi:10.1155/2017/ 5310924

Wang L, Liu Y, Stratigopoulos G, Panigrahi S, Sui L, Zhang Y, Leduc CA, Glover HJ, De Rosa MC, Burnett LC, et al. 2021. Bardet–Biedl syndrome proteins regulate intracellular signaling and neuronal function in patient-specific iPSC-derived neurons. *J Clin Invest* 131: e146287. doi:10 .1172/JCI146287

Webb TR, Parfitt DA, Gardner JC, Martinez A, Bevilacqua D, Davidson AE, Zito I, Thiselton DL, Ressa JHC, Apergi M, et al. 2012. Deep intronic mutation in OFD1, identified by targeted genomic next-generation sequencing, causes a severe form of X-linked retinitis pigmentosa (RP23). *Hum Mol Genet* **21:** 3647–3654. doi:10.1093/hmg/dds194

Weihbrecht K, Goar WA, Carter CS, Sheffield VC, Seo S. 2018. Genotypic and phenotypic characterization of the Sdccag8Tn(sb-Tyr)2161B.CA1C2Ove mouse model. *PLoS ONE* **13:** e0192755. doi:10.1371/journal.pone.0192755

Wright AF, Chakarova CF, Abd El-Aziz MM, Bhattacharya SS. 2010. Photoreceptor degeneration: genetic and mechanistic dissection of a complex trait. *Nat Rev Genet* **11:** 273–284. doi:10.1038/nrg2717

Yang S, Bahl K, Chou HT, Woodsmith J, Stelzl U, Walz T, Nachury MV. 2020. Near-atomic structures of the BBSome reveal the basis for BBSome activation and binding to GPCR cargoes. *eLife* **9:** e55954. doi:10.7554/eLife.55954

Yen HJ, Tayeh MK, Mullins RF, Stone EM, Sheffield VC, Slusarski DC. 2006. Bardet–Biedl syndrome genes are important in retrograde intracellular trafficking and Kupffer's vesicle cilia function. *Hum Mol Genet* **15:** 667–677. doi:10.1093/hmg/ddi468

Zaghloul NA, Katsanis N. 2009. Mechanistic insights into Bardet–Biedl syndrome, a model ciliopathy. *J Clin Invest* **119:** 428–437. doi:10.1172/JCI37041

Zhang Q, Nishimura D, Seo S, Vogel T, Morgan DA, Searby C, Bugge K, Stone EM, Rahmouni K, Sheffield VC. 2011. Bardet–Biedl syndrome 3 (Bbs3) knockout mouse model reveals common BBS-associated phenotypes and Bbs3 unique phenotypes. *Proc Natl Acad Sci* **108:** 20678–20683. doi:10.1073/pnas.1113220108

Zhang Q, Nishimura D, Vogel T, Shao J, Swiderski R, Yin T, Searby C, Carter CS, Kim G, Bugge K, et al. 2013. BBS7 is required for BBSome formation and its absence in mice results in Bardet-Biedl syndrome phenotypes and selective abnormalities in membrane protein trafficking. *J Cell Sci* **126:** 2372–2380. doi:10.1242/jcs.111740

Zhang Y, Liu H, Li W, Zhang Z, Shang X, Zhang D, Li Y, Zhang S, Liu J, Hess RA, et al. 2017. Intraflagellar transporter protein (IFT27), an IFT25 binding partner, is essential for male fertility and spermiogenesis in mice. *Dev Biol* **432:** 125–139. doi:10.1016/j.ydbio.2017.09.023

Ziegler WH, Lüdiger S, Hassan F, Georgiadis ME, Swolana K, Khera A, Mertens A, Franke D, Wohlgemuth K, Dahmer-Heath M, et al. 2022. Primary URECs: a source to better understand the pathology of renal tubular epithelia in pediatric hereditary cystic kidney diseases. *Orphanet J Rare Dis* **17:** 122. doi:10.1186/s13023-022-02265-1

Canine and Feline Models of Inherited Retinal Diseases

Simon M. Petersen-Jones and András M. Komáromy

Department of Small Animal Clinical Sciences, College of Veterinary Medicine, Michigan State University, East Lansing, Michigan 48824, USA

Correspondence: peter315@msu.edu

Naturally occurring inherited retinal diseases (IRDs) in cats and dogs provide a rich source of potential models for human IRDs. In many cases, the phenotypes between the species with mutations of the homologous genes are very similar. Both cats and dogs have a high-acuity retinal region, the area centralis, an equivalent to the human macula, with tightly packed photoreceptors and higher cone density. This and the similarity in globe size to that of humans means these large animal models provide information not obtainable from rodent models. The established cat and dog models include those for Leber congenital amaurosis, retinitis pigmentosa (including recessive, dominant, and X-linked forms), achromatopsia, Best disease, congenital stationary night blindness and other synaptic dysfunctions, *RDH5*-associated retinopathy, and Stargardt disease. Several of these models have proven to be important in the development of translational therapies such as gene-augmentation therapies. Advances have been made in editing the canine genome, which necessitated overcoming challenges presented by the specifics of canine reproduction. Feline genome editing presents fewer challenges. We can anticipate the generation of specific cat and dog IRD models by genome editing in the future.

Spontaneously occurring inherited retinal diseases (IRDs) in companion animals that recapitulate human IRDs have been recognized for over one century (Magnusson 1911). More detailed studies starting from the 1950s have further strengthened the comparative aspects of these conditions (Parry 1953). Certain common breeding practices (line breeding, intensive use of "popular" sires) tend to expose recessively inherited traits that may be present in the population. Therefore, the majority of cat and dog IRDs are recessive, although dominant and X-linked conditions have also been identified. Dogs and cats with spontaneous IRDs present opportunities to understand and treat conditions in a model species with a human-sized eye and retinal regions with high photoreceptor density allowing high-acuity vision. This is in contrast with rodent models that have a small eye, are nocturnal, and do not have a retinal region for high-acuity vision. The high-acuity retinal region, known as the area centralis, is analogous to the human macula (Mowat et al. 2008). Peak cone density in the center of the canine area centralis approaches that of humans (Beltran et al. 2014). In some instances, these large animal models may recapitulate the analogous human condition much more closely than the rodent models.

With advances in genomic studies, excellent annotated genomes of dog and cat are available, and the tools are in place for identification of the mutations underlying hereditary conditions in these species. In addition to identifying potential models for translational purposes, this work is also important for allowing the animal breeders to use genetic testing to eliminate these conditions, thus improving the health of future dog and cat populations. Studies performed with colonies of dogs and cats with IRD have been valuable for the further understanding of disease mechanisms, development, and testing of translational therapies, and, in some instances, even the identification of previously unknown genes.

In this review, we will consider the IRDs under the category of the human condition that they mimic. These include Leber congenital amaurosis (LCA), retinitis pigmentosa (RP) (including the cone-rod dystrophies), achromatopsia (ACHM), congenital stationary night blindness (CSNB), and miscellaneous conditions such as Best disease and Stargardt disease. We will only discuss those conditions where a colony has been established for study and therapeutic testing. There are many other mutations that have been identified in different dog breeds where colonies have not been established, but genetic testing has been introduced to allow them to be bred out of the pet population. These are covered in other reviews (Miyadera et al. 2012; Bunel et al. 2019; Winkler et al. 2020). The accompanying tables list the genes and mutations identified within them.

LEBER CONGENITAL AMAUROSIS (LCA) MODELS

RPE65-LCA

Groundbreaking proof-of-concept gene-augmentation studies in a dog model of RPE65-LCA were first reported in 2001 (Table 1; Acland et al. 2001). Subsequently, the same and other

groups used the dog model to further study adeno-associated viral (AAV) gene-augmentation therapy (Narfström et al. 2003; Le Meur et al. 2007; Bainbridge et al. 2015). The initial dog studies were important steps toward three different human clinical trials and occurred prior to a mouse model being used. One of these trials led to the first United States Food and Drug Administration (FDA)-approved gene-augmentation therapy (Russell et al. 2017). The RPE65 mutation was identified in the Briard breed with a retinopathy that had been studied extensively (Narfström et al. 1989; Wrigstad et al. 1994) before the causal gene mutation was identified (Veske et al. 1999). Studies using this dog model have been the subject of other review articles (Petersen-Jones et al. 2012).

NPHP5

More recently, gene therapy in NPHP5 (also known as IQCB1) mutant dogs has been reported (Aguirre et al. 2021). NPHP5 is a ciliary protein, and the resulting IRD is categorized as a ciliopathy. Variants in genes expressed at the photoreceptor connecting cilium are an important cause of IRDs. The effect of ciliary gene mutations on the function of cilia in other cell types can result in a range of syndromic phenotypes, which may be embryonic lethal, and cause CNS and renal disease as well as photoreceptor degeneration. NPHP5-mutant dogs (American pit bull terriers) have a nonsyndromic condition but with a severe retinal phenotype with a failure of cone outer segment development and stunted rod outer segments. This developmental abnormality is followed by a more rapid rod loss and relative sparing of central cones that are nonfunctional (Downs et al. 2016). This phenotype is similar to that described for human patients. Gene-augmentation therapy results in functional rescue and structural preservation showing translational promise (Aguirre et al. 2021).

CRX

A cat model with a mutation in the transcription factor CRX has been identified (Menotti-Raymond et al. 2010). CRX plays an important

Table 1. Models for Leber congenital amaurosis (LCA)

Gene	Species	Mutation	Mode of inheritance	Studies	Comments	Key references
AIPL1 (Aryl Hydrocarbon Receptor Interacting Protein-Like 1)	Cat	c.577C > T, p.Arg193Ter	Autosomal-recessive	Characterization	Severe phenotype with no detectable photoreceptor function and a rapid degeneration; AIPL1 is a chaperone for PDE6	Rah et al. 2005; Lyons et al. 2016
CEP290 (Centrosomal Protein 290)	Cat	c.6960 + 9T > G, p.Ile2321AlafsTer3	Autosomal-recessive	Characterization	Ciliopathy but milder phenotype than most human subjects; the intronic mutation introduces a stronger splice site causing a frameshift; some wild-type protein is still produced	Narfström 1985; Menotti-Raymond et al. 2007
CRX Cone-Rod Homeobox	Cat	c.546delC, p.Pro185LysfsTer2	Autosomal-dominant	Characterization	Retinal transcription factor; phenotype mimics human LCA-*CRX*; mutant allele has a dominant-negative effect	Leon and Curtis 1990; Menotti-Raymond et al. 2010; Occelli et al. 2016
NPHP5 Nephrocystin-5 (also IQ Motif Containing B1: IQCB1)	Dog	c.952-953insC, p.Ser319IlefsTer13	Autosomal-recessive	Characterization and gene therapy	Ciliopathy; severe early-onset; early loss of rods with retention of central retinal cones that lack function	Downs et al. 2016; Aguirre et al. 2021
RD3 (RD3 Regulator Of GUCY2D)	Dog	c.418_419ins[22]	Autosomal-recessive	Characterization	RD3 is important for guanylate cyclase trafficking; results in a severe early-onset rod-cone dystrophy	Santos-Anderson et al. 1980; Kukekova et al. 2009
RPE65 (Retinoid Isomerohydrolase RPE65)	Dog	c.487_490delAAGA, p.Lys154LeufsTer53	Autosomal-recessive	Characterization and gene therapy	RPE65 has a major role in the visual cycle; proof-of-concept gene therapy in the dog model led to human clinical trials and an FDA-approved product	Narfström and Wrigstad 1999; Acland et al. 2001
STK38L (Serine/Threonine Kinase 38-Like)	Dog	c.299_300ins [218;285_299], p.Lys63_Glu103del	Autosomal-recessive	Characterization	STK38L has involvement in photoreceptor development inherited retinal disease (IRD) patients have not been identified with mutations in *STK38L*	Goldstein et al. 2010

role in the maturation of photoreceptors and also their maintenance in adults (Furukawa et al. 1997; Hennig et al. 2008). In humans, most mutations lead to a dominant LCA phenotype, although cone-rod dystrophy and RP phenotypes have also been described (Rivolta et al. 2001). Mechanistic classification of the various *CRX* mutations has been proposed (Tran and Chen 2014). Based on this classification, the feline mutation is a class III mutation. This class of mutations have an antimorphic frameshift or nonsense mutation with intact DNA binding. The affected cats show overexpression of the mutant allele that is believed to bind the CRX recognition site present in many photoreceptor gene promoters without activating transcription (Occelli et al. 2016).

CEP290

CEP290 is another ciliary gene. A cat IRD with a *CEP290* mutation has been characterized (Narfström 1983; Narfström and Nilsson 1989). The phenotype of patients with *CEP290* mutations ranges from those with severe syndromic conditions to those with a retina-only phenotype, most typically an LCA. The cat phenotype is milder with variable age-of-onset and rate of progression. The mutation is intronic, creating a strong alternative splice site that, when used, results in a 4-base-pair extension of exon 50 with a resulting premature stop codon (Menotti-Raymond et al. 2007). Use of the introduced splice site truncates the predicted protein by 159 residues. The comparably mild phenotype compared to human patients may suggest that either a truncated product is produced that has some function and/or the original splice site is still used to a certain extent resulting in some normal gene product (Minella et al. 2018). The *CEP290* mutation was identified in Abyssinian cats but is also present in several other cat breeds.

RD3

A spontaneous early-onset retinal degeneration was studied in collies. The photoreceptor outer segments failed to develop to maturity and degenerated relatively rapidly (classified as a rod-cone dysplasia) (Santos-Anderson et al. 1980).

Studies identified a 22-bp insertion in the *RD3* gene (also known as *C1orf36*), making this a dog model for *RD3*-LCA (Kukekova et al. 2009).

RETINITIS PIGMENTOSA MODELS

CNGB1

A dog model with a truncating mutation in *CNGB1* has been identified in the Papillon breed (Table 2). Homozygous mutant dogs develop a relatively slow rod photoreceptor degeneration mimicking *CNGB1*-RP (Winkler et al. 2013). Gene-augmentation therapy with a construct targeting photoreceptors rescues the dog phenotype and halts retinal degeneration (Fig. 1; Petersen-Jones et al. 2018). This, along with the relatively slow photoreceptor degeneration, makes this an attractive target for gene augmentation. The affected dogs show some desensitized residual rod responses on ERG that is likely due to homomeric CNGA1 channels in the rod outer segments (Petersen-Jones et al. 2022).

PDE6A

A dog model with a *PDE6A* mutation has been described (Petersen-Jones et al. 1999; Tuntivanich et al. 2009). The phenotype is of a halt in the maturation of rod outer segments and a complete lack of rod function. There is a rapid rod photoreceptor degeneration with a slower secondary loss of rods. Similar to RP, there is central retinal preservation. Human subjects have night blindness from childhood and a progressive loss of visual fields with central retinal preservation (Kuehlewein et al. 2020, 2022). The dog phenotype mimics the human condition, although photoreceptor degeneration in the dog may be somewhat more rapid. The phenotype in the dog was shown to be similar to that of the *PDE6B* dog (see below). Subretinal AAV gene-augmentation therapy rescued the canine phenotype, restoring rod vision and electroretinographic responses when performed prior to advanced rod loss (Fig. 2; Occelli et al. 2017). Rods in treated retinal regions extended normal-appearing outer segments and both rod and

Table 2. Selected models for retinitis pigmentosa (RP)

Gene	Species	Mutation	Mode of inheritance	Studies	Comments	Key references
CNGB1 (Cyclic Nucleotide Gated Channel Subunit β1)	Dog	c.2387delA;2389_2390insAGCTAC, p.Ser791ArgfsTer2	Autosomal-recessive	Characterization and gene therapy	Rod outer segment cGMP-gated channel gene; relatively slow rod loss with even slower secondary cone loss provides a wide window for successful gene augmentation	Winkler et al. 2013; Petersen-Jones et al. 2018
PDE6A (Phosphodiesterase 6A)	Dog	c.1939delA, p.Asn616ThrfsTer39	Autosomal-recessive	Characterization and gene therapy	Rod phototransduction gene; early-onset with rapid rod death; most human subjects appear to have a milder phenotype than the dog model	Petersen-Jones et al. 1999; Tuntivanich et al. 2009; Occelli et al. 2017
PDE6B (Phosphodiesterase 6B)	Dog	*Rcd1*-c.2420G > A, p.Trp807Ter; c.2404_2406delAAC, p.Asn802del	Autosomal-recessive	Characterization and gene therapy	Rod phototransduction gene; early-onset with rapid rod death; *Rcd1* was first canine inherited retinal disease (IRD) to be identified and studied in detail	Suber et al. 1993; Petit et al. 2012; Goldstein et al. 2013; Pichard et al. 2016
RHO (Rhodopsin)	Dog	c.11C > G, p.Thr4Arg	Autosomal-dominant	Characterization and gene therapy	Rod phototransduction gene; phenotype is of a class B1 *RHO* mutation—very sensitive to light damage	Kijas et al. 2002; Cideciyan et al. 2005; Iwabe et al. 2016; Sudharsan et al. 2017; Cideciyan et al. 2018
RPGR (Retinitis Pigmentosa GTPase Regulator)	Dog	XLPRA1: c.1028-1032delGAGAA XLPRA2: c.1084-1085delGA	X-linked	Characterization and gene therapy	Ciliopathy; severity of phenotype varies between the different mutations, which are both ORF15 microdeletions; XLPRA1 has a later onset and XLPRA2 has an early and severe phenotype	Zangerl et al. 2002; Zhang et al. 2002; Beltran et al. 2012, 2015, 2017
RPGRIP1 (RPGR Interacting Protein 1)	Dog	CFA15: g.8228_8229insA29GGAAGCAACAGGATG	Autosomal-recessive	Characterization and gene therapy	Ciliopathy; presence of two modifying loci suggested	Mellersh et al. 2006; Lheriteau et al. 2014; Forman et al. 2016; Miyadera et al. 2018

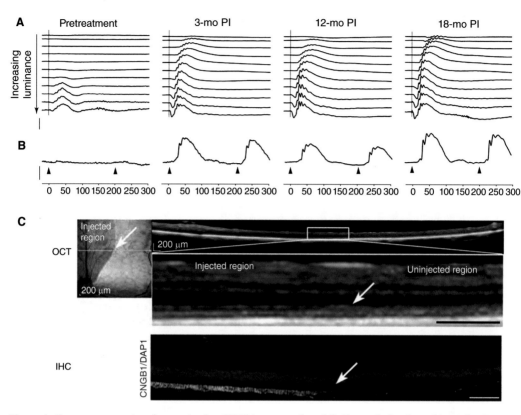

Figure 1. Gene-augmentation therapy in the *CNGB1*-mutant dog. (*A*) Shows dark-adapted ERG luminance: response series. Note that, prior to treatment, there is only a response to the stronger (higher luminance) flash stimuli. Following gene-augmentation therapy, a normal-appearing, rod-mediated response is restored and maintained for the study period. (*B*) Shows 5-Hz rod-mediated flicker. This is not present prior to therapy and is restored by therapy. (*C*) OCT imaging across the treated region shows improvement of the appearance of the zones representing the inner and outer segments in the treated region. IHC shows *CNGB1* expression in the treated region, with normal-appearing photoreceptors. Scale bars, 200 μm (*top*); 100 μm (*bottom*).

cone preservation was achieved and maintained for several years (Occelli et al. 2020).

PDE6B

Four different *PDE6B* mutations have been identified in dogs and two maintained as colonies for study. The rod-cone dysplasia type 1 (*rcd1*) Irish setter dog was first reported in the 1940s (Hodgman et al. 1949) and was the first dog RP model for which the causal mutation was found (Suber et al. 1993). Subsequently, American Staffordshire terriers with an early-onset IRD were used to form a colony for study and found to have a *PDE6B* mutation (Goldstein et al. 2013). The phenotype of the *rcd1*-dog,

which has a nonsense mutation, has been studied in detail (Aguirre and Rubin 1975b). Homozygous dogs have a severe phenotype in which full maturation of both rod and cone outer segments was halted in conjunction with accumulation of high levels of retinal cyclic GMP due to a failure of rod phototransduction (Aguirre et al. 1978). Gene therapy using an AAV construct delivered subretinally was shown to restore rod function and preserve photoreceptors in the *rcd1* dog (Petit et al. 2012; Pichard et al. 2016).

RHO

A dominant canine *rhodopsin* (*RHO*) mutation has been identified and studied in detail (Kijas

 Cite this article as *Cold Spring Harb Perspect Med* doi: 10.1101/cshperspect.a041286

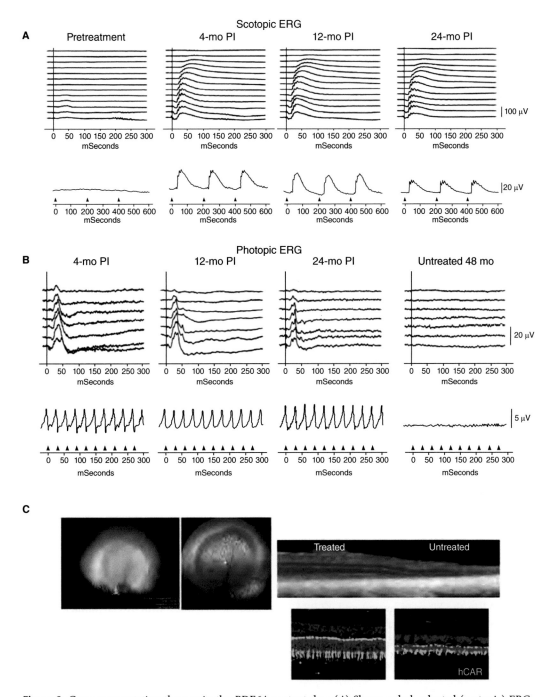

Figure 2. Gene-augmentation therapy in the *PDE6A*-mutant dog. (*A*) Shows a dark-adapted (scotopic) ERG luminance:response series and rod flicker responses. Note the restoration of rod response following gene-augmentation therapy. (*B*) Light-adapted (photopic) ERG responses are maintained in the treated eye. (*C*) Color fundus image and cSLO IR image of a treated eye showing preservation of a normal-appearing retina in the treated retinal region. The OCT shows the junction between treated and untreated retinal regions showing preservation in the treated area. The IHC images show cones labeled with human cone arrestin antibody in the treated (*left* image) and untreated (*right* image) retinal regions showing improved and preserved cone photoreceptor structure in the treated region.

et al. 2002). An interesting feature of the phenotype is the sensitivity of the mutant dog retina to light exposure (Cideciyan et al. 2005; Iwabe et al. 2016; Sudharsan et al. 2017). The mutated protein is transported to the rod outer segments in similar amounts to the wild-type protein, which is a feature of type-B *RHO* mutations. Although the mutant protein triggers phototransduction, it is responsible for photoreceptor degeneration in proportion to environmental light exposure. Similar light sensitivity has also been shown in mouse models with specific *RHO* mutations and suspected in some *RHO*-RP patients. The light-sensitive patients are classified as having a type-B1 phenotype (mutant rod opsin is trafficked to the outer segments and has a deleterious effect) (Cideciyan et al. 1998). A therapeutic approach was selected that consisted of a "knockdown" of the mutant transcript using an shRNA combined with introduction of a rod opsin construct resistant to the shRNA in a single construct (Cideciyan et al. 2018). The shRNA selected was also shown in vitro to act against some common human *RHO* mutations, including the commonest human rod opsin mutation, Pro23His (Cideciyan et al. 2018). This study provides proof-of-concept for combined knockdown/replacement therapy for retinal dystrophies associated with expression of a deleterious allele.

RPGR

Spontaneously occurring X-linked photoreceptor degeneration has been identified in dogs due to mutations in *RPGR*: X-linked PRA type 1 (*XLPRA1* in the Siberian husky) and *XLPRA2* (originating in the miniature schnauzer; Murgiano et al. 2019). In both *XLPRA1* and 2, microdeletions were identified in the ORF15 region of *RPGR* (Zangerl et al. 2002; Zhang et al. 2002). This region of the gene is a mutation hotspot in human subjects with *RPGR*-RP (Vervoort et al. 2000). The disease severity between the two forms varies considerably, with *XLPRA1* being juvenile in onset and slowly progressive while *XLPRA2* is early in onset and rapidly progressive (Beltran et al. 2012). Gene-augmentation therapy has been successful in slowing degeneration

in both dog models (Beltran et al. 2012, 2015, 2017).

RPGRIP1

A colony of dogs with an early-onset progressive retinal degeneration were found to harbor an insert in the *RPGRIP1* gene (Mellersh et al. 2006). However, identification of dogs in the pet population with the same mutation and yet a lack of retinal degeneration provided some doubt as to the significance of the insertion (Miyadera et al. 2009; Das et al. 2017). Further studies identified the importance of a second locus, which consisted of a deletion involving *MAP9* (Forman et al. 2016). The presence of the mutation at the second locus resulted in an earlier disease onset. The condition was classified as a cone-rod dystrophy, and the clinical picture is further complicated by mapping of a third locus that also appears to act as a phenotype modifier predominantly influencing cone function (Miyadera et al. 2018). *RPGRIP1* mutations in humans result in LCA or cone-rod dystrophy (Zahid et al. 2018).

Using dogs obtained from the initial closed colony, which had a consistent phenotype, gene therapy to introduce a normal copy of the canine *RPGRIP1* gene delivered using subretinal AAV vectors rescued the phenotype (Lhériteau et al. 2014).

OTHER RP MODELS

Mutations in several other genes have been identified in pet dogs with IRDs mimicking RP. Some have been established as laboratory colonies allowing further study of the phenotypes. This has led to the identification of different functional and histopathological changes.

In one instance, a very common mutation present across several dog breeds was identified and studied and found to be in a previously undescribed retinal gene. The condition in dogs was termed progressive rod-cone degeneration (*prcd*) (Aguirre et al. 1982). Following identification of the novel gene, it was named *PRCD* after the canine condition and mutations in the human homolog shown to be a cause of recessive RP (Zangerl et al. 2006).

ACHROMATOPSIA (ACHM) MODELS

ACHM, also referred to as rod monochromacy or total color blindness, has been identified in several dog breeds (Table 3). The classic ACHM phenotype becomes evident at 8–12 wk, soon after retinal differentiation is completed (Rubin 1971a,b; Aguirre and Rubin 1974, 1975a; Komáromy et al. 2013; Yeh et al. 2013; Dixon 2016). Affected puppies show severe visual impairment under photopic light conditions, while visual performance under scotopic conditions remains normal. Nystagmus and photophobia are less common in dogs than in humans with ACHM. Clinical ophthalmic examination is unremarkable with no detectable retinal degenerative changes, probably because dogs do not have a "cone-only" fovea. Diagnosis is confirmed by the absence or severe reduction of photopic ERG responses (Aguirre and Rubin 1975a; Komáromy et al. 2010, 2013; Yeh et al.

2013; Tanaka et al. 2015; Dixon 2016). Histologically, affected cones show progressive degeneration of their outer segments, followed by loss of inner segments and the entire cone photoreceptor cell (Aguirre and Rubin 1974; Komáromy et al. 2013). To date, all known forms of canine ACHM are channelopathies caused by mutations in either *CNGA3* or *CNGB3* (Sidjanin et al. 2002; Tanaka et al. 2015). This is important from a translational aspect since up to 90% of human ACHM patients are affected by mutations in the same two genes (Kohl et al. 2005; Mayer et al. 2017; Felden et al. 2019; Michalakis et al. 2022).

CNGA3

Two independent forms of canine *CNGA3*-ACHM have been identified and characterized in pet dogs, a missense mutation and an in-frame 3-base-pair deletion (Tanaka et al. 2015; Dixon 2016). To date, no gene therapy has been performed in these dogs, mainly because their discovery lagged behind the development and

Table 3. Models for achromatopsia

Gene	Species	Mutation	Mode of inheritance	Studies	Comments	Key references
CNGA3 (Cyclic Nucleotide-Gated Channel Subunit α3)	Dog	c.1270C > T, p.Arg424Trp c.1931_1933delTGG, p.Val644del	Autosomal-recessive	Characterization	Cone cGMP-gated channel gene; two separate mutations identified—phenotype similar	Tanaka et al. 2015; Dixon 2016
CNGB3 (Cyclic Nucleotide-Gated Channel Subunit β3)	Dog	c.784G > A, p.Asp262Asn CFA29:g.35,699,378-36,104,197del, c.0	Autosomal-recessive	Characterization and gene therapy	Cone cGMP-gated channel gene; two separate mutations identified in different dog breeds with similar phenotypes; gene therapy restoration of cone function is successful in younger dogs	Sidjanin et al. 2002; Yeh et al. 2013

use of the *CNGA3*-mutant sheep model (Banin et al. 2015; Gootwine et al. 2017a,b; Ofri et al. 2018).

CNGB3

Two canine forms of *CNGB3*-ACHM with identical phenotypes have been identified: one in Alaskan malamutes with a 404,820-bp genomic deletion and the other in German shorthaired pointers with an Asp262Asn missense mutation (Sidjanin et al. 2002; Yeh et al. 2013). Subretinal AAV-mediated *CNGB3* gene-augmentation therapy has been performed successfully in both models (Fig. 3), although treatment failed if conducted at ≥6 mo of age, most likely because cone outer segments were too degenerated (Komáromy et al. 2010; Ye et al. 2017). Cone outer segment deconstruction by intravitreal bolus injection of ciliary neurotrophic factor (CNTF) resulted in improved treatment outcomes of AAV gene therapy in older dogs (Komáromy et al. 2013).

MISCELLANEOUS MODELS

BEST1-Related Dystrophies

Three distinct mutations have been identified in the canine *BEST1* gene and result in similar clinical phenotypes as in human patients (Table 4). The first, identified in mastiff breeds, is a premature stop mutation located in the first coding exon of *cBEST1* (Guziewicz et al. 2007, 2011); the second, in the coton de Tulear, is a missense change (Guziewicz et al. 2007, 2011); and the third, in the Lapponian herder, is a frameshift mutation combined with a missense variation, which results in a truncation of the BEST1 carboxyl terminus (Zangerl et al. 2010). Based on the mutations, these autosomal-recessive traits and clinical phenotypes are referred to as canine multifocal retinopathy 1 (*cmr1*), *cmr2*, and *cmr3*, respectively (Guziewicz et al. 2017). They are characterized by a predilection of multifocal subretinal lesions, also affecting the canine macula-like area centralis (Guziewicz et al. 2017). These retina-wide RPE–PR microdetachments contract with dark adaptation and ex-

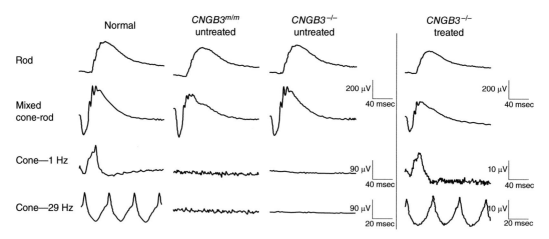

Figure 3. Normal rod function and loss of cone function in *CNGB3^{m/m}*- and *CNGB3^{−/−}*-mutant dogs and short-term restoration of cone ERG signals following a single subretinal treatment with rAAV5-PR2.1-*hCNGB3*. Representative ERG traces evoked by full-field white flashes under dark-adapted (rod and mixed cone-rod responses) and light-adapted (cone 1 Hz and 29 Hz) conditions are shown. Compared to an age-matched normal *wildtype* dog, the treated eye of the *CNGB3^{−/−}* dog showed restoration of cone function as elicited by single and 29-Hz flicker light flashes 7 wk after subretinal injection. The smaller amplitude of the restored cone function compared to the normal dog can be explained by the fact that the subretinal bleb covered ~30% of the entire retina. (*CNGB3^{−/−}*) Homozygous for genomic deletion, (*CNGB3^{m/m}*) homozygous for Asp262Asn missense mutation. (Figure from Komáromy et al. 2010; reprinted, with permission, from Oxford University Press © 2010.)

Cite this article as *Cold Spring Harb Perspect Med* doi: 10.1101/cshperspect.a041286

Table 4. Models for miscellaneous inherited retinal diseases (IRDs)

Disease	Gene	Species	Mutation	Mode of inheritance	Studies	Comments	Key references
Best disease	*BEST1* (Bestrophin 1)	Dog	cmr1: c.73C>T, p.Arg25Ter; cmr2: c.482G>A, p.Gly161Asp; cmr3: c.C1388del and c.1466G>T, p.Pro463fs and p.Gly489Val	Autosomal-recessive	Characterization and gene therapy	*BEST1*-RPE channel gene; three separate mutations in different dog breeds; the disease mechanism differs between cmr3 and the other two forms; phenotype is similar	Guziewicz et al. 2007, 2011, 2017, 2018; Zangerl et al. 2010
Complete congenital stationary night blindness (CSNB)	*LRIT3* (Leucine-Rich Repeat, Ig-Like And Transmembrane Domains 3)	Dog	c.762_763delG, p.Lys246AsnfsTer5	Autosomal-recessive	Characterization and gene therapy	Photoreceptor/ON bipolar synapse gene; recapitulates a complete CSNB phenotype with loss of ON pathway responses but retention of OFF pathway responses	Kondo et al. 2015; Das et al. 2019
Incomplete CSNB2 or LCA	*CABP4* (Calcium-Binding Protein 4)	Dog	Not reported	Autosomal-recessive	Characterization and gene therapy	Photoreceptor synapse gene; condition in dog is not stationary—they develop a progressive retinal degeneration	Beckwith-Cohen et al. 2022
RDH5-retinopathy	*RDH5* (Retinol Dehydrogenase 5)	Cat	c.542G>T, p.Gly181Val	Autosomal-recessive	Characterization	Visual cycle gene; cat model shows slow rod recovery and "macular" degeneration; in humans results in slow rod recovery and appearance of white fleck retinal lesions—hence fundus albipunctatus	Occelli et al. 2021

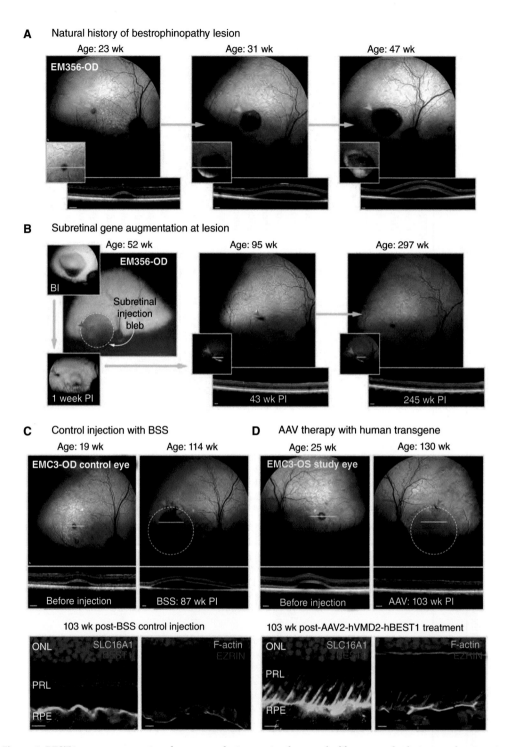

Figure 4. *BEST1* gene-augmentation therapy results in sustained reversal of foveomacular lesions and restoration of RPE–PR interface structure. (*A*) Natural history of the central subretinal detachment documented by in vivo imaging in the right eye of a compound heterozygous (c.73C > T/1388delC) dog with bestrophinopathy (cBest) at three time points. (*Legend continues on following page.*)

pand with exposure to light (Guziewicz et al. 2018). Subretinal AAV-mediated *BEST1* gene-augmentation therapy was performed successfully in the three genotypes *cmr1*, *cmr3*, and *cmr1/cmr3*, reversing both the clinically detectable subretinal lesions and the diffuse microdetachments (Fig. 4; Guziewicz et al. 2018).

Photoreceptor to Bipolar Cell Connectivity Disorders

Two models with mutations involving photoreceptor to bipolar cell connectivity have more recently been reported. The first is a dog CSNB model identified in beagles with a mutation in *LRIT3* (Das et al. 2019). The resulting lack of rod ERG b-wave with no detected retinal degeneration mimicked the human phenotype (Kondo et al. 2015). There is currently some debate about the precise site of *LRIT3* expression (Hasan et al. 2019). However, gene-augmentation therapy with a promoter intended to drive expression in bipolar cells (short *GRM6*) partially restored the ERG b-wave and improved vision under scotopic conditions (Miyadera et al. 2022). *LRIT3* mutations are reported to be a cause of complete CSNB in human patients (Zeitz et al. 2013). Another spontaneous no ERG b-wave canine model in whippets (Somma et al. 2017) has been identified

and is associated with a mutation in *CABP4* (Beckwith-Cohen et al. 2022). *CABP4* mutations in humans result in a loss of night vision with categorization varying from CSNB to LCA (Zeitz et al. 2006; Aldahmesh et al. 2010). Gene-augmentation therapy was successful in restoring a rod b-wave and improving vision in mutant dogs (Beckwith-Cohen et al. 2022).

RDH5-Associated Retinopathy

Recently, we have reported on a spontaneous cat model with a loss-of-function mutation in *RDH5* (Occelli et al. 2022). RDH5 is the final enzyme in the visual (retinoid) cycle for regeneration of 11-*cis*-retinal in the RPE. Human subjects with *RDH5* loss-of function mutations have very delayed recovery of rod function following light exposure. Most patients also develop white retinal spots and are thus categorized as having fundus albipunctatus. A subset of patients develops macular degeneration suggesting cone impairment as well as rod functional abnormalities. *RDH5* knockout mice fail to recapitulate the human phenotype, whereas the large-animal cat model shows many of the features (Fig. 5). These include a very delayed rod ERG recovery following exposure to a standard rod-suppressing light. Additionally, a

---

Figure 4. (*Continued*) A series of representative near-infrared reflectance (NIR) images demonstrate the evolution of the focal lesion (green arrowhead) in the canine macula from the vitelliform stage (*left*) through early pseudohypopyon (*middle*) to an advanced pseudohypopyon stage (*right*). (*A*) (*insets*) Autofluorescence and OCT images. (*B*) Subretinal injection with AAV2-canine *BEST1* (1.5E10 vg/mL) was performed in the eye shown in *A* at 52 wk of age, entirely encompassing the lesion depicted in the fundus photograph before injection (BI) (*left, upper inset*). The subretinal bleb area is denoted by the dashed circle. The treated eye showed ophthalmoscopic resolution of lesion 1 wk postinjection (PI) (*left, lower inset*); however, confirmatory OCT scans were not available at this age. Images acquired at 43 (*middle*) and 245 wk (*right*) PI document sustained reversal of the central lesion and fully reattached retina within the treated area. (*B*) (*middle and right, insets*) Autofluorescence and OCT images. Scale bars, 200 μm. (*C,D*) Restoration of RPE–photoreceptor interface structure post-AAV-human *BEST1* treatment in the cBest (homozygous c.73C > T) model in comparison with control. (*Upper*) NIR images exhibiting early vitelliform lesions shown at ages 19 and 25 wk. Both eyes were injected at 27 wk of age with either balanced salt solution (BSS) or AAV2-human *BEST1* (2E11 vg/mL). Bleb boundaries are marked by dashed circles; the locations of corresponding OCT scans cut through the subretinal lesions before injection or through the matching locations mapped PI are marked by green horizontal lines; retinotomy sites are indicated by blue arrowheads. Scale bars, 200 μm (*C,D*). (*Lower*) Confocal fluorescence images of IHC assessment of AAV-h*BEST1*- or BSS-injected eyes; in contrast to the BSS control eye (*C*), cytoskeleton rescue and restoration of RPE–PR interface structure are shown in AAV-treated retina 103-wk PI (*D*). Scale bars, 10 μm. Retinas are immunolabeled with anti-BEST1 (red) and anti-SLC16A1 (green). EM356-OD, EMC3-OD, and EMC3-OS designate the individual animal and eye. (All panels in figure reprinted from Guziewicz et al. 2018 under Creative Commons Attribution-NonCommercial-NoDerivatives License 4.0 (CC BY-NC-ND).)

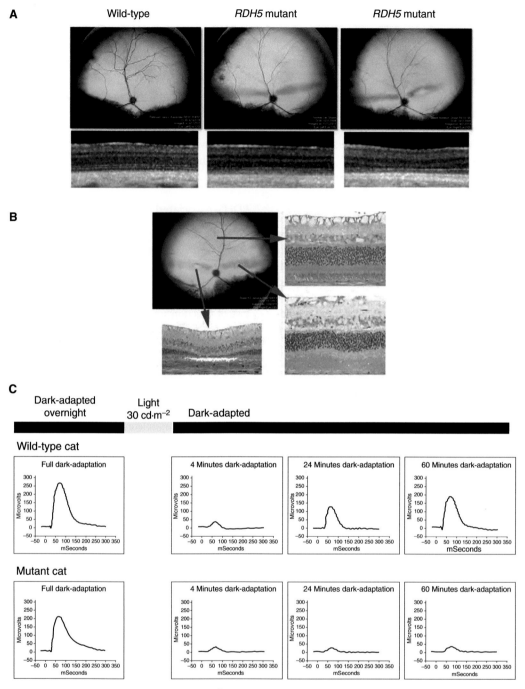

Standard ISCEV rod stimulus: 0.01 cd·s·m⁻²

Figure 5. Phenotype of the *RDH5*-mutant cat. (*A*) Shows color fundus image of the left eye for a wild-type and two stages of retinal changes in an affected cat. Note the hyporeflective horizontal lesion that follows the area centralis/visual streak (1 yr of age); by 4.5 yr of age, a region of hyperreflectivity is seen in the area centralis indicative of retinal thinning. The corresponding OCT images through the area centralis are shown *beneath*. At 1 yr of age, the affected cat has loss of definition of the zones representing the inner/outer segments. At 4.5 yr of age, thinning of the outer retina is marked. (*B*) Plastic sections through the indicated retinal regions. Away from the area centralis/visual streak morphology appears normal. The area centralis region shows marked outer retinal thinning. The section from the visual streak shows lengthening and distortion of the outer segments, which results in the hyporeflective lesion visible on fundus examination. (*C*) A comparison of recovery of rod ERG function following exposure to a rod-suppressing light for 10 min following dark adaptation. Over the 60 min, there was virtually no recovery of rod responses in the mutant cat.

subset of the mutant cats develop degeneration in the macula-equivalent area centralis (region of high cone and rod density for high-acuity vision) (Occelli et al. 2022). These features provide the opportunity to study key aspects of *RDH5*-retinopathy in a large animal model.

SUMMARY

Following the introduction of FDA-approved gene therapy for *RPE65*-LCA, several other gene-therapy approaches are planned or are in clinical trials. Large animal models are becoming more widely used for developing and testing such therapies. The advantages of a large eye coupled with a high-acuity retinal region make these attractive species to use. Although the models are dependent on the occurrence of spontaneous mutations, there are likely several potentially valuable models that will probably be identified in the future. One such potentially important model is the *ABCA4*-mutant dog (Mäkeläinen et al. 2019), which could fill an unmet need for an animal model that recapitulates the important features of Stargardt disease.

Identification of spontaneously occurring gene mutations is now easier thanks to advances in canine and feline genomics and improvement in the reference genome sequences. The species-specific reproductive system in dogs has made producing genetically modified dogs challenging. Recently, however, some successes have been reported (Zou et al. 2015; Feng et al. 2018; Kim et al. 2022). These may lead to genome-edited dog IRD models. While a genetically modified cat has not yet been reported, advances have been made since the first cat cloning was reported in 2002 (Shin et al. 2002). Recent reports suggest a genome-edited cat may soon be produced with a specific cat allergen gene, which is proposed to be responsible for human allergies to domestic cats, knocked out, thus making it hypoallergenic for humans (Brackett et al. 2022).

REFERENCES

Acland GM, Aguirre GD, Ray J, Zhang Q, Aleman TS, Cideciyan AV, Pearce-Kelling SE, Anand V, Zeng Y, Maguire AM, et al. 2001. Gene therapy restores vision in a canine model of childhood blindness. *Nat Genet* **28:** 92–95.

Aguirre GD, Rubin LF. 1974. Pathology of hemeralopia in the Alaskan malamute dog. *Invest Ophthalmol Vis Sci* **13:** 231–235.

Aguirre GD, Rubin LF. 1975a. The electroretinogram in dogs with inherited cone degeneration. *Invest Ophthalmol Vis Sci* **14:** 840–847.

Aguirre GD, Rubin LF. 1975b. Rod-cone dysplasia (progressive retinal atrophy) in Irish setters. *J Am Vet Med Assoc* **166:** 157–164.

Aguirre GD, Farber D, Lolley R, Fletcher RT, Chader GJ. 1978. Rod-cone dysplasia in Irish setters: a defect in cyclic GMP metabolism in visual cells. *Science* **201:** 1133–1134. doi:10.1126/science.210508

Aguirre GD, Alligood J, O'Brien P, Buyukmihci N. 1982. Pathogenesis of progressive rod-cone degeneration in miniature poodles. *Invest Ophthalmol Vis Sci* **23:** 610–630.

Aguirre GD, Cideciyan AV, Dufour VL, Ripolles-García A, Sudharsan R, Swider M, Nikonov R, Iwabe S, Boye SL, Hauswirth WW, et al. 2021. Gene therapy reforms photoreceptor structure and restores vision in *NPHP5*-associated Leber congenital amaurosis. *Mol Ther* **29:** 2456–2468. doi:10.1016/j.ymthe.2021.03.021

Aldahmesh MA, Al-Owain M, Alqahtani F, Hazzaa S, Alkuraya FS. 2010. A null mutation in CABP4 causes Leber's congenital amaurosis-like phenotype. *Mol Vis* **16:** 207–212.

Bainbridge JW, Mehat MS, Sundaram V, Robbie SJ, Barker SE, Ripamonti C, Georgiadis A, Mowat FM, Beattie SG, Gardner PJ, et al. 2015. Long-term effect of gene therapy on Leber's congenital amaurosis. *N Engl J Med* **372:** 1887–1897. doi:10.1056/NEJMoa1414221

Banin E, Gootwine E, Obolensky A, Ezra-Elia R, Ejzenberg A, Zelinger L, Honig H, Rosov A, Yamin E, Sharon D, et al. 2015. Gene augmentation therapy restores retinal function and visual behavior in a sheep model of *CNGA3* achromatopsia. *Mol Ther* **23:** 1423–1433. doi:10.1038/mt.2015.114

Beckwith-Cohen B, Winkler PA, Occelli LM, Sun K, Montiani-Ferreira F, Marinho LF, Lee A, Parys M, Hauswirth WW, Petersen-Jones S. 2022. Gene augmentation therapy restores vision in a CaBP4-mutant canine model of cone-rod synaptic disorder. *Invest Ophthalmol Vis Sci* **63:** 1108–1108.

Beltran WA, Cideciyan AV, Lewin AS, Iwabe S, Khanna H, Sumaroka A, Chiodo VA, Fajardo DS, Román AJ, Deng WT, et al. 2012. Gene therapy rescues photoreceptor blindness in dogs and paves the way for treating human X-linked retinitis pigmentosa. *Proc Natl Acad Sci* **109:** 2132–2137. doi:10.1073/pnas.1118847109

Beltran WA, Cideciyan AV, Guziewicz KE, Iwabe S, Swider M, Scott EM, Savina SV, Ruthel G, Stefano F, Zhang L, et al. 2014. Canine retina has a primate fovea-like bouquet of cone photoreceptors which is affected by inherited macular degenerations. *PLoS ONE* **9:** e90390. doi:10.1371/journal.pone.0090390

Beltran WA, Cideciyan AV, Iwabe S, Swider M, Kosyk MS, McDaid K, Martynyuk I, Ying GS, Shaffer J, Deng WT, et al. 2015. Successful arrest of photoreceptor and vision loss expands the therapeutic window of retinal gene therapy to later stages of disease. *Proc Natl Acad Sci* **112**: E5844–E5853. doi:10.1073/pnas.1509914112

Beltran WA, Cideciyan AV, Boye SE, Ye GJ, Iwabe S, Dufour VL, Marinho LF, Swider M, Kosyk MS, Sha J, et al. 2017. Optimization of retinal gene therapy for X-linked retinitis pigmentosa due to *RPGR* mutations. *Mol Ther* **25**: 1866–1880. doi:10.1016/j.ymthe.2017.05.004

Brackett NF, Davis BW, Adli M, Pomés A, Chapman MD. 2022. Evolutionary biology and gene editing of cat allergen, Fel d 1. *CRISPR J* **5**: 213–223. doi:10.1089/crispr.2021.0101

Bunel M, Chaudieu G, Hamel C, Lagoutte L, Manes G, Botherel N, Brabet P, Pilorge P, André C, Quignon P. 2019. Natural models for retinitis pigmentosa: progressive retinal atrophy in dog breeds. *Hum Genet* **138**: 441–453. doi:10.1007/s00439-019-01999-6

Cideciyan AV, Hood DC, Huang Y, Banin E, Li ZY, Stone EM, Milam AH, Jacobson SG. 1998. Disease sequence from mutant *rhodopsin* allele to rod and cone photoreceptor degeneration in man. *Proc Natl Acad Sci* **95**: 7103–7108. doi:10.1073/pnas.95.12.7103

Cideciyan AV, Jacobson SG, Aleman TS, Gu D, Pearce-Kelling SE, Sumaroka A, Acland GM, Aguirre GD. 2005. In vivo dynamics of retinal injury and repair in the *rhodopsin* mutant dog model of human retinitis pigmentosa. *Proc Natl Acad Sci* **102**: 5233–5238. doi:10.1073/pnas.0408892102

Cideciyan AV, Sudharsan R, Dufour VL, Massengill MT, Iwabe S, Swider M, Lisi B, Sumaroka A, Marinho LF, Appelbaum T, et al. 2018. Mutation-independent rhodopsin gene therapy by knockdown and replacement with a single AAV vector. *Proc Natl Acad Sci* **115**: E8547–E8556. doi:10.1073/pnas.1805055115

Das RG, Marinho FP, Iwabe S, Santana E, McDaid KS, Aguirre GD, Miyadera K. 2017. Variabilities in retinal function and structure in a canine model of cone-rod dystrophy associated with *RPGRIP1* support multigenic etiology. *Sci Rep* **7**: 1–15. doi: 10.1038/s41598-017-13112-w

Das RG, Becker D, Jagannathan V, Goldstein O, Santana E, Carlin K, Sudharsan R, Leeb T, Nishizawa Y, Kondo M, et al. 2019. Genome-wide association study and whole-genome sequencing identify a deletion in *LRIT3* associated with canine congenital stationary night blindness. *Sci Rep* **9**: 14166. doi:10.1038/s41598-019-50573-7

Dixon CJ. 2016. Achromatopsia in three sibling Labrador retrievers in the UK. *Vet Ophthalmol* **19**: 68–72. doi:10.1111/vop.12265

Downs LM, Scott EM, Cideciyan AV, Iwabe S, Dufour V, Gardiner KL, Genini S, Marinho LF, Sumaroka A, Kosyk MS, et al. 2016. Overlap of abnormal photoreceptor development and progressive degeneration in Leber congenital amaurosis caused by *NPHP5* mutation. *Hum Mol Genet* **25**: 4211–4226. doi:10.1093/hmg/ddw254

Felden J, Baumann B, Ali M, Audo I, Ayuso C, Bocquet B, Casteels I, Garcia-Sandoval B, Jacobson SG, Jurklies B, et al. 2019. Mutation spectrum and clinical investigation of achromatopsia patients with mutations in the *GNAT2* gene. *Hum Mutat* **40**: 1145–1155.

Feng C, Wang X, Shi H, Yan Q, Zheng M, Li J, Zhang Q, Qin Y, Zhong Y, Mi J, et al. 2018. Generation of ApoE deficient dogs via combination of embryo injection of CRISPR/

Cas9 with somatic cell nuclear transfer. *J Genet Genomics* **45**: 47–50. doi:10.1016/j.jgg.2017.11.003

Forman OP, Hitti RJ, Boursnell M, Miyadera K, Sargan D, Mellersh C. 2016. Canine genome assembly correction facilitates identification of a *MAP9* deletion as a potential age of onset modifier for *RPGRIP1*-associated canine retinal degeneration. *Mamm Genome* **27**: 237–245. doi:10.1007/s00335-016-9627-x

Furukawa T, Morrow EM, Cepko CL. 1997. *Crx*, a novel otx-like homeobox gene, shows photoreceptor-specific expression and regulates photoreceptor differentiation. *Cell* **91**: 531–541. doi:10.1016/S0092-8674(00)80439-0

Goldstein O, Kukekova AV, Aguirre GD, Acland GM. 2010. Exonic SINE insertion in STK38L causes canine early retinal degeneration (*erd*). *Genomics* **96**: 362–368. doi:10.1016/j.ygeno.2010.09.003

Goldstein O, Mezey JG, Schweitzer PA, Boyko AR, Gao C, Bustamante CD, Jordan JA, Aguirre GD, Acland GM. 2013. *IQCB1* and *PDE6B* mutations cause similar early onset retinal degenerations in two closely related terrier dog breeds. *Invest Ophthalmol Vis Sci* **54**: 7005–7019. doi:10.1167/iovs.13-12915

Gootwine E, Abu-Siam M, Obolensky A, Rosov A, Honig H, Nitzan T, Shirak A, Ezra-Elia R, Yamin E, Banin E, et al. 2017a. Gene augmentation therapy for a missense substitution in the cGMP-binding domain of ovine *CNGA3* gene restores vision in day-blind sheep. *Invest Ophthalmol Vis Sci* **58**: 1577–1584. doi:10.1167/iovs.16-20986

Gootwine E, Ofri R, Banin E, Obolensky A, Averbukh E, Ezra-Elia R, Ross M, Honig H, Rosov A, Yamin E, et al. 2017b. Safety and efficacy evaluation of rAAV2tYF-PR1.7-*hCNGA3* vector delivered by subretinal injection in CNGA3 mutant achromatopsia sheep. *Hum Gene Ther Clin Dev* **28**: 96–107. doi:10.1089/humc.2017.028

Guziewicz KE, Zangerl B, Lindauer SJ, Mullins RF, Sandmeyer LS, Grahn BH, Stone EM, Acland GM, Aguirre GD. 2007. Bestrophin gene mutations cause canine multifocal retinopathy: a novel animal model for best disease. *Invest Ophthalmol Vis Sci* **48**: 1959–1967. doi:10.1167/iovs.06-1374

Guziewicz KE, Slavik J, Lindauer SJ, Aguirre GD, Zangerl B. 2011. Molecular consequences of *BEST1* gene mutations in canine multifocal retinopathy predict functional implications for human bestrophinopathies. *Invest Ophthalmol Vis Sci* **52**: 4497–4505. doi:10.1167/iovs.10-6385

Guziewicz KE, Sinha D, Gómez NM, Zorych K, Dutrow EV, Dhingra A, Mullins RF, Stone EM, Gamm DM, Boesze-Battaglia K, et al. 2017. Bestrophinopathy: an RPE-photoreceptor interface disease. *Prog Retin Eye Res* **58**: 70–88. doi:10.1016/j.preteyeres.2017.01.005

Guziewicz KE, Cideciyan AV, Beltran WA, Komáromy AM, Dufour VL, Swider M, Iwabe S, Sumaroka A, Kendrick BT, Ruthel G, et al. 2018. *BEST1* gene therapy corrects a diffuse retina-wide microdetachment modulated by light exposure. *Proc Natl Acad Sci* **115**: E2839–E2848. doi:10.1073/pnas.1720662115

Hasan N, Pangeni G, Cobb CA, Ray TA, Nettesheim ER, Ertel KJ, Lipinski DM, McCall MA, Gregg RG. 2019. Presynaptic expression of LRIT3 transsynaptically organizes the postsynaptic glutamate signaling complex containing TRPM1. *Cell Rep* **27**: 3107–3116.e3. doi:10.1016/j.celrep.2019.05.056

 Cite this article as *Cold Spring Harb Perspect Med* doi: 10.1101/cshperspect.a041286

Hennig AK, Peng GH, Chen S. 2008. Regulation of photoreceptor gene expression by Crx-associated transcription factor network. *Brain Res* **1192:** 114–133. doi:10.1016/j.brainres.2007.06.036

Hodgman SFJ, Parry HB, Rasbridge WJ, Steel JD. 1949. Progressive retinal atrophy in dogs. I: The disease in Irish setters (red). *Veterinary Record* **61:** 185–190.

Iwabe S, Ying GS, Aguirre GD, Beltran WA. 2016. Assessment of visual function and retinal structure following acute light exposure in the light sensitive T4R rhodopsin mutant dog. *Exp Eye Res* **146:** 341–353. doi:10.1016/j.exer.2016.04.006

Kijas JW, Cideciyan AV, Aleman TS, Pianta MJ, Pearce-Kelling SE, Miller BJ, Jacobson SG, Aguirre GD, Acland GM. 2002. Naturally occurring *rhodopsin* mutation in the dog causes retinal dysfunction and degeneration mimicking human dominant retinitis pigmentosa. *Proc Natl Acad Sci* **99:** 6328–6333. doi:10.1073/pnas.082714499

Kim DE, Lee JH, Ji KB, Park KS, Kil TY, Koo O, Kim MK. 2022. Generation of genome-edited dogs by somatic cell nuclear transfer. *BMC Biotechnol* **22:** 19. doi:10.1186/s12896-022-00749-3

Kohl S, Varsanyi B, Antunes GA, Baumann B, Hoyng CB, Jägle H, Rosenberg T, Kellner U, Lorenz B, Salati R, et al. 2005. *CNGB3* mutations account for 50% of all cases with autosomal recessive achromatopsia. *Eur J Hum Genet* **13:** 302–308. doi:10.1038/sj.ejhg.5201269

Komáromy AM, Alexander JJ, Rowlan JS, Garcia MM, Chiodo VA, Kaya A, Tanaka JC, Acland GM, Hauswirth WW, Aguirre GD. 2010. Gene therapy rescues cone function in congenital achromatopsia. *Hum Mol Genet* **19:** 2581–2593. doi:10.1093/hmg/ddq136

Komáromy AM, Rowlan JS, Corr AT, Reinstein SL, Boye SL, Cooper AE, Gonzalez A, Levy B, Wen R, Hauswirth WW, et al. 2013. Transient photoreceptor deconstruction by CNTF enhances rAAV-mediated cone functional rescue in late stage *CNGB3*-achromatopsia. *Mol Ther* **21:** 1131–1141. doi:10.1038/mt.2013.50

Kondo M, Das G, Imai R, Santana E, Nakashita T, Imawaka M, Ueda K, Ohtsuka H, Sakai K, Aihara T, et al. 2015. A naturally occurring canine model of autosomal recessive congenital stationary night blindness. *PLoS ONE* **10:** e0137072. doi:10.1371/journal.pone.0137072

Kuehlewein L, Zobor D, Andreasson SO, Ayuso C, Banfi S, Bocquet B, Bernd AS, Biskup S, Boon CJF, Downes SM, et al. 2020. Clinical phenotype and course of *PDE6A*-associated retinitis pigmentosa disease, characterized in preparation for a gene supplementation trial. *JAMA Ophthalmol* **138:** 1241–1250. doi:10.1001/jamaophthalmol.2020.4206

Kuehlewein L, Straßer T, Blumenstock G, Stingl K, Fischer MD, Wilhelm B, Zrenner E, Wissinger B, Kohl S, Weisschuh N, et al. 2022. Central visual function and genotype–phenotype correlations in *PDE6A*-associated retinitis pigmentosa. *Invest Ophthalmol Vis Sci* **63:** 9–9. doi:10.1167/iovs.63.5.9

Kukekova AV, Goldstein O, Johnson JL, Richardson MA, Pearce-Kelling SE, Swaroop A, Friedman JS, Aguirre GD, Acland GM. 2009. Canine *RD3* mutation establishes rod-cone dysplasia type 2 (*rcd2*) as ortholog of human and murine *rd3*. *Mamm Genome* **20:** 109–123. doi:10.1007/s00335-008-9163-4

Le Meur G, Stieger K, Smith AJ, Weber M, Deschamps JY, Nivard D, Mendes-Madeira A, Provost N, Péréon Y, Cherel Y, et al. 2007. Restoration of vision in RPE65-deficient briard dogs using an AAV serotype 4 vector that specifically targets the retinal pigmented epithelium. *Gene Ther* **14:** 292–303. doi:10.1038/sj.gt.3302861

Leon A, Curtis R. 1990. Autosomal dominant rod-cone dysplasia in the *Rdy* cat 1. Light and electron microscopic findings. *Exp Eye Res* **51:** 361–381. doi:10.1016/0014-4835(90)90149-O

Lhériteau E, Petit L, Weber M, Le Meur G, Deschamps JY, Libeau L, Mendes-Madeira A, Guihal C, François A, Guyon R, et al. 2014. Successful gene therapy in the RPGRIP1-deficient dog: a large model of cone-rod dystrophy. *Mol Ther* **22:** 265–277. doi:10.1038/mt.2013.232

Lyons LA, Creighton EK, Alhaddad H, Beale HC, Grahn RA, Rah H, Maggs DJ, Helps CR, Gandolfi B. 2016. Whole genome sequencing in cats, identifies new models for blindness in AIPL1 and somite segmentation in HES7. *BMC Genomics* **17:** 265. doi:10.1186/s12864-016-2595-4

Magnusson H. 1911. Über retinitis pigmentosa und konsinguinität beim hunde. *Arch Vergl Ophthalmol* **2:** 147–163.

Mäkeläinen S, Gòdia M, Hellsand M, Viluma A, Hahn D, Makdoumi K, Zeiss CJ, Mellersh C, Ricketts SL, Narfström K, et al. 2019. An ABCA4 loss-of-function mutation causes a canine form of Stargardt disease. *PLoS Genet* **15:** e1007873. doi:10.1371/journal.pgen.1007873

Mayer AK, Van Cauwenbergh C, Rother C, Baumann B, Reuter P, De Baere E, Wissinger B, Kohl S; ACHM Study Group. 2017. *CNGB3* mutation spectrum including copy number variations in 552 achromatopsia patients. *Hum Mutat* **38:** 1579–1591. doi:10.1002/humu.23311

Mellersh CS, Boursnell ME, Pettitt L, Ryder EJ, Holmes NG, Grafham D, Forman OP, Sampson J, Barnett KC, Blanton S, et al. 2006. Canine *RPGRIP1* mutation establishes cone-rod dystrophy in miniature longhaired dachshunds as a homologue of human Leber congenital amaurosis. *Genomics* **88:** 293–301. doi:10.1016/j.ygeno.2006.05.004

Menotti-Raymond M, David VA, Schaffer AA, Stephens R, Wells D, Kumar-Singh R, O'Brien SJ, Narfström K. 2007. Mutation in *CEP290* discovered for cat model of human retinal degeneration. *J Heredity* **98:** 211–220. doi:10.1093/jhered/esm019

Menotti-Raymond M, Deckman KH, David V, Myrkalo J, O'Brien SJ, Narfström K. 2010. Mutation discovered in a feline model of human congenital retinal blinding disease. *Invest Ophthalmol Vis Sci* **51:** 2852–2859. doi:10.1167/iovs.09-4261

Michalakis S, Gerhardt M, Rudolph G, Priglinger S, Priglinger C. 2022. Achromatopsia: genetics and gene therapy. *Mol Diagn Ther* **26:** 51–59. doi:10.1007/s40291-021-00565-z

Minella AL, Occelli LM, Narfstrom K, Petersen-Jones SM. 2018. Central retinal preservation in rdAc cats. *Vet Ophthalmol* **21:** 224–232.

Miyadera K, Kato K, Aguirre-Hernandez J, Tokuriki T, Morimoto K, Busse C, Barnett K, Holmes N, Ogawa H, Sasaki N, et al. 2009. Phenotypic variation and genotype-phenotype discordance in canine cone-rod dystrophy with an *RPGRIP1* mutation. *Mol Vis* **15:** 2287–2305.

Miyadera K, Acland GM, Aguirre GD. 2012. Genetic and phenotypic variations of inherited retinal diseases in dogs: the power of within- and across-breed studies. *Mamm Genome* **23:** 40–61. doi:10.1007/s00335-011-9361-3

Miyadera K, Murgiano L, Spector C, Marinho FP, Dufour V, Das RG, Brooks M, Swaroop A, Aguirre GD. 2018. Isolated population helps tease out a third locus underlying a multigenic form of canine *RPGRIP1* cone-rod dystrophy. *Invest Ophthalmol Vis Sci* **59:** 1438–1438.

Miyadera K, Santana E, Roszak K, Iffrig S, Visel M, Iwabe S, Boyd RF, Bartoe JT, Sato Y, Gray A, et al. 2022. Targeting ON-bipolar cells by AAV gene therapy stably reverses *LRIT3*-congenital stationary night blindness. *Proc Natl Acad Sci* **119:** e2117038119. doi:10.1073/pnas.2117038119

Mowat FM, Petersen-Jones SM, Williamson H, Williams DL, Luthert PJ, Ali RR, Bainbridge JW. 2008. Topographical characterization of cone photoreceptors and the area centralis of the canine retina. *Mol Vis* **14:** 2518–2527.

Murgiano L, Becker D, Torjman D, Niggel JK, Milano A, Cullen C, Feng R, Wang F, Jagannathan V, Pearce-Kelling S, et al. 2019. Complex structural *PPT1* variant associated with non-syndromic canine retinal degeneration. *G3 (Bethesda)* **9:** 425–437. doi:10.1534/g3.118.200859

Narfström K. 1983. Hereditary progressive retinal atrophy in the Abyssinian cat. *J Heredity* **74:** 273–276. doi:10.1093/oxfordjournals.jhered.a109782

Narfström K. 1985. Progressive retinal atrophy in the Abyssinian cat. Clinical characteristics. *Invest Ophthalmol Vis Sci* **26:** 193–200.

Narfström K, Nilsson SE. 1989. Morphological findings during retinal development and maturation in hereditary rod-cone degeneration in Abyssinian cats. *Exp Eye Res* **49:** 611–628. doi:10.1016/S0014-4835(89)80058-2

Narfström K, Wrigstad A. 1999. Clinical, electrophysiological and morphological changes in a case of hereditary retinal degeneration in the Papillon dog. *Vet Ophthalmol* **2:** 67–74. doi:10.1046/j.1463-5224.1999.00049.x

Narfström K, Wrigstad A, Nilsson SE. 1989. The Briard dog: a new animal model of congenital stationary night blindness. *Br J Ophthalmol* **73:** 750–756. doi:10.1136/bjo.73.9.750

Narfström K, Bragadóttir R, Redmond TM, Rakoczy PE, van VT, Bruun A. 2003. Functional and structural evaluation after AAV.RPE65 gene transfer in the canine model of Leber's congenital amaurosis. *Adv Exp Med Biol* **533:** 423–430. doi:10.1007/978-1-4615-0067-4_54

Occelli LM, Tran NM, Narfström K, Chen S, Petersen-Jones SM. 2016. crx^rdy^ cat: a large animal model for *CRX*-associated Leber congenital amaurosis. *Invest Ophthalmol Vis Sci* **57:** 3780–3792. doi:10.1167/iovs.16-19444

Occelli LM, Schön C, Seeliger MW, Biel M, Michalakis S, Petersen-Jones S; RD-CURE Consortium. 2017. Gene supplementation rescues rod function and preserves photoreceptor and retinal morphology in dogs, leading the way toward treating human *PDE6A*-retinitis pigmentosa. *Hum Gene Ther* **28:** 1189–1201. doi:10.1089/hum.2017.155

Occelli LM, Michalakis S, Biel M; RD-Cure Consortium; Petersen-Jones SM. 2020. Gene augmentation therapy in a large animal model of *PDE6A*-retinitis pigmentosa results in functional and structural rescue for at least 2.5 years. *Invest Ophthalmol Vis Sci* **61:** 1913–1913.

Occelli LM, Daruwalla A, De Silva SR, Winkler PA, Sun K, Pasmanter N, Minella A, Querubin J, Lyons LA, Consortium L, et al. 2022. A large animal model of *RDH5*-associated retinopathy recapitulates important features of the human phenotype. *Hum Mol Genet* **31:** 1263–1277. doi:10.1093/hmg/ddab316

Ofri R, Averbukh E, Ezra-Elia R, Ross M, Honig H, Obolensky A, Rosov A, Hauswirth WW, Gootwine E, Banin E. 2018. Six years and counting: restoration of photopic retinal function and visual behavior following gene augmentation therapy in a sheep model of *CNGA3* achromatopsia. *Hum Gene Ther* **29:** 1376–1386. doi:10.1089/hum.2018.076

Parry HB. 1953. Degenerations of the dog retina. II: Generalized progressive atrophy of hereditary origin. *Br J Ophthalmol* **37:** 487–502. doi:10.1136/bjo.37.8.487

Petersen-Jones SM, Entz DD, Sargan DR. 1999. cGMP phosphodiesterase-α mutation causes progressive retinal atrophy in the Cardigan Welsh corgi dog. *Invest Ophthalmol Vis Sci* **40:** 1637–1644.

Petersen-Jones SM, Annear MJ, Bartoe JT, Mowat FM, Barker SE, Smith AJ, Bainbridge JW, Ali RR. 2012. Gene augmentation trials using the Rpe65-deficient dog: contributions towards development and refinement of human clinical trials. *Adv Exp Med Biol* **723:** 177–182. doi:10.1007/978-1-4614-0631-0_24

Petersen-Jones SM, Occelli LM, Winkler PA, Lee W, Sparrow JR, Tsukikawa M, Boye SL, Chiodo V, Capasso JE, Becirovic E, et al. 2018. Patients and animal models of CNGβ1-deficient retinitis pigmentosa support gene augmentation approach. *J Clin Invest* **128:** 190–206. doi:10.1172/JCI95161

Petersen-Jones SM, Pasmanter N, Occelli LM, Querubin JR, Winkler PA. 2022. Residual rod function in *CNGB1* mutant dogs. *Doc Ophthalmol* **145:** 237–246.

Petit L, Lhériteau E, Weber M, Le Meur G, Deschamps JY, Provost N, Mendes-Madeira A, Libeau L, Guihal C, Colle MA, et al. 2012. Restoration of vision in the pde6β-deficient dog, a large animal model of rod-cone dystrophy. *Mol Ther* **20:** 2019–2030. doi:10.1038/mt.2012.134

Pichard V, Provost N, Mendes-Madeira A, Libeau L, Hulin P, Tshilenge KT, Biget M, Ameline B, Deschamps JY, Weber M, et al. 2016. AAV-mediated gene therapy halts retinal degeneration in PDE6β-deficient dogs. *Mol Ther* **24:** 867–876. doi:10.1038/mt.2016.37

Rah H, Maggs DJ, Blankenship TN, Narfström K, Lyons LA. 2005. Early-onset, autosomal recessive, progressive retinal atrophy in Persian cats. *Invest Ophthalmol Vis Sci* **46:** 1742–1747. doi:10.1167/iovs.04-1019

Rivolta C, Berson EL, Dryja TP. 2001. Dominant Leber congenital amaurosis, cone-rod degeneration, and retinitis pigmentosa caused by mutant versions of the transcription factor CRX. *Hum Mutat* **18:** 488–498. doi:10.1002/humu.1226

Rubin LF. 1971a. Clinical features of hemeralopia in the adult Alaskan malamute. *J Am Vet Med Assoc* **158:** 1696.

Rubin LF. 1971b. Hemeralopia in Alaskan malamute pups. *J Am Vet Med Assoc* **158:** 1699.

Russell S, Bennett J, Wellman JA, Chung DC, Yu ZF, Tillman A, Wittes J, Pappas J, Elci O, McCague S, et al. 2017. Efficacy and safety of voretigene neparvovec (AAV2-hRPE65v2) in patients with *RPE65*-mediated inherited

Cite this article as *Cold Spring Harb Perspect Med* doi: 10.1101/cshperspect.a041286

retinal dystrophy: a randomised, controlled, open-label, phase 3 trial. *Lancet* **390**: 849–860. doi:10.1016/S0140-6736(17)31868-8

Santos-Anderson RM, Tso M, Wolf ED. 1980. An inherited retinopathy in collies: a light and electron microscopic study. *Invest Ophthalmol Vis Sci* **19**: 1282–1294.

Shin T, Kraemer D, Pryor J, Liu L, Rugila J, Howe L, Buck S, Murphy K, Lyons L, Westhusin M. 2002. A cat cloned by nuclear transplantation. *Nature* **415**: 859. doi:10.1038/nature723

Sidjanin DJ, Lowe JK, McElwee JL, Milne BS, Phippen TM, Sargan DR, Aguirre GD, Acland GM, Ostrander EA. 2002. Canine *CNGB3* mutations establish cone degeneration as orthologous to the human achromatopsia locus *ACHM3*. *Hum Mol Genet* **11**: 1823–1833. doi:10.1093/hmg/11.16.1823

Somma AT, Duque Moreno JC, Sato MT, Rodrigues BD, Bacellar-Galdino M, Occelli LM, Petersen-Jones SM, Montiani-Ferreira F. 2017. Characterization of a novel form of progressive retinal atrophy in whippet dogs: a clinical, electroretinographic, and breeding study. *Vet Ophthalmol* **20**: 450–459. doi:10.1111/vop.12448

Suber ML, Pittler SJ, Quin N, Wright GC, Holcombe N, Lee RH, Craft CM, Lolley RN, Baehr W, Hurwitz RL. 1993. Irish setter dogs affected with rod/cone dysplasia contain a nonsense mutation in the rod cGMP phosphodiesterase β-subunit gene. *Proc Natl Acad Sci* **90**: 3968–3972. doi:10.1073/pnas.90.9.3968

Sudharsan R, Simone KM, Anderson NP, Aguirre GD, Beltran WA. 2017. Acute and protracted cell death in light-induced retinal degeneration in the canine model of rhodopsin autosomal dominant retinitis pigmentosa. *Invest Ophthalmol Vis Sci* **58**: 270–281. doi:10.1167/iovs.16-20749

Tanaka N, Dutrow EV, Miyadera K, Delemotte L, MacDermaid CM, Reinstein SL, Crumley WR, Dixon CJ, Casal ML, Klein ML, et al. 2015. Canine *CNGA3* gene mutations provide novel insights into human achromatopsia-associated channelopathies and treatment. *PLoS ONE* **10**: e0138943. doi:10.1371/journal.pone.0138943

Tran NM, Chen S. 2014. Mechanisms of blindness: animal models provide insight into distinct *CRX*-associated retinopathies. *Dev Dyn* **243**: 1153–1166. doi:10.1002/dvdy.24151

Tuntivanich N, Pittler SJ, Fischer AJ, Omar G, Kiupel M, Weber A, Yao S, Steibel JP, Khan NW, Petersen-Jones SM. 2009. Characterization of a canine model of autosomal recessive retinitis pigmentosa due to a *PDE6A* mutation. *Invest Ophthalmol Vis Sci* **50**: 801–813. doi:10.1167/iovs.08-2562

Vervoort R, Lennon A, Bird AC, Tulloch B, Axton R, Miano MG, Meindl A, Meitinger T, Ciccodicola A, Wright AF. 2000. Mutational hot spot within a new *RPGR* exon in X-linked retinitis pigmentosa. *Nat Genet* **25**: 462–466. doi:10.1038/78182

Veske A, Nilsson SE, Narfström K, Gal A. 1999. Retinal dystrophy of Swedish briard/briard–beagle dogs is due to a 4-bp deletion in *RPE65*. *Genomics* **57**: 57–61. doi:10.1006/geno.1999.5754

Winkler PA, Ekenstedt KJ, Occelli LM, Frattaroli AV, Bartoe JT, Venta PJ, Petersen-Jones SM. 2013. A large animal model for *CNGB1* autosomal recessive retinitis pigmentosa. *PLoS ONE* **8**: e72229. doi:10.1371/journal.pone.0072229

Winkler PA, Occelli LM, Petersen-Jones SM. 2020. Large animal models of inherited retinal degenerations: a review. *Cells* **9**: 882. doi:10.3390/cells9040882

Wrigstad A, Narfström K, Nilsson SE. 1994. Slowly progressive changes of the retina and retinal pigment epithelium in briard dogs with hereditary retinal dystrophy. A morphological study. *Doc Ophthalmol* **87**: 337–354. doi:10.1007/BF01203343

Ye GJ, Komáromy AM, Zeiss C, Calcedo R, Harman CD, Koehl KL, Stewart GA, Iwabe S, Chiodo VA, Hauswirth WW, et al. 2017. Safety and efficacy of AAV5 vectors expressing human or canine CNGB3 in *CNGB3*-mutant dogs. *Hum Gene Ther Clin Dev* **28**: 197–207. doi:10.1089/humc.2017.125

Yeh CY, Goldstein O, Kukekova AV, Holley D, Knollinger AM, Huson HJ, Pearce-Kelling SE, Acland GM, Komáromy AM. 2013. Genomic deletion of *CNGB3* is identical by descent in multiple canine breeds and causes achromatopsia. *BMC Genet* **14**: 27. doi:10.1186/1471-2156-14-27

Zahid S, Branham K, Schlegel D, Pennesi ME, Michaelides M, Heckenlively J, Jayasundera T. 2018. RPGRIP1. In *Retinal dystrophy gene atlas*, pp. 243–244. Springer, New York.

Zangerl B, Zhang Q, Johnson J, Acland G, Aguirre G. 2002. Independent origin of three microdeletions in RPGR exon ORF15 of canids. *Invest Ophthalmol Vis Sci* **43**: 3674.

Zangerl B, Goldstein O, Philp AR, Lindauer SJ, Pearce-Kelling SE, Mullins RF, Graphodatsky AS, Ripoll D, Felix JS, Stone E, et al. 2006. Identical mutation in a novel retinal gene causes progressive rod-cone degeneration in dogs and retinitis pigmentosa in humans. *Genomics* **88**: 551–563. doi:10.1016/j.ygeno.2006.07.007

Zangerl B, Wickstrom K, Slavik J, Lindauer SJ, Ahonen S, Schelling C, Lohi H, Guziewicz KE, Aguirre GD. 2010. Assessment of canine *BEST1* variations identifies new mutations and establishes an independent bestrophinopathy model (*cmr3*). *Mol Vis* **16**: 2791–2804.

Zeitz C, Kloeckener-Gruissem B, Forster U, Kohl S, Magyar I, Wissinger B, Mátyás G, Borruat FX, Schorderet DF, Zrenner E, et al. 2006. Mutations in *CABP4*, the gene encoding the Ca^{2+}-binding protein 4, cause autosomal recessive night blindness. *Am J Hum Genet* **79**: 657–667. doi:10.1086/508067

Zeitz C, Jacobson SG, Hamel CP, Bujakowska K, Neuillé M, Orhan E, Zanlonghi X, Lancelot ME, Michiels C, Schwartz SB, et al. 2013. Whole-exome sequencing identifies *LRIT3* mutations as a cause of autosomal-recessive complete congenital stationary night blindness. *Am J Hum Genet* **92**: 67–75. doi:10.1016/j.ajhg.2012.10.023

Zhang Q, Acland GM, Wu WX, Johnson JL, Pearce-Kelling S, Tulloch B, Vervoort R, Wright AF, Aguirre GD. 2002. Different *RPGR* exon ORF15 mutations in *Canids* provide insights into photoreceptor cell degeneration. *Hum Mol Genet* **11**: 993–1003. doi:10.1093/hmg/11.9.993

Zou Q, Wang X, Liu Y, Ouyang Z, Long H, Wei S, Xin J, Zhao B, Lai S, Shen J, et al. 2015. Generation of gene-target dogs using CRISPR/Cas9 system. *J Mol Cell Biol* **7**: 580–583. doi:10.1093/jmcb/mjv061

Pig Models in Retinal Research and Retinal Disease

Maureen A. McCall

Departments of Ophthalmology & Visual Sciences and Anatomical Sciences & Neurobiology, University of Louisville, Louisville, Kentucky 40202, USA

Correspondence: mo.mccall@louisville.edu

The pig has been used as a large animal model in biomedical research for many years and its use continues to increase because induced mutations phenocopy several inherited human diseases. In addition, they are continuous breeders, can be propagated by artificial insemination, have large litter sizes (on the order of mice), and can be genetically manipulated using all of the techniques that are currently available in mice. The pioneering work of Petters and colleagues set the stage for the use of the pig as a model of inherited retinal disease. In the last 10 years, the pig has become a model of choice where specific disease-causing mutations that are not phenocopied in rodents need to be studied and therapeutic approaches explored. The pig is not only used for retinal eye disease but also for the study of the cornea and lens. This review attempts to show how broad the use of the pig has become and how it has contributed to the assessment of treatments for eye disease. In the last 10 years, there have been several reviews that included the use of the pig in biomedical research (see body of the review) that included information about retinal disease. None directly discuss the use of the pig as an animal model for retinal diseases, including inherited diseases, where a single genetic mutation has been identified or for multifactorial diseases such as glaucoma and diabetic retinopathy. Although the pig is used to explore diseases of the cornea and lens, this review focuses on how and why the pig, as a large animal model, is useful for research in neural retinal disease and its treatment.

The focus of this review is to describe how the pig has been used as a model of human disease and, in light of that, how it can be used as an emerging model in the future. Because of the use of the pig in agriculture, many aspects of pig anatomy, physiology, metabolism, immunity, and cognition have been well described. This background has been used in the creation and use of the pig in general biomedical research.

These data provide significant background about the pig that is relevant to its use in retinal research, and as an emerging model of retinal disease. The review is organized around the areas of commonality between the pig and human and how they positively impact the future of the pig as a model of retinal disease. The article does not serve as a comparison between pigs and other species that also are used in retinal research. These comparisons are only mentioned when relevant to why the pig could be an improvement over other currently used species.

PHYSICAL CHARACTERISTICS OF THE PIG EYE

There are many aspects of the pig including its eye and retina that make it ideal as a model to characterize disease natural history, as well as to develop and evaluate various therapeutics and surgical devices. The pig's overall body size from birth to maturity is similar to human (Hou et al. 2022). In addition to larger domestic pigs, a variety of strains that are even smaller at maturity are available (Panepinto et al. 1983). Although domestic piglets are smaller than full-term human infants at birth (MA McCall, unpubl.; pig mean ~1.3 kg/~3 lb), they grow quickly and then track human weight gain through to about 7 mo of age, when the majority of pigs attain a weight of ~100 kg (Fig. 1). Comparisons of sizes of various pig strains used in biomedical research can be found in Gutierrez et al. (2015).

EYE SIZE AND RETINAL MORPHOLOGY

Eye size and growth are similar between pig and human (for reviews, see Bertschinger et al. 2008; Middleton 2010; Sanchez et al. 2011). For example, the neonatal pig eye is ~17 mm to ~25 mm

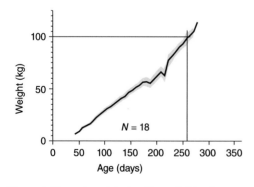

Figure 1. Pigs gain weight in a linear fashion between about P50 through P250. The solid lines define the age × weight when animals can be group housed. When pigs reach 100 kg, they must be housed singly, and this may cause problems related to space in the vivarium.

in diameter (Fig. 2). These similarities translate into several benefits for eye and retinal research. The pig is used in easily translated therapeutic dosing in young infants through mature patients (Liu et al. 2014; Turner et al. 2016; Lansing et al. 2018; Vrolyk et al. 2020). The eye size similarity to human is used to develop surgical or transplantation procedures (Sørensen et al. 2012; McAllister et al. 2013; Kim et al. 2015; de Smet et al. 2016; Soler et al. 2017; Vecino et al. 2018; Palácios et al. 2019; Sørensen 2019; Bantseev et al. 2020; Han et al. 2022; Li et al. 2022a,d) as well as subretinal or intravitreal dosing of therapeutic drugs/agents (Cehofski et al. 2018, 2022; Bantseev et al. 2020; Olsen et al. 2020). Finally, the similarity in eye size and the presence of a visual streak provides the ability to develop and test tools for eye/retinal surgery (Bergeles et al. 2011; Brant Fernandes et al. 2016; Fernandes et al. 2017; Gatto et al. 2021), determine biodistribution, as well as indwelling devices (e.g., prosthetics) (for reviews, see Bertschinger et al. 2008; Ivastinovic et al. 2010, 2012; Bosse et al. 2011; Kelly et al. 2011; Zhao et al. 2012; Waschkowski et al. 2013; Adekunle et al. 2015; Noda et al. 2015; Lohmann et al. 2019; Chen et al. 2020; Choi et al. 2020; Maya-Vetencourt et al. 2020; Shire et al. 2020; Vu et al. 2022), scaffolds (Fujie et al. 2014; Popelka et al. 2015; Peng et al. 2016; Gonzalez-Calle et al. 2018; Thompson et al. 2019; Gandhi et al. 2020; Wendland et al. 2021), or cell transplants (Li et al. 2009; Fjord-Larsen et al. 2010; Koss et al. 2016; García Delgado et al. 2019; Kashani et al. 2019; Sharma et al. 2019; Stanzel et al. 2019).

While the pig does not have a fovea like humans and some nonhuman primates, it has a visual streak with high cone densities ranging from 20,000 to 35,000/mm^2 (Fig. 3; Hendrickson and Hicks, 2002). The streak runs across the horizontal meridian of the eye from nasal to temporal retina and is ~7 mm in the superior to inferior direction (pink). Its inferior edge runs through the optic disc (OD). There are two small areas, nasal and temporal, that contain the highest cone density (black). On the temporal side, one area is ~2.5 mm temporal to the OD. On the nasal side, the other area is ~6 mm nasal to the disc; both are located just superior to the disc. Whether these areas are similar to the macula/fovea has

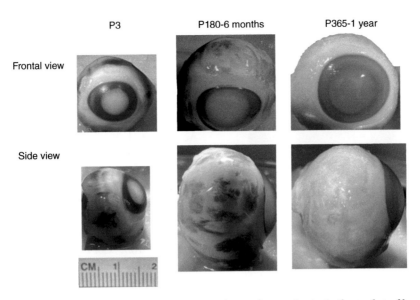

Figure 2. Pig eye size changes from birth to 1 year. At each age, the eye size is similar to that of humans. This feature, as well as the similar vasculature and the absence of a tapetum, makes the pig eye most similar to human, with the exception of nonhuman primates.

not been, but should be, explored. The pig retina has both a larger overall number of cones compared to human, 17–20 versus 5 million (Curcio et al. 1990; Hendrickson and Hicks 2002) and a higher cone:rod ratio (Packer et al. 1989; Hendrickson and Hicks 2002). The pig is a dichromat with medium (556 nm) and short (439 nm) wavelength cones (Szél et al. 1988; Neitz and Jacobs 1989). Figure 4 shows the morphology of pig rods and cones at postnatal day 90.

The retinal ganglion cell–packing density mirrors the cone densities (Garcá et al. 2005), and there have been several studies characterizing their morphology (Hebel 1976; Peichl et al. 1987; Garcia et al. 2002; Ruiz-Ederra et al. 2003; Veiga-Crespo et al. 2013; Pereiro et al. 2020). Two recent studies examined the morphologies of pig retinal ganglion cells (Veiga-Crespo et al. 2013) and the distributions of retinal ganglion cells with small, medium, and large somas (Garcá et al. 2005). The majority of cells with small somas are found within the streak (Garcá et al. 2005) and the morphology of these cells has counterparts in the mouse and rabbit retina (Veiga-Crespo et al. 2013). Even with these results, it is still not clear what the morphology of the ganglion cells is in areas with the highest density. As such, we still do not

know whether there is a midget system in the pig. Further, the remaining retinal circuitry at any location in the retina has not been thoroughly examined and should be a priority in the future (Fig. 5).

RETINAL DEVELOPMENT

There have been a variety of studies that have characterized the fetal and postnatal development and expression patterns of proteins related to specific retinal cell types in the pig from as early as fetal day 39 (Ghosh and Arner 2010) through to mid- and late gestation (Wang et al. 2014) and postnatal development (Guduric-Fuchs et al. 2009). There is a review of the pre- and postnatal development of the eye that compares across several species and includes human, nonhuman primate, pig, dog, rat, and mouse (Van Cruchten et al. 2017). There is general agreement that the pig retina is primarily composed of neuroblasts that express Pax6, although the retinal ganglion cell layer is beginning to form and Brn3B[+] retinal ganglion cells are clearly evident at ~E65. Recoverin[+] cells are found in the outer portion of the neuroblastic layer as early as E50, presumably marking the emerging cone photoreceptors.

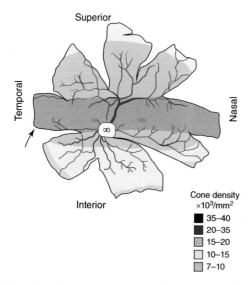

Figure 3. The distribution of cone density in the adult pig retina relative to its vascular pattern. The visual streak (pink) stretches from nasal to temporal margins and is approximately 7 mm from inferior to superior and begins directly above the optic disc (OD). There are two areas, one in nasal and one temporal to the OD that have the highest cone density (gray). Note that the inferior retina (yellow) has very low cone density compared to the superior (green) retina. (Figure adapted from Hendrickson and Hicks 2002, with permission from Elsevier Science © 2002.)

L-/M- and S-opsin expression arises at about E85 at about the same time, and rhodopsin expression is evident (Wang et al. 2014). At birth, the pig retina is fully differentiated; the mature lamination pattern is present as are the markers for the major cell classes of the inner retina (see summary in Fig. 5; Guduric-Fuchs et al. 2009). Further, retinal function matures (using the ERG) between P30 and P60 (Fig. 6). The pig, like nonhuman primates and human babies, are born with their eyes open and can process visual information. Like the pig, retinal function becomes more mature with age.

METABOLIC SIMILARITIES MAKE THE PIG A GOOD MODEL OF DIABETIC RETINOPATHY

Metabolic similarities also allow for the development of several pig models of diabetes (for reviews, see Lai and Lo 2013; Ludwig et al.

2020; also see Lee et al. 2010; King et al. 2011; Hein et al. 2012; Pepper et al. 2013; Guo et al. 2015; Acharya et al. 2017; Kleinwort et al. 2017; Umeyama et al. 2017; Bulc et al. 2020; Ludwig et al. 2020; Niu et al. 2020, 2022). Several of these pig models document aspects of diabetic retinopathy (Hein et al. 2012; Renner et al. 2016; Acharya et al. 2017; Kleinwort et al. 2017; Bek 2019; Nagaya et al. 2020). One in particular is the Ossabaw pig, which can be fed a Western diet to produce diabetes that includes the early signs of diabetic retinopathy as well as changes in the corneal stroma (Fig. 7; Lim et al. 2018; Sinha et al. 2021). These pigs are commercially available from CorVus Biomedical (corvus-biomed.org). These pigs also have highly pigmented retinal pigment epithelial (RPE) cells, which may be of use for laser or other chemical treatments.

There are models where certain aspects of diabetic retinopathy have been evaluated and used to evaluate treatments (for reviews, see Renner et al. 2016; Kleinwort et al. 2017; Zettler et al. 2020). Ocular manifestations of diabetes in

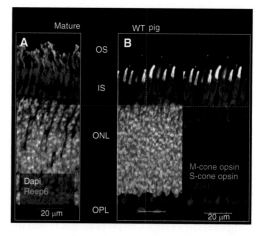

Figure 4. Confocal images of rods (A) and cones (B) in the mature wild-type (WT) pig retina. Rod morphology can be demonstrated using Reep6 (green; gift of Anand Swaroop), and rhodopsin expression (magenta) is localized to the tips of the rod outer segments (OS). Cone morphology can be demonstrated using GNAT2 (magenta; gift of James Hurley) and the expression of M- or S-opsin is localized to the tips of the cone OS. (IS) Inner segment, (ONL) outer nuclear layer, (OPL) outer plexiform layer.

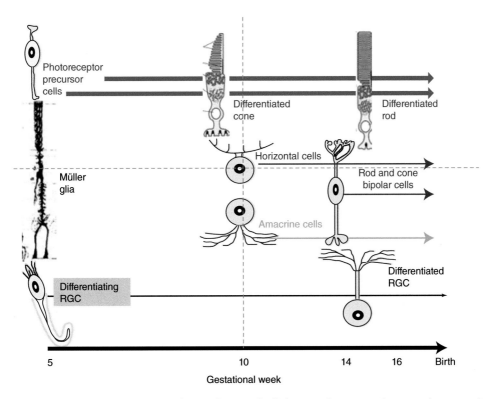

Figure 5. Diagram of the differentiation of particular retinal cell classes in the pigs as a function of gestational age. Gestation is completed at about 16 weeks. The differentiation pattern of cells in the pig retina is similar to most mammals and the timing is similar to humans. At birth, pigs like humans are born with their eyes open and can use their vision to navigate around their pen. (RGC) Retinal ganglion cell.

pig models has been reviewed in Zettler et al. (2020) and include cataracts in INSC[94Y] (Kleinert et al. 2018) and in HNF1A[P231fsinsC] transgenic pigs, as well as streptozotocin (STZ) or diet-induced diabetic pigs (Chen et al. 2009; Niu et al. 2020). Similarly, there are many publications that show the similarities between diabetic pig models and human vasculature changes such as retinal hemorrhage, cotton-wool spots, and central edema in HNF1A[P231fsinsC] (Kleinwort et al. 2017). Changes in retinal layer thickness, cell density, Müller cell morphology, microglia, and in the expression of cone arrestin have been reported in diabetic pigs (Acharya et al. 2017; Kleinwort et al. 2017; Nagaya et al. 2020; Renner 2020). Despite these in-depth investigations of the ocular and retinal phenotypes in diabetic pig models, there appears to be no research into how these manifestations alter retinal function or in visual behavior, even though

there are clear indications in diabetic rodent models (Aung et al. 2014; Pardue et al. 2014; Moore-Dotson et al. 2016; Kim et al. 2018; Allen et al. 2019, 2020; Moore-Dotson and Eggers 2019; Eggers and Carreon 2020; Flood et al. 2020, 2022).

Immune System in Retinal Transplants and Viral-Mediated Gene Therapy in the Pig

Similarities in the pig and human metabolic rates, immune systems, as well as organ physiology are well documented in part because of the potential to use the pig in xenotransplantation. The immune system of the pig also has been well studied (for a recent review, see Pabst 2020). In brief, after primate and mouse immune systems, the pig is the next-best characterized, and its immune system is estimated as 80% similar to human (Dawson et al. 2011). The similarities between pig and

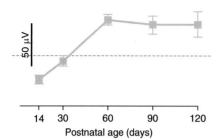

WT pig scotopic ERG development

50 μV

14   30   60   90   120

Postnatal age (days)

Figure 6. Wild-type (WT) rod-isolated retinal function (measured by the dark-adapted full-field electroretinogram) (flash = 0.01 cd·sec/m²) is immature at birth and the b-wave amplitude increases and plateaus by P60. (Figure adapted from Fernandez de Castro et al. 2014, with permission from the Association for Research in Vision & Ophthalmology [ARVO] © 2014.) This maturation is also found for the cone-evoked response (see Fig. 8).

human across the different types of immune cells are described in detail in Pabst (2020). As a result, the pig offers a wide range of established methods and tools for assessing inflammation and toxicology (see descriptions in Summerfield 2009; Bode et al. 2010; Forster et al. 2010a,b).

Successful pig solid organ transplantation to humans is yet to be realized, although many genetically modified pigs have been produced to reduce rejection (for reviews, see Deng et al. 2022; Denner 2022; Mueller and Denner 2022; Shahab et al. 2022; Sykes and Sachs 2022). Human corneal transplants, like in other organs, are not readily available, and pig corneas are being preprocessed (decellularization and/or cross-linking) to produce cell-free tissue for transplantation to humans, and are tolerated because the tissue poses no risk for rejection (for reviews, see Kim et al. 2014; Lamm et al. 2014; Kim and Hara 2015; Isidan et al. 2019, 2021; Song and Pan 2019; Islam et al. 2021; Santillo et al. 2021; Yoon et al. 2021; Li et al. 2022b). Together, the impetus to create new genetically modified pigs and engineered tissue holds hope for the use of pig cells and organs for human transplantation.

The in-depth comparisons of pig and human immune systems also arise because of the potential to use pig in regeneration and in

screening of new drugs for retinal and other diseases and for immunotoxicity. As a result, this growing literature can be referenced when a pig is used to screen inflammatory response or toxicology to drugs, virus, or other molecules injected subretinally or intravitreally for treatment of retinal disease. All of these studies/resources, enhance the ability to use the pig for the study of immune responses after any retinal manipulation. Two recent studies used pigs to evaluate immune reaction after allogenic transplantation into the subretinal space. The most recent assessed allogenic transplantation of porcine fetal retinal progenitor cells (pRPCs) into the pig subretinal space (Abud et al. 2022). Without immunosuppression, GFP⁺ pRPCs survived for 12 wk. In only small numbers of host CD45⁺ cells, a marker immune system activation was present, and their numbers correlated with the numbers of transplanted progenitor cells. Further, no host immune response was found in a variety of somatic tissue samples. Another study used induced pluripotent stem cell–derived RPE cells in a similar allogenic transplantation approach (Sohn et al. 2015). However, these investigators found elevated IL-12 levels in the vitreous (note, not sampled in Abud et al. 2022), as well as CD45⁺ cells in retinal tissue. The cause for these contrasting results warrants further study in the future.

With respect to gene therapy, the most common vector system for ocular gene therapy is adeno-associated virus (AAV). As with transplantation, immune response to AAV delivery both intravitreally and subretinally has been studied in a variety of animal models (for review, see Bucher et al. 2021). There is increasing evidence that AAV can cause both local and systemic immune or inflammatory responses in many species (Ren et al. 2022) including dogs (Boyd et al. 2016; Ye et al. 2017). These reactions can be directed against the AAV capsid protein, the vector DNA, the promoter, or the transgene itself, and also have been reported to result from impurities included as a byproduct of the manufacturing process of virus (Bucher et al. 2021; Hamilton and Wright 2021). In our hands in the pig, inflammatory ocular responses develop primarily when the AAV viral titer is high (>1 × 10¹¹ viral

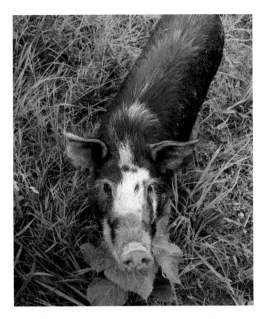

Figure 7. A young Ossabaw pig. (Figure from Aerin Telcontar and reprinted under the Creative Commons Attribution-Share Alike 4.0 International License.)

genomes [vg]/eye), and we have not observed a difference in the frequency of inflammation induced by subretinal versus intravitreal, although we have not performed parametric studies to date (MA McCall, unpubl.).

AAV vectors trigger an immune response via the binding of Toll-like receptors (TLR2 or TLR9), and a motif that contains a cytosine nucleotide is followed by a guanine nucleotide in the linear sequence of bases along its $5' \rightarrow 3'$ direction (CpG). As a test of this hypothesis, we (Chan et al. 2019, 2021) used a strategy to block TLR9 activation. We engineered a short TLR9 inhibitory sequence (TLR9i) and incorporated it into the vector genome. The construct was evaluated both in vitro and in vivo in mice. As a test of its efficacy in the pig eye, similarly, we engineered and injected subretinally a version with the inflammation-inhibiting oligonucleotide (AAV8.GFP.io2) into wild-type (WT) pigs (4×10^{11} vg/eye). Controls were injected with AAV8.GFP without io2. At 6 wk postinjection (wpi), the morphology of cone outer segments was degraded in all five of the AAV8.GFP eyes, whereas cone outer segments

were more similar to vehicle or uninjected controls in AAV8.GFP.io2-injected contralateral eyes (Chan et al. 2019). In all eyes, changes were noted in the outer retinal layers using sdOCT b-scans, although in AAV8.GFP.io2 eyes, damage was both less severe and laminar changes at 2 wpi were resolving at 6 wpi (the last time point studied). Finally, AAV8.GFP stimulated robust microglial infiltration into the outer nuclear layer and elevated the number of CD8$^+$ T cells infiltrated into the neural retina. Neither of these hallmarks of an inflammatory response were found in eyes treated with AAV8.GFP.io2, indicating that the Toll-like receptor 9 likely plays a role in an inflammatory response when the retina is challenged by an AAV. Inclusion of these blocking sequences may be beneficial if viral vector therapies do produce an immune response.

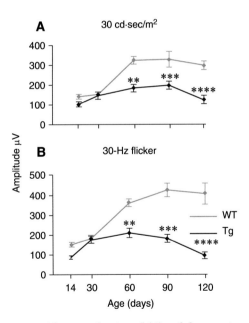

Figure 8. The cone-dominated (*A*) and the cone-isolated 30-Hz flicker (*B*) responses mature similarly in wild-type (WT) and TgP23H littermates to at least P30 and then begin to diverge, with the WT cone response reaching maturity between P60 and P90. To establish statistical differences, an *n* of 10 to 12 animals were included in the data sets. (Figure adapted from Fernandez de Castro et al. 2014, with permission from the Association for Research in Vision & Ophthalmology [ARVO] © 2014.)

Husbandry and Genetic Manipulations in the Pig

Pig breeding is highly standardized and can be accomplished by natural or artificial insemination. Pigs are sexually mature at ~6 mo of age. The estrous cycle is about 24 d and a sow reenters estrus 4–7 d after a litter is weaned (Soede et al. 2011). Gestation time is 114 d, litter sizes are large (on average 12 piglets), and a sow can produce two to three litters per year. All of these factors make pigs a practical large animal model for research compared with other species, where offspring size can be extremely small, gestation times considerably longer, and estrus occurs less frequently. This is particularly true when large cohorts of genetically modified animals are needed to track the natural history of disease (e.g., Petters et al. 1997; Li et al. 1998; Fernandez de Castro et al. 2014; Scott et al. 2014) or for examination of therapeutic strategies, where statistical power requires at least five to six pigs per experimental group (as in Fig. 8, where we tracked the changes in cone function in a transgenic P23H hRho pig model of autosomal-dominant retinitis pigmentosa [RP]).

Current Molecular Manipulations Are Available to Create Pig Models of Disease— Pigs Can Be Genetically Engineered Using Methods Available in Other Species

The pig has been the focus of the development of molecular genetic manipulation first because of agricultural needs (Wells and Prather 2017) and following upon that as a large animal model for diseases (for review, see Whitworth et al. 2022). As mentioned above, because the pig resembles the human in size, anatomy, physiology, and immune system, there are many cases in which the pig recapitulates the human phenotype where genetically engineered mice fall short. For example, cystic fibrosis, neurofibromatosis, diabetes, and Batten's disease, among others, have been much more accurately recapitulated in pigs (Rogers et al. 2008; Welsh et al. 2009; Beraldi et al. 2015; Kleinwort et al. 2017; Isakson et al. 2018; White et al. 2018; Swier et al. 2022). In addition, neurodegenerative diseases that require longer life spans (e.g., Huntington's [Yan et al. 2018] or Alzheimer's [Jakobsen et al. 2016; Andersen et al. 2022]) or brain morphology similar to human (e.g., traumatic brain injury [TBI]) are challenging in rodents and, again, many models do not recapitulate the human disease manifestation. The pig has been shown to be better suited to the study of these diseases (for thorough reviews, see Hoffe and Holahan 2019; Yang et al. 2021) and tests of their visual as well as cognitive abilities have been developed (Murphy et al. 2013). All of these models and the assays for visually guided behavior are suitable for characterizing pig models of retinal dysfunction. The largest resource for genetically modified pig models is the National Swine Resource and Research Center (NSRRC) at the University of Missouri (nsrrc.missouri.edu). The NSRRC assists with the growing need for pig models by providing a list of current and future strains and provides consulting regarding the creation of new pig models.

Transgenic Pig Models of Retinal Disease

Three transgenic pig models of RP have been published. The first expressed a mutant pig rhodopsin transgene, with a Pro346Leu mutation. The effects of its expression were well characterized, and these pigs were used in both transplantation and gene-editing strategies (Petters et al. 1997; Tso et al. 1997; Li et al. 1998; Banin et al. 1999; Blackmon et al. 2000; Huang et al. 2000; Peng et al. 2000; Ghosh et al. 2004; Kraft et al. 2005; Ng et al. 2008; Sommer et al. 2011; Klassen et al. 2012). Two transgenic pig models have been created that express a human mutant gene. The first expresses the P23H human rhodopsin gene and its natural history of photoreceptor dysfunction was characterized over several founder lines (Ross et al. 2012). Subsequently, the natural history of one line, 53-1, has been characterized in detail showing the time line of both altered rod photoreceptor number and morphology as well as rod photoreceptor dysfunction (Ross et al. 2012; Fernandez de Castro et al. 2014; Scott et al. 2014, 2015). More recently, we have tracked the morphology of the rods and cones in these pigs (Fig. 9). The third is a pig model of cone-rod dystrophy (GUCY2D) created via lentiviral trans-

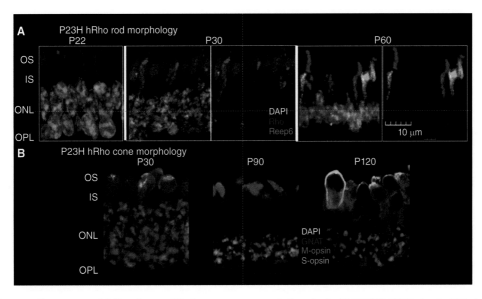

Figure 9. Changes in rod (*A*) and cone (*B*) photoreceptor morphology in the TgP23H hRHO pig. At P22, there remain many rods with rhodopsin expression (magenta) in their outer segments (OS). With time, the number of rods with rhodopsin expression decline and the number of rods (labeled with REEP6, green) also decline, albeit more slowly. (*B*) Similarly, cone morphology (GNAT2, magenta) changes with age and the outer/inner segment (OS/IS) morphology becomes bulbous. Cone opsin expression remains past P120. (ONL) Outer nuclear layer, (OPL) outer plexiform layer.

genesis (Kostic et al. 2013). Here, too, heterogeneity of RP among the founders was characterized but no further manipulations have been reported.

Retinal Gene Editing, the Creation of Pig Models of Retinal Disease

Genetically manipulated pigs are now created with somatic cell nuclear transfer (SCNT) using cells that have been genetically modified with one of several nucleases (Ryu et al. 2018). The first used zinc finger nucleases (ZFNs). This approach was rapidly replaced by transcription activator-like effector nucleases (TALENs) as the approach was shown more successful. Most recently by clustered regularly interspaced short palindromic repeats/CRISPR-associated 9 (CRISPR-Cas9), gene editing has replaced these less-efficient editors, and the CRISPR-Cas9 system is continuously being enhanced to improve editing efficiency and specificity.

There are many reviews of the various iterations using CRISPR-Cas9 to create mutant pig models, and that information will not be covered here (Gao et al. 2021; Ratner et al. 2021; Yang et al. 2021; Zhang et al. 2021; Javaid et al. 2022; Shahab et al. 2022; Stirm et al. 2022; Sykes and Sachs 2022; Yin et al. 2022). The numbers of CRISPR-Cas9-generated pig models of disease continue to grow within the last 5 years. Two models of type 2 diabetes (Zou et al. 2019; Li et al. 2022c) have been published, although neither has had ocular changes characterized, to determine whether they could be useful models for diabetic retinopathy. A pig model of USH1C in which the harmonin gene was targeted shows a retinal phenotype (Grotz et al. 2022) as does a pig model of Batten disease (Swier et al. 2022). A pig harboring a natural mutation Myo7 has been described (Derks et al. 2021), but again no retinal phenotype reported. In a pig model of USH3 (mutated clarin1), biallelic heterozygous mutants have both a hearing deficit and a retinal phenotype (A Dinculescu and MA McCall, unpubl.). Each of these new models represents an example of pig model that recapitulated a human disease, whereas the equivalent mouse models failed this crucial test. With these

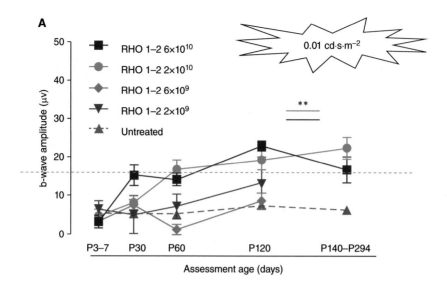

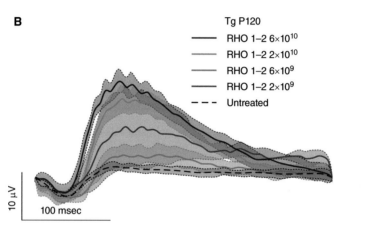

Figure 10. Rod-isolated response. (*A*) When the TgP23H retina is treated at P3 with the meganuclease, Rho1-2, which selectively targets human rhodopsin P23H sequence, rod-isolated responses are produced (no isolated rod response is evoked in untreated Tg retina) and the b-wave amplitude increases as a function of time postinjection. (*B*) There appears to be a plateau in the b-wave between P120 and P294. We have not observed any decline through 1 yr of age in treated retinas.

recent successes, it is likely that more pig models of retinal disease will be created.

Retinal Gene Therapy, the Treatment of Pig Models of Retinal Disease

Several thorough and thoughtful reviews of retinal gene therapy have been published (Bonillo et al. 2022; Leroy et al. 2022), in particular the most recently published review devoted to ge-

nome editing in the eye (Suh et al. 2022). The majority of evaluations of gene therapy in the retina continue to be performed in the mouse or in cells in culture with toxicity evaluated in non-human primates. As described above, there are many drawbacks to the use of mice. In many cases, mouse models do not copy the human phenotype, the eye size makes it difficult to predict the volume and titer/concentration of the therapeutic agent, and the size differential makes it equally difficult to predict the size of the treatment area in the large human eye. Finally, the significant difference in the distribution and density of rods and cones in mice versus humans also makes predictions of the efficacy of treatments difficult. While the nonhuman primates are very appropriate for toxicity evaluations and they could solve these dilemmas, they are a diminishing resource, and ethical concerns make their use as a testing model problematic. The pig and its eye and retina fill many of the gaps left by the mouse for a preclinical animal model. The widespread availability and the ease with which models of disease can be made, not to mention their litter sizes, make the pig an exceptional model for the assessment of therapeutic efficacy. We have used the Tg P23H hRHO pig to assess the efficacy of gene-editing therapies that target the human mutant gene. One successful example are our experiments evaluating a meganuclease (Rho1-2) that targets the human P23H rhodopsin gene. Figures 10 and 11 show that this approach has great potential for translation to the clinic. AAV-mediated delivery of Rho1-2 produces a scotopic response in the Tg retina

where none could be evoked (Fig. 10) and restores/maintains rods with normal morphology and correctly localized rhodopsin expression (Fig. 11).

As more pig models of retinal disease are made and characterized, the prediction is that the pig will become the model of choice for retinal gene therapy. While the engineering of pig models is now well established, there are still gaps in our knowledge. The field needs the complete and fully annotated pig genome, which is well underway. We need academic facilities with the training in pig husbandry and assessment of retinal structure and function to help retinal scientists to characterize and evaluate treatments. We need partnerships with biotechnology and the NIH to provide support for this work, which is more costly than mice, but that will surely lead to new and cutting-edge therapeutic approaches that go beyond AAV or lentivirus delivery and are safer than these viral delivery approaches.

The pig is not the sole model that will be useful in gene therapy evaluations. It will not replace the mouse or the zebrafish as initial screening tools that have faster generation times

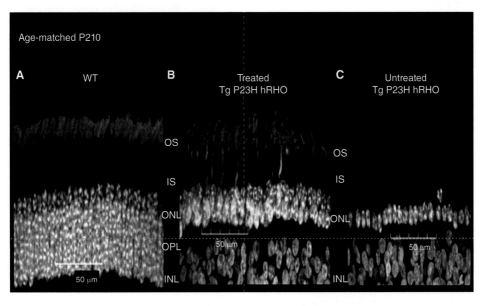

Figure 11. Treatment with Rho1-2 also rescues rod photoreceptor morphology. (*A*) Wild-type (WT) pig retina. (*B*) Age-matched Tg P23H hRHO retina treated with Rho1-2 meganuclease at P3. (*C*) Age-matched untreated Tg P23H hRHO retina. Rhodopsin (magenta), Reep6 (green). (OS) Outer segment, (IS) inner segment, (ONL) outer nuclear layer, (OPL) outer plexiform layer.

and are cheaper to generate. However, as a large animal model for retinal diseases, this review shows that the pig has many advantages as therapies and for evaluation of toxicity and biodistribution as these approaches are advanced to the last stage of preclinical testing.

ACKNOWLEDGMENTS

Funding from the Kentucky Lions Eye Research Chair, Foundation for Fighting Blindness, Jewish Heritage Foundation for Research Excellence, and NIH NEI R01 026158, 032645.

REFERENCES

Abud MB, Baranov P, Patel S, Hicks CA, Isaac DLC, Louzada RN, Dromel P, Singh D, Sinden J, Ávila MP, et al. 2022. In vivo study to assess dosage of allogeneic pig retinal progenitor cells: long-term survival, engraftment, differentiation and safety. *J Cell Mol Med* **26:** 3254–3268. doi:10.1111/jcmm.17332

Acharya NK, Qi X, Goldwaser EL, Godsey GA, Wu H, Kosciuk MC, Freeman TA, Macphee CH, Wilensky RL, Venkataraman V, et al. 2017. Retinal pathology is associated with increased blood-retina barrier permeability in a diabetic and hypercholesterolaemic pig model: beneficial effects of the LpPLA(2) inhibitor Darapladib. *Diab Vasc Dis Res* **14:** 200–213. doi:10.1177/1479164116683149

Adekunle AN, Adkins A, Wang W, Kaplan HJ, De Castro JF, Lee SJ, Huie P, Palanker D, Mccall M, Pardue MT. 2015. Integration of perforated subretinal prostheses with retinal tissue. *Transl Vis Sci Technol* **4:** 5. doi:10.1167/tvst.4.4.5

Allen RS, Feola A, Motz CT, Ottensmeyer AL, Chesler KC, Dunn R, Thulé PM, Pardue MT. 2019. Retinal deficits precede cognitive and motor deficits in a rat model of type II diabetes. *Invest Ophthalmol Vis Sci* **60:** 123–133. doi:10.1167/iovs.18-25110

Allen RS, Bales K, Feola A, Pardue MT. 2020. In vivo structural assessments of ocular disease in rodent models using optical coherence tomography. *J Vis Exp* doi:10.3791/61588

Andersen OM, Bøgh N, Landau AM, Pløen GG, Jensen AMG, Monti G, Ulhøi BP, Nyengaard JR, Jacobsen KR, Jørgensen MM, et al. 2022. A genetically modified minipig model for Alzheimer's disease with SORL1 haploinsufficiency. *Cell Rep Med* **3:** 100740. doi:10.1016/j.xcrm.2022.100740

Aung MH, Park HN, Han MK, Obertone TS, Abey J, Aseem F, Thule PM, Iuvone PM, Pardue MT. 2014. Dopamine deficiency contributes to early visual dysfunction in a rodent model of type 1 diabetes. *J Neurosci* **34:** 726–736. doi:10.1523/JNEUROSCI.3483-13.2014

Banin E, Cideciyan AV, Aleman TS, Petters RM, Wong F, Milam AH, Jacobson SG. 1999. Retinal rod photoreceptor-specific gene mutation perturbs cone pathway development. *Neuron* **23:** 549–557. doi:10.1016/S0896-6273(00)80807-7

Bantseev V, Schuetz C, Booler HS, Horvath J, Hovaten K, Erickson S, Bentley E, Nork TM, Freeman WR, Stewart JM, et al. 2020. Evaluation of surgical factors affecting vitreous hemorrhage following port delivery system with ranibizumab implant insertion in a minipig model. *Retina* **40:** 1520–1528. doi:10.1097/IAE.0000000000002614

Bek T. 2019. Translational research in retinal vascular disease. An approach. *Acta Ophthalmol* **97:** 441–450. doi:10.1111/aos.14045

Beraldi R, Chan CH, Rogers CS, Kovács AD, Meyerholz DK, Trantzas C, Lambertz AM, Darbro BW, Weber KL, White KA, et al. 2015. A novel porcine model of ataxia telangiectasia reproduces neurological features and motor deficits of human disease. *Hum Mol Genet* **24:** 6473–6484. doi:10.1093/hmg/ddv356

Bergeles C, Kummer MP, Kratochvil BE, Framme C, Nelson BJ. 2011. Steerable intravitreal inserts for drug delivery: in vitro and ex vivo mobility experiments. *Med Image Comput Comput Assist Inter* **14:** 33–40. doi:10.1007/978-3-642-23623-5_5

Bertschinger DR, Beknazar E, Simonutti M, Safran AB, Sahel JA, Rosolen SG, Picaud S, Salzmann J. 2008. A review of in vivo animal studies in retinal prosthesis research. *Graefes Arch Clin Exp Ophthalmol* **246:** 1505–1517. doi:10.1007/s00417-008-0891-7

Blackmon SM, Peng YW, Hao Y, Moon SJ, Oliveira LB, Tatebayashi M, Petters RM, Wong F. 2000. Early loss of synaptic protein PSD-95 from rod terminals of rhodopsin P347L transgenic porcine retina. *Brain Res* **885:** 53–61. doi:10.1016/S0006-8993(00)02928-0

Bode G, Clausing P, Gervais F, Loegsted J, Luft J, Nogues V, Sims J. 2010. The utility of the minipig as an animal model in regulatory toxicology. *J Pharmacol Toxicol Methods* **62:** 196–220. doi:10.1016/j.vascn.2010.05.009

Bonillo M, Pfromm J, Fischer MD. 2022. Challenges to gene editing approaches in the retina. *Klin Monbl Augenheilkd* **239:** 275–283. doi:10.1055/a-1757-9810

Bosse B, Zrenner E, Wilke R. 2011. Standard ERG equipment can be used to monitor functionality of retinal implants. *Annu Int Conf IEEE Eng Med Biol Soc* **2011:** 1089–1092. doi:10.1109/IEMBS.2011.6090254

Boyd RF, Boye SL, Conlon TJ, Erger KE, Sledge DG, Langohr IM, Hauswirth WW, Komáromy AM, Boye SE, Petersen-Jones SM, et al. 2016. Reduced retinal transduction and enhanced transgene-directed immunogenicity with intravitreal delivery of rAAV following posterior vitrectomy in dogs. *Gene Ther* **23:** 548–556. doi:10.1038/gt.2016.31

Brant Fernandes RA, Koss MJ, Falabella P, Stefanini FR, Maia M, Diniz B, Ribeiro R, Hu Y, Hinton D, Clegg DO, et al. 2016. An innovative surgical technique for subretinal transplantation of human embryonic stem cell-derived retinal pigmented epithelium in Yucatan mini pigs: preliminary results. *Ophthalmic Surg Lasers Imaging Retina* **47:** 342–351. doi:10.3928/23258160-20160324-07

Bucher K, Rodríguez-Bocanegra E, Dauletbekov D, Fischer MD. 2021. Immune responses to retinal gene therapy using adeno-associated viral vectors—implications for treatment success and safety. *Prog Retin Eye Res* **83:** 100915. doi:10.1016/j.preteyeres.2020.100915

Bulc M, Całka J, Palus K. 2020. Effect of streptozotocin-inducted diabetes on the pathophysiology of enteric neurons in the small intestine based on the porcine diabetes model. *Int J Mol Sci* 21: 2047. doi:10.3390/ijms21062047

Cehofski LJ, Kruse A, Magnusdottir SO, Alsing AN, Nielsen JE, Kirkeby S, Honoré B, Vorum H. 2018. Dexamethasone intravitreal implant downregulates PDGFR-α and upregulates caveolin-1 in experimental branch retinal vein occlusion. *Exp Eye Res* 171: 174–182. doi:10.1016/j.exer.2018.02.029

Cehofski LJ, Kruse A, Mæng MO, Sejergaard BF, Schlosser A, Sorensen GL, Grauslund J, Honoré B, Vorum H. 2022. Dexamethasone intravitreal implant is active at the molecular level eight weeks after implantation in experimental central retinal vein occlusion. *Molecules* 27: 5687. doi:10.3390/molecules27175687

Chan YK, Wang S, Letizia A, Chan Y, Lim E, Graveline A, Verdera HC, Alphonse P, Xue Y, Chiang J, et al. 2019. *Reducing AAV-mediated immune responses and pathology in a subretinal pig model by engineering the vector genome,* Vol. 27, p. 298. Cell, Cambridge, MA.

Chan YK, Wang SK, Chu CJ, Copland DA, Letizia AJ, Costa Verdera H, Chiang JJ, Sethi M, Wang MK, Neidermyer WJ, et al. 2021. Engineering adeno-associated viral vectors to evade innate immune and inflammatory responses. *Sci Transl Med* 13: eabd3438. doi:10.1126/scitranslmed.abd3438

Chen H, Liu YQ, Li CH, Guo XM, Huang LJ. 2009. The susceptibility of three strains of Chinese minipigs to diet-induced type 2 diabetes mellitus. *Lab Anim (NY)* 38: 355–363. doi:10.1038/laban1109-355

Chen J, Poulaki V, Kim SJ, Eldred WD, Kane S, Gingerich M, Shire DB, Jensen R, Dewalt G, Kaplan HJ, et al. 2020. Implantation and extraction of penetrating electrode arrays in minipig retinas. *Transl Vis Sci Technol* 9: 19. doi:10.1167/tvst.9.5.19

Choi KE, Anh VTQ, Seo HW, Kim N, Kim S, Kim SW. 2020. Ab-interno surgical technique for the implantation of a wireless subretinal prosthesis in mini-pigs. *Sci Rep* 10: 18507. doi:10.1038/s41598-020-75579-4

Curcio CA, Sloan KR, Kalina RE, Hendrickson AE. 1990. Human photoreceptor topography. *J Comp Neurol* 292: 497–523. doi:10.1002/cne.902920402

Dawson HD. 2011. Comparative assessment of the pig, mouse, and human genomes: a structural and functional analysis of genes involved in immunity. In *The minipig in biomedical research* (ed. McAnulty PA, Dayan A, Hastings KH, Ganderup N-C). CRC, Boca Raton, FL.

Deng J, Yang L, Wang Z, Ouyang H, Yu H, Yuan H, Pang D. 2022. Advance of genetically modified pigs in xeno-transplantation. *Front Cell Dev Biol* 10: 1033197. doi:10.3389/fcell.2022.1033197

Denner J. 2022. Virus safety of xenotransplantation. *Viruses* 14: 1926. doi:10.3390/v14091926

Derks MFL, Megens HJ, Giacomini WL, Groenen MAM, Lopes MS. 2021. A natural knockout of the MYO7A gene leads to pre-weaning mortality in pigs. *Anim Genet* 52: 514–517. doi:10.1111/age.13068

De Smet MD, Stassen JM, Meenink TC, Janssens T, Vanheukelom V, Naus GJ, Beelen MJ, Jonckx B. 2016. Release of experimental retinal vein occlusions by direct intralumi-nal injection of ocriplasmin. *Br J Ophthalmol* 100: 1742–1746. doi:10.1136/bjophthalmol-2016-309190

Eggers ED, Carreon TA. 2020. The effects of early diabetes on inner retinal neurons. *Vis Neurosci* 37: E006. doi:10.1017/S095252382000005X

Fernandes RAB, Stefanini FR, Falabella P, Koss MJ, Wells T, Diniz B, Ribeiro R, Schor P, Maia M, Penha FM, et al. 2017. Development of a new tissue injector for subretinal transplantation of human embryonic stem cell derived retinal pigmented epithelium. *Int J Retina Vitreous* 3: 41. doi:10.1186/s40942-017-0095-6

Fernandez De Castro JP, Scott PA, Fransen JW, Demas J, Demarco PJ, Kaplan HJ, Mccall MA. 2014. Cone photoreceptors develop normally in the absence of functional rod photoreceptors in a transgenic swine model of retinitis pigmentosa. *Invest Ophthalmol Vis Sci* 55: 2460–2468. doi:10.1167/iovs.13-13724

Fjord-Larsen L, Kusk P, Tornøe J, Juliusson B, Torp M, Bjarkam CR, Nielsen MS, Handberg A, Sørensen JC, Wahlberg LU. 2010. Long-term delivery of nerve growth factor by encapsulated cell biodelivery in the Göttingen minipig basal forebrain. *Mol Ther* 18: 2164–2172. doi:10.1038/mt.2010.154

Flood MD, Wellington AJ, Cruz LA, Eggers ED. 2020. Early diabetes impairs ON sustained ganglion cell light responses and adaptation without cell death or dopamine insensitivity. *Exp Eye Res* 200: 108223. doi:10.1016/j.exer.2020.108223

Flood MD, Wellington AJ, Eggers ED. 2022. Impaired light adaptation of ON-sustained ganglion cells in early diabetes is attributable to diminished response to dopamine D4 receptor activation. *Invest Ophthalmol Vis Sci* 63: 33. doi:10.1167/iovs.63.1.33

Forster R, Bode G, Ellegaard L, Van Der Laan JW. 2010a. The RETHINK project—minipigs as models for the toxicity testing of new medicines and chemicals: an impact assessment. *J Pharmacol Toxicol Methods* 62: 158–159. doi:10.1016/j.vascn.2010.05.003

Forster R, Bode G, Ellegaard L, Van Der Laan JW. 2010b. The RETHINK project on minipigs in the toxicity testing of new medicines and chemicals: conclusions and recommendations. *J Pharmacol Toxicol Methods* 62: 236–242. doi:10.1016/j.vascn.2010.05.008

Fujie T, Mori Y, Ito S, Nishizawa M, Bae H, Nagai N, Onami H, Abe T, Khademhosseini A, Kaji H. 2014. Micropatterned polymeric nanosheets for local delivery of an engineered epithelial monolayer. *Adv Mater* 26: 1699–1705. doi:10.1002/adma.201304183

Gandhi JK, Mano F, Iezzi R Jr, Lobue SA, Holman BH, Fautsch MP, Olsen TW, Pulido JS, Marmorstein AD. 2020. Fibrin hydrogels are safe, degradable scaffolds for sub-retinal implantation. *PLoS ONE* 15: e0227641. doi:10.1371/journal.pone.0227641

Gao M, Zhu X, Yang G, Bao J, Bu H. 2021. CRISPR/Cas9-mediated gene editing in porcine models for medical research. *DNA Cell Biol* 40: 1462–1475. doi:10.1089/dna.2020.6474

Garcá M, Ruiz-Ederra J, Hernandez-Barbachano H, Vecino E. 2005. Topography of pig retinal ganglion cells. *J Comp Neurol* 486: 361–372. doi:10.1002/cne.20516

García Delgado AB, De La Cerda B, Alba Amador J, Valdés Sánchez ML, Fernández-Muñoz B, Relimpio López I,

Rodríguez De La Rúa E, Lloret AD, Calado SM, Sánchez Pernaute R, et al. 2019. Subretinal transplant of induced pluripotent stem cell-derived retinal pigment epithelium on nanostructured fibrin-agarose. *Tissue Eng Part A* **25**: 799–808. doi:10.1089/ten.tea.2019.0007

Garcia M, Forster V, Hicks D, Vecino E. 2002. Effects of Müller glia on cell survival and neuritogenesis in adult porcine retina in vitro. *Invest Ophthalmol Vis Sci* **43**: 3735–3743.

Gatto C, Romano MR, Giurgola L, Ferrara M, Ragazzi E, D'Amato Tothova J. 2021. Ex vivo evaluation of retinal cytotoxicity after the use of multiple medical devices in pars plana vitrectomy in porcine eyes. *Exp Eye Res* **213**: 108837. doi:10.1016/j.exer.2021.108837

Ghosh F, Arner K. 2010. Cell type differentiation dynamics in the developing porcine retina. *Dev Neurosci* **32**: 47–58. doi:10.1159/000261704

Ghosh F, Wong F, Johansson K, Bruun A, Petters RM. 2004. Transplantation of full-thickness retina in the rhodopsin transgenic pig. *Retina* **24**: 98–109. doi:10.1097/00006982-200402000-00014

Gonzalez-Calle A, Brant R, Diniz B, Swenson S, Markland F, Humayun MS, Weiland JD. 2018. Disintegrin-integrin binding for attachment of polymer substrate to the retina. *J Clin Exp Ophthalmol* **9**: 752. doi:10.4172/2155-9570.1000752

Grotz S, Schäfer J, Wunderlich KA, Ellederova Z, Auch H, Bähr A, Runa-Vochozkova P, Fadl J, Arnold V, Ardan T, et al. 2022. Early disruption of photoreceptor cell architecture and loss of vision in a humanized pig model of usher syndromes. *EMBO Mol Med* **14**: e14817. doi:10.15252/emmm.202114817

Guduric-Fuchs J, Ringland LJ, Gu P, Dellett M, Archer DB, Cogliati T. 2009. Immunohistochemical study of pig retinal development. *Mol Vis* **15**: 1915–1928.

Guo Q, Zhu HY, Jin L, Gao QS, Kang JD, Cui CD, Yin XJ. 2015. Production of cloned Wuzhishan miniature pigs and application for alloxan toxicity test. *Anim Biotechnol* **26**: 292–297. doi:10.1080/10495398.2015.1025957

Gutierrez K, Dicks N, Glanzner WG, Agellon LB, Bordignon V. 2015. Efficacy of the porcine species in biomedical research. *Front Genet* **6**: 293. doi:10.3389/fgene.2015.00293

Hamilton BA, Wright JF. 2021. Challenges posed by immune responses to AAV vectors: addressing root causes. *Front Immunol* **12**: 675897. doi:10.3389/fimmu.2021.675897

Han IC, Bohrer LR, Gibson-Corley KN, Wiley LA, Shrestha A, Harman BE, Jiao C, Sohn EH, Wendland R, Allen BN, et al. 2022. Biocompatibility of human induced pluripotent stem cell-derived retinal progenitor cell grafts in immunocompromised rats. *Cell Transplant* **31**: 9636897221104451. doi:10.1177/09636897221104451

Hebel R. 1976. Distribution of retinal ganglion cells in five mammalian species (pig, sheep, ox, horse, dog). *Anat Embryol (Berl)* **150**: 45–51.

Hein TW, Potts LB, Xu W, Yuen JZ, Kuo L. 2012. Temporal development of retinal arteriolar endothelial dysfunction in porcine type 1 diabetes. *Invest Ophthalmol Vis Sci* **53**: 7943–7949. doi:10.1167/iovs.12-11005

Hendrickson A, Hicks D. 2002. Distribution and density of medium- and short-wavelength selective cones in the do-

mestic pig retina. *Exp Eye Res* **74**: 435–444. doi:10.1006/exer.2002.1181

Hoffe B, Holahan MR. 2019. The use of pigs as a translational model for studying neurodegenerative diseases. *Front Physiol* **10**: 838. doi:10.3389/fphys.2019.00838

Hou N, Du X, Wu S. 2022. Advances in pig models of human diseases. *Animal Model Exp Med* **5**: 141–152. doi:10.1002/ame2.12223

Huang Y, Cideciyan AV, Alemán TS, Banin E, Huang J, Syed NA, Petters RM, Wong F, Milam AH, Jacobson SG. 2000. Optical coherence tomography (OCT) abnormalities in rhodopsin mutant transgenic swine with retinal degeneration. *Exp Eye Res* **70**: 247–251. doi:10.1006/exer.1999.0793

Isakson SH, Rizzardi AE, Coutts AW, Carlson DF, Kirstein MN, Fisher J, Vitte J, Williams KB, Pluhar GE, Dahiya S, et al. 2018. Genetically engineered minipigs model the major clinical features of human neurofibromatosis type 1. *Commun Biol* **1**: 158. doi:10.1038/s42003-018-0163-y

Isidan A, Liu S, Li P, Lashmet M, Smith LJ, Hara H, Cooper DKC, Ekser B. 2019. Decellularization methods for developing porcine corneal xenografts and future perspectives. *Xenotransplantation* **26**: e12564. doi:10.1111/xen.12564

Isidan A, Liu S, Chen AM, Zhang W, Li P, Smith LJ, Hara H, Cooper DKC, Ekser B. 2021. Comparison of porcine corneal decellularization methods and importance of preserving corneal limbus through decellularization. *PLoS ONE* **16**: e0243682. doi:10.1371/journal.pone.0243682

Islam R, Islam MM, Nilsson PH, Mohlin C, Hagen KT, Paschalis EI, Woods RL, Bhowmick SC, Dohlman CH, Espevik T, et al. 2021. Combined blockade of complement C5 and TLR co-receptor CD14 synergistically inhibits pig-to-human corneal xenograft induced innate inflammatory responses. *Acta Biomater* **127**: 169–179. doi:10.1016/j.actbio.2021.03.047

Ivastinovic D, Langmann G, Nemetz W, Hornig R, Richard G, Velikay-Parel M. 2010. Clinical stability of a new method for fixation and explanation of epiretinal implants. *Acta Ophthalmol* **88**: e285–e286. doi:10.1111/j.1755-3768.2009.01694.x

Ivastinovic D, Langmann G, Asslaber M, Georgi T, Wedrich A, Velikay-Parel M. 2012. Distribution of glial fibrillary acidic protein accumulation after retinal tack insertion for intraocular fixation of epiretinal implants. *Acta Ophthalmol* **90**: e416–e417. doi:10.1111/j.1755-3768.2011.02321.x

Jakobsen JE, Johansen MG, Schmidt M, Liu Y, Li R, Callesen H, Melnikova M, Habekost M, Matrone C, Bouter Y, et al. 2016. Expression of the Alzheimer's disease mutations AβPP695sw and PSEN1M146I in double-transgenic Göttingen minipigs. *J Alzheimers Dis* **53**: 1617–1630. doi:10.3233/JAD-160408

Javaid D, Ganie SY, Hajam YA, Reshi MS. 2022. CRISPR/Cas9 system: a reliable and facile genome editing tool in modern biology. *Mol Biol Rep* **49**: 12133–12150. doi:10.1007/s11033-022-07880-6

Kashani AH, Martynova A, Koss M, Brant R, Zhu DH, Lebkowski J, Hinton D, Clegg D, Humayun MS. 2019. Subretinal implantation of a human embryonic stem cell-derived retinal pigment epithelium monolayer in a porcine model. *Adv Exp Med Biol* **1185**: 569–574. doi:10.1007/978-3-030-27378-1_93

Kelly SK, Shire DB, Chen J, Doyle P, Gingerich MD, Cogan SF, Drohan WA, Behan S, Theogarajan L, Wyatt JL, et al. 2011. A hermetic wireless subretinal neurostimulator for vision prostheses. *IEEE Trans Biomed Eng* **58:** 3197–3205. doi:10.1109/TBME.2011.2165713

Kim MK, Hara H. 2015. Current status of corneal xenotransplantation. *Int J Surg* **23:** 255–260. doi:10.1016/j.ijsu.2015.07.685

Kim MK, Choi HJ, Kwon I, Pierson RN III, Cooper DK, Soulillou JP, O'connell PJ, Vabres B, Maeda N, Hara H, et al. 2014. The international xenotransplantation association consensus statement on conditions for undertaking clinical trials of xenocorneal transplantation. *Xenotransplantation* **21:** 420–430. doi:10.1111/xen.12129

Kim YJ, Park SH, Choi KS. 2015. Fluctuation of infusion pressure during microincision vitrectomy using the constellation vision system. *Retina* **35:** 2529–2536. doi:10.1097/IAE.0000000000000625

Kim MK, Aung MH, Mees L, Olson DE, Pozdeyev N, Iuvone PM, Thule PM, Pardue MT. 2018. Dopamine deficiency mediates early rod-driven inner retinal dysfunction in diabetic mice. *Invest Ophthalmol Vis Sci* **59:** 572–581. doi:10.1167/iovs.17-22692

King JL, Mason JO III, Cartner SC, Guidry C. 2011. The influence of alloxan-induced diabetes on Müller cell contraction-promoting activities in vitreous. *Invest Ophthalmol Vis Sci* **52:** 7485–7491. doi:10.1167/iovs.11-7781

Klassen H, Kiilgaard JF, Warfvinge K, Samuel MS, Prather RS, Wong F, Petters RM, La Cour M, Young MJ. 2012. Photoreceptor differentiation following transplantation of allogeneic retinal progenitor cells to the dystrophic rhodopsin Pro347Leu transgenic pig. *Stem Cells Int* **2012:** 939801. doi:10.1155/2012/939801

Kleinert M, Clemmensen C, Hofmann SM, Moore MC, Renner S, Woods SC, Huypens P, Beckers J, De Angelis MH, Schürmann A, et al. 2018. Animal models of obesity and diabetes mellitus. *Nat Rev Endocrinol* **14:** 140–162. doi:10.1038/nrendo.2017.161

Kleinwort KJH, Amann B, Hauck SM, Hirmer S, Blutke A, Renner S, Uhl PB, Lutterberg K, Sekundo W, Wolf E, et al. 2017. Retinopathy with central oedema in an INS (C94Y) transgenic pig model of long-term diabetes. *Diabetologia* **60:** 1541–1549. doi:10.1007/s00125-017-4290-7

Koss MJ, Falabella P, Stefanini FR, Pfister M, Thomas BB, Kashani AH, Brant R, Zhu D, Clegg DO, Hinton DR, et al. 2016. Subretinal implantation of a monolayer of human embryonic stem cell-derived retinal pigment epithelium: a feasibility and safety study in Yucatán minipigs. *Graefes Arch Clin Exp Ophthalmol* **254:** 1553–1565. doi:10.1007/s00417-016-3386-y

Kostic C, Lillico SG, Crippa SV, Grandchamp N, Pilet H, Philippe S, Lu Z, King TJ, Mallet J, Sarkis C, et al. 2013. Rapid cohort generation and analysis of disease spectrum of large animal model of cone dystrophy. *PLoS ONE* **8:** e71363. doi:10.1371/journal.pone.0071363

Kraft TW, Allen D, Petters RM, Hao Y, Peng YW, Wong F. 2005. Altered light responses of single rod photoreceptors in transgenic pigs expressing P347L or P347S rhodopsin. *Mol Vis* **11:** 1246–1256.

Lai AK, Lo AC. 2013. Animal models of diabetic retinopathy: summary and comparison. *J Diabetes Res* **2013:** 106594. doi:10.1155/2013/106594

Lamm V, Hara H, Mammen A, Dhaliwal D, Cooper DK. 2014. Corneal blindness and xenotransplantation. *Xenotransplantation* **21:** 99–114. doi:10.1111/xen.12082

Lansing M, Sauvé Y, Dimopoulos I, Field CJ, Suh M, Wizzard P, Goruk S, Lim D, Muto M, Wales P, et al. 2018. Parenteral lipid dose restriction with soy oil, not fish oil, preserves retinal function in neonatal piglets. *JPEN J Parenter Enteral Nutr* **42:** 1177–1184. doi:10.1002/jpen.1145

Lee SE, Ma W, Rattigan EM, Aleshin A, Chen L, Johnson LL, D'agati VD, Schmidt AM, Barile GR. 2010. Ultrastructural features of retinal capillary basement membrane thickening in diabetic swine. *Ultrastruct Pathol* **34:** 35–41. doi:10.3109/01913120903308583

Leroy BP, Fischer MD, Flannery JG, MacLaren RE, Dalkara D, Scholl HPN, Chung DC, Spera C, Viriato D, Banhazi J. 2022. Gene therapy for inherited retinal disease: long-term durability of effect. *Ophthalmic Res* doi:10.1159/000526317

Li ZY, Wong F, Chang JH, Possin DE, Hao Y, Petters RM, Milam AH. 1998. Rhodopsin transgenic pigs as a model for human retinitis pigmentosa. *Invest Ophthalmol Vis Sci* **39:** 808–819.

Li SY, Yin ZQ, Chen SJ, Chen LF, Liu Y. 2009. Rescue from light-induced retinal degeneration by human fetal retinal transplantation in minipigs. *Curr Eye Res* **34:** 523–535. doi:10.1080/02713680902936148

Li KV, Flores-Bellver M, Aparicio-Domingo S, Petrash C, Cobb H, Chen C, Canto-Soler MV, Mathias MT. 2022a. A surgical kit for stem cell-derived retinal pigment epithelium transplants: collection, transportation, and subretinal delivery. *Front Cell Dev Biol* **10:** 813538. doi:10.3389/fcell.2022.813538

Li X, Huang Y, Liang Q, Li G, Feng S, Song Y, Zhang Y, Wang L, Jie Y, Pan Z. 2022b. Local immunosuppression in Wuzhishan pig to Rhesus monkey Descemet's stripping automated endothelial keratoplasty: an innovative method to promote the survival of xenografts. *Ophthalmic Res* **65:** 196–209. doi:10.1159/000521193

Li Y, Wang H, Chen H, Liao Y, Gou S, Yan Q, Zhuang Z, Li H, Wang J, Suo Y, et al. 2022c. Generation of a genetically modified pig model with CREBRF(R457Q) variant. *FASEB J* **36:** e22611. doi:10.1096/fj.202201117

Li Z, Fu P, Wei BT, Wang J, Li AL, Li MJ, Bian GB. 2022d. An automatic drug injection device with spatial micro-force perception guided by an microscopic image for robot-assisted ophthalmic surgery. *Front Robot AI* **9:** 913930. doi:10.3389/frobt.2022.913930

Lim RR, Grant DG, Olver TD, Padilla J, Czajkowski AM, Schnurbusch TR, Mohan RR, Hainsworth DP, Walters EM, Chaurasia SS. 2018. Young Ossabaw pigs fed a Western diet exhibit early signs of diabetic retinopathy. *Invest Ophthalmol Vis Sci* **59:** 2325–2338. doi:10.1167/iovs.17-23616

Liu L, Bartke N, Van Daele H, Lawrence P, Qin X, Park HG, Kothapalli K, Windust A, Bindels J, Wang Z, et al. 2014. Higher efficacy of dietary DHA provided as a phospholipid than as a triglyceride for brain DHA accretion in neonatal piglets. *J Lipid Res* **55:** 531–539. doi:10.1194/jlr.M045930

Lohmann TK, Haiss F, Schaffrath K, Schnitzler AC, Waschkowski F, Barz C, Van Der Meer AM, Werner C, Johnen S,

Laube T, et al. 2019. The very large electrode array for retinal stimulation (VLARS)—A concept study. *J Neural Eng* **16:** 066031. doi:10.1088/1741-2552/ab4113

Ludwig B, Wolf E, Schönmann U, Ludwig S. 2020. Large animal models of diabetes. *Methods Mol Biol* **2128:** 115–134. doi:10.1007/978-1-0716-0385-7_9

Maya-Vetencourt JF, Di Marco S, Mete M, Di Paolo M, Ventrella D, Barone F, Elmi A, Manfredi G, Desii A, Sannita WG, et al. 2020. Biocompatibility of a conjugated polymer retinal prosthesis in the domestic pig. *Front Bioeng Biotechnol* **8:** 579141. doi:10.3389/fbioe.2020.579141

McAllister IL, Vijayasekaran S, Xia W, Yu DY. 2013. Evaluation of the ability of a photocoagulator to rupture the retinal vein and Bruch's membrane for potential vein bypass in retinal vein occlusion. *Ophthalmic Surg Lasers Imaging Retina* **44:** 268–273. doi:10.3928/23258160-20130503-10

Middleton S. 2010. Porcine ophthalmology. *Vet Clin North Am Food Anim Pract* **26:** 557–572. doi:10.1016/j.cvfa.2010.09.002

Moore-Dotson JM, Eggers ED. 2019. Reductions in calcium signaling limit inhibition to diabetic retinal rod bipolar cells. *Invest Ophthalmol Vis Sci* **60:** 4063–4073. doi:10.1167/iovs.19-27137

Moore-Dotson JM, Beckman JJ, Mazade RE, Hoon M, Bernstein AS, Romero-Aleshire MJ, Brooks HL, Eggers ED. 2016. Early retinal neuronal dysfunction in diabetic mice: reduced light-evoked inhibition increases rod pathway signaling. *Invest Ophthalmol Vis Sci* **57:** 1418–1430. doi:10.1167/iovs.15-17999

Mueller NJ, Denner J. 2022. Porcine cytomegalovirus/porcine roseolovirus (PCMV/PRV): a threat for xenotransplantation? *Xenotransplantation* **29:** e12775. doi:10.1111/xen.12775

Murphy E, Kraak L, Nordquist RE, Van Der Staay FJ. 2013. Successive and conditional discrimination learning in pigs. *Anim Cogn* **16:** 883–893. doi:10.1007/s10071-013-0621-3

Nagaya M, Hasegawa K, Watanabe M, Nakano K, Okamoto K, Yamada T, Uchikura A, Osafune K, Yokota H, Nagaoka T, et al. 2020. Genetically engineered pigs manifesting pancreatic agenesis with severe diabetes. *BMJ Open Diabetes Res Care* **8:** e001792. doi:10.1136/bmjdrc-2020-001792

Neitz J, Jacobs GH. 1989. Spectral sensitivity of cones in an ungulate. *Vis Neurosci* **2:** 97–100. doi:10.1017/S0952523800011949

Ng YF, Chan HH, Chu PH, To CH, Gilger BC, Petters RM, Wong F. 2008. Multifocal electroretinogram in rhodopsin P347L transgenic pigs. *Invest Ophthalmol Vis Sci* **49:** 2208–2215. doi:10.1167/iovs.07-1159

Niu M, Liu Y, Xiang L, Zhao Y, Yuan J, Jia Y, Dai X, Chen H. 2020. Long-term case study of a Wuzhishan miniature pig with diabetes. *Animal Model Exp Med* **3:** 22–31. doi:10.1002/ame2.12098

Niu M, Zhao Y, Xiang L, Jia Y, Yuan J, Dai X, Chen H. 2022. 16S rRNA gene sequencing analysis of gut microbiome in a mini-pig diabetes model. *Animal Model Exp Med* **5:** 81–88. doi:10.1002/ame2.12202

Noda T, Fujisawa T, Kawasaki R, Tashiro H, Takehara H, Sasagawa K, Tokuda T, Ohta J. 2015. Fabrication and functional demonstration of a smart electrode with a built-in CMOS microchip for neural stimulation of a retinal prosthesis. *Annu Int Conf IEEE Eng Med Biol Soc* **2015:** 3355–3358. doi:10.1109/EMBC.2015.7319111

Olsen TW, Dyer RB, Mano F, Boatright JH, Chrenek MA, Paley D, Wabner K, Schmit J, Chae JB, Sellers JT, et al. 2020. Drug tissue distribution of TUDCA from a biodegradable suprachoroidal implant versus intravitreal or systemic delivery in the pig model. *Transl Vis Sci Technol* **9:** 11. doi:10.1167/tvst.9.6.11

Pabst R. 2020. The pig as a model for immunology research. *Cell Tissue Res* **380:** 287–304. doi:10.1007/s00441-020-03206-9

Packer O, Hendrickson AE, Curcio CA. 1989. Photoreceptor topography of the retina in the adult pigtail macaque (*Macaca nemestrina*). *J Comp Neurol* **288:** 165–183. doi:10.1002/cne.902880113

Palácios RM, De Carvalho ACM, Maia M, Caiado RR, Camilo DAG, Farah ME. 2019. An experimental and clinical study on the initial experiences of Brazilian vitreoretinal surgeons with heads-up surgery. *Graefes Arch Clin Exp Ophthalmol* **257:** 473–483. doi:10.1007/s00417-019-04246-w

Panepinto LM, Phillips RW, Norden S, Pryor PC, Cox R. 1983. A comfortable, minimum stress method of restraint for Yucatan miniature swine. *Lab Anim Sci* **33:** 95–97.

Pardue MT, Barnes CS, Kim MK, Aung MH, Amarnath R, Olson DE, Thulé PM. 2014. Rodent hyperglycemia-induced inner retinal deficits are mirrored in human diabetes. *Transl Vis Sci Technol* **3:** 6. doi:10.1167/tvst.3.3.6

Peichl L, Ott H, Boycott BB. 1987. α Ganglion cells in mammalian retinae. *Proc R Soc Lond B Biol Sci* **231:** 169–197. doi:10.1098/rspb.1987.0040

Peng YW, Hao Y, Petters RM, Wong F. 2000. Ectopic synaptogenesis in the mammalian retina caused by rod photoreceptor-specific mutations. *Nat Neurosci* **3:** 1121–1127. doi:10.1038/80639

Peng CH, Chuang JH, Wang ML, Jhan YY, Chien KH, Chung YC, Hung KH, Chang CC, Lee CK, Tseng WL, et al. 2016. Laminin modification subretinal bio-scaffold remodels retinal pigment epithelium-driven microenvironment in vitro and in vivo. *Oncotarget* **7:** 64631–64648. doi:10.18632/oncotarget.11502

Pepper AR, Welch I, Bruni A, Macgillivary A, Mazzuca DM, White DJ, Wall W. 2013. Establishment of a stringent large animal model of insulin-dependent diabetes for islet autotransplantation: combination of pancreatectomy and streptozotocin. *Pancreas* **42:** 329–338. doi:10.1097/MPA.0b013e318264bcdd

Pereiro X, Ruzafa N, Urcola JH, Sharma SC, Vecino E. 2020. Differential distribution of RBPMS in pig, rat, and human retina after damage. *Int J Mol Sci* **21:** 9330. doi:10.3390/ijms21239330

Petters RM, Alexander CA, Wells KD, Collins EB, Sommer JR, Blanton MR, Rojas G, Hao Y, Flowers WL, Banin E, et al. 1997. Genetically engineered large animal model for studying cone photoreceptor survival and degeneration in retinitis pigmentosa. *Nat Biotechnol* **15:** 965–970. doi:10.1038/nbt1097-965

Popelka Š, Studenovská H, Abelová L, Ardan T, Studený P, Straňák Z, Klíma J, Dvořánková B, Kotek J, Hodan J, et al. 2015. A frame-supported ultrathin electrospun polymer membrane for transplantation of retinal pigment epithe-

Cite this article as *Cold Spring Harb Perspect Med* doi: 10.1101/cshperspect.a041296

lial cells. *Biomed Mater* **10**: 045022. doi:10.1088/1748-6041/10/4/045022

Ratner LD, La Motta GE, Briski O, Salamone DF, Fernandez-Martin R. 2021. Practical approaches for knock-out gene editing in pigs. *Front Genet* **11**: 617850. doi:10.3389/fgene.2020.617850

Ren D, Fisson S, Dalkara D, Ail D. 2022. Immune responses to gene editing by viral and non-viral delivery vectors used in retinal gene therapy. *Pharmaceutics* **14**: 1973. doi:10.3390/pharmaceutics14091973

Renner S, Dobenecker B, Blutke A, Zöls S, Wanke R, Ritzmann M, Wolf E. 2016. Comparative aspects of rodent and nonrodent animal models for mechanistic and translational diabetes research. *Theriogenology* **86**: 406–421. doi:10.1016/j.theriogenology.2016.04.055

Rogers CS, Stoltz DA, Meyerholz DK, Ostedgaard LS, Rokhlina T, Taft PJ, Rogan MP, Pezzulo AA, Karp PH, Itani OA, et al. 2008. Disruption of the CFTR gene produces a model of cystic fibrosis in newborn pigs. *Science* **321**: 1837–1841. doi:10.1126/science.1163600

Ross JW, Fernandez De Castro JP, Zhao J, Samuel M, Walters E, Rios C, Bray-Ward P, Jones BW, Marc RE, Wang W, et al. 2012. Generation of an inbred miniature pig model of retinitis pigmentosa. *Invest Ophthalmol Vis Sci* **53**: 501–507. doi:10.1167/iovs.11-8784

Ruiz-Ederra J, Hitchcock PF, Vecino E. 2003. Two classes of astrocytes in the adult human and pig retina in terms of their expression of high affinity NGF receptor (TrkA). *Neurosci Lett* **337**: 127–130. doi:10.1016/s0304-3940(02)01322-8

Ryu J, Prather RS, Lee K. 2018. Use of gene-editing technology to introduce targeted modifications in pigs. *J Anim Sci Biotechnol* **9**: 5. doi:10.1186/s40104-017-0228-7

Sanchez I, Martin R, Ussa F, Fernandez-Bueno I. 2011. The parameters of the porcine eyeball. *Graefes Arch Clin Exp Ophthalmol* **249**: 475–482. doi:10.1007/s00417-011-1617-9

Santillo D, Mathieson I, Corsi F, Göllner R, Guandalini A. 2021. The use of acellular porcine corneal stroma xenograft (BioCorneaVet™) for the treatment of deep stromal and full thickness corneal defects: a retrospective study of 40 cases (2019–2021). *Vet Ophthalmol* **24**: 469–483. doi:10.1111/vop.12927

Scott PA, Fernandez De Castro JP, Kaplan HJ, McCall MA. 2014. A Pro23His mutation alters prenatal rod photoreceptor morphology in a transgenic swine model of retinitis pigmentosa. *Invest Ophthalmol Vis Sci* **55**: 2452–2459. doi:10.1167/iovs.13-13723

Scott PA, Kaplan HJ, McCall MA. 2015. Prenatal exposure to curcumin protects rod photoreceptors in a transgenic Pro23His swine model of retinitis pigmentosa. *Transl Vis Sci Technol* **4**: 5. doi:10.1167/tvst.4.5.5

Shahab M, Din NU, Shahab N. 2022. Genetically engineered porcine organs for human xenotransplantation. *Cureus* **14**: e29089. doi:10.7759/cureus.29089

Sharma R, Khristov V, Rising A, Jha BS, Dejene R, Hotaling N, Li Y, Stoddard J, Stankewicz C, Wan Q, et al. 2019. Clinical-grade stem cell-derived retinal pigment epithelium patch rescues retinal degeneration in rodents and pigs. *Sci Transl Med* **11**: eaat5580. doi:10.1126/scitranslmed.aat5580

Shire DB, Gingerich MD, Wong PI, Skvarla M, Cogan SF, Chen J, Wang W, Rizzo JF. 2020. Micro-fabrication of components for a high-density sub-retinal visual prosthesis. *Micromachines (Basel)* **11**: 944. doi:10.3390/mi11100944

Sinha NR, Balne PK, Bunyak F, Hofmann AC, Lim RR, Mohan RR, Chaurasia SS. 2021. Collagen matrix perturbations in corneal stroma of Ossabaw mini pigs with type 2 diabetes. *Mol Vis* **27**: 666–678.

Soede NM, Langendijk P, Kemp B. 2011. Reproductive cycles in pigs. *Anim Reprod Sci* **124**: 251–258. doi:10.1016/j.anireprosci.2011.02.025

Sohn EH, Jiao C, Kaalberg E, Cranston C, Mullins RF, Stone EM, Tucker BA. 2015. Allogenic iPSC-derived RPE cell transplants induce immune response in pigs: a pilot study. *Sci Rep* **5**: 11791. doi:10.1038/srep11791

Soler VJ, Laurent C, Sakr F, Regnier A, Tricoire C, Cases O, Kozyraki R, Douet JY, Pagot-Mathis V. 2017. Preliminary study of the safety and efficacy of medium-chain triglycerides for use as an intraocular tamponading agent in minipigs. *Graefes Arch Clin Exp Ophthalmol* **255**: 1593–1604. doi:10.1007/s00417-017-3695-9

Sommer JR, Wong F, Petters RM. 2011. Phenotypic stability of Pro347Leu rhodopsin transgenic pigs as indicated by photoreceptor cell degeneration. *Transgenic Res* **20**: 1391–1395. doi:10.1007/s11248-011-9491-0

Song YW, Pan ZQ. 2019. Reducing porcine corneal graft rejection, with an emphasis on porcine endogenous retrovirus transmission safety: a review. *Int J Ophthalmol* **12**: 324–332.

Sørensen NB. 2019. Subretinal surgery: functional and histological consequences of entry into the subretinal space. *Acta Ophthalmol* **97**: 1–23. doi:10.1111/aos.14249

Sørensen NF, Ejstrup R, Svahn TF, Sander B, Kiilgaard J, La Cour M. 2012. The effect of subretinal viscoelastics on the porcine retinal function. *Graefes Arch Clin Exp Ophthalmol* **250**: 79–86. doi:10.1007/s00417-011-1782-x

Stanzel B, Ader M, Liu Z, Amaral J, Aguirre LIR, Rickmann A, Barathi VA, Tan GSW, Degreif A, Al-Nawaiseh S, et al. 2019. Surgical approaches for cell therapeutics delivery to the retinal pigment epithelium and retina. *Adv Exp Med Biol* **1186**: 141–170. doi:10.1007/978-3-030-28471-8_6

Stirm M, Fonteyne LM, Shashikadze B, Stöckl JB, Kurome M, Keßler B, Zakhartchenko V, Kemter E, Blum H, Arnold GJ, et al. 2022. Pig models for Duchenne muscular dystrophy—from disease mechanisms to validation of new diagnostic and therapeutic concepts. *Neuromuscul Disord* **32**: 543–556. doi:10.1016/j.nmd.2022.04.005

Suh S, Choi EH, Raguram A, Liu DR, Palczewski K. 2022. Precision genome editing in the eye. *Proc Natl Acad Sci* **119**: e2210104119. doi:10.1073/pnas.2210104119

Summerfield A. 2009. Special issue on porcine immunology: an introduction from the guest editor. *Dev Comp Immunol* **33**: 265–266. doi:10.1016/j.dci.2008.07.014

Swier VJ, White KA, Johnson TB, Sieren JC, Johnson HJ, Knoernschild K, Wang X, Rohret FA, Rogers CS, Pearce DA, et al. 2022. A novel porcine model of CLN2 Batten disease that recapitulates patient phenotypes. *Neurotherapeutics* **19**: 1905–1919. doi:10.1007/s13311-022-01296-7

Sykes M, Sachs DH. 2022. Progress in xenotransplantation: overcoming immune barriers. *Nat Rev Nephrol* **18:** 745–761. doi:10.1038/s41581-022-00624-6

Szél A, Diamantstein T, Röhlich P. 1988. Identification of the blue-sensitive cones in the mammalian retina by anti-visual pigment antibody. *J Comp Neurol* **273:** 593–602. doi:10.1002/cne.902730413

Thompson JR, Worthington KS, Green BJ, Mullin NK, Jiao C, Kaalberg EE, Wiley LA, Han IC, Russell SR, Sohn EH, et al. 2019. Two-photon polymerized poly(caprolactone) retinal cell delivery scaffolds and their systemic and retinal biocompatibility. *Acta Biomater* **94:** 204–218. doi:10.1016/j.actbio.2019.04.057

Tso MO, Li WW, Zhang C, Lam TT, Hao Y, Petters RM, Wong F. 1997. A pathologic study of degeneration of the rod and cone populations of the rhodopsin Pro347Leu transgenic pigs. *Trans Am Ophthalmol Soc* **95:** 467–479; discussion 479–483.

Turner JM, Sauvé Y, Suh M, Wales PW, Wizzard P, Goruk S, Field CJ. 2016. A third-generation lipid emulsion that contains n-3 long-chain PUFAs preserves retinal function in parenterally fed neonatal piglets. *J Nutr* **146:** 2260–2266. doi:10.3945/jn.116.237669

Umeyama K, Nakajima M, Yokoo T, Nagaya M, Nagashima H. 2017. Diabetic phenotype of transgenic pigs introduced by dominant-negative mutant hepatocyte nuclear factor 1α. *J Diabetes Complications* **31:** 796–803. doi:10.1016/j.jdiacomp.2017.01.025

Van Cruchten S, Vrolyk V, Perron Lepage MF, Baudon M, Voute H, Schoofs S, Haruna J, Benoit-Biancamano MO, Ruot B, Allegaert K. 2017. Pre- and postnatal development of the eye: a species comparison. *Birth Defects Res* **109:** 1540–1567. doi:10.1002/bdr2.1100

Vecino E, Urcola H, Bayon A, Sharma SC. 2018. Ocular hypertension/glaucoma in minipigs: episcleral veins cauterization and microbead occlusion methods. *Methods Mol Biol* **1695:** 41–48. doi:10.1007/978-1-4939-7407-8_4

Veiga-Crespo P, Del Rio P, Blindert M, Ueffing M, Hauck SM, Vecino E. 2013. Phenotypic map of porcine retinal ganglion cells. *Mol Vis* **19:** 904–916.

Vrolyk V, Desmarais MJ, Lambert D, Haruna J, Benoit-Biancamano MO. 2020. Neonatal and juvenile ocular development in Göttingen minipigs and domestic pigs: a histomorphological and immunohistochemical study. *Vet Pathol* **57:** 889–914. doi:10.1177/0300985820954551

Vu QA, Seo HW, Choi KE, Kim N, Kang YN, Lee J, Park SH, Kim JT, Kim S, Kim SW. 2022. Structural changes in the retina after implantation of subretinal three-dimensional implants in mini pigs. *Front Neurosci* **16:** 1010445. doi:10.3389/fnins.2022.1010445

Wang W, Zhou L, Lee SJ, Liu Y, Fernandez De Castro J, Emery D, Vukmanic E, Kaplan HJ, Dean DC. 2014. Swine cone and rod precursors arise sequentially and display sequential and transient integration and differentiation potential following transplantation. *Invest Ophthalmol Vis Sci* **55:** 301–309. doi:10.1167/iovs.13-12600

Waschkowski F, Brockmann C, Laube T, Mokwa W, Roessler G, Walter P. 2013. Development of a very large array for retinal stimulation. *Annu Int Conf IEEE Eng Med Biol Soc* **2013:** 2748–2751. doi:10.1109/EMBC.2013.6610109

Wells KD, Prather RS. 2017. Genome-editing technologies to improve research, reproduction, and production in pigs. *Mol Reprod Dev* **84:** 1012–1017. doi:10.1002/mrd.22812

Welsh MJ, Rogers CS, Stoltz DA, Meyerholz DK, Prather RS. 2009. Development of a porcine model of cystic fibrosis. *Trans Am Clin Climatol Assoc* **120:** 149–162.

Wendland RJ, Jiao C, Russell SR, Han IC, Wiley LA, Tucker BA, Sohn EH, Worthington KS. 2021. The effect of retinal scaffold modulus on performance during surgical handling. *Exp Eye Res* **207:** 108566. doi:10.1016/j.exer.2021.108566

White KA, Swier VJ, Cain JT, Kohlmeyer JL, Meyerholz DK, Tanas MR, Uthoff J, Hammond E, Li H, Rohret FA, et al. 2018. A porcine model of neurofibromatosis type 1 that mimics the human disease. *JCI Insight* **3:** e120402. doi:10.1172/jci.insight.120402

Whitworth KM, Green JA, Redel BK, Geisert RD, Lee K, Telugu BP, Wells KD, Prather RS. 2022. Improvements in pig agriculture through gene editing. *CABI Agric Biosci* **3:** 41. doi:10.1186/s43170-022-00111-9

Yan S, Tu Z, Liu Z, Fan N, Yang H, Yang S, Yang W, Zhao Y, Ouyang Z, Lai C, et al. 2018. A Huntingtin knockin pig model recapitulates features of selective neurodegeneration in Huntington's disease. *Cell* **173:** 989–1002.e13. doi:10.1016/j.cell.2018.03.005

Yang W, Chen X, Li S, Li XJ. 2021. Genetically modified large animal models for investigating neurodegenerative diseases. *Cell Biosci* **11:** 218. doi:10.1186/s13578-021-00729-8

Ye GJ, Komáromy AM, Zeiss C, Calcedo R, Harman CD, Koehl KL, Stewart GA, Iwabe S, Chiodo VA, Hauswirth WW, et al. 2017. Safety and efficacy of AAV5 vectors expressing human or canine CNGB3 in CNGB3-mutant dogs. *Hum Gene Ther Clin Dev* **28:** 197–207. doi:10.1089/humc.2017.125

Yin P, Li S, Li XJ, Yang W. 2022. New pathogenic insights from large animal models of neurodegenerative diseases. *Protein Cell* **13:** 707–720. doi:10.1007/s13238-022-00912-8

Yoon CH, Choi HJ, Kim MK. 2021. Corneal xenotransplantation: where are we standing? *Prog Retin Eye Res* **80:** 100876. doi:10.1016/j.preteyeres.2020.100876

Zettler S, Renner S, Kemter E, Hinrichs A, Klymiuk N, Backman M, Riedel EO, Mueller C, Streckel E, Braun-Reichhart C, et al. 2020. A decade of experience with genetically tailored pig models for diabetes and metabolic research. *Anim Reprod* **17:** e20200064. doi:10.1590/1984-3143-AR2020-0064

Zhang J, Khazalwa EM, Abkallo HM, Zhou Y, Nie X, Ruan J, Zhao C, Wang J, Xu J, Li X, et al. 2021. The advancements, challenges, and future implications of the CRISPR/Cas9 system in swine research. *J Genet Genomics* **48:** 347–360. doi:10.1016/j.jgg.2021.03.015

Zhao Y, Nandra M, Yu CC, Tai YC. 2012. High performance 3-coil wireless power transfer system for the 512-electrode epiretinal prosthesis. *Annu Int Conf IEEE Eng Med Biol Soc* **2012:** 6583–6586.

Zou X, Ouyang H, Yu T, Chen X, Pang D, Tang X, Chen C. 2019. Preparation of a new type 2 diabetic miniature pig model via the CRISPR/Cas9 system. *Cell Death Dis* **10:** 823. doi:10.1038/s41419-019-2056-5

Toward Retinal Organoids in High-Throughput

Stefan Erich Spirig[1,2] and Magdalena Renner[1,2]

[1]Institute of Molecular and Clinical Ophthalmology Basel, Basel, Switzerland

[2]Department of Ophthalmology, University of Basel, Basel, Switzerland

Correspondence: magdalena.renner@iob.ch

Human retinal organoids recapitulate the cellular diversity, arrangement, gene expression, and functional aspects of the human retina. Protocols to generate human retinal organoids from pluripotent stem cells are typically labor intensive, include many manual handling steps, and the organoids need to be maintained for several months until they mature. To generate large numbers of human retinal organoids for therapy development and screening purposes, scaling up retinal organoid production, maintenance, and analysis is of utmost importance. In this review, we discuss strategies to increase the number of high-quality retinal organoids while reducing manual handling steps. We further review different approaches to analyze thousands of retinal organoids with currently available technologies and point to challenges that still await to be overcome both in culture and analysis of retinal organoids.

Organoids are three-dimensional cellular ensembles of multiple organ-specific cell types. The cell types are grouped and spatially organized similarly to an organ and recapitulate specific functions of that organ (Lancaster and Knoblich 2014b; Clevers 2016; Paşca et al. 2022). Organoids can be generated in vitro from different types of stem cells, such as organ-restricted adult stem cells or pluripotent stem cells (PSCs). Adult organ stem cells isolated from biopsies have the capacity to generate organoids resembling the source organ (e.g., intestinal organoids) (Clevers 2016; Kim et al. 2020). PSCs with the potential to differentiate into most cell types of the body can be subdivided into embryonic stem cells, derived from the inner cell mass of preimplantation embryos, and induced pluripotent stem cells (iPSCs), reprogrammed from adult cells such as fibroblasts or blood mononu-

clear cells (Liu et al. 2020; Yamanaka 2020). All these stem cells are presently being used to produce organoids that mimic different organs of the whole body (Clevers 2016; Kim et al. 2020). The organoids vary greatly in size and complexity according to the diverse nature of the tissues they model. As an example, intestinal organoids that are already used for high-throughput applications such as drug screenings (Lukonin et al. 2020) are rather small (on average 100 μm), develop relatively quickly (differentiated cells are present 5–7 d after plating), and typically contain less than 10 different cell types (Boonekamp et al. 2020; Pleguezuelos-Manzano et al. 2020). On the other hand, organoids of the central nervous system, such as cerebral and retinal organoids, are quite large (more than 1 mm), develop slowly (during 2–9 mo), and can include more than 40 different cell types arranged in a complex manner (Lancaster et al. 2013; Lancaster and Knoblich 2014a; Cowan et al. 2020; He et al. 2022).

Organoids as model systems built from human cells are a promising new tool for studying human development and disease in vitro. Source cells with a disease mutation can be used to generate patient-specific disease models, either by reprogramming patient cells to iPSCs or by introducing a precise patient mutation into control iPSCs by genome engineering. Patient-specific disease models allow not only the study of mechanisms of human disease in an unprecedented manner but also the testing of therapies such as gene therapy, small-molecule drugs, or oligonucleotides (Afanasyeva et al. 2021; Zhang et al. 2021a).

While studying organ development and disease phenotypes may require just a few dozen organoids, screening for novel drugs, for example, necessitates the generation of thousands of organoids in a high-throughput manner. However, this is easier said than done. The complex differentiation protocols to generate organoids typically include many manual handling steps. The maximum differentiation state may be reached only after weeks or months of culture, and the random 3D organization of organoids with high variability in size and shape is a problem for automated analysis. Hence, novel approaches to the culture and analysis of organoids in a high-throughput manner must be found. This review addresses this need in the context of human retinal organoids.

HUMAN RETINAL ORGANOIDS AS A MODEL SYSTEM

Retinal Organoids Mimic the Development of Human Retina

Retinal organoids were first generated by the group of Sasai from mouse embryonic stem cells (Eiraku et al. 2011) and shortly thereafter from human PSCs (Meyer et al. 2011; Nakano et al. 2012). Mouse retinal organoids develop in just a few weeks while human retinal organoids reach comparable stages of development only after several months (Llonch et al. 2018), reflecting the

difference in the developmental rates of mice and humans. Several studies have shown that human retinal organoids mature at a rate comparable to the developing human retina, in terms of gene-expression profiles, cell-type generation, and morphological properties (Cowan et al. 2020; Lu et al. 2020; Sridhar et al. 2020; Kim et al. 2023).

Comparison of Retinal Organoids to Human Retina, Validating Them as a Model System

The human retina is a highly complex organ of more than 100 cell types with different morphologies, functions, and gene-expression profiles (Masland 2012; Zeng and Sanes 2017). Cell bodies in the human retina are arranged in three nuclear layers: the outer nuclear, inner nuclear, and ganglion cell layer. Photoreceptor cell bodies are located in the outer nuclear layer, horizontal, bipolar, amacrine, and Müller cells in the inner nuclear layer, and amacrine and ganglion cells in the ganglion cell layer. Synaptic connections between cells of adjacent nuclear layers are established in the outer- and inner-plexiform layers, respectively (Masland 2012). Finally, photoreceptors of the neural retina are in close contact with retinal pigment epithelial cells, which are important for photoreceptor function (Strauss 2005; Sparrrow et al. 2010).

Validation of retinal organoids as a model of the human retina depends on several criteria, namely, the presence of retinal cell types, their correct arrangement, responses to light, and synaptic transmission (Lancaster and Knoblich 2014b). The major retinal cell classes (photoreceptors, horizontal-, bipolar-, amacrine-, ganglion- and Müller cells) have been identified immunohistochemically in organoids generated with several different culture protocols (Zhong et al. 2014; Capowski et al. 2018). Photoreceptors were typically found on the outside of the organoids, while other cell types were located more internally. Only recently were we able to generate five-layered retinal organoids with three nuclear and two synaptic layers and to confirm the correct localization of organoid cell classes within the appropriate layers by comparisons to the adult retina by immunostaining (Cowan et al. 2020).

Cite this article as *Cold Spring Harb Perspect Med* doi: 10.1101/cshperspect.a041275

Moreover, organoid photoreceptors are light sensitive and able to transmit light responses via synapses to second- or third-order cells (Zhong et al. 2014; Cowan et al. 2020; Saha et al. 2022). Single-cell genomics confirmed the presence of all major retinal cell classes in retinal organoids and a high similarity of organoid cell types to those of the human retina (Kim et al. 2023).

By comparing organoids to healthy, light-responsive human retina (fovea and periphery), we furthermore validated the expression of many disease-associated genes in the same cell types as in human adult retina (Cowan et al. 2020). Thus, existing retinal organoids can be accepted as models for the human retina that recapitulate aspects of cell-type diversity, arrangement, gene expression, and function.

Retinal organoids, however, can still be improved as they currently lack some cell types and anatomical features of the human retina. Organoid photoreceptors are currently missing contact with retinal pigment epithelium, which is often present in isolated patches on retinal organoids. Microfluidic chips have been developed to establish contact of retinal pigment epithelium with photoreceptor outer segments (Achberger et al. 2019). Additionally, efforts are ongoing to integrate missing microglia and blood vessels into retinal organoids, respectively (Gao et al. 2022; Chichagova et al. 2023; Li et al. 2023). Further, retinal organoids lack an optic nerve because ganglion cells are lost in mature retinal organoids. Therefore, they are typically not connected to brain structures targeted by retinal ganglion cell axons (Zhong et al. 2014; Cowan et al. 2020). In assemblies of retinal and brain organoids, axonal projections toward brain structures have been described (Fligor et al. 2021; Fernando et al. 2022). Finally, retinal organoids resemble more the retinal periphery and, although cone-rich organoids and organoids with some anatomical characteristics of the fovea-parafovea region have been described, organoids containing a fovea or organoids of fovea identity still await publication (Kim et al. 2019; Cowan et al. 2020; Völkner et al. 2022). Organoid (co-)culture modifications toward a more complete retina model are promising, but need to become more robust, reproducible, and auto-

mation friendly for high-throughput applications.

RETINAL ORGANOIDS FOR THERAPY DEVELOPMENT

The treatment of retinal diseases requires a deep understanding of the mechanisms and genes involved. Many genes are associated with inherited retinal degeneration, where mutations in a single gene can lead to deterioration or even complete loss of vision, and different mutations in the same gene can result in different clinical phenotypes (RetNet, the Retinal Information Network). Certain genes are associated with specific retinal diseases and some of these genes are important for the function of specific cell types (Berger et al. 2010).

Only recently has single-cell RNA sequencing of the healthy human retina allowed comprehensive identification of the cell types that express known disease-associated genes. Expression of these genes is often restricted to one or a few cell types (Cowan et al. 2020), and, thus, in many cases, the treatment of retinal diseases will be cell-type specific.

There are currently four main approaches to the therapy of retinal diseases: gene therapy, optogenetic vision restoration, cell therapy, and small molecule treatment. First, gene therapy aims to introduce a functional copy of the mutated gene into the impacted cells using viral vectors or to repair the mutation with genome-engineering tools. To prevent side-effects on cell types that do not express the disease-relevant gene, entry of the virus or expression of the virus cargo should be cell-type specific. Organoids produced in large numbers will help identify viral vector variants with affinity to specific cell types, as well as to screen for cell-type-specific expression of the virus cargo mediated by promoter elements (Gonzalez-Cordero et al. 2018; Jüttner et al. 2019; Tornabene et al. 2019; Garita-Hernandez et al. 2020; Völkner et al. 2021; McClements et al. 2022; Tso et al. 2023). Furthermore, organoids could be used to optimize new gene-editing tools such as base editing, prime editing (da Costa et al. 2021), small oligos (Dulla et al. 2018), or homology-directed repair to repair disease mutations (Gallego et al. 2020; Pasquini et al. 2020). Gene therapy needs to be adapted to individual mutations and more than 250 genes are associated with inherited retinal diseases (RetNet). Several gene-therapy approaches are already in clinical trials (clinicaltrials.gov) and *Luxturna* to treat RPE65-based retinal degeneration has been approved (Russell et al. 2017).

Second, artificial stimulation of the retina by optogenetic tools (Boyden et al. 2005) can be first tested and optimized in retinal organoids (Garita-Hernandez et al. 2018). Although it has been shown that retinal organoids contain functional synapses transmitting signals from photoreceptors to second- and third-order cells (Cowan et al. 2020), it is still unclear to what extent retinal circuits are present in organoids (Fathi et al. 2021).

Third, cell therapy aims to replace degenerated cells in patients and the cells for transplantation could be purified from retinal organoids. However, the functional integration of photoreceptors, for example, into existing retinal circuits is a challenge (Llonch et al. 2018).

Fourth, small-molecule treatments aim to slow or prevent retinal degeneration. The small-molecule drugs are usually applied systemically or via intravitreal injection and they can easily target the entire retina (Maneu et al. 2022). However, these drugs are not usually cell-type specific and may also interfere with healthy cells. This can be modeled by first applying the compound to the organoid culture medium. To identify small-molecule drugs with the desired effect, typically thousands of chemical compounds are tested in parallel in several replicates and this would require the generation of many thousand retinal organoids. Due to the present technical limitations, high-throughput, small-molecule screens have not yet been performed on human retinal organoids. However, initial attempts at large-scale screens have been made using simpler organoid models: Lukonin et al. have published results of a screen of 2789 compounds that used approximately 450,000 intestinal organoids (Lukonin et al. 2020). Tumor biopsies can also be cultured under organoid growth conditions and have been used for drug screenings. These models can facilitate personalized medicine by testing the response of an individual's specific tumor to various treatments, allowing for the selection of the optimal treatment option (Aboulkheyr Es et al. 2018).

Finally, the toxicology of treatments developed for medical conditions not primarily affecting the eye needs to be studied early in drug development. Several compounds such as thioridazine or tamoxifen can cause severe damage to the retina under high dosage (Corradetti et al. 2019). Retinal organoids can be used to screen for negative effects of potential drugs on the retina (Fig. 1; Dorgau et al. 2022).

SCALING UP RETINAL ORGANOID NUMBERS

Organoids can be generated from patient cells or from cells in which precise disease mutations have been introduced by genome engineering. Such retinal organoids have been used already in studies to elucidate disease phenotypes and the mechanisms of disease, as well as to test targeted therapies (Zhang et al. 2021a) and a small number of compounds (Dorgau et al. 2022). Relatively few organoids in the range of several dozen are sufficient for these types of studies. Studies like high-throughput compound screens with the aim to produce and analyze organoids in the range of thousands have not yet been conducted due to the limitations of both organoid culture and analysis that need to be overcome.

TOWARD HIGH-THROUGHPUT ORGANOID CULTURE

Although various protocols for organoid generation exist, they are mostly based on common principles (Zhang et al. 2021b) and can be divided into several steps. First, iPSCs are subjected to neural induction to initiate differentiation of a neural identity. Second, eye-field development is induced and, third, retina tissue is harvested and cultured floating in 3D for further development and differentiation during several months. Each of these steps is a bottleneck because they are each typically associated with time-consuming manual procedures that limit the rate at which organoids can be handled.

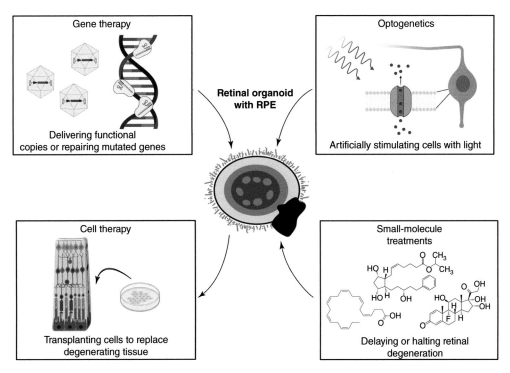

Figure 1. Main therapeutic approaches for retinal diseases that can be tested on retinal organoids. Organoids can also be a source of cells for transplantation in cell therapy. In the *center* of the figure is an illustration of a retinal organoid with a black bud of retinal pigment epithelium (RPE) attached to it. (Figure created with BioRender.com.)

Furthermore, the efficacies of each of these steps vary and the success rate of each procedure needs to be maximized to generate organoids in large numbers. In short, high-throughput culture of organoids requires the optimizing of organoid variability and numbers and the reduction of labor-intensive manual handling.

Given that the differentiation time-course of retinal organoids resembles that of the human retina in utero, optimal retinal organoid culture should closely mimic human embryonic development. During embryonic development, the neural tube gives rise at its anterior end to the forebrain, midbrain, and hindbrain. The forebrain gives rise to the optic vesicles that further develop into retina. Several publications have reported that PSC lines differ in their capacity to form retinal organoids (Capowski et al. 2018; Wang et al. 2018; Mellough et al. 2019; Rashidi et al. 2022). Indeed, a common by-product of retinal organoid differentiation are brain organoids

without retina (Meyer et al. 2011; Fernando et al. 2022). Similarly to retinal organoids, different PSC lines when subjected to differentiation into cerebral organoids form different parts of the forebrain, such as dorsal forebrain, ventral forebrain, and retina, which suggests that the ratio of tissues generated is cell-line dependent (Kanton et al. 2019).

Hence, choosing an appropriate cell line is the first step toward high-throughput generation of retinal organoids. Some protocols add growth factors or small molecules to improve differentiation into retina, but here again the responses to both can be cell-line dependent and each line needs to be optimized (Chichagova et al. 2020; Regent et al. 2022). Most protocols perform neural induction on embryoid bodies (EBs), which are small clumps of PSCs aggregated in 3D. The size of the EBs can influence the efficiency of retinal organoid generation and some cell lines only form retinal organoids efficiently from EBs of a particular size (Mellough et al. 2019; Cowan et al. 2020). EB size can be regulated by seeding individualized PSCs at defined numbers into the round bottom cavity of a cell-culture dish (Choi et al. 2010; Cowan et al. 2020). Traditionally, this is performed in low-attachment U-bottom or V-bottom 96-well plates (Nakano et al. 2012) with one EB per well. However, these plates are expensive, feeding requires large amounts of medium, and several thousand PSCs per well need to be seeded for efficient EB formation. More high-throughput-friendly EBs can be formed in hydrogel microwell arrays (Cowan et al. 2020; Decembrini et al. 2020; Rashidi et al. 2022). The molds to prepare agarose microwell arrays are commercially available, reusable, and take up to 256 EBs that can easily be cultured in a standard multiwell plate. For two PSC lines that generate five-layered human retina, we have shown that EBs generated from only a few hundred cells lead to higher yields of retina tissue than seeding more than a thousand cells per microwell. Using agarose microwells, up to 4000 organoids can be generated from a single well of a six-well plate of iPSCs (Cowan et al. 2020), thus allowing high-throughput organoid production. Some protocols perform neural induction on PSCs in 2D without EB formation (Singh et al. 2015), but this requires many wells of evenly seeded PSCs to produce thousands of retinal organoids.

For differentiation into the eye field, EBs are either maintained in 3D in the presence of growth factors and extracellular matrix components (Nakano et al. 2012; Rashidi et al. 2022) or they are plated on Matrigel-coated dishes (Zhong et al. 2014). Most protocols require isolation of retina tissue from floating 3D aggregates or from Matrigel plates by manual microdissection. This step is not only time consuming and very challenging technically, but it also leads to discarding of retina that cannot be identified morphologically or handled within a reasonable amount of time. However, detaching the entire content of the Matrigel plate by scraping allows complete harvesting of all retina tissue from each plate (Cowan et al. 2020; Regent et al. 2020). Avoiding manual microdissection is the second critical step toward high-throughput production of retinal organoids.

Even though AMASS (agarose microwell-assisted seeding and scraping) allows the production of thousands of retinal organoids (Cowan et al. 2020), many further manual steps need to be eliminated for high-throughput organoid culture. One of these is the changing of organoid culture media several times per week during up to 38 wk of development, depending on the time point chosen for analysis. Given free-floating cultures in low-attachment 10-cm dishes, automatizing media exchange would require highly advanced and potentially custom-built robotic equipment that is currently not available in most academic laboratories. It has been suggested to culture organoids in bioreactors; although this seems to be beneficial for early organoid development, it is damaging to older organoids that contain fragile structures such as photoreceptor outer segments (Ovando-Roche et al. 2018).

A further challenge to producing thousands of organoids is the inefficiency of organoid differentiation itself, where a percentage of the 3D aggregates will not contain retina. Hence, these organoids need to be excluded from experiments or the number of replicates needs to be increased.

For many procedures, such as drug testing, imaging-based readouts, or transduction with gene therapy vectors, retinal organoids must be singularized in wells of multiwell plates. This involves labor-intensive manual intervention to transfer organoids to an assay plate that may also be subject to bias when selecting organoids for inclusion in an experiment that must meet certain quality criteria, such as the presence of retina. Automatizing this step to allow experiments on thousands of retinal organoids, for example in a drug screen, would require a custom-built machine that uses artificial intelligence to assess organoid quality and to sort them into assay plates without reducing organoid viability or disrupting fragile outer segments. Such an algorithm has been successfully developed to assess the quality of mouse retinal organoids (Kegeles et al. 2020).

Organoid Morphology

Optimal organoids for accurate high-throughput screening should be consistent in size, regular in shape, and include only retina. However, retinal organoids obtained by scraping typically contain several buds of retina as well as further buds of nonretinal identity that do not negatively impact retina development. The retina within the buds may be regularly organized in layers but the size, number, and shape of the buds differ greatly from organoid to organoid. Furthermore, retinal organoids are not perfectly round and on their long axis can reach diameters from one to three millimeters. In a high-throughput experiment such as a drug screen, the inconsistent sizes of the organoids may influence the outcome. Because of their relatively large size, retinal organoids do not fit into 1536-well plates and only barely into 384-well plates, where media consumption and thus viability may differ according to size and so may potentially influence experiment outcome.

Culture Time

Human retinal organoids in culture reach stages in which their cell types are comparable to adult retinal cells at around 30 wk of organoid development (Cowan et al. 2020). Although it has been reported that human retinal organoids can be cryopreserved (Nakano et al. 2012; Reichman et al. 2017), it remains to be shown whether cryopreserved organoids retain a layered structure with at least a defined photoreceptor layer and inner nuclear layer with viable cells. Thus, at present, cultures cannot be paused and experiments need to be strictly planned many months in advance. This long culture time brings the risk of losing organoids from events such as contamination, equipment failure, and supply-chain interruptions, or due to human error. The long culture time also places pressure on laboratory space that may limit the number of organoids that can be cultured. Thus, organoid analysis time points need careful selection to balance the required degree of organoid maturation against the shortest possible culture time. Ways to increase the rate of organoid development without severely impacting organoid quality have so far proven elusive. One possible solution for some experiments is to use organoids from primates, which develop faster in accor-

dance with the shorter gestation times of the animals (Fig. 2; Jacobo Lopez et al. 2022).

High-Throughput Organoid Analysis

Although organoids are open to analysis by a wide range of routine assays, depending on the scientific question, the analysis of thousands of retinal organoids remains a challenge.

Imaging

The most widely used readouts for retinal organoids are imaging based. Although retinal organoids are 3D model systems, phenotype analysis is often performed by immunohistochemistry on thin sections of fixed tissue. This can produce data on positioning and the abundance of cell types and antigens, but each stained section shows the state at only one time point. Since organoid size and cell-type composition are not constant, reliable comparison of sections may be difficult, especially when the differences in phenotype are small.

Preparing organoid sections for imaging is a labor-intensive, low-throughput manual task. However, cultured murine retinal organoids in arrays of hydrogel milliwells allowed imaging of individual organoids at different time points. Furthermore, milliwell arrays containing organoids can be embedded for thin sectioning and arrayed immunohistochemical analyses (Decembrini et al. 2020). This method has yet to be tested on human retinal organoids.

Using tissue-clearing methods, retinal organoids can be stained and imaged without sectioning and the associated sectioning problems, but this may complicate data analysis and image acquisition (Reichman et al. 2017; Cora et al. 2019). However, tissue clearing and 3D analysis are becoming more automation friendly and could be adapted for retinal organoids (Ueda et al. 2020).

Live Imaging

A more scalable approach is to use live imaging. This allows analysis of an organoid over several time points and, thus, comparison of each or-

	Challenges	Toward high-throughput organoid generation
iPSC colonies 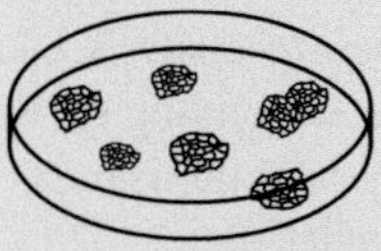	Not all iPSCs generate retinal organoids efficiently	Select iPSC line with high capacity to form retinal organoids
Neural induction 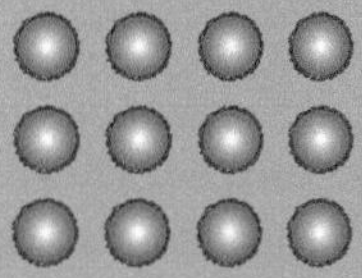	EB size can influence differentiation into retina	Optimize retina yield by: Controlling EB size in microwell arrays Optimizing EB size for optimal yield of retina
Eye-field formation 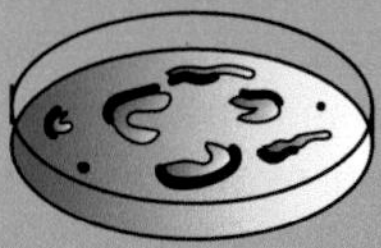	Eye-field formation could be favored over other CNS areas by some cell lines	Adding small molecules may improve differentiation into retina, needs optimization for each cell line
Retina harvest 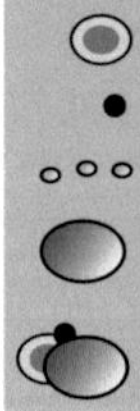 ○ Retina structure ● RPE ○ ○ ○ Debris Nonretinal brain tissue Retina–brain organoids	Harvesting of retina from culture plate that contains heterogeneous tissue Scraping yields mix of tissue identities	Retina harvest by checkerboard scraping + fast + easy + high-throughput + suited for automation + no selection bias + no retina left behind on plate for trashing Optimize EB size to obtain high percentage of aggregates with retina Brain tissue attached to retina does not negatively impact retina development
Retina maturation 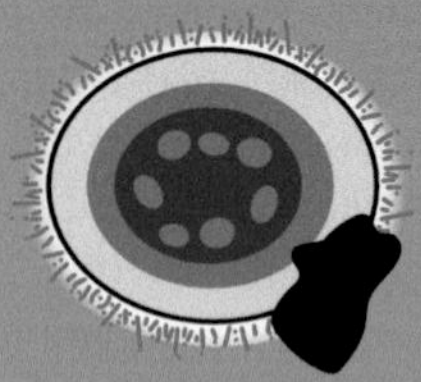	- Culture up to 38 weeks - Frequent media changes necessary - Quality control - Freezing organoids not efficient, experiments cannot be paused - Expensive supplements - Sensitive to accidents, equipment failure, human error - Placing organoids in assay plates	Automate: - Plate handling and media exchange - Selection of high-quality retinal organoids for further culture or for experiments - Placing of organoids into assay plates

Figure 2. Challenges of retinal organoid culture and measures to increase throughput. Each step of the cultivation process requires careful optimization. (iPSC) Induced pluripotent stem cells, (EB) embryoid body, (CNS) central nervous system, (RPE) retinal pigment epithelium.

ganoid before the onset of a phenotype or the administration of a treatment. The data analysis then is more robust. Several imaging techniques have been used to characterize retinal organoids. Methods like phase contrast, differential interference contrast, or standard brightfield imaging of organoids can assess overall viability and the quality of the tissue (Browne et al. 2017). This is suitable for high-throughput screening experiments but only a limited amount of information can be drawn from these images.

The analysis of organoids in which fluorophores are expressed cell-type specifically retrieves additional information at the cell-type level. This can be carried out with engineered stem cell lines or after delivery of a transgene to more developed organoids.

Engineering stem cell lines to carry reporter genes and their differentiation into retinal organoids has been successful and may be a useful tool to study individual cell types in a high-throughput manner (Vergara et al. 2017; Phillips et al. 2018; Lam et al. 2020; Jones et al. 2022; Nazlamova et al. 2022). A common approach is to engineer a fluorophore gene into the locus of a cell-type-specific gene and so to couple the fluorophore expression pattern to that of the cell-type-specific gene. This leads to uniform labeling of a specific cell type. However, this process is very time consuming since proper validation of the line can only be achieved after the full development of the organoid. Tagging cell-type-specific genes with a fluorophore may also lead to undesired effects on gene expression and the development of that cell type. This would be particularly troublesome when patient-derived organoids are used. Furthermore, gene editing of PSCs can cause off-target mutations and hence influence differentiation efficiency, making it more difficult to generate organoids for high-throughput applications. A simpler approach is to deliver the fluorophore transgene into more developed organoids.

Although transfection can be used for organoids (Lancaster et al. 2013; Fujii et al. 2015), the use of a viral vector as a delivery vehicle is more common. In efforts to use retinal organoids as preclinical models for gene therapy, several groups have shown that transduction of organoids using adeno-associated viral vectors is a feasible way to label a multitude of cell types. These vectors in combination with cell-type-specific promoter elements can label specific cell types in mature retinal organoids (Gonzalez-Cordero et al. 2018; Völkner et al. 2021; McClements et al. 2022; Tso et al. 2023). One disadvantage of viral delivery is that transduction efficiency may vary between organoids and be a further source of variability in high-throughput applications.

Although promising, live imaging of organoids for high-throughput applications also comes with certain problems. Retinal organoids are inherently opaque, and light from the imagers used for screening may fail to completely penetrate; this will lead to an asymmetric readout. This might be acceptable if the organoids stay in the same orientation during an experiment. However, minor turbulence in the medium (e.g., during media change) can result in movement of the organoid that exposes a different part of the tissue and makes comparisons between time points unreliable. Anchoring of retinal organoids and maintaining a sufficient supply of nutrients need to be addressed.

Molecular Assays

Common 2D cell-culture assays can be adapted for retinal organoids. Western blots, qPCR, flow cytometry, as well as recent "omic" technologies such as transcriptomics, epigenomics, or proteomics have been used to study organoids (Afanasyeva et al. 2021). These assays can be performed on entire organoids or on organoids dissociated into single cells. Modified versions of whole-organoid RNA sequencing can be explored as scalable readouts. The difficulty of these assays is to retain cell-type-specific information when applied to high-throughput applications. Analysis of single or sorted cells retains information about cell types but loses information about cell positioning. Dissociation of organoids to single cells must avoid reducing cell viability, and the dissociation of large quantities of organoids simultaneously is very challenging.

Molecular assays typically used for high-throughput screening, such as luminescence, fluorescence, or colorimetric assays, have yet to be explored in the context of retinal organoids.

An alternative to high-throughput screens that test just one condition per retinal organoid are pooled screening assays that combine several perturbations inside a single organoid. For example, CRISPR screening can modulate the expression of different genes in individual cells within a single organoid and the effects can be read out by single-cell RNA sequencing (Ungricht et al. 2022). Relatively few organoids are required for pooled screens but they yield information about changes in gene expression in a large number of cells.

Functional Assays

The capacity to recapitulate some of the functions of an organ is a key feature of organoid biology. Functional assays, such as patch clamp recordings (Meyer et al. 2011; Zhong et al. 2014; Deng et al. 2018; Li et al. 2021), multielectrode array recordings (Buskin et al. 2018; Hallam et al. 2018; Chichagova et al. 2023), and calcium imaging (Cowan et al. 2020), have been applied to retinal organoids. This has revealed that organoid photoreceptors are intrinsically light sensitive and transmit visual input information through synapses to inner nuclear cells, similarly to the human retina.

Functional assays like patch-clamping are not feasible as a high-throughput readout due to the extensive manual work required to measure just a few cells. Scaling up multielectrode array-based assays is becoming more feasible and has been applied to cerebral organoids (Durens et al. 2020). This may be adaptable for retinal organoids; however, multielectrode arrays would not allow comparison of cell types but could be used to study responses of ganglion cells as the only spiking cells in the retina. Current drawbacks of MEA recordings to study retinal ganglion cells in retinal organoids are the loss of retinal ganglion cells in organoids aged more than 20 wk (Buskin et al. 2018; Fligor et al. 2021) and the internal location of the retinal ganglion cells.

Calcium imaging may be the most sensitive functional assay for screening applications since it is based on live imaging and the expression of

the calcium sensor can be targeted to certain cell types. Combining calcium imaging with visual stimulation in larger screens would require specialized equipment and sophisticated data analysis.

While many different assays are available for studying retinal organoids, very few of them are suitable for high-throughput applications. The challenge is to choose a readout that minimizes manual handling time per organoid and that, ideally, can be automated without loss of information at a cell-type level. A simple and clear readout is the essential basis of any high-throughput screening (Fig. 3).

DISCUSSION

Retinal organoids are a new and powerful tool to study retinal biology, development, and disease. Their use as preclinical models to test new therapeutic approaches, especially in high-throughput, could revolutionize drug and therapy research of retinal diseases.

For reliable use in screening, several features of retinal organoid cultures need to be optimized and they must become more automation friendly. The production of thousands of retinal organoids is mostly theoretical at present but is essential for high-throughput screening. In addition, most differentiation protocols rely on expensive supplements, and more cost-efficient alternatives are necessary for routine high-throughput organoid screens. Another significant challenge is to sort out genuine organoids from other cell aggregates that might form and so to ensure reliable organoid quality throughout a screen.

Finding suitable phenotypes for high-throughput screening is also a challenge, as most reported disease-modeling phenotypes are monitored by transcriptome changes or immunohistochemistry (Chirco et al. 2021; Kruczek et al. 2021; Chahine Karam et al. 2022; Völkner et al. 2022). These phenotypes need to be adapted in some way and/or other more screening-friendly phenotypes sought to test and screen therapies on diseased organoids. Improvements in both organoid throughput in culture and the analysis of retinal organoids are important not only for high-throughput screening of organoids but also

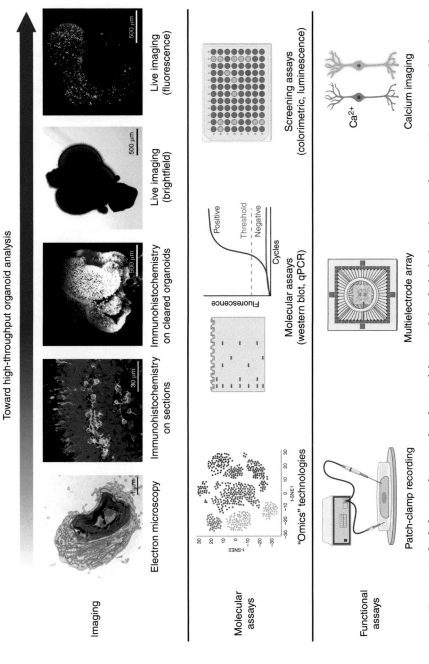

Figure 3. Methods for retinal organoid analysis and their suitability for high-throughput applications. Some imaging-based, molecular, or functional assays can be more easily adapted for analyzing high numbers of retinal organoids (*right* side of figure). (Figure created with BioRender.com.)

to facilitate the generation of high-quality retinal organoids for research that exploits this exciting new model.

ACKNOWLEDGMENTS

We thank Patrick King for English proofreading, and Pierre Balmer, Veronica Moreno, and Alvaro Herrero for their helpful suggestions on the manuscript.

REFERENCES

Aboulkheyr Es H, Montazeri L, Aref AR, Vosough M, Baharvand H. 2018. Personalized cancer medicine: an organoid approach. *Trends Biotechnol* **36:** 358–371. doi:10.1016/j.tibtech.2017.12.005

Achberger K, Probst C, Haderspeck J, Bolz S, Rogal J, Chuchuy J, Nikolova M, Cora V, Antkowiak L, Haq W, et al. 2019. Merging organoid and organ-on-a-chip technology to generate complex multi-layer tissue models in a human retina-on-a-chip platform. *eLife* **8:** e46188. doi:10.7554/eLife.46188

Afanasyeva TAV, Corral-Serrano JC, Garanto A, Roepman R, Cheetham ME, Collin RWJ. 2021. A look into retinal organoids: methods, analytical techniques, and applications. *Cell Mol Life Sci* **78:** 6505–6532. doi:10.1007/s00018-021-03917-4

Berger W, Kloeckener-Gruissem B, Neidhardt J. 2010. The molecular basis of human retinal and vitreoretinal diseases. *Prog Retin Eye Res* **29:** 335–375. doi:10.1016/j.preteyeres.2010.03.004

Boonekamp KE, Dayton TL, Clevers H. 2020. Intestinal organoids as tools for enriching and studying specific and rare cell types: advances and future directions. *J Mol Cell Biol* **12:** 562–568. doi:10.1093/jmcb/mjaa034

Boyden ES, Zhang F, Bamberg E, Nagel G, Deisseroth K. 2005. Millisecond-timescale, genetically targeted optical control of neural activity. *Nat Neurosci* **8:** 1263–1268. doi:10.1038/nn1525

Browne AW, Arnesano C, Harutyunyan N, Khuu T, Martinez JC, Pollack HA, Koos DS, Lee TC, Fraser SE, Moats RA, et al. 2017. Structural and functional characterization of human stem-cell-derived retinal organoids by live imaging. *Invest Ophthalmol Vis Sci* **58:** 3311–3318.

Buskin A, Zhu L, Chichagova V, Basu B, Mozaffari-Jovin S, Dolan D, Droop A, Collin J, Bronstein R, Mehrotra S, et al. 2018. Disrupted alternative splicing for genes implicated in splicing and ciliogenesis causes PRPF31 retinitis pigmentosa. *Nat Commun* **9:** 4234. doi:10.1038/s41467-018-06448-y

Capowski EE, Samimi K, Mayerl SJ, Phillips MJ, Pinilla I, Howden SE, Saha J, Jansen AD, Edwards KL, Jager LD, et al. 2018. Reproducibility and staging of 3D human retinal organoids across multiple pluripotent stem cell lines. *Development* **146:** dev.171686. doi:10.1242/dev.171686

Chahine Karam F, Loi TH, Ma A, Nash BM, Grigg JR, Parekh D, Riley LG, Farnsworth E, Bennetts B, Gonzalez-Cor-

dero A, et al. 2022. Human iPSC-derived retinal organoids and retinal pigment epithelium for novel intronic RPGR variant assessment for therapy suitability. *J Pers Med* **12:** 502. doi:10.3390/jpm12030502

Chichagova V, Hilgen G, Ghareeb A, Georgiou M, Carter M, Sernagor E, Lako M, Armstrong L. 2020. Human iPSC differentiation to retinal organoids in response to IGF1 and BMP4 activation is line- and method-dependent. *Stem Cells* **38:** 195–201. doi:10.1002/stem.3116

Chichagova V, Georgiou M, Carter M, Dorgau B, Hilgen G, Collin J, Queen R, Chung G, Ajeian J, Moya-Molina M, et al. 2023. Incorporating microglia-like cells in human induced pluripotent stem cell-derived retinal organoids. *J Cell Mol Med* **27:** 435–445. doi:10.1111/jcmm.17670

Chirco KR, Chew S, Moore AT, Duncan JL, Lamba DA. 2021. Allele-specific gene editing to rescue dominant CRX-associated LCA7 phenotypes in a retinal organoid model. *Stem Cell Rep* **16:** 2690–2702. doi:10.1016/j.stemcr.2021.09.007

Choi YY, Chung BG, Lee DH, Khademhosseini A, Kim JH, Lee SH. 2010. Controlled-size embryoid body formation in concave microwell arrays. *Biomaterials* **31:** 4296–4303. doi:10.1016/j.biomaterials.2010.01.115

Clevers H. 2016. Modeling development and disease with organoids. *Cell* **165:** 1586–1597. doi:10.1016/j.cell.2016.05.082

Cora V, Haderspeck J, Antkowiak L, Mattheus U, Neckel P, Mack A, Bolz S, Ueffing M, Pashkovskaia N, Achberger K, et al. 2019. A cleared view on retinal organoids. *Cells* **8:** 391. doi:10.3390/cells8050391

Corradetti G, Violanti S, Au A, Sarraf D. 2019. Wide field retinal imaging and the detection of drug associated retinal toxicity. *Int J Retina Vitr* **5:** 26. doi:10.1186/s40942-019-0172-0

Cowan CS, Renner M, De Gennaro M, Gross-Scherf B, Goldblum D, Hou Y, Munz M, Rodrigues TM, Krol J, Szikra T, et al. 2020. Cell types of the human retina and its organoids at single-cell resolution. *Cell* **182:** 1623–1640.e34. doi:10.1016/j.cell.2020.08.013

da Costa BL, Levi SR, Eulau E, Tsai YT, Quinn PMJ. 2021. Prime editing for inherited retinal diseases. *Front Genome Ed* **3:** 775330. doi:10.3389/fgeed.2021.775330

Decembrini S, Hoehnel S, Brandenberg N, Arsenijevic Y, Lutolf MP. 2020. Hydrogel-based milliwell arrays for standardized and scalable retinal organoid cultures. *Sci Rep* **10:** 10275. doi:10.1038/s41598-020-67012-7

Deng WL, Gao ML, Lei XL, Lv JN, Zhao H, He KW, Xia XX, Li LY, Chen YC, Li YP, et al. 2018. Gene correction reverses ciliopathy and photoreceptor loss in iPSC-derived retinal organoids from retinitis pigmentosa patients. *Stem Cell Rep* **10:** 1267–1281. doi:10.1016/j.stemcr.2018.02.003

Dorgau B, Georgiou M, Chaudhary A, Moya-Molina M, Collin J, Queen R, Hilgen G, Davey T, Hewitt P, Schmitt M, et al. 2022. Human retinal organoids provide a suitable tool for toxicological investigations: a comprehensive validation using drugs and compounds affecting the retina. *Stem Cells Transl Med* **11:** 159–177. doi:10.1093/stcltm/szab010

Dulla K, Aguila M, Lane A, Jovanovic K, Parfitt DA, Schulkens I, Chan HL, Schmidt I, Beumer W, Vorthoren L, et al. 2018. Splice-modulating oligonucleotide QR-110 restores CEP290 mRNA and function in human c.2991-

Cite this article as *Cold Spring Harb Perspect Med* doi: 10.1101/cshperspect.a041275

+1655A>G LCA10 models. *Mol Ther Nucleic Acids* **12**: 730–740. doi:10.1016/j.omtn.2018.07.010

Durens M, Nestor J, Williams M, Herold K, Niescier RF, Lunden JW, Phillips AW, Lin Y-C, Dykxhoorn DM, Nestor MW. 2020. High-throughput screening of human induced pluripotent stem cell-derived brain organoids. *J Neurosci Methods* **335**: 108627. doi:10.1016/j.jneumeth.2020.108627

Eiraku M, Takata N, Ishibashi H, Kawada M, Sakakura E, Okuda S, Sekiguchi K, Adachi T, Sasai Y. 2011. Self-organizing optic-cup morphogenesis in three-dimensional culture. *Nature* **472**: 51–56. doi:10.1038/nature09941

Fathi M, Ross CT, Hosseinzadeh Z. 2021. Functional 3-dimensional retinal organoids: technological progress and existing challenges. *Front Neurosci* **15**: 668857. doi:10.3389/fnins.2021.668857

Fernando M, Lee S, Wark JR, Xiao D, Lim BY, O'Hara-Wright M, Kim HJ, Smith GC, Wong T, Teber ET, et al. 2022. Differentiation of brain and retinal organoids from confluent cultures of pluripotent stem cells connected by nerve-like axonal projections of optic origin. *Stem Cell Rep* **17**: 1476–1492. doi:10.1016/j.stemcr.2022.04.003

Fligor CM, Lavekar SS, Harkin J, Shields PK, VanderWall KB, Huang KC, Gomes C, Meyer JS. 2021. Extension of retinofugal projections in an assembled model of human pluripotent stem cell-derived organoids. *Stem Cell Rep* **16**: 2228–2241. doi:10.1016/j.stemcr.2021.05.009

Fujii M, Matano M, Nanki K, Sato T. 2015. Efficient genetic engineering of human intestinal organoids using electroporation. *Nat Protoc* **10**: 1474–1485. doi:10.1038/nprot.2015.088

Gallego C, Gonçalves MAFV, Wijnholds J. 2020. Novel therapeutic approaches for the treatment of retinal degenerative diseases: focus on CRISPR/Cas-based gene editing. *Front Neurosci* **14**: 838. doi:10.3389/fnins.2020.00838

Gao ML, Zhang X, Han F, Xu J, Yu SJ, Jin K, Jin ZB. 2022. Functional microglia derived from human pluripotent stem cells empower retinal organs. *Sci China Life Sci* **65**: 1057–1071. doi:10.1007/s11427-021-2086-0

Garita-Hernandez M, Guibbal L, Toualbi L, Routet F, Chaffiol A, Winckler C, Harinquet M, Robert C, Fouquet S, Bellow S, et al. 2018. Optogenetic light sensors in human retinal organoids. *Front Neurosci* **12**: 789. doi:10.3389/fnins.2018.00789

Garita-Hernandez M, Routet F, Guibbal L, Khabou H, Toualbi L, Riancho L, Reichman S, Duebel J, Sahel JA, Goureau O, et al. 2020. AAV-mediated gene delivery to 3d retinal organoids derived from human induced pluripotent stem cells. *Int J Mol Sci* **21**: 994. doi:10.3390/ijms21030994

Gonzalez-Cordero A, Goh D, Kruczek K, Naeem A, Fernando M, Kleine Holthaus SM, Takaaki M, Blackford SJI, Kloc M, Agundez L, et al. 2018. Assessment of AAV vector tropisms for mouse and human pluripotent stem cell–derived RPE and photoreceptor cells. *Hum Gene Ther* **29**: 1124–1139. doi:10.1089/hum.2018.027

Hallam D, Hilgen G, Dorgau B, Zhu L, Yu M, Bojic S, Hewitt P, Schmitt M, Uteng M, Kustermann S, et al. 2018. Human-induced pluripotent stem cells generate light responsive retinal organoids with variable and nutrient-dependent efficiency. *Stem Cells* **36**: 1535–1551. doi:10.1002/stem.2883

He Z, Maynard A, Jain A, Gerber T, Petri R, Lin HC, Santel M, Ly K, Dupré JS, Sidow L, et al. 2022. Lineage recording in human cerebral organoids. *Nat Methods* **19**: 90–99. doi:10.1038/s41592-021-01344-8

Jacobo Lopez A, Kim S, Qian X, Rogers J, Stout JT, Thomasy SM, La Torre A, Chen R, Moshiri A. 2022. Retinal organoids derived from rhesus macaque iPSCs undergo accelerated differentiation compared to human stem cells. *Cell Prolif* **55**: e13198. doi:10.1111/cpr.13198

Jones MK, Agarwal D, Mazo KW, Chopra M, Jurlina SL, Dash N, Xu Q, Ogata AR, Chow M, Hill AD, et al. 2022. Chromatin accessibility and transcriptional differences in human stem cell-derived early-stage retinal organoids. *Cells* **11**: 3412. doi:10.3390/cells11213412

Jüttner J, Szabo A, Gross-Scherf B, Morikawa RK, Rompani SB, Hantz P, Szikra T, Esposti F, Cowan CS, Bharioke A, et al. 2019. Targeting neuronal and glial cell types with synthetic promoter AAVs in mice, non-human primates and humans. *Nat Neurosci* **22**: 1345–1356. doi:10.1038/s41593-019-0431-2

Kanton S, Boyle MJ, He Z, Santel M, Weigert A, Sanchís-Calleja F, Guijarro P, Sidow L, Fleck JS, Han D, et al. 2019. Organoid single-cell genomic atlas uncovers human-specific features of brain development. *Nature* **574**: 418–422. doi:10.1038/s41586-019-1654-9

Kegeles E, Naumov A, Karpulevich EA, Volchkov P, Baranov P. 2020. Convolutional neural networks can predict retinal differentiation in retinal organoids. *Front Cell Neurosci* **14**: 171. doi:10.3389/fncel.2020.00171

Kim S, Lowe A, Dharmat R, Lee S, Owen LA, Wang J, Shakoor A, Li Y, Morgan DJ, Hejazi AA, et al. 2019. Generation, transcriptome profiling, and functional validation of cone-rich human retinal organoids. *Proc Natl Acad Sci* **116**: 10824–10833. doi:10.1073/pnas.1901572116

Kim J, Koo BK, Knoblich JA. 2020. Human organoids: model systems for human biology and medicine. *Nat Rev Mol Cell Biol* **21**: 571–584. doi:10.1038/s41580-020-0259-3

Kim HJ, O'Hara-Wright M, Kim D, Loi TH, Lim BY, Jamieson RV, Gonzalez-Cordero A, Yang P. 2023. Comprehensive characterization of fetal and mature retinal cell identity to assess the fidelity of retinal organoids. *Stem Cell Rep* **18**: 175–189. doi:10.1016/j.stemcr.2022.12.002

Kruczek K, Qu Z, Gentry J, Fadl BR, Gieser L, Hiriyanna S, Batz Z, Samant M, Samanta A, Chu CJ, et al. 2021. Gene therapy of dominant CRX-Leber congenital amaurosis using patient stem cell-derived retinal organoids. *Stem Cell Rep* **16**: 252–263. doi:10.1016/j.stemcr.2020.12.018

Lam PT, Gutierrez C, Del Rio-Tsonis K, Robinson ML. 2020. Generation of a retina reporter hiPSC line to label progenitor, ganglion, and photoreceptor cell types. *Transl Vis Sci Technol* **9**: 21. doi:10.1167/tvst.9.3.21

Lancaster MA, Knoblich JA. 2014a. Generation of cerebral organoids from human pluripotent stem cells. *Nat Protoc* **9**: 2329–2340. doi:10.1038/nprot.2014.158

Lancaster MA, Knoblich JA. 2014b. Organogenesis in a dish: modeling development and disease using organoid technologies. *Science* **345**: 1247125. doi:10.1126/science.1247125

Lancaster MA, Renner M, Martin C-A, Wenzel D, Bicknell LS, Hurles ME, Homfray T, Penninger JM, Jackson AP, Knoblich JA. 2013. Cerebral organoids model human brain development and microcephaly. *Nature* **501**: 373–379. doi:10.1038/nature12517

Li L, Zhao H, Xie H, Akhtar T, Yao Y, Cai Y, Dong K, Gu Y, Bao J, Chen J, et al. 2021. Electrophysiological characterization of photoreceptor-like cells in human inducible pluripotent stem cell-derived retinal organoids during in vitro maturation. *Stem Cells* **39**: 959–974. doi:10.1002/stem.3363

Li M, Gao L, Zhao L, Zou T, Xu H. 2023. Toward the next generation of vascularized human neural organoids. *Med Res Rev* **43**: 31–54. doi:10.1002/med.21922

Liu G, David BT, Trawczynski M, Fessler RG. 2020. Advances in pluripotent stem cells: history, mechanisms, technologies, and applications. *Stem Cell Rev Rep* **16**: 3–32. doi:10.1007/s12015-019-09935-x

Llonch S, Carido M, Ader M. 2018. Organoid technology for retinal repair. *Dev Biol* **433**: 132–143. doi:10.1016/j.ydbio.2017.09.028

Lu Y, Shiau F, Yi W, Lu S, Wu Q, Pearson JD, Kallman A, Zhong S, Hoang T, Zuo Z, et al. 2020. Single-cell analysis of human retina identifies evolutionarily conserved and species-specific mechanisms controlling development. *Dev Cell* **53**: 473–491.e9. doi:10.1016/j.devcel.2020.04.009

Lukonin I, Serra D, Challet Meylan L, Volkmann K, Baaten J, Zhao R, Meeusen S, Colman K, Maurer F, Stadler MB, et al. 2020. Phenotypic landscape of intestinal organoid regeneration. *Nature* **586**: 275–280. doi:10.1038/s41586-020-2776-9

Maneu V, Lax P, De Diego AMG, Cuenca N, García AG. 2022. Combined drug triads for synergic neuroprotection in retinal degeneration. *Biomed Pharmacother* **149**: 112911. doi:10.1016/j.biopha.2022.112911

Masland RH. 2012. The neuronal organization of the retina. *Neuron* **76**: 266–280. doi:10.1016/j.neuron.2012.10.002

McClements ME, Steward H, Atkin W, Goode EA, Gándara C, Chichagova V, MacLaren RE. 2022. Tropism of AAV vectors in photoreceptor-like cells of human iPSC-derived retinal organoids. *Transl Vis Sci Technol* **11**: 3. doi:10.1167/tvst.11.4.3

Mellough CB, Collin J, Queen R, Hilgen G, Dorgau B, Zerti D, Felemban M, White K, Sernagor E, Lako M. 2019. Systematic comparison of retinal organoid differentiation from human pluripotent stem cells reveals stage specific, cell line, and methodological differences. *Stem Cells Transl Med* **8**: 694–706. doi:10.1002/sctm.18-0267

Meyer JS, Howden SE, Wallace KA, Verhoeven AD, Wright LS, Capowski EE, Pinilla I, Martin JM, Tian S, Stewart R, et al. 2011. Optic vesicle-like structures derived from human pluripotent stem cells facilitate a customized approach to retinal disease treatment. *Stem Cells* **29**: 1206–1218. doi:10.1002/stem.674

Nakano T, Ando S, Takata N, Kawada M, Muguruma K, Sekiguchi K, Saito K, Yonemura S, Eiraku M, Sasai Y. 2012. Self-formation of optic cups and storable stratified neural retina from human ESCs. *Cell Stem Cell* **10**: 771–785. doi:10.1016/j.stem.2012.05.009

Nazlamova L, Cassidy EJ, Sowden JC, Lotery A, Lakowski J. 2022. Generation of a cone photoreceptor-specific GNGT2 reporter line in human pluripotent stem cells. *Stem Cells* **40**: 190–203. doi:10.1093/stmcls/sxab015

Ovando-Roche P, West EL, Branch MJ, Sampson RD, Fernando M, Munro P, Georgiadis A, Rizzi M, Kloc M,

Naeem A, et al. 2018. Use of bioreactors for culturing human retinal organoids improves photoreceptor yields. *Stem Cell Res Ther* **9**: 156. doi:10.1186/s13287-018-0907-0

Paşca SP, Arlotta P, Bateup HS, Camp JG, Cappello S, Gage FH, Knoblich JA, Kriegstein AR, Lancaster MA, Ming GL, et al. 2022. A nomenclature consensus for nervous system organoids and assembloids. *Nature* **609**: 907–910. doi:10.1038/s41586-022-05219-6

Pasquini G, Cora V, Swiersy A, Achberger K, Antkowiak L, Müller B, Wimmer T, Fraschka SAK, Casadei N, Ueffing M, et al. 2020. Using transcriptomic analysis to assess double-strand break repair activity: towards precise in vivo genome editing. *Int J Mol Sci* **21**: 1380. doi:10.3390/ijms21041380

Phillips MJ, Capowski EE, Petersen A, Jansen AD, Barlow K, Edwards KL, Gamm DM. 2018. Generation of a rod-specific NRL reporter line in human pluripotent stem cells. *Sci Rep* **8**: 2370. doi:10.1038/s41598-018-20813-3

Pleguezuelos-Manzano C, Puschhof J, den Brink S, Geurts V, Beumer J, Clevers H. 2020. Establishment and culture of human intestinal organoids derived from adult stem cells. *Curr Protoc Immunol* **130**: e106. doi:10.1002/cpim.106

Rashidi H, Leong YC, Venner K, Pramod H, Fei Q-Z, Jones OJR, Moulding D, Sowden JC. 2022. Generation of 3D retinal tissue from human pluripotent stem cells using a directed small molecule-based serum-free microwell platform. *Sci Rep* **12**: 6646. doi:10.1038/s41598-022-10540-1

Regent F, Chen HY, Kelley RA, Qu Z, Swaroop A, Li T. 2020. A simple and efficient method for generating human retinal organoids. *Mol Vis* **26**: 97–105.

Regent F, Batz Z, Kelley RA, Gieser L, Swaroop A, Chen HY, Li T. 2022. Nicotinamide promotes formation of retinal organoids from human pluripotent stem cells via enhanced neural cell fate commitment. *Front Cell Neurosci* **16**: 878351. doi:10.3389/fncel.2022.878351

Reichman S, Slembrouck A, Gagliardi G, Chaffiol A, Terray A, Nanteau C, Potey A, Belle M, Rabesandratana O, Duebel J, et al. 2017. Generation of storable retinal organoids and retinal pigmented epithelium from adherent human iPS cells in xeno-free and feeder-free conditions. *Stem Cells* **35**: 1176–1188. doi:10.1002/stem.2586

Russell S, Bennett J, Wellman JA, Chung DC, Yu ZF, Tillman A, Wittes J, Pappas J, Elci O, McCague S, et al. 2017. Efficacy and safety of voretigene neparvovec (AAV2-hRPE65v2) in patients with RPE65-mediated inherited retinal dystrophy: a randomised, controlled, open-label, phase 3 trial. *The Lancet* **390**: 849–860. doi:10.1016/S0140-6736(17)31868-8

Saha A, Capowski E, Fernandez Zepeda MA, Nelson EC, Gamm DM, Sinha R. 2022. Cone photoreceptors in human stem cell-derived retinal organoids demonstrate intrinsic light responses that mimic those of primate fovea. *Cell Stem Cell* **29**: 460–471.e3. doi:10.1016/j.stem.2022.01.002

Singh RK, Mallela RK, Cornuet PK, Reifler AN, Chervenak AP, West MD, Wong KY, Nasonkin IO. 2015. Characterization of three-dimensional retinal tissue derived from human embryonic stem cells in adherent monolayer cultures. *Stem Cells Dev* **24**: 2778–2795. doi:10.1089/scd.2015.0144

Sparrrow RJ, Hicks DP, Hamel C. 2010. The retinal pigment epithelium in health and disease. *Curr Mol Med* **10:** 802–823. doi:10.2174/156652410793937813

Sridhar A, Hoshino A, Finkbeiner CR, Chitsazan A, Dai L, Haugan AK, Eschenbacher KM, Jackson DL, Trapnell C, Bermingham-McDonogh O, et al. 2020. Single-cell transcriptomic comparison of human fetal retina, hPSC-derived retinal organoids, and long-term retinal cultures. *Cell Rep* **30:** 1644–1659.e4. doi:10.1016/j.celrep.2020.01.007

Strauss O. 2005. The retinal pigment epithelium in visual function. *Physiol Rev* **85:** 845–881. doi:10.1152/physrev.00021.2004

Tornabene P, Trapani I, Minopoli R, Centrulo M, Lupo M, de Simone S, Tiberi P, Dell'Aquila F, Marrocco E, Iodice C, et al. 2019. Intein-mediated protein *trans*-splicing expands adeno-associated virus transfer capacity in the retina. *Sci Transl Med* **11:** eaav4523. doi:10.1126/scitranslmed.aav4523

Tso A, da Costa BL, Fehnel A, Levi SR, Jenny LA, Ragi SD, Li Y, Quinn PMJ. 2023. Generation of human iPSC-derived retinal organoids for assessment of AAV-mediated gene delivery. In *Retinitis pigmentosa* (ed. Tsang SH, Quinn PMJ), Vol. 2560, Methods in molecular biology, pp. 287–302. Springer, New York.

Ueda HR, Ertürk A, Chung K, Gradinaru V, Chédotal A, Tomancak P, Keller PJ. 2020. Tissue clearing and its applications in neuroscience. *Nat Rev Neurosci* **21:** 61–79. doi:10.1038/s41583-019-0250-1

Ungricht R, Guibbal L, Lasbennes MC, Orsini V, Beibel M, Waldt A, Cuttat R, Carbone W, Basler A, Roma G, et al. 2022. Genome-wide screening in human kidney organoids identifies developmental and disease-related aspects of nephrogenesis. *Cell Stem Cell* **29:** 160–175.e7. doi:10.1016/j.stem.2021.11.001

Vergara MN, Flores-Bellver M, Aparicio-Domingo S, McNally M, Wahlin KJ, Saxena MT, Mumm JS, Canto-Soler MV. 2017. Enabling quantitative screening in retinal organoids: 3D automated reporter quantification technology (3D-ARQ). *Development* **144:** 3698–3705. doi:10.1242/dev.146290

Völkner M, Pavlou M, Büning H, Michalakis S, Karl MO. 2021. Optimized adeno-associated virus vectors for efficient transduction of human retinal organoids. *Hum Gene Ther* **32:** 694–706. doi:10.1089/hum.2020.321

Völkner M, Wagner F, Steinheuer LM, Carido M, Kurth T, Yazbeck A, Schor J, Wieneke S, Ebner LJA, Del Toro Runzer C, et al. 2022. HBEGF-TNF induce a complex outer retinal pathology with photoreceptor cell extrusion in human organoids. *Nat Commun* **13:** 6183. doi:10.1038/s41467-022-33848-y

Wang L, Hiler D, Xu B, AlDiri I, Chen X, Zhou X, Griffiths L, Valentine M, Shirinifard A, Sablauer A, et al. 2018. Retinal cell type DNA methylation and histone modifications predict reprogramming efficiency and retinogenesis in 3D organoid cultures. *Cell Rep* **22:** 2601–2614. doi:10.1016/j.celrep.2018.01.075

Yamanaka S. 2020. Pluripotent stem cell-based cell therapy—promise and challenges. *Cell Stem Cell* **27:** 523–531. doi:10.1016/j.stem.2020.09.014

Zeng H, Sanes JR. 2017. Neuronal cell-type classification: challenges, opportunities and the path forward. *Nat Rev Neurosci* **18:** 530–546. doi:10.1038/nrn.2017.85

Zhang X, Wang W, Jin ZB. 2021a. Retinal organoids as models for development and diseases. *Cell Regen* **10:** 33. doi:10.1186/s13619-021-00097-1

Zhang Z, Xu Z, Yuan F, Jin K, Xiang M. 2021b. Retinal organoid technology: where are we now? *Int J Mol Sci* **22:** 10244. doi:10.3390/ijms221910244

Zhong X, Gutierrez C, Xue T, Hampton C, Vergara MN, Cao L-H, Peters A, Park TS, Zambidis ET, Meyer JS, et al. 2014. Generation of three-dimensional retinal tissue with functional photoreceptors from human iPSCs. *Nat Commun* **5:** 4047. doi:10.1038/ncomms5047

Overview of Retinal Gene Therapy: Current Status and Future Challenges

Jean Bennett

Center for Advanced Retinal and Ocular Therapeutics, University of Pennsylvania Perelman School of Medicine, Philadelphia, Pennsylvania 19104, USA

Correspondence: jebennet@pennmedicine.upenn.edu

The success of the first Food and Drug Administration (FDA)- and European Medicines Agency (EMA)-approved gene therapy for genetic disease, voretigene neparovovec-rzyl, (Luxturna) has helped pave the way for development of retinal gene therapies to target other genetic and acquired forms of blindness. Gene therapy trials are now taking place in multiple continents and numerous countries, they use several different gene transfer reagents ("vectors"), studies have used several different routes of administration, and different strategies are being tested in interventional studies with promising results. The future has never been brighter for individuals with retinal degeneration. Here and in the literature cited below, we summarize the state-of-the-art of retinal gene therapy and consider some of the questions and challenges that lie ahead.

It was not long ago that individuals newly diagnosed with retinal degeneration were told that there was nothing that could be done. They were often told that they were destined to a life of worsening vision and ultimately total blindness. Patients were then referred to occupational therapy specialists and to programs that could provide mobility training (use of a "blind cane") and/or to organizations that provided "seeing eye" dogs. Low vision expertise is still invaluable for such patients. However, progress in genetic characterization of different forms of retinal disease over the past three decades has led to an improved understanding of the pathogenetic mechanisms and excellent genotype/phenotype correlations. Animal models have been identified or engineered for many of the different genetic forms of retinal degeneration. As

gene transfer reagents ("vectors") were developed, it became appropriate to make the first attempts to intervene on a genetic basis. The initial studies involved a gene-augmentation approach, where a wild-type copy of the disease-causing gene was delivered to the target cells. This led to the first U.S. Food and Drug Administration (FDA)-approved gene therapy reagent targeting a genetic disease, an adeno-associated virus (AAV) serotype 2 (AAV2) gene-augmentation vector. This AAV targets a form of congenital blindness, Leber congenital amaurosis (LCA) caused by bi-allelic loss-of-function *RPE65* mutations, and was approved by the U.S. FDA in 2017 (see Bennett and Maguire 2022; Reape and High 2022). The reagent, voretigene neparvovec-rzyl (Luxturna), was approved shortly thereafter (2018) in the European

Union. The success of Luxturna has helped pave the way for development of gene therapies to target other genetic and acquired forms of blindness. Gene therapy trials are now taking place in multiple continents and numerous countries, several different gene transfer reagents ("vectors") have been tested and "de-risked" in human retinas, studies have used several different routes of administration, and different strategies are being tested in interventional studies with promising results. The future has never been brighter for individuals with retinal degeneration. Here we summarize the state-of-the-art of retinal gene therapy and consider some of the questions and challenges that remain.

VECTORS AND GENE THERAPY

There has been tremendous growth of the vector toolkit available to test gene-based therapies. Initial studies in small and large animals relied on vector-mediated delivery of reporter genes to elucidate the characteristics of one vector versus another (Bennett et al. 1994; Li et al. 1994; Allocca et al. 2007; Lebherz et al. 2008; Vandenberghe et al. 2011; Ramachandran et al. 2017). The first studies used recombinant adenovirus, a DNA vector developed initially due to its promise in targeting the pulmonary epithelium for treatment of cystic fibrosis. Recombinant adenovirus provided the first opportunity to deliver

early-onset and high levels of transgene expression in animal models but were then largely abandoned for applications to retinal degenerative disease due to the much greater advantages of recombinant AAV. AAV is relatively benign immunologically, especially at the doses and anatomic sites used for retinal applications. AAV also transduces retinal cells efficiently. Thus, applications using AAV have increased over the past decade (Fig. 1). Adenovirus continues to be tested in a few clinical trials, although its applications are largely restricted to retinoblastoma, where its potent immunologic characteristics and high and early-onset levels of expression might be useful in clearing tumor cells (Fig. 1).

AAV serotype 2, AAV2, was first tested in the retinas of animal models in 1997 (Bennett et al. 1997; Flannery et al. 1997). AAV2 targets both retinal pigmented epithelium (RPE) and photoreceptors efficiently after subretinal injection and the transduction details can be altered by packaging in different (or modified) capsid serotypes or capsids generated by evolutionary or in silico design (see Auricchio et al. 2001; Lebherz et al. 2008; Dalkara et al. 2013; Zinn et al. 2015; Zin et al. 2022). RNA-containing viral vectors (lentiviral vectors) were also developed and were shown to target RPE cells efficiently and, in some cases, photoreceptors (Auricchio et al. 2001; Kong et al. 2008). Lentiviral vectors with modified envelopes have been used in several

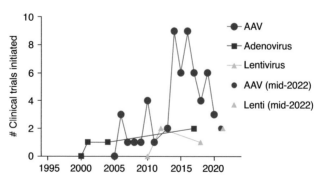

Figure 1. Viral vectors used over time in retinal gene therapy clinical trials. The year indicates when an interventional trial was first posted on clinicaltrials.gov. (Not all trials enrolled subjects immediately after the post; however, the majority started enrollment within a year. These trials continue for years. In some cases, there were several clinical trials initiated using the same vector [for example, choroideremia in 2015]. Long-term follow-up studies were excluded.) Data points for 2022 are indicated separately (as of mid-2022) since the year is still in progress.

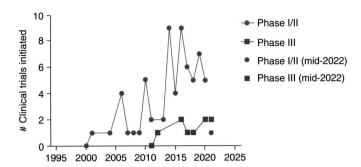

Figure 2. Number of phase I/II versus phase III retinal gene therapy clinical trials using viral vectors over time. The year indicates when the trial was first posted on clinicaltrials.gov. Phase I/II includes trials that were listed as either phase I or phase II (as well as combined phase I/II trials). Phase III includes trials that were listed as either phase II/III or phase III. (Not all trials enrolled subjects immediately after the post; however, the majority started enrollment within a year. These trials continue for years. Long-term follow-up studies were excluded.) Data points for 2022 are indicated separately (as of mid-2022) since the year is still in progress.

different clinical trials (Fig. 1). Lentiviral vectors, unlike adenoviral or AAV vectors, integrate efficiently into the host cell DNA, which may increase durability of expression but which also raises safety concerns. However, progress has been made in limiting the potential of lentiviral integration adjacent to proto-oncogenes. Further, the ability to image the retina facilitates monitoring for potential neoplastic changes.

Transduction characteristics, the temporal and spatial expression patterns of transgenes after delivery of the vector, are dependent on the surgical approach and the dose. Subretinal injection exposes the cells lining the subretinal space. In the neural retina, these are cone and rod photoreceptors, and Müller cells. The RPE lines the other side of the subretinal space. AAV2 readily infects RPE cells and so this was a natural choice for studies targeting the *RPE65* form of LCA. AAV4 and AAV5 target RPE cells as well and so these vectors have also been used in *RPE65* studies (Duong et al. 2016; Georgiadis et al. 2016; Le Meur et al. 2018).

A number of vectors also transduce photoreceptors efficiently after subretinal injection. AAV5, AAV8, and AAV9 each transduce photoreceptors more efficiently than AAV2 and are thus being used (or considered for use) in clinical trials (Vandenberghe et al. 2011; Ramachandran et al. 2017). Transduction efficiency can also be increased by modifying tyrosine residues in the capsid, as done by Zhong et al. (2008), and

tyrosine mutant capsids are also being used in clinical trials.

CURRENT CLINICAL TARGETS FOR RETINAL GENE THERAPY

The development of Luxturna created a path with which to conduct retinal gene-augmentation studies for other genetic and acquired blinding diseases. The positive results also fueled the interest of academic groups, small biotechnology companies, and also large pharmaceutical entities. This resulted in an increased number of phase I/II and then phase III retinal gene therapy trials over the past decade (Fig. 2).[1] Disease targets using a gene-augmentation approach include achromatopsia, several different forms of autosomal recessive (AR) retinitis pigmentosa (RP), X-linked (XL) RP due to retinitis pigmentosa GTPase regulator (RPGR) mutations, XL retinoschisis, and choroideremia. The results have inspired patients with other orphan retinal diseases to band together and lobby for treatment for "their" particular gene/mutation. The path used to develop *RPE65* gene therapy is also being used to develop and test a

---

[1]In some cases, several different trials targeting the same gene/mutation (and even using the same vector) were initiated simultaneously. This is particularly apparent in studies of choroideremia where several different centers ran contemporaneous clinical trials using the same vector.

variety of other gene therapy strategies for treatment of other human retinal diseases, including delivery of mitochondrial genes, gene-editing molecules, antisense RNA, decoy receptors, metabolic support, and even genes aiming to render cells other than photoreceptors light-sensitive ("optogenetic" therapy).

The studies of mitochondrial diseases rely on the fact that intravitreal injection of particular recombinant viruses, such as AAV2, leads to transduction of ganglion cells and/or Müller glia (Dudus et al. 1999; Bennett et al. 2000). Since ganglion cells contribute to the structure of the optic nerve, AAV2 has been used in gene therapy studies targeting the mitochondrial disorder, Leber's hereditary optic neuropathy (LHON). AAV2 and AAV8 have also been used through intravitreal injection to transform inner retinal and anterior segment cells into factories with which to secrete various therapeutic proteins (such as vascular endothelium growth factor [VEGF] antagonists, and retinoschisin for XL retinoschisis). An AAV generated through evolutionary design to transduce photoreceptors after intravitreal injection, AAV7m8, also happens to target ganglion cells efficiently (Grishanin et al. 2019). AAV7m8 is thus employed in clinical trials to test efficacy of a VEGF antagonist in neovascular age-related macular degeneration (nAMD). Regardless of the AAV capsid serotype under study, there is a higher incidence of inflammation after intravitreal injection of high dose AAV than after subretinal injection.

Antisense oligonucleotides (AONs) have recently been evaluated for their ability to alter transcription and translation of some of the more common genes/mutations leading to inherited retinal disease, including an insertion of a pseudo-exon in an intronic site in *CEP290* (c.2991 + 1655A>G), the gene encoding Centrosomal protein, 290 kD. The *CEP290* cDNA (nearly 8 kb) is one of the disease-causing genes whose cDNA is larger than the AAV maximum cargo capacity of 4.8 kb. Because AAV cannot accommadate the intact CEP290 cDNA, alternative strategies are particularly attractive. The idea of using AONs to treat retinal disease was not new. In fact, nearly a decade before *CEP290* mutations had been identified as a cause of LCA

(den Hollander et al. 2006), the AON named Vitravene (fomivirsen) had been approved by the U.S. FDA (Fig. 3). This therapy for cytomegalovirus retinitis was used in patients with human immunodeficiency virus (HIV) infection from 1998 through the 2000s.[2]

The AON used for CEP290 mutations (Sepofarsen), is more fully phosphorothioated than Vitravene to protect against degradation and it also has 2'-*O*-methyl-modified RNA oligonucleotides. Sepofarsen can efficiently restore splicing and increase protein levels in vitro for the common *CEP290* mutation (Dulla et al. 2018). Because AONs penetrate the retina, they are delivered by intravitreal injection, an office procedure. However, since the compound has a limited half-life, repeat injections are required. Initial results of early phase studies were promising (Cideciyan et al. 2019). However, a Sepofarsen phase 3 clinical trial targeting LCA-CEP290 did not meet the primary end point, although some aspects of visual function improved significantly (Russell et al. 2022). The company sponsoring the studies, ProQR, has evaluated AONs for this blinding disease and others, including ARRP caused by *USH2A* exon 13 mutations (which cause ARRP) and autosomal-dominant (AD) RP caused by a common rhodopsin mutation (P23H) (Fig. 3).

CURRENT QUESTIONS AND CHALLENGES FOR RETINAL GENE THERAPY

Route of Administration

To increase the access to retinal gene therapy and to reduce the risks associated with subretinal injection (general anesthesia and surgical complications), it would be desirable to deliver the reagent through a common office procedure, such as intravitreal injection. As described above, there are several disease targets that may be addressed effectively by AAV through intravitreal administration. These include LHON (see Chen and Yu-Wai-Man 2022),

---

[2]Vitravene is not prescribed as frequently now thanks to highly active antiretroviral therapy (HAART). The Vitravene AONs were modified to enhance stability with a phosphorothioate backbone.

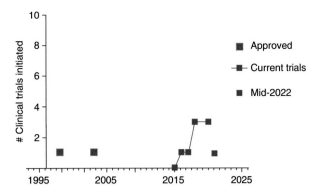

Figure 3. Number of retinal gene therapy clinical trials using antisense oligonucleotide (AON) reagents over time. The year indicates when the trial was first posted on clinicaltrials.gov except that the points for 1998 and 2004 indicate years of U.S. Food and Drug Administration (FDA) approvals for Vitravene and Macugen, respectively. (Not all trials enrolled subjects immediately after the posting; however, the majority started enrollment within a year.) The data point for 2022 is indicated separately since the year is still in progress.

retinoschisis (Ku et al. 2022), nAMD, and some approaches for optogenetic therapy (Roska 2022; Stefanov and Flannery 2022).

There are other diseases where intravitreal injection will not suffice. Preclinical *RPE65* studies using the naturally occurring Briard dog model showed that subretinal delivery of AAV2. RPE65 resulted in rescue of retinal and visual function. Intravitreal delivery of a similar dose did not (Acland et al. 2001). Subsequent studies in affected mice and dogs and unaffected monkeys confirmed the fact that delivery to the subretinal space was required for transduction of outer retinal cells and therefore efficacy of the reagent (in the affected dogs). Clinical trials for *RPE65* deficiency thus employed subretinal injection.

As with *RPE65* deficiency, many of the recent gene therapy clinical studies targeting cells in the outer retina (choroideremia [see Yusuf and Mac-Laren 2022], XLRP [see Hashem et al. 2022], achromatopsia [see Banin 2022], etc.) also use subretinal delivery. While retina surgeons at large medical centers are now comfortable with subretinal injection, it would be advantageous to be able to deliver through an office procedure. This is particularly true for diseases affecting millions of patients, such as nAMD or diabetic retinopathy. The suprachoroidal space is an attractive target as it can be accessed in an office procedure and this route may result in delivery of vector to the outer retina. Thus, efforts are underway to test suprachoroidal delivery in gene therapy clinical trials. It will be interesting to learn whether suprachoroidal delivery results in the desired amount of transgene expression in the target cells and also whether this is safe from inflammatory and immunologic perspectives.

Vector Design

As described above and also by Zin et al. (2022), development of new vectors, including those generated by evolutionary design, may result in safer and more efficient gene transfer. Additional strategies may help address the "large gene problem" (i.e., the fact that AAV has limited cargo capacity and cannot deliver large transgene cassettes such as those containing *USH2A*, *ABCA4*, or *CEP290*) (see above). For gene-augmentation strategies targeting those particular genes, it may be necessary to incorporate trans-splicing strategies or to use dual vectors. Availability of retinal organoids (see Zack 2022) may assist in developing such endeavors.

Gain-of-Function Mutations

Designs of studies targeting loss-of-function mutations are relatively simple. Those targeting gain-of-function mutations are far more complex. Lewin and Smith (2022) have developed strategies such as knockdown of the mutant allele together with delivery of a "hardened" cDNA for treating

ADRP due to rhodopsin mutations. Gene-editing strategies could also be employed to treat gain-of-function mutations (see Ling et al. 2022).

Gene-Agnostic Approaches

Although there has been great progress in developing strategies that can target specific genes and mutations, there are hundreds of retinal disease-causing genes. It will be extremely costly (in both time and money) to develop a strategy targeting each specific gene. Further, in many patients, the disease-causing gene has not been identified. Therefore, the approaches described by Léveillard (2022) and Cepko (2022) to manipulate metabolic pathways to maintain the health of the retina as long as possible hold great importance.

For diseases that have advanced so far that gene augmentation would not be effective (i.e., the primary cell type has degenerated and thus cannot be treated with gene therapy), it may be necessary to render other second- or third-order retinal neurons light-sensitive. These approaches are described by Roska (2022) and Stefanov and Flannery (2022), respectively.

CONCLUDING REMARKS: THE FUTURE OF RETINAL GENE THERAPY RPE65 EXPERIENCE AND EXTRAPOLATION TO OTHER RETINAL DISEASES

The past two decades have seen tremendous growth in development and acceptance of retinal gene therapy. The first viral vector-delivered gene therapy, Luxturna, has been approved and is used to treat a previously untreatable disease. Two different antisense RNA molecules have already been approved for treatment of retinal disease and several more are in late-stage clinical trials. So far, these new AONs appear even more stable than predicted.

Meanwhile, a different strategy, gene editing using recombinant AAV-mediated delivery of CRISPR along with the guide RNA (Stefanidakis et al. 2019), is being applied to individuals with the common *CEP290* intronic mutation. The retina is the first organ to be the target for an in vivo gene-editing approach in humans. If safe and successful, this will pave the way for other in vivo gene-editing studies in humans such as those described by Ling et al. (2022).

Approaches with which to target late stages of disease using gene therapy are now also under evaluation. Many of these studies have fueled the steady increases (save for the dip during the covid-19 pandemic lockdown year, 2020) in initiation of phase I–III gene therapy clinical trials incorporating AAV (Figs. 1 and 2). Gene-augmentation therapy requires the presence of the primary disease-causing cells. If those cells have degenerated, what can be done? Several groups are now studying optogenetic therapy in clinical trials. Dr. Zhuo-Hua Pan and colleagues used rAAV vectors to deliver a microbial rhodopsin, channelrhodopsin-2 (ChR2), to ganglion cells of an animal model of RP and demonstrated restoration of visual responses (Bi et al. 2006). This work led to initiation of a phase I/II clinical trial (sponsored by Allergan/AbbVie) using intravitreal delivery of AAV2 (clinicaltrials.gov, NCT02556736, initiated 2015). A second study (clinicaltrials.gov, NCT03326336) was inspired by results from a large set of preclinical studies in animal models, postmortem retinas, and induced pluripotent stem cell (iPSC)-derived retinas (Fradot et al. 2011; Busskamp et al. 2012; Garita-Hernandez et al. 2018). This optogenetic gene therapy clinical trial sponsored by GenSight Biologics (clinicaltrials.gov: NCT03326336, initiated in 2018) is the first to use a red-shifted channelrhodopsin variant (ChrimsonR) delivery with the AAV serotype AAV7m8 and use of goggles to fine-tune the light stimuli. It is also the first to report preliminary efficacy (as well as safety) data (clinicaltrials.gov) indicating that virus-mediated delivery of an optogenetic molecule can restore some visual function in a human (Sahel et al. 2021a) (see also gensight-biologics.com). A third optogenetic gene therapy approach delivers a "multi-characteristic" opsin (vMCO-I) (Wright et al. 2017a,b) to retinal ganglion cells using AAV2. These studies, sponsored by Nanoscope Therapeutics, have been (and are being) carried out in individuals with RP and with Stargardt disease (clinicaltrials.gov: NCT04945772 initiated 2021 and NCT05417126 initiated 2022, respectively).

There are also now several large programs evaluating anti-neovascular gene therapy. Drugs such as aflibercept and ranibizumab that bind vascular endothelial growth factor (VEGF) thereby inhibiting neovascularization are effective if injected repeatedly. The goal of delivering them through a gene therapy vector is to enable a one-time treatment. Initial trials by Avalanche Biotechnologies used AAV2-mediated delivery of a soluble receptor of VEGF, S-Flt-1 (Constable et al. 2016; Scaria et al. 2017). In recent years, aflibercept and ranibizumab themselves have been "vectorized" and are being tested (see for example trials sponsored by Adverum and REGENXBIO; clinicaltrials.gov: NCT03748784 and NCT05407636, respectively). Progress in developing a one-time treatment for nAMD, could serve as the rationale to test the reagent in other retinal neovascular diseases, which also affect millions of people, such as diabetic retinopathy or retinopathy of prematurity.

In summary, these are exciting times for retinal gene therapy! An approach that started as an effort to develop a treatment for a small number of patients with an ultrarare inherited disease is in the process of being expanded to try to improve vision and quality of life for many more people. As the studies proceed, tools will be developed (including reagents, potency assays, etc.) that will fuel the entire enterprise. In addition, we will learn more about critical aspects of gene therapy, including the benefits and limitations of viral vectors, AONs, gene editing, routes of delivery, and immune responses. Simultaneously, additional more appropriate and noninvasive outcome measures will be developed. When retinal gene therapy trials were first initiated in 2007, the only approved outcome measure for new ophthalmic drugs was a visual acuity measure: performance reading the eye chart. There are other aspects besides visual acuity that are clinically meaningful. Further, many patients have such poor vision at baseline that they cannot even see an eye chart. There is a need for measures that can measure other improvements in functional vision. The multi-luminance mobility test described by Chung et al. (2018) (see also Reape and High 2022) is one such example of the type of outcome measure required. Another measure that has been shown to be useful in quantifying visual function and that could be implemented more widely in the future is "StreetLab," an artificial environment designed to test visual function in an artificial street, an apartment, and in a driving simulation (Sahel et al. 2021b). It may also be possible to harness high-resolution anatomic measures as surrogates for improvement in visual function, for example, measures of the ellipsoid zone using optical coherence tomography (Sahel et al. 2021b). Finally, it will also be important to develop and include rehabilitation strategies so that visually impaired individuals can learn how to best use their new-found vision. Environments such as "StreetLab" could be reproduced so that more patients had access to vision rehabilitation centers. With the progress in development of virtual reality devices, it may also be possible to deliver rehabilitation headsets directly to patients' homes. Continued caution and stepwise progress will lead us to a point where the treatments under development will become even more effective and we no longer have to tell our patients "There is nothing we can do to treat your blindness."

COMPETING INTEREST STATEMENT

J.B. is a coauthor on intellectual property describing the gene therapy for RPE65 deficiency but waived any potential financial gain in 2002.

ACKNOWLEDGMENTS

I am deeply grateful to my collaborators and colleagues and the patients in our clinical trials for sharing the passion of developing treatments for currently untreatable blinding diseases. J.B. is supported by the F.M. Kirby Foundation and Center for Advanced Retinal and Ocular Therapeutics (CAROT), University of Pennsylvania.

REFERENCES

*Reference is also in this subject collection.

Acland GM, Aguirre GD, Ray J, Zhang Q, Aleman TS, Cideciyan AV, Pearce-Kelling SE, Anand V, Zeng Y, Maguire AM, et al. 2001. Gene therapy restores vision in a canine model of childhood blindness. *Nat Genet* **28**: 92–95.

Allocca M, Mussolino C, Garcia-Hoyos M, Sanges D, Iodice C, Petrillo M, Vandenberghe LH, Wilson JM, Marigo V, Surace EM, et al. 2007. Novel adeno-associated virus serotypes efficiently transduce murine photoreceptors. *J Virol* **81:** 11372–11380. doi:10.1128/JVI.01327-07

Auricchio A, Kobinger G, Anand V, Hildinger M, O'Connor E, Maguire AM, Wilson JM, Bennett J. 2001. Exchange of surface proteins impacts on viral vector cellular specificity and transduction characteristics: the retina as a model. *Hum Mol Genet* **10:** 3075–3081. doi:10.1093/hmg/10.26 .3075

* Banin E. 2022. Achromatopsia. *Cold Spring Harb Perspect Med* doi:10.1101/cshperspect.a041281

* Bennett J, Maguire AM. 2022. Lessons learned from the development of the first FDA-approved gene therapy drug, voretigene neparvovec-rzyl. *Cold Spring Harb Perspect Med* doi:10.1101/cshperspect.a41307

Bennett J, Wilson J, Sun D, Forbes B, Maguire A. 1994. Adenovirus vector-mediated in vivo gene transfer into adult murine retina. *Invest Ophthalmol Vis Sci* **35:** 2535–2542.

Bennett J, Duan D, Engelhardt JF, Maguire AM. 1997. Real-time, noninvasive in vivo assessment of adeno-associated virus-mediated retinal transduction. *Invest Ophthalmol Vis Sci* **38:** 2857–2863.

Bennett J, Anand V, Acland GM, Maguire AM. 2000. Cross-species comparison of in vivo reporter gene expression after recombinant adeno-associated virus-mediated retinal transduction. *Methods Enzymol* **316:** 777–789. doi:10 .1016/S0076-6879(00)16762-X

Bi A, Cui J, Ma YP, Olshevskaya E, Pu M, Dizhoor AM, Pan ZH. 2006. Ectopic expression of a microbial-type rhodopsin restores visual responses in mice with photoreceptor degeneration. *Neuron* **50:** 23–33. doi:10.1016/j.neuron .2006.02.026

Busskamp V, Picaud S, Sahel JA, Roska B. 2012. Optogenetic therapy for retinitis pigmentosa. *Gene Ther* **19:** 169–175. doi:10.1038/gt.2011.155

* Cepko C. 2022. Glucose metabolism. *Cold Spring Harb Perspect Med* doi:10.1101/cshperspect.a041289

* Chen BS, Yu-Wai-Man P. 2022. From bench to bedside—delivering gene therapy for Leber hereditary optic neuropathy. *Cold Spring Harb Perspect Med* **12:** a041282. doi:10.1101/cshperspect.a041282

Chung DC, McCague S, Yu ZF, Thill S, DiStefano-Pappas J, Bennett J, Cross D, Marshall K, Wellman J, High KA. 2018. Novel mobility test to assess functional vision in patients with inherited retinal dystrophies. *Clin Exp Ophthalmol* **46:** 247–259. doi:10.1111/ceo.13022

Cideciyan AV, Jacobson SG, Drack AV, Ho AC, Charng J, Garafalo AV, Roman AJ, Sumaroka A, Han IC, Hochstedler MD, et al. 2019. Effect of an intravitreal antisense oligonucleotide on vision in Leber congenital amaurosis due to a photoreceptor cilium defect. *Nat Med* **25:** 225–228. doi:10.1038/s41591-018-0295-0

Constable IJ, Pierce CM, Lai CM, Magno AL, Degli-Esposti MA, French MA, McAllister IL, Butler S, Barone SB, Schwartz SD, et al. 2016. Phase 2a randomized clinical trial: safety and post hoc analysis of subretinal rAAV. sFLT-1 for wet age-related macular degeneration. *EBioMedicine* **14:** 168–175. doi:10.1016/j.ebiom.2016.11.016

Dalkara D, Byrne LC, Klimczak RR, Visel M, Yin L, Merigan WH, Flannery JG, Schaffer DV. 2013. In vivo–directed evolution of a new adeno-associated virus for therapeutic outer retinal gene delivery from the vitreous. *Sci Transl Med* **5:** 189ra176. doi:10.1126/scitranslmed.3005708

den Hollander AI, Koenekoop RK, Yzer S, Lopez I, Arends ML, Voesenek KE, Zonneveld MN, Strom TM, Meitinger T, Brunner HG, et al. 2006. Mutations in the CEP290 (NPHP6) gene are a frequent cause of Leber congenital amaurosis. *Am J Hum Genet* **79:** 556–561. doi:10.1086/ 507318

Dudus L, Anand V, Acland G, Chen SJ, Wilson J, Fisher K, Maguire A, Bennett J. 1999. Persistent transgene product in retina, optic nerve and brain after intraocular injection of rAAV. *Vis Res* **39:** 2545–2553. doi:10.1016/S0042-6989 (98)00308-3

Dulla K, Aguila M, Lane A, Jovanovic K, Parfitt DA, Schulkens I, Chan HL, Schmidt I, Beumer W, Vorthoren L, et al. 2018. Splice-modulating oligonucleotide QR-110 restores CEP290 mRNA and function in human c.2991 + 1655A>G LCA10 models. *Mol Ther Nucleic Acids* **12:** 730–740. doi:10.1016/j.omtn.2018.07.010

Duong T, Vasireddy V, Merkel C, Bennicelli J, Bennett J. 2016. 556. Comparative in vitro transduction efficiency of AAV vector serotypes 1–9 in different cellular models. *Mol Ther* **24:** S222–S223. doi:10.1016/S1525-0016(16) 33364-0

Flannery JG, Zolotukhin S, Vaquero MI, LaVail MM, Muzyczka N, Hauswirth WW. 1997. Efficient photoreceptor-targeted gene expression in vivo by recombinant adeno-associated virus. *Proc Natl Acad Sci* **94:** 6916–6921. doi:10 .1073/pnas.94.13.6916

Fradot M, Busskamp V, Forster V, Cronin T, Léveillard T, Bennett J, Sahel JA, Roska B, Picaud S. 2011. Gene therapy in ophthalmology: validation on cultured retinal cells and explants from postmortem human eyes. *Hum Gene Ther* **22:** 587–593. doi:10.1089/hum.2010.157

Garita-Hernandez M, Guibbal L, Toualbi L, Routet F, Chaffiol A, Winckler C, Harinquet M, Robert C, Fouquet S, Bellow S, et al. 2018. Optogenetic light sensors in human retinal organoids. *Front Neurosci* **12:** 789. doi:10.3389/ fnins.2018.00789

Georgiadis A, Duran Y, Ribeiro J, Abelleira-Hervas L, Robbie SJ, Sünkel-Laing B, Fourali S, Gonzalez-Cordero A, Cristante E, Michaelides M, et al. 2016. Development of an optimized AAV2/5 gene therapy vector for Leber congenital amaurosis owing to defects in RPE65. *Gene Ther* **23:** 857–862. doi:10.1038/gt.2016.66

Grishanin R, Vuillemenot B, Sharma P, Keravala A, Greengard J, Gelfman C, Blumenkrantz M, Lawrence M, Hu W, Kiss S, et al. 2019. Preclinical evaluation of ADVM-022, a novel gene therapy approach to treating wet age-related macular degeneration. *Mol Ther* **27:** 118–129. doi:10 .1016/j.ymthe.2018.11.003

* Hashem SA, Georgiou M, Ali RR, Michaelides M. 2022. *RPGR*-related retinopathy: clinical features, molecular genetics, and gene replacement therapy. *Cold Spring Harb Perspect Med* doi:10.1101/cshperspect.a041280

Kong J, Kim SR, Binley K, Pata I, Doi K, Mannik J, Zernant-Rajang N, Kan O, Iqball S, Naylor S, et al. 2008. Correction of the disease phenotype in the mouse model of Stargardt disease by lentiviral gene therapy. *Gene Ther* **15**: 1311–1320. doi:10.1038/gt.2008.78

* Ku CA, Bush RA, Wei LW, Sieving PA. 2022. X-linked retinoschisis. *Cold Spring Harb Perspect Med* doi:10.1101/cshperspect.a41288

Lebherz C, Maguire A, Tang W, Bennett J, Wilson JM. 2008. Novel AAV serotypes for improved ocular gene transfer. *J Gene Med* **10**: 375–382. doi:10.1002/jgm.1126

Le Meur G, Lebranchu P, Billaud F, Adjali O, Schmitt S, Bézieau S, Péréon Y, Valabregue R, Ivan C, Darmon C, et al. 2018. Safety and long-term efficacy of AAV4 gene therapy in patients with RPE65 Leber congenital amaurosis. *Mol Ther* **26**: 256–268. doi:10.1016/j.ymthe.2017.09.014

* Léveillard T. 2022. Gene-independent approaches: neuroprotection. *Cold Spring Harb Perspect Med* doi:10.1101/cshperspect.a041284

* Lewin AS, Smith WC. 2022. Gene therapy for rhodopsin mutations. *Cold Spring Harb Perspect Med* **12**: a041283. doi:10.1101/cshperspect.a041283

Li T, Adamian M, Roof DJ, Berson EL, Dryja TP, Roessler BJ, Davidson BL. 1994. In vivo transfer of a reporter gene to the retina mediated by an adenoviral vector. *Invest Ophthalmol Vis Sci* **35**: 2543–2549.

* Ling J, Jenny LA, Zhou A, Tsang SH. 2022. Therapeutic gene editing in inherited retinal disorders. *Cold Spring Harb Perspect Med* doi:10.1101/cshperspect.a041292

Ramachandran PS, Lee V, Wei Z, Song JY, Casal G, Cronin T, Willett K, Huckfeldt R, Morgan JI, Aleman TS, et al. 2017. Evaluation of dose and safety of AAV7m8 and AAV8BP2 in the non-human primate retina. *Hum Gene Ther* **28**: 154–167. doi:10.1089/hum.2016.111

* Reape KZ, High KA. 2022. Trial by "firsts": clinical trial design and regulatory considerations in the development and approval of the first AAV gene therapy product in the US. *Cold Spring Harb Perspect Med* doi:10.1101/cshperspect.a041312

* Roska B. 2022. Optogenetics. *Cold Spring Harb Perspect Med* doi:10.1101/cshperspect.a41290

Russell SR, Drack AV, Cideciyan AV, Jacobson SG, Leroy BP, Van Cauwenbergh C, Ho AC, Dumitrescu AV, Han IC, Martin M, et al. 2022. Intravitreal antisense oligonucleotide sepofarsen in Leber congenital amaurosis type 10: a phase 1b/2 trial. *Nat Med* **28**: 1014–1021. doi:10.1038/s41591-022-01755-w

Sahel JA, Boulanger-Scemama E, Pagot C, Arleo A, Galluppi F, Martel JN, Esposti SD, Delaux A, de Saint Aubert JB, de Montleau C, et al. 2021a. Partial recovery of visual function in a blind patient after optogenetic therapy. *Nat Med* **28**: 1014–1021.

Sahel JA, Grieve K, Pagot C, Authié C, Mohand-Said S, Paques M, Audo I, Becker K, Chaumet-Riffaud AE, Azoulay L, et al. 2021b. Assessing photoreceptor status in retinal dystrophies: from high-resolution imaging to functional vision. *Am J Ophthalmol* **230**: 12–47. doi:10.1016/j.ajo.2021.04.013

Scaria A, Heier J, Campochiaro P, Purvis A, Delacono C, LeHalpere A, Deslandes JY, Buggage R. 2017. Preliminary results of a phase 1, open-label, multi-center, dose-escalating, safety and tolerability study of a single intravitreal injection of AAV2-sFLT01 in patients with neovascular age-related macular degeneration. American Society of Cell and Gene Therapy, Washington, DC.

Stefanidakis M, Maeder M, Bounoutas G, Yudkoff C, Chao H, Giannoukos G, Ciulla D, Marco E, Samuelsson S, Wilson C, et al. 2019. Efficient in vivo editing of CEP290 IVS26 by EDIT-101 as a novel therapeutic for the treatment of Leber congenital amaurosis 10. *Invest Opthalmol Vis Sci* **59**: 385.

* Stefanov A, Flannery JG. 2022. A systematic review of optogenetic vision restoration: history, challenges, and new inventions from bench to bedside. *Cold Spring Harb Perspect Med* doi:10.1101/cshperspect.a41304

Vandenberghe L, Bell P, Maguire A, Cearley C, Xiao R, Calcedo R, Wang L, Castle M, Maguire A, Grant R, et al. 2011. Dosage thresholds for AAV2 and AAV8 photoreceptor gene therapy in monkey. *Sci Transl Med* **3**: a54. doi:10.1126/scitranslmed.3002103

Wright W, Gajjeraman S, Batabyal S, Pradhan S, Bhattacharya S, Mahapatra V, Tripathy A, Mohanty S. 2017a. Erratum: publisher's note: restoring vision in mice with retinal degeneration using multicharacteristic opsin. *Neurophotonics* **4**: 049801.

Wright W, Gajjeraman S, Batabyal S, Pradhan S, Bhattacharya S, Mahapatra V, Tripathy A, Mohanty S. 2017b. Restoring vision in mice with retinal degeneration using multicharacteristic opsin. *Neurophotonics* **4**: 041505.

* Yusuf IH, MacLaren RE. 2022. Choroideremia: towards regulatory approval of retinal gene therapy. *Cold Spring Harb Perspect Med* doi:10.1101/cshperspect.a041279

* Zack D. 2022. New medical therapies. *Cold Spring Harb Perspect Med* doi:10.1101/cshperspect.a041313

Zhong L, Li B, Mah CS, Govindasamy L, Agbandje-McKenna M, Cooper M, Herzog RW, Zolotukhin I, Warrington KH Jr, Weigel-Van Aken KA, et al. 2008. Next generation of adeno-associated virus 2 vectors: point mutations in tyrosines lead to high-efficiency transduction at lower doses. *Proc Natl Acad Sci* **105**: 7827–7832. doi:10.1073/pnas.0802866105

* Zin EA, Ozturk BE, Dalkara D, Byrne LC. 2022. Developing new vectors for retinal gene therapy. *Cold Spring Harb Perspect Med* doi:10.1101/cshperspect.a041291

Zinn E, Pacouret S, Khaychuk V, Turunen HT, Carvalho LS, Andres-Mateos E, Shah S, Shelke R, Maurer AC, Plovie E, et al. 2015. In silico reconstruction of the viral evolutionary lineage yields a potent gene therapy vector. *Cell Rep* **12**: 1056–1068. doi:10.1016/j.celrep.2015.07.019

Lessons Learned from the Development of the First FDA-Approved Gene Therapy Drug, Voretigene Neparvovec-rzyl

Jean Bennett[1,2] and Albert M. Maguire[1,2,3]

[1]Scheie Eye Institute at the Perelman Center for Advanced Medicine, Philadelphia, Pennsylvania 19104, USA

[2]Center for Advanced Retinal and Ocular Therapeutics, University of Pennsylvania Perelman School of Medicine, Philadelphia, Pennsylvania 19104, USA

[3]Division of Ophthalmology at the Children's Hospital of Philadelphia of the Department of Ophthalmology, University of Pennsylvania, Philadelphia, Pennsylvania 19102, USA

Correspondence: jebennet@pennmedicine.upenn.edu

In the 5 years following U.S. Food and Drug Administration (FDA) approval of the first gene therapy reagent approved to treat a genetic disease, voretigene neparvovec-rzyl (Luxturna), retinal disease clinics, hospital pharmacies, operating rooms, and even health insurance entities around the world have incorporated gene therapy as a standard procedure. The success of Luxturna has helped pave the way to establish a template for developing other gene therapy reagents that promise to restore sight or halt the progression of photoreceptor cell loss in both inherited and acquired retinal diseases. Here we review lessons learned from development of a gene therapy drug for *RPE65* disease and how these lessons may expedite the development of additional treatments for previously untreatable blinding conditions.

The first gene therapy reagent to be administered directly in vivo to treat genetic disease was approved by the U.S. Food and Drug Administration (FDA) in 2017, a recombinant adeno-associated virus carrying the wild-type cDNA encoding the retinal pigmented epithelium (RPE) 65 kDa protein, RPE65. This reagent, voretigene neparvovec-rzyl (Luxturna), and known as AAV2-hRPE65v2 during development and clinical trials, was approved by the European Medicines Agency (EMA) the following year and has since been approved in numerous other countries and on multiple continents.

The reagent is an adeno-associated virus serotype 2 (AAV2) vector that delivers the human *RPE65* cDNA to the retina in patients with inherited retinal degeneration (Leber congenital amaurosis type 2 [LCA2]) due to biallelic *RPE65* mutations.

This drug is administered at Centers of Excellence in those various countries by surgeons who have been trained to perform the subretinal injection procedure necessary to deliver the reagent. This procedure places the AAV reagent in direct contact with the diseased RPE cells. Prior to this time, subretinal injection procedures had only been used infrequently in clinical care as part of a method to treat choroidal neovascularization and complications thereof (e.g., acute subretinal hemorrhage in the macula).

Learnings from the development of Luxturna and the de-risking of delivery of AAV vectors to the subretinal space (at least up to 1.5E11 vector genomes [vg]) have since been applied to carry out preclinical and clinical studies aiming to develop gene-based treatments for dozens of other genetic and acquired blinding retinal diseases. The positive results have fueled studies in small biotechnology companies as well as large pharmaceutical entities. The results have inspired patients with other orphan retinal diseases to band together and lobby for treatment for their particular "gene." There are now more than a dozen different gene augmentation trials at various stages in progress that have adapted a similar approach as that used for RPE65 to treat other forms of retinal degeneration. The path used to develop RPE65 gene therapy is also being used to test a variety of other gene therapy strategies for human retinal disease treatment, including delivery of decoy receptors, gene-editing molecules, antisense RNA, mitochondrial genes, and even genes aiming to render cells other than photoreceptors light-sensitive ("optogenetic" therapy). The RPE65 experience has also been applied to the development of gene-based therapies for other neurologic diseases. The second gene therapy product approved by the FDA for a genetic disease (spinal muscular atrophy) was Zolgensma (Onasemnogene abeparvovec, approved in 2020). Gene therapy clinical trials are in progress for a variety of other inherited central nervous system (CNS) diseases, including several forms of mucopolysaccharidosis, and diseases such as Canavan and Batten disease. Several of these diseases have retinal manifestations and so it is possible that these gene therapies will be applied intraocularly as well. Gene therapy studies are also planned entailing delivery to the cochlea to test treatments for genetic forms of deafness.

Here we look at some of the concerns and challenges faced in developing RPE65 gene therapy and how the lessons learned may influence development of additional gene therapies. We also review some of the questions that remain and consider how the experiences from prior studies may influence the development of additional treatments for these previously untreatable blinding diseases.

ROUTE OF ADMINISTRATION

When we initiated preclinical RPE65 studies using the naturally occurring Briard dog model, we showed that subretinal delivery of AAV2.RPE65 resulted in rescue of retinal and visual function. Intravitreal delivery of a similar dose did not (subsequent studies in affected mice and dogs and unaffected monkeys confirmed the fact that delivery to the subretinal space was required for transduction of outer retinal cells and, therefore, efficacy of the reagent [in the affected dogs]). Intravitreal delivery of AAV2 resulted in transduction of ganglion cells but not cells in the outer retina and thus there is no efficacy in this disease (expression after intravitreal injection was seen not only in ganglion cells within the retina, but also throughout the axons composing the optic nerve, optic chiasm, and all the way to the first-order synapse in the lateral geniculate). Transduction of the visual pathway after intravitreal injection of AAV2 was not a surprise for us as we had previously observed this phenomenon (Dudus et al. 1999; Bennett et al. 2000; Vandenberghe et al. 2011).[4]

When planning our formal RPE65 preclinical safety and toxicity studies, we postulated that one of the potential complications of RPE65 gene therapy would be failed subretinal injection with inadvertent delivery of the AAV2.hRPE65v2 reagent to the vitreous. We postulated that a potential surgical complication, leakage of the gene therapy reagent from the retinotomy site, could potentially also expose the vitreal cavity. Although the planned human subretinal surgery included vitrectomy and air–fluid exchange,

---

[4]It took us 2 years to publish the first observation of ganglion cell and visual tract transduction after intravitreal injection (Dudus et al. 1999). After submission to multiple high-impact journals and reviews, the results were eventually published in *Vision Research*. The results remain important as witnessed by the fact that, since then, intravitreal injection has been used to target ganglion cells in preclinical and clinical studies (e.g., Guy et al. 2017; Cukras et al. 2018; Bouquet et al. 2019).

which would reduce the exposure to the cells lining the vitreous cavity, an exposure could potentially result in inflammation or inadvertent transduction of ganglion cells or anterior segment structures. Thus, we included high-dose intravitreal injections as well as subretinal injections in our good laboratory practice (GLP) toxicity studies even though the planned delivery route in humans was subretinal. This design incorporating the "worst case scenario" is one that we and others have adopted in risk evaluation of gene therapy reagents for other inherited retinal degenerations. We also noted that some recombinant viral vectors delivered intravitreally at high doses cause inflammation, whereas the same doses injected subretinally are benign (Anand et al. 2002). Success in generating AAV vectors that can penetrate through the retina and target outer retinal cells after intravitreal injection (without resulting in inflammation) or delivery of particular vectors to the suprachoroidal space to transduce outer retinal cells will require additional evaluation of these sites of application effect.

RETINAL DISEASE DOSING EXTRAPOLATIONS FROM ANIMALS TO HUMANS ARE NOT STRAIGHTFORWARD

The eyes of animals of different species differ considerably from each other anatomically and there are thus many considerations in extrapolating doses from one species to another (Fig. 1). For example, the lens of rodents occupies the bulk of the vitreous cavity while lenses of dogs and primates do not, eyes of some species are more spherical than others, the weight of the eye and the volume of vitreous fluid differ from species to species, there are different blood supplies in eyes of different species, and the surgical approach in one species will differ from that in another due to anatomical considerations. Of considerable importance is that animals other than primates lack a true macular retina.

One can approximate the size differences between eyes of different species as a rough guide for comparative studies, but this does not take into account some of the anatomic considerations listed above or the fact that there are differences in photoreceptor composition between eyes of different species (for example, the presence of a macula in primates only, the fact that rod photoreceptors predominate over cones [10:1] in the mouse retina, or the focal area of increased cone density in the canine retina [the area centralis]). In addition, in some animal models, the reagent is most likely to be therapeutic if it is administered very early in development. For treatment of the *LCA5* form of LCA, for example, efficacy is observed by treating the mouse at postnatal day 4 when the eye is a fraction of the size of an adult mouse eye (Fig. 1; Song et al. 2018). This time point in the mouse, at which there are retinal progenitor cells but no differentiated photoreceptors, is roughly equivalent to the first trimester of pregnancy in a human.

A similarity between the retinas of each species is that after subretinal injection, the area of the retina exposed to a designated amount of the test reagent (AAV, in this case) can be approximated according to the volume of fluid injected. By increasing the volume of solution, one increases the area of retina (as well as the number of cells) exposed to the vector. Since the number of RPE or photoreceptor cells in different species of humans/animals is known or can be estimated and the total dose of the reagent is known, and since

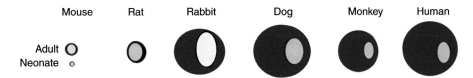

Figure 1. Comparative anatomy. Approximate differences in sizes of the eye and lens in species commonly used for preclinical testing compared to the human eye. The size of the eye and percentage occupied by the lens are factors that dictate the route of delivery and the volume (and thus virus dose) that can be administered. Figure created from data derived from Faqui (2016) and Dejneka et al. (2004), and measurements made in the Bennett laboratory.

the volume of solution that is injected can be measured, one can estimate the number of viral particles exposed to each cell (an approximate multiplicity of infection [MOI]). Although the regulatory bodies currently prefer to review data in terms of total dose delivered, estimates of MOI may be more relevant in terms of treating retinal disease than measurements of total dose. We carried out calculations on potential effects of MOI on safety and efficacy, which increased our confidence in the final dose selections used in our phase 1–3 clinical trials for *RPE65* deficiency. Such data may aid in decisions for final dose selection in upcoming clinical trials. A sample dosing exercise for a hypothetical gene therapy clinical trial for a retinal degenerative disease is shown in Figure 2. Due to the epithelial structure of the retina with high surface-to-volume ratio, pharmacodynamics may differ considerably as compared to other organs (e.g., liver or muscle).

ADHERENCE AND SAFETY CHARACTERISTICS OF THE DELIVERY DEVICE WITH RESPECT TO AAV

As mandated by the FDA, we conducted studies of the compatibility of the subretinal injection

devices we planned to use in our clinical trials with the test reagent, AAV2.hRPE65v2. We did not detect any safety concerns with respect to changes in pH, particulates, or endotoxin levels after incubating and delivering our AAV through those injection devices in the laboratory. However, we were surprised at the extent of loss of vector to the "inert" surfaces of the injection device and/or tubing. Up to 80% of the vector was lost due to binding to the inner surfaces of the device (Fig. 3). This propelled us to test and then incorporate a nonionic surfactant, Pluronic F68 (PF68; poloxamer 188) into our AAV product (Bennicelli et al. 2008). In the presence of 0.001% PF68, the full dose of vector is delivered through the device. Inclusion of PF68 at this concentration did not result in toxicity. This important addition has been incorporated in delivery of AAV in numerous other clinical trials (e.g., Patrício et al. 2020; Aleman et al. 2022).

IMPORTANCE OF ASSESSING PROPORTION OF "FULL" VS. "EMPTY" AAV CAPSIDS IN CLINICAL STUDIES

The protocol that our manufacturing team used to generate both research grade and clinical grade

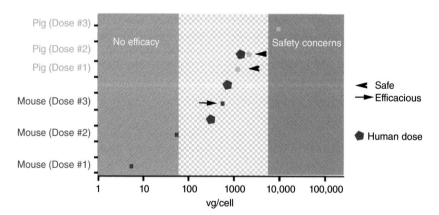

Figure 2. Dose extrapolation exercise. Hypothetical data using efficacy in an affected mouse model and toxicity in an unaffected large animal (pig) model to select doses to be used in a phase 1 human clinical trial. Efficacy in the mouse (blue squares) requires subretinal administration of Dose #3 (arrow). (Approximate dose [vg] per cell is calculated based the known number of cells in retinas of different species and the area of retina that is targeted. The area targeted is a function of volume injected.) Meanwhile, in the pig (green squares), there is safety (no observed adverse effect level [NOAEL]) at Doses #1 and #2 (arrowheads). Signs of toxicity appear at Dose #3. Proposed human doses (red polygons) would span a region where there is efficacy in mice and safety in pigs. Typically, a phase 1 gene therapy safety study uses three doses. One would want to avoid doses in which there is a slim chance of efficacy or a high chance of toxicity.

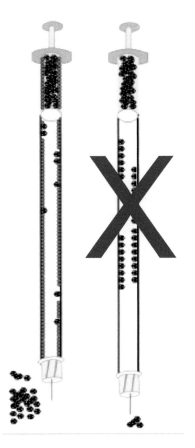

Figure 3. Accurate dosing of adeno-associated virus (AAV), devices, and surfactant. When AAV is loaded into an injection device, up to 80% of the particles bind to the "inert" surfaces of the device, thus making accurate dosing difficult. Bennicelli et al. (2008) showed that addition of a small amount of surfactant (Pluronic F68), prevents this binding and allows accurate dosing. (X) Syringe lacking surfactant.

AAV incorporated cesium chloride (CsCl) gradient ultracentrifugation to separate out the heavier transgene cassette-containing ("full") AAV capsids from those that were empty (Fig. 4). This is a critical step because the empty capsids do not confer any potential rescue effect. There is no potential gain by exposing the recipient to empty AAV capsids. In fact, this can only be undesirable or even harmful on an immunologic basis (Timmers et al. 2020). Empty capsids have the potential of increasing innate or adaptive immune responses to the vector. In other studies, systemic administration of empty capsids was shown to

contribute to hepatic transaminase elevations in mice (Gao et al. 2014). Our AAV2.hRPE65v2 product contained <5% empty capsids.

AAV manufacturing protocols have advanced since the time we generated our initial good manufacturing practice (GMP) AAV preparations in 2007 and many AAV manufacturing groups have replaced CsCl gradient centrifugation with other purification methods. We suspect, however, that some of the differences in outcomes between different clinical trials could be due to the ratio of full:empty AAV capsids. Of course, there are other potential contaminants of AAV preparations that are likely to be of equal or even higher concern with respect to toxicity, including retained nucleic acid fragments derived from the manufacturing process that are partially copurified with the vectors (Wright 2014). The bottom line is that the "full" capsid AAV preparation should be as pure as possible and that the details thereof be collected so that they can be used in the future to correlate vector characteristics with safety and efficacy. This is an important consideration in choosing a vector core, which will provide the reagent for testing and clinical application.

THE POWER OF COLLABORATORS, PATIENTS, AND SOCIAL MEDIA

When we received the federal and institutional regulatory approvals allowing us to enroll our first subject in the Children's Hospital of Philadelphia (CHOP) RPE65 gene therapy trial in mid-2007, we were surprised to find that there were no U.S.-based patients available for us to invite. Many patients who had been diagnosed with LCA had not been genotyped and thus would not meet the inclusion requirement of biallelic *RPE65* mutations. Others were known only to particular specialists who were planning or conducting separate competing investigations. At that point in time, there were few laboratories carrying out genetic screens on patient samples and even fewer that were approved to give clinical laboratory improvement amendment (CLIA) genetic diagnoses. There was no incentive to conduct CLIA testing as insurance did not cover the costs (since there were no ap-

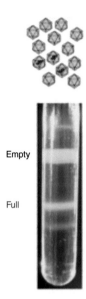

Figure 4. A variable that can affect the success (and potentially the safety) of gene therapy is the ratio of "full" (transgene-containing adeno-associated virus [AAV] capsids) versus "empty" (capsids alone) in the test reagent. Shown is the appearance of bands representing empty and full capsids after centrifugation of an AAV preparation on a cesium chloride (CsCl) gradient. The band containing "full" capsids can be isolated from that containing "empties." Image provided by Dr. Shangzhen Zhou.

proved treatments available). Dr. Edwin Stone had previously predicted the need for such a service and established the John and Marcia Carver Nonprofit Genetic Testing Laboratory (University of Iowa). We took advantage of a long-standing collaboration with colleagues at the Second University of Naples, Italy, Drs. Simonelli, Auricchio, Banfi, Testa, and Rossi. Dr. Francesca Simonelli, a retinal degeneration specialist with a large referral practice covering most of Italy, had already been conducting genotype–phenotype studies. She had sent blood samples to her molecular genetics colleague, Dr. Banfi (Telethon Institute of Genetics and Medicine [TIGEM]) and he had readily identified more than half a dozen individuals with biallelic *RPE65* mutations who, from Dr. Simonelli's perspective, were good candidates for our studies. Because Dr. Banfi's testing had not been done with CLIA standards, we shipped additional blood

samples to the Carver laboratory for CLIA verification. Testing there readily confirmed that this was *RPE65* disease and provided the necessary official documentation.

Dr. Simonelli informed her RPE65 patients about our study and they were eager to participate. At that time, prior to initiation of any human retinal gene therapy trial in the United States, there were many unknowns about safety of the reagent and potential complications. Since Dr. Simonelli's patients lived in Italy, we were concerned that it would be risky to send treated patients back after intervention without access to immediate follow-up. The concerns were addressed when Dr. Simonelli offered to become the principal investigator of a second site for our study, a site in Naples. She and her team would establish baseline and follow-up visits in duplicate with the ones that we planned at CHOP. A contract research organization confirmed that Dr. Simonelli possessed the clinical equipment that was necessary. We supplied the equipment to be used for exploratory measures.[5] The surgical administration of the vector would occur only at CHOP, however. Not only would the subjects have care in both Italy and the United States, but all of the clinical testing would be duplicated, thus adding validity and statistical power to the data. This led to the enrollment of the first four subjects in our clinical trial, all Italian. By the time we were ready to enroll the additional subjects in our phase 1 study, specialists in Mexico, Belgium, and the United States (including Drs. Villanueva, LeRoy, Fulton, and Traboulsi) had genotyped and referred patients.[6]

By the time we were ready to initiate our phase 3 studies in 2013, social media had become popular and readily accessible. Information had become available about the positive safety and

---

[5]Delivery of duplicate exploratory materials was itself no small feat. One of us (J.B.) made several trips hand-delivering (and negotiating with customs agents and airport security teams) pupillometers, computers, mobility courses, and cameras and training team members on their operation and data capture.

[6]Two of the individuals from Mexico had traveled by oxcart from their farm to the airport. They experienced many "firsts" on this trip, including the airplane trip, eating at a restaurant, and sleeping on a bed (instead of a hammock).

efficacy results derived from our phase 1 and follow-on studies and families started contacting us directly. Connections and announcements were shared through Facebook and other social media. Patients from as far away as New Zealand and India contacted us directly, including an individual in the western United States who heard about our studies when picking up their "Seeing Eye" dog. (We even had numerous queries from pet owners who wanted to bring their beloved dogs or cats to our clinic to receive gene therapy for various eye diseases.) Meanwhile, patients and families set up their own (gene-specific) patient online advocate groups and held fundraisers, education sessions, and meetings where patients and their families could meet scientists and clinicians, learn about the latest results and technology, and even be genotyped. Numerous inspirational stories were also shared on these venues, including one RPE65 patient's successful competitions on *America's Got Talent* and *American Idol* (www.goldderby.com/article/2022/christian-guardino-agt-golden-buzzer-american-idol)! A benefit of the growth in social media has been that patients with even ultra-rare genetic disorders have banded together, educated one another, and are lobbying for treatments for their own specific diseases. Many of these individuals have volunteered to participate in ancillary studies that could one day support an interventional study (such as natural history studies, evaluations of novel outcome measures, etc.). They know that these individual studies will not give them direct benefit, but they are committed to the mission to find treatments for blindness. One downside of the social media interface is the sharing of unofficial data—good or bad—before critical review and publication. This can sometimes lead to rapid dissemination of inaccurate and confusing misinformation and serve as a distraction from carefully conducted research.

RPE65 VARIANTS AND PREDICTIONS OF EFFICACY

It was important prior to enrolling a subject in a clinical trial and for treatment with Luxturna to understand the likelihood that the RPE65 variants detected are actual disease-causing mutations and not just benign variants. If they are benign variants, then the individual is exposed to unnecessary risks (anesthesia, subretinal injection, etc.) and stands no chance of benefit. In many cases, there are clear indications of the likelihood that one particular RPE65 variant will be disease-causing (vs. benign polymorphisms). These indications come from segregation analyses, the locations of the nucleic acid changes with respect to the RPE65 isomerohydrolase protein, a molecule that was identified and characterized by T. Michael Redmond (Redmond and Hamel 2000; Redmond et al. 2005), and from mutation prediction software such as PolyPhen2 and SIFT. Typically, it is not difficult to conduct such analyses. However, in particular instances, there may be variants of unknown significance (VUS). Examples of such situations are (1) evaluating an adopted child with no known biologic relatives, (2) discovering a nonpaternity issue when doing segregation studies, or (3) discovering a de novo mutation. In such cases, additional analyses are warranted. Yang et al. described an in vitro mutagenesis approach for verifying mutational pathogenicity before administering gene therapy (Yang et al. 2019). In a series of four pediatric patients, new compound heterozygous or homozygous RPE65 variants were identified with unknown significance. These mutations were incorporated into the RPE65 protein in the laboratory and the enzymatic activity of the modified protein was tested and shown to be abolished. This served as determination that the variants were indeed disease-causing. The subjects were treated with Luxturna and each one showed benefit, the definitive evidence that their mutations were disease-causing.

PREEXISTING HUMORAL ANTI-AAV2-NEUTRALIZING ANTIBODIES DO NOT PREVENT EFFICACY AFTER SUBRETINAL INJECTION

When we initiated our phase 1 RPE65 gene therapy clinical trial at CHOP, we did not know whether it would be safe to include subjects who had been immunized previously to wild-type AAV. Evidence that individuals had previous exposure was manifested by presence of serum antibody titers to the AAV2 capsid. Many individuals are exposed to wild-type AAV2 in childhood (Calcedo and Wilson 2016). Would such individuals benefit from the intervention or would transduction be blocked by neutralizing antibodies? Would an enhanced immune response result in toxicity? Anti-AAV2 Nabs have a prevalence of 30%–40% in the population but this percentage varies geographically (Blacklow et al. 1968; Chirmule et al. 1999; Louis Jeune et al. 2013). In Africa, for example, prevalence can be as high as 60% (Calcedo et al. 2009). We decided to exclude participants who had anti-AAV2-neutralizing antibodies (Nabs) >1:1000 in our phase 1 studies. (Two such individuals were the Mexican children who lived on a farm —see footnote 6.) The exclusion cut-off number was selected based on prior experience with systemic delivery of AAV2 in hemophilia human gene therapy studies.

After we completed our phase 1 studies, we approached the FDA to ask whether it would be appropriate to use the contralateral uninjected eye as a control in planned phase 3 studies. They said no, that both eyes must be injected. Based on traditional biostatistics designs used in FDA-approved trials, it was determined that subjects, not eyes or organs, should be used as controls. In addition, it was felt that many clinicians would attempt to treat the second eye once the drug was approved. We had learned from our preclinical and clinical studies that unilateral subretinal injection would elicit systemic NAbs to AAV2. However, we did not know whether these would preclude a repeat injection to the contralateral eye. We were thus tasked to evaluate the safety of contralateral eye AAV2.hRPE65v2 administration. We carried out preclinical studies in affected dogs and unaffected nonhuman primates whereby we delivered a high dose of AAV subretinally and subsequently treated the contralateral eye, also with the high dose, at the time point when the immune response would be maximal. We also immunized the nonhuman primates (NHPs) systemically with AAV prior to subretinal injection to mimic a situation where humans would have high titer-neutralizing antibodies. Finally, we evaluated anti-AAV2 antibody levels in intraocular fluid and sera of individuals (unaffected with *RPE65* mutations)

receiving cataract surgery to determine whether high levels of serum antibodies correlated with high levels of intraocular fluid antibodies.

We found that it was safe to carry out subretinal injections of 1.5E11vg AAV2.hRPE65v2 in animals that had preexisting anti-AAV2 NAbs and that it was safe to readminister 1.5E11vg AAV2.hRPE65v2 to the contralateral eyes of animals even when immune responses were maximal (Amado et al. 2010). We also found that intraocular fluid in humans is sequestered from antibodies that are present in the circulation. Similarly, intraocular fluid of animals is sequestered from humoral antibodies, at least until that eye is directly exposed to AAV2. We thus proceeded cautiously to readminister AAV2. hRPE65v2 to the contralateral eyes of our phase 1 subjects in a follow-on study. We found that subretinal readministration to the contralateral eye was safe and that it led to the same level of improvement in retinal and visual function as in the initially injected eye (Bennett et al. 2012, 2016). We eliminated the exclusion requirement relating to presence of humoral anti-AAV2 NAbs in our phase 3 clinical trial.

There were no instances of inflammation due to the vector in phase 3 regardless of level of anti-AAV2 NAbs. Currently, treatment of individuals with Luxturna is agnostic as to their AAV2 immune status. Additional laboratory studies support the safety of repeat subretinal injection to the initially injected eye (Weed et al. 2019), although that has not been tested yet in humans with *RPE65* disease. This again is different than the experience in nonocular disease where readministration may not be beneficial.

It should be noted that administration of AAV to the intravitreal cavity is not necessarily as safe from an antibody perspective as subretinal injection. Intravitreal administration of high-dose AAV (and of other viral vectors) is more likely to result in inflammation, perhaps because some AAVs target anterior segment structures (see above) (Anand et al. 2002; Lebherz et al. 2008; Ramachandran et al. 2017). Inflammation was encountered after intravitreal injection of AAV8 in a trial for X-linked retinoschisis (sponsor: National Eye Institute [NEI]/National Institutes of Health [NIH]), in some subjects treated with AAV2 in trials for Leber hereditary optic neuropathy (GenSight Biologics), and in subjects treated with ADVM-022, AAV7m8 delivering the cDNA encoding aflibercept (Adverum Biotechnologies) (Cukras et al. 2018; Bouquet et al. 2019; Adverum Biotechnologies 2020). The Adverum clinical trial now excludes individuals with serum Nabs >1:125 (https://investors.adverum.com/events-and-presentations/default.aspx). Going forward, it will also be important to conduct analyses of the association of cellular immune responses with intravitreal inflammation to be able to fully understand and then derisk this route of delivery.

PREVENTING VERTICAL TRANSMISSION

One of the main concerns of the FDA in early studies was whether vector injected subretinally might contact and infect systemic sites. A particular concern was whether the vector would expose the gonads (testis and ovaries), infect sperm or eggs, and thus be carried to the next generation at fertilization. None of our laboratory or GLP preclinical data, obtained after delivering AAV subretinally, supported this possibility. Nevertheless, we were required to tell all of the subjects (including 8-year-old children) in our phase 1 studies that they must use contraception for at least a year after surgery. When we met with regulatory authorities to discuss some proposed readministration studies, we were surprised when the FDA ethicists told us that we were impinging upon our subject's liberties. Our follow-on studies and phase 3 trial allowed individuals the freedom to decide on their own whether they were going to use contraception 4 months after vector delivery.

TRIALS AND TRIBULATIONS WITH OUTCOME MEASURES

In our initial studies using three affected Briard dogs and then in subsequent studies using affected dogs of different ages and with different AAV formulations and transgenes, we used a variety of outcome measures to evaluate successful restoration of vision. There were a number of noninvasive measures that appeared informative including electroretinograms (ERGs) (Acland et al. 2001, 2005; Bennicelli et al. 2008), pupillometry (Acland et al. 2005), nystagmus testing (Jacobs et al. 2006, 2009; Bennicelli et al. 2008), and navigation through a maze in dim light (Acland et al. 2001; Bennicelli et al. 2008). ERGs and pupillary light responses (PLRs) also improved when mice were later treated with AAV2.hRPE65v2 (Jacobson et al. 2005a; Bennicelli et al. 2008). We thus incorporated all of these as exploratory measures in our phase 1 gene therapy clinical trial at CHOP. In that phase 1 study, only one eye (the worse seeing eye) was treated with AAV2.RPE65v2, so that were able to compare results in treated versus untreated (control) eyes.

Notably, the only outcome measure that was *not useful* in humans was the ERG. This measure had been robust in the affected dogs and, in fact, had been used to support the dosing strategy implemented in three different RPE65 gene therapy clinical trials (National Institutes of Health Recombinant DNA Advisory Committee (RAC) 2005a,b; Bainbridge et al. 2008). The other measures, including pupillometry, nystagmus testing, and navigation, gave robust results in our phase 1 clinical trial at CHOP.

At baseline, PLRs were flat (i.e., pupils did not constrict when exposed to light). PLRs showed improvement in all subjects as early as 8 days postinjection (Bennett et al. 2012). Because the PLR is consensual, when the treated eye was exposed to light, both pupils constricted. In contrast, when the untreated eye was exposed to light, neither pupil constricted. The amplitudes of constriction correlated with the intensity of the light stimuli. The effect was analogous to what is seen clinically as an afferent pupillary defect (APD)—with one eye responding to light but the other not. However, in this case, the APD was in the untreated eye. This measure provided the first objective data indicating that the intervention was effective (Maguire et al. 2008, 2009). Later, when we carried out a follow-on study where the contralateral eye was treated, the PLR was restored in both eyes and the "APD" disappeared (Ashtari et al. 2011; Bennett et al. 2012, 2016).

Improved ocular gaze fixation was also found with nystagmus testing. In fact, improved ocular stability may have been reflected by a trend in improvement in visual acuity (VA) in the untreated eyes (Maguire et al. 2008). However, like the affected dogs, not all human subjects had severe baseline nystagmus. The severity of nystagmus is also affected by level of alertness and by various medications, and so was not pursued further.

Ability to navigate independently using eyesight alone seemed like a "real-world" outcome to pursue. We had shown that blind dogs had improved ability to navigate in dim environments after gene therapy. Similar results were found in our phase 1 RPE65 subjects. At baseline, these individuals had difficulty navigating quickly and accurately through a physical obstacle course, particularly in dim light. After treatment, the individuals were able to avoid collisions with obstacles and walk quickly to the exit of the obstacle course using their treated eye. Their performance was unchanged using their untreated eye.

After we reported the promising initial results of our phase 1 clinical trial for RPE65 deficiency in a packed ballroom at the annual meeting of Association for Research in Vision and Ophthalmology (ARVO) in 2008, the last question from the audience was, "Why weren't you able to record full-field ERGs?" We still do not know the answer to this question. We tried to record multifocal ERGs and did see some signal in the injected area of one subject's retina, but this was not something we could reproduce in additional subjects (Simonelli et al. 2010). The fact that full-field ERGs were restored in animal models but not humans may be related to the differences in *RPE65* mutations. The affected dogs were all homozygous for a four-nucleotide (AAGA) deletion, which produces a frameshift, and a premature stop codon (Aguirre et al. 1998; Veske et al. 1999). Affected mice either had an engineered knockout of *Rpe65* (Redmond and Hamel 2000) or a spontaneous nonsense mutation in exon 3 of the *Rpe65* gene (Pang et al. 2005). In contrast, the humans suffered from a variety of compound heterozygous and homozygous mutations but none had the same changes found in the affected Briards (or mice). An alternative explanation may be that

ERG restoration in animals may have been due to the developmental age at which the animals were treated. In most of the canine and murine studies, animals were treated early in life (typically 4 months for the Briard and 1 month for the mouse) (Acland et al. 2001; Bennicelli et al. 2008). The equivalent human age would be very early childhood. It may not be possible to restore full-field ERGs in human until infants are enrolled. Since Luxturna is now approved for use in children 1 year and older, we may be able to test this hypothesis.

Ultimately, the FDA informed us that for drug approval, a metric reflecting a "clinically meaningful improvement" was required, in other words, some measure of activity of daily living. We standardized and validated a multi-luminance mobility test (MLMT) to be able to grade speed and accuracy of navigation under specified illuminance levels (Chung et al. 2018). Performance using both eyes together and each eye individually was recorded by video and results analyzed by a reading center. The results showed robust improvement of functional vision and correlated with other clinical measures (full-field light sensitivity, visual fields) and a modified visual function questionnaire (Russell et al. 2017; Maguire et al. 2021b). The MLMT was viewed favorably with respect to the clinically meaningful requirement. A physical test similar to the MLMT (Ora-VNC test, Andover, MA) is now used to videotape and measure functional vision in other gene therapy clinical trials for inherited retinal degeneration. In the future, it may be possible to simplify the task of assessing the impact of gene therapy (or other interventions) on functional vision through the use of virtual reality–based testing (Aleman et al. 2021). Such a system can facilitate conduct of the test and allow the test to be tailored to different retinal diseases. Further, automated scoring of the tests can allow rapid and objective readouts without the risk of disclosing personal identifiers.

DO PROSPECTS FOR BENEFIT CHANGE WITH AGE?

Our preclinical ERG data from animal models indicated that benefit was greatest in young animals in both mice and dogs. Restoration of retinal function was far greater and a larger percentage of animals responded in cohorts of 2- to 4-month-old mice than in cohorts of elderly (>15-month-old) mice. Similarly, ERG responses were better after treatment of puppies than of middle-aged dogs (Jacobson et al. 2005b). We therefore proposed to include children in our phase 1 clinical trial. Because children had not previously been enrolled in gene therapy clinical trials for nonlethal diseases, our proposal was selected for a full meeting of the NIH Recombinant DNA Advisory Committee (RAC). Because the gene therapy administration involves anesthesia and surgery, it presents more than a minor increase over minimal risk. Therefore, according to the Code of Federal Regulations (21 C.F.R. 50.52, 2013), prior to initiating a study in children, evidence must be provided that administration of the study agent provides a prospect of direct benefit. Therefore, the traditional preference to enroll adults first strongly applied. We explained our rationale for pediatric enrollment and dose selection, which included possible efficacy at the low dose with a plan to test for safety and efficacy first in adults and then enroll children (ages 8 and over). The RAC unanimously approved our plan. Interestingly, once our study was approved to enroll pediatric subjects, other retinal gene therapy clinical trials were grandfathered in. We did indeed demonstrate dramatic efficacy in children but perhaps what was even more surprising, is that we saw efficacy even in middle-aged adults with advanced disease. The improvements were generally more difficult to measure using standard measures of visual function (such as VA) because there were only islands of remaining viable photoreceptors. Interestingly, functional magnetic resonance imaging (fMRI) documented increased blood flow to the regions of visual cortex predicted to be activated after AAV delivery to the relevant portion of the retina (Ashtari et al. 2011, 2015; Bennett et al. 2016). There were even structural benefits (myelination) that accompanied the functional benefits (Ashtari et al. 2015). The findings revealed that even though the visual pathway had not been used for decades in these "blind" individuals, the "wiring" was present and could be employed if responsiveness to retinal stimulatory input was reestablished.

Because of the small number of individuals enrolled in phase 3 studies ($n = 29$), any analysis of age effect is statistically underpowered. Because of this and the numerous other variables involved, we have not yet definitively determined whether the intervention is more effective and durable in children versus adults, but this is a question that is being examined. There are now post-approval reports, however, of excellent outcomes in both young and middle-aged subjects (Deng et al. 2022; Sengillo et al. 2022). Thus, the morphology of the retina seems to be a better predictor of outcomes than age. However, if the retina is "corrected" too late in life, the individual may not be able to benefit from vision because of amblyopia (i.e., the brain may not recognize information delivered from the retina).

SURGICAL CONSIDERATIONS AND POST-MARKETING EXPERIENCE

Prior to conducting the multicenter phase 3 RPE65 clinical trial, experiences in the numerous animal studies and in human subjects were assimilated to generate a detailed standard operating procedure to maximize safety and potential benefit. The protocol specified the dose, volume, and distance away from the fovea (to minimize stress on this vulnerable area). After FDA approval, Spark Therapeutics instituted a subretinal injection training program that incorporated many of the details that we had previously shared with Novartis in a subretinal injection manual (www.med.upenn.edu/carot/assets/user-content/documents/sr-training-package-final.pdf). Board-certified retina surgeons were provided didactic and hands-on wet laboratory training and were then qualified to participate in Centers of Excellence qualified to administer Luxturna.

A number of groups have subsequently reported some of their results—a step that is invaluable in terms of sharing both positive and negative experiences. Some report the first experiences in their respective countries with a limited number of patients (Testa et al. 2021; Ferraz Sallum et al. 2022; Kortüm et al. 2022; Kwak et al. 2022).

Others report results in a series of patients. Most investigators report improved retinal and visual function within the first year consistent with clinical trial results (Deng et al. 2022; Stingl et al. 2022). Gange et al. (2022) report progressive perifoveal chorioretinal atrophy (at the injection site) after surgery in 80% of eyes with some showing scotomas related to the atrophy. Sengillo et al. (2022) treated 41 patients, 25 of which were pediatric. They reported improved VA in the pediatric patients, a trend seen in our original study group (Russell et al. 2017).

One detail becomes apparent in reviewing the different post-marketing study results is that the different surgeons have varied the surgical technique, including whether or not to make a pre-bleb with balanced salt solution, where to place the bleb, whether or not to incorporate optical coherence tomography (OCT) into the subretinal injection procedure, whether or not to make multiple blebs, when to treat the second eye, etc. We previously reported a two-step procedure whereby two injections are placed distant from the fovea and then the bleb is allowed to "roll" into the fovea via gravity after fluid–air exchange (Maguire et al. 2021a). Testa et al. (2021) delayed injection of the second eye to 45 days, apparently due to a retinal hemorrhage complication in the first eye. Previously the maximum recommended interval between injection of the first and second eye was 18 days. One wonders whether this increase in time between the first and second injection and other variables in the different studies will affect the overall results. So far, most reports still indicate that inflammatory responses are minimal. We encourage different groups to publish any and all details of their studies (including any leakage from the retinotomy site into the vitreous, difficulties in raising the bleb, or other complications) so that the field (and patients) can benefit.[7]

It will be particularly interesting to learn whether there is more benefit when the intervention is administered in infants and toddlers than in older individuals. The phase 3 studies were open to individuals age 3 and over. However, the youngest individual who received intervention in this study was 4 years old. The EMA and FDA surprised us by allowing children as young as 1 year old to be treated. So far, we have heard of at least a couple of 2-year-olds who have been treated: one by Sengillo et al. (2022) and one by our team at CHOP. Both individuals have responded well to gene therapy. Of course, it is challenging to obtain quantitative measures of retinal visual function in such young patients, particularly at baseline. Perhaps there will be restoration of full-field ERGs in these individuals (see above). Alternatively, as they get older, it may be possible to compare responses in treated versus untreated portions of their retinas to assess the effect of age on treatment outcomes.

CONCLUDING REMARKS: THE *RPE65* EXPERIENCE AND EXTRAPOLATION TO OTHER INHERITED RETINAL DEGENERATIONS

Luxturna introduced the concept of a one-time gene-based treatment for a previously untreatable disease to patients and to physicians. With the progress in identification of disease-causing genes and mutations, other retinal diseases are now being explored as targets for gene therapy. Antisense and gene editing strategies now complement gene augmentation approaches. Gene therapy studies have expanded to include disease and neurosensory pathways as targets. There are now programs evaluating anti-neovascular and optogenetic gene therapy and there is a company planning a gene-based treatment for inherited retinal degeneration that is agnostic to the disease-causing gene/mutation. As the field proceeds, we learn more about the promise and limitations of delivery vehicles, safety limits and immune response. The retina has become a very attractive target for gene therapy given the advantages inherent in this tissue (e.g., immunologic, anatomic, statistical design, etc). The challenge at present is to move stepwise and cautiously to de-risk new strategies so that we can continue to

---

[7] A recent review of retinal gene therapy clinical trial listings on clinicaltrials.gov reveals that more than half of the 19 trials labeled as "complete," there is no associated publication. We believe that companies running gene therapy (and other) clinical trials should report their findings so that others avoid repeating unsuccessful or potentially harmful studies.

bring new and durable treatment options for devastating diseases.

COMPETING INTEREST STATEMENT

J.B. and A.M.M. are coauthors on intellectual property describing the gene therapy for RPE65 deficiency but waived any potential financial gain in 2002.

ACKNOWLEDGMENTS

We are deeply grateful to the families and patients for their participation in our studies leading up to approval of voretigene neparvovec-rzyl. It has also been an honor to work with our extraordinarily talented and kind teammates in carrying out *RPE65* preclinical and clinical studies. We thank Dr. Zhao for providing the image used in Figure 4.

Authors are supported by the F.M. Kirby Foundation and Center for Advanced Retinal and Ocular Therapeutics (CAROT), University of Pennsylvania.

REFERENCES

Acland GM, Aguirre GD, Ray J, Zhang Q, Aleman TS, Cideciyan AV, Pearce-Kelling SE, Anand V, Zeng Y, Maguire AM, et al. 2001. Gene therapy restores vision in a canine model of childhood blindness. *Nat Genet* **28**: 92–95.

Acland GM, Aguirre GD, Bennett J, Aleman TS, Cideciyan AV, Bennicelli J, Dejneka NS, Pearce-Kelling SE, Maguire AM, Palczewski K, et al. 2005. Long-term restoration of rod and cone vision by single dose rAAV-mediated gene transfer to the retina in a canine model of childhood blindness. *Mol Ther* **12**: 1072–1082. doi:10.1016/j.ymthe.2005.08.008

Adverum Biotechnologies 2020. Adverum biotechnologies reports additional clinical data from first cohort of OPTIC Phase 1 Trial of ADVM-022 intravitreal gene therapy for Wet AMD at the Atlantic Coast Retina Club Macula 20/20 Annual Meeting. *GlobeNewswire*, January 11, 2020. https://www.globenewswire.com/news-release/2020/01/11/1969182/0/en/Adverum-Biotechnologies-Reports-Additional-Clinical-Data-from-First-Cohort-of-OPTIC-Phase-1-Trial-of-ADVM-022-Intravitreal-Gene-Therapy-for-Wet-AMD-at-the-Atlantic-Coast-Retina-Clu.html

Aguirre G, Baldwin V, Pearce-Kelling S, Narfstrom K, Ray K, Acland G. 1998. Congenital stationary night blindness in the dog: common mutation in the RPE65 gene indicates founder effect. *Mol Vis* **4**: 23.

Aleman TS, Miller AJ, Maguire KH, Aleman EM, Serrano LW, O'Connor KB, Bedoukian EC, Leroy BP, Maguire AM, Bennett J. 2021. A virtual reality orientation and mobility test for inherited retinal degenerations: testing a proof-of-concept after gene therapy. *Clin Ophthalmol* **15**: 939–952. doi:10.2147/OPTH.S292527

Aleman TS, Huckfeldt RM, Serrano LW, Pearson DJ, Vergilio GK, McCague S, Marshall KA, Ashtari M, Doan TM, Weigel-DiFranco CA, et al. 2022. AAV2-hCHM subretinal delivery to the macula in choroideremia: two year interim results of an ongoing phase I/II gene therapy trial. *Ophthalmology* doi:10.1016/j.ophtha.2022.06.006

Amado D, Mingozzi F, Hui D, Bennicelli J, Wei Z, Chen Y, Bote E, Grant R, Golden J, Narfstrom K, et al. 2010. Safety and efficacy of subretinal readministration of a viral vector in large animals to treat congenital blindness. *Sci Transl Med* **2**: 21ra16. doi:10.1126/scitranslmed.3000659

Anand V, Duffy B, Yang Z, Dejneka NS, Maguire AM, Bennett J. 2002. A deviant immune response to viral proteins and transgene product is generated on subretinal administration of adenovirus and adeno-associated virus. *Mol Ther* **5**: 125–132. doi:10.1006/mthe.2002.0525

Ashtari M, Cyckowski LL, Monroe JF, Marshall KA, Chung DC, Auricchio A, Simonelli F, Leroy BP, Maguire AM, Shindler KS, et al. 2011. The human visual cortex responds to gene therapy-mediated recovery of retinal function. *J Clin Invest* **121**: 2160–2168. doi:10.1172/JCI57377

Ashtari M, Zhang H, Cook PA, Cyckowski LL, Shindler KS, Marshall KA, Aravand P, Vossough A, Gee JC, Maguire AM, et al. 2015. Plasticity of the human visual system after retinal gene therapy in patients with Leber's congenital amaurosis. *Sci Transl Med* **7**: 296ra110. doi:10.1126/scitranslmed.aaa8791

Bainbridge JW, Smith AJ, Barker SS, Robbie S, Henderson R, Balaggan K, Viswanathan A, Holder GE, Stockman A, Tyler N, et al. 2008. Effect of gene therapy on visual function in Leber's congenital amaurosis. *N Engl J Med* **358**: 2231–2239. doi:10.1056/NEJMoa0802268

Bennett J, Anand V, Acland GM, Maguire AM. 2000. Cross-species comparison of in vivo reporter gene expression after recombinant adeno-associated virus-mediated retinal transduction. *Methods Enzymol* **316**: 777–789. doi:10.1016/S0076-6879(00)16762-X

Bennett J, Ashtari M, Wellman J, Marshall KA, Cyckowski LL, Chung DC, McCague S, Pierce EA, Chen Y, Bennicelli JL, et al. 2012. AAV2 gene therapy readministration in three adults with congenital blindness. *Sci Transl Med* **4**: 120ra115. doi:10.1126/scitranslmed.3002865

Bennett J, Wellman J, Marshall KA, McCague S, Ashtari M, DiStefano-Pappas J, Elci OU, Chung DC, Sun J, Wright JF, et al. 2016. Safety and durability of effect of contralateral-eye administration of AAV2 gene therapy in patients with childhood-onset blindness caused by RPE65 mutations: a follow-on phase 1 trial. *Lancet* **388**: 661–672. doi:10.1016/S0140-6736(16)30371-3

Bennicelli J, Wright JF, Komaromy A, Jacobs JB, Hauck B, Zelenaia O, Mingozzi F, Hui D, Chung D, Rex TS, et al. 2008. Reversal of blindness in animal models of Leber congenital amaurosis using optimized AAV2-mediated gene transfer. *Mol Ther* **16**: 458–465. doi:10.1038/sj.mt.6300389

Blacklow NR, Hoggan MD, Kapikian AZ, Austin GJ, Rowe WP. 1968. Epidemiology of adenovirus-associated virus infection in a nursery population. *Am J Epidemiol* **88**: 368–378. doi:10.1093/oxfordjournals.aje.a120897

Bouquet C, Vignal Clermont C, Galy A, Fitoussi S, Blouin L, Munk MR, Valero S, Meunier S, Katz B, Sahel JA, et al. 2019. Immune response and intraocular inflammation in patients with Leber hereditary optic neuropathy treated with intravitreal injection of recombinant adeno-associated virus 2 carrying the *ND4* gene: a secondary analysis of a phase 1/2 clinical trial. *JAMA Ophthalmol* 137: 399–406. doi:10.1001/jamaophthalmol.2018.6902

Calcedo R, Wilson JM. 2016. AAV natural infection induces broad cross-neutralizing antibody responses to multiple AAV serotypes in chimpanzees. *Hum Gene Ther Clin Dev* 27: 79–82. doi:10.1089/humc.2016.048

Calcedo R, Vandenberghe LH, Gao G, Lin J, Wilson JM. 2009. Worldwide epidemiology of neutralizing antibodies to adeno-associated viruses. *J Infect Dis* 199: 381–390. doi:10.1086/595830

Chirmule N, Propert K, Magosin S, Qian Y, Qian R, Wilson J. 1999. Immune responses to adenovirus and adeno-associated virus in humans. *Gene Ther* 6: 1574–1583. doi:10.1038/sj.gt.3300994

Chung DC, McCague S, Yu ZF, Thill S, DiStefano-Pappas J, Bennett J, Cross D, Marshall K, Wellman J, High KA. 2018. Novel mobility test to assess functional vision in patients with inherited retinal dystrophies. *Clin Exp Ophthalmol* 46: 247–259. doi:10.1111/ceo.13022

Cukras C, Wiley HE, Jeffrey BG, Sen HN, Turriff A, Zeng Y, Vijayasarathy C, Marangoni D, Ziccardi L, Kjellstrom S, et al. 2018. Retinal AAV8-RS1 gene therapy for X-linked retinoschisis: initial findings from a phase I/IIa trial by intravitreal delivery. *Mol Ther* 26: 2282–2294. doi:10.1016/j.ymthe.2018.05.025

Dejneka N, Surace E, Aleman T, Cideciyan A, Lyubarsky A, Savchenko A, Redmond T, Tang W, Wei Z, Rex T, et al. 2004. In utero gene therapy rescues vision in a murine model of congenital blindness. *Mol Ther* 9: 182–188. doi:10.1016/j.ymthe.2003.11.013

Deng C, Zhao PY, Branham K, Schlegel D, Fahim AT, Jayasundera TK, Khan N, Besirli CG. 2022. Real-world outcomes of voretigene neparvovec treatment in pediatric patients with RPE65-associated Leber congenital amaurosis. *Graefes Arch Clin Exp Ophthalmol* 260: 1543–1550. doi:10.1007/s00417-021-05508-2

Dudus L, Anand V, Acland G, Chen SJ, Wilson J, Fisher K, Maguire A, Bennett J. 1999. Persistent transgene product in retina, optic nerve and brain after intraocular injection of rAAV. *Vis Res* 39: 2545–2553. doi:10.1016/S0042-6989(98)00308-3

Faqui AS. 2016. *A comprehensive guide to toxicology in nonclinical drug development*, 2nd ed. Academic, Cambridge, MA.

Ferraz Sallum JM, Godoy J, Kondo A, Kutner JM, Vasconcelos H, Maia A. 2022. The first gene therapy for *RPE65* biallelic dystrophy with voretigene neparvovec-rzyl in Brazil. *Ophthalmic Genet* doi:10.1080/13816810.2022.2053995

Gange WS, Sisk RA, Besirli CG, Lee TC, Havunjian M, Schwartz H, Borchert M, Sengillo JD, Mendoza C, Berrocal AM, et al. 2022. Perifoveal chorioretinal atrophy after subretinal voretigene neparvovec-rzyl for RPE65-mediated Leber congenital amaurosis. *Ophthalmol Retina* 6: 58–64. doi:10.1016/j.oret.2021.03.016

Gao K, Li M, Zhong L, Su Q, Li J, Li S, He R, Zhang Y, Hendricks G, Wang J, et al. 2014. Empty virions in AAV8 vector preparations reduce transduction efficiency and may cause total viral particle dose-limiting side-effects. *Mol Ther Methods Clin Dev* 1: 20139.

Guy J, Feuer WJ, Davis JL, Porciatti V, Gonzalez PJ, Koilkonda RD, Yuan H, Hauswirth WW, Lam BL. 2017. Gene therapy for Leber hereditary optic neuropathy: low- and medium-dose visual results. *Ophthalmology* 124: 1621–1634. doi:10.1016/j.ophtha.2017.05.016

Jacobs J, Dell'Osso L, Hertle R, Acland G, Bennett J. 2006. Eye movement recordings as an effectiveness indicator of gene therapy in *RPE65*-deficient canines: implications for the ocular motor system. *Invest Ophthalmol Vis Sci* 47: 2865–2875. doi:10.1167/iovs.05-1233

Jacobs JB, Dell'Osso LF, Wang ZI, Acland GM, Bennett J. 2009. Using the NAFX to measure the effectiveness over time of gene therapy in canine LCA. *Invest Ophthalmol Vis Sci* 50: 4685–4692. doi:10.1167/iovs.09-3387

Jacobson S, Aleman T, Cideciyan A, Sumaroka A, Schwartz S, Windsor E, Traboulsi E, Heon E, Pittler S, Milam A, et al. 2005a. Identifying photoreceptors in blind eyes caused by *RPE65* mutations: prerequisite for human gene therapy success. *Proc Natl Acad Sci* 102: 6177–6182. doi:10.1073/pnas.0500646102

Jacobson SG, Aleman TS, Cideciyan AV, Sumaroka A, Schwartz SB, Windsor EA, Traboulsi EI, Heon E, Pittler SJ, Milam AH, et al. 2005b. Identifying photoreceptors in blind eyes caused by *RPE65* mutations: prerequisite for human gene therapy success. *Proc Natl Acad Sci* 102: 6177–6182. doi:10.1073/pnas.0500646102

Kortüm FC, Kempf M, Jung R, Kohl S, Ott S, Kortuem C, Sting K, Stingl K. 2022. Short term morphological rescue of the fovea after gene therapy with voretigene neparvovec. *Acta Ophthalmol* 100: e807–e812. doi:10.1111/aos.14990

Kwak JJ, Kim HR, Byeon SH. 2022. Short-term outcomes of the first in vivo gene therapy for RPE65-mediated retinitis pigmentosa. *Yonsei Med J* 63: 701–705. doi:10.3349/ymj.2022.63.7.701

Lebherz C, Maguire A, Tang W, Bennett J, Wilson JM. 2008. Novel AAV serotypes for improved ocular gene transfer. *J Gene Med* 10: 375–382. doi:10.1002/jgm.1126

Louis Jeune V, Joergensen JA, Hajjar RJ, Weber T. 2013. Preexisting anti-adeno-associated virus antibodies as a challenge in AAV gene therapy. *Hum Gene Ther Methods* 24: 59–67. doi:10.1089/hgtb.2012.243

Maguire AM, Simonelli F, Pierce EA, Pugh EN Jr, Mingozzi F, Bennicelli J, Banfi S, Marshall KA, Testa F, Surace EM, et al. 2008. Safety and efficacy of gene transfer for Leber's congenital amaurosis. *N Engl J Med* 358: 2240–2248. doi:10.1056/NEJMoa0802315

Maguire AM, High KA, Auricchio A, Wright JF, Pierce EA, Testa F, Mingozzi F, Bennicelli JL, Ying GS, Rossi S, et al. 2009. Age-dependent effects of RPE65 gene therapy for Leber's congenital amaurosis: a phase 1 dose-escalation trial. *Lancet* 374: 1597–1605. doi:10.1016/S0140-6736(09)61836-5

Maguire AM, Bennett J, Aleman EM, Leroy BP, Aleman TS. 2021a. Clinical perspective: treating RPE65-associated retinal dystrophy. *Mol Ther* 29: 442–463. doi:10.1016/j.ymthe.2020.11.029

Maguire AM, Russell S, Chung DC, Yu ZF, Tillman A, Drack AV, Simonelli F, Leroy BP, Reape KZ, High KA, et al. 2021b. Durability of voretigene neparvovec for biallelic RPE65-mediated inherited retinal disease: phase 3 results at 3 and 4 years. *Ophthalmology* **128:** 1460–1468. doi:10.1016/j.ophtha.2021.03.031

National Institutes of Health Recombinant DNA Advisory Committee (RAC). 2005a. Discussion of human gene transfer protocol #0410-677: a phase I trial of ocular subretinal injection of a recombinant adeno-associated virus (rAAV-*RPE65*) gene vector in patients with retinal disease due to *RPE65* mutations. In *Recombinant DNA Advisory Committee (RAC) 100th Meeting.* Bethesda, MD. https://osp.od.nih.gov/wp-content/uploads/RAC_Minutes_Jun_2005.pdf

National Institutes of Health Recombinant DNA Advisory Committee (RAC). 2005b. Discussion of human gene transfer protocol #0510-740: a phase I safety study in subjects with Leber congenital amaurosis (LCA) using adeno-associated viral vector to deliver the gene for human RPE65 into the retinal pigment epithelium (RPE). In *Recombinant DNA Advisory Committee (RAC) 102nd Meeting.* NIH, Bethesda, MD. https://osp.od.nih.gov//wp-content/uploads/RAC_Minutes_Dec_2005.pdf

Pang JJ, Chang B, Hawes NL, Hurd RE, Davisson MT, Li J, Noorwez SM, Malhotra R, McDowell JH, Kaushal S, et al. 2005. Retinal degeneration 12 (rd12): a new, spontaneously arising mouse model for human Leber congenital amaurosis (LCA). *Mol Vis* **11:** 152–162.

Patrício MI, Cox CI, Blue C, Barnard AR, Martinez-Fernandez de la Camara C, MacLaren RE. 2020. Inclusion of PF68 surfactant improves stability of rAAV titer when passed through a surgical device used in retinal gene therapy. *Mol Ther Methods Clin Dev* **17:** 99–106. doi:10.1016/j.omtm.2019.11.005

Ramachandran PS, Lee V, Wei Z, Song JY, Casal G, Cronin T, Willett K, Huckfeldt R, Morgan JI, Aleman TS, et al. 2017. Evaluation of dose and safety of AAV7m8 and AAV8BP2 in the non-human primate retina. *Hum Gene Ther* **28:** 154–167. doi:10.1089/hum.2016.111

Redmond T, Hamel C. 2000. Genetic analysis of RPE65: from human disease to mouse model. *Methods Enzymol* **316:** 705–724. doi:10.1016/S0076-6879(00)16758-8

Redmond T, Poliakov E, Yu S, Tsai J, Lu Z, Gentleman S. 2005. Mutation of key residues of RPE65 abolishes its enzymatic role as isomerohydrolase in the visual cycle. *Proc Natl Acad Sci* **102:** 13658–13663. doi:10.1073/pnas.0504167102

Russell S, Bennett J, Wellman JA, Chung DC, Yu ZF, Tillman A, Wittes J, Pappas J, Elci O, McCague S, et al. 2017. Efficacy and safety of voretigene neparvovec (AAV2-hRPE65v2) in patients with RPE65-mediated inherited retinal dystrophy: a randomised, controlled, open-label, phase 3 trial. *Lancet* **390:** 849–860. doi:10.1016/S0140-6736(17)31868-8

Sengillo JD, Gregori NZ, Sisk RA, Weng CY, Berrocal AM, Davis JL, Mendoza-Santiesteban CE, Zheng DD, Feuer WJ, Lam BL. 2022. Visual acuity, retinal morphology, and patients' perceptions after voretigene neparvovec-rzyl therapy for RPE65-associated retinal disease. *Ophthalmol Retina* **6:** 273–283. doi:10.1016/j.oret.2021.11.005

Simonelli F, Maguire AM, Testa F, Pierce EA, Mingozzi F, Bennicelli JL, Rossi S, Marshall K, Banfi S, Surace EM, et al. 2010. Gene therapy for Leber's congenital amaurosis is safe and effective through 1.5 years after vector administration. *Mol Ther* **18:** 643–650. doi:10.1038/mt.2009.277

Song JY, Aravand P, Nikonov S, Leo L, Lyubarsky A, Bennicelli JL, Pan J, Wei Z, Shpylchak I, Herrera P, et al. 2018. Amelioration of neurosensory structure and function in animal and cellular models of a congenital blindness. *Mol Ther* **26:** 1581–1593. doi:10.1016/j.ymthe.2018.03.015

Stingl K, Kempf M, Bartz-Schmidt KU, Dimopoulos S, Reichel F, Jung R, Kelbsch C, Kohl S, Kortüm FC, Nasser F, et al. 2022. Spatial and temporal resolution of the photoreceptors rescue dynamics after treatment with voretigene neparvovec. *Br J Ophthalmol* **106:** 831–838. doi:10.1136/bjophthalmol-2020-318286

Testa F, Melillo P, Della Corte M, Di Iorio V, Brunetti-Pierri R, Citro A, Ferrara M, Karali M, Annibale R, Banfi S, et al. 2021. Voretigene neparvovec gene therapy in clinical practice: treatment of the first two Italian pediatric patients. *Transl Vis Sci Technol* **10:** 11. doi:10.1167/tvst.10.10.11

Timmers AM, Newmark JA, Turunen HT, Farivar T, Liu J, Song C, Ye GJ, Pennock S, Gaskin C, Knop DR, et al. 2020. Ocular inflammatory response to intravitreal injection of adeno-associated virus vector: relative contribution of genome and capsid. *Hum Gene Ther* **31:** 80–89. doi:10.1089/hum.2019.144

Vandenberghe L, Bell P, Maguire A, Cearley C, Xiao R, Calcedo R, Wang L, Castle M, Maguire A, Grant R, et al. 2011. Dosage thresholds for AAV2 and AAV8 photoreceptor gene therapy in monkey. *Sci Transl Med* **3:** 88ra54. doi:10.1126/scitranslmed.3002103

Veske A, Nilsson S, Narfström K, Gal A. 1999. Retinal dystrophy of Swedish Briard/Briard-beagle dogs is due to a 4-bp deletion in RPE65. *Genomics* **57:** 57–61. doi:10.1006/geno.1999.5754

Weed L, Ammar MJ, Zhou S, Wei Z, Serrano LW, Sun J, Lee V, Maguire AM, Bennett J, Aleman TS. 2019. Safety of same-eye subretinal sequential readministration of AAV2-hRPE65v2 in non-human primates. *Mol Ther Methods Clin Dev* **15:** 133–148. doi:10.1016/j.omtm.2019.08.011

Wright JF. 2014. AAV empty capsids: for better or for worse? *Mol Ther* **22:** 1–2. doi:10.1038/mt.2013.268

Yang U, Gentleman S, Gai X, Gorin MB, Borchert MS, Lee TC, Villanueva A, Koenekoop R, Maguire AM, Bennett J, et al. 2019. Utility of in vitro mutagenesis of RPE65 protein for verification of mutational pathogenicity before gene therapy. *JAMA Ophthalmol* **137:** 1381–1388. doi:10.1001/jamaophthalmol.2019.3914

Trial by "Firsts": Clinical Trial Design and Regulatory Considerations in the Development and Approval of the First AAV Gene Therapy Product in the United States

Kathleen Z. Reape[1] and Katherine A. High[2]

Spark Therapeutics, Philadelphia, Pennsylvania 19104, USA

Correspondence: kzreape@gmail.com; khigh@askbio.com

Given the therapeutic potential of supplying a normal copy of a mutant gene to the correct target tissue, gene therapy holds extraordinary promise for the treatment of genetic disease. Like other novel classes of therapeutics however, gene therapies must overcome a range of clinical, regulatory, and manufacturing hurdles to reach regulatory approval. This paper reviews key aspects of clinical trial design, development, and evaluation of a novel primary end point, and regulatory interactions that resulted in the first approval by the U.S. Food and Drug Administration (FDA) of an adeno-associated virus (AAV) gene therapy product.

While there have been some recent successes, it remains a significant challenge to bring innovative, advanced gene and cell therapies to market, particularly for rare diseases with no currently available treatment options. During the development process, these novel medicines face major clinical, regulatory, and manufacturing hurdles that must be overcome for these therapeutic options to become available to patients. Early and continuous planning, as well as frequent involvement, discussion, and integration of input from regulators, investigators, experts, and patients and their families, is fundamental to the success of any clinical program, but is especially crucial for an innovative therapy.

In 2017, the U.S. Food and Drug Administration (FDA) approval of voretigene-neparvovec-rzyl (VN) (Luxturna), an AAV (adeno-associated virus) vector-based gene therapy for the treatment of individuals with confirmed biallelic *RPE65* mutation-associated retinal dystrophy, represented the culmination of over two decades of research and development. This was the first gene therapy for a genetic disease to be fully approved in the both the United States and the European Union (2018).

---

[1]Present address: Akouos Therapeutics, Boston, Massachusetts 02210.

[2]Present address: Asklepios BioPharmaceuticals, Philadelphia, Pennsylvania 19104; Perelman School of Medicine, University of Pennsylvania, Philadelphia, Pennsylvania 19104.

The VN clinical development program may serve as a model for other innovative therapies. Using the VN program as a "case study," this review will discuss important considerations and "lessons learned" that may be relevant to expediting development of advanced therapies, with a focus on clinical and regulatory insights. Findings from the individual clinical trials comprising the VN clinical development program have been published previously (Maguire et al. 2008, 2009, 2019, 2021; Simonelli et al. 2010; Bennett et al. 2012, 2016; Testa et al. 2013; Ashtari et al. 2017; Russell et al. 2017; Chung et al. 2018, 2019) and will be briefly summarized here.

OVERALL CLINICAL DEVELOPMENT PROGRAM

The VN clinical program enrolled a total of 43 individuals with *RPE65* mutations, with 41 individuals receiving a range of doses in three clinical trials: a dose-escalation phase 1 study (Study 101; Maguire et al. 2009) with unilateral administration to the worse-seeing eye; a second phase 1 study (Study 102; Bennett et al. 2016) in the same participants with unilateral administration of the highest dose tested in the previous study to the contralateral eye, after at least 1 year of follow-up from the first administration; and an open-label, randomized, controlled phase 3 study (Study 301; Russell et al. 2017) in which those individuals initially randomized to the control group could cross over to intervention after a 1-year observation period. All participants who received at least one dose of VN in either the phase 1 or phase 3 clinical trials were subsequently enrolled in an ongoing companion long-term follow-up (LTFU) protocol (LTFU study; Maguire et al. 2019, 2021) for a planned total of 15 years of follow-up post-administration.

In addition, since a novel primary end point (the multi-luminance mobility test [MLMT]) was used in the phase 3 pivotal trial, a non-interventional validation study of this test instrument was conducted (Chung et al. 2018). The purpose of this supportive study was to determine whether the MLMT could reliably detect changes in functional vision (defined as a measure of how a person functions in a visually dependent activity) over time in individuals with inherited retinal disorders (IRDs), identify a range of performance, and differentiate between normal-sighted and low vision participants.

To better understand the clinical course of individuals with *RPE65* mutation-associated retinal dystrophy, a retrospective natural history study was also performed (Chung et al. 2019). As this is a rare condition, limited historical data characterizing the natural progression existed, and, at the time, genetic testing was relatively new and far from being universally implemented. A further complication (secondary to the lack of genetic testing) was that much of the available historical data were confounded by the use of multiple nonspecific clinical descriptors (e.g., retinitis pigmentosa, Leber's congenital amaurosis, etc.) that were inconsistently applied, rather than using specific molecular genetic diagnoses (e.g., *RPE65* mutation-associated retinal dystrophy).

All three clinical trials (Studies 101, 102, and 301) enrolled individuals with confirmed biallelic *RPE65* mutations. The phase 1 studies were designed primarily to assess the safety and tolerability of subretinal administration of VN, and secondarily to evaluate a number of efficacy measures, to inform the design of the phase 3 clinical trial. In the phase 3 trial, individuals were randomized in a 2:1 fashion to either the intervention group (1.5E11 vector genomes [vg] VN administered bilaterally, at least 7–14 days apart) or the control group and were followed for 1 year. After completing 1 year of observation, control participants were allowed to cross over and receive bilateral administration of VN.

TRIAL DESIGN

The open-label randomized controlled phase 3 trial (Russell et al. 2017) served as the pivotal study to evaluate safety and efficacy. The safety data obtained from the phase 1 clinical trials enabled the expansion of the enrollment criteria in phase 3 to include individuals with less severe degrees of vision loss and children as young as age 3. This allowed for a broader and more representative population of individuals with *RPE65* mutation-associated retinal dystrophy (who could potentially benefit from VN) to participate in the phase 3 clinical trial.

Achieving an optimal trial design for the pivotal phase 3 study necessitated overcoming a number of clinical and regulatory challenges encountered in the setting of a new class of therapeutics for a rare disease with no existing treatment options. For these novel compounds, a customized development approach is needed. Crucial decisions for the phase 3 study included the choice of comparator, the duration of the observation period, and the selection of primary and secondary end points, all in the setting of an ultra-rare disease with a small patient population and a lack of natural history data.

A clear limitation in the design of the phase 3 study was the dearth of available natural history data. Consisting mostly of case reports or small series from single institutions, these data were not sufficient to support the use of historical controls as a comparator to the clinical course following administration of the investigational product. This stands in contrast to other more prevalent and more well-characterized single gene disorders such as spinal muscular atrophy type 1 (Kolb et al. 2017; U.S. FDA 2019b).

Use of the contralateral uninjected eye in the same participant was also considered as a potential control. Disease progression is generally symmetric (Lorenz et al. 2000), so the contralateral uninjected eye, with the same mutation in the same stage of degeneration, is perhaps the ideal scientific control. In discussions with ophthalmologists and regulators, however, this consideration was rejected for two major reasons. First, a large discrepancy in vision between two eyes in the same individual for a prolonged period of time (e.g., 1 year) may lead to complications including amblyopia and disruptions to central visual pathways, impacting binocular vision, particularly in young children (Bradfield 2013). Second, since the two eye injections would occur near simultaneously in clinical practice to avoid these complications, the use of a non-interventional contralateral control eye would fail to assess product performance as it would be used clinically.

A randomized controlled trial design thus appeared to be the best choice for the phase 3 study

(Fig. 1). Use of a non-interventional control group posed some challenges, however, and steps were taken to minimize any perceived burden of being randomized to control, with its potential negative impact on enrollment. A 2:1 randomization scheme was implemented to give participants a greater chance at being assigned to the intervention group. Further, at the end of the 1-year period of observation, all participants in the control group were offered the opportunity to cross over and receive the intervention. All agreed and their results recapitulated the results of the original intervention group, thus serving as a second "confirmatory" trial within the original trial. This was a unique feature of the phase 3 design, afforded all participants access to the investigational product, and was effective at providing confirmatory evidence without expanding the required number of participants or conducting a separate, second phase 3 trial, both of which would have likely resulted in an extended development timeline and delayed approval.

Another point of discussion was the optimal duration of the non-interventional observation period. *RPE65*-associated retinal dystrophy is a progressive disease and any excessive delay in administering a potentially therapeutic intervention contributes to further vision loss that cannot be restored. Based on nonclinical findings and the results observed in the two phase 1 trials, an early and robust treatment effect was anticipated, with improvement being demonstrated as early as 30 days after administration. Given the progressive nature of this condition and its impact on pediatric patients, it was proposed that the duration of the observation period should be 6 months; however, the final trial design incorporated an observation period of 1 year to evaluate safety and efficacy, consistent with most conventional pivotal clinical trial designs.

RPE65 is expressed in the retinal pigment epithelial (RPE) cells and is a key enzyme involved in the visual cycle and the regeneration of 11-*cis*-retinal (Fig. 2). Despite the biochemical disruption of the visual cycle and progressive vision loss, the retinal anatomy is preserved for a prolonged period; it is this preservation that provides a path forward for therapeutic intervention with gene therapy.

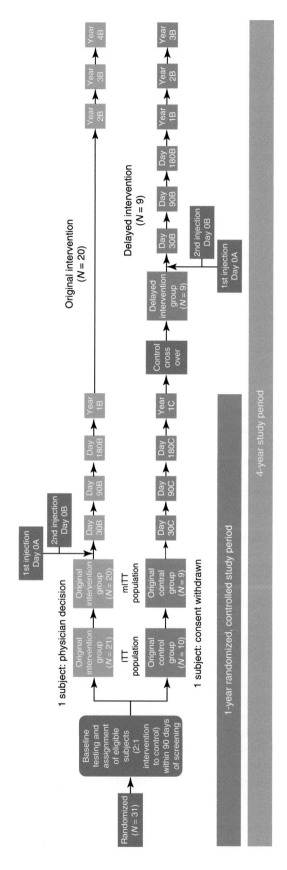

Figure 1. Phase 3 and long-term follow-up study design. (ITT) Intent-to-treat population. (Figure reprinted from Maguire et al. 2021 under the terms of a Creative Commons license CC BY-NC-ND 4.0.)

Cite this article as *Cold Spring Harb Perspect Med* doi: 10.1101/cshperspect.a041312

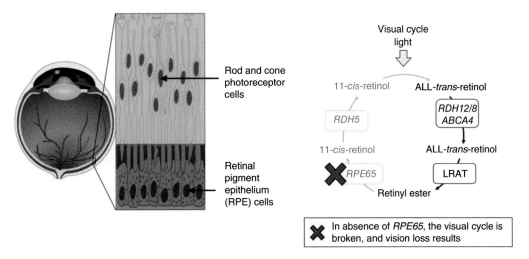

Figure 2. Role of *RPE65* in the visual cycle. (Reprinted from Cellular, Tissue and Gene Therapies Advisory Committee October 12, 2017. Meeting Briefing Document, Spark Therapeutics, Luxturna. Full document freely available for download at www.fda.gov/media/108385/download, U.S. FDA 2017a.)

The absence of the enzyme leads to accumulation of toxic precursors and damage to the RPE cells, and thus inevitably to the photoreceptors, leading to progressive loss of vision. The rod photoreceptors are affected primarily, resulting in diminished peripheral vision and the inability to see in dim light (nyctalopia, a clinical hallmark of this disorder). Some children are diagnosed in infancy, while others may enter school in a sighted classroom, but by the second decade of life, virtually all those affected have profound visual impairment (Chung et al. 2019). Individuals with *RPE65*-mutation-associated retinal dystrophy have difficulty performing activities even in normal daytime lighting and are severely limited in orientation and navigation in dim light settings. A 2011 FDA Advisory Committee (U.S. FDA 2011) convened to discuss cellular and gene therapy trials for the treatment of retinal disorders, concluded that a need existed for novel end points to be specifically tailored to a disease and its clinical deficits. The committee also recommended the use of multiple tools to assess visual function and functional vision, and to consider patient-reported outcomes related to daily activities.

Most ophthalmic assessments, such as visual acuity (VA) or visual fields (VFs) measure visual function, or how the eyes perform (either individually or together). In contrast, functional vision describes how an individual performs in vision-related activities, such as reading and navigation. Patients with biallelic *RPE65* mutations have diminished VA and VF, accompanied by nyctalopia, all of which impact functional vision. Based on the recommendations of the 2011 FDA Advisory Committee, as well as discussions with regulators, it was determined that the phase 3 trial for VN should have a primary end point that was a measure of functional vision and took into account a specific major clinical deficit associated with *RPE65* mutation-associated retinal dystrophy (i.e., nyctalopia). Of note, mobility tests have been previously used as measures of functional vision, but none of those in common use integrated dependence on the level of environmental illumination into the testing. Measures of visual function were also collected as secondary and exploratory end points, including full-field light sensitivity threshold (FST) testing, VA, and VF. Other exploratory end points included questionnaire-based patient and parent-reported assessments of visual function and community-based functional vision assessments performed in the home setting by low vision rehabilitation specialists. Patient and parent input were critical in adapting the visual function questionnaire so that it was meaningful to a pediatric population and in designing relevant community-based assessment components.

The goal of selecting efficacy end points was to evaluate the participants' visual function and functional vision over a range of parameters in a quantifiable manner that could be compared pre- and post-intervention. The combination of a novel, clinically relevant functional vision end point (the multi-luminance mobility test), along with more conventional visual function end points (VA, FST, VF) and patient-reported outcomes, provided a rigorous method of evaluating the efficacy of VN. At both the study level, and at the level of individual participants, the findings across all of the different types of end points were consistent and reinforced each other, demonstrating a robust treatment effect and lending credence to the novel end point.

NOVEL PRIMARY END POINT

A challenge in the setting of this rod-mediated condition was the absence of well-studied, validated end points that integrated standardized, controlled changes in the level of illumination into the test method. Existing tests of functional vision and/or mobility did not consider light levels, and did not adequately address the effects of illumination on speed and accuracy of performance in a standardized manner. In addition, based on the patient population with biallelic *RPE65* mutations, the test would have to be one that could be performed easily across a wide age range (i.e., very young children to adults).

The MLMT is an assessment that requires a participant to navigate a course independently and accurately within a time limit under varying lighting conditions (Fig. 3). The range and specific light levels were selected to be representative of illuminated environments commonly encountered in everyday life. In fact, during the design and refinement of the MLMT, real-world measurements of illumination levels using a light meter were obtained in a range of indoor and outdoor environments (e.g., outdoor parking lot at night, shopping mall, stairwell). Seven different light levels were tested, ranging from a low level of 1 lux to a maximal level of 400 lux. A key learning regarding the light levels was related to

the intervals between each level. While the gradations in lux levels represented illumination in real-world settings, the intervals between them were not consistently the same. The seven light levels tested in phase 3 were 1 lux, 4 lux, 10 lux, 50 lux, 125 lux, 250 lux, and 400 lux. Based on the scoring algorithm, the sponsor considered an improvement in one or more light levels clinically meaningful, although the magnitude of improvement (in lux) between light levels was not evenly spaced. In retrospect, in constructing the MLMT, the light levels across the range might have been separated by equal intervals (i.e., half-log gradations between each level) to improve ease of interpretation of the test. However, the statistical analysis of the data relied on relative changes in light levels in the intervention group compared to the control group, making the magnitude of the change from one level to the next moot. Moreover, as most participants demonstrated improvement of greater than one light level and/or improvement to the lowest light level, the small variability in changes between light levels had negligible impact on conclusions regarding efficacy.

As the results of the MLMT would serve as the primary efficacy end point in the phase 3 clinical trial, a great deal of effort was put forth to ensure the highest possible degree of rigor and standardization in both the conduct of the assessment and the interpretation of the results. A lighting engineer was consulted in the construction of a dedicated testing room at each clinical site and permanent lighting was installed overhead with careful attention to the minimization of shadows or other artifacts on the mobility course. To further standardize the lighting for the MLMT, the light levels were measured daily, using calibrated light meters at five different points on the course, prior to initiating any test runs (Russell et al. 2017).

A total of 12 different standardized courses were developed and presented in a randomized fashion to minimize any potential learning effect. Each course had the same number of blocks, turns, and obstacles. A "practice" MLMT course (not used for test runs) was used to familiarize participants with how to perform the test.

Each test run was videotaped for evaluation and scoring. A central independent panel of

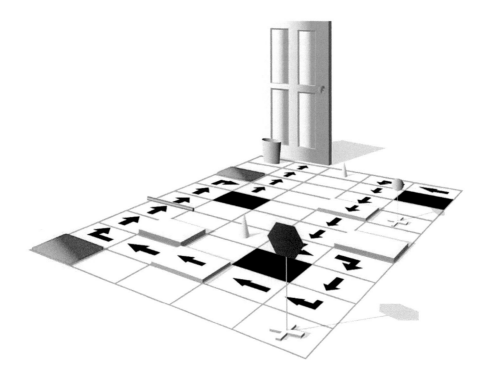

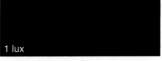

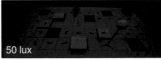

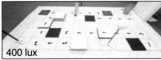

Light levels	Examples
1 lux	Moonless summer night; indoor nightlight
4 lux	Cloudless night with half moon; parking lot at night
10 lux	1 hour after sunset in city; bus stop at night
50 lux	Outdoor train station at night; inside of lighted stairwell
125 lux	30 minutes before sunrise; interior of train/bus at night
250 lux	Interior of elevator or office hallway
400 lux	Office environment or food court

Light meter: National Institute of Standards and Technology–calibrated.
Extech model #EA33 light meters used to provide examples and to set/verify specified light levels used for mobility testing.

Figure 3. Multi-luminance mobility test (MLMT) and light levels. (Reprinted from Cellular, Tissue and Gene Therapies Advisory Committee October 12, 2017. Meeting Briefing Document, Spark Therapeutics, Luxturna. Full document freely available for download at www.fda.gov/media/108385/download, U.S. FDA 2017a.)

graders (trained by low-vision specialists) viewed each test run video and scored each for both accuracy and time, following a clearly defined scoring protocol. Two graders individually scored each video and an additional grader adjudicated in the case of disagreement. The videos were filtered so that the light levels being tested were not readily apparent to the viewer. Videos were presented in a randomized fashion and graders were masked as to clinical site, study visit, participant, and group assignment. As an additional quality control measure, 10% of videos from the prior quarter were randomly selected and presented for re-grading throughout the course of the study. Statistics on the more than 4000 videos graded during the phase 1 and phase 3 clinical trials, the mobility test validation study (MTVS) (vide infra), and the LTFU study demonstrated a very high degree of concordance across all evaluated components (e.g., time to completion, number of errors) of the MLMT (U.S. FDA 2017b; Chung et al. 2018).

A separate study (MTVS) was conducted in 54 children and adults (28 with low vision and history of an IRD and 26 normal-sighted individuals) to determine the performance characteristics of the MLMT (Chung et al. 2018), specifically whether the MLMT could detect changes in functional vision over time in participants with IRDs and whether it could differentiate normal-sighted individuals from those with low vision. Further, the study defined relationships between MLMT performance and measures of visual function. One-third of the participants with low vision showed a decline in performance over the year of observation. This finding strikes at the heart of clinical equipoise for the randomized controlled trial, but was unknown at the time of phase 3 trial initiation. Earlier availability of this data may have bolstered arguments for a shortened observation period for the control cohort and an earlier cross over to intervention at 6 months rather than 1 year. The validation study also demonstrated that the MLMT could differentiate low vision from normal-sighted populations, and, among low-vision individuals, could identify a range of performance levels and track declines in performance over time. Another key aspect of the MTVS was that it allowed definition of the relationship

between MLMT performance and VF and VA. Specifically, a cut-off effect was observed; those with VA better than 0.5 logMAR (or 20/63 Snellen equivalent) had passing performance on the mobility test, whereas those with worse VA showed a range of performance. A cut-off effect was also observed for Goldmann VFs, with those with VF < 500 sum total degrees exhibiting a range of performance on the mobility test, whereas those with VF > 500 sum total degrees typically passed the mobility test.

There were two major shortcomings of the MLMT. Although designed for children, it was too complex for very young children and toddlers. In the phase 3 clinical trial, the youngest child who could understand and properly execute the MLMT was 4 years old. The second major challenge was the presence of a ceiling effect. There were a number of individuals who entered the phase 3 trial able to pass at 4 lux (i.e., the second-lowest light level). Based on the design of the study, they could only potentially achieve a maximal improvement of one light level. Technically, it was not possible to conduct the MLMT at illumination levels below 1 lux, as this was a limitation of the video cameras being used to record the test runs; light levels below 1 lux were too dark to record evaluable videos. Overall, however, the MLMT was an important and reliable instrument for measuring functional vision, and it directly addressed a major clinical deficit (i.e., nyctalopia) that was relevant to individuals with *RPE65* mutation-associated retinal dystrophy.

This novel end point was developed and refined from phase 1 to phase 3 in dialogue with regulators and is now described in the FDA guidance document for gene therapy for IRDs (U.S. FDA 2020) as an example of a clinically meaningful novel primary efficacy end point that was developed in collaboration with the FDA. It addressed a specific clinical feature of this disease, a mobility test sensitive to levels of environmental illumination.

SECONDARY AND EXPLORATORY END POINTS CONFIRM PRIMARY

By design, the MLMT incorporates input from VA, VF, and light sensitivity (FST); together, these inputs enable an individual to navigate independently, accurately, and at a reasonable pace across a range of environmental illuminations. Perhaps not surprisingly then, most of the secondary and exploratory end points (including VA, VF, and FST) tended to confirm the results observed for the primary MLMT end point. It is unusual in clinical trials to encounter the consistency of the treatment effect across a range of end points that was observed with VN. The results were highly consistent, even across studies. For example, the increase in VF among those who received the intervention in phase 3 crossed the threshold that was defined in the MLMT validation study as that required for improved performance, supporting the contribution of VF to performance as measured by the MLMT (Russell et al. 2017; Chung et al. 2018).

This high degree of internal consistency is at least partly attributable to the mechanism of action. The clinical findings in individuals with *RPE65* mutation-associated retinal dystrophy are the result of the RPE65 enzyme deficiency, and the subsequent breakdown of the visual cycle. When RPE65 activity is restored by subretinal administration of VN, the visual cycle resumes, retinal cells remain viable and continue to function, and most of the visual measures improve. Since there is little heterogeneity in the mechanistic pathophysiology of the disease, resumption of near normal to normal physiology and the treatment response is similar across end points and among individuals.

FST was selected as the first secondary efficacy end point. Similar to the changes in light levels observed on the MLMT (a test of functional vision), FST (a measure of visual function) demonstrated improvement in light sensitivity for each individual eye. Further, FST, with a dynamic range that extends to light levels far lower than 1 lux, could differentiate among those participants who experienced an improvement of one light level on the MLMT and may have encountered a "ceiling effect." Among controls with one light level improvement, the corresponding gains in FST were far less than what was observed in those with one light level MLMT improvement (to 1 lux) in the intervention group.

There was also good correlation between the primary end point (MLMT) and the FST. The MLMT was designed primarily as a research tool and was not intended to be implemented into general clinical practice. Because of the correlation between the more conventional measure (the FST) and the novel primary end point measure (the MLMT), the FST was used in the commercial setting to confirm clinical improvement for "pay for performance" agreements with insurers. Novel one-time therapies pose challenges for reimbursement, which are beyond the scope of this review; however, the correlation between the FST and MLMT was a key component enabling innovative and clinically important approaches to reimbursement (Spark Therapeutics 2018). Since the development timeline is long, foresight is needed to anticipate what payers may be looking for in the future, and to ensure that sufficient health economic measures are integrated into the development plan, particularly when no precedents exist.

For clinical studies in rare disease, it is prudent to include a wide range of end points, selected based on the underlying pathophysiology of the disease and the mechanism of action of the intervention and to include conventional measures as well as more novel approaches when warranted. A mixture of both subjective and objective end points is desirable. Observations from phase 1 trials can be used to refine instruments and evaluations, and to select and rank efficacy end points for the pivotal study.

FDA ADVISORY COMMITTEE DISCUSSIONS

Even after clinical trials have been completed and findings appear to be straightforward, it is important to continue interactions with regulators, investigators, and patients and their families. The FDA requested an Advisory Committee Meeting for VN (U.S. FDA 2017c), convening a panel of external experts in October 2017 to review the clinical program, safety and efficacy findings, and to make a nonbinding recommendation regarding approval. The discussion at this meeting yielded some important insights that were later incorporated into the VN package insert. Typically, the labeling language for a product tends to reflect the conditions and population that were represented in its phase 3 clinical trial. In this case, the external experts recognized the rarity of the condition and actually recommended expansion of labeling language beyond the criteria set forth in the clinical trial to allow flexibility in identifying eligible recipients and to expand the eligible patient population.

A major point of discussion was the retinal thickness as measured by optical coherence tomography (OCT). In the phase 3 trial, the requirement specified a thickness of 100 μm or greater. This was a surrogate measure indicative of retinal viability, but it was not a specific measure of viable cells. The discussion among the Advisory Committee focused on "real world" situations. For example, are individuals with measurements of 95 or 99 μm really at greater risk from the administration procedure? If so, should they be excluded from receiving VN? The discussants recommended flexibility and the labeling language reads that "Patients must have viable retinal cells as determined by the treating physician(s)" (Luxturna 2017).

A second example included the age range of recipients. As previously noted, the youngest participant in the phase 3 clinical trial was 4 years old. The protocol allowed for children as young as 3 to be enrolled, but there were no individuals at that age with the attentive skills necessary to complete the MLMT. Mechanistically, VN would not perform differently in very young children, and the dose does not need to be adjusted for age or weight. Since this is a progressive degenerative disease, a delay in treatment results in the loss of more retinal cells, so there is an advantage to treating this condition as early as possible. The Advisory Committee focused its discussion on the most appropriate youngest age for administration. The decisive factor in the discussion was the timing of retinal growth and cell division. Since AAV vector DNA is stabilized predominantly in a non-integrated form, cell division results in gradual loss of the donated DNA. Thus, introduction into a population of dividing cells could result in a gradually declining percentage of transduced cells, essentially "diluting" out the effects of the transgene. If a child is treated when still very young, and the

retinal cells are actively dividing, the treatment effect may not be durable. This was noted to be primarily an efficacy concern, rather than a safety concern. Generally, it was acknowledged that retinal growth and cell division should be complete by ~8 months, so it would be reasonable to allow administration to children as young as 1 year of age; this is the language that was included in the Luxturna package insert (Luxturna 2017).

The strength of the clinical findings, both efficacy and safety, along with the recommendations of external experts, allowed for VN to become a treatment option for a broader range of individuals than those included in the clinical trials and expanded the population that could potentially benefit from this gene therapy.

NATURAL HISTORY STUDY

A natural history study is a planned observational study intended to track the course of a disease, with the aim of identifying factors (e.g., demographic, genetic, environmental, etc.) that correlate with disease development and outcomes (U.S. FDA 2019a). Knowledge of the natural history of a rare condition is important in informing and planning all stages of drug development. As part of the clinical development plan for VN, a retrospective natural history chart review was conducted (Chung et al. 2019) and included data from 70 patients with *RPE65* mutation-associated retinal dystrophy.

The primary parameters analyzed were VA and VF. Age was used as a surrogate for time, so that all individual data points could be included in the analysis. On average, cross-sectional data demonstrated that VA, although markedly impaired, was fairly stable during the first decade of life; VA began to decrease around the ages of 15–20, with a rapid decline after the age of 20. By the age of 18, more than half of this cohort met the criteria for "legal blindness" in the United States, as defined by the VA of the better eye (U.S. Social Security Administration, n.d.). Similar changes were seen with VF, although there were fewer evaluable assessments. VF decline appeared to be more linear and gradual than VA loss, although at around age 14–15 years, on average, the degree of impairment began to exceed the "legal blindness" criteria for this parameter in the United States (U.S. Social Security Administration, n.d.). Natural history findings demonstrated symmetrical progression, as well as the presence of nyctalopia in a majority of patients. Almost three-quarters (74.3%) of participants reported issues with navigation and mobility, providing support for the selection of the MLMT as the primary efficacy end point in phase 3.

More than 20 distinct clinical diagnoses were reported for these 70 individuals with confirmed biallelic *RPE65* mutations, with some having multiple clinical diagnoses. Additionally, a total of 56 unique *RPE65* mutations were observed. No clear correlation was observed between specific *RPE65* mutations and clinical diagnosis, onset, severity, or rate of progression. The findings of heterogeneity among clinical diagnoses and lack of a consistent genotype–phenotype correlation underscore the need for genetic testing and molecular diagnosis to accurately identify patients who might benefit from VN.

CONCLUSIONS

There are several aspects of the VN development program that have general applicability to rare disease and/or gene therapy clinical trials. First, a conservative approach to first-in-human trials is warranted. This involves carefully defining the phase 1 participant population and then expanding the enrollment criteria to include a broader population in a phase 3 clinical trial, once safety (and often preliminary efficacy) has been established. Second, as the range of conditions that may be amenable to gene therapy expands, the process of developing and validating novel, clinically meaningful, and quantifiable end points will be an important component of clinical trials, as many diseases will have no available treatment options. Finally, the cohesiveness of the clinical data is important. In the VN clinical trial, the end points all reinforced each other and the totality of the data made sense physiologically, providing additional support for the efficacy of the intervention.

Careful consideration of all these factors and early input from experts in the field, investigators, patients and their families, and regulators

may facilitate the development of a robust clinical program, accelerate clinical development, and potentially lead to increased availability of more advanced therapies for patients.

REFERENCES

Ashtari M, Nikonova ES, Marshall KA, Young GJ, Aravand P, Pan W, Ying GS, Willett AE, Mahmoudian M, Maguire AM, et al. 2017. The role of the human visual cortex in assessment of the long-term durability of retinal gene therapy in follow-on RPE65 clinical trial patients. *Ophthalmology* **124:** 873–883. doi:10.1016/j.ophtha.2017.01.029

Bennett J, Ashtari M, Wellman J, Marshall KA, Cyckowski LL, Chung DC, McCague S, Pierce EA, Chen Y, Bennicelli JL, et al. 2012. AAV2 gene therapy readministration in three adults with congenital blindness. *Sci Transl Med* **4:** 120ra15. doi:10.1126/scitranslmed.3002865

Bennett J, Wellman J, Marshall KA. 2016. Safety and durability of effect of contralateral-eye administration of AAV2 gene therapy in patients with childhood-onset blindness caused by RPE65 mutations: a follow-on phase 1 trial. *Lancet* **388:** 661–672. doi:10.1016/S0140-6736(16)30371-3

Bradfield Y. 2013. Identification and treatment of amblyopia. *Am Fam Physician* **87:** 348–352.

Chung DC, McCague S, Yu ZF, Thill S, DiStefano-Pappas J, Bennett J, Cross D, Marshall K, Wellman J, High KA. 2018. Novel mobility test to assess functional vision in patients with inherited retinal dystrophies. *Clin Exp Ophthalmol* **46:** 247–259. doi:10.1111/ceo.13022

Chung DC, Bertelsen M, Lorenz B, Pennesi ME, Leroy BP, Hamel CP, Pierce E, Sallum J, Larsen M, Stieger K, et al. 2019. The natural history of inherited retinal dystrophy due to biallelic mutations in the *RPE65* gene. *Am J Ophthalmol* **199:** 58–70. doi:10.1016/j.ajo.2018.09.024

Kolb SJ, Coffey CS, Yankey JW, Krosschell K, Arnold WD, Rutkove SB, Swoboda KJ, Reyna SP, Sakonju A, Darras BT, et al. 2017. Natural history of infantile-onset spinal muscular atrophy. *Ann Neurol* **82:** 883–891. doi:10.1002/ana.25101

Lorenz B, Gyürüs P, Preising M, Bremser D, Gu S, Andrassi M, Gerth C, Gal A. 2000. Early-onset severe rod-cone dystrophy in young children with RPE65 mutations. *Invest Ophthalmol Vis Sci* **41:** 2735–2742.

Luxturna (voretigene neparvovec-rzyl) U.S. full prescribing information. 2017. Available at http://sparktx.com/LUXTURNA_US_Prescribing_Information.pdf [accessed February 5, 2022].

Maguire AM, Simonelli F, Pierce EA, Pugh EN, Mingozzi F, Bennicelli J, Banfi S, Marshall KA, Testa F, Surace EM, et al. 2008. Safety and efficacy of gene transfer for Leber's congenital amaurosis. *N Engl J Med* **358:** 2240–2248. doi:10.1056/NEJMoa0802315

Maguire AM, High KA, Auricchio A, Wright JF, Pierce EA, Testa F, Mingozzi F, Bennicelli JL, Ying GS, Rossi S, et al. 2009. Age-dependent effects of RPE65 gene therapy for Leber's congenital amaurosis: a phase 1 dose-escalation trial. *Lancet* **374:** 1597–1605. doi:10.1016/S0140-6736(09)61836-5

Maguire AM, Russell S, Wellman JA, Chung DC, Yu ZF, Tillman A, Wittes J, Pappas J, Elci O, Marshall KA, et al. 2019. Efficacy, safety, and durability of voretigene neparvovec-rzyl in *RPE65* mutation–associated inherited retinal dystrophy: results of phase 1 and 3 trials. *Ophthalmology* **126:** 1273–1285. doi:10.1016/j.ophtha.2019.06.017

Maguire AM, Russell S, Chung DC, Yu ZF, Tillman A, Drack AV, Simonelli F, Leroy BP, Reape KZ, et al. 2021. Durability of voretigene neparvovec for biallelic *RPE65*-mediated inherited retinal disease-phase 3 results at 3 and 4 years. *Ophthalmology* **128:** 1460–1468. doi:10.1016/j.ophtha.2021.03.031

Russell S, Bennett J, Wellman JA, Chung DC, Yu ZF, Tillman A, Wittes J, Pappas J, Elci O, McCague S, et al. 2017. Efficacy and safety of voretigene neparvovec (AAV2-hRPE65v2) in patients with *RPE65*-mediated inherited retinal dystrophy: a randomised, controlled, open-label, phase 3 trial. *Lancet* **390:** 849–860. doi:10.1016/S0140-6736(17)31868-8

Simonelli F, Maguire AM, Testa F, Pierce EA, Mingozzi F, Bennicelli JL, Rossi S, Marshall K, Banfi S, Surace EM, et al. 2010. Gene therapy for Leber's congenital amaurosis is safe and effective through 1.5 years after vector administration. *Mol Ther* **18:** 643–650. doi:10.1038/mt.2009.277

Spark Therapeutics. 2018. Spark therapeutics announces first-of-their-kind programs to improve patient access to Luxturna (voretigene neparvovec-rzyl), a one-time gene therapy treatment. Available at https://sparktx.com/press_releases/spark-therapeutics-announces-first-of-their-kind-programs-to-improve-patient-access-to-luxturna-voretigene-neparvovec-rzyl-a-one-time-gene-therapy-treatment [accessed February 5, 2022].

Testa F, Maguire AM, Rossi S, Pierce EA, Melillo P, Marshall K, Banfi S, Surace EM, Sun J, Acerra C, et al. 2013. Three-year follow-up after unilateral subretinal delivery of adeno-associated virus in patients with Leber congenital amaurosis type 2. *Ophthalmology* **120:** 1283–1291. doi:10.1016/j.ophtha.2012.11.048

U.S. FDA. 2011. Cellular, Tissue and Gene Therapies Advisory Committee, June 29, 2011. Available at http://wayback.archive-it.org/7993/20170113010817/http://www.fda.gov/downloads/AdvisoryCommittees/CommitteesMeetingMaterials/BloodVaccinesandOtherBiologics/CellularTissueandGeneTherapiesAdvisoryCommittee/UCM267068.pdf [accessed February 5, 2022].

U.S. FDA. 2017a. Cellular, Tissue and Gene Therapies Advisory Committee, October 12, 2017. Meeting Briefing Document, Spark Therapeutics, Luxturna. Available at https://www.fda.gov/media/108385/download [accessed February 5, 2022].

U.S. FDA. 2017b. Cellular, Tissue and Gene Therapies Advisory Committee, October 12, 2017. FDA Briefing Document. Available at https://www.fda.gov/media/108375/download

U.S. FDA. 2017c. Cellular, Tissue and Gene Therapies Advisory Committee, October 12, 2017. Meeting Transcript. Available at https://www.fda.gov/media/109384/download [accessed February 5, 2022].

U.S. FDA. 2019a. Rare diseases: natural history studies for drug development. Draft Guidance for Industry 2019. Available at https://www.fda.gov/regulatory-information/search-fda-guidance-documents/rare-diseases-natural-history-studies-drug-development [accessed February 5, 2022].

U.S. FDA. 2019b. Summary basis for regulatory action. Zolgensma, May 24, 2019. Available at https://www.fda.gov/media/127961/download [accessed July 1, 2022].

U.S. FDA. 2020. Human gene therapy for retinal disorders. Guidance for Industry, January 2020. Available at https://www.fda.gov/regulatory-information/search-fda-guidance-documents/human-gene-therapy-retinal-disorders [accessed May 5, 2022].

U.S. Social Security Administration. n.d. Disability evaluation under social security: special senses and speech-adult. Available at https://www.ssa.gov/disability/professionals/bluebook/2.00-SpecialSensesandSpeech-Adult.htm#2_02 [accessed May 5, 2022].

Developing New Vectors for Retinal Gene Therapy

Emilia A. Zin,[1] Bilge E. Ozturk,[2] Deniz Dalkara,[1] and Leah C. Byrne[2,3,4]

[1]Sorbonne Université, INSERM, CNRS, Institut de la Vision, F-75012 Paris, France

[2]Department of Ophthalmology, University of Pittsburgh, Pittsburgh, Pennsylvania 15213, USA

[3]Department of Neurobiology, University of Pittsburgh, Pittsburgh, Pennsylvania 15213, USA

[4]Department of Bioengineering, University of Pittsburgh, Pittsburgh, Pennsylvania 15213, USA

Correspondence: deniz.dalkara@gmail.com; lbyrne@pitt.edu

Since their discovery over 55 years ago, adeno-associated virus (AAV) vectors have become powerful tools for experimental and therapeutic in vivo gene delivery, particularly in the retina. Increasing knowledge of AAV structure and biology has propelled forward the development of engineered AAV vectors with improved abilities for gene delivery. However, major obstacles to safe and efficient therapeutic gene delivery remain, including tropism, inefficient and untargeted gene delivery, and limited carrying capacity. Additional improvements to AAV vectors will be required to achieve therapeutic benefit while avoiding safety issues. In this review, we provide an overview of recent methods for engineering-enhanced AAV capsids, as well as remaining challenges that must be overcome to achieve optimized therapeutic gene delivery in the eye.

ADENO-ASSOCIATED VIRAL VECTORS FOR RETINAL GENE THERAPY

Simultaneous advances in genetics, natural history studies, and gene delivery have resulted in the advancement of gene therapy. Gene therapy is rapidly becoming a promising option to treat inherited and complex retinal diseases. However, for recent advances to translate into clinically meaningful outcomes, noninvasive and precise gene delivery tools are required to efficiently deliver genes to affected cell types and to prevent, contain, or reverse the course of retinal diseases. Adeno-associated virus (AAV) vectors are the gold standard for gene delivery in the retina. However, accumulating evidence suggests that methods beyond the classical approaches of biomining and rational design will be required to fully understand AAV biology and to create sufficiently effective gene delivery vectors. To this end, new approaches have been developed to make AAVs more efficient, including high-throughput screening and machine learning (ML)-guided capsid development. Here, we discuss obstacles to AAV development in the context of intricate intraocular spaces, and we describe bioengineering methods that can be applied to overcome these challenges.

STRUCTURE OF AAV

AAVs are single-stranded DNA viruses, part of the Parvoviridae family, and within the Dependoparvovirus genus (Hastie and Samulski 2015). To replicate, AAVs require the presence of adenovirus, herpesvirus, or papilloma virus genes (McPherson et al. 1985; Weindler and Heilbronn 1991; Cotmore et al. 2019).

AAVs are small (25 nm) with a genome of 4700 base pairs containing three open-reading frames and two viral genes—*rep* (replication) and *cap* (capsid)—that encode nonstructural, structural, assembly-activating proteins (AAPs), and membrane-associated accessory proteins (MAAPs). The open reading frames are flanked by two inverted terminal repeats (ITRs). ITRs have an essential role in inducing transgene expression, vector production, and cell transduction, and they can form hairpin structures by self-annealing (Buller and Rose 1978; Wistuba et al. 1995; Sonntag et al. 2010). The *rep* gene encodes four regulatory proteins—Rep78, Rep68, Rep52, and Rep40—that play a role in AAV genome replication and virion assembly. The *cap* gene encodes three structural virion proteins, VP1, VP2, and VP3, which form the capsid with the help of the AAP. VPs are generated through alternative splicing and the use of an alternate translational start codon (ACG) (Srivastava et al. 1983). Therefore, VP1, VP2, and VP3 share a common carboxyl terminus.

The AAV capsid consists of 60 virion proteins, comprising a mixture of VP1, VP2, and VP3 at a 1:1:10 estimated ratio, organized in T = 1 icosahedral symmetry (Xie et al. 2002; Govindasamy et al. 2006). VP3 has a molecular weight of 59–61 kDa and its sequence is shared among all VPs. VP2 has a molecular weight of 64–67 kDa. VP1 has a molecular weight of 79–82 kDa and a unique 137 aa amino-terminal region (VP1u), which is critical for successful infection. Although VP3 is capable of forming the capsid by itself, the VP1/VP2 common region, as well as VP1u, are important for nuclear localization,

genome release, and endosomal trafficking and escape.

WHY AAV?

AAV was first discovered over 55 years ago (Atchison et al. 1965), and has since become the main viral vector currently used in gene therapy clinical trials. AAV's potential for safely delivering genetic cargo was first demonstrated in the 1980s, when the virus's wild-type genes were removed and substituted with a transgene (Samulski et al. 1987). In the subsequent 35 years, AAV has been continuously optimized to perform the task of delivering therapeutic genes to target cells.

With the removal of the *rep* and *cap* genes, AAV is incapable of replicating in host cells, even in the presence of adenovirus or herpesvirus. Replication incompetency, along with comparatively low immunogenicity, make AAV an attractive gene therapy vector. AAV has successfully been used as a gene vector in animal models for the past three decades. Furthermore, it has been the viral vector of choice for many clinical trials over the last decade, especially for inherited retinal diseases. Thirteen naturally occurring serotypes of AAV (AAV1 to AAV13) each possess different cell tropisms (Bulcha et al. 2021). This naturally occurring toolbox of AAV vectors, with varying rates of transduction and immunogenicity, comprises a range of options for gene delivery vectors. AAV capsid proteins may also be tailored through engineering, which has resulted in 100s of additional AAV variants with unique tropisms. Furthermore, AAV can package a double-stranded, self-complimentary AAV (scAAV) genome instead of a single-stranded construct, speeding up the rate of protein expression by bypassing the complimentary strand synthesis (McCarty et al. 2001). Additionally, a large variety of AAV-compatible promoters and regulatory sequences are available, making AAV a highly customizable vector.

Besides AAV, additional viral vectors have been used for gene therapy in the eye. Adenovirus has a carrying capacity of 37,000 base pairs, accommodating large transgenes. However, the high immunogenic response to adenovirus leads to potentially adverse effects and unknown transduction rates. Furthermore, clearance of transgene-encoded protein results in short-lived therapeutic effects. Lentiviruses have also been used, and they have an 8000 base pair carrying capacity. Their genetic cargo undergoes random integration into the host cell genome, which has mixed outcomes, as random integration can have deleterious effects. While genomic integration is attractive for cells with a high mitotic index, the retina is a postmitotic tissue. Importantly, adenovirus and lentivirus have very limited tropism for photoreceptors compared to AAVs. For these reasons, AAV is the preferred viral vector for gene delivery in the retina.

OBSTACLES TO BE OVERCOME

Despite its promise for treating diseases affecting tissues across the body, numerous obstacles prevent the effective translation of AAV-mediated gene therapies to the clinic (Fig. 1). The most significant limitations of AAV vectors include limited tropism for affected cell types, limited diffusion of the vector across structural barriers such as the inner limiting membrane (ILM), limited carrying capacity and inability to efficiently package large cargos, and immune response to the capsid or gene product delivered, as well as inactivation through neutralizing antibodies (NABs).

Limited Tropism

To date, over 13 naturally occurring serotypes and more than 100 AAV variants have been identified (Kotterman and Schaffer 2014). The tropism of natural serotypes is generally broad, and AAV vectors with the capacity to specifically target retinal cell types are currently lacking (Fig. 1A; Petrs-Silva and Linden 2013; Kotterman and Schaffer 2014). Transduction specificity and efficiency is determined and limited by affinity to receptors (Gao et al. 2005; Vandenberghe et al. 2011), as well as the route of administration. Subretinal injection behind the retina results in varying levels of photoreceptor and retinal pigment epithelium (RPE) transduc-tion, depending on the AAV serotype used, with poor transduction in the inner retinal cells (Lipinski et al. 2013; Trapani et al. 2014). Subretinal injections are invasive, risky procedures that often require vitrectomies, and they are incapable of transducing the entire retinal surface due to localized delivery and limited lateral spread (Khabou et al. 2018b; Boye et al. 2020). Intravitreal injections, on the other hand, result in better transduction of cells within the inner retina and cover a larger surface area, but they also result in limited transduction in photoreceptors and RPE cells due to structural barriers that prevent diffusion, including the ILM (Fig. 1B; Dalkara et al. 2009; Trapani et al. 2014). Suprachoroidal injections, a recently developed approach involving injection with microneedles into a potential space between the choroid and the sclera, have been investigated as a potentially less invasive approach to delivering vectors to the outer retina (Yiu et al. 2020). However, suprachoroidal injections have limited ability to target the central retina and macula of large animals and have been linked to adverse immune reactions.

Penetrating the Inner Limiting Membrane

The adult retina is insulated from the vitreous body by the ILM, which histologically defines the border between the retina and the vitreous humor. The ILM is essential for normal eye development, but it is dispensable in adults, and ILM removal is considered beneficial for patients undergoing macular hole surgery. The ILM contains a thick layer of glycans in the primate retina, including heparan sulfate (HS), which is known to be essential for the binding of AAV2 and 3 to the ILM. Binding to proteoglycans prevents AAV dilution in the vitreous volume, but the benefit of binding to this proteoglycan is also a hindrance, as it may act as a sink, impeding AAV entry into the retina (Dalkara et al. 2009). This is evident from retinal gene delivery experiments in primate eyes that show high transduction rates in areas of the retina where the ILM is thinnest or injections under the ILM (Gamlin et al. 2019).

Several methods of enzymatic or surgical disruption of the ILM have been tested as a

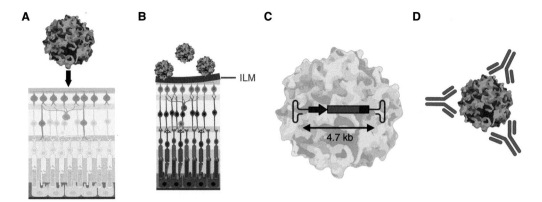

Figure 1. Obstacles preventing efficient retinal gene therapies. (*A*) Limited tropism. (*B*) Limited diffusion across barriers. (ILM) Inner limiting membrane. (*C*) Limited carrying capacity. Adeno-associated virus (AAV) vectors can package up to 4.7 kb, aside from the inverted terminal repeat (ITR) sequences. (*D*) Immune response. (Figure was created with BioRender.com.)

method to enhance AAV access to the retina from the vitreous (Dalkara et al. 2009; Cehajic-Kapetanovic et al. 2010); however, these methods have intrinsic risks that restrict their development for clinical use. Others have attempted injections under the ILM as a means to provide better access to the retina using AAVs (Gamlin et al. 2019). Of note, the ILM is disrupted as part of the natural history of diseases involving photoreceptor degeneration, potentially offering the possibility to overcome this physical barrier more easily in later stages of retinal degenerative diseases (Kolstad et al. 2010; Vacca et al. 2014). Capsid engineering has also been used to create variants with altered ILM interaction, leading to improved transduction (Dalkara et al. 2013; Byrne et al. 2020; Öztürk et al. 2021).

Small Packaging Capacity

An important challenge in AAV-mediated retinal gene therapy is the delivery of large genes that exceed the carrying capacity of AAV (Fig. 1C). Some strategies to overcome this obstacle include modifying the genetic payload, including gene truncation, and in vivo genome editing.

The use of dual vectors has also emerged as a promising approach to overcome the limited carrying capacity of AAVs. By dividing the open reading frame into multiple vectors, the transgene can be split into halves; each half is pack-

aged independently in single vectors that can reassemble once the dual AAV vectors coinfect the same cell. A range of strategies have been used to reassemble and form the full-length expression cassette, including homologous recombination and *trans*-splicing. Studies in the retina have demonstrated examples of each of these approaches in vitro and in vivo; however, low efficiency and the production of truncated protein products remain important concerns for clinical use (Colella et al. 2014; Dyka et al. 2014; Trapani et al. 2014, 2015). To ensure efficient protein production, a cell should be infected with equal ratios of each half of the divided message. Random infection rates cause the formation of truncated protein products, and while the inclusion of microRNA (miR) target sites in the gene transcript has previously been shown to effectively reduce the production of truncated proteins (Karali et al. 2011), a decrease in the efficiency of protein expression remains a limitation of the approach.

Neutralizing Antibodies/Immune Response

AAV immunogenicity is a complex problem, and it is dependent on several factors including serotype, transgene expression, organ of interest, and dosage (Fig. 1D). The route of vector administration to the retina also influences immune response (Kotterman et al. 2015). AAVs administered via subretinal injection are less exposed to the immune system, and subretinal injections in one eye can be followed by additional injection in the other eye (Li et al. 2008b; Bennett et al. 2016). Subretinal injections have, however, been associated with retinal thinning when performed under the fovea, and this approach may not be appropriate in fragile, damaged retinas (Bennett et al. 2016). Intravitreal injections are less invasive, and have been used to deliver AAV pan-retinally (Ali et al. 1998). However, intravitreal injections are associated with increased potential for immune response due to access to the systemic circulation and transduction of cells in the anterior segment of the eye. Intravitreal delivery is also made more difficult through dilution that occurs in the vitreous, and the diffusion distance from the ILM to outer nuclear layer (ONL) that must be overcome to achieve an effective therapeutic effect, thus requiring higher viral doses and increasing the chance of triggering an immune response. Similarly, suprachoroidal injections are also associated with significant immune response and loss of transgene expression in nonhuman primates (NHPs), likely as a result of delivery of AAV to the circulatory system (Yiu et al. 2020).

The understanding of the factors contributing to AAV-induced inflammation is currently incomplete (Ail et al. 2022). These factors include the preexistence of serum antibodies against AAVs, and the generation of new antibodies in response to the AAV capsid or transgene after intraocular injections. Binding antibodies (BABs) and a subset of BABs called NABs block AAV transduction locally and systemically.

A dose-dependent increase in BABs and NABs has been documented in ocular gene therapies, across serotypes and modes of injection. Recent work also suggests a correlation between serum BAB levels with clinical grading of inflammation, especially at high doses. Notably, immune reactions to AAV are strongly dependent on capsid dosage; dose sparing through the use of more efficient engineered capsids and strong cell-type-specific promoters can be sufficient to avoid inflammation (Khabou et al. 2018a; Ail et al. 2022). Moreover, when well-

tolerated doses are used, the route of administration does not seem to strongly influence the rise of binding and NABs to AAVs (Ail et al. 2022).

Although immunosuppression can partially mitigate cellular and humoral responses induced by vector administration in naive patients, preexisting NABs continue to present challenges for efficient gene delivery, particularly from intravitreal and suprachoroidal routes. Additional approaches to circumventing NABs include shielding AAV particles from antibodies by covalent attachment of polymers to the viral capsid, encapsulation of vectors inside biomaterials, or by engineered capsid variants that evade recognition by anti-AAV antibodies present in the human population (Bartel et al. 2011).

APPROACHES TO AAV ENGINEERING

In recent decades, a spectrum of approaches has been pursued to develop AAVs with improved properties that enable more effective therapies (Fig. 2). Biomining has been used to search for naturally occurring serotypes with better tropism for human tissue types. Rational mutagenesis of naturally occurring serotypes has sought to build on our increasing knowledge of AAV biology to create efficient vectors. High-throughput screening approaches, including screening of ancestral sequences, directed evolution, and single-cell RNA-seq AAV engineering (scAAVengr) screening have been used to identify promising capsids from pools of mutant capsids. Furthermore, in silico design, artificial intelligence (AI) and ML have also been applied to AAVs, accelerating the speed of capsid discovery for gene therapy. As a result of these efforts, newly engineered capsids, including rationally designed capsids and capsids designed through directed evolution are currently in use in ongoing clinical trials.

Biomining

Soon after its discovery, AAV was considered as a promising viral vector for gene delivery, and methods to overcome obstacles to efficient transduction were begun. Biomining, one early

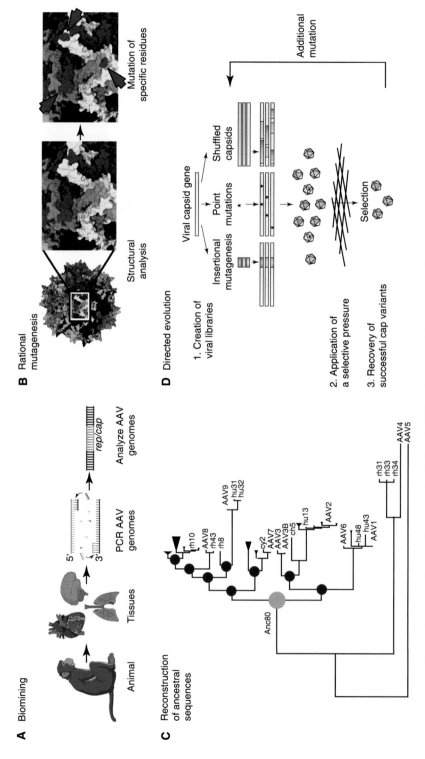

Figure 2. Approaches to adeno-associated virus (AAV) engineering. (*A*) Biomining. (*B*) Rational mutagenesis. (*C*) Reconstruction and screening of ancestral AAVs. (*D*) Directed evolution. (*E*) Single-cell RNA-seq AAV engineering (scAAVengr). (*F*) In silico design, artificial intelligence (AI), and machine learning. (PCR) Polymerase chain reaction. (Figure was created with BioRender.com.)

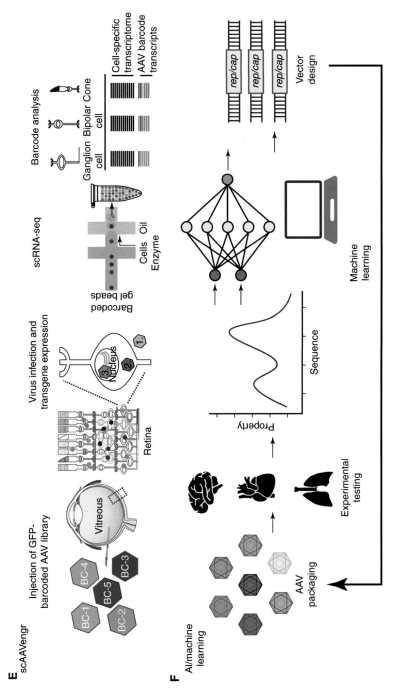

Figure 2. (*See facing page for legend.*)

approach to AAV development (Fig. 2A), involves the identification of naturally occurring serotypes with potentially better characteristics as gene delivery vectors. AAV1 to AAV6 were the first AAV serotypes identified (Gao et al. 2005). All AAV serotypes but AAV5 were first found as contaminants of adenovirus preparations, while AAV5 was found in a human condylomatous wart. Biomining in simian viral preparations resulted in 10 AAV variants with 96% homology to AAV1 or AAV6. However, only two of these variants showed different tropisms for human cancer cell lines when compared to either AAV1 or 6 (Schmidt et al. 2006).

In the absence of adenovirus or herpesvirus, AAV establishes latent infections either through integrating into chromosome 19 or by forming stable episomes. It was hypothesized that additional undescribed endogenous AAV variants could thus be recovered from human and NHP tissues (Gao et al. 2005; Schmidt et al. 2006). Polymerase chain reaction (PCR) was used to amplify the *cap* gene, which was then sequenced (Gao et al. 2005). Over 100 novel AAV variants, separated in different clades, have since been described (Gao et al. 2004; Mietzsch et al. 2021). Of these, 55 were from human cells and 55 were from NHPs. Twenty-five AAV variants were initially screened in vivo in mouse models. Of note, AAV8, AAV9, and AAVrh.10 were identified as interesting variants for gene therapy, with higher transduction efficiencies in murine hepatocytes or lung when compared to AAV2. AAV8 is currently employed in clinical trials for several retinal degenerative diseases, as it has improved infectivity of photoreceptors when delivered subretinally compared to AAV2 (Vandenberghe et al. 2011). AAV9 and AAVrh.10 are the serotypes of choice in several trials targeting the central nervous system.

Rational Mutagenesis

Crystal structures of AAV capsids have been determined for many AAV serotypes in the past decades (Mietzsch et al. 2019), leading to deeper understanding of the structural basis for receptor binding, tropism, and transduction efficien-

cy. This information has in turn influenced strategies for rational design and modification of the capsid (Fig. 2B). AAV2 is the best studied serotype due to its early discovery and successful implementation in gene delivery, making it more amenable to rational design.

The amino acid residues involved in HS binding (R484, R487, K532, R585, and R588) have been extensively modified (Boye et al. 2016) as have key residues responsible for ubiquitination upon cell entry (Zhong et al. 2008; Petrs-Silva et al. 2009, 2011). Rational design of the AAV capsid has been explored for the purpose of avoiding proteasomal degradation and enhancing transduction efficiencies. Substitution of surface-exposed tyrosine, threonine, and serine residues, which are phosphorylated as part of the ubiquitin-dependent proteasomal degradation process, prevents this process. Surface-exposed tyrosine-to-phenylalanine (Y-F), threonine-to-valine (T-V), or serine-to-valine (S-V) mutations (or a combination thereof) increase transduction efficiency in several tissues and organs, including the retina (Kay et al. 2013). AAV1 was given the ability to bind HS through the addition of a single E531K mutation, resulting in a vector with a similar tropism as AAV6, with the ability to infect the retina from intravitreal injections in mice (Wu et al. 2006; Woodard et al. 2016). However, similar attempts to graft AAV2 HS-binding residues onto other vectors such as AAV5 and AAV8 did not impart the ability to transduce the retina from the vitreous. This result demonstrates the complexity of the factors influencing AAV tropism in a complex structure such as the retina, and the difficulty in attempting to engineer AAV through a rational approach.

Ancestral Screening

Improvements in phylogenetic analysis, DNA sequencing, and synthesis have permitted the reconstruction of ancestral proteins, including AAV capsids. Using statistical and ML methods, applied to an analysis of extant AAVs, groups have sought to infer and reconstruct theoretical ancestral capsid sequences. Instead of analyzing a single estimated ancestral sequence, two groups have built libraries of predicted sequences that would represent putative ancestral AAVs at specific phylogenetic nodes (Fig. 2C; Santiago-Ortiz et al. 2015; Zinn et al. 2015).

One group analyzed the node that encompassed the ancestor of AAV1, AAV6, and AAV7 (Santiago-Ortiz et al. 2015), to determine whether ancestral AAVs had broad or specific tropisms, and whether ancestral AAVs might be more stable than their ancestors, making them better suited as the starting material for directed evolution studies. AAV1 and AAV6 have therapeutic relevance, while AAV7 is known for its relative resistance to NABs. Ancestral variants from the screen were stable, and showed promiscuous rather than specific infectivity profiles. The authors therefore suggested that a hypothesized increase in mutational tolerance and evolvability of this library might be harnessed in directed evolution studies.

Meanwhile, another group (Zinn et al. 2015) focused on the node representing a hypothetical ancestor of AAVs 1–3 and 6–9, called Anc80, to determine whether ancestral AAVs might be more stable, more infectious, or whether the seroprevalence for NABs against this ancestral variant might be lower in the modern human population. In silico phylogenetic and statistical modeling was used to predict putative ancestral sequences of the AAV capsid protein. A library of predicted AAV capsid sequences was then synthesized and screened in HEK cells. From this screen, the Anc80L65 clone was chosen for further analysis, and was shown to outperform other vectors in photoreceptor cells. Further lack of toxicity and desirable immune reactivity showed that a combination of in silico analysis and library selection can be a useful method for assessing AAV vector properties and discovering therapeutically relevant variants.

High-Throughput Approaches to Engineering AAVs

A range of high-throughput strategies have been exploited to create new capsids over the past decade. Directed evolution (Fig. 2D) is a method involving the introduction of mutations in the *cap* gene to yield highly diverse AAV libraries.

Selective pressure is then applied to enrich for novel variants with enhanced properties. Techniques for the introduction of mutations include the insertion of random peptide sequences into a defined location on the capsid, incorporation of peptide sequences into random locations in the *cap* gene, error-prone PCR and site-directed mutagenesis, and gene shuffling, which generates chimeric AAV capsids by fragmentation of the cap gene (Müller et al. 2003; Maheshri et al. 2006; Perabo et al. 2006a,b; Grimm et al. 2008). The creation of high-quality and highly diverse libraries, which thoroughly explore possible sequence space, are key to the identification of novel AAV variants with new abilities.

scAAVengr

Accurate, quantitative comparisons of the efficiency and tropism of newly engineered vectors are challenging. Large numbers of animals are typically required to characterize the performance of variants, and variation between animals and injections lead to inaccurate comparisons. These challenges are compounded in valuable large animal models such as primates, in which there is large variability between animals. Recently, an scAAVengr pipeline was developed for rapid, quantitative in vivo comparison of transgene expression in retinal cells from newly engineered AAV capsid variants across all different cell types in a tissue in parallel, and in the same animals (Fig. 2E; Öztürk et al. 2021; Xi et al. 2022). scAAVengr uses single-cell RNA-seq to identify single cells by marker gene expression, and simultaneously quantify the ability of AAV variants to drive gene expression in those cells at the single-cell level based on quantification of transgenes. The scAAVengr single-cell RNA-seq pipeline allows for highly quantitative, direct evaluation of the multiple lead candidates across all cell types in a tissue, which is critical for understanding the clinical potential of a vector.

In Silico Design, AI, and Machine Learning

Directed evolution is a high-throughput protein engineering method applicable to AAV capsids; however, the overall success rate in these screens can be low because of the complex relationship between capsid structure and the AAV transduction pathway and the many aspects of AAV structure and function that must be simultaneously optimized. High-throughput screening methodologies can be aided by in silico design and ML (Fig. 2F). ML refers to algorithmic approaches that enable automatic learning. ML allows for rules for vector design to be established directly from input data. Training data can be acquired through deep sequencing of viral libraries.

Recently, ML was used to guide capsid engineering and to interrogate AAV biology (Ogden et al. 2019). The effects of mutations across all 735 amino acid positions, including all synonymous codons for each amino acid, were analyzed to enable detection of noncoding elements. Single-codon insertions and deletions, as well as control wild-type AAV2 sequences and stop codon substitutions were also included. Based on the analysis of resulting variants, the authors predicted that an additive model built from this data would approximate the fitness of nearby variants with multiple mutations. It was hypothesized that this approach would thereby enable the design of functional variants with higher throughput than rational design and improved efficiency compared to random mutagenesis. 1271 variants were designed and tested by measuring liver biodistribution in mice. The set of AAVs designed through the ML model included a higher fraction of mutants targeted to the liver, compared to a control set of vectors with random mutations, demonstrating that machine-guided design is a valuable approach to create higher percentages of viable mutants. These methods may enable rapid and systematic optimization of AAV capsids that might have been undetectable or lost using other less informed screening efforts.

Next Generation AAVs in the Clinic

Next-generation AAVs with enhanced properties have the potential to improve clinical outcomes. A recent meta-analysis of AAV usage in clinical settings (Au et al. 2022) found that six different capsid types were used in clinical trials for eye disorders, with the majority of clinical trials using natural AAV2. The other two natural AAVs used in clinical trials are AAV5 and AAV8. Recent clinical trials are using engineered serotypes including AAV2TYF (Zhong et al. 2008), 7m8 (Dalkara et al. 2013), and 4D-R100 (Kotterman et al. 2021). AAV2TYF, a tyrosine-to-phenylalanine mutant, was designed to avoid proteasome degradation (Zhong et al. 2008). This vector has been used in three different clinical trials (NCT03316560, NCT02599922, NCT0241666 22). 7m8, which has been used in four clinical trials (NCT03748784, NCT04418427, NCT0464 5212, NCT03326336), was designed through directed evolution, and its capsid carries a 10–amino acid insertion that enables greater transduction via intravitreal injection. 4D-R100 was also optimized through directed evolution, and it is being used in two clinical trials (NCT04483440, NCT04517149).

Promoters and *cis*-Regulatory Elements

While generating efficient AAV capsid variants is key to the optimization of gene delivery, promoters and other *cis*-regulatory elements that flank the transgene also define the therapeutic outcome by regulating gene expression. Promoters are sequences located at the 5′ end of the transgene and drive gene expression. Often simply referred to as "promoters," they are frequently a combination of transcriptional start site, promoter, enhancer, and regulatory sequences (Gray et al. 2011). RNA polymerase attaches itself to a promoter, while enhancers are sequences upstream or downstream of promoters that regulate gene expression. As the packaging capacity of AAV is limited, AAV-compatible promoters condense these functions in short fragments, often between ~200 and 2000 bp long.

Promoters can be ubiquitous or cell-specific, and define which infected cells will express a transgene. Ubiquitous promoters, such as the cytomegalovirus (CMV) early enhancer/promoter or the synthetic CAG promoter, can drive strong gene expression in all cell types. On the other hand, cell-specific promoters can be used to target one or more cells (Khani et al. 2007; Planul and Dalkara 2017). The specificity of promoters is essential to tailor targeted expression. Promoter specificity is influenced by viral dose, injection route, the state of the retina, the species in which the promoter is used, and capsid tropism (Khabou et al. 2018a).

The search for efficient, cell-specific promoters has led to extensive efforts such as the Pleiades Promoter Project (Portales-Casamar et al. 2010), the retina-specific synthetic promoter search by Botond Roska's team (Jüttner et al. 2019), and a recently described method that identified Müller glia and amacrine cell-specific promoters (Lin et al. 2022). These projects have developed a wide range of synthetic promoters with varying abilities to target specific cell types. Furthermore, several of these studies have shown that promoters can have unexpected off-target transgene expression in unwanted cell types, which may be a source of toxicity. Promoters with excellent cell specificity may not drive high transgene expression levels, and so efficiency must also be taken into consideration.

An array of promoters restrict expression of transgenes to specific cell types in the retina. For example, the RPE65 promoter (Meur et al. 2007), the VMD2 promoter (Alexander and Hauswirth 2008; Conlon et al. 2013; Guziewicz et al. 2013), and the CD365 promoter (Sutanto et al. 2005) drive expression in RPE cells following subretinal injection in rodents. The hRK or GRK1 promoter has been used to drive expression in photoreceptors from subretinal injections in mice and pigs (Khani et al. 2007; Boye et al. 2010; Zou et al. 2011; Manfredi et al. 2013). pR2.1 and pR1.7 promoters have been used to drive expression in cones in mice, rats, ferrets, guinea pigs, and macaques (Li et al. 2008a; Ye et al. 2016). And Grm6, 4xGRm6, In4s-In3-200En-mGluR500P, and Ple22 promoters drive expression in bipolar cells in mice and marmosets via subretinal and intravitreal injection (Doroudchi et al. 2011; Cronin et al. 2014; de Leeuw et al. 2014; Gaub et al. 2014; Macé et al. 2015; Scalabrino et al. 2015; Lu et al. 2016).

The choice of *cis*-regulatory elements can also affect toxicity. A previous study in mice has shown that ubiquitous promoters such as CMV and CAG, as well as one RPE-specific promoter (Best1), were correlated to ocular toxicity (Xiong et al. 2019). These results indicate that promoters should be screened for toxic effects before being employed in therapeutic studies.

CONCLUDING REMARKS

Over the past several decades, significant progress has been made in the design of next-generation AAVs with enhanced abilities to deliver therapeutic genes to the retina. AAVs are the gold standard for gene delivery, although efficient and specific gene delivery remains a key bottleneck in the development of gene therapies. Significant shortcomings remain, including tropism, limited carrying capacity, and immunogenicity. A range of approaches have been implemented and have shown promise in engineering new variants with desirable properties, including rational design, high-throughput screening, and ML. Together, these approaches may yield a toolbox of AAV vectors capable of targeting each of the cell types affected by the range of retinal diseases that exist.

ACKNOWLEDGMENTS

Figures were created with BioRender (BioRender .com). This work was supported by the ERC H2020 FET OPEN NEUROPA project under grant agreement No. 863214 (D.D.), the Institut National de la Santé et de la Recherche Médicale (INSERM), Sorbonne Université, The Foundation Fighting Blindness, Agence National de Recherche (ANR) RHU Light4Deaf, *LabEx LIFESENSES (ANR-10-LABX-65), and *IHU FOReSIGHT (ANR18-IAHU-01). E.A.Z. is supported by the Paris Region Fellowship Programme, Île-de-France (374397). We also acknowledge support from National Institutes of Health (NIH) CORE Grant P30 EY08098 to the University of Pittsburgh Department of Ophthalmology, from the Eye and Ear Foundation of Pittsburgh, and from an unrestricted grant from Research to Prevent Blindness, New York, NY. Funding to L.C.B. was provided by the UPMC Immune Transplant and Therapy Center, the NIH (UG3MH120094), Foundation Fighting Blindness, and Research to Prevent Blindness.

REFERENCES

Ail D, Ren D, Brazhnikova E, Nouvel-Jaillard C, Bertin S, Mirashrafi SB, Fisson S, Dalkara D. 2022. Systemic and local immune responses to intraocular AAV vector administration in non-human primates. *Mol Ther Methods Clin Dev* **24**: 306–316. doi:10.1016/j.omtm.2022.01.011

Alexander JJ, Hauswirth WW. 2008. Prospects for retinal cone-targeted gene therapy. *Drug News Perspect* **21**: 267–271. doi:10.1358/dnp.2008.21.5.1223972

Ali RR, Reichel MB, Alwis MD, Kanuga N, Kinnon C, Levinsky RJ, Hunt DM, Bhattacharya SS, Thrasher AJ. 1998. Adeno-associated virus gene transfer to mouse retina. *Hum Gene Ther* **9**: 81–86. doi:10.1089/hum.1998.9.1-81

Atchison RW, Casto BC, Hammon W. 1965. Adenovirus-associated defective virus particles. *Science* **149**: 754–756. doi:10.1126/science.149.3685.754

Au HKE, Isalan M, Mielcarek M. 2022. Gene therapy advances: a meta-analysis of AAV usage in clinical settings. *Front Med (Lausanne)* **8**: 809118.

Bennett J, Wellman J, Marshall KA, McCague S, Ashtari M, DiStefano-Pappas J, Elci OU, Chung DC, Sun J, Wright JF, et al. 2016. Safety and durability of effect of contralateral-eye administration of AAV2 gene therapy in patients with childhood-onset blindness caused by RPE65 mutations: a follow-on phase 1 trial. *Lancet* **388**: 661–672. doi:10.1016/S0140-6736(16)30371-3

Boye SE, Boye SL, Pang J, Ryals R, Everhart D, Umino Y, Neeley AW, Besharse J, Barlow R, Hauswirth WW. 2010. Functional and behavioral restoration of vision by gene therapy in the guanylate cyclase-1 (GC1) knockout mouse. *PLoS ONE* **5**: e11306. doi:10.1371/journal.pone.0011306

Boye SL, Bennett A, Scalabrino ML, McCullough KT, Vliet KV, Choudhury S, Ruan Q, Peterson J, Agbandje-McKenna M, Boye SE. 2016. Impact of heparan sulfate binding on transduction of retina by recombinant adeno-associated virus vectors. *J Virol* **90**: 4215–4231. doi:10.1128/JVI.00200-16

Boye SL, Choudhury S, Crosson S, Pasquale GD, Afione S, Mellen R, Makal V, Calabro KR, Fajardo D, Peterson J, et al. 2020. Novel AAV44.9-based vectors display exceptional characteristics for retinal gene therapy. *Mol Ther* **28**: 1464–1478. doi:10.1016/j.ymthe.2020.04.002

Bulcha JT, Wang Y, Ma H, Tai PWL, Gao G. 2021. Viral vector platforms within the gene therapy landscape. *Signal Transduct Target Ther* **6**: 53. doi:10.1038/s41392-021-00487-6

Buller RM, Rose JA. 1978. Characterization of adenovirus-associated virus-induced polypeptides in KB cells. *J Virol* **25**: 331–338. doi:10.1128/jvi.25.1.331-338.1978

Byrne LC, Day TP, Visel M, Fortuny C, Dalkara D, Merigan WH, Schaffer DV, Flannery JG. 2020. In vivo directed evolution of adeno-associated virus in the primate retina. *JCI Insight* **5**: e135112. doi:10.1172/jci.insight.135112

Cehajic-Kapetanovic J, Goff MML, Allen A, Lucas RJ, Bishop PN. 2010. Glycosidic enzymes enhance retinal transduction following intravitreal delivery of AAV2. *Mol Vis* **17**: 1771–1783.

Colella P, Trapani I, Cesi G, Sommella A, Manfredi A, Puppo A, Iodice C, Rossi S, Simonelli F, Giunti M, et al. 2014. Efficient gene delivery to the cone-enriched pig retina by dual AAV vectors. *Gene Ther* **21**: 450–456. doi:10.1038/gt.2014.8

Conlon TJ, Deng WT, Erger K, Cossette T, Pang J, Ryals R, Clément N, Cleaver B, McDoom I, Boye SE, et al. 2013. Preclinical potency and safety studies of an AAV2-mediated gene therapy vector for the treatment of *MERTK* associated retinitis pigmentosa. *Hum Gene Ther Clin Dev* **24**: 23–28. doi:10.1089/humc.2013.037

Cotmore SF, Agbandje-McKenna M, Canuti M, Chiorini JA, Eis-Hubinger AM, Hughes J, Mietzsch M, Modha S, Ogliastro M, Pénzes JJ, et al. 2019. ICTV virus taxonomy profile: Parvoviridae. *J Gen Virol* **100**: 367–368. doi:10.1099/jgv.0.001212

Cronin T, Vandenberghe LH, Hantz P, Juttner J, Reimann A, Kacsó A-E, Huckfeldt RM, Busskamp V, Kohler H, Lagali PS, et al. 2014. Efficient transduction and optogenetic stimulation of retinal bipolar cells by a synthetic adeno-associated virus capsid and promoter. *EMBO Mol Med* **6**: 1175–1190. doi:10.15252/emmm.201404077

Dalkara D, Kolstad KD, Caporale N, Visel M, Klimczak RR, Schaffer DV, Flannery JG. 2009. Inner limiting membrane barriers to AAV-mediated retinal transduction from the vitreous. *Mol Ther* **17**: 2096–2102. doi:10.1038/mt.2009.181

Dalkara D, Byrne LC, Klimczak RR, Visel M, Yin L, Merigan WH, Flannery JG, Schaffer DV. 2013. In vivo-directed evolution of a new adeno-associated virus for therapeutic outer retinal gene delivery from the vitreous. *Sci Transl Med* **5**: 189ra76. doi:10.1126/scitranslmed.3005708

de Leeuw CN, Dyka FM, Boye SL, Laprise S, Zhou M, Chou AY, Borretta L, McInerny SC, Banks KG, Portales-Casamar E, et al. 2014. Targeted CNS delivery using human minipromoters and demonstrated compatibility with adeno-associated viral vectors. *Mol Ther Methods* **1**: 5.

Doroudchi MM, Greenberg KP, Liu J, Silka KA, Boyden ES, Lockridge JA, Arman AC, Janani R, Boye SE, Boye SL, et al. 2011. Virally delivered channelrhodopsin-2 safely and effectively restores visual function in multiple mouse models of blindness. *Mol Ther* **19**: 1220–1229. doi:10.1038/mt.2011.69

Dyka FM, Boye SL, Chiodo VA, Hauswirth WW, Boye SE. 2014. Dual adeno-associated virus vectors result in efficient in vitro and in vivo expression of an oversized gene, MYO7A. *Hum Gene Ther Method* **25**: 166–177. doi:10.1089/hgtb.2013.212

Gamlin PD, Alexander JJ, Boye SL, Witherspoon CD, Boye SE. 2019. SubILM injection of AAV for gene delivery to the retina. *Methods Mol Biol* **1950**: 249–262. doi:10.1007/978-1-4939-9139-6_14

Gao G, Vandenberghe LH, Alvira MR, Lu Y, Calcedo R, Zhou X, Wilson JM. 2004. Clades of adeno-associated viruses are widely disseminated in human tissues. *J Virol* **78**: 6381–6388. doi:10.1128/JVI.78.12.6381-6388.2004

Gao G, Vandenberghe L, Wilson J. 2005. New recombinant serotypes of AAV vectors. *Curr Gene Ther* **5**: 285–297. doi:10.2174/1566523054065057

Gaub BM, Berry MH, Holt AE, Reiner A, Kienzler MA, Dolgova N, Nikonov S, Aguirre GD, Beltran WA, Flannery JG, et al. 2014. Restoration of visual function by expression of a light-gated mammalian ion channel in retinal ganglion cells or ON-bipolar cells. *Proc Natl*

Cite this article as *Cold Spring Harb Perspect Med* doi: 10.1101/cshperspect.a041291

Acad Sci **111:** E5574–E5583. doi:10.1073/pnas.1315034111

Govindasamy L, Padron E, McKenna R, Muzyczka N, Kaludov N, Chiorini JA, Agbandje-McKenna M. 2006. Structurally mapping the diverse phenotype of adeno-associated virus serotype 4. *J Virol* **80:** 11556–11570. doi:10.1128/JVI.01536-06

Gray SJ, Foti SB, Schwartz JW, Bachaboina L, Taylor-Blake B, Coleman J, Ehlers MD, Zylka MJ, McCown TJ, Samulski RJ. 2011. Optimizing promoters for recombinant adeno-associated virus-mediated gene expression in the peripheral and central nervous system using self-complementary vectors. *Hum Gene Ther* **22:** 1143–1153. doi:10.1089/hum.2010.245

Grimm D, Lee JS, Wang L, Desai T, Akache B, Storm TA, Kay MA. 2008. In vitro and in vivo gene therapy vector evolution via multispecies interbreeding and retargeting of adeno-associated viruses. *J Virol* **82:** 5887–5911. doi:10.1128/JVI.00254-08

Guziewicz KE, Zangerl B, Komáromy AM, Iwabe S, Chiodo VA, Boye SL, Hauswirth WW, Beltran WA, Aguirre GD. 2013. Recombinant AAV-mediated BEST1 transfer to the retinal pigment epithelium: analysis of serotype-dependent retinal effects. *PLoS ONE* **8:** e75666. doi:10.1371/journal.pone.0075666

Hastie E, Samulski RJ. 2015. Recombinant adeno-associated virus vectors in the treatment of rare diseases. *Expert Opin Orphan Drugs* **3:** 675–689. doi:10.1517/21678707.2015.1039511

Jüttner J, Szabo A, Gross-Scherf B, Morikawa RK, Rompani SB, Hantz P, Szikra T, Esposti F, Cowan CS, Bharioke A, et al. 2019. Targeting neuronal and glial cell types with synthetic promoter AAVs in mice, non-human primates and humans. *Nat Neurosci* **22:** 1345–1356. doi:10.1038/s41593-019-0431-2

Karali M, Manfredi A, Puppo A, Marrocco E, Gargiulo A, Allocca M, Corte MD, Rossi S, Giunti M, Bacci ML, et al. 2011. MicroRNA-restricted transgene expression in the retina. *PLoS ONE* **6:** e22166. doi:10.1371/journal.pone.0022166

Kay CN, Ryals RC, Aslanidi GV, Min SH, Ruan Q, Sun J, Dyka FM, Kasuga D, Ayala AE, Vliet KV, et al. 2013. Targeting photoreceptors via intravitreal delivery using novel, capsid-mutated AAV vectors. *PLoS ONE* **8:** e62097. doi:10.1371/journal.pone.0062097

Khabou H, Cordeau C, Pacot L, Fisson S, Dalkara D. 2018a. Dosage thresholds and influence of transgene cassette in adeno-associated virus-related toxicity. *Hum Gene Ther* **29:** 1235–1241. doi:10.1089/hum.2018.144

Khabou H, Garita-Hernandez M, Chaffiol A, Reichman S, Jaillard C, Brazhnikova E, Bertin S, Forster V, Desrosiers M, Winckler C, et al. 2018b. Noninvasive gene delivery to foveal cones for vision restoration. *JCI Insight* **3:** e96029. doi:10.1172/jci.insight.96029

Khani SC, Pawlyk BS, Bulgakov OV, Kasperek E, Young JE, Adamian M, Sun X, Smith AJ, Ali RR, Li T. 2007. AAV-mediated expression targeting of rod and cone photoreceptors with a human rhodopsin kinase promoter. *Invest Ophth Vis Sci* **48:** 3954–3961. doi:10.1167/iovs.07-0257

Kolstad KD, Dalkara D, Guerin K, Visel M, Hoffmann N, Schaffer DV, Flannery JG. 2010. Changes in adeno-associated virus-mediated gene delivery in retinal degenera-tion. *Hum Gene Ther* **21:** 571–578. doi:10.1089/hum.2009.194

Kotterman MA, Schaffer DV. 2014. Engineering adeno-associated viruses for clinical gene therapy. *Nat Rev Genet* **15:** 445–451. doi:10.1038/nrg3742

Kotterman MA, Yin L, Strazzeri JM, Flannery JG, Merigan WH, Schaffer DV. 2015. Antibody neutralization poses a barrier to intravitreal adeno-associated viral vector gene delivery to non-human primates. *Gene Ther* **22:** 116–126. doi:10.1038/gt.2014.115

Kotterman M, Beliakoff G, Croze R, Vazin T, Schmitt C, Szymanski P, Leong M, Quezada M, Holt J, Barglow K, et al. 2021. Directed evolution of AAV targeting primate retina by intravitreal injection identifies R100, a variant demonstrating robust gene delivery and therapeutic efficacy in non-human primates. bioRxiv doi:10.1101/2021.06.24.449775

Li Q, Timmers AM, Guy J, Pang J, Hauswirth WW. 2008a. Cone-specific expression using a human red opsin promoter in recombinant AAV. *Vision Res* **48:** 332–338. doi:10.1016/j.visres.2007.07.026

Li W, Kong F, Li X, Dai X, Liu X, Zheng Q, Wu R, Zhou X, Lü F, Chang B, et al. 2008b. Gene therapy following subretinal AAV5 vector delivery is not affected by a previous intravitreal AAV5 vector administration in the partner eye. *Mol Vis* **15:** 267–275.

Lin C-H, Sun Y, Chan CSY, Wu M-R, Gu L, Davis AE, Gu B, Zhang W, Tanasa B, Zhong LR, et al. 2022. Identification of *cis*-regulatory modules for adeno-associated virus-based cell type-specific targeting in the retina and brain. *J Biol Chem* **298:** 101674. doi:10.1016/j.jbc.2022.101674

Lipinski DM, Thake M, MacLaren RE. 2013. Clinical applications of retinal gene therapy. *Prog Retin Eye Res* **32:** 22–47. doi:10.1016/j.preteyeres.2012.09.001

Lu Q, Ganjawala T, Ivanova E, Cheng J, Troilo D, Pan ZH. 2016. AAV-mediated transduction and targeting of retinal bipolar cells with improved mGluR6 promoters in rodents and primates. *Gene Ther* **23:** 680–689. doi:10.1038/gt.2016.42

Macé E, Caplette R, Marre O, Sengupta A, Chaffiol A, Barbe P, Desrosiers M, Bamberg E, Sahel JA, Picaud S, et al. 2015. Targeting channelrhodopsin-2 to ON-bipolar cells with vitreally administered AAV restores ON and OFF visual responses in blind mice. *Mol Ther* **23:** 7–16. doi:10.1038/mt.2014.154

Maheshri N, Koerber JT, Kaspar BK, Schaffer DV. 2006. Directed evolution of adeno-associated virus yields enhanced gene delivery vectors. *Nat Biotechnol* **24:** 198–204. doi:10.1038/nbt1182

Manfredi A, Marrocco E, Puppo A, Cesi G, Sommella A, Corte MD, Rossi S, Giunti M, Craft CM, Bacci ML, et al. 2013. Combined rod and cone transduction by adeno-associated virus 2/8. *Hum Gene Ther* **24:** 982–992. doi:10.1089/hum.2013.154

McCarty DM, Monahan PE, Samulski RJ. 2001. Self-complementary recombinant adeno-associated virus (scAAV) vectors promote efficient transduction independently of DNA synthesis. *Gene Ther* **8:** 1248–1254. doi:10.1038/sj.gt.3301514

McPherson RA, Rosenthal LJ, Rose JA. 1985. Human cytomegalovirus completely helps adeno-associated virus replication. *Virology* **147**: 217–222. doi:10.1016/0042-6822 (85)90243-0

Meur GL, Stieger K, Smith AJ, Weber M, Deschamps JY, Nivard D, Mendes-Madeira A, Provost N, Péréon Y, Cherel Y, et al. 2007. Restoration of vision in RPE65-deficient Briard dogs using an AAV serotype 4 vector that specifically targets the retinal pigmented epithelium. *Gene Ther* **14**: 292–303. doi:10.1038/sj.gt.3302861

Mietzsch M, Pénzes JJ, Agbandje-McKenna M. 2019. Twenty-five years of structural parvovirology. *Viruses* **11**: 362. doi:10.3390/v11040362

Mietzsch M, Jose A, Chipman P, Bhattacharya N, Daneshparvar N, McKenna R, Agbandje-McKenna M. 2021. Completion of the AAV structural atlas: serotype capsid structures reveals clade-specific features. *Viruses* **13**: 101. doi:10.3390/v13010101

Müller OJ, Kaul F, Weitzman MD, Pasqualini R, Arap W, Kleinschmidt JA, Trepel M. 2003. Random peptide libraries displayed on adeno-associated virus to select for targeted gene therapy vectors. *Nat Biotechnol* **21**: 1040–1046. doi:10.1038/nbt856

Ogden PJ, Kelsic ED, Sinai S, Church GM. 2019. Comprehensive AAV capsid fitness landscape reveals a viral gene and enables machine-guided design. *Science* **366**: 1139–1143. doi:10.1126/science.aaw2900

Öztürk BE, Johnson ME, Kleyman M, Turunç S, He J, Jabalameli S, Xi Z, Visel M, Dufour VL, Iwabe S, et al. 2021. scAAVengr, a transcriptome-based pipeline for quantitative ranking of engineered AAVs with single-cell resolution. *eLife* **10**: e64175. doi:10.7554/eLife.64175

Perabo L, Endell J, King S, Lux K, Goldnau D, Hallek M, Büning H. 2006a. Combinatorial engineering of a gene therapy vector: directed evolution of adeno-associated virus. *J Gene Med* **8**: 155–162. doi:10.1002/jgm.849

Perabo L, Goldnau D, White K, Endell J, Boucas J, Humme S, Work LM, Janicki H, Hallek M, Baker AH, et al. 2006b. Heparan sulfate proteoglycan binding properties of adeno-associated virus retargeting mutants and consequences for their in vivo tropism. *J Virol* **80**: 7265–7269. doi:10.1128/JVI.00076-06

Petrs-Silva H, Linden R. 2013. Advances in recombinant adeno-associated viral vectors for gene delivery. *Curr Gene Ther* **13**: 335–345. doi:10.2174/1566523211313 6660028

Petrs-Silva H, Dinculescu A, Li Q, Min SH, Chiodo V, Pang JJ, Zhong L, Zolotukhin S, Srivastava A, Lewin AS, et al. 2009. High-efficiency transduction of the mouse retina by tyrosine-mutant AAV serotype vectors. *Mol Ther* **17**: 463–471. doi:10.1038/mt.2008.269

Petrs-Silva H, Dinculescu A, Li Q, Deng WT, Pang J, Min SH, Chiodo V, Neeley AW, Govindasamy L, Bennett A, et al. 2011. Novel properties of tyrosine-mutant AAV2 vectors in the mouse retina. *Mol Ther* **19**: 293–301. doi:10.1038/mt.2010.234

Planul A, Dalkara D. 2017. Vectors and gene delivery to the retina. *Annu Rev Vis Sci* **3**: 121–140. doi:10.1146/annurev-vision-102016-061413

Portales-Casamar E, Swanson DJ, Liu L, de Leeuw CN, Banks KG, Sui SJH, Fulton DL, Ali J, Amirabbasi M, Arenillas DJ, et al. 2010. A regulatory toolbox of Mini-Promoters to drive selective expression in the brain. *Proc Natl Acad Sci* **107**: 16589–16594. doi:10.1073/pnas .1009158107

Samulski RJ, Chang LS, Shenk T. 1987. A recombinant plasmid from which an infectious adeno-associated virus genome can be excised in vitro and its use to study viral replication. *J Virol* **61**: 3096–3101. doi:10.1128/jvi.61.10 .3096-3101.1987

Santiago-Ortiz J, Ojala DS, Westesson O, Weinstein JR, Wong SY, Steinsapir A, Kumar S, Holmes I, Schaffer DV. 2015. AAV ancestral reconstruction library enables selection of broadly infectious viral variants. *Gene Ther* **22**: 934–946. doi:10.1038/gt.2015.74

Scalabrino ML, Boye SL, Fransen KMH, Noel JM, Dyka FM, Min SH, Ruan Q, Leeuw CND, Simpson EM, Gregg RG, et al. 2015. Intravitreal delivery of a novel AAV vector targets ON bipolar cells and restores visual function in a mouse model of complete congenital stationary night blindness. *Hum Mol Genet* **24**: 6229–6239. doi:10.1093/ hmg/ddv341

Schmidt M, Grot E, Cervenka P, Wainer S, Buck C, Chiorini JA. 2006. Identification and characterization of novel adeno-associated virus isolates in ATCC virus stocks. *J Virol* **80**: 5082–5085. doi:10.1128/JVI.80.10.5082-5085.2006

Sonntag F, Schmidt K, Kleinschmidt JA. 2010. A viral assembly factor promotes AAV2 capsid formation in the nucleolus. *Proc Natl Acad Sci* **107**: 10220–10225. doi:10.1073/ pnas.1001673107

Srivastava A, Lusby EW, Berns KI. 1983. Nucleotide sequence and organization of the adeno-associated virus 2 genome. *J Virol* **45**: 555–564. doi:10.1128/jvi.45.2.555-564.1983

Sutanto EN, Zhang D, Lai YKY, Shen W-Y, Rakoczy EP. 2005. Development and evaluation of the specificity of a cathepsin D proximal promoter in the eye. *Curr Eye Res* **30**: 53–61. doi:10.1080/02713680490894298

Trapani I, Colella P, Sommella A, Iodice C, Cesi G, de Simone S, Marrocco E, Rossi S, Giunti M, Palfi A, et al. 2014. Effective delivery of large genes to the retina by dual AAV vectors. *EMBO Mol Med* **6**: 194–211. doi:10.1002/emmm .201302948

Trapani I, Toriello E, de Simone S, Colella P, Iodice C, Polishchuk EV, Sommella A, Colecchi L, Rossi S, Simonelli F, et al. 2015. Improved dual AAV vectors with reduced expression of truncated proteins are safe and effective in the retina of a mouse model of Stargardt disease. *Hum Mol Genet* **24**: 6811–6825. doi:10.1093/hmg/ddv386

Vacca O, Darche M, Schaffer DV, Flannery JG, Sahel J-A, Rendon A, Dalkara D. 2014. AAV-mediated gene delivery in Dp71-null mouse model with compromised barriers. *Glia* **62**: 468–476. doi:10.1002/glia.22617

Vandenberghe LH, Bell P, Maguire AM, Cearley CN, Xiao R, Calcedo R, Wang L, Castle MJ, Maguire AC, Grant R, et al. 2011. Dosage thresholds for AAV2 and AAV8 photoreceptor gene therapy in monkey. *Sci Transl Med* **3**: 88ra54. doi:10.1126/scitranslmed.3002103

Weindler FW, Heilbronn R. 1991. A subset of herpes simplex virus replication genes provides helper functions for productive adeno-associated virus replication. *J Virol* **65**: 2476–2483. doi:10.1128/jvi.65.5.2476-2483.1991

Wistuba A, Weger S, Kern A, Kleinschmidt JA. 1995. Intermediates of adeno-associated virus type 2 assembly: identification of soluble complexes containing Rep and Cap

Cite this article as *Cold Spring Harb Perspect Med* doi: 10.1101/cshperspect.a041291

proteins. *J Virol* **69:** 5311–5319. doi:10.1128/jvi.69.9 .5311-5319.1995

Woodard KT, Liang KJ, Bennett WC, Samulski RJ. 2016. Heparan sulfate binding promotes accumulation of intra-vitreally delivered adeno-associated viral vectors at the retina for enhanced transduction but weakly influences tropism. *J Virol* **90:** 9878–9888. doi:10.1128/JVI.01568-16

Wu Z, Asokan A, Grieger JC, Govindasamy L, Agbandje-McKenna M, Samulski RJ. 2006. Single amino acid changes can influence titer, heparin binding, and tissue tropism in different adeno-associated virus serotypes. *J Virol* **80:** 11393–11397. doi:10.1128/JVI.01288-06

Xi Z, Öztürk BE, Johnson ME, Turunç S, Stauffer WR, Byrne LC. 2022. Quantitative single-cell transcriptome-based ranking of engineered AAVs in human retinal explants. *Mol Ther Methods* **25:** 476–489.

Xie Q, Bu W, Bhatia S, Hare J, Somasundaram T, Azzi A, Chapman MS. 2002. The atomic structure of adeno-associated virus (AAV-2), a vector for human gene therapy. *Proc Natl Acad Sci* **99:** 10405–10410. doi:10.1073/pnas .162250899

Xiong W, Wu DM, Xue Y, Wang SK, Chung MJ, Ji X, Rana P, Zhao SR, Mai S, Cepko CL. 2019. AAV *cis*-regulatory sequences are correlated with ocular toxicity. *Proc Natl Acad Sci* **116:** 5785–5794. doi:10.1073/pnas.1821000116

Ye G-J, Budzynski E, Sonnentag P, Nork TM, Sheibani N, Gurel Z, Boye SL, Peterson JJ, Boye SE, Hauswirth WW, et al. 2016. Cone-specific promoters for gene therapy of achromatopsia and other retinal diseases. *Hum Gene Ther* **27:** 72–82. doi:10.1089/hum.2015.130

Yiu G, Chung SH, Mollhoff IN, Nguyen UT, Thomasy SM, Yoo J, Taraborelli D, Noronha G. 2020. Suprachoroidal and subretinal injections of AAV using transscleral microneedles for retinal gene delivery in nonhuman primates. *Mol Ther Methods Clin Dev* **16:** 179–191.

Zhong L, Li B, Mah CS, Govindasamy L, Agbandje-McKenna M, Cooper M, Herzog RW, Zolotukhin I, Warrington KH, Aken KAWV, et al. 2008. Next generation of adeno-associated virus 2 vectors: point mutations in tyrosines lead to high-efficiency transduction at lower doses. *Proc Natl Acad Sci* **105:** 7827–7832. doi:10.1073/pnas.080 2866105

Zinn E, Pacouret S, Khaychuk V, Turunen HT, Carvalho LS, Andres-Mateos E, Shah S, Shelke R, Maurer AC, Plovie E, et al. 2015. In silico reconstruction of the viral evolutionary lineage yields a potent gene therapy vector. *Cell Rep* **12:** 1056–1068. doi:10.1016/j.celrep .2015.07.019

Zou J, Luo L, Shen Z, Chiodo VA, Ambati BK, Hauswirth WW, Yang J. 2011. Whirlin replacement restores the formation of the USH2 protein complex in whirlin knockout photoreceptors. *Invest Ophth Vis Sci* **52:** 2343–2351. doi:10.1167/iovs.10-6141

Immunology of Retinitis Pigmentosa and Gene Therapy–Associated Uveitis

Paul Yang,[1] Debarshi Mustafi,[2,3,4] and Kathryn L. Pepple[2]

[1]Casey Eye Institute, Oregon Health & Science University, Portland, Oregan 97239, USA

[2]Department of Ophthalmology, Roger and Karalis Johnson Retina Center, University of Washington, Seattle, Washington 98109, USA

[3]Brotman Baty Institute for Precision Medicine, Seattle, Washington 98109, USA

[4]Department of Ophthalmology, Seattle Children's Hospital, Seattle, Washington 98109, USA

Correspondence: yangp@ohsu.edu; kpepple@uw.edu

The underlying immune state of inherited retinal degenerations (IRDs) and retinitis pigmentosa (RP) has been an emerging area of interest, wherein the consequences have never been greater given the widespread recognition of gene therapy–associated uveitis (GTU) in gene therapy clinical trials. Whereas some evidence suggests that the adaptive immune system may play a role, the majority of studies indicate that the innate immune system is likely the primary driver of neuroinflammation in RP. During retinal degeneration, discrete mechanisms activate resident microglia and promote infiltrating macrophages that can either be protective or detrimental to photoreceptor cell death. This persistent stimulation of innate immunity, overlaid by the introduction of viral antigens as part of gene therapy, has the potential to trigger a complex microglia/macrophage-driven proinflammatory state. A better understanding of the immune pathophysiology in IRD and GTU will be necessary to improve the success of developing novel treatments for IRDs.

A HISTORY OF INFLAMMATION IN RETINITIS PIGMENTOSA

Inherited retinal degenerations (IRDs) are a heterogeneous group of predominantly monogenic disorders that result in retinal dysfunction and/or outer retinal degeneration (Daiger et al. 1998; Verbakel et al. 2018). Retinitis pigmentosa (RP) is the most common IRD with a prevalence of 1:4000, and is one of the leading causes of vision loss in the developed world (Hartong et al. 2006). Inflammation has long been suspected to be a component of RP. Indeed, the etymology of "retinitis" is indicative of the historical association of RP with inflammation of the retina. The many clinical biomarkers of inflammation in RP that are frequently observed contribute to this association, including vitreous cells, cystoid macular edema (CME), vascular sheathing, as well as retinal and vascular leakage on fluorescein angiography (Fetkenhour et al. 1977; Spalton et al. 1978; Pruett 1983; Heckenlively et al. 1985; Newsome 1986; Porta et al. 1992; van den Born et al. 1994;

Yoshida et al. 2013a). Following these clinical observations, a series of studies on peripheral blood lymphocytes from RP patients was performed in the 1980s that suggested an association between retinal degeneration and altered immune reactivity. The results, however, were tenuous and, over time, superseded by the discovery of the first causative gene for RP in 1990 (Dryja et al. 1990). Subsequent studies in RP shifted away from inflammation and toward gene discovery. With improvements in genetic testing technology and patient access over the past three decades (Mustafi et al. 2022), over 80 genes for RP and more than 300 IRD genes have been identified (Verbakel et al. 2018). Whereas the pendulum for research into the etiology of RP has decidedly shifted from inflammation to genetics, it is becoming clear that immune-mediated damage may be a critical component of cell death in RP and other IRDs.

Much of the evidence for immune-mediated damage or neuroinflammation in RP comes from studies in the rodent models of retinal degeneration that were developed to elucidate the primary mechanisms of genotype-specific photoreceptor degeneration in RP. The concept of immune-mediated damage or neuroinflammation as a secondary mechanism of neuronal cell death is not unique as it has been linked to well-known neurodegenerative conditions of the central nervous system (CNS) such as Alzheimer's and Parkinson's disease (Choi et al. 2021; Muzio et al. 2021). While innate and adaptive immune systems are intimately connected, and activation of one arm of the immune system generally implies involvement of the other, the growing body of literature indicates that innate immunity likely plays a greater role in RP-associated neuroinflammation. Multiple innate signaling pathways, effector cells, and soluble mediators activated by dead and dying photoreceptors have been shown to intensify photoreceptor degeneration and may be associated with clinical signs of inflammation (Murakami et al. 2020). In this review, we will provide an overview of the known and hypothesized mechanisms of retinal degeneration–associated neuroinflammation and their roles in RP pathogenesis. We will also discuss the possible impact of the underlying immune state of IRDs on retinal gene therapy and gene therapy–associated uveitis (GTU).

THE ADAPTIVE IMMUNE SYSTEM IN RP

A search for immune mechanisms involved in RP began during the era when powerful in vitro and in vivo tools to dissect T- and B-cell function in human disease were first being developed. In parallel lines of research, T lymphocytes were rapidly identified as important mediators of other inflammatory eye diseases such as uveitis (Caspi 2011). However, despite efforts that began in the 1980s, evidence that adaptive immune responses directly contribute to neuroinflammation and photoreceptor cell death in RP remains limited (for review, see Adamus 2021). Provocative results from early studies included T cells collected from patients with RP that demonstrated autoreactivity against soluble retinal antigens (Char et al. 1974; Brinkman et al. 1980; Heredia et al. 1981; Kumar et al. 1983; Newsome and Nussenblatt 1984; Chant et al. 1985; Heckenlively et al. 1985) and the presence of both T and B cells within vitreous biopsies from patients with RP (Newsome and Michels 1988). Together, these early studies suggested that the adaptive immune system in RP may be sensitized to retinal antigens and important in disease pathogenesis. Thus, the hypothesis that adaptive immunity plays a significant role in disease pathogenesis remains controversial as other investigators were not able to confirm the presence of any specific anamnestic response to retinal S antigen (also known as rod arrestin) in additional cohorts of RP patients (Benezra et al. 1984; Hendricks and Fishman 1985, 1986). Additionally, antiretinal autoantibodies are not found in all RP patients and can also be positive in normal control patients (Shimazaki et al. 2008). Other controversial findings of altered adaptive immune function that were not repeatable among different studies of patients with RP include elevated serum IgM levels, diminished lymphocyte production of interferon γ (IFN-γ), diminished monocyte expression of class II major histocompatibility (HLA-DR) antigens, and low-normal lymphocyte count and circulating immune complexes (Rahi 1973;

Spalton et al. 1978; Spiro et al. 1978; Hooks et al. 1983; Galbraith and Fudenberg 1984; García-Calderón et al. 1984; Detrick et al. 1985; Hendricks and Fishman 1985, 1986, 1987; Newsome et al. 1988). One potential reason for the inconsistencies within and between cohorts of RP patients may be the heterogeneous nature of the disease. It is possible that antiretinal adaptive immune responses may be more common in certain RP genotypes or only develop during specific phases in the course of retinal degeneration. As genetic testing for RP was not yet available in the 1980s, the genotype-specific data was not collected in these studies. One study in 1999 did show a correlation between the presence of CME and antiretinal antibodies in patients with RP, although the strength of the antiretinal antibody activity was not necessarily correlated with the severity of the CME or systemic autoimmune conditions (Heckenlively et al. 1999). However, the etiology of CME in RP has yet to be elucidated and it is not known whether the correlation found by Heckenlively et al. was simply a mutual consequence of a breakdown in the blood–retinal barrier (BRB). While the majority of patients in this study were skewed toward simplex RP, it is unknown whether this was due to sampling bias or a preponderance of CME in these patients. More recently, two studies using the serum of patients with RP provided some indirect evidence of adaptive as well as innate immune reactivity in retinal degeneration (Okita et al. 2020; Koyanagi et al. 2018). The authors showed that patients with RP had elevated levels of interleukin (IL)-8 (CXCL8) and regulated activation of normal T-cell-expressed and secreted (RANTES), which can be expressed by macrophages and monocytes, and play a role in chemotaxis of T cells, among other leukocytes. High-sensitivity C-reactive protein (hs-CRP) was also found to be elevated and correlated with a deterioration in the patient's visual field (Koyanagi et al. 2018). However, these data do not distinguish between causality versus sequelae of retinal degeneration, and provide only limited evidence that there may be a generalized (i.e., not retina-specific) reactivity of the systemic immune response in patients with RP. Finally, histopathology studies in human cadaver eyes

with RP have not identified retinal lymphocyte infiltration, a key hallmark of a tissue-specific adaptive autoimmune response, but rather observed microglia/macrophage infiltration into the photoreceptor layer (Gupta et al. 2003; Marc et al. 2003). Similar findings in the retina of multiple rodent models of RP have shifted the focus toward innate immune reactivity in retinal degeneration (Roque et al. 1996; Hughes et al. 2003; Zeiss and Johnson 2004; Zeng et al. 2005; Wang et al. 2013; Aredo et al. 2015; Zhao et al. 2015; Blank et al. 2018; Lew et al. 2020). Thus, the evidence for adaptive immunity in animal models of RP has been scant with the exception of two studies showing that memory T-cell activation may play a significant role in Royal College of Surgeons (RCS) rats (*Mertk* mutation) (Adamus et al. 2012; Kyger et al. 2013). Adamus and colleagues showed that systemic treatment with recombinant T-cell receptor ligand (RTL) immunotherapy, which tolerizes antigen-specific T cells to specific retinal proteins, delays photoreceptor degeneration in this rat model of RP. However, RTL immunotherapy is also known to inhibit microglia activation (Sinha et al. 2010), which limits the interpretation of these results as proof of a significant T-lymphocyte response in RP. In summary, the evidence for adaptive immune reactivity in RP is limited, and additional studies in patients and animal models will be required to evaluate its existence and potential impact on retinal degeneration.

THE INNATE IMMUNE SYSTEM IN RP

The innate immune system uses pattern recognition receptors (PRRs) not only to rapidly defend against microbial infections via the detection of pathogen-associated molecular patterns (PAMPs), but also to respond to noninfectious stimuli released during tissue damage or degeneration (Janeway and Medzhitov 2002). Even in the absence of infection, damage-associated molecular patterns (DAMPs) released from dead or dying cells can be potent activators of local inflammation that lead to additional local tissue injury. Once activated, innate immune cells shape adaptive immune responses through antigen presentation and cytokine production. Many aspects of innate immunity have been implicated in CNS neurodegenerative diseases with important pathogenic roles being identified for activated tissue-resident and blood-derived macrophages (Choi et al. 2021; Muzio et al. 2021). Thus, it is not surprising that microglia have been the focus of many studies with regard to neuroinflammation in RP.

In the healthy neuroretina, the innate immune system includes barriers such as an intact blood–retinal barrier (BRB) as well as the cellular and secreted factors that act to recognize and remove harmful pathogens and cellular debris without causing sight-threatening inflammation. In addition to forming the outer BRB, the retinal pigment epithelium (RPE) is well established as one of the most important cell types mediating ocular immune deviation (also known as immune privilege) by modulating the phenotypes and responses of inflammatory cells recruited to the retina (Keino et al. 2018; Taylor et al. 2021). Moreover, it is becoming evident that resident microglia, peripherally derived macrophages, and macroglia (Müller cells and astrocytes) collectively contribute to and modulate retinal neuroinflammation (Reichenbach and Bringmann 2020). In the following sections, we will summarize the evidence that support a mechanistic role for innate immunity in the pathogenesis of neuroinflammation in RP.

INNATE INTERCELLULAR SIGNALING

There is growing evidence showing that bidirectional communication among microglia, Müller cells, RPE, and photoreceptors is not only important in normal retinal homeostasis, but also plays a critical role in retinal degeneration (Rashid et al. 2019; Karlen et al. 2020). For example, the chemokine fractalkine (CX3CL1) is a neuroimmune modulator expressed by CNS neurons and the retina as a membrane-bound or soluble ligand, and its receptor, CX3CR1, is expressed by microglia (Wolf et al. 2013; Zabel et al. 2016). The CX3CL1-CX3CR1 signaling pathway has been shown to be a key immune regulator that mitigates microglial activation and phagocytosis in the rd10 mouse (*Pde6b* mutation) model of RP (Peng et al. 2014; Zabel et al. 2016; Roche et al. 2017). For example, genetic ablation of

CX3CR1 increased microglia/macrophage infiltration into the outer nuclear layer and accelerated photoreceptor degeneration (Peng et al. 2014). In addition, in vitro studies show that activated microglia can induce Müller cells to up-regulate glial cell line–derived neurotrophic factor (GDNF) and leukemia inhibitory factor (LIF), which are both neuroprotective to photoreceptors (Wang et al. 2011). The up-regulation of LIF expression by Müller cells has also been shown with in vivo experiments in VPP mice (*Rho* mutations) (Joly et al. 2008). Joly et al. confirmed the neuroprotective effect of LIF by showing that retinal degeneration was accelerated in VPP mice that lacked LIF due to genetic ablation. On the other hand, prior to any biomarkers of early or late apoptosis (caspase-3, cleaved PARP, or TUNEL), it has been shown that mutant rod photoreceptors from rd10 mice express phosphatidylserine (PS), which is recognized by microglia during phagocytosis initiation and presumably invites active phagocytosis of stressed rod photoreceptors (Zhao et al. 2015). While PS expression may potentiate precocious microglia-mediated photoreceptor cell death, Zhao et al. concluded that additional signals are likely required to trigger microglia phagocytosis during retinal degeneration. Indeed, PS is not unique to RP as it also mediates other essential microglia-mediated functions such as synaptic pruning during normal CNS neurodevelopment (Scott-Hewitt et al. 2020). In contrast, microglia that have migrated to the subretinal space in the $Rho^{P23H/wt}$ mouse model of RP have also been shown to interact with the RPE in a neuroprotective manner by promoting interdigitation of RPE microvilli with photoreceptor outer segments (O'Koren et al. 2019). While it is becoming clear that the innate immune response to retinal degeneration is modulated by a complex network of intercellular signals that are still being elucidated, one of the major triggers is likely DAMP molecules.

DAMAGE-ASSOCIATED MOLECULAR PATTERNS

DAMP molecules released from damaged or dead cells likely act synergistically with PS and other factors to trigger microglial activation (Tang et al. 2012; Mahaling et al. 2022). The innate immune system uses PRRs to recognize DAMPs, which can be derived from the extracellular matrix, plasma membrane, endoplasmic reticulum, mitochondria, cytoplasm, and nucleus of damaged retinal cells. In the degenerating retina, activation of PRRs such as Toll-like receptor (TLR)2 and 4 and nucleotide-binding oligomerization domain-like receptor pyrin domain 3 (NLRP3) has been reported, and a number of DAMPs have been identified/proposed that could trigger local inflammation and contribute to disease progression in RP (Kohno et al. 2013; Syeda et al. 2015; Viringipurampeer et al. 2016; Appelbaum et al. 2017; Sudharsan et al. 2017; Garces et al. 2020; Olivares-González et al. 2020). The list of DAMPs includes (1) high-mobility group box 1 (HMGB1), (2) heparan sulfate and chondroitin sulfate proteoglycans (HSPGs and CSPGs), (3) heat shock protein 70 (HSP70), and (4) β-amyloid. HMGB1 is an intracellular nuclear protein that is released into the extracellular space under conditions of stress or cell death (Scaffidi et al. 2002). The level of HMGB1 was found to be significantly elevated in the vitreous from patients with RP, and hypothesized to be released during programmed necrosis of photoreceptors (Murakami et al. 2015). HSPGs and CSPGs are components of the plasma membrane specific to the inner limiting membrane of the retina (Murillo-Lopez et al. 1991; Yanagishita and Hascall 1992). Retinal cultures from a mouse (rd also known as rd1 mice; *Pde6b* nonsense mutation) and rat model of RP (RCS rat; *Mertk* mutation) showed secretions that were most pronounced for HSPG after photoreceptor degeneration (Landers et al. 1994). Heat shock protein 70 is part of a family of molecular chaperones that prevent protein aggregation and are neuroprotective during cell stress (Furukawa and Koriyama 2016). Up-regulation of HSP70 has been observed in RPE cells from RP mice with a mutation in the *Prpf31* gene (Valdés-Sánchez et al. 2020). β-Amyloid deposition is typically associated with neurodegenerative diseases and thought to be pathologically derived from membrane-spanning amyloid precursor protein (APP) (Sisodia et al. 1990). While β-amyloid was not detected in the retina from patients with RP, there was an elevated level of APP immunoreactivity in the RPE cells (Löffler et al. 1995). Data demonstrating functional consequences associated with the presence of these DAMPs is lacking so their direct contribution to retinal degeneration is not yet fully understood.

RESIDENT MICROGLIA VERSUS PERIPHERALLY DERIVED MACROPHAGES

While there are many different ways an underlying genetic mutation causing RP leads to cellular dysfunction, photoreceptor and RPE cell death is the final common end point. In RP, photoreceptor cell death can occur by multiple mechanisms including apoptosis, regulated necrosis, and autophagy (Newton and Megaw 2020; Power et al. 2020). The intersection of these cell death pathways and activation of innate immunity is still not fully understood, but even when cell death occurs by the relatively noninflammatory process of apoptosis, immune function is required to clear the cellular debris (Chang et al. 1993). In the retina, this function is primarily provided by the retinal microglia. Microglia are resident immune cells of the retina that are uniquely derived from early mesodermal tissue and reside in the synaptic inner retinal layers with a stellate phenotype (Milam et al. 1998). In addition to providing immune surveillance, microglia also play a vital role in synaptic homeostasis and cross talk among Müller cells, RPE, and photoreceptors (Karlen et al. 2020). In both human and rodent studies of retinal degeneration in RP, it has been shown that photoreceptor cell death triggers the activation of microglia. Once activated, the microglia change in morphology and migrate from the plexiform layers to the photoreceptor outer nuclear layer and subretinal space (Thanos 1992; Gupta et al. 2003; Hughes et al. 2003; Marc et al. 2003; Zeiss and Johnson 2004; Zeng et al. 2005; Wang et al. 2013; Aredo et al. 2015; Zhao et al. 2015). Histopathologic evidence shows that these activated microglia contain rhodopsin-positive cytoplasmic inclusions, which confirms their role in removing the cellular debris of rod photoreceptor degeneration (Gupta et al. 2003). Müller cells have also been shown to phagocytose dead rod photoreceptors, contributing to a concerted effort to clear potentially inflammatory debris during the course of retinal degeneration (Sakami et al. 2019).

Despite the beneficial function of removing cellular debris following photoreceptor cell death, there is mounting evidence that retinal microglia may also play a role in hastening retinal degeneration. Initial evidence was first provided by experiments in RCS rats (*Mertk* mutation) showing that resident microglia migrated to the outer retina and phagocytosed dead photoreceptors during the onset of retinal degeneration (Thanos et al. 1996; Roque et al. 1999). These results were subsequently confirmed in multiple rodent models of RP, which demonstrated microglial activation preceding or coincident with structural photoreceptor cell death or apoptosis (Roque et al. 1996; Hughes et al. 2003; Zeiss and Johnson 2004; Zeng et al. 2005; Wang et al. 2013; Aredo et al. 2015; Zhao et al. 2015; Blank et al. 2018; Lew et al. 2020). In a landmark study using live-cell imaging, the theory that retinal microglia could exacerbate retinal degeneration was confirmed when active microglia were observed to infiltrate the outer retina and phagocytose nonapoptotic rod photoreceptors in rd10 mice (*Pde6b* mutation) (Zhao et al. 2015). By distinguishing resident microglia and infiltrating macrophages with different color fluorescent proteins driven by the expression of CX3CR1 and CCR2, respectively, Zhao et al. concluded that resident microglia were the primary source of the observed phagocytic behavior. Furthermore, the authors also showed that pharmacologic inhibition of phagocytosis or genetic ablation of resident microglia was effective in reducing photoreceptor degeneration. However, resident microglia have been shown to be necessary for the long-term maintenance of synaptic function and integrity in C57BL/6J wild-type adult mouse (Wang et al. 2016), which indicate that indiscriminate ablation of resident microglia will likely have unintended negative consequences. Taken together, these studies show that while resident microglia play an essential role in the homeostasis of the neurosensory retina and clear potentially inflammatory debris during retinal degeneration,

activated microglia can also exacerbate photoreceptor cell death by phagocytosing stressed photoreceptors.

In addition to the resident retinal microglia, multiple studies in RP models have shown that bone marrow–derived (BMD) peripheral monocytes cross the BRB into the degenerating neuroretina and rapidly differentiate into macrophages (for review, see Jin et al. 2017; Karlen et al. 2020). Once in the retina, these BMD macrophages are phenotypically difficult to distinguish from resident microglia without the use of lineage-tracing strategies (Jin et al. 2017; Karlen et al. 2020). As the main effector function of a macrophage is to drive inflammation and clear infectious pathogens, their presence in the degenerating retina has implicated them in neuroinflammation. Two studies attempted to clarify the role of infiltrating macrophages on retinal degeneration in rd10 mice by inhibiting retinal recruitment of BMD monocytes via various strategies (Sasahara et al. 2008; Guo et al. 2012). Sasahara and colleagues used either intravitreal injections of antibodies against stromal-derived factor 1 (SDF-1) or systemic depletion of myeloid progenitors using clodronate liposome. Guo et al. developed an rd10 mouse strain with a genetic knockout of the CCR2 receptor. Whereas reduction of monocyte recruitment using genetic ablation of CCR2 reduced retinal degeneration, the use of intravitreal anti-SDF-1 antibodies or systemic monocyte depletion actually exacerbated retinal degeneration. These studies suggest that the SDF-1/CXCR4 pathway for the recruitment of monocytes is neuroprotective, whereas the monocyte chemoattractant protein 1 (MCP-1)/CCR2 pathway is proinflammatory. Diffuse ablation of systemic monocytes with clodronate liposome probably had a net negative impact due to dysregulation of these two pathways. Moreover, clodronate liposome may also have cross-reactivity for both macrophages and activated microglia, which confounds interpretation of the results (Graykowski and Cudaback 2021). In summary, BMD monocytes appear to play a complex role during retinal degeneration wherein discrete mechanisms promote infiltrating macrophages that can either be protective or detrimental to photoreceptor cell death.

THE SPECTRUM OF MICROGLIA/ MACROPHAGE PHENOTYPES

In the degenerating retina, it appears that both resident microglia and infiltrating macrophages can be activated and recruited to develop either a neuroprotective housekeeping or proinflammatory neurotoxic phenotype. Traditionally, it is thought that microglia and macrophages can be activated to a neurotoxic M1 phenotype (classically activated) or neuroprotective M2 phenotype (alternatively activated); however, this dichotomy is now regarded as an oversimplification (Hu et al. 2015). It is more likely that subpopulations of microglia/macrophages exist with overlapping M1/M2 functionality. It is unknown exactly what series of retinal circumstances favors one phenotype over the other, but factors that alter the cytokine milieu and other cues in the retinal microenvironment are likely involved. For example, extracellular factors in the CNS that promote the M1 phenotype include tumor necrosis factor α (TNF-α), IL-1, IL-6, lipocalin-2, and IFN-γ, whereas the M2 phenotype is promoted by transforming growth factor β (TGF-β), IL-4, IL-10, IL-25, bone morphogenetic protein 7, galectin-1, and substance P (Hu et al. 2015).

The M1 phenotype is associated with oxidative stress, immune stimulation, and production of the following proinflammatory factors in the CNS: TNF-α, inducible nitric oxide synthase (iNOS), IL-1, IL-6, IL-12, and IL-23 (Hu et al. 2015). Elevated TNF-α and nitric oxide (NO) levels can cause direct photoreceptor cytotoxicity and cell death (Olivares-González et al. 2020; Toma et al. 2021). Activated microglia in rd1, rd7 (*Nr2e3* mutation), rd8 (*Crb1* mutation), rd10, and *Cngb1*$^{-/-}$ (*Cngb1* knockout) mice, and P23H (*Rho* mutation) rats secrete proinflammatory cytokines that can accelerate retinal degeneration, which include TNF-α, IL-1β, and IL-6 (Zeng et al. 2005; Guo et al. 2012; Wang et al. 2013, 2020; Yoshida et al. 2013b; Aredo et al. 2015; Zhao et al. 2015; Noailles et al. 2016; Blank et al. 2018). Indeed, genetic knockdown of TNF-α in T17M mice (*Rho* mutation) delayed photoreceptor degeneration (Rana et al. 2017). Inducible nitric oxide synthase, which

catalyzes production of NO, was shown to be expressed by subretinal microglia and macrophages during retinal degeneration in rd8 mice (Aredo et al. 2015). Other signs of immune activation in degenerating retinas include the expression of microglia and macrophage chemoattractants such as MCP-1(CCL2) and RANTES (CCL5) in rd1, rd10, and *Mertk*$^{-/-}$ (*Mertk* knockout) mice, and P23H and RCS (*Mertk* mutation) rats (Zeng et al. 2005; Guo et al. 2012; Yoshida et al. 2013b; Noailles et al. 2016; Lew et al. 2020). Lew et al. showed that in *Mertk*$^{-/-}$ mice and RCS rats, elevated levels of retinal RANTES mRNA was detectable at a time when retinal structure and function were normal, preceding microglia migration by ~6 d and peak photoreceptor cell death by ~11 d. In patients with RP, analysis of aqueous and vitreous fluid also support the presence of an M1 microglia/ macrophage-associated chronic inflammatory state as evidenced by abnormal elevations in the following cytokine and chemokine levels: IL-1α, IL-1β, IL-6, IL-8, TNF-α, IFN-γ, MCP-1, and RANTES (Yoshida et al. 2013a; Lu et al. 2020). In a paired aqueous-serum study, intraocular levels of IL-6 and MCP-1 were found to be higher in the aqueous than serum from patients with RP, which suggests that neuroinflammation in RP may be associated with proinflammatory signals from the innate immune system within the retina (Ten Berge et al. 2019).

Polarization of microglia and macrophages toward the M1 phenotype in the CNS (Yang et al. 2013; Liu et al. 2018) is facilitated by signaling through the TLR and IL-1 receptor (IL-1R) wherein the myeloid differentiation factor 88 (MyD88) is an important adaptor molecule. Activation of the TLR/MyD88 and IL-1R/ MyD88 pathway has been implicated in favoring the M1 phenotype in the rd1, rd10, and *Abca4*$^{-/-}$ *Rdh8*$^{-/-}$ (*Abca4 Rdh8* double-knockout) mice and canine models of RP (Kohno et al. 2013; Syeda et al. 2015; Appelbaum et al. 2017; Garces et al. 2020). Knocking out or blocking MyD88 reduces photoreceptor cell death in rd1 and rd10 mice, respectively (Syeda et al. 2015; Garces et al. 2020). In the rd1/*MyD88*$^{-/-}$ mice, TNF-α expression was also reduced. In the rd10 mice injected with MyD88 inhibitors, there was reduced microglia and macrophage migration to the outer retina and increased expression of arginase 1 (Arg1), a biomarker for the M2 phenotype. Expression of an important inflammation-associated transcription factor, nuclear factor κ light-chain enhancer of activated B cells (NF-κB), is also up-regulated during retinal degeneration in the RPE/subretinal microglia/macrophages isolates of rd8 mice and whole retinas of $Cngb1^{-/-}$ mice, which suggests this pathway may also be important for cytotoxic microglia activation (Aredo et al. 2015; Blank et al. 2017).

The M2 phenotype is associated with phagocytic debris clearance, secretion of neurotrophic factors, mitigation of inflammation, and expression of the following anti-inflammatory factors in the CNS: TGF-β, IL-4, IL-10, and IL-1R antagonists (Hu et al. 2015). TGF-β signaling was found to be neuroprotective during retinal degeneration in rd1, rd10, $Rho^{-/-}$ (Rho knockout), and VPP mice (Wang et al. 2020; Bielmeier et al. 2022). In vitro studies also showed that addition of TGF-β reduced the propensity of Müller cells from RCS rats to secrete TNF-α and NO (Cotinet et al. 1997). In vivo studies that overexpress TGF-β1 using adeno-associated virus (AAV)-mediated gene therapy in rd1 mice showed that the neuroprotection was specific to cone photoreceptors and likely mediated by microglia (Wang et al. 2020). When resident microglia were chemically depleted, the benefit of TGF-β1 overexpression was abrogated. In a study of ocular fluid in patients with RP, Yoshida et al. observed elevated levels of IL-10, which is associated with the M2 phenotype (Yoshida et al. 2013a; Hu et al. 2015). Taken together, the cytokine profiles found in these animal and human studies appear to be skewed toward neuroinflammation and the M1 phenotype, although anti-inflammatory protective cytokines were also observed, underscoring the complexity of the innate immune system in RP.

IMMUNOSUPPRESSION AND IMMUNOMODULATION IN RP

Given that the evidence thus far suggests that activated microglia and macrophage subgroups in RP may exhibit a maladaptive proinflamma-tory response, there have been a number of studies examining the effects of different pharmacologic immunosuppressive or immunomodulatory agents in animal models of RP. One of the first studies of immunosuppression was performed in RCS (Mertk mutation) and S334ter-4 (Rho mutation) rats, wherein intravitreal fluocinolone acetonide implants were found to reduce photoreceptor degeneration and microglial activation (Glybina et al. 2009, 2010). These two studies suggest that corticosteroids may inhibit microglia and macrophage-mediated neuroinflammation during retinal degeneration. Indeed, it has been shown that CNS microglia express specific glucocorticoid receptors (Sierra et al. 2008), and corticosteroids suppress the ability of activated CNS microglia to produce iNOS, NO, and TNF-α, which are known to mediate neurotoxicity (Drew and Chavis 2000; Golde et al. 2003). While synthetic corticosteroids have long been the gold standard anti-inflammatory drug for treating numerous inflammatory and autoimmune conditions, their long-term use for chronic conditions is limited by a wide range of serious side-effects (Ramamoorthy and Cidlowski 2016). More recently, sustained release intravitreal corticosteroids, which avoid systemic side effects, have been approved for the treatment of diabetic macular edema and noninfectious posterior uveitis (Abdulla et al. 2022; Ehlers et al. 2022). However, the risks of glaucoma and cataract may still outweigh the potential benefits in RP given that the expected benefit is not a gain of function, but rather a slower decline in vision loss over decades that would require repeated injections.

To avoid corticosteroid-associated side-effects, two of the most commonly used steroid-sparing immunomodulators have been explored in animal models of RP: the antimetabolite, mycophenolate mofetil (MMF), and the anti-TNF-α biologic agent, adalimumab. Yang et al. recently showed that systemic administration of MMF potently slowed retinal degeneration and reduced microglial/macrophage activation in the rd10 and rd1 mouse models of RP (Yang et al. 2020). Classically, MMF is known to suppress lymphocyte proliferation by reducing purine synthesis via the reversible inhibition of inosine monophosphate dehydrogenase (IMPDH) (Allison and Eugui 2000), but it has also been shown to inhibit CNS microglia activation and migration (Dehghani et al. 2003, 2010; Ebrahimi et al. 2012; Kleine et al. 2022). However, Yang et al. also showed that the suppression of purine synthesis by MMF produces neuroprotection that is upstream to microglia activation via the mitigation of cGMP photoreceptor cytotoxicity, an alternative pathway for cell death for certain genotypes of RP (Arango-Gonzalez et al. 2014). Alternatively, adalimumab is a monoclonal antibody that has a very specific mechanism of action: to bind and block TNF-α (Mirshahi et al. 2012), which is an inflammatory cytokine secreted by the neurotoxic M1 microglia/macrophage phenotype, as discussed in the previous section. In rd10 mice, both intravitreal or systemic delivery of adalimumab delayed photoreceptor cell death, microglia and Müller cell activation, and decreased expression of TNF-α (Martínez-Fernández de la Cámara et al. 2015; Olivares-González et al. 2020). These results further support the theory that M1 microglia/macrophages play a significant role in retinal degeneration. Clinically, the safety and efficacy of intravitreal anti-TNF-α remains to be proven (Pascual-Camps et al. 2014; Leal et al. 2018), but systemically delivered adalimumab is FDA-approved for noninfectious uveitis. Although the long-term use of MMF and anti-TNF-α has already been proven safe and effective for treatment of other inflammatory eye diseases (Daniel et al. 2010; Mirshahi et al. 2012), the benefit-to-risk ratio of systemic immune suppression in IRDs remains to be determined given the course of retinal degeneration that would require decades of treatment for a lifetime.

Other nontraditional anti-inflammatory agents that are not typically regarded as immunomodulators have also shown promise in animal models of RP. Both norgestrel and minocycline have been shown to slow retinal degeneration and reduce microglial activation in rd10 mice (Peng et al. 2014; Roche et al. 2016, 2017, 2018). In addition, minocycline was shown to be neuroprotective in five other models of RP: rds (*Prph2* mutation) mice, *Mertk*$^{-/-}$ mice, *Rho*$^{-/-}$ mice, P23H rat, and RCS rat (Hughes et al. 2004;

Di Pierdomenico et al. 2018; Terauchi et al. 2021; Ozaki et al. 2022). Although minocycline is primarily a second-generation tetracycline antibiotic, it also has antiapoptotic and anti-inflammatory properties in neurodegenerative diseases (Peng et al. 2014; Möller et al. 2016). Similarly, norgestrel, a synthetic progesterone analog, also has many potential mechanisms of action that include the up-regulation of growth factors, reducing excitotoxicity, and suppressing microglia and macrophage activation (Pardue and Allen 2018). Moreover, the neuroprotective effect of norgestrel has been shown to be dependent on the up-regulation of CX3CR1 signaling in retinal microglia (Peng et al. 2014; Roche et al. 2016, 2017). Tauroursodeoxycholic acid (TUDCA), which has neuroprotective properties, has been shown to reduce retinal degeneration in multiple rodent models (rd1, rd10, Bbs1, and *Lrat*$^{-/-}$ mice) and also inhibit microglia activation and migration in P23H rats and *Rpgr* conditional knockout mice (Boatright et al. 2006; Phillips et al. 2008; Fernández-Sánchez et al. 2011, 2022; Oveson et al. 2011; Drack et al. 2012; Zhang et al. 2012, 2019; Noailles et al. 2014; Lawson et al. 2016).

IMMUNE RESPONSE TO VIRAL VECTOR–ASSOCIATED GENE THERAPY

The FDA approval of the first retinal gene therapy in 2017 for patients with retinal dystrophy associated with biallelic mutations in *RPE65* (Maguire et al. 2021) and subsequent explosion in the number of clinical trials in the pipeline for other genotypes have demonstrated the importance of gene therapy for the treatment of IRDs. With over 30 gene therapy clinical trials in the works for various IRDs (Thompson et al. 2020), it is increasingly important to not only understand the pathophysiology of the retinal degeneration, but also any associated immune-mediated responses to therapy. Clinical signs of GTU have included anterior chamber cells and flare, keratic precipitates, vitritis, panuveitis, and choroidal scarring or atrophy (Gange et al. 2022; for review, see Bucher et al. 2021). The following risk factors for GTU have been identified in preclinical studies and human clinical trials: higher viral dose (≥1e11 vg/eye), impurities such as empty viral capsids in the gene therapy product, delivery by the intravitreal rather than subretinal route, and use of ubiquitous promoters and certain nonmammalian transgenes (Xiong et al. 2019; Bucher et al. 2021; Timmers et al. 2020; Chan et al. 2021a; Mehta et al. 2021). Emerging considerations also include the contribution of host-specific factors such as the baseline immune state of IRD (Mishra et al. 2021; Vijayasarathy et al. 2021). Fortunately, the majority of reports in human subjects indicate that GTU is typically mild, transient, and responsive to treatment with topical and oral corticosteroids. However, despite treatment with corticosteroids, some eyes have experienced serious adverse events (Kuzmin et al. 2021) including vision loss attributed to severe inflammatory responses (Bainbridge et al. 2015; Wilson et al. 2017; Adverum Biotechnologies 2021) or required chronic immunosuppression for persistent uveitis (Pennesi et al. 2022). These adverse events have heightened the need to better understand the underlying pathophysiology of GTU to minimize the risks and develop better treatments.

Both systemic and local steroids have been used for treatment of incident inflammation following gene therapy administration (Cukras et al. 2018; Bouquet et al. 2019). As the risk of inflammation from gene therapy administration became more widely appreciated, clinical trial protocols began to include prophylactic perioperative oral and/or periocular steroid treatment. Corticosteroids appear to be more effective in suppressing acute signs of inflammation following subretinal compared to intravitreal delivery; however, high viral genomes administered by either route can still provoke inflammation despite corticosteroid prophylaxis (Bucher et al. 2021; Supplemental Figures 18 and 19 in Chan et al. 2021b). Due the risks of systemic and local corticosteroids (Suhler et al. 2017; Valdes and Sobrin 2020), alternative and additional methods of immune modulation have been used in both animal model studies and human clinical trials to improve inflammation prevention (Byrne et al. 2020; Mishra et al. 2021). Corticosteroid dose, duration of treatment, and the incorporation of alternative immune modulating drugs vary widely across clinical trials as the optimal approach remains to be determined. Ultimately, different approaches may be needed to best address the combined differences in the underlying neuroinflammatory state of a given IRD and the inflammatory response to different gene therapy products.

The primary routes of gene therapy administration for retinal disease are intravitreal, subretinal, or suprachoroidal injection (Ochakovski et al. 2017; Ding et al. 2019; Shen et al. 2020; Yiu et al. 2020). Each approach has pros and cons ranging from complexity of the procedure, access to target tissues, and risk of eliciting undesirable immune responses. The subretinal route generates less clinically evident uveitis and systemic humoral responses against AAV capsid than intravitreal injection (Li et al. 2008; Reichel et al. 2018), but serum antibody responses continue to be a widely used biomarker for correlation with variables driving ocular inflammation (Ail et al. 2022). One proposed explanation for this observation is that lower viral doses are delivered and sequestered within the subretinal bleb, which limits off-target transduction of nonretinal tissues and antigen-presenting cells found in the choroid, ciliary body, and iris, thereby limiting activation of the local and systemic immune system against gene therapy–associated antigens (Streilein 2003; McMenamin et al. 2019). Additionally, the RPE provides many cell surface ligands and secreted factors that enforce a state of local immune tolerance (Taylor et al. 2021). Therefore, the subretinal space is likely an area of immune deviation that is more tolerant and can harbor higher doses of AAV before a local inflammatory response is elicited. However, some of these theoretical benefits of the subretinal approach are being reconsidered in light of new data. First, reflux from the subretinal bleb into the vitreous has been demonstrated in human eyes using intraoperative OCT (Davis et al. 2019; Vasconcelos et al. 2020). Second, animal studies indicate that gene therapy can overwhelm tolerizing mechanisms of the subretinal space. Using flow cytometry, Chandler et al. demonstrated that subretinal injections in wild-type mice led to the accumulation of intraretinal CD45[+] cells, including CD4[+]

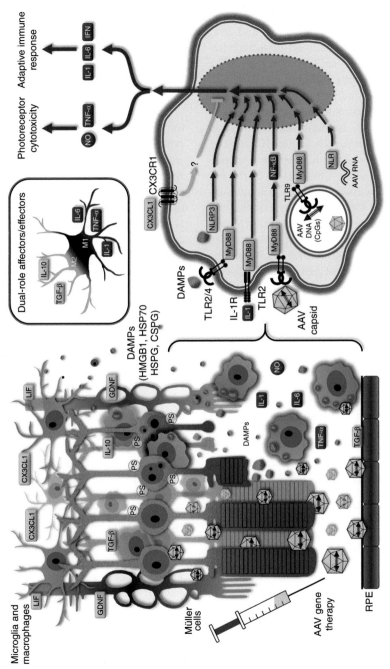

Figure 1. (*See following page for legend.*)

and CD8[+] T cells, indicating that the systemic immune system is fully capable of responding to subretinal gene therapy despite injection into this relatively immunologically privileged space (Chandler et al. 2021). Furthermore, these results demonstrated a similar number and array of CD45[+] cells as were identified following intravitreal injections in mice (Tummala et al. 2021), suggesting that despite minimal signs of clinical inflammation, any administration of gene therapy with AAV vectors to the eye stimulates an immune response. Immunohistochemistry in large animal models, such as pigs (Chan et al. 2021b) and nonhuman primate models (Timmers et al. 2020; Chung et al. 2021), has also identified activation of local glia and infiltration of CD3[+] T cells following subretinal injection, confirming immune recognition of subretinal gene therapy across multiple mammalian species. The clinical significance of this immune reaction to the efficacy of gene therapy delivered by subretinal injection remains to be determined. However, results from studies using AAV-mediated gene therapy for the treatment of hemophilia raise the possibility that immune recognition can carry the risk of T-cell-mediated killing of transduced cells (Manno et al. 2006). At this time, there is no clinical or experimental evidence that T-cell cytotoxicity occurs following administration of ocular gene therapy. But this mechanism or other forms of cell death (apoptosis, pyroptosis, or necroptosis) could be responsible for the perifoveal chorioretinal atrophy that occurs months to years postoperatively in a small proportion of patients who have received subretinal gene therapy for *RPE65*-associated retinal dystrophy (Gange et al. 2022). In addition, exacerbation of RPE atrophy has also been reported in a phase 1/2 clinical trial using a lentiviral vector for subretinal gene therapy in patients with *ABCA4*-associated retinal dystrophy (Parker et al. 2022), suggesting that the underlying mechanisms of RPE toxicity or immune damage are not limited to AAV vectors.

Compared to subretinal administration, intravitreal vector administration more frequently exhibits a stronger dose-dependent association with GTU (Bucher et al. 2021; Chan et al. 2021b; Ail et al. 2022). The specific mechanisms responsible for GTU remain to be proven, but extrapolation from other studies in experimental models of ocular infection and autoimmune uveitis suggests that AAV capsid and genomic material activate uveal-resident, antigen-presenting cells such as dendritic cells and microglia/macrophages through innate immune receptors (Fig. 1). TLR9 detects viral DNA by recognition of the phosphodiester backbone of DNA and is enhanced by the presence of unmethylated cytosine-phosphate-guanine (CpG) motifs (Haas et al. 2008; Rogers et al. 2011). TLR2 has also been implicated in sensing the AAV capsid (Hösel et al. 2012). Both TLR2 and TLR9 signal through the downstream adaptor protein MyD88 to induce the expression of type 1 interferons and proinflammatory cytokines, which, in turn, activate local inflammation and prime the adaptive immune response (Zhu et al. 2009).

Figure 1. The innate immune response to photoreceptor degeneration and adeno-associated virus (AAV) gene therapy. As photoreceptors degenerate, damage-associated molecular patterns (DAMPs) are liberated and phosphatidylserine (PS) is expressed on stressed photoreceptors, which likely act in concert to trigger resident microglia activation and bone-derived macrophage infiltration. DAMPs can be composed of HMGB1, heparan sulfate and chondroitin sulfate proteoglycans (HSPGs and CSPGs), and heat shock protein 70 (HSP70). The innate immune response is modulated by intercellular signaling that involves the microglia/macrophages, Müller cells, retinal pigment epithelium (RPE), and photoreceptors. Neuroprotective factors include chemokine fractalkine (CX3CL1), transforming growth factor β (TGF-β), IL-10, glial cell line–derived neurotrophic factor (GDNF), and leukemia inhibitory factor (LIF). Proinflammatory factors include IL-1, IL-6, tumor necrosis factor α (TNF-α), and nitric oxide (NO). The pattern-recognition receptors for DAMPs and AAV antigens include Toll-like receptor (TLR) and nucleotide-binding oligomerization domain-like receptor (NLR). Microglia also express receptors for IL-1 (IL-1R) and CX3CL1 (CX3CR1). Myeloid differentiating factor 88 (MyD88) is an important adaptor molecule for the TLR and IL-1 pathways. Ultimately, microglia can be activated to a proinflammatory M1 phenotype that expresses TNF-α and NO, which are cyotototic, as well as IL-1, IL-6, and interferon (IFN), which promote an adaptive immune response. (NLRP3) NLR pyrin domain 3.

TLR9 is not only important for innate recognition of AAV vectors, but its activation also influences the development of antitransgene T-cell responses in experimental models (Ashley et al. 2019). Moreover, vectors engineered to inhibit TLR9 signaling can significantly decrease inflammation in mouse and pig models, but are less effective in preventing inflammation in nonhuman primate models (Chan et al. 2021b). While these results make inhibition of innate signaling at the time of gene therapy administration an attractive target for potential therapeutic intervention, neutralizing antibodies can still be generated in MyD88-deficient animals, indicating that alternative pathways are sufficient for generating adaptive immune responses to AAV vectors (Rogers et al. 2015).

The increased appreciation for the incidence and severity of GTU has grown in proportion to the number of gene therapy trials and participants involved. In parallel, the possibility has been raised that inflammation may be more common in certain patient populations due to disease-associated risk factors yet to be identified (Adverum Biotechnologies 2021). The susceptibility of different forms of IRD to develop an underlying proinflammatory state is now an area of active interest, as discussed extensively in this review with regard to RP. Another example is the retinoschisin (RS1) knockout mouse model of X-linked retinoschisis (XLRS), wherein bulk RNA-seq on retinal tissues has identified marked up-regulation of multiple immune response pathway genes consistent with a microglia-driven proinflammatory state in degenerating retina (Vijayasarathy et al. 2021). Remarkably, gene replacement with AAV8-RS1 in this mouse model not only rescued retinal structure and function, but it also induced the microglia toward an immune quiescent state. However, in the gene therapy clinical trial for XLRS using an intravitreal injection of the same vector, dose-related GTU was observed in 44% of patients and structural/functional rescue of the retina was not generally observed (Cukras et al. 2018). After gene therapy, serum studies showed a dose-related increase in anti-AAV8 antibodies, but antibodies against the gene product, RS1, were not detected. A follow-up study of the serum and peripheral blood mononuclear cell samples from the same subjects revealed elevated proinflammatory cytokines and elevated baseline CD4/CD8 T-cell ratios, which was modestly correlated with GTU (Mishra et al. 2021). The authors conclude that the degenerating retina in XLRS may prime the immune system for an inflammatory response to AAV transduction, which may reduce the efficacy of gene therapy. These studies underscore the need to better understand the underlying immune state of different IRDs, especially in the context of the risk for GTU and reduced therapeutic potential of AAV-associated gene therapy.

CONCLUSION

Although the genetic etiology of IRD is well established, the underlying immune state of IRDs and especially the role of the innate immune system to exacerbate photoreceptor degeneration in RP has been an emerging area of interest for the past several decades. The consequences of understanding the role of the immune system in IRDs has never been greater, especially given the increasingly widespread recognition of GTU in gene therapy clinical trials and its potential impact on meeting safety and efficacy end points. While some evidence suggests that the adaptive immune system may play a role, the majority of the studies indicate that the innate immune system is likely the primary driver of neuroinflammation and GTU. During retinal degeneration and GTU, TLRs and NLRs work in concert to recognize DAMPs liberated from photoreceptor cell death and viral vector–associated PAMPs (AAV capsid, DNA, and RNA). It is possible that the persistent stimulation of DAMPs in IRDs, overlaid by the introduction of PAMPs as part of gene therapy, has the potential to exacerbate a complex microglia/macrophage-driven proinflammatory state with an uncertain outcome. Clearly, additional work developing models of IRD in nonhuman primates that recapitulate the human immune system and use new technologies such as induced pluripotent stem cell (iPSC)-derived microglia (Abud et al. 2017) and single-cell RNA sequencing of pathological microglia (Gosselin et al. 2017) will be necessary to provide further insights into this evolving field. By improving our understanding of the innate immune system in IRD and GTU, novel strategies can be developed to treat both the immune pathophysiology of IRDs and improve the success of gene therapy clinical trials in IRDs.

ACKNOWLEDGMENTS

We acknowledge funding sources from the NIH R01EY030431 (K.L.P.), University of Washington (UW) vision research core grant (NEI P30EY01730), Oregon Health and Science (OHSU) core grant (NEI P30EY010572), unrestricted departmental grants from Research to Prevent Blindness (UW, Oregon Health Sciences University [OHSU]), career development ment award from Research to Prevent Blindness (K.L.P.), the Graham Siddall uveitis research fund (K.L.P.), and the Foundation Fighting Blindness TRAP1 Award TA-NMT-0521-0803-OHSU-TRAP (P.Y.).

REFERENCES

Abdulla D, Ali Y, Menezo V, Taylor SRJ. 2022. The use of sustained release intravitreal steroid implants in non-infectious uveitis affecting the posterior segment of the eye. *Ophthalmol Ther* 11: 479–487. doi:10.1007/s40123-022-00456-4

Abud EM, Ramirez RN, Martinez ES, Healy LM, Nguyen CHH, Newman SA, Yeromin AV, Scarfone VM, Marsh SE, Fimbres C, et al. 2017. iPSC-derived human microglia-like cells to study neurological diseases. *Neuron* 94: 278–293.e9. doi:10.1016/j.neuron.2017.03.042

Adamus G. 2021. Importance of autoimmune responses in progression of retinal degeneration initiated by gene mutations. *Front Med* 8: 672444. doi:10.3389/fmed.2021.672444

Adamus G, Wang S, Kyger M, Worley A, Lu B, Burrows GG. 2012. Systemic immunotherapy delays photoreceptor cell loss and prevents vascular pathology in Royal College of Surgeons rats. *Mol Vis* 18: 2323–2337.

Adverum Biotechnologies. 2021. Adverum provides update on ADVM-022 and the INFINITY trial in patients with diabetic macular edema. https://www.globenewswire.com/news-release/2021/07/22/2267699/32452/en/Adverum-Provides-Update-on-ADVM-022-and-the-INFINITY-Trial-in-Patients-with-Diabetic-Macular-Edema.html [accessed May 17, 2022].

Ail D, Ren D, Brazhnikova E, Nouvel-Jaillard C, Bertin S, Mirashrafi SB, Fisson S, Dalkara D. 2022. Systemic and local immune responses to intraocular AAV vector administration in non-human primates. *Mol Ther Methods Clin Dev* 24: 306–316. doi:10.1016/j.omtm.2022.01.011

Allison AC, Eugui EM. 2000. Mycophenolate mofetil and its mechanisms of action. *Immunopharmacology* 47: 85–118. doi:10.1016/S0162-3109(00)00188-0

Appelbaum T, Santana E, Aguirre GD. 2017. Strong upregulation of inflammatory genes accompanies photoreceptor demise in canine models of retinal degeneration. *PLoS ONE* 12: e0177224. doi:10.1371/journal.pone.0177224

Arango-Gonzalez B, Trifunović D, Sahaboglu A, Kranz K, Michalakis S, Farinelli P, Koch S, Koch F, Cottet S, Janssen-Bienhold U, et al. 2014. Identification of a common non-apoptotic cell death mechanism in hereditary retinal degeneration. *PLoS ONE* 9: e112142. doi:10.1371/journal.pone.0112142

Aredo B, Zhang K, Chen X, Wang CXZ, Li T, Ufret-Vincenty RL. 2015. Differences in the distribution, phenotype and gene expression of subretinal microglia/macrophages in C57BL/6N (Crb1rd8/rd8) versus C57BL6/J (Crb1wt/wt) mice. *J Neuroinflammation* 12: 6. doi:10.1186/s12974-014-0221-4

Ashley SN, Somanathan S, Giles AR, Wilson JM. 2019. TLR9 signaling mediates adaptive immunity following systemic AAV gene therapy. *Cell Immunol* 346: 103997. doi:10.1016/j.cellimm.2019.103997

Bainbridge JW, Mehat MS, Sundaram V, Robbie SJ, Barker SE, Ripamonti C, Georgiadis A, Mowat FM, Beattie SG, Gardner PJ, et al. 2015. Long-term effect of gene therapy on Leber's congenital amaurosis. *N Engl J Med* 372: 1887–1897. doi:10.1056/NEJMoa1414221

Benezra D, Gery I, Chan CC, Nussen-Blatt RB, Palestine AG, Kaiser-Kupfer M, Maftzir G, Peer J. 1984. Cellular and humoral immune parameters among patients with retinitis pigmentosa and other retinal disorders. *Ophthalmic Paediatr Genet* 4: 193–197. doi:10.3109/13816818409006121

Bielmeier CB, Schmitt SI, Kleefeldt N, Boneva SK, Schlecht A, Vallon M, Tamm ER, Hillenkamp J, Ergün S, Neueder A, et al. 2022. Deficiency in retinal TGFβ signaling aggravates neurodegeneration by modulating pro-apoptotic and MAP kinase pathways. *Int J Mol Sci* 23: 2626. doi:10.3390/ijms23052626

Blank T, Goldmann T, Koch M, Amann L, Schön C, Bonin M, Pang S, Prinz M, Burnet M, Wagner JE, et al. 2018. Early microglia activation precedes photoreceptor degeneration in a mouse model of CNGB1-linked retinitis pigmentosa. *Front Immunol* 8: 1930. doi:10.3389/fimmu.2017.01930

Boatright JH, Moring AG, McElroy C, Phillips MJ, Do VT, Chang B, Hawes NL, Boyd AP, Sidney SS, Stewart RE, et al. 2006. Tool from ancient pharmacopoeia prevents vision loss. *Mol Vis* 12: 1706–1714.

Bouquet C, Clermont CV, Galy A, Fitoussi S, Blouin L, Munk MR, Valero S, Meunier S, Katz B, Sahel JA, et al. 2019. Immune response and intraocular inflammation in patients with Leber hereditary optic neuropathy treated with intravitreal injection of recombinant adeno-associated virus 2 carrying the *ND4* gene: a secondary analysis of a phase 1/2 clinical trial. *JAMA Ophthalmol* 137: 399–406. doi:10.1001/jamaophthalmol.2018.6902

Brinkman CJ, Pinckers AJ, Broekhuyse RM. 1980. Immune reactivity to different retinal antigens in patients suffering from retinitis pigmentosa. *Invest Ophthalmol Vis Sci* **19**: 743–750.

Bucher K, Rodríguez-Bocanegra E, Dauletbekov D, Dominik Fischer M. 2021. Immune responses to retinal gene therapy using adeno-associated viral vectors—implications for treatment success and safety. *Prog Retin Eye Res* **83**: 100915. doi:10.1016/j.preteyeres.2020.100915

Byrne LC, Day TP, Visel M, Strazzeri JA, Fortuny C, Dalkara D, Merigan WH, Schaffer DV, Flannery JG. 2020. In vivo-directed evolution of adeno-associated virus in the primate retina. *JCI Insight* **5**: e135112. doi:10.1172/jci.insight .135112

Caspi RR. 2011. Understanding autoimmune uveitis through animal models the Friedenwald Lecture. *Invest Ophthalmol Vis Sci* **52**: 1873–1879. doi:10.1167/iovs.10-6909

Chan YK, Dick AD, Hall SM, Langmann T, Scribner CL, Mansfield BC, Group OGTIW Others. 2021a. Inflammation in viral vector-mediated ocular gene therapy: a review and report from a workshop hosted by the foundation fighting blindness, 9/2020. *Transl Vis Sci Technol* **10**: 3.

Chan YK, Wang SK, Chu CJ, Copland DA, Letizia AJ, Verdera HC, Chiang JJ, Sethi M, Wang MK, Neidermyer WJ, et al. 2021b. Engineering adeno-associated viral vectors to evade innate immune and inflammatory responses. *Sci Transl Med* **13**: eabd3438. doi:10.1126/scitranslmed. abd3438

Chandler LC, McClements ME, Yusuf IH, Martinez-Fernandez de la Camara C, MacLaren RE, Xue K. 2021. Characterizing the cellular immune response to subretinal AAV gene therapy in the murine retina. *Mol Ther Methods Clin Dev* **22**: 52–65. doi:10.1016/j.omtm.2021 .05.011

Chang GQ, Hao Y, Wong F. 1993. Apoptosis: final common pathway of photoreceptor death in *rd*, *rds*, and mutant mice. *Neuron* **11**: 595–605. doi:10.1016/0896-6273(93) 90072-Y

Chant SM, Heckenlively J, Meyers-Elliott RH. 1985. Autoimmunity in hereditary retinal degeneration. I: Basic studies. *Br J Ophthalmol* **69**: 19–24. doi:10.1136/ bjo.69.1.19

Char DH, Bergsma DR, Rabson AS, Albert DM, Herberman RB. 1974. Cell-mediated immunity to retinal antigens in patients with pigmentary retinal degenerations. *Invest Ophthalmol* **13**: 198–203.

Choi S, Guo L, Cordeiro MF. 2021. Retinal and brain microglia in multiple sclerosis and neurodegeneration. *Cells* **10**: 1507. doi:10.3390/cells10061507

Chung SH, Mollhoff IN, Mishra A, Sin T-N, Ngo T, Ciulla T, Sieving P, Thomasy SM, Yiu G. 2021. Host immune responses after suprachoroidal delivery of AAV8 in nonhuman primate eyes. *Hum Gene Ther* **32**: 682–693. doi:10 .1089/hum.2020.281

Cotinet A, Goureau O, Hicks D, Thillaye-Goldenberg B, de Kozak Y. 1997. Tumor necrosis factor and nitric oxide production by retinal Müller glial cells from rats exhibiting inherited retinal dystrophy. *Glia* **20**: 59–69. doi:10 .1002/(SICI)1098-1136(199705)20:1<59::AID-GLIA6>3 .0.CO;2-0

Cukras C, Wiley HE, Jeffrey BG, Sen HN, Turriff A, Zeng Y, Vijayasarathy C, Marangoni D, Ziccardi L, Kjellstrom S, et al. 2018. Retinal AAV8-RS1 gene therapy for X-linked

retinoschisis: initial findings from a phase I/IIa trial by intravitreal delivery. *Mol Ther* **26**: 2282–2294. doi:10 .1016/j.ymthe.2018.05.025

Daiger S, Rossiter BJF, Greenberg J, Christoffels A, Hide W. 1998. Data services and software for identifying genes and mutations causing retinal degeneration. *Invest Ophthalmol Vis Sci* **39**: S295.

Daniel E, Thorne JE, Newcomb CW, Pujari SS, Kaçmaz RO, Levy-Clarke GA, Nussenblatt RB, Rosenbaum JT, Suhler EB, Foster CS, et al. 2010. Mycophenolate mofetil for ocular inflammation. *Am J Ophthalmol* **149**: 423–432. e2. doi:10.1016/j.ajo.2009.09.026

Davis JL, Gregori NZ, MacLaren RE, Lam BL. 2019. Surgical technique for subretinal gene therapy in humans with inherited retinal degeneration. *Retina* **39**(Suppl 1): S2–S8. doi:10.1097/IAE.0000000000002609

Dehghani F, Hischebeth GTR, Wirjatijasa F, Kohl A, Korf H-W, Hailer NP. 2003. The immunosuppressant mycophenolate mofetil attenuates neuronal damage after excitotoxic injury in hippocampal slice cultures. *Eur J Neurosci* **18**: 1061–1072. doi:10.1046/j.1460-9568.2003.02821.x

Dehghani F, Sayan M, Conrad A, Evers J, Ghadban C, Blaheta R, Korf HW, Hailer NP. 2010. Inhibition of microglial and astrocytic inflammatory responses by the immunosuppressant mycophenolate mofetil. *Neuropathol Appl Neurobiol* **36**: 598–611. doi:10.1111/j.1365-2990.2010 .01104.x

Detrick B, Newsome DA, Percopo CM, Hooks JJ. 1985. Class II antigen expression and γ interferon modulation of monocytes and retinal pigment epithelial cells from patients with retinitis pigmentosa. *Clin Immunol Immunopathol* **36**: 201–211. doi:10.1016/0090-1229(85)90121-7

Ding K, Shen J, Hafiz Z, Hackett SF, Silva RLE, Khan M, Lorenc VE, Chen D, Chadha R, Zhang M, et al. 2019. AAV8-vectored suprachoroidal gene transfer produces widespread ocular transgene expression. *J Clin Invest* **129**: 4901–4911. doi:10.1172/JCI129085

Di Pierdomenico J, Scholz R, Valiente-Soriano FJ, Sánchez-Migallón MC, Vidal-Sanz M, Langmann T, Agudo-Barriuso M, García-Ayuso D, Villegas-Pérez MP. 2018. Neuroprotective effects of FGF2 and minocycline in two animal models of inherited retinal degeneration. *Invest Ophthalmol Vis Sci* **59**: 4392–4403. doi:10.1167/iovs.18-24621

Drack AV, Dumitrescu AV, Bhattarai S, Gratie D, Stone EM, Mullins R, Sheffield VC. 2012. TUDCA slows retinal degeneration in two different mouse models of retinitis pigmentosa and prevents obesity in Bardet-Biedl syndrome type 1 mice. *Invest Ophthalmol Vis Sci* **53**: 100–106. doi:10 .1167/iovs.11-8544

Drew PD, Chavis JA. 2000. Inhibition of microglial cell activation by cortisol. *Brain Res Bull* **52**: 391–396. doi:10 .1016/S0361-9230(00)00275-6

Dryja TP, McGee TL, Reichel E, Hahn LB, Cowley GS, Yandell DW, Sandberg MA, Berson EL. 1990. A point mutation of the rhodopsin gene in one form of retinitis pigmentosa. *Nature* **343**: 364–366. doi:10.1038/343364a0

Ebrahimi F, Koch M, Pieroh P, Ghadban C, Hobusch C, Bechmann I, Dehghani F. 2012. Time dependent neuroprotection of mycophenolate mofetil: effects on temporal dynamics in glial proliferation, apoptosis, and scar formation. *J Neuroinflammation* **9:** 89. doi:10.1186/1742-2094-9-89

Ehlers JP, Yeh S, Maguire MG, Smith JR, Mruthyunjaya P, Jain N, Kim LA, Weng CY, Flaxel CJ, Schoenberger SD, et al. 2022. Intravitreal pharmacotherapies for diabetic macular edema: a report by the American Academy of Ophthalmology. *Ophthalmology* **129:** 88–99. doi:10.1016/j .ophtha.2021.07.009

Fernández-Sánchez L, Lax P, Pinilla I, Martín-Nieto J, Cuenca N. 2011. Tauroursodeoxycholic acid prevents retinal degeneration in transgenic P23H rats. *Invest Ophthalmol Vis Sci* **52:** 4998–5008. doi:10.1167/iovs.11-7496

Fernández-Sánchez L, Albertos-Arranz H, Ortuño-Lizarán I, Lax P, Cuenca N. 2022. Neuroprotective effects of tauroursodexicholic acid involves vascular and glial changes in retinitis pigmentosa model. *Front Neuroanat* **16:** 858073. doi:10.3389/fnana.2022.858073

Fetkenhour CL, Choromokos E, Weinstein J, Shoch D. 1977. Cystoid macular edema in retinitis pigmentosa. *Trans Sect Ophthalmol Am Acad Ophthalmol Otolaryngol* **83:** OP515–21.

Furukawa A, Koriyama Y. 2016. A role of heat shock protein 70 in photoreceptor cell death: potential as a novel therapeutic target in retinal degeneration. *CNS Neurosci Ther* **22:** 7–14. doi:10.1111/cns.12471

Galbraith GM, Fudenberg HH. 1984. One subset of patients with retinitis pigmentosa has immunologic defects. *Clin Immunol Immunopathol* **31:** 254–260. doi:10.1016/0090-1229(84)90245-9

Gange WS, Sisk RA, Besirli CG, Lee TC, Havunjian M, Schwartz H, Borchert M, Sengillo JD, Mendoza C, Berrocal AM, et al. 2022. Perifoveal chorioretinal atrophy after subretinal voretigene neparvovec-rzyl for RPE65-mediated Leber congenital amaurosis. *Ophthalmol Retina* **6:** 58–64. doi:10.1016/j.oret.2021.03.016

Garces K, Carmy T, Illiano P, Brambilla R, Hackam AS. 2020. Increased neuroprotective microglia and photoreceptor survival in the retina from a peptide inhibitor of myeloid differentiation factor 88 (MyD88). *J Mol Neurosci* **70:** 968–980. doi:10.1007/s12031-020-01503-0

García-Calderón PA, Engel P, Cols N, Heredia García CD. 1984. Immune complexes in retinitis pigmentosa. *Ophthalmic Paediatr Genet* **4:** 199–202. doi:10.3109/1381 6818409006122

Glybina IV, Kennedy A, Ashton P, Abrams GW, Iezzi R. 2009. Photoreceptor neuroprotection in RCS rats via low-dose intravitreal sustained-delivery of fluocinolone acetonide. *Invest Ophthalmol Vis Sci* **50:** 4847–4857. doi:10.1167/iovs.08-2831

Glybina IV, Kennedy A, Ashton P, Abrams GW, Iezzi R. 2010. Intravitreous delivery of the corticosteroid fluocinolone acetonide attenuates retinal degeneration in S334ter-4 rats. *Invest Ophthalmol Vis Sci* **51:** 4243–4252. doi:10.1167/iovs.09-4492

Golde S, Coles A, Lindquist JA, Compston A. 2003. Decreased iNOS synthesis mediates dexamethasone-induced protection of neurons from inflammatory injury in vitro. *Eur J Neurosci* **18:** 2527–2537. doi:10.1046/j .1460-9568.2003.02917.x

Gosselin D, Skola D, Coufal NG, Holtman IR, Schlachetzki JCM, Sajti E, Jaeger BN, O'Connor C, Fitzpatrick C, Pasillas MP, et al. 2017. An environment-dependent tran-

scriptional network specifies human microglia identity. *Science* **356:** eaal3222. doi:10.1126/science.aal3222

Graykowski D, Cudaback E. 2021. Don't know what you got till it's gone: microglial depletion and neurodegeneration. *Neural Regeneration Res* **16:** 1921–1927. doi:10.4103/ 1673-5374.308078

Guo C, Otani A, Oishi A, Kojima H, Makiyama Y, Nakagawa S, Yoshimura N. 2012. Knockout of ccr2 alleviates photoreceptor cell death in a model of retinitis pigmentosa. *Exp Eye Res* **104:** 39–47. doi:10.1016/j.exer.2012.08.013

Gupta N, Brown KE, Milam AH. 2003. Activated microglia in human retinitis pigmentosa, late-onset retinal degeneration, and age-related macular degeneration. *Exp Eye Res* **76:** 463–471. doi:10.1016/S0014-4835(02)00332-9

Haas T, Metzger J, Schmitz F, Heit A, Müller T, Latz E, Wagner H. 2008. The DNA sugar backbone 2′ deoxyribose determines Toll-like receptor 9 activation. *Immunity* **28:** 315–323. doi:10.1016/j.immuni.2008.01.013

Hartong DT, Berson EL, Dryja TP. 2006. Retinitis pigmentosa. *Lancet* **368:** 1795–1809. doi:10.1016/S0140-6736 (06)69740-7

Heckenlively JR, Solish AM, Chant SM, Meyers-Elliott RH. 1985. Autoimmunity in hereditary retinal degenerations. II: Clinical studies: antiretinal antibodies and fluorescein angiogram findings. *Retina* **5:** 256–257. doi:10.1097/ 00006982-198500540-00016

Hendricks RL, Fishman GA. 1985. Lymphocyte subpopulations and S-antigen reactivity in retinitis pigmentosa. *Arch Ophthalmol* **103:** 61–65. doi:10.1001/archopht .1985.01050010065021

Hendricks RL, Fishman GA. 1986. Cellular immune function of patients with retinitis pigmentosa. *Invest Ophthalmol Vis Sci* **27:** 356–363.

Hendricks RL, Fishman GA. 1987. Interferon-γ production and HLA-DR expression in patients with retinitis pigmentosa. *Exp Eye Res* **45:** 923–931. doi:10.1016/S0014-4835(87)80106-9

Heredia CD, Vich JM, Huguet J, García-Calderón JV, García-Calderón PA. 1981. Altered cellular immunity and suppressor cell activity in patients with primary retinitis pigmentosa. *Br J Ophthalmol* **65:** 850–854. doi:10.1136/ bjo.65.12.850

Hooks JJ, Geis S, Detrick-Hooks B, Newsome DA. 1983. Retinitis pigmentosa associated with a defect in the production of interferon-γ. *Am J Ophthalmol* **96:** 755–758. doi:10.1016/s0002-9394(14)71920-8

Hösel M, Broxtermann M, Janicki H, Esser K, Arzberger S, Hartmann P, Gillen S, Kleeff J, Stabenow D, Odenthal M, et al. 2012. Toll-like receptor 2-mediated innate immune response in human nonparenchymal liver cells toward adeno-associated viral vectors. *Hepatology* **55:** 287–297. doi:10.1002/hep.24625

Hu X, Leak RK, Shi Y, Suenaga J, Gao Y, Zheng P, Chen J. 2015. Microglial and macrophage polarization—new prospects for brain repair. *Nat Rev Neurol* **11:** 56–64. doi:10.1038/nrneurol.2014.207

Hughes EH, Schlichtenbrede FC, Murphy CC, Sarra GM, Luthert PJ, Ali RR, Dick AD. 2003. Generation of activated sialoadhesin-positive microglia during retinal degeneration. *Invest Ophthalmol Vis Sci* **44:** 2229–2234. doi:10 .1167/iovs.02-0824

Hughes EH, Schlichtenbrede FC, Murphy CC, Broderick C, van Rooijen N, Ali RR, Dick AD. 2004. Minocycline delays photoreceptor death in the rds mouse through a microglia-independent mechanism. *Exp Eye Res* 78: 1077–1084. doi:10.1016/j.exer.2004.02.002

Janeway CA Jr, Medzhitov R. 2002. Innate immune recognition. *Annu Rev Immunol* 20: 197–216. doi:10.1146/annurev.immunol.20.083001.084359

Jin N, Gao L, Fan X, Xu H. 2017. Friend or foe? Resident microglia vs bone marrow-derived microglia and their roles in the retinal degeneration. *Mol Neurobiol* 54: 4094–4112. doi:10.1007/s12035-016-9960-9

Joly S, Lange C, Thiersch M, Samardzija M, Grimm C. 2008. Leukemia inhibitory factor extends the lifespan of injured photoreceptors in vivo. *J Neurosci* 28: 13765–13774. doi:10.1523/JNEUROSCI.5114-08.2008

Karlen SJ, Miller EB, Burns ME. 2020. Microglia activation and inflammation during the death of mammalian photoreceptors. *Annu Rev Vis Sci* 6: 149–169. doi:10.1146/annurev-vision-121219-081730

Keino H, Horie S, Sugita S. 2018. Immune privilege and eye-derived T-regulatory cells. *J Immunol Res* 2018: 1679197. doi:10.1155/2018/1679197

Kleine J, Hohmann U, Hohmann T, Ghadban C, Schmidt M, Laabs S, Alessandri B, Dehghani F. 2022. Microglia-dependent and independent brain cytoprotective effects of mycophenolate mofetil during neuronal damage. *Front Aging Neurosci* 14: 863598. doi:10.3389/fnagi.2022.863598

Kohno H, Chen Y, Kevany BM, Pearlman E, Miyagi M, Maeda T, Palczewski K, Maeda A. 2013. Photoreceptor proteins initiate microglial activation via Toll-like receptor 4 in retinal degeneration mediated by all-trans-retinal. *J Biol Chem* 288: 15326–15341. doi:10.1074/jbc.M112.448712

Koyanagi Y, Murakami Y, Funatsu J, Akiyama M, Nakatake S, Fujiwara K, Tachibana T, Nakao S, Hisatomi T, Yoshida S, et al. 2018. Optical coherence tomography angiography of the macular microvasculature changes in retinitis pigmentosa. *Acta Ophthalmol* 96: e59–e67. doi:10.1111/aos.13475

Kumar M, Gupta RM, Nema HV. 1983. Role of autoimmunity in retinitis pigmentosa. *Ann Ophthalmol* 15: 838–840.

Kuzmin DA, Shutova MV, Johnston NR, Smith OP, Fedorin VV, Kukushkin YS, van der Loo JCM, Johnstone EC. 2021. The clinical landscape for AAV gene therapies. *Nat Rev Drug Discov* 20: 173–174. doi:10.1038/d41573-021-00017-7

Kyger M, Worley A, Adamus G. 2013. Autoimmune responses against photoreceptor antigens during retinal degeneration and their role in macrophage recruitment into retinas of RCS rats. *J Neuroimmunol* 254: 91–100. doi:10.1016/j.jneuroim.2012.10.007

Landers RA, Rayborn ME, Myers KM, Hollyfield JG. 1994. Increased retinal synthesis of heparan sulfate proteoglycan and HNK-1 glycoproteins following photoreceptor degeneration. *J Neurochem* 63: 737–750. doi:10.1046/j.1471-4159.1994.63020737.x

Lawson EC, Bhatia SK, Han MK, Aung MH, Ciavatta V, Boatright JH, Pardue MT. 2016. Tauroursodeoxycholic acid protects retinal function and structure in rd1 mice.

Adv Exp Med Biol 854: 431–436. doi:10.1007/978-3-319-17121-0_57

Leal I, Rodrigues FB, Sousa DC, Romão VC, Duarte GS, Carreño E, Dick AD, Marques-Neves C, Costa J, Fonseca JE. 2018. Efficacy and safety of intravitreal anti-tumour necrosis factor drugs in adults with non-infectious uveitis—a systematic review. *Acta Ophthalmol* 96: e665–e675. doi:10.1111/aos.13699

Lew DS, Mazzoni F, Finnemann SC. 2020. Microglia inhibition delays retinal degeneration due to MerTK phagocytosis receptor deficiency. *Front Immunol* 11: 1463. doi:10.3389/fimmu.2020.01463

Li Q, Miller R, Han PY, Pang J, Dinculescu A, Chiodo V, Hauswirth WW. 2008. Intraocular route of AAV2 vector administration defines humoral immune response and therapeutic potential. *Mol Vis* 14: 1760–1769.

Liu JT, Wu SX, Zhang H, Kuang F. 2018. Inhibition of MyD88 signaling skews microglia/macrophage polarization and attenuates neuronal apoptosis in the hippocampus after status epilepticus in mice. *Neurotherapeutics* 15: 1093–1111. doi:10.1007/s13311-018-0653-0

Löffler KU, Edward DP, Tso MO. 1995. Immunoreactivity against tau, amyloid precursor protein, and β-amyloid in the human retina. *Invest Ophthalmol Vis Sci* 36: 24–31.

Lu B, Yin H, Tang Q, Wang W, Luo C, Chen X, Zhang X, Lai K, Xu J, Chen X, et al. 2020. Multiple cytokine analyses of aqueous humor from the patients with retinitis pigmentosa. *Cytokine* 127: 154943. doi:10.1016/j.cyto.2019.154943

Maguire AM, Russell S, Chung DC, Yu ZF, Tillman A, Drack AV, Simonelli F, Leroy BP, Reape KZ, High KA, et al. 2021. Durability of voretigene neparvovec for biallelic RPE65-mediated inherited retinal disease: phase 3 results at 3 and 4 years. *Ophthalmology* 128: 1460–1468. doi:10.1016/j.ophtha.2021.03.031

Mahaling B, Low SWY, Beck M, Kumar D, Ahmed S, Connor TB, Ahmad B, Chaurasia SS. 2022. Damage-associated molecular patterns (DAMPs) in retinal disorders. *Int J Mol Sci* 23: 2591. doi:10.3390/ijms23052591

Manno CS, Pierce GF, Arruda VR, Glader B, Ragni M, Rasko JJ, Ozelo MC, Hoots K, Blatt P, Konkle B, et al. 2006. Successful transduction of liver in hemophilia by AAV-factor IX and limitations imposed by the host immune response. *Nat Med* 12: 342–347. doi:10.1038/nm1358

Marc RE, Jones BW, Watt CB, Strettoi E. 2003. Neural remodeling in retinal degeneration. *Prog Retin Eye Res* 22: 607–655. doi:10.1016/S1350-9462(03)00039-9

Martínez-Fernández de la Cámara C, Hernández-Pinto AM, Olivares-González L, Cuevas-Martín C, Sánchez-Aragó M, Hervás D, Salom D, Cuezva JM, de la Rosa EJ, Millán JM, et al. 2015. Adalimumab reduces photoreceptor cell death in a mouse model of retinal degeneration. *Sci Rep* 5: 11764. doi:10.1038/srep11764

McMenamin PG, Saban DR, Dando SJ. 2019. Immune cells in the retina and choroid: two different tissue environments that require different defenses and surveillance. *Prog Retin Eye Res* 70: 85–98. doi:10.1016/j.preteyeres.2018.12.002

Mehta N, Robbins DA, Yiu G. 2021. Ocular inflammation and treatment emergent adverse events in retinal gene therapy. *Int Ophthalmol Clin* 61: 151–177. doi:10.1097/IIO.0000000000000366

Milam AH, Li ZY, Fariss RN. 1998. Histopathology of the human retina in retinitis pigmentosa. *Prog Retin Eye Res* **17:** 175–205. doi:10.1016/S1350-9462(97)00012-8

Mirshahi A, Hoehn R, Lorenz K, Kramann C, Baatz H. 2012. Anti-tumor necrosis factor α for retinal diseases: current knowledge and future concepts. *J Ophthalmic Vis Res* **7:** 39–44.

Mishra A, Vijayasarathy C, Cukras CA, Wiley HE, Sen HN, Zeng Y, Wei LL, Sieving PA. 2021. Immune function in X-linked retinoschisis subjects in an AAV8-RS1 phase I/IIa gene therapy trial. *Mol Ther* **29:** 2030–2040. doi:10.1016/j.ymthe.2021.02.013

Möller T, Bard F, Bhattacharya A, Biber K, Campbell B, Dale E, Eder C, Gan L, Garden GA, Hughes ZA, et al. 2016. Critical data-based re-evaluation of minocycline as a putative specific microglia inhibitor. *Glia* **64:** 1788–1794. doi:10.1002/glia.23007

Murakami Y, Ikeda Y, Nakatake S, Tachibana T, Fujiwara K, Yoshida N, Notomi S, Nakao S, Hisatomi T, Miller JW, et al. 2015. Necrotic enlargement of cone photoreceptor cells and the release of high-mobility group box-1 in retinitis pigmentosa. *Cell Death Discov* **1:** 15058. doi:10.1038/cddiscovery.2015.58

Murakami Y, Ishikawa K, Nakao S, Sonoda KH. 2020. Innate immune response in retinal homeostasis and inflammatory disorders. *Prog Retin Eye Res* **74:** 100778. doi:10.1016/j.preteyeres.2019.100778

Murillo-Lopez F, Politi L, Adler R, Hewitt AT. 1991. Proteoglycan synthesis in cultures of murine retinal neurons and photoreceptors. *Cell Mol Neurobiol* **11:** 579–591. doi:10.1007/BF00741447

Mustafi D, Hisama FM, Huey J, Chao JR. 2022. The current state of genetic testing platforms for inherited retinal diseases. *Ophthalmol Retina* **6:** 702–710. doi:10.1016/j.oret.2022.03.011

Muzio L, Viotti A, Martino G. 2021. Microglia in neuroinflammation and neurodegeneration: from understanding to therapy. *Front Neurosci* **15:** 742065. doi:10.3389/fnins.2021.742065

Newsome DA. 1986. Retinal fluorescein leakage in retinitis pigmentosa. *Am J Ophthalmol* **101:** 354–360. doi:10.1016/0002-9394(86)90831-7

Newsome DA, Michels RG. 1988. Detection of lymphocytes in the vitreous gel of patients with retinitis pigmentosa. *Am J Ophthalmol* **105:** 596–602. doi:10.1016/0002-9394(88)90050-5

Newsome DA, Nussenblatt RB. 1984. Retinal S antigen reactivity in patients with retinitis pigmentosa and Usher's syndrome. *Retina* **4:** 195–199. doi:10.1097/00006982-198400430-00012

Newsome DA, Quinn TC, Hess AD, Pitha-Rowe PM. 1988. Cellular immune status in retinitis pigmentosa. *Ophthalmology* **95:** 1696–1703. doi:10.1016/S0161-6420(88)32965-9

Newton F, Megaw R. 2020. Mechanisms of photoreceptor death in retinitis pigmentosa. *Genes (Basel)* **11:** 1120. doi:10.3390/genes11101120

Noailles A, Fernández-Sánchez L, Lax P, Cuenca N. 2014. Microglia activation in a model of retinal degeneration and TUDCA neuroprotective effects. *J Neuroinflammation* **11:** 186. doi:10.1186/s12974-014-0186-3

Noailles A, Maneu V, Campello L, Gómez-Vicente V, Lax P, Cuenca N. 2016. Persistent inflammatory state after photoreceptor loss in an animal model of retinal degeneration. *Sci Rep* **6:** 33356. doi:10.1038/srep33356

Ochakovski GA, Bartz-Schmidt KU, Fischer MD. 2017. Retinal gene therapy: surgical vector delivery in the translation to clinical trials. *Front Neurosci* **11:** 174. doi:10.3389/fnins.2017.00174

Okita A, Murakami Y, Shimokawa S, Funatsu J, Fujiwara K, Nakatake S, Koyanagi Y, Akiyama M, Takeda A, Hisatomi T, et al. 2020. Changes of serum inflammatory molecules and their relationships with visual function in retinitis pigmentosa. *Invest Ophthalmol Vis Sci* **61:** 30. doi:10.1167/iovs.61.11.30

O'Koren EG, Yu C, Klingeborn M, Wong AYW, Prigge CL, Mathew R, Kalnitsky J, Msallam RA, Silvin A, Kay JN, et al. 2019. Microglial function is distinct in different anatomical locations during retinal homeostasis and degeneration. *Immunity* **50:** 723–737.e7. doi:10.1016/j.immuni.2019.02.007

Olivares-González L, Velasco S, Millán JM, Rodrigo R. 2020. Intravitreal administration of adalimumab delays retinal degeneration in rd10 mice. *FASEB J* **34:** 13839–13861. doi:10.1096/fj.202000044RR

Oveson BC, Iwase T, Hackett SF, Lee SY, Usui S, Sedlak TW, Snyder SH, Campochiaro PA, Sung JU. 2011. Constituents of vile, bilirubin and TUDCA, protect against oxidative stress-induced retinal degeneration. *J Neurochem* **116:** 144–153. doi:10.1111/j.1471-4159.2010.07092.x

Ozaki E, Delaney C, Campbell M, Doyle SL. 2022. Minocycline suppresses disease-associated microglia (DAM) in a model of photoreceptor cell degeneration. *Exp Eye Res* **217:** 108953. doi:10.1016/j.exer.2022.108953

Pardue MT, Allen RS. 2018. Neuroprotective strategies for retinal disease. *Prog Retin Eye Res* **65:** 50–76. doi:10.1016/j.preteyeres.2018.02.002

Parker MA, Erker LR, Audo I, Choi D, Mohand-Said S, Sestakauskas K, Benoit P, Appelqvist T, Krahmer M, Séguat-Prévost C, et al. 2022. Three-year safety results of SAR422459 (EIAV-ABCA4) gene therapy in patients with ABCA4-associated Stargardt disease: an open-label dose-escalation phase I/IIa clinical trial, cohorts 1-5. *Am J Ophthalmol* **240:** 285–301. doi:10.1016/j.ajo.2022.02.013

Pascual-Camps I, Hernández-Martínez P, Monje-Fernández L, Dolz-Marco R, Gallego-Pinazo R, Wu L, Arévalo JF, Díaz-Llopis M. 2014. Update on intravitreal anti-tumor necrosis factor α therapies for ocular disorders. *J Ophthalmic Inflamm Infect* **4:** 26. doi:10.1186/s12348-014-0026-8

Peng B, Xiao J, Wang K, So KF, Tipoe GL, Lin B. 2014. Suppression of microglial activation is neuroprotective in a mouse model of human retinitis pigmentosa. *J Neurosci* **34:** 8139–8150. doi:10.1523/JNEUROSCI.5200-13.2014

Pennesi ME, Yang P, Birch DG, Weng CY, Moore AT, Iannaccone A, Comander JI, Jayasundera T, Chulay T; XLRS-001 Study Group. 2022. Intravitreal delivery of rAAV2-tYF-CB-hRS1 vector for gene augmentation therapy in patients with X-linked retinoschisis: 1-year clinical results. *Ophthalmol Retina* **6:** 1130–1144. doi:10.1016/j.oret.2022.06.013

Phillips MJ, Walker TA, Choi HY, Faulkner AE, Kim MK, Sidney SS, Boyd AP, Nickerson JM, Boatright JH, Pardue

MT. 2008. Tauroursodeoxycholic acid preservation of photoreceptor structure and function in the rd10 mouse through postnatal day 30. *Invest Ophthalmol Vis Sci* **49**: 2148–2155. doi:10.1167/iovs.07-1012

Porta A, Pierrottet C, Aschero M, Orzalesi N. 1992. Preserved para-arteriolar retinal pigment epithelium retinitis pigmentosa. *Am J Ophthalmol* **113**: 161–164. doi:10.1016/S0002-9394(14)71528-4

Power M, Das S, Schütze K, Marigo V, Ekström P, Paquet-Durand F. 2020. Cellular mechanisms of hereditary photoreceptor degeneration—focus on cGMP. *Prog Retin Eye Res* **74**: 100772. doi:10.1016/j.preteyeres.2019.07.005

Pruett RC. 1983. Retinitis pigmentosa: clinical observations and correlations. *Trans Am Ophthalmol Soc* **81**: 693–735.

Rahi AH. 1973. Autoimmunity and the retina. II: Raised serum IgM levels in retinitis pigmentosa. *Br J Ophthalmol* **57**: 904–909. doi:10.1136/bjo.57.12.904

Ramamoorthy S, Cidlowski JA. 2016. Corticosteroids: mechanisms of action in health and disease. *Rheum Dis Clin North Am* **42**: 15–31. doi:10.1016/j.rdc.2015.08.002

Rana T, Kotla P, Fullard R, Gorbatyuk M. 2017. TNFa knockdown in the retina promotes cone survival in a mouse model of autosomal dominant retinitis pigmentosa. *Biochim Biophys Acta Mol Basis Dis* **1863**: 92–102. doi:10.1016/j.bbadis.2016.10.008

Rashid K, Akhtar-Schaefer I, Langmann T. 2019. Microglia in retinal degeneration. *Front Immunol* **10**: 1975. doi:10.3389/fimmu.2019.01975

Reichel FF, Peters T, Wilhelm B, Biel M, Ueffing M, Wissinger B, Bartz-Schmidt KU, Klein R, Michalakis S, Fischer MD, et al. 2018. Humoral immune response after intravitreal but not after subretinal AAV8 in primates and patients. *Invest Ophthalmol Vis Sci* **59**: 1910–1915. doi:10.1167/iovs.17-22494

Reichenbach A, Bringmann A. 2020. Glia of the human retina. *Glia* **68**: 768–796. doi:10.1002/glia.23727

Roche SL, Wyse-Jackson AC, Gómez-Vicente V, Lax P, Ruiz-Lopez AM, Byrne AM, Cuenca N, Cotter TG. 2016. Progesterone attenuates microglial-driven retinal degeneration and stimulates protective fractalkine-CX3CR1 signaling. *PLoS ONE* **11**: e0165197. doi:10.1371/journal.pone.0165197

Roche SL, Wyse-Jackson AC, Ruiz-Lopez AM, Byrne AM, Cotter TG. 2017. Fractalkine-CX3CR1 signaling is critical for progesterone-mediated neuroprotection in the retina. *Sci Rep* **7**: 43067. doi:10.1038/srep43067

Roche SL, Ruiz-Lopez AM, Moloney JN, Byrne AM, Cotter TG. 2018. Microglial-induced Müller cell gliosis is attenuated by progesterone in a mouse model of retinitis pigmentosa. *Glia* **66**: 295–310. doi:10.1002/glia.23243

Rogers GL, Martino AT, Aslanidi GV, Jayandharan GR, Srivastava A, Herzog RW. 2011. Innate immune responses to AAV vectors. *Front Microbiol* **2**: 194. doi:10.3389/fmicb.2011.00194

Rogers GL, Suzuki M, Zolotukhin I, Markusic DM, Morel LM, Lee B, Ertl HCJ, Herzog RW. 2015. Unique roles of TLR9- and MyD88-dependent and -independent pathways in adaptive immune responses to AAV-mediated gene transfer. *J Innate Immun* **7**: 302–314. doi:10.1159/000369273

Roque RS, Imperial CJ, Caldwell RB. 1996. Microglial cells invade the outer retina as photoreceptors degenerate in royal college of surgeons rats. *Invest Ophthalmol Vis Sci* **37**: 196–203.

Roque RS, Rosales AA, Jingjing L, Agarwal N, Al-Ubaidi MR. 1999. Retina-derived microglial cells induce photoreceptor cell death in vitro. *Brain Res* **836**: 110–119. doi:10.1016/S0006-8993(99)01625-X

Sakami S, Imanishi Y, Palczewski K. 2019. Müller glia phagocytose dead photoreceptor cells in a mouse model of retinal degenerative disease. *FASEB J* **33**: 3680–3692. doi:10.1096/fj.201801662R

Sasahara M, Otani A, Oishi A, Kojima H, Yodoi Y, Kameda T, Nakamura H, Yoshimura N. 2008. Activation of bone marrow-derived microglia promotes photoreceptor survival in inherited retinal degeneration. *Am J Pathol* **172**: 1693–1703. doi:10.2353/ajpath.2008.080024

Scaffidi P, Misteli T, Bianchi ME. 2002. Release of chromatin protein HMGB1 by necrotic cells triggers inflammation. *Nature* **418**: 191–195. doi:10.1038/nature00858

Scott-Hewitt N, Perrucci F, Morini R, Erreni M, Mahoney M, Witkowska A, Carey A, Faggiani E, Schuetz LT, Mason S, et al. 2020. Local externalization of phosphatidylserine mediates developmental synaptic pruning by microglia. *EMBO J* **39**: e105380. doi:10.15252/embj.2020105380

Shen J, Kim J, Tzeng SY, Ding K, Hafiz Z, Long D, Wang J, Green JJ, Campochiaro PA. 2020. Suprachoroidal gene transfer with nonviral nanoparticles. *Sci Adv* **6**: eaba1606. doi:10.1126/sciadv.aba1606

Shimazaki K, Jirawuthiworavong GV, Heckenlively JR, Gordon LK. 2008. Frequency of anti-retinal antibodies in normal human serum. *J Neuroophthalmol* **28**: 5–11. doi:10.1097/WNO.0b013e318167549f

Sierra A, Gottfried-Blackmore A, Milner TA, McEwen BS, Bulloch K. 2008. Steroid hormone receptor expression and function in microglia. *Glia* **56**: 659–674. doi:10.1002/glia.20644

Sinha S, Miller L, Subramanian S, McCarty OJT, Proctor T, Meza-Romero R, Huan J, Burrows GG, Vandenbark AA, Offner H. 2010. Binding of recombinant T cell receptor ligands (RTL) to antigen presenting cells prevents upregulation of CD11b and inhibits T cell activation and transfer of experimental autoimmune encephalomyelitis. *J Neuroimmunol* **225**: 52–61. doi:10.1016/j.jneuroim.2010.04.013

Sisodia SS, Koo EH, Beyreuther K, Unterbeck A, Price DL. 1990. Evidence that β-amyloid protein in Alzheimer's disease is not derived by normal processing. *Science* **248**: 492–495. doi:10.1126/science.1691865

Spalton DJ, Rahi AH, Bird AC. 1978. Immunological studies in retinitis pigmentosa associated with retinal vascular leakage. *Br J Ophthalmol* **62**: 183–187. doi:10.1136/bjo.62.3.183

Spiro R, Weleber R, Kimberling W. 1978. Serum IgM in retinitis pigmentosa: a genetic study. *Clin Genet* **13**: 295–304. doi:10.1111/j.1399-0004.1978.tb01184.x

Streilein JW. 2003. Ocular immune privilege: the eye takes a dim but practical view of immunity and inflammation. *J Leukoc Biol* **74**: 179–185. doi:10.1189/jlb.1102574

Sudharsan R, Beiting DP, Aguirre GD, Beltran WA. 2017. Involvement of innate immune system in late stages of inherited photoreceptor degeneration. *Sci Rep* **7**: 17897. doi:10.1038/s41598-017-18236-7

Suhler EB, Thorne JE, Mittal M, Betts KA, Tari S, Camez A, Bao Y, Joshi A. 2017. Corticosteroid-related adverse events systematically increase with corticosteroid dose in noninfectious intermediate, posterior, or panuveitis: post hoc analyses from the VISUAL-1 and VISUAL-2 trials. *Ophthalmology* **124**: 1799–1807. doi:10.1016/j.ophtha.2017.06.017

Syeda S, Patel AK, Lee T, Hackam AS. 2015. Reduced photoreceptor death and improved retinal function during retinal degeneration in mice lacking innate immunity adaptor protein MyD88. *Exp Neurol* **267**: 1–12. doi:10.1016/j.expneurol.2015.02.027

Tang D, Kang R, Coyne CB, Zeh HJ, Lotze MT. 2012. PAMPs and DAMPs: signal 0s that spur autophagy and immunity. *Immunol Rev* **249**: 158–175. doi:10.1111/j.1600-065X.2012.01146.x

Taylor AW, Hsu S, Ng TF. 2021. The role of retinal pigment epithelial cells in regulation of macrophages/microglial cells in retinal immunobiology. *Front Immunol* **12**: 724601. doi:10.3389/fimmu.2021.724601

Ten Berge JC, Fazil Z, van den Born I, Wolfs RCW, Schreurs MWJ, Dik WA, Rothova A. 2019. Intraocular cytokine profile and autoimmune reactions in retinitis pigmentosa, age-related macular degeneration, glaucoma and cataract. *Acta Ophthalmol* **97**: 185–192. doi:10.1111/aos.13899

Terauchi R, Kohno H, Watanabe S, Saito S, Watanabe A, Nakano T. 2021. Minocycline decreases CCR2-positive monocytes in the retina and ameliorates photoreceptor degeneration in a mouse model of retinitis pigmentosa. *PLoS ONE* **16**: e0239108. doi:10.1371/journal.pone.0239108

Thanos S. 1992. Sick photoreceptors attract activated microglia from the ganglion cell layer: a model to study the inflammatory cascades in rats with inherited retinal dystrophy. *Brain Res* **588**: 21–28. doi:10.1016/0006-8993(92)91340-K

Thanos S, Moore S, Hong Y-M. 1996. Retinal microglia. *Prog Retin Eye Res* **15**: 331–361. doi:10.1016/1350-9462(96)00006-7

Thompson DA, Iannaccone A, Ali RR, Arshavsky VY, Audo I, Bainbridge JWB, Besirli CG, Birch DG, Branham KE, Cideciyan AV, et al. 2020. Advancing clinical trials for inherited retinal diseases: recommendations from the Second Monaciano Symposium. *Transl Vis Sci Technol* **9**: 2–2. doi:10.1167/tvst.9.7.2

Timmers AM, Newmark JA, Turunen HT, Farivar T, Liu J, Song C, Ye GJ, Pennock S, Gaskin C, Knop DR, et al. 2020. Ocular inflammatory response to intravitreal injection of adeno-associated virus vector: relative contribution of genome and capsid. *Hum Gene Ther* **31**: 80–89. doi:10.1089/hum.2019.144

Toma C, De Cillà S, Palumbo A, Garhwal DP, Grossini E. 2021. Oxidative and nitrosative stress in age-related macular degeneration: a review of their role in different stages of disease. *Antioxidants (Basel)* **10**: 653. doi:10.3390/antiox10050653

Tummala G, Crain A, Rowlan J, Pepple KL. 2021. Characterization of gene therapy associated uveitis following intravitreal adeno-associated virus injection in mice. *Invest Ophthalmol Vis Sci* **62**: 41. doi:10.1167/iovs.62.2.41

Valdes LM, Sobrin L. 2020. Uveitis therapy: the corticosteroid options. *Drugs* **80**: 765–773. doi:10.1007/s40265-020-01314-y

Valdés-Sánchez L, Calado SM, de la Cerda B, Aramburu A, García-Delgado AB, Massalini S, Montero-Sánchez A, Bhatia V, Rodríguez-Bocanegra E, Diez-Lloret A, et al. 2020. Retinal pigment epithelium degeneration caused by aggregation of PRPF31 and the role of HSP70 family of proteins. *Mol Med* **26**: 1. doi:10.1186/s10020-019-0124-z

van den Born LI, van Soest S, van Schooneveld MJ, Riemslag FC, de Jong PT, Bleeker-Wagemakers EM. 1994. Autosomal recessive retinitis pigmentosa with preserved para-arteriolar retinal pigment epithelium. *Am J Ophthalmol* **118**: 430–439. doi:10.1016/S0002-9394(14)75792-7

Vasconcelos HM Jr, Lujan BJ, Pennesi ME, Yang P, Lauer AK. 2020. Intraoperative optical coherence tomographic findings in patients undergoing subretinal gene therapy surgery. *Int J Retina Vitreous* **6**: 13. doi:10.1186/s40942-020-00216-1

Verbakel SK, van Huet RAC, Boon CJF, den Hollander AI, Collin RWJ, Klaver CCW, Hoyng CB, Roepman R, Klevering BJ. 2018. Non-syndromic retinitis pigmentosa. *Prog Retin Eye Res* **66**: 157–186. doi:10.1016/j.preteyeres.2018.03.005

Vijayasarathy C, Zeng Y, Brooks MJ, Fariss RN, Sieving PA. 2021. Genetic rescue of X-linked retinoschisis mouse ($Rs1^{-/y}$) retina induces quiescence of the retinal microglial inflammatory state following AAV8-*RS1* gene transfer and identifies gene networks underlying retinal recovery. *Hum Gene Ther* **32**: 667–681. doi:10.1089/hum.2020.213

Viringipurampeer IA, Metcalfe AL, Bashar AE, Sivak O, Yanai A, Mohammadi Z, Moritz OL, Gregory-Evans CY, Gregory-Evans K. 2016. NLRP3 inflammasome activation drives bystander cone photoreceptor cell death in a P23H rhodopsin model of retinal degeneration. *Hum Mol Genet* **25**: 1501–1516. doi:10.1093/hmg/ddw029

Wang M, Ma W, Zhao L, Fariss RN, Wong WT. 2011. Adaptive Müller cell responses to microglial activation mediate neuroprotection and coordinate inflammation in the retina. *J Neuroinflammation* **8**: 173. doi:10.1186/1742-2094-8-173

Wang NK, Lai CC, Liu CH, Yeh LK, Chou CL, Kong J, Nagasaki T, Tsang SH, Chien CL. 2013. Origin of fundus hyperautofluorescent spots and their role in retinal degeneration in a mouse model of Goldmann–Favre syndrome. *Dis Model Mech* **6**: 1113–1122.

Wang X, Zhao L, Zhang J, Fariss RN, Ma W, Kretschmer F, Wang M, Qian HH, Badea TC, Diamond JS, et al. 2016. Requirement for microglia for the maintenance of synaptic function and integrity in the mature retina. *J Neurosci* **36**: 2827–2842. doi:10.1523/JNEUROSCI.3575-15.2016

Wang SK, Xue Y, Cepko CL. 2020. Microglia modulation by TGF-β1 protects cones in mouse models of retinal degeneration. *J Clin Invest* **130**: 4360–4369.

Wilson DJ, Sahel JA, Weleber RG, Erker LR, Lauer AK, Stout T, Audo IS, Mohand-Said S, Barale PO, Titeux L, et al. 2017. One year results of a phase I/IIa study of SAR422459 in patients with Stargardt macular degeneration (SMD). *Invest Ophthalmol Vis Sci* **58**: 3385–3385.

Wolf Y, Yona S, Kim KW, Jung S. 2013. Microglia, seen from the CX3CR1 angle. *Front Cell Neurosci* **7**: 26. doi:10.3389/fncel.2013.00026

Xiong W, Wu DM, Xue Y, Wang SK, Chung MJ, Ji X, Rana P, Zhao SR, Mai S, Cepko CL. 2019. AAV *cis*-regulatory sequences are correlated with ocular toxicity. *Proc Natl Acad Sci* **116**: 5785–5794. doi:10.1073/pnas.1821000116

Yanagishita M, Hascall VC. 1992. Cell surface heparan sulfate proteoglycans. *J Biol Chem* **267**: 9451–9454. doi:10.1016/S0021-9258(19)50108-9

Yang Y, Zhang R, Xia F, Zou T, Huang A, Xiong S, Zhang J. 2013. LPS converts Gr-1+CD115+ myeloid-derived suppressor cells from M2 to M1 via P38 MAPK. *Exp Cell Res* **319**: 1774–1783. doi:10.1016/j.yexcr.2013.05.007

Yang P, Lockard R, Titus H, Hiblar J, Weller K, Wafai D, Weleber RG, Duvoisin RM, Morgans CW, Pennesi ME. 2020. Suppression of cGMP-dependent photoreceptor cytotoxicity with mycophenolate is neuroprotective in murine models of retinitis pigmentosa. *Invest Ophthalmol Vis Sci* **61**: 25. doi:10.1167/iovs.61.10.25

Yiu G, Chung SH, Mollhoff IN, Nguyen UT, Thomasy SM, Yoo J, Taraborelli D, Noronha G. 2020. Suprachoroidal and subretinal injections of AAV using transscleral microneedles for retinal gene delivery in nonhuman primates. *Mol Ther Methods Clin Dev* **16**: 179–191. doi:10.1016/j.omtm.2020.01.002

Yoshida N, Ikeda Y, Notomi S, Ishikawa K, Murakami Y, Hisatomi T, Enaida H, Ishibashi T. 2013a. Clinical evidence of sustained chronic inflammatory reaction in retinitis pigmentosa. *Ophthalmology* **120**: 100–105. doi:10.1016/j.ophtha.2012.07.006

Yoshida N, Ikeda Y, Notomi S, Ishikawa K, Murakami Y, Hisatomi T, Enaida H, Ishibashi T. 2013b. Laboratory evidence of sustained chronic inflammatory reaction in

retinitis pigmentosa. *Ophthalmology* **120**: e5–e12. doi:10.1016/j.ophtha.2012.07.008

Zabel MK, Zhao L, Zhang Y, Gonzalez SR, Ma W, Wang X, Fariss RN, Wong WT. 2016. Microglial phagocytosis and activation underlying photoreceptor degeneration is regulated by CX3CL1-CX3CR1 signaling in a mouse model of retinitis pigmentosa. *Glia* **64**: 1479–1491. doi:10.1002/glia.23016

Zeiss CJ, Johnson EA. 2004. Proliferation of microglia, but not photoreceptors, in the outer nuclear layer of the *rd-1* mouse. *Invest Ophthalmol Vis Sci* **45**: 971–976. doi:10.1167/iovs.03-0301

Zeng HY, Zhu XA, Zhang C, Yang LP, Wu LM, Tso MOM. 2005. Identification of sequential events and factors associated with microglial activation, migration, and cytotoxicity in retinal degeneration in *rd* mice. *Invest Ophthalmol Vis Sci* **46**: 2992–2999. doi:10.1167/iovs.05-0118

Zhang T, Baehr W, Fu Y. 2012. Chemical chaperone TUDCA preserves cone photoreceptors in a mouse model of Leber congenital amaurosis. *Invest Ophthalmol Vis Sci* **53**: 3349–3356. doi:10.1167/iovs.12-9851

Zhang X, Shahani U, Reilly J, Shu X. 2019. Disease mechanisms and neuroprotection by tauroursodeoxycholic acid in *Rpgr* knockout mice. *J Cell Physiol* **234**: 18801–18812. doi:10.1002/jcp.28519

Zhao L, Zabel MK, Wang X, Ma W, Shah P, Fariss RN, Qian H, Parkhurst CN, Gan WB, Wong WT. 2015. Microglial phagocytosis of living photoreceptors contributes to inherited retinal degeneration. *EMBO Mol Med* **7**: 1179–1197. doi:10.15252/emmm.201505298

Zhu J, Huang X, Yang Y. 2009. The TLR9-MyD88 pathway is critical for adaptive immune responses to adeno-associated virus gene therapy vectors in mice. *J Clin Investn* **119**: 2388–2398. doi:10.1172/jci37607

Choroideremia: Toward Regulatory Approval of Retinal Gene Therapy

Imran H. Yusuf[1,2] and Robert E. MacLaren[1,2]

[1]Nuffield Laboratory of Ophthalmology, Department of Clinical Neurosciences, University of Oxford, John Radcliffe Hospital, Oxford OX3 9DU, United Kingdom

[2]Oxford Eye Hospital, John Radcliffe Hospital, Oxford University Hospitals NHS Foundation Trust, Oxford OX3 9DU, United Kingdom

Correspondence: enquiries@ndcn.ox.ac.uk

Choroideremia is an X-linked inherited retinal degeneration characterized by primary centripetal degeneration of the retinal pigment epithelium (RPE), with secondary degeneration of the choroid and retina. Affected individuals experience reduced night vision in early adulthood with blindness in late middle age. The underlying *CHM* gene encodes REP1, a protein involved in the prenylation of Rab GTPases essential for intracellular vesicle trafficking. Adeno-associated viral gene therapy has demonstrated some benefit in clinical trials for choroideremia. However, challenges remain in gaining regulatory approval. Choroideremia is slowly progressive, which presents difficulties in demonstrating benefit over short pivotal clinical trials that usually run for 1–2 years. Improvements in visual acuity are particularly challenging due to the initial negative effects of surgical detachment of the fovea. Despite these challenges, great progress toward a treatment has been made since choroideremia was first described in 1872.

Choroideremia is rare X-linked recessive inherited retinal degeneration resulting from mutations in the *CHM* gene on the long arm of the X chromosome (Xq21.2) (OMIM: 300390) (Cremers et al. 1990a,b,c). The disease affects approximately one in 50,000 males, although may be more common in Finland (~1 in 40,000) (Sankila et al. 1992). *CHM* encodes REP1 (Rab escort-binding protein 1), a molecule essential for the prenylation, posttranslational modification, and chaperone of proteins involved in intracellular vesicle trafficking (Gordiyenko et al. 2010). In the retinal pigment epithelium (RPE), REP1 knockdown has been shown to affect the clearance of endocytosed photoreceptor outer segment discs through inhibition of late phagosome–lysosome fusion events in vitro (Gordiyenko et al. 2010). This is likely to form a major mechanism of primary RPE toxicity in choroideremia. Although REP1 is ubiquitously expressed, mutations in *CHM* result in nonsyndromic retinal degeneration, which may be in part explained by compensatory expression of REP2 in other tissues encoded by the *CHML* gene: an X-derived intronless retrogene present on chromosome

1q42, with a high degree of homology to *REP1* (Seabra 1996).

In ancient Greek, khórion (χόρῐον) denotes membrane or skin with erēmíā (ἐρημίᾱ) denoting a desert, barren wilderness, or otherwise desolate area. Thus, choroideremia was originally named on the presumption that the choroid was the primary site of degeneration based on the characteristic fundoscopic appearances, as first described in 1872 by Ludwig Mauthner (Mauthner 1872). The other historic description for choroideremia was tapetochoroidal dystrophy, which refers to the yellow, tapetal-like reflex observed in patients with advanced disease. Choroideremia was originally considered a developmental and stationary disorder. However, these assumptions—and that of the choroid being the primary site of degeneration—have all since been refuted. Nonetheless, recent evidence suggests mild choroidal thinning on OCT imaging in affected individuals, consistent with a mild developmental abnormality of the choroid (Xue et al. 2016).

The dominant early symptoms of nyctalopia and constricted visual fields relate to involvement of the RPE with functional deficits in the canonical rod visual cycle hosted by the RPE. The cone visual cycle, in contrast, may be regenerated by Müller cells and other RPE-independent mechanisms (Muniz et al. 2007). The genetic basis of choroideremia was identified relatively early through positional cloning in 1990, supported by the characteristic clinical phenotype, disease severity, and X-linked inheritance (Cremers et al. 1990c). Over 350 disease-associated mutations have been described in the *CHM* gene, most of which are null, or presumed functional nulls, resulting in the absence or functional abrogation of REP1 (Han et al. 2021). Given the small size of the *CHM* cDNA (1.96 kb), the slowly progressive nature of choroideremia, easily identifiable clinical phenotype and inheritance pattern, and the absence of amblyopia and/or significant developmental abnormalities, choroideremia has been an ideal candidate for adeno-associated viral (AAV) retinal gene therapy as a therapeutic approach.

This review focuses on the challenges in gaining regulatory approval of retinal gene ther-

apy vectors for choroideremia. To contextualize these discussions, we first summarize the current understanding of clinical phenotype from multimodal retinal imaging studies, and discuss their relevance to the natural history of disease, patient selection for clinical trials, and end points in the assessment of treatment efficacy. Recent findings from pivotal retinal gene therapy clinical trials for choroideremia are summarized (Table 1), followed by a detailed discussion in the challenges toward regulatory approval of the first therapy. In particular, the slow nature of retinal degeneration in choroideremia creates challenges in detecting a benefit over a short pivotal clinical trial. An improvement in best-corrected visual acuity (BCVA) is only possible in patients with advanced disease where efficacy may be limited by RPE dysfunction and degeneration at or around the fovea. Moreover, the effect of surgical detachment of the fovea, necessary for the transduction of the foveal RPE, cannot easily be controlled for in clinical trials. Furthermore, disease-related variability in key outcome measures may obscure therapeutic signals in clinical trials. These challenges can, in part, be overcome and the approval of the first therapy for choroideremia is expected in the near future, 150 years after the first description of the disease.

CLINICAL PHENOTYPE

Affected males with choroideremia present with night blindness in childhood due to the effects of peripheral RPE degeneration on the rod visual cycle and subsequent rod cell death. In early disease, midperipheral retinal degeneration may be identified on clinical examination with retinal thinning and pigment clumping. The visual field becomes progressively constricted as centripetal degeneration of the RPE, retina, and choroid progresses toward the fovea (Fig. 1). Although choroideremia may be clinically misclassified as retinitis pigmentosa (RP) in early disease, as Mauthner observed (Mauthner 1872), the retinal vessels are not constricted and the optic disc is not atrophic due to the associated choroidal degeneration, which prevents retinal hyperoxia and subsequent vaso-

Cite this article as *Cold Spring Harb Perspect Med* doi: 10.1101/cshperspect.a041279

Table 1. Summary of interventional retinal gene therapy clinical trials for choroideremia

Trial	Vector and dose	Phase	Baseline characteristics	Follow-up	Center	References
Nightstar/Biogen NCT01461213 2011–2018	rAAV2.REP1 $0.6–1.0 \times 10^{10}$	1/2	23–89 Early Treatment Diabetic Retinopathy Study (ETDRS) letters 6.4–13.0 db $n = 6$	6 mo	University of Oxford, UK	MacLaren et al. 2014 Noted that patients with advanced choroideremia had the most significant visual acuity gains
	rAAV2.REP1 $0.6–1.0 \times 10^{10}$	1/2	23–89 ETDRS letters 6.4–13.0 db $n = 6$	3.5 yr	University of Oxford, UK	Edwards et al. 2016 Treatment effects sustained to 3.5 yr
	rAAV2.REP1 $1.0 \times 10^{10} – 1.0 \times 10^{11}$	1/2	23–89 ETDRS letters $n = 14$	2–5 yr	University of Oxford, UK	Xue et al. 2018 Treatment effects sustained to 5 yr, including three study eyes that gained >3 lines of vision (additional data: Simunovic et al. 2016; Xue et al. 2016)
STAR study Nightstar/Biogen NCT03496012 2017–2020	rAAV2.REP 1.0×10^{10} 1.0×10^{11} Untreated	3	34–73 ETDRS $n = 169$	1 yr	International, multicenter 18 centers	Data not published (Biogen press release, Biogen 2021)
GEMINI study Nightstar/Biogen NCT03507686 2017–2022	rAAV2.REP1 1.0×10^{11}	2	$n = 60$ $>/= 34$ letters	2 yr	International, multicenter six centers	Data not published
University of Oxford REGENERATE NCT02407678 2016–2021	rAAV2.REP1	2	$n = 30$ $>/= 34$ letters	2 yr	University of Oxford and Moorfields Eye Hospital, UK	Data not published
Nightstar/Biogen SOLSTICE NCT03584165 2018–2027	rAAV2.REP1 rAAV8.RPGR	Follow-up	$n =$ up to 440 Observational long-term follow-up study	5 yr	International, multicenter 18 centers	Data not published

Continued

Table 1. *Continued*

Trial	Vector and dose	Phase	Baseline characteristics	Follow-up	Center	References
THOR study Tübingen NCT02671539 2016–2018	rAAV2.REP1 1×10^{11}	2	$n = 6$ ETDRS 35–75 letters	2 yr	Tübingen, Germany	Fischer et al. 2019 Improvements versus controls over 24 mo in best-corrected visual acuity (BCVA) and microperimetry (MP) but not statistically significant Fischer et al. 2020 After 12-mo, one participant gained 17 letters
Spark Therapeutics NCT02341807 2015–2022	AAV2.hCHM Doses not stated	1/2	$n = 15$ ETDRS > 35 letters Central field <30°	5 yr	USA three sites	Data not published
4D Molecular Therapeutics NCT04483440 2020–2023	Intravitreal 4D-110 AAV.hCHM	1	$n = 15$ ETDRS >/= 34 letters	6 mo	USA two sites	Data not published
Foundation Fighting Blindness, Canada NCT02077361 2015–2025	rAAV2.REP1 (as used in NCT01461213)	1/2	$n = 6$	2 yr	Alberta, Canada	Dimopoulos et al. 2018
Bascom Palmer, Florida NCT02553135 2015–2018	AAV2.REP1 10×10^{11}	2	$n = 6$ ETDRS 35–75 letters	2 yr	Bascom Palmer, Miami, USA	Lam et al. 2019 Supports BCVA as an outcome measure in advanced choroideremia

Cite this article as *Cold Spring Harb Perspect Med* doi: 10.1101/cshperspect.a041279

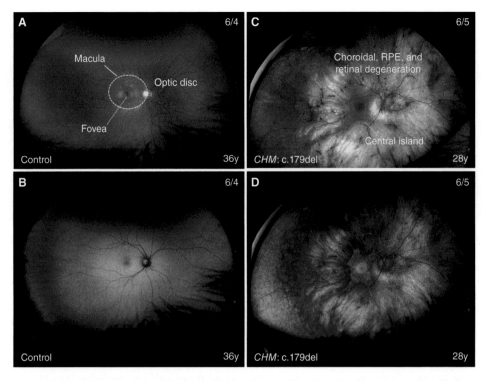

Figure 1. Retinal appearance in choroideremia. (*C,D*) A 28-yr-old male with a hemizygous frameshifting mutation in *CHM* (c.179delA) who presented with nyctalopia in childhood. Pseudocolor retinal imaging demonstrates midperipheral RPE, retinal, and choroidal degeneration exposing the pale underlying sclera, and deep choroidal vessels. Centripetal degeneration preserves a central island of retinal pigment epithelium (RPE) and retina; foveal preservation typically sustains an excellent visual acuity until late in the disease. Although pigment migration may be identified in the midperiphery, in contrast to retinitis pigmentosa (RP), choroidal degeneration prevents secondary retinal vascular attenuation. Fundus autofluorescence (FAF) imaging more clearly defines the central island of residual RPE with scalloped edges typical of choroideremia. The fovea is typically threatened from degeneration of the nasal side of the central island (Jolly et al. 2017), which may be due to the temporal displacement of the fovea on the optical axis. (*A,B*) A healthy control is shown for comparison. Widefield pseudocolor and autofluorescence images are shown (Optos, Dunfermline, UK).

constriction seen in RP. Optical coherence tomography (OCT) imaging (Fig. 2) reveals RPE loss at the leading edge of the degeneration with loss of outer retina and choriocapillaris thereafter. Absolute scotomas are present in retinal locations where the RPE and retina have degenerated. Typically, by the third decade, a central island of residual retinal tissue with scalloped edges remains, which undergoes exponential decay over time (Aylward et al. 2018). Central visual function, such as BCVA and mesopic microperimetry within the fovea and parafovea are well preserved, or normal, until late in the disease (Figs. 2 and 3). In a proportion of individuals, short-wavelength autofluorescence (SW-AF) imaging demonstrates a mottled RPE surrounding a central smooth zone where photoreceptor morphology is better preserved, validating the mottled zone as a degenerative feature of both the RPE and retina (Stevanovic et al. 2020). Color vision in choroideremia is typically lost along the tritan axis in early disease, as estimated by the Cambridge Color Test, correlating well with visual acuity (Seitz et al. 2018). Encroachment of the degeneration on the fovea is followed by a reduction in visual acuity, with visual decline accelerating between the age of 30 and 40 years (Bozkaya et al. 2022),

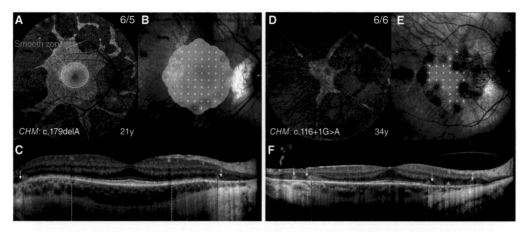

Figure 2. Clinical features of early choroideremia. (*A*) A central island of retinal pigment epithelium (RPE), retina, and choroid typically develops in the third decade in males with a frameshifting mutation in *CHM*, although visual acuity is preserved initially. On short-wavelength autofluorescence (SW-AF) imaging, a mottled zone is observed on the peripheries of the island with a smooth zone in the center in early disease stages. On optical coherence tomography (OCT) imaging, the mottled zone manifests as incomplete choroidal transmission (blue dashed line (*C*) with complete choroidal transmission identifying the peripheral limits of RPE atrophy (red dashed line). Moreover, the ellipsoid zone appears discontinuous over the mottled RPE. Retinal sensitivity falls on the edges of the central island as the degeneration progresses centripetally (*B*). Choroidal and photoreceptor degeneration most likely occur secondary to RPE degeneration, since the choroid (green arrowheads) and photoreceptors (white arrows) are present beyond the limits of RPE atrophy on OCT imaging (*C,F*). With advancing disease and a reduction in size of the remaining island, the smooth zone may be lost (*D*) with choroidal transmission seen under the fovea (*F*). Loss of the RPE and overlying retina results in absolute scotomas on microperimetry seen outside of the central island (*E*). Outer retinal tubulations are seen on OCT imaging (yellow arrows, *F*) in the degenerate outer retina. Schisis within the macula (blue arrowhead, *F*) and epiretinal membrane may develop as nonspecific effects of retinal degeneration.

and blindness in the fifth to sixth decade of life. Outer retinal tubulations are present in >90% of individuals (Xue et al. 2016); schisis within the retina is often seen in late disease (Fig. 3).

Although isolated *CHM* mutations result in nonsyndromic retinal degeneration, recent evidence suggests that systemic lipid metabolism may be affected (Cunha et al. 2021). However, it is unclear as to whether serum lipids and cardiovascular disease risk are higher in choroideremia patients compared to age-matched controls.

Differential Diagnosis

For nonsyndromic individuals with a choroideremia-like phenotype without mutations in the *CHM* gene, sequencing of the *RPE65* gene may identify a specific dominant mutation (D477G) that may phenocopy as choroideremia through a presumed dominant-negative disease mecha-

nism (Table 2; Bowne et al. 2011). Individuals in this group typically become symptomatic in early adulthood with nyctalopia and central visual disturbance, with severe visual loss at 40–70 years of age (Hull et al. 2016; Jauregui et al. 2020; Kiang et al. 2020). Heterozygous null mutations in *RGR* and a specific missense mutation in *RHO* have been reported with choroideremia-like phenotypes in separate pedigrees (Audo et al. 2010; Ba-Abbad et al. 2018). Other nonsyndromic differential diagnoses of choroideremia include progressive bifocal chorioretinal atrophy. Nongenetic causes include acquired disease due to extensive peripheral retinal ablative procedures, such as cryotherapy or drug toxicity, such as from thioridazine use.

For individuals with syndromic features and a choroideremia-like retinal phenotype, consideration should be given to a chromosomal deletion involving flanking genes at the *CHM* locus, or a

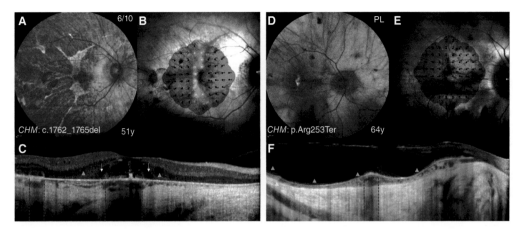

Figure 3. Clinical features of late choroideremia. (*A,B*) With advanced disease, the central island degenerates further, associated with a reduction in visual acuity and foveal sensitivity with foveal encroachment. Optical coherence tomography (OCT) and autofluorescence imaging confirm retinal pigment epithelium (RPE) loss (red dashed lines, *C*), and complete choroidal degeneration (yellow arrowhead). Schisis cavities within the retina may progress and extend to the peripheral retina (blue arrowheads, *C,F*). (*D,E*) In end-stage disease, RPE remnants may remain with perception of light vision and minimal retinal sensitivity before loss of the island results in total blindness.

deletion at the tip of the long arm of the X chromosome. Learning difficulties and deafness are recurrent syndromic features associated with chromosomal deletions involving the *CHM* gene (Cremers et al. 1989; Merry et al. 1989; Hildebrand et al. 2007; Poloschek et al. 2008; Iossa et al. 2015; Liang et al. 2017). Short stature secondary to hypogonadotrophic hypogonadism with ataxia due to cerebellar vermis hypoplasia, spastic paraplegia, and/or learning difficulties should raise suspicions of Oliver–MacFarlane syndrome caused by mutations in *PNPLA6* (Table 2; Kmoch et al. 2015; O'Neil et al. 2019; Wu et al. 2021). A further differential for a syndromic child with a choroideremia-like retinal appearance includes Alagille syndrome, associated with mutations in *JAG1* in 90% of affected individuals. However, severe systemic disease including biliary atresia and congenital heart disease may dominate the clinical picture, particularly as visual acuity is well preserved in early life. A choroideremia-like phenotype may be evident in Danon disease (Taylor and Adler 1993) in which mutations in lysosome-associated membrane protein-2 (*LAMP-2*), expressed in the RPE (Thompson et al. 2016; Fukushima et al. 2020), produce midperipheral pigmentary change associated with hyperreflective foci in the outer

nuclear layer on OCT imaging (Hasegawa et al. 2022). *LAMP-2*, present on the X chromosome, is an important constituent of the lysosomal membrane involved in autophagy within the RPE. Systemic manifestations of Danon disease include cardiomyopathy (hypertrophic in males and dilated in females) and generalized myopathy with many patients requiring cardiac transplantation (Taylor and Adler 1993).

Table 2. Differential diagnosis of choroideremia

Nonsyndromic

Gyrate atrophy (*OAT*)

Dominant mutation in *RPE65* (D477G)

Progressive bifocal chorioretinal atrophy (locus: *6q14-16*)

Excessive cryotherapy, or other ablative procedures

Drug toxicity (i.e., thioridazine)

Rhodopsin mutation (M207R) (Audo et al. 2010)

Dominant RGR mutation (haploinsufficiency) (Ba-Abbad et al. 2018)

Syndromic

Deletion on the X chromosome, involving *CHM*

Oliver–MacFarlane syndrome (*PNPLA6*)

Alagille syndrome (*JAG1*)

Danon disease (*LAMP2*)

Female Carriers

Female carriers of choroideremia were recognized long before confirmation of the *CHM* gene on the X chromosome in 1990 in affected individuals. Initial reports noted peripheral retinal pigmentation in female carriers (François 1971) with phenotypic heterogeneity (Forsius et al. 1977). In 1986, a description of 126 female carriers identified symptoms in ~7%, although 40% had visual field changes and 33% abnormal dark adaptation (Kärnä 1986). Full-field electroretinography was found to be affected in ~15%

of carriers (Sieving et al. 1986). Disease is slowly progressive in carriers with marked variability, although visual acuity is typically well preserved (Kärnä 1986). FAF imaging may detect subtle mottling of the RPE in the absence of manifest fundoscopic signs (Ortiz-Ramirez et al. 2020), and other multimodal retinal imaging techniques may be supportive (Ma et al. 2017; Paavo et al. 2019; Corvi et al. 2020; Murro et al. 2020).

Four main carrier phenotypes are recognized based on multimodal retinal imaging findings: Fine, Coarse, Geographic, and Male-pattern (Fig. 4; De Silva et al. 2021). The variable clinical

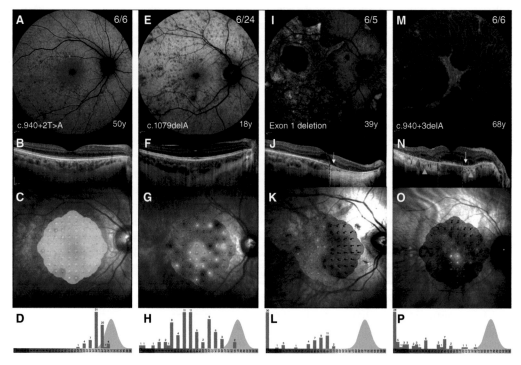

Figure 4. Multimodal retinal imaging features in four female *CHM* carriers. The retinal phenotype in female carriers of *CHM* mutations is dependent on the embryonic stage and the skew of X-inactivation, the specific variant, age, and other modifiers. (*A–D*) Fine, (*E–H*) Coarse, (*I–L*) Geographic, and (*M–P*) Male pattern choroideremia carrier phenotypes are described. Initially, fine patchy (*A*) hypoautofluorescence may be identified with a normal appearance of the retinal layers on OCT. An individual with a coarse mottled pattern shows streaks of choroidal hypertransmission on OCT imaging (*F*), suggesting patchy disease of the RPE, and reduced retinal sensitivity (*G–H*). With progressive disease, focal loss of RPE results in geographic atrophy, characterized by loss of autofluorescent signal (*I*), choroidal hypertransmission on OCT imaging (*J*, dashed red line), and absolute scotoma on microperimetry (*K–L*). Note that preserved retina has a coarse appearance and reduced function. Further degeneration may result in a male phenotype with an island of residual RPE at the posterior pole with overlying retina (*N*) that may be sufficient to support a visual acuity of 6/6 if the fovea is preserved. As in affected males, the choroid (green arrowheads) and retina (white arrow) is preserved beyond the area of remaining RPE.

phenotypes are determined by the stage and pattern of X chromosomal inactivation that occurs in mammals through heterochromatin packaging, as described originally by Mary Lyons (Lyon 1961). In human embryonic development, X-inactivation occurs around the blastocyst stage, and remains fixed throughout the life of the cell and all descendant cells. In female carriers, skewed inactivation of the X chromosome containing the wild-type *CHM* allele in the early blastocyst stage may result in severe, male pattern disease, since most or all RPE cells are affected. Later inactivation may result in a geographic pattern where localized clonal expansion of affected RPE cells manifests clinically in coalescing patches of RPE atrophy. A fine or coarse granular or mottled appearance on FAF imaging may represent later X-inactivation, whereby normal and abnormal RPE cells are juxtaposed throughout the retina. Moreover, different patterns of X-inactivation between RPE lineages may underpin interocular asymmetry in carrier females. Accordingly, while some carrier females remain asymptomatic, others may exhibit a more severe disease phenotype similar to that observed in affected males (Jauregui et al. 2019). Note that these patterns are distinct from carriers of X-linked RP where radial streaks are apparent from migration of affected and unaffected photoreceptors during development, and X-linked albinism where a "mud-splattered" fundus secondary to mosaicism of the melanosomes in affected and unaffected RPE cells is observed with radial streaks in the periphery (Wu et al. 2018). Bruch's membrane degeneration in a choroideremia carrier may be complicated by choroidal neovascularization (Wavre-Shapton et al. 2013; Ang et al. 2021).

Although mosaicism of the X chromosome may be determined from peripheral white blood cells, the cell lineages are distinct from those relevant to X-linked inherited degenerations, which affect the retina and RPE. It has been assumed that skewed X-inactivation (>80% inactivation of the healthy X chromosome) (Ørstavik 2006) may lead to male pattern phenotypes of X-linked diseases. However, a study of 12 female carriers of disease-associated *CHM* alleles found no correlation between disease severity and skewed lyonization of the wild-type *CHM* allele (Perez-Cano

et al. 2009). These assays are complicated by age-dependent skewed X-inactivation in peripheral blood, which increases after the age of 55 years (Ørstavik 2006). An extreme demonstration of severe, male pattern choroideremia in a female carrier has been reported in the context of Turner's syndrome—monosomy of the X chromosome in females (Cheng et al. 2018).

CLINICAL GENETICS

The familial nature and male predominance of choroideremia was appreciated from early reports, with X-linked inheritance suggested in 1942 by Goedbloed (Goedbloed 1942). The locus harboring the *CHM* gene was provisionally assigned to Xq13-21 (Lewis et al. 1985; Nussbaum et al. 1985; Schwartz et al. 1986), and further narrowed thereafter to Xq21 (Cremers et al. 1987, 1989; Nussbaum et al. 1987; Sankila et al. 1990) with the underlying *CHM* gene identified as the genetic cause of choroideremia (Xq21.2) through positioning cloning in 1990 (Cremers et al. 1990c). The *CHM* gene encodes REP1, a protein of 653 amino acids that is ubiquitously expressed in human tissues. More than 350 mutations in *CHM* have been identified (as summarized in detail by Han et al. 2021), all of which are presumed to abrogate or reduce the biological function of REP1, either due to reduced expression and/or reduced chaperone or prenylation activity. Most exonic mutations are truncating with only six missense mutations presumed to act as functional nulls (Han et al. 2021). The low number of missense mutations in *CHM* is striking and supports the known primary function of REP1 as a chaperone protein, whose function can be compensated for in nonocular tissues by REP2 with a 95% sequence homology. Numerous intronic mutations and large deletions have been identified, together accounting for ~33% of pathogenic variants (Han et al. 2021). The large number of reported deletions in *CHM* may be explained by a weak selection pressure due to compensation in other tissues by REP2 and the relatively late onset of end-stage disease in affected males (i.e., after the age of reproduction). Molecular genetic testing is typically undertaken through next-generation sequencing of exons and intron–exon boundaries. However, several pathogenic deep intronic mutations have been identified, which may require direct sequencing of the gene if the clinical suspicion is high. Moreover, the detection of large deletions, insertions, duplications, and rearrangements may require multiplex ligation-dependent probe amplification (MLPA), which together may account for as many as 14% of mutations (Han et al. 2021). Additional variants have been described affecting highly conserved sequences within the *CHM* promoter (Vaché et al. 2019). Since most pathological mutations in *CHM* are functional nulls, there is only limited evidence for correlation between genotype and phenotype (Simunovic et al. 2016). The large number of unique variants in *CHM* further

supports gene therapy as the leading therapeutic strategy. Other strategies are reviewed in detail elsewhere (Cehajic Kapetanovic et al. 2019a,b; Han et al. 2021).

DISEASE MECHANISM

CHM encodes REP1, which functions in the posttranslational modification of proteins through prenylation, a process by which covalent lipid (hydrophobic) prenyl molecules are attached to the carboxyl terminus of a protein to facilitate attachment to intracellular membranes (Fig. 5). Specifically, REP1 facilitates the transfer of a geranylgeranyl group by GGTases to Rab GTPases, a superfamily of Ras G-proteins involved in intracellular vesicle trafficking. The absence of REP1 has been associated with the re-

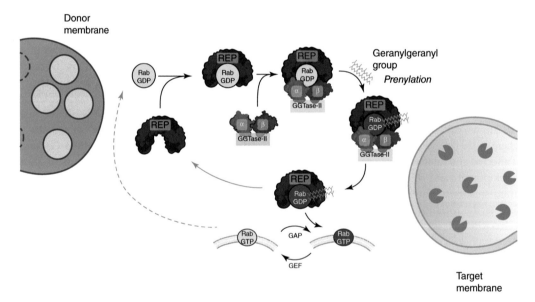

Figure 5. REP1 function within the retinal pigment epithelium (RPE). The *CHM* gene encodes REP1, which functions as a geranylgeranyl transferase in the prenylation posttranslational modification of Rab proteins, escorting them to their cellular targets. Prenyl molecules are attached to the carboxyl-terminus Rab proteins, facilitating their attachment to cell membranes. The REP cycle shows the escort of Rab GDP by REP1, the addition of α- and β-subunits through GGTase-II, and the addition of a geranylgeranyl group to the carboxyl terminus of the Rab protein (prenylation), which facilitates membrane attachment. In the RPE, shed outer segment discs from photoreceptors are continually phagocytosed by the RPE, fused to endosomes to form the late phagosome, and later fused with lysosomes to form the phagolysosome toward the basolateral RPE membrane where a low pH facilitates degradation. The ablation of REP1 has been shown to delay phagosome maturation and clearance of photoreceptor outer segments, with accumulation of debris within the RPE, which is the probable mechanism underlying primary RPE cell death in choroideremia. In the retina, REP1 is known to interact primarily with Rab27a and others to facilitate prenylation, which in turn coordinates inward movement of the phagolysosome.

duced prenylation of several Rabs (Seabra et al. 1995). In addition, REP1 is responsible for escorting Rab proteins through the cytoplasm to their target membrane.

In the RPE, efficient phagocytosis of shed photoreceptor outer segments is critical for the maintenance of homeostasis. The Rab family of GTPases is involved in phagosome maturation within the RPE, whereby phagocytosed outer segments fuse with endosomes and lysosomes to form mature phagolysosomes (Kwon and Freeman 2020). Two independent studies identified RPE dysfunction and degeneration following ablation or silencing of *CHM* associated with alterations in phagocytic and secretory pathways within the RPE (Gordiyenko et al. 2010; Wavre-Shapton et al. 2013). Furthermore, restoration of the human transgene to *CHM*-deficient iPSC-derived RPE cells restored prenylation, vesicle trafficking, and phagocytosis (Duong et al. 2018). Multimodal imaging studies in affected patients (Figs. 2 and 3) show RPE atrophy at the leading edge of degeneration, followed thereafter by loss of the outer retina and choriocapillaris. However, the pathophysiology of disease is likely to be more complex. Conditional knockout models using inducible and tissue-specific Cre expression showed independent degeneration of RPE and photoreceptors that involved different subsets of Rab proteins (Tolmachova et al. 2006). Independent degeneration of photoreceptors and early loss of choriocapillaris perfusion within preserved RPE have also been observed in choroideremia patients (Jacobson et al. 2006; Foote et al. 2019). Loss of the rod photoreceptor outer segments prior to RPE loss may in part explain early loss of rod function observed in patients with choroideremia (Aleman et al. 2017).

Although there are observations of photoreceptor defects in animal models that appear independent of RPE degeneration (Tolmachova et al. 2006), overall, the evidence supports the RPE as the most likely primary site of degeneration in choroideremia. Delays in phagosome maturation and photoreceptor outer segment clearance with consequent accumulation of debris within the RPE are the most likely pathogenic mechanisms for cellular

toxicity, although others, such as deficits in melanosome trafficking have been suggested (Hume et al. 2001). Other proteins involved in the prenylation pathway do not appear to influence disease progression in affected individuals when evaluated ex vivo (e.g., *CHML*, *RABGGTB*, *RAB27A*), nor do their levels of expression differ from controls (Fry et al. 2021). However, prenylation of Rabs (e.g., RAB27A and RAB6A) may be assessed in vitro as a functional assay for assessing the potency of AAV vectors, regardless of the specific *CHM* mutation (Patrício et al. 2018).

REP1 is ubiquitously expressed and, in nonhuman primates, its absence is embryonically lethal (Tolmachova et al. 2006; Moosajee et al. 2009). It is unclear why mutations in *CHM* result in nonsyndromic retinal degeneration. However, in humans, the X-derived retrogene, REP2, presents as cDNA (i.e., without introns) on chromosome 1 as the *CHML* gene bears a 95% sequence homology to REP1 and may provide a compensatory mechanism in nonocular tissues facilitated by other Rabs (Cremers et al. 1994). Rab27a is preferentially prenylated by REP1 and is particularly important for retinal function (Larijani et al. 2003). However, it is unclear whether nonsyndromic retinal degeneration occurs due to altered activity of specific Rab(s), or whether the RPE is particularly susceptible to long-term abnormalities of intracellular vesicle trafficking.

RPE degeneration appears to affect the midperipheral retina early in choroideremia. This observation may be explained by the relatively high metabolic demands on the RPE in the midperipheral retina, which forms a watershed zone in which the relative density of photoreceptors to RPE cells is highest across the retina (5000 RPE cells per mm^2 at the fovea; 2500 per mm^2 in the peripheral retina). In choroideremia and other primary RPE diseases, such as gyrate atrophy, the midperipheral RPE and retina is affected first, followed by progressive RPE degeneration, which then progresses centripetally and contiguously. This observation might also explain why the foveal encroachment in late disease occurs initially on the nasal side of the island (Figs. 2 and 4–6).

CLINICAL TRIALS

Table 1 lists the interventional clinical trials of retinal gene therapy for choroideremia, with a summary of study characteristics, key findings, and references to published data. The most advanced clinical program is the STAR study (NightStaRx/Biogen; NCT03496012), a pivotal international phase 3 clinical trial, which evaluated the effect of subretinal AAV2.REP1 over 12 mo in individuals with advanced choroideremia (34–73 ETDRS letters). Although primary and secondary end points were not met in this study (Biogen press release, Biogen 2021), a trend to clinical benefit aligned in the treatment group across all end points, narrowly missing statistical significance following Bonferroni correction. However, there is as yet nothing in the public domain to suggest that the sponsor is intending to negotiate with the U.S. FDA on whether the marginal clinical data might be sufficient to justify some form of limited approval. It is likely that a further phase 3 clinical trial will be undertaken, which may benefit from observations made during the STAR study, including refinements in study design, such as vector dose, surgical technique, and consideration of novel end points. These modifications may help to overcome the challenges in gaining regulatory approval of retinal gene therapy for choroideremia, which will be considered in detail.

CHALLENGES IN THE REGULATORY APPROVAL OF GENE THERAPY FOR CHOROIDEREMIA

The principal challenges in the approval of the first gene therapy for choroideremia are (1) the short duration of pivotal clinical trials for a very slow degeneration; (2) a requirement for visual acuity improvement necessitates the inclusion of patients with late disease because this is when the acuity begins to drop; (3) the need for surgical detachment of the fovea for transduction of the subfoveal RPE—a process that in itself will have a detrimental effect on visual acuity that is not seen in noninterventional controls; and (4)

the transduction of dysfunctional RPE cells in patients with late disease. These challenges are a consequence, primarily, of the thresholds required to satisfy regulators and the costs of running clinical trials. In preclinical studies, which are not subject to the same constraints, retinal gene therapy, in general, has been shown to be most effective when delivered in the early stages of disease when a greater number of target cells are available, with therapeutic efficacy demonstrated over a relatively longer period.

Short Duration of Clinical Trials

Inherited retinal degenerations are individually rare, often slowly progressive, and may have ocular asymmetry. These characteristics alone present challenges in the demonstration of benefit during short pivotal clinical trials, which are typically 1–2 years in duration, given that degeneration in the control (untreated) eyes is slow. This often means that sustained improvement of visual function in a proportion of participants is necessary to show a clinically and statistically significant difference between treatment groups for regulatory approval. For retinal gene therapy, which for the most part aims to prevent further visual loss through the prevention of cell death of transduced target cells, this is a somewhat burdensome objective. Moreover, visual improvement may not be possible for all genetic causes of retinal degeneration, which vary in terms of the primary affected cell type, the type of protein (e.g., visual cycle, structural, ciliary, phototransduction), the speed of retinal degeneration, and age of onset. The length of clinical trials in retinal gene therapy is generally restricted due to the associated costs. However, a conditional approval enabling longer-term observations prior to final approval may circumvent the challenge with evaluation of gene therapy for slow retinal degenerations, as discussed in more detail below.

The Inclusion of Patients with Late Choroideremia

The central, key functional outcome measure in clinical trials in ophthalmology remains BCVA, with the degree of improvement defined in terms of letter or lines of improvement on the ETDRS chart. These outcome measures have become standard in the assessment of efficacy of interventions (e.g., anti–vascular endothelial growth factor [VEGF] injections) for the major acquired macular disorders (e.g., age-related macular degeneration, diabetic macular edema) where significant, short-term visual benefits are expected. However, the pathobiology and natural history of these late-onset acquired disorders are distinct from inherited retinal degenerations, as are the therapies used to address them. Moreover, BCVA represents a high-contrast stimulus, which is an imperfect measure of a patient's visual function. For the Nightstar/Biogen STAR phase 3 clinical trial, the threshold for approval predesignated by the FDA as the primary end point was a three-line (15-letter) gain in a significantly greater proportion of patients compared with the control group. Choroideremia patients (Figs. 2 and 3) typically maintain visual acuity until late in the disease. Therefore, gains in BCVA require the inclusion of late-stage patients whose central vision has dropped to between 35–73 ETDRS letters (to allow headroom to gain 15 letters—88 letters is better than 6/6 or 20/20). Conversely, below 35 letters (6/60 or 20/200), fixation becomes unreliable and visual acuity readings become inconsistent. This group typically exhibits significant central RPE dysfunction and degeneration—the target cell for transduction in choroideremia (such as the patient in Fig. 3)—which may not be optimal for effective transduction. The inclusion of patients with late disease is therefore a consequence of the current accepted regulatory practice, rather than what is generally accepted as optimal in the field of retinal gene therapy—that is, to treat early in the disease process to maximize the therapeutic effect.

Surgical Detachment of the Fovea

Since BCVA is the primary outcome measure in most clinical trials, transduction of foveal cones is a key strategy in retinal gene therapy that often necessitates surgical detachment of the fovea following subretinal injection. The

visual thresholds for approval must be achieved despite any adverse structural and functional effects related to the maneuver—an effect that cannot easily be controlled for in clinical trials of subretinal gene therapy due to the associated surgical risks. Surgical detachment of photoreceptors may lead to short-term structural and functional changes within the retina as seen in animal models (Kyhn et al. 2008; Secondi et al. 2012) and in human patients treated with gene therapy (Aleman et al. 2022), which may offset early therapeutic signals in clinical trials. While mild foveal dysfunction with a loss of a few letters of visual acuity may be perfectly acceptable in the context of giving a sight-saving gene therapy treatment, this becomes an issue when the visual acuity gains being chased in a pivotal trial are only marginal. Therefore, in the early postoperative period, retinal function in the region of the bleb/retinal detachment may be worse than measured at baseline. Moreover, focal loss of the RPE is typically apparent at retinotomy sites following the delivery subretinal gene therapy, an effect that should be compensated for in relevant methods of analysis when compared to control eyes (e.g., microperimetry and FAF) across short trials. Consequently, treated eyes must achieve greater effective functional improvements to compensate for the effect of retinal detachment in the absence of a paired control intervention. Further research may help to quantify the structural and functional effects of early surgical retinal detachment within the bleb margin, although this may vary depending on the underlying gene. For subretinal gene therapy, these further data may support the modification of thresholds for approval by the regulators to account for these effects.

RPE Dysfunction in Late Disease

Individuals with late choroideremia are preferentially selected for clinical trials (Table 1) to avoid a ceiling effect that prevents measurable improvements in BCVA. At this late stage, the residual island of RPE is usually mottled, with or without a central smooth zone on FAF imaging (Fig. 3). Mottled RPE has been further associated with photoreceptor abnormalities on OCT imaging (Stevanovic et al. 2020). These observations support structural degeneration of the remaining RPE in late choroideremia, the primary target cell in retinal gene therapy. It is unclear whether dysfunctional RPE in late choroideremia can be transduced as efficiently as the RPE in early disease or within the smooth zone. In preclinical studies, carrier female mice ($Chm^{-/WT}$) were typically injected at 3–4 wk, without assessments of the effects on REP1 expression following AAV2. REP1 injection in later disease (Tolmachova et al. 2013). Mechanisms of RPE cell death in choroideremia may be REP1-independent in later stages, and therefore not retrievable by REP1 transgene replacement. Furthermore, dosing may be more challenging in late disease where the effective multiplicity of infection (MOI) may be high as fewer remaining, dysfunctional RPE cells remain, which receive a high dose of AAV. The late application of gene therapy may therefore affect the predictability and efficiency of transduction. There are no direct in vitro studies comparing the efficiency of AAV transduction in RPE cell lines with or without degenerative features or toxic insults. However, a comparison of the relative efficacy of retinal gene therapy in preserving vision in subjects with early disease versus late disease may help to answer this question.

Gene therapy for choroideremia aims to restore REP1 function and prenylation activity to the remaining RPE cells, thereby preventing or slowing RPE cell death, and secondary photoreceptor and choroidal degeneration. Substantial improvements in visual acuity in later-stage choroideremia patients suggest that RPE function is improved following subfoveal retinal gene therapy, where it is presumed that restoration of RPE prenylation and intracellular vesicle trafficking improves the function of foveal cones. It is unclear whether the dysfunctional RPE is able to express the REP1 transgene as efficiently. Consequently, the extent to which gene therapy can rescue dysfunctional RPE within the remaining central island of residual tissue is unclear, and whether this varies between the smooth and mottled zones on FAF imaging.

TOWARD REGULATORY APPROVAL

Novel End Points

The FDA emphasizes the importance of functional benefits for the approval of gene therapy vectors for inherited retinal degeneration. Although BCVA is the most recognized functional outcome measure, improvements in BCVA are not always possible in IRDs: this may relate to amblyopia, and/or photoreceptor or RPE degeneration at the fovea. In choroideremia, visual acuity is lost in late disease and the aim of gene therapy is early intervention to preserve the maximum visual function over the long term. In early choroideremia, visual acuity is well preserved (Fig. 2), and a ceiling effect means that alternative functional end points must be sought for clinical trials. Since rod function is lost early in the disease course, end points that evaluate rod function may be supportive. Scotopic microperimetry is a novel end point that measures differential rod and cone sensitivities within the macula—typically targeted in subretinal gene therapy vector delivery (Taylor et al. 2022). In the pivotal clinical trial of *RPE65* gene therapy, the multiluminance mobility test (MLMT) was used as a primary outcome measure that was accepted by the FDA in the process of regulatory approval. However, the MLMT is not relevant to many other retinal degenerations, which may not affect the visual cycle with a profound effect on scotopic visual function. Microperimetry is a key functional outcome measure in many retinal gene therapy clinical trials, permitting a point-wise assessment of macular sensitivity (Pfau et al. 2021). However, in choroideremia, the decay of the central island may lead to precipitous drops in measured retinal sensitivity. Moreover, the retinal locations analyzed on repeat assessment are not perfectly consistent, which may lead to variability (i.e., when retinal function is assessed over a blood vessel). A key technique for development is the accurate mapping of microperimetry plots so that sequential assessments test identical retinal locations and to link microperimetry assessments to structural retinal imaging techniques, such as FAF imaging, to reduce variability between assessments and subjects.

A qualitative difference in the RPE has been noted in the central island in the majority of patients with choroideremia on SW-AF imaging (Stevanovic et al. 2020). Centripetal degeneration results in a mottled zone of degenerating RPE with a more preserved smooth zone centrally with healthier appearing RPE (Fig. 2). A significant difference in the continuity of the ellipsoid zone was observed in mottled versus smooth zone on SW-AF imaging, suggesting indirectly that photoreceptor degeneration is more pronounced over the mottled zone. This suggests the possibility of using the smooth RPE zone (e.g., changes in size and/or retinal sensitivity) as an outcome measure following retinal gene therapy. The objective definition of the smooth and mottled zones on FAF may be further aided by near-infrared autofluorescence (NIR-AF) imaging since the area of the NIR-AF signal appears to broadly match that of the smooth zone on SW-AF imaging (Fig. 6), although this requires further validation. In support of this suggestion, choroideremia patients may be categorized based on NIR-AF patterns, which appear to correlate with other structural measures of degeneration on OCT imaging (Birtel et al. 2019).

Modification of the Process of Regulatory Approval

In general, the difficulty in gaining approvals for novel therapeutics for inherited retinal degenerations by the regulators (e.g., FDA) may necessitate reconsideration of the pathway to regulatory approval that recognizes the slowly progressive nature of IRDs. Pivotal clinical trials are expensive to run; 3–5-year studies would be financially prohibitive, although far more likely to demonstrate the requisite functional benefits. An alternative pathway to approval may be that if safety is demonstrated in a phase 3 study over 1–2 years, with trends toward functional benefit, a period of conditional approval could be granted by the regulators, allowing sponsors to collect

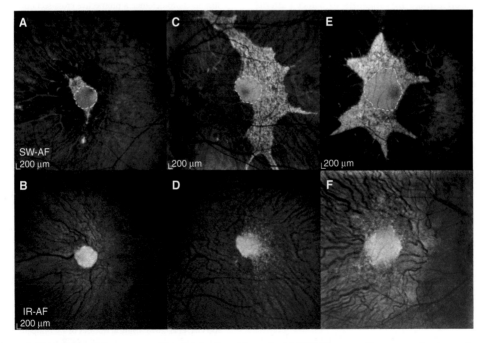

Figure 6. Near-infrared fluorescence imaging in choroideremia. (*A,C,E*) The smooth zone on short-wavelength autofluorescence maps to residual signal on near-infrared autofluorescence imaging in three patients with choroideremia. (*B,D,F*) Note that the limits of the central zone on infrared autofluorescence (IR-AF) correspond closely to the approximate boundaries of the smooth zone (yellow dashed line) as seen on short-wavelength autofluorescence (SW-AF) imaging.

longer-term data that can then be reviewed by the regulators prior to final approval.

This approach may change the paradigm of patient selection for clinical trials across different forms of retinal degeneration. In the case of choroideremia, this change would support the inclusion of patients with early disease who have a greater number of target RPE cells and may have a better long-term prognosis following intervention. The effective MOI would be more predictable on early-stage patients, potentially reducing variability between subjects. In late disease, the rescue of dysfunctional target cells may result in an improvement in visual function that typically plateaus once nonoptimally transduced cells, which may contribute to retinal function in the early postoperative period, die. In early disease, this phenomenon may be relevant only to RPE cells at the edge of the remaining island. A clear therapeutic effect could be shown through preservation of the island while the central island in the control eye undergoes exponential decay (Aylward et al. 2018). The current regulatory prerequisites encourage investigators to select patients and doses based on what might show the greatest functional benefit over the shorter term, so that other groups may benefit following approval. However, these may not be the same groups that would otherwise be chosen for clinical trial participation if long-term preservation of vision was the goal. Reform of the process of regulatory approval of gene therapy vectors may benefit patients by focusing patient selection around long-term functional improvements, which would probably be favored by patient groups.

CONCLUDING REMARKS

Choroideremia is an untreatable blinding disease due to mutations in the *CHM* gene. Significant advances have been made in describing the genetic basis and molecular pathophysiology of the disease, with more than 350 mutations described. A pivotal phase 3 clinical trial of retinal gene therapy for choroideremia showed clear therapeutic benefits, although it fell short of the thresholds for regulatory approval. In this review, we summarize the challenges in gaining approval for gene therapy investigational medi-

cal products for slow inherited retinal degenerations such as choroideremia and suggest novel end points that might be supportive. Despite these challenges, the approval of the first therapy for choroideremia is expected in the near future, 150 years after the first clinical description of the disease by Mauthner in 1872.

COMPETING INTEREST STATEMENT

R.E.M. is a named inventor on a patent for choroideremia gene therapy owned by the University of Oxford.

ACKNOWLEDGMENTS

R.E.M. is a consultant to Biogen Inc.

REFERENCES

Aleman TS, Han G, Serrano LW, Fuerst NM, Charlson ES, Pearson DJ, Chung DC, Traband A, Pan W, Ying GS, et al. 2017. Natural history of the central structural abnormalities in choroideremia: a prospective cross-sectional study. *Ophthalmology* **124:** 359–373. doi:10.1016/j.ophtha.2016.10.022

Aleman TS, Huckfeldt RM, Serrano LW, Pearson DJ, Vergilio GK, McCague S, Marshall KA, Ashtari M, Doan TM, Weigel-DiFranco CA, et al. 2022. Adeno-associated virus serotype 2-hCHM subretinal delivery to the macula in choroideremia: two-year interim results of an ongoing phase I/II gene therapy trial. *Ophthalmology* **129:** 1177–1191. doi:10.1016/j.ophtha.2022.06.006

Ang JL, Wright AF, Dhillon B, Cackett P. 2021. Choroidal neovascularisation in a predicted female choroideraemia carrier treated with intravitreal anti-vascular endothelial growth factor. *Euro J Ophthalmol* **31:** 4–10. doi:10.1177/1120672120965495

Audo I, Friedrich A, Mohand-Saïd S, Lancelot ME, Antonio A, Moskova-Doumanova V, Poch O, Bhattacharya S, Sahel JA, Zeitz C. 2010. An unusual retinal phenotype associated with a novel mutation in RHO. *Arch Ophthal* **128:** 1036–1045. doi:10.1001/archophthalmol.2010.162

Aylward JW, Xue K, Patrício MI, Jolly JK, Wood JC, Brett J, Jasani KM, MacLaren RE. 2018. Retinal degeneration in choroideremia follows an exponential decay function. *Ophthalmology* **125:** 1122–1124. doi:10.1016/j.ophtha.2018.02.004

Ba-Abbad R, Leys M, Wang X, Chakarova C, Waseem N, Carss KJ, Raymond FL, Bujakowska KM, Pierce EA, Mahroo OA, et al. 2018. Clinical features of a retinopathy associated with a dominant allele of the *RGR* gene. *Invest Ophthalmol Vis Sci* **59:** 4812–4820. doi:10.1167/iovs.18-25061

Biogen. 2021. Biogen announces topline results from Phase 3 Gene Therapy Study in Choroideremia. https://investors.biogen.com/news-releases/news-release-details/biogen-announces-topline-results-phase-3-gene-therapy-study

Birtel J, Salvetti AP, Jolly JK, Xue K, Gliem M, Müller PL, Holz FG, MacLaren RE, Charbel Issa P. 2019. Near-infrared autofluorescence in choroideremia: anatomic and functional correlations. *Arch Ophthal* **199:** 19–27.

Bowne SJ, Humphries MM, Sullivan LS, Kenna PF, Tam LC, Kiang AS, Campbell M, Weinstock GM, Koboldt DC, Ding L, et al. 2011. A dominant mutation in RPE65 identified by whole-exome sequencing causes retinitis pigmentosa with choroidal involvement. *Eur J Hum Genet* **19:** 1074–1081. doi:10.1038/ejhg.2011.86

Bozkaya D, Zou H, Lu C, Tsao NW, Lam BL. 2022. Bilateral visual acuity decline in males with choroideremia: a pooled, cross-sectional meta-analysis. *BMC Ophthalmol* **22:** 29. doi:10.1186/s12886-022-02250-z

Cehajic Kapetanovic J, Barnard AR, MacLaren RE. 2019a. Molecular therapies for choroideremia. *Genes (Basel)* **10:** 738. doi:10.3390/genes10100738

Cehajic Kapetanovic J, Patrício MI, MacLaren RE. 2019b. Progress in the development of novel therapies for choroideremia. *Expert Rev Ophthalmol* **14:** 277–285. doi:10.1080/17469899.2019.1699406

Cheng JL, Farnsworth K, Bernstein PS. 2018. Choroideremia in a woman with turner syndrome. *JAMA Ophthalmol* **136:** 1076–1078. doi:10.1001/jamaophthalmol.2018.2630

Corvi F, Corradetti G, Wong A, Eng JG, Sadda S. 2022. Peripheral optical coherence tomography findings in a choroideremia carrier. *Retin Cases Brief Rep* **16:** 766–769. doi:10.1097/ICB.0000000000001109

Cremers FP, Brunsmann F, van de Pol TJ, Pawlowitzki IH, Paulsen K, Wieringa B, Ropers HH. 1987. Deletion of the DXS165 locus in patients with classical choroideremia. *Clin Genet* **32:** 421–423. doi:10.1111/j.1399-0004.1987.tb03166.x

Cremers FP, van de Pol DJ, Diergaarde PJ, Wieringa B, Nussbaum RL, Schwartz M, Ropers HH. 1989. Physical fine mapping of the choroideremia locus using Xq21 deletions associated with complex syndromes. *Genomics* **4:** 41–46. doi:10.1016/0888-7543(89)90312-1

Cremers FP, Brunsmann F, Berger W, van Kerkhoff EP, van de Pol TJ, Wieringa B, Pawlowitzki IH, Ropers HH. 1990a. Cloning of the breakpoints of a deletion associated with choroideremia. *Hum Genet* **86:** 61–64. doi:10.1007/BF00205174

Cremers FP, Sankila EM, Brunsmann F, Jay M, Jay B, Wright A, Pinckers AJ, Schwartz M, van de Pol DJ, Wieringa B, et al. 1990b. Deletions in patients with classical choroideremia vary in size from 45 kb to several megabases. *Am J Hum Genet* **47:** 622–628.

Cremers FP, van de Pol DJ, van Kerkhoff LP, Wieringa B, Ropers HH. 1990c. Cloning of a gene that is rearranged in patients with choroideraemia. *Nature* **347:** 674–677. doi:10.1038/347674a0

Cremers FP, Armstrong SA, Seabra MC, Brown MS, Goldstein JL. 1994. REP-2, a Rab escort protein encoded by the choroideremia-like gene. *J Biol Chem* **269:** 2111–2117. doi:10.1016/S0021-9258(17)42142-9

Cunha DL, Richardson R, Tracey-White D, Abbouda A, Mitsios A, Horneffer-van der Sluis V, Takis P, Owen N, Skinner J, Welch AA, et al. 2021. REP1 deficiency causes systemic dysfunction of lipid metabolism and oxidative stress in choroideremia. *JCI Insight* **6:** e146934. doi:10.1172/jci.insight.146934

De Silva SR, Arno G, Robson AG, Fakin A, Pontikos N, Mohamed MD, Bird AC, Moore AT, Michaelides M, Webster AR, et al. 2021. The X-linked retinopathies: physiological insights, pathogenic mechanisms, phenotypic features and novel therapies. *Prog Retin Eye Res* **82:** 100898. doi:10.1016/j.preteyeres.2020.100898

Dimopoulos IS, Hoang SC, Radziwon A, Binczyk NM, Seabra MC, MacLaren RE, Somani R, Tennant MTS, MacDonald IM. 2018. Two-year results after AAV2-mediated gene therapy for choroideremia: the Alberta experience. *Am J Ophthalmol* **193:** 130–142. doi:10.1016/j.ajo.2018.06.011

Duong TT, Vasireddy V, Ramachandran P, Herrera PS, Leo L, Merkel C, Bennett J, Mills JA. 2018. Use of induced pluripotent stem cell models to probe the pathogenesis of choroideremia and to develop a potential treatment. *Stem Cell Res* **27:** 140–150. doi:10.1016/j.scr.2018.01.009

Edwards TL, Jolly JK, Groppe M, Barnard AR, Cottriall CL, Tolmachova T, Black GC, Webster AR, Lotery AJ, Holder GE, et al. 2016. Visual acuity after retinal gene therapy for choroideremia. *N Engl J Med* **374:** 1996–1998. doi:10.1056/NEJMc1509501

Fischer MD, Ochakovski GA, Beier B, Seitz IP, Vaheb Y, Kortuem C, Reichel FFL, Kuehlewein L, Kahle NA, Peters T, et al. 2019. Efficacy and safety of retinal gene therapy using adeno-associated virus vector for patients with choroideremia: a randomized clinical trial. *JAMA Ophthalmol* **137:** 1247–1254. doi:10.1001/jamaophthalmol.2019.3278

Fischer MD, Ochakovski GA, Beier B, Seitz IP, Vaheb Y, Kortuem C, Reichel FFL, Kuehlewein L, Kahle NA, Peters T, et al. 2020. Changes in retinal sensitivity after gene therapy in choroideremia. *Retina* **40:** 160–168. doi:10.1097/IAE.0000000000002360

Foote KG, Rinella N, Tang J, Bensaid N, Zhou H, Zhang Q, Wang RK, Porco TC, Roorda A, Duncan JL. 2019. Cone structure persists beyond margins of short-wavelength autofluorescence in choroideremia. *Invest Ophthalmol Vis Sci* **60:** 4931–4942. doi:10.1167/iovs.19-27979

Forsius H, Hyvärinen L, Nieminen H, Flower R. 1977. Fluorescein and indocyanine green fluorescence angiography in study of affected males and in female carriers with choroidermia. A preliminary report. *Acta Ophthalmol* **55:** 459–470. doi:10.1111/j.1755-3768.1977.tb06123.x

François J. 1971. Sex-linked chorioretinal heredodegenerations. *Birth Defects Orig Artic Ser* **7:** 99–116.

Fry LE, Patrício MI, Jolly JK, Xue K, MacLaren RE. 2021. Expression of Rab prenylation pathway genes and relation to disease progression in choroideremia. *Transl Vis Sci Technol* **10:** 12. doi:10.1167/tvst.10.8.12

Fukushima M, Inoue T, Miyai T, Obata R. 2020. Retinal dystrophy associated with Danon disease and pathogenic mechanism through LAMP2-mutated retinal pigment epithelium. *Euro J Ophthalmol* **30:** 570–578. doi:10.1177/1120672119832183

Goedbloed J. 1942. Mode of inheritance in chorioideremia. *Ophthalmologica* **104:** 308–315. doi:10.1159/000300062

Gordiyenko NV, Fariss RN, Zhi C, MacDonald IM. 2010. Silencing of the *CHM* gene alters phagocytic and secretory pathways in the retinal pigment epithelium. *Invest Ophthalmol Vis Sci* **51:** 1143–1150. doi:10.1167/iovs.09-4117

Han RC, Fry LE, Kantor A, McClements ME, Xue K, MacLaren RE. 2021. Is subretinal AAV gene replacement still the only viable treatment option for choroideremia? *Expert Opin Orphan Drugs* **9:** 13–24. doi:10.1080/21678707.2021.1882300

Hasegawa A, Noda K, Fujiya A, Hirooka K, Anzai T, Ishida S. 2022. Outer retinal abnormalities in a patient with Danon disease. *Retinal Cases Brief Rep* **16:** 619–621. doi:10.1097/ICB.0000000000001043

Hildebrand MS, de Silva MG, Tan TY, Rose E, Nishimura C, Tolmachova T, Hulett JM, White SM, Silver J, Bahlo M, et al. 2007. Molecular characterization of a novel X-linked syndrome involving developmental delay and deafness. *Am J Med Genet A* **143A:** 2564–2575. doi:10.1002/ajmg.a.31995

Hull S, Mukherjee R, Holder GE, Moore AT, Webster AR. 2016. The clinical features of retinal disease due to a dominant mutation in RPE65. *Mol Vis* **22:** 626–635.

Hume AN, Collinson LM, Rapak A, Gomes AQ, Hopkins CR, Seabra MC. 2001. Rab27a regulates the peripheral distribution of melanosomes in melanocytes. *J Cell Biol* **152:** 795–808. doi:10.1083/jcb.152.4.795

Iossa S, Costa V, Corvino V, Auletta G, Barruffo L, Cappellani S, Ceglia C, Cennamo G, D'Adamo AP, D'Amico A, et al. 2015. Phenotypic and genetic characterization of a family carrying two Xq21.1-21.3 interstitial deletions associated with syndromic hearing loss. *Mol Cytogenet* **8:** 18. doi:10.1186/s13039-015-0120-0

Jacobson SG, Cideciyan AV, Sumaroka A, Aleman TS, Schwartz SB, Windsor EA, Roman AJ, Stone EM, MacDonald IM. 2006. Remodeling of the human retina in choroideremia: rab escort protein 1 (*REP-1*) mutations. *Invest Ophthalmol Vis Sci* **47:** 4113–4120. doi:10.1167/iovs.06-0424

Jauregui R, Park KS, Tanaka AJ, Cho A, Paavo M, Zernant J, Francis JH, Allikmets R, Sparrow JR, Tsang SH. 2019. Spectrum of disease severity and phenotype in choroideremia carriers. *Am J Ophthalmol* **207:** 77–86. doi:10.1016/j.ajo.2019.06.002

Jauregui R, Cho A, Oh JK, Tanaka AJ, Sparrow JR, Tsang SH. 2020. Phenotypic expansion of autosomal dominant retinitis pigmentosa associated with the D477G mutation in RPE65. *Cold Spring Harb Mol Case Stud* **6:** a004952. doi:10.1101/mcs.a004952

Jolly JK, Xue K, Edwards TL, Groppe M, MacLaren RE. 2017. Characterizing the natural history of visual function in choroideremia using microperimetry and multimodal retinal imaging. *Invest Ophthalmol Vis Sci* **58:** 5575–5583. doi:10.1167/iovs.17-22486

Kärnä J. 1986. Choroideremia. A clinical and genetic study of 84 Finnish patients and 126 female carriers. *Acta Ophthalmol Suppl* **176:** 1–68.

Kiang AS, Kenna PF, Humphries MM, Ozaki E, Koenekoop RK, Campbell M, Farrar GJ, Humphries P. 2020. Properties and therapeutic implications of an enigmatic D477G RPE65 variant associated with autosomal dominant retinitis pigmentosa. *Genes (Basel)* **11:** 1420. doi:10.3390/genes11121420

Kmoch S, Majewski J, Ramamurthy V, Cao S, Fahiminiya S, Ren H, MacDonald IM, Lopez I, Sun V, Keser V, et al. 2015. Mutations in PNPLA6 are linked to photoreceptor degeneration and various forms of childhood blindness. *Nat Commun* **6:** 5614. doi:10.1038/ncomms6614

Kwon W, Freeman SA. 2020. Phagocytosis by the retinal pigment epithelium: recognition, resolution, recycling. *Front Immunol* **11:** 604205. doi:10.3389/fimmu.2020.604205

Kyhn MV, Kiilgaard JF, Lopez AG, Scherfig E, Prause JU, la Cour M. 2008. Functional implications of short-term retinal detachment in porcine eyes: study by multifocal electroretinography. *Acta Ophthalmol* **86:** 18–25. doi:10.1111/j.1600-0420.2007.00983.x

Lam BL, Davis JL, Gregori NZ, MacLaren RE, Girach A, Verriotto JD, Rodriguez B, Rosa PR, Zhang X, Feuer WJ. 2019. Choroideremia gene therapy phase 2 clinical trial: 24-month results. *Am J Ophthalmol* **197:** 65–73. doi:10.1016/j.ajo.2018.09.012

Larijani B, Hume AN, Tarafder AK, Seabra MC. 2003. Multiple factors contribute to inefficient prenylation of Rab27a in Rab prenylation diseases. *J Biol Chem* **278:** 46798–46804. doi:10.1074/jbc.M307799200

Lewis RA, Nussbaum RL, Ferrell R. 1985. Mapping X-linked ophthalmic diseases. Provisional assignment of the locus for choroideremia to Xq13-q24. *Ophthalmology* **92:** 800–806. doi:10.1016/S0161-6420(85)33956-8

Liang S, Jiang N, Li S, Jiang X, Yu D. 2017. A maternally inherited 8.05 Mb Xq21 deletion associated with choroideremia, deafness, and mental retardation syndrome in a male patient. *Mol Cytogenet* **10:** 23. doi:10.1186/s13039-017-0324-6

Lyon MF. 1961. Gene action in the X-chromosome of the mouse (*Mus musculus* L). *Nature* **190:** 372–373. doi:10.1038/190372a0

Ma KK, Lin J, Boudreault K, Chen RW, Tsang SH. 2017. Phenotyping choroideremia and its carrier state with multimodal imaging techniques. *Retin Cases Brief Rep* **11**(Suppl 1): S178–S181.

MacLaren RE, Groppe M, Barnard AR, Cottriall CL, Tolmachova T, Seymour L, Clark KR, During MJ, Cremers FP, Black GC, et al. 2014. Retinal gene therapy in patients with choroideremia: initial findings from a phase 1/2 clinical trial. *Lancet* **383:** 1129–1137. doi:10.1016/S0140-6736(13)62117-0

Mauthner L. 1872. Ein fall von choroideremie. *Ber Naturwissensch-med Ver Inssbruck* **2:** 191–197.

Merry DE, Lesko JG, Sosnoski DM, Lewis RA, Lubinsky M, Trask B, van den Engh G, Collins FS, Nussbaum RL. 1989. Choroideremia and deafness with stapes fixation: a contiguous gene deletion syndrome in Xq21. *Am J Hum Genet* **45:** 530–540.

Moosajee M, Tulloch M, Baron RA, Gregory-Evans CY, Pereira-Leal JB, Seabra MC. 2009. Single *choroideremia* gene in nonmammalian vertebrates explains early embryonic lethality of the zebrafish model of choroideremia. *Invest Ophthalmol Vis Sci* **50:** 3009–3016. doi:10.1167/iovs.08-2755

Muniz A, Villazana-Espinoza ET, Hatch AL, Trevino SG, Allen DM, Tsin AT. 2007. A novel cone visual cycle in the cone-dominated retina. *Exp Eye Res* **85:** 175–184. doi:10.1016/j.exer.2007.05.003

Murro V, Mucciolo DP, Giorgio D, Sodi A, Passerini I, Virgili G, Rizzo S. 2020. Optical coherence tomography angiography (OCT-A) in choroideremia (CHM) carriers. *Ophthalmic Genet* **41:** 146–151. doi:10.1080/13816810.2020.1747086

Nussbaum RL, Lewis RA, Lesko JG, Ferrell R. 1985. Choroideremia is linked to the restriction fragment length polymorphism DXYS1 at XQ13-21. *Am J Hum Genet* **37**: 473–481.

Nussbaum RL, Lesko JG, Lewis RA, Ledbetter SA, Ledbetter DH. 1987. Isolation of anonymous DNA sequences from within a submicroscopic X chromosomal deletion in a patient with choroideremia, deafness, and mental retardation. *Proc Natl Acad Sci* **84**: 6521–6525. doi:10.1073/pnas.84.18.6521

O'Neil E, Serrano L, Scoles D, Cunningham KE, Han G, Chiang J, Bennett J, Aleman TS. 2019. Detailed retinal phenotype of Boucher–Neuhäuser syndrome associated with mutations in *PNPLA6* mimicking choroideremia. *Ophthalmic Genet* **40**: 267–275. doi:10.1080/13816810.2019.1605392

Ørstavik KH. 2006. Skewed X inactivation in healthy individuals and in different diseases. *Acta Paediatr Suppl* **95**: 24–29. doi:10.1080/08035320600618783

Ortiz-Ramirez GY, Villanueva-Mendoza C, Zenteno Ruiz JC, Reyes M, Cortés-González V. 2020. Autofluorescence in female carriers with choroideremia: a familial case with a novel mutation in the *CHM* gene. *Ophthalmic Genet* **41**: 625–628. doi:10.1080/13816810.2020.1810283

Paavo M, Carvalho JRL Jr, Lee W, Sengillo JD, Tsang SH, Sparrow JR. 2019. Patterns and intensities of near-infrared and short-wavelength fundus autofluorescence in choroideremia probands and carriers. *Invest Ophthalmol Vis Sci* **60**: 3752–3761. doi:10.1167/iovs.19-27366

Patrício MI, Barnard AR, Cox CI, Blue C, MacLaren RE. 2018. The biological activity of AAV vectors for choroideremia gene therapy can be measured by in vitro prenylation of RAB6A. *Mol Ther Methods Clin Dev* **9**: 288–295. doi:10.1016/j.omtm.2018.03.009

Perez-Cano HJ, Garnica-Hayashi RE, Zenteno JC. 2009. *CHM* gene molecular analysis and X-chromosome inactivation pattern determination in two families with choroideremia. *Am J Med Genet A Part A* **149a**: 2134–2140. doi:10.1002/ajmg.a.32727

Pfau M, Jolly JK, Wu Z, Denniss J, Lad EM, Guymer RH, Fleckenstein M, Holz FG, Schmitz-Valckenberg S. 2021. Fundus-controlled perimetry (microperimetry): application as outcome measure in clinical trials. *Prog Retin Eye Res* **82**: 100907. doi:10.1016/j.preteyeres.2020.100907

Poloschek CM, Kloeckener-Gruissem B, Hansen LL, Bach M, Berger W. 2008. Syndromic choroideremia: sublocalization of phenotypes associated with Martin–Probst deafness mental retardation syndrome. *Invest Ophthalmol Vis Sci* **49**: 4096–4104. doi:10.1167/iovs.08-2044

Sankila EM, Bruns GA, Schwartz M, Nikoskelainen E, Niebuhr E, Hodgson SV, Wright AF, de la Chapelle A. 1990. DXS26 (HU16) is located in Xq21.1. *Hum Genet* **85**: 117–120. doi:10.1007/BF00276335

Sankila EM, Tolvanen R, van den Hurk JA, Cremers FP, de la Chapelle A. 1992. Aberrant splicing of the CHM gene is a significant cause of choroideremia. *Nat Genet* **1**: 109–113. doi:10.1038/ng0592-109

Schwartz M, Rosenberg T, Niebuhr E, Lundsteen C, Sardemann H, Andersen O, Yang HM, Lamm LU. 1986. Choroideremia: further evidence for assignment of the locus to Xq13-Xq21. *Hum Genet* **74**: 449–452. doi:10.1007/BF00280505

Seabra MC. 1996. New insights into the pathogenesis of choroideremia: a tale of two REPs. *Ophthalmic Genet* **17**: 43–46. doi:10.3109/13816819609057869

Seabra MC, Ho YK, Anant JS. 1995. Deficient geranylgeranylation of Ram/Rab27 in choroideremia. *J Biol Chem* **270**: 24420–24427. doi:10.1074/jbc.270.41.24420

Secondi R, Kong J, Blonska AM, Staurenghi G, Sparrow JR. 2012. Fundus autofluorescence findings in a mouse model of retinal detachment. *Invest Ophthalmol Vis Sci* **53**: 5190–5197. doi:10.1167/iovs.12-9672

Seitz IP, Jolly JK, Dominik Fischer M, Simunovic MP. 2018. Colour discrimination ellipses in choroideremia. *Graefes Arch Clin Exp Ophthalmol* **256**: 665–673. doi:10.1007/s00417-018-3921-0

Sieving PA, Niffenegger JH, Berson EL. 1986. Electroretinographic findings in selected pedigrees with choroideremia. *Am J Ophthalmol* **101**: 361–367. doi:10.1016/0002-9394(86)90832-9

Simunovic MP, Jolly JK, Xue K, Edwards TL, Groppe M, Downes SM, MacLaren RE. 2016. The spectrum of CHM gene mutations in choroideremia and their relationship to clinical phenotype. *Invest Ophthalmol Vis Sci* **57**: 6033–6039. doi:10.1167/iovs.16-20230

Stevanovic M, Cehajic Kapetanovic J, Jolly JK, MacLaren RE. 2020. A distinct retinal pigment epithelial cell autofluorescence pattern in choroideremia predicts early involvement of overlying photoreceptors. *Acta Ophthalmol* **98**: e322–e327. doi:10.1111/aos.14281

Taylor MRG, Adler ED. 1993. Danon disease. In *Genereviews* (ed. Adam MP, Ardinger HH, Pagon RA, Wallace SE, Bean LJH, Gripp KW, Mirzaa GM, Amemiya A). University of Washington, Seattle.

Taylor LJ, Josan AS, Pfau M, Simunovic MP, Jolly JK. 2022. Scotopic microperimetry: evolution, applications and future directions. *Clin Exp Optom* **105**: 793–800. doi:10.1080/08164622.2021.2023477

Thompson DA, Constable PA, Liasis A, Walters B, Esteban MT. 2016. The physiology of the retinal pigment epithelium in Danon disease. *Retina* **36**: 629–638. doi:10.1097/IAE.0000000000000736

Tolmachova T, Anders R, Abrink M, Bugeon L, Dallman MJ, Futter CE, Ramalho JS, Tonagel F, Tanimoto N, Seeliger MW, et al. 2006. Independent degeneration of photoreceptors and retinal pigment epithelium in conditional knockout mouse models of choroideremia. *J Clin Invest* **116**: 386–394. doi:10.1172/JCI26617

Tolmachova T, Tolmachov OE, Barnard AR, de Silva SR, Lipinski DM, Walker NJ, Maclaren RE, Seabra MC. 2013. Functional expression of Rab escort protein 1 following AAV2-mediated gene delivery in the retina of choroideremia mice and human cells ex vivo. *J Mol Med* **91**: 825–837. doi:10.1007/s00109-013-1006-4

Vache C, Torriano S, Faugère V, Erkilic N, Baux D, Garcia-Garcia G, Hamel CP, Meunier I, Zanlonghi X, Koenig M, et al. 2019. Pathogenicity of novel atypical variants leading to choroideremia as determined by functional analyses. *Hum Mutat* **40**: 31–35. doi:10.1002/humu.23671

Wavre-Shapton ST, Tolmachova T, Lopes da Silva M, Futter CE, Seabra MC. 2013. Conditional ablation of the choroideremia gene causes age-related changes in mouse retinal pigment epithelium. *PLoS ONE* **8:** e57769. doi:10.1371/journal.pone.0057769

Wu AL, Wang JP, Tseng YJ, Liu L, Kang YC, Chen KJ, Chao AN, Yeh LK, Chen TL, Hwang YS, et al. 2018. Multimodal imaging of mosaic retinopathy in carriers of hereditary x-linked recessive diseases. *Retina* **38:** 1047–1057. doi:10.1097/IAE.0000000000001629

Wu S, Sun Z, Zhu T, Weleber RG, Yang P, Wei X, Pennesi ME, Sui R. 2021. Novel variants in PNPLA6 causing syndromic retinal dystrophy. *Exp Eye Res* **202:** 108327. doi:10.1016/j.exer.2020.108327

Xue K, Oldani M, Jolly JK, Edwards TL, Groppe M, Downes SM, MacLaren RE. 2016. Correlation of optical coherence tomography and autofluorescence in the outer retina and choroid of patients with choroideremia. *Invest Ophthalmol Vis Sci* **57:** 3674–3684. doi:10.1167/iovs.15-18364

Xue K, Jolly JK, Barnard AR, Rudenko A, Salvetti AP, Patrício MI, Edwards TL, Groppe M, Orlans HO, Tolmachova T, et al. 2018. Beneficial effects on vision in patients undergoing retinal gene therapy for choroideremia. *Nat Med* **24:** 1507–1512. doi:10.1038/s41591-018-0185-5

RPGR-Related Retinopathy: Clinical Features, Molecular Genetics, and Gene Replacement Therapy

Shaima Awadh Hashem,[1,2] Michalis Georgiou,[1,2,3] Robin R. Ali,[1,2,4] and Michel Michaelides[1,2]

[1]UCL Institute of Ophthalmology, University College London, London EC1V 9EL, United Kingdom

[2]Moorfields Eye Hospital NHS Foundation Trust, London EC1V 2PD, United Kingdom

[3]Jones Eye Institute, University of Arkansas for Medical Sciences, Little Rock, Arkansas 72205, USA

[4]Centre for Cell and Gene Therapy, King's College London, London WC2R 2LS, United Kingdom

Correspondence: michel.michaelides@ucl.ac.uk

Retinitis pigmentosa GTPase regulator (*RPGR*) gene variants are the predominant cause of X-linked retinitis pigmentosa (XLRP) and a common cause of cone-rod dystrophy (CORD). XLRP presents as early as the first decade of life, with impaired night vision and constriction of peripheral visual field and rapid progression, eventually leading to blindness. In this review, we present *RPGR* gene structure and function, molecular genetics, animal models, *RPGR*-associated phenotypes and highlight emerging potential treatments such as gene-replacement therapy.

Retinitis pigmentosa GTPase regulator (*RPGR*) gene variants are the predominant cause of X-linked retinitis pigmentosa (XLRP), accounting for 70%–80% of cases (Tee et al. 2016). The other less common causes of XLRP are retinitis pigmentosa 2 (*RP2*) and 23 (*RP23* or *OFD1*) (Branham et al. 2012; Webb et al. 2012). *RPGR* XLRP is one of the most severe forms of rod-cone dystrophy (RCD), in terms of the early age of onset and rate of degeneration. Typically, symptoms include abnormal night vision and peripheral visual field constriction, leading to visual impairment by the fourth decade of life.

In male patients, the retinal degeneration is particularly severe and shows rapid progression, while the phenotype of *RPGR* female carriers can be variable, ranging from early-onset severe disease to most commonly being asymptomatic or mildly symptomatic in later life (Georgiou et al. 2021a). Skewed inactivation of the X-chromosome in females is suggested to be the molecular basis of the variable phenotype (Wu et al. 2010). Female carriers usually have a radial pattern tapetal-like reflex (TLR) originating from the fovea, often more visible on fundus autofluorescence imaging (FAF).

More rarely, *RPGR* variants can cause cone-rod dystrophy (CORD), which presents in the second to fourth decade of life and is characterized by early central degeneration of the cones, reduced visual acuity, photophobia, and myopia (Thiadens et al. 2011).

Cite this article as *Cold Spring Harb Perspect Med* doi: 10.1101/cshperspect.a041280

RPGR PHENOTYPES AND CLINICAL FEATURES

A range of phenotypes are caused by *RPGR* pathogenic variants, which includes RCD (also known as RPGR-associated RP), early-onset severe retinal dystrophy (EOSRD), CORD, cone dystrophy (COD), macular atrophy, and syndromic XLRP. The most common presenting conditions, RCD and CORD, are described below.

RPGR-ASSOCIATED ROD-CONE DYSTROPHY

XLRP is the most common phenotype associated with *RPGR*. It is also one of the most severe forms, in which patients present with nyctalopia as early as in the first decade and progress to blindness in their thirties or forties (Sandberg et al. 2007). Electrophysiological changes are detected in childhood, as well as myopia and retinal abnormalities (Flaxel et al. 1999).

On retinal examination, affected males have an accumulation of pigment that reflects the byproduct of photoreceptor outer segment and retinal pigment epithelium (RPE) degeneration (Fig. 1). Changes in the photoreceptor layer are readily documented and monitored over time with optical coherence tomography (OCT), in the form of disruption in the ellipsoid zone (EZ) (Fig. 1). This disruption starts typically in the rod-dense region at the retinal periphery and progresses gradually toward the center of the fovea. A mean rate of EZ decline of 0.67 mm^2 was documented in 38 RPGR RP patients using en face images of the macular OCT volume scans (Tee et al. 2019).

Functional disease progression using retinal sensitivity decline has been reported with static perimetry (Tee et al. 2018). Microperimetry (MP) testing has also documented objective assessment of retinal sensitivity change over time and may, in addition to static perimetry, be valuable in assessing gene therapy outcomes. In a recent report, MP testing was performed in 76 individuals (53 adults, 23 children) with *RPGR* retinopathy, who were followed for 2.8 yr. Strong correlation of the baseline best corrected visual acuity (BCVA) and contrast sensitivity (CS) with the mean sensitivity (MS) and volumetric indices was statistically significant, while the rate of progression in the ORF15 genotype subgroup was comparable to that of the subgroup with disease-causing variants in exons 1 to 14. Most patients investigated in the study lost retinal sensitivity rapidly during their second and third decades of life (Anikina et al. 2022). A faster progression rate in younger affected males was also documented by following up the constriction of the parafoveal hyperautofluorescent ring, which is reported in the majority of *RPGR* RP patients (Tee et al. 2019).

Adaptive optics scanning light ophthalmoscopy (AOSLO) imaging enables in vivo noninvasive visualization of the cone mosaic (Georgiou et al. 2018) with the good repeatability previously reported in *RPGR*-XLRP (Tanna et al. 2017). AOSLO may provide new insights into possible mechanisms of cone vision loss in patients with retinal degeneration and a more rapid trial readout.

RPGR-ASSOCIATED COD AND CORD

RPGR variants are responsible for 1%–2% of all cases of COD and CORD phenotypes (Gill et al. 2019). These are progressive phenotypes that present in the second to fourth decade of life and primarily affect cones, albeit in the first instance. Patients initially experience symptoms of central visual field defects, reduced visual acuity and color vision, and photophobia (Vervoort et al. 2000; Ebenezer et al. 2005). Although ophthalmoscopic findings are often most evident at the macula, symptoms (and signs) of rod involvement occur in the majority of patients over time (Michaelides et al. 2006). Patients with XLCORD/COD typically also present with moderate-to-high myopia. A correlation between higher rates of vision loss and greater degrees of myopia has been previously described (Talib et al. 2019).

XLCORD patients classically harbor *RPGR* ORF15 variants that are frequently located 3′ to the highly repetitive region; while OFR15 variants that are located 5′ typically lead to RCD (RP) (Michaelides et al. 2006; Branham et al. 2012). However, exceptions have been reported,

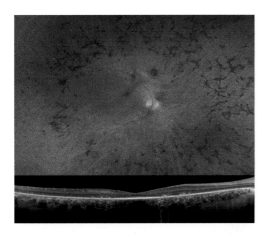

Figure 1. Retinitis pigmentosa GTPase regulator (*RPGR*)-associated rod-cone dystrophy. Color fundus photograph of the right eye of a 29-yr-old patient with *RPGR*-associated retinitis pigmentosa showing extensive peripheral retinal bone spicule pigmentation and atrophy (*top*); and optical coherence tomography (*bottom*) showing macular thinning and loss of outer retinal architecture peripherally, with relative preservation centrally.

including in an *RPGR* XLCORD pedigree with a frameshift insertion detected 5′ to the repetitive region of ORF15 (Mears et al. 2000).

On fundoscopy, a range of macular changes are observed, from mild disturbance of the RPE to severe chorioretinal atrophy. FAF imaging may identify a parafoveal hyperautofluorescent ring, which unlike those in RP, increase in size with disease progression, associated with worsening amplitude of pattern electroretinogram P50 (Robson et al. 2008a,b).

OCT typically shows early foveal EZ disruption, which is usually followed by increasing gradual disruption extending into the periphery (Fig. 2).

FEMALE CARRIERS

RPGR carriers are frequently asymptomatic or mildly affected (Ebenezer et al. 2005). Only a minority exhibit severe RP/EOSRD or CORD (Georgiou et al. 2021a). However, on examination, 40% of female carriers have the typical XLRP macular TLR, which is best seen with FAF, but can also be seen clinically. It appears

in the posterior pole as a hyperreflective radial spoke-like pattern with a golden sheen (Fig. 3; Talib et al. 2018, 2019). Cellular imaging of the TLR areas in carriers of *RPGR*-associated retinopathy showed increased rod photoreceptor reflectivity on confocal AOSLO and reduced cone photoreceptor densities. Moreover, increased reflectivity of the outer retinal bands was documented in the parafoveal TLR areas on OCT (inner segment EZ and outer segment interdigitation zone) (Kalitzeos et al. 2019). It was suggested that mosaicism, to an extent, could be responsible for the heterogeneity seen in carriers (Talib et al. 2018).

RPGR-ASSOCIATED SYNDROMIC CILIOPATHY

Ciliopathies are a group of genetic conditions caused by defects in cilia, which is currently an established cause of retinal dystrophy due to the important role of retinal proteins in cilia main-

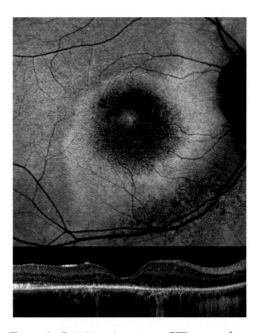

Figure 2. Retinitis pigmentosa GTPase regulator (*RPGR*)-associated cone-rod dystrophy. Fundus autofluorescence image (*top*) showing parafoveal hyperautofluorescent ring with corresponding ellipsoid zone disruption on optical coherence tomography (*below*).

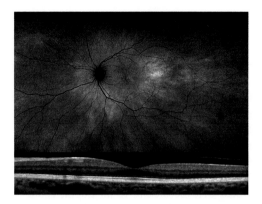

Figure 3. Retinal imaging in a female retinitis pigmentosa GTPase regulator (*RPGR*) retinopathy carrier. Fundus autofluorescence image of the left eye of an asymptomatic 45-yr-old female carrier showing a radial pattern "tapetal" reflex. Optical coherence tomography of the right eye shows preserved retinal lamination (*below*).

tenance and function (Wheway et al. 2014). Clinical evidence of *RPGR*'s role in cilia function is highlighted by certain disease-causing variants resulting in patients with *RPGR* XLRP also having hearing impairment, respiratory tract infection, and bronchiectasis (Zito et al. 2003). It is believed that ORF15 may not be involved in extraocular *RPGR* phenotypes, as all variants reported to date are in exons 1–14 (Tee et al. 2016).

MOLECULAR GENETICS

The *RPGR* gene is located on the short arm of the X chromosome and is responsible for the expression of at least 21 alternative transcripts. This gene consists of 19 exons and encodes a protein product of 90 kDa. Exons 2–11 coding for the amino terminus, which is highly similar to regulator of chromosome condensation 1 (RCC1) (Shu et al. 2007). RCC1 is a well-characterized protein that plays a role in nucleocytoplasmic transport and cell division regulation (Hadjebi et al. 2008). All proteins known to directly interact with RPGR do so through the regulator of chromosome and condensation-like domain (RLD), and all known splice-site variants of *RPGR* contain the RLD domain (Georgiou et al. 2021b).

To date, more than 300 *RPGR* variants have been identified with the majority present in the guanine-cytosine-rich mutational hotspot open reading frame15 (ORF15). *RPGR* isoforms are formed from posttranslational modification (He et al. 2008) and alternative splicing (Yan et al. 1998; Kirschner et al. 1999). *RPGR* isoforms are expressed in multiple tissues including the kidney, testis, lung, and retina, with *RPGR* OFR15 being the major isoform expressed in the retina (Vervoort et al. 2000). The majority of pathogenic variants affecting the retina are identified in the *RPGR* OFR15 isoform (Sharon et al. 2000).

RPGR STRUCTURE AND FUNCTION

In the retina, RPGR is typically found in the photoreceptor-connecting cilium (Hong et al. 2003) and consists of an RCC1-like domain at the amino terminus, and the ORF15 at the carboxy terminal, which still has no known predicted function. Previous studies have identified an RPGR protein-interaction network (Hong et al. 2001; Vervoort and Wright 2002; Hadjebi et al. 2008; Murga-Zamalloa et al. 2010), and suggested that RPGR-interacting protein (RPGRIP1) contributed to RPGR localization at the connecting cilia (Hong et al. 2001). Regulation of intercellular protein transport between the photoreceptor inner and outer segments (Hong et al. 2001), as well as maintaining correct location and concentration of opsin, is achieved when RPGR is bound to the connecting cilia. Multiple other proteins interact with RPGR, such as whirlin, maintenance of chromosomes 1 and 3 proteins, rod cyclic guanosine monophosphate phosphodiesterase (subunit δ), nephrocystin-5, and structural GTPase Rab8A (Hong et al. 2000; Beltran et al. 2006; Nemet et al. 2015; Tee et al. 2016).

In a murine RPGR knockout model, mislocalization of opsin with ensuing degeneration was reported (Hong et al. 2000). An RPGR-deficient mouse model showed that the connecting cilium is structurally not affected (Khanna et al. 2005; Shu et al. 2005). More recently, an important posttranslational modification has been identified, namely, glutamylation, which is necessary to enable RPGR function as a regulator of photoreceptor ciliary transport (Kapetanovic et al. 2019).

RPGR ANIMAL MODELS

The Siberian husky canine breed has two naturally occurring *RPGR* ORF15 disease-causing variants that result in distinct phenotypes. A 5-nucleotide deletion in *RPGR* ORF15 (del1028-1032) leads to a premature stop codon and truncation of 230 residues, resulting in X-linked progressive retinal atrophy 1 (XLPRA1) secondary to loss of RPGR function (Zhang et al. 2002). This phenotype is characterized by gradual post-developmental photoreceptor degeneration, affecting rods more than cones, which is in keeping with human RP, but with slower progression. OCT shows normal outer nuclear layer (ONL) thickness up to 28 wk of age, while from 56 wk of age, ONL thickness starts to thin in the inferior retina, while initially remaining preserved at the visual streak (Beltran et al. 2012).

The more severe phenotype, XLPRA2, is caused by a two-nucleotide deletion in ORF15 (del1084-1085), downstream to the first, resulting in frameshift and the inclusion of 34 basic amino acids with truncation of 161 residues (Zhang et al. 2002). A generalized decrease in ONL thickness is shown on OCT that is more profound in the center than the periphery (Beltran et al. 2012). In XLRPA2, an accumulation of abnormal protein product in the endoplasmic reticulum was suggested to cause the rapid course and early disease onset from around 5 wk, affecting rods and cones (Zhang et al. 2002; Beltran et al. 2006).

Three mouse models of RPGR deficiency exist; one mouse model was designed from the deletion of RPGR exons 4–6 (Hong et al. 2000). This model, 20 d after birth, has shown reduced rhodopsin levels in rods and mislocalization of cone opsin to inner segments, nuclear, and synaptic regions. However, electroretinography (ERG) was within normal limits. After 6 mo, degeneration was documented with photoreceptor loss, but the connecting cilia remained distinguishable (Hong et al. 2000).

A naturally occurring RPGR-deficient murine model is the retinal degeneration 9 (Rd9) strain of mice. RPGRORF15 levels are undetectable in the retina of affected male mice, which is caused by duplication of a 32-base pair in ORF15 that leads to a truncated protein product (Thompson et al. 2012). Deletion of exon 1 has resulted in another RPGR-deficient model (Huang et al. 2012), with a similar phenotype to the aforementioned murine model.

Transgenic mice have been generated with mutant RPGR ORF15 into RPGR knockout backgrounds and wild-type (Hong et al. 2004), which are very similar to XLPRA2, but differ from the RPGR-null mice in being more severe (Hong and Li 2002).

Photoreceptor rescue has been reported in both murine and canine models with adeno-associated virus (AAV) gene augmentation (Hong et al. 2005; Beltran et al. 2012; Pawlyk et al. 2016). In a canine model, late retinal degeneration arrest was documented, which suggested a wide therapeutic window (Beltran et al. 2015). ORF15 DNA sequence variations were noticed in this AAV vector and are likely caused by the repetitive purine nucleotides (Deng et al. 2015). This inherent mutability has been addressed with codon optimization (Fischer et al. 2017) and repetitive sequence abbreviation (Hong et al. 2005; Pawlyk et al. 2016).

Structural and functional defects were detected in transgenic mice that were engineered with multiple copies of *RPGR* in their genome, where the copies of *RPGR* were proportionate to the disease severity (Brunner et al. 2008). Mice that carried 8–10 copies had no sperm flagella detected, while other mice with 4–5 copies had lower sperm levels. These observations are relevant when considering the potential deleterious effects of *RPGR* overexpression (Georgiou et al. 2021b).

TREATMENT PRINCIPLES

The management of *RPGR*-related retinopathy remains supportive, with treatment being available only for complications, such as cataract and cystoid macular edema.

Different treatment approaches have been explored aiming to improve vision or halt/slow disease progression. Neuroprotection and dietary supplements of high doses of vitamin A and docosahexaenoic acid (DHA) were investigated in previous trials, and neither modality showed visual therapeutic benefits (Berson et al. 1993, 2004; Hoffman et al. 2004; Birch et al. 2013). Gene-replacement therapy is becoming a promising treatment option, which is currently being investigated in phase 1/2 and phase 3 trials following success in multiple animal models (Beltran et al. 2012, 2015; Pawlyk et al. 2016).

Retinal prosthesis, such as The Argus II retinal system (Second Sight Medical Products) is another approach that has been explored to aid blind or severely visually impaired patients with RP (Ho et al. 2015). Argus II retinal prosthesis, also called "Bionic eye," was FDA-approved in 2013 (Greenemeier 2013) to be used by RP patients aged above 25 yr, with vision level of light perception or no light perception in both eyes and previous history of vision; it has now been discontinued. Other approaches for advanced visual loss include optogenetics and stem cell therapies (see Pavlou and Reh 2022; Stefanov and Flannery 2022; Zin et al. 2022; Monville et al. 2023).

GENE-REPLACEMENT THERAPY

With the evolution in genetics over the last 20 yr, gene-replacement trials are now significantly facilitated by the application of engineered viruses as vectors introducing functional genetic material. AAV is the vector of choice for retinal gene therapy given its small size, is non-pathogenic in humans, has weaker postinjection immune response, and is simple and amendable to engineering (Naso et al. 2017).

Delivery of subretinal AAV gene therapy has been performed in three phase 1/2 clinical trials (NCT03316560, NCT03252847, and NCT03116 113) as well as in an ongoing phase 3 clinical trial (NCT04671433) (Table 1), whereas NCT0451 7149 is a phase 1/2 trial of a single intravitreal injection of AAV-RPGR.

NCT03116113 consisted of a dose escalation phase where 18 patients received subretinal AAV8 encoding codon-optimized human RPGR (AAV-coRPGR) and were followed for 6 mo. The early findings included subretinal inflammation in some patients, which was steroid responsive, with the study achieving the prespecified safety endpoint. Retinal sensitivity improvement on mesopic MP was recorded in six patients at 1 mo, which was variably sustained throughout the follow-up period (Dufour et al. 2020).

Safety and efficacy of AAV5-RPGR is investigated in NCT03252847. The primary end point of this clinical trial was to accomplish absence of safety events, while the secondary measures are the improvement of vision, retinal sensitivity, vision-guided mobility, and better quality of life, assessed using quality-of-life (QOL) questionnaires. The 1-yr results from the dose-escalation phase were presented ($n =$ 10, AAO 2020 and ARVO 2022) and described well-tolerated AAV5-RPGR, static perimetry, and MP improvements in addition to enhanced vision-guided mobility (Georgiou et al. 2021b).

The number of patients to acquire clinically relevant hematology and chemistry adverse events is the primary outcome of NCT033 16560, which investigates rAAV2tYF-GRK1-RPGR. The change from baseline in vision by ETDRS, perimetry, retinal structure, and QOL questionnaires are the secondary outcome measures of the trial. The reported results of the

Table 1. Retinitis pigmentosa GTPase regulator (RPGR) gene therapy clinical trials

Clinicaltrials.gov identifier	Intervention	Transgene details	Phase
NCT03252847	AAV5-RPGR	Shortened ORF15	I/II
NCT03116113	AAV8.GRK1.RPGR	Codon-optimized	I/II
NCT03316560	AAV2tYF.GRK1.RPGR	Codon-optimized	I/II
NCT04517149	AAV-RPGR (4D-125)	Codon-optimized	I/II
NCT04671433	AAV5-RPGR	Shortened ORF15	III

dose-escalation phase identified improvements in retinal sensitivity on MP.

In NCT04517149, safety and efficacy are investigated by a single intravitreal injection of AAV-RPGR at two dose levels (Georgiou et al. 2021c).

The favorable results observed at the low and intermediate doses in terms of both safety and efficacy are being further investigated in a randomized controlled phase 3 clinical trial (NCT04671433), which raises the anticipation and hopes for establishing a possible treatment in the near future.

CONCLUDING REMARKS AND FUTURE PROSPECTS

Inherited retinal diseases carry undeniable disease burden (Liew et al. 2014; Galvin et al. 2020). Recent advances in both genetic engineering and retinal imaging are contributing to the rapid progress in the field of inherited retinal disease. *RPGR*-associated disease is at the severe end of the phenotypic spectrum, leading to progressive vision loss and eventual blindness. Multiple novel approaches are under investigation aiming for vision restoration and to halt/slow degeneration.

Gene editing and posttranscriptional regulation, as in clustered regularly interspaced short palindromic repeats (CRISPR) and their associated enzyme (Cas), antisense oligonucleotides (AON), stem cell therapies, retinal implants, and optogenetics are all currently being investigated in the search for a cure for RP (refer to Ling et al. 2022; Palanker 2022; Stefanov and Flannery 2022). The promising positive safety and efficacy results of gene therapy in phase 1/2 have supported the advancement of an *RPGR* XLRP gene-replacement therapy, raising the anticipation for ongoing and upcoming phase 3 clinical trials, hoping to result in the long-awaited approved treatment for *RPGR* RP.

REFERENCES

*Reference is also in this subject collection.

Anikina E, Georgiou M, Tee J, Webster AR, Weleber RG, Michaelides M. 2022. Characterization of retinal function using microperimetry-derived metrics in both adults and children with RPGR-associated retinopathy. *Am J Ophthalmol* 234: 81–90. doi:10.1016/j.ajo.2021.07.018

Beltran WA, Hammond P, Acland GM, Aguirre GD. 2006. A frameshift mutation in *RPGR* exon ORF15 causes photoreceptor degeneration and inner retina remodeling in a model of X-linked retinitis pigmentosa. *Invest Ophthalmol Vis Sci* 47: 1669–1681. doi:10.1167/iovs.05-0845

Beltran WA, Cideciyan A, Lewin AS, Iwabe S, Khanna H, Sumaroka A, Chiodo VA, Fajardo DS, Román AJ, Deng WT, et al. 2012. Gene therapy rescues photoreceptor blindness in dogs and paves the way for treating human X-linked retinitis pigmentosa. *Proc Natl Acad Sci* 109: 2132–2137. doi:10.1073/pnas.1118847109

Beltran WA, Cideciyan A, Iwabe S, Swider M, Kosyk MS, McDaid K, Martynyuk I, Ying GS, Shaffer J, Deng WT, et al. 2015. Successful arrest of photoreceptor and vision loss expands the therapeutic window of retinal gene therapy to later stages of disease. *Proc Natl Acad Sci* 112: E5844–E5853. doi:10.1073/pnas.1509914112

Berson EL, Rosner B, Sandberg MA, Hayes KC, Nicholson BW, Weigel Difranco C, Willett W. 1993. A randomized trial of vitamin A and vitamin E supplementation for retinitis pigmentosa. *Arch Opthalmol* 111: 761–772. doi:10.1001/archopht.1993.01090060049022

Berson EL, Rosner B, Sandberg MA, Weigel-DiFranco C, Moser A, Brockhurst RJ, Hayes KC, Johnson CA, Anderson EJ, Gaudio AR, et al. 2004. Clinical trial of docosahexaenoic acid in patients with retinitis pigmentosa receiving vitamin A treatment. *Arch Opthalmol* 122: 1297–1305. doi:10.1001/archopht.122.9.1297

Birch DG, Weleber RG, Duncan JL, Jaffe GJ, Tao W. 2013. Randomized trial of ciliary neurotrophic factor delivered by encapsulated cell intraocular implants for retinitis pigmentosa. *Am J Ophthalmol* 156: 283–292.e1. doi:10.1016/j.ajo.2013.03.021

Branham K, Othman M, Brumm M, Karoukis AJ, Atmaca-Sonmez P, Yashar BM, Schwartz SB, Stover NB, Trzupek K, Wheaton D, et al. 2012. Mutations in *RPGR* and *RP2* account for 15% of males with simplex retinal degenerative disease. *Invest Ophthalmol Vis Sci* 53: 8232–8237. doi:10.1167/iovs.12-11025

Brunner S, Colman D, Travis AJ, Luhmann UFO, Shi W, Feil S, Imsand C, Nelson J, Grimm C, Rülicke T, et al. 2008. Overexpression of RPGR leads to male infertility in mice due to defects in flagellar assembly. *Biol Reprod* 79: 608–617. doi:10.1095/biolreprod.107.067454

Deng WT, Dyka FM, Dinculescu A, Li J, Zhu P, Chiodo VA, Boye SL, Conlon TJ, Erger K, Cossette T, et al. 2015. Stability and safety of an AAV vector for treating RPGR-ORF15 X-linked retinitis pigmentosa. *Hum Gene Ther* 26: 593–602. doi:10.1089/hum.2015.035

Dufour VL, Cideciyan AV, Ye GJ, Song C, Timmers A, Habecker PL, Pan W, Weinstein NM, Swider M, Durham AC, et al. 2020. Toxicity and efficacy evaluation of an adeno-associated virus vector expressing codon-optimized RPGR delivered by subretinal injection in a canine model of X-linked retinitis pigmentosa. *Hum Gene Ther* 31: 253–267. doi:10.1089/hum.2019.297

Ebenezer ND, Michaelides M, Jenkins SA, Audo I, Webster AR, Cheetham ME, Stockman A, Maher ER, Ainsworth JR, Yates JR, et al. 2005. Identification of novel *RPGR* ORF15 mutations in X-linked progressive cone-rod dystrophy (XLCORD) families. *Invest Ophthalmol Vis Sci* **46:** 1891–1898. doi:10.1167/iovs.04-1482

Fischer MD, McClements ME, Martinez-Fernandez de la Camara C, Bellingrath JS, Dauletbekov D, Ramsden SC, Hickey DG, Barnard AR, MacLaren RE. 2017. Codon-optimized RPGR improves stability and efficacy of AAV8 gene therapy in two mouse models of X-linked retinitis pigmentosa. *Mol Ther* **25:** 1854–1865. doi:10.1016/j.ymthe.2017.05.005

Flaxel CJ, Jay M, Thiselton DL, Nayudu M, Hardcastle AJ, Wright A, Bird AC. 1999. Difference between RP2 and RP3 phenotypes in X linked retinitis pigmentosa. *Br J Ophthalmol* **83:** 1144–1148. doi:10.1136/bjo.83.10.1144

Galvin O, Chi G, Brady L, Hippert C, Rubido MDV, Daly A, Michaelides M. 2020. The impact of inherited retinal diseases in the Republic of Ireland (ROI) and the United Kingdom (UK) from a cost-of-illness perspective. *Clin Ophthalmol* **14:** 707–719. doi:10.2147/OPTH.S241928

Georgiou M, Kalitzeos A, Patterson EJ, Dubra A, Carroll J, Michaelides M. 2018. Adaptive optics imaging of inherited retinal diseases. *Br J Ophthalmol* **102:** 1028–1035. doi:10.1136/bjophthalmol-2017-311328

Georgiou M, Ali N, Yang E, Grewal PS, Rotsos T, Pontikos N, Robson AG, Michaelides M. 2021a. Extending the phenotypic spectrum of PRPF8, PRPH2, RP1 and RPGR, and the genotypic spectrum of early-onset severe retinal dystrophy. *Orphanet J Rare Dis* **16:** 1–11. doi:10.1186/s13023-021-01759-8

Georgiou M, Awadh Hashem S, Daich Varela M, Michaelides M. 2021b. Gene therapy in X-linked retinitis pigmentosa due to defects in RPGR. *Int Ophthalmol Clin* **61:** 97–108. doi:10.1097/IIO.0000000000000384

Georgiou M, Fujinami K, Michaelides M. 2021c. Inherited retinal diseases: therapeutics, clinical trials and end points —A review. *Clin Exp Ophthalmol* **49:** 270–288. doi:10.1111/ceo.13917

Gill JS, Georgiou M, Kalitzeos A, Moore AT, Michaelides M. 2019. Progressive cone and cone-rod dystrophies: clinical features, molecular genetics and prospects for therapy. *Br J Ophthalmol* **103:** 711–720. doi:10.1136/bjophthalmol-2018-313278

Greenemeier L. 2013. FDA approves first retinal implant. *Nature* https://doi.org/10.1038/nature.2013.12439

Hadjebi O, Casas-Terradellas E, Garcia-Gonzalo FR, Rosa JL. 2008. The RCC1 superfamily: from genes, to function, to disease. *Biochim Biophys Acta* **1783:** 1467–1479. doi:10.1016/j.bbamcr.2008.03.015

He S, Parapuram SK, Hurd TW, Behnam B, Margolis B, Swaroop A, Khanna H. 2008. Retinitis pigmentosa GTPase regulator (RPGR) protein isoforms in mammalian retina: insights into X-linked retinitis pigmentosa and associated ciliopathies. *Vision Res* **48:** 366–376. doi:10.1016/j.visres.2007.08.005

Ho AC, Humayun MS, Dorn JD, da Cruz L, Dagnelie G, Handa J, Barale PO, Sahel JA, Stanga PE, Hafezi F, et al. 2015. Long-term results from an epiretinal prosthesis to restore sight to the blind. *Ophthalmology* **122:** 1547–1554. doi:10.1016/j.ophtha.2015.04.032

Hoffman DR, Locke KG, Wheaton DH, Fish GE, Spencer R, Birch DG. 2004. A randomized, placebo-controlled clinical trial of docosahexaenoic acid supplementation for X-

linked retinitis pigmentosa. *Am J Ophthalmol* **137:** 704–718.

Hong DH, Li T. 2002. Complex expression pattern of RPGR reveals a role for purine-rich exonic splicing enhancers. *Invest Ophthalmol Vis Sci* **43:** 3373–3382.

Hong DH, Pawlyk BS, Shang J, Sandberg MA, Berson EL, Li T. 2000. A retinitis pigmentosa GTPase regulator (RPGR)-deficient mouse model for X-linked retinitis pigmentosa (RP3). *Proc Natl Acad Sci* **97:** 3649–3654. doi:10.1073/pnas.97.7.3649

Hong DH, Yue G, Adamian M, Li T. 2001. Retinitis pigmentosa GTPase regulator (RPGR)-interacting protein is stably associated with the photoreceptor ciliary axoneme and anchors RPGR to the connecting cilium. *J Biol Chem* **276:** 12091–12099. doi:10.1074/jbc.M009351200

Hong DH, Pawlyk B, Sokolov M, Strissel KJ, Yang J, Tulloch B, Wright AF, Arshavsky VY, Li T. 2003. RPGR isoforms in photoreceptor connecting cilia and the transitional zone of motile cilia. *Invest Ophthalmol Vis Sci* **44:** 2413–2421. doi:10.1167/iovs.02-1206

Hong DH, Pawlyk BS, Adamian M, Li T. 2004. Dominant, gain-of-function mutant produced by truncation of RPGR. *Invest Ophthalmol Vis Sci* **45:** 36–41. doi:10.1167/iovs.03-0787

Hong DH, Pawlyk BS, Adamian M, Sandberg MA, Li T. 2005. A single, abbreviated RPGR-ORF15 variant reconstitutes RPGR function in vivo. *Invest Ophthalmol Vis Sci* **46:** 435–441. doi:10.1167/iovs.04-1065

Huang WC, Wright AF, Roman AJ, Cideciyan AV, Manson FD, Gewaily DY, Schwartz SB, Sadigh S, Limberis MP, Bell P, et al. 2012. RPGR-associated retinal degeneration in human X-linked RP and a murine model. *Invest Ophthalmol Vis Sci* **53:** 5594–5608. doi:10.1167/iovs.12-10070

Kalitzeos A, Samra R, Kasilian M, Tee JJL, Strampe M, Langlo C, Webster AR, Dubra A, Carroll J, Michaelides M. 2019. Cellular imaging of the tapetal-like reflex in carriers of RPGR-associated retinopathy. *Retina* **39:** 570–580. doi:10.1097/IAE.0000000000001965

Kapetanovic JC, McClements ME, de la Camara CM-F, Maclaren RE. 2019. Molecular strategies for RPGR gene therapy. *Genes (Basel)* **10:** 674. doi:10.3390/genes10090674

Khanna H, Hurd TW, Lillo C, Shu X, Parapuram SK, He S, Akimoto M, Wright AF, Margolis B, Williams DS, et al. 2005. RPGR-ORF15, which is mutated in retinitis pigmentosa, associates with SMC1, SMC3, and microtubule transport proteins. *J Biol Chem* **280:** 33580–33587. doi:10.1074/jbc.M505827200

Kirschner R, Rosenberg T, Schultz-Heienbrok R, Lenzner S, Feil S, Roepman R, Cremers FPM, Ropers HH, Berger W. 1999. RPGR transcription studies in mouse and human tissues reveal a retina-specific isoform that is disrupted in a patient with X-linked retinitis pigmentosa. *Hum Mol Genet* **8:** 1571–1578. doi:10.1093/hmg/8.8.1571

* Ling J, Jenny LA, Zhou A, Tsang SH. 2022. Therapeutic gene editing in inherited retinal disorders. *Cold Spring Harb Perspect Med* doi:10.1101/cshperspect.a041292

Liew G, Michaelides M, Bunce C. 2014. A comparison of the causes of blindness certifications in England and Wales in working age adults (16–64 years), 1999–2000 with 2009–2010. *BMJ Open* **4:** e004015. doi:10.1136/bmjopen-2013-004015

Mears AJ, Hiriyanna S, Vervoort R, Yashar B, Gieser L, Fahrner S, Daiger SP, Heckenlively JR, Sieving PA, Wright AF, et al. 2000. Remapping of the RP15 locus for X-linked cone-rod degeneration to Xp11.4-p21.1, and identification of a de novo insertion in the RPGR exon ORF15. *Am J Hum Genet* **67**: 1000–1003. doi:10.1086/303091

Michaelides M, Hardcastle AJ, Hunt DM, Moore AT. 2006. Progressive cone and cone-rod dystrophies: phenotypes and underlying molecular genetic basis. *Survey Ophthalmol* **51**: 232–258. doi:10.1016/j.survophthal.2006.02.007

* Monville C, Goureau O, Ben M'Barek K. 2023. Photoreceptor cell replacement using pluripotent stem cells: current knowledge and remaining questions. *Cold Spring Harb Perspect Med* **13**: a041309. doi:10.1101/cshperspect.a041309

Murga-Zamalloa C, Swaroop A, Khanna H. 2010. Multiprotein complexes of retinitis pigmentosa GTPase regulator (RPGR), a ciliary protein mutated in X-linked retinitis pigmentosa (XLRP). *Adv Exp Med Biol* **664**: 105–114. doi:10.1007/978-1-4419-1399-9_13

Naso MF, Tomkowicz B, Perry WL, Strohl WR. 2017. Adeno-associated virus (AAV) as a vector for gene therapy. *BioDrugs* **31**: 317–334. doi:10.1007/s40259-017-0234-5

Nemet I, Ropelewski P, Imanishi Y. 2015. Rhodopsin trafficking and mistrafficking: signals, molecular components, and mechanisms. *Prog Mol Biol Transl Sci* **132**: 39–71. doi:10.1016/bs.pmbts.2015.02.007

* Palanker D. 2022. Electronic retinal prostheses. *Cold Spring Harb Perspect Med* doi:10.1101/cshperspect.a041525

* Pavlou M, Reh TA. 2022. Cell-based therapies: strategies for regeneration. *Cold Spring Harb Perspect Med* doi:10.1101/cshperspect.a041306

Pawlyk BS, Bulgakov O, Sun X, Adamian M, Shu X, Smith AJ, Berson EL, Ali RR, Khani S, Wright AF, et al. 2016. Photoreceptor rescue by an abbreviated human RPGR gene in a murine model of X-linked retinitis pigmentosa. *Gene Ther* **23**: 196–204. doi:10.1038/gt.2015.93

Robson AG, Michaelides M, Luong VA, Holder GE, Bird AC, Webster AR, Moore AT, Fitzke FW. 2008a. Functional correlates of fundus autofluorescence abnormalities in patients with *RPGR* or *RIMS1* mutations causing cone or cone–rod dystrophy. *Br J Ophthal* **92**: 95–102. doi:10.1136/bjo.2007.124008

Robson AG, Michaelides M, Saihan Z, Bird AC, Webster AR, Moore AT, Fitzke FW, Holder GE. 2008b. Functional characteristics of patients with retinal dystrophy that manifest abnormal parafoveal annuli of high density fundus autofluorescence; a review and update. *Doc Ophthalmol* **116**: 79–89. doi:10.1007/s10633-007-9087-4

Sandberg MA, Rosner B, Weigel-DiFranco C, Dryja TP, Berson EL. 2007. Disease course of patients with X-linked retinitis pigmentosa due to *RPGR* gene mutations. *Invest Ophthalmol Vis Sci* **48**: 1298–1304. doi:10.1167/iovs.06-0971

Sharon D, Bruns GAP, McGee TL, Sandberg MA, Berson EL, Dryja TP. 2000. X-linked retinitis pigmentosa: mutation spectrum of the RPGR and RP2 genes and correlation with visual function. *Invest Ophthalmol Vis Sci* **41**: 2712–2721.

Shu X, Fry AM, Tulloch B, Manson FDC, Crabb JW, Khanna H, Faragher AJ, Lennon A, He S, Trojan P, et al. 2005. RPGR ORF15 isoform co-localizes with RPGRIP1 at centrioles and basal bodies and interacts with nucleophosmin. *Hum Mol Genet* **14**: 1183–1197. doi:10.1093/hmg/ddi129

Shu X, Black GC, Rice JM, Hart-Holden N, Jones A, O'Grady A, Ramsden S, Wright AF. 2007. RPGR mutation analysis and disease: an update. *Hum Mutat* **28**: 322–328. doi:10.1002/humu.20461

* Stefanov A, Flannery JG. 2022. A systematic review of optogenetic vision restoration: history, challenges, and new inventions from bench to bedside. *Cold Spring Harb Perspect Med* doi:10.1101/cshperspect.a041304

Talib M, van Schooneveld MJ, van Cauwenbergh C, Wijnholds J, ten Brink JB, Florijn RJ, Schalij-Delfos NE, Dagnelie G, van Genderen MM, de Baere E, et al. 2018. The spectrum of structural and functional abnormalities in female carriers of pathogenic variants in the *RPGR* gene. *Invest Ophthalmol Vis Sci* **59**: 4123–4133. doi:10.1167/iovs.17-23453

Talib M, van Schooneveld MJ, Thiadens AA, Fiocco M, Wijnholds J, Florijn RJ, Schalij-Delfos NE, van Genderen MM, Putter H, Cremers FPM, et al. 2019. Clinical and genetic characteristics of male patients with RPGR-associated retinal dystrophies: a long-term follow-up study. *Retina* **39**: 1186–1199. doi:10.1097/IAE.0000000000002125

Tanna P, Kasilian M, Strauss R, Tee J, Kalitzeos A, Tarima S, Visotcky A, Dubra A, Carroll J, Michaelides M. 2017. Reliability and repeatability of cone density measurements in patients with Stargardt disease and *RPGR*-associated retinopathy. *Invest Ophthalmol Vis Sci* **58**: 3608–3615. doi:10.1167/iovs.17-21904

Tee JJL, Smith AJ, Hardcastle AJ, Michaelides M. 2016. *RPGR*-associated retinopathy: clinical features, molecular genetics, animal models and therapeutic options. *Br J Ophthalmol* **100**: 1022–1027. doi:10.1136/bjophthalmol-2015-307698

Tee JJL, Yang Y, Kalitzeos A, Webster A, Bainbridge J, Weleber RG, Michaelides M. 2018. Characterization of visual function, interocular variability and progression using static perimetry–derived metrics in *RPGR*-associated retinopathy. *Invest Ophthalmol Vis Sci* **59**: 2422–2436. doi:10.1167/iovs.17-23739

Tee JJL, Yang Y, Kalitzeos A, Webster A, Bainbridge J, Michaelides M. 2019. Natural history study of retinal structure, progression, and symmetry using ellipzoid zone metrics in RPGR-associated retinopathy. *Am J Ophthalmol* **198**: 111–123. doi:10.1016/j.ajo.2018.10.003

Thiadens AAHJ, Soerjoesing GG, Florijn RJ, Tjiam AG, den Hollander AI, van den Born LI, Riemslag FC, Bergen AAB, Klaver CCW. 2011. Clinical course of cone dystrophy caused by mutations in the RPGR gene. *Graefes Arch Clin Exp Ophthalmol* **249**: 1527–1535. doi:10.1007/s00417-011-1789-3

Thompson DA, Khan NW, Othman MI, Chang B, Jia L, Grahek G, Wu Z, Hiriyanna S, Nellissery J, Li T, et al. 2012. Rd9 is a naturally occurring mouse model of a common form of retinitis pigmentosa caused by mutations in RPGR-ORF15. *PLoS ONE* **7**: e35865. doi:10.1371/journal.pone.0035865

Vervoort R, Wright AF. 2002. Mutations of *RPGR* in X-linked retinitis pigmentosa (RP3). *Hum Mutat* **19**: 486–500. doi:10.1002/humu.10057

Vervoort R, Lennon A, Bird AC, Tulloch B, Axton R, Miano MG, Meindl A, Meitinger T, Ciccodicola A, Wright AF. 2000. Mutational hot spot within a new RPGR exon in X-linked retinitis pigmentosa. *Nat Genet* **25**: 462–466. doi:10.1038/78182

Webb TR, Parfitt DA, Gardner JC, Martinez A, Bevilacqua D, Davidson AE, Zito I, Thiselton DL, Ressa JHC, Apergi M, et al. 2012. Deep intronic mutation in OFD1, identified by targeted genomic next-generation sequencing, causes a severe form of X-linked retinitis pigmentosa (RP23). *Hum Mol Genet* **21**: 3647–3654. doi:10.1093/hmg/dds194

Wheway G, Parry DA, Johnson CA. 2014. The role of primary cilia in the development and disease of the retina. *Organogenesis* **10**: 69–85. doi:10.4161/org.26710

Wu DM, Khanna H, Atmaca-Sonmez P, Sieving PA, Branham K, Othman M, Swaroop A, Daiger SP, Heckenlively JR. 2010. Long-term follow-up of a family with dominant X-linked retinitis pigmentosa. *Eye* **24**: 764–774. doi:10.1038/eye.2009.270

Yan D, Swain PK, Breuer D, Tucker RM, Wu W, Fujita R, Rehemtulla A, Burke D, Swaroop A. 1998. Biochemical characterization and subcellular localization of the mouse retinitis pigmentosa GTPase regulator (mRpgr). *J Biol Chem* **273**: 19656–19663. doi:10.1074/jbc.273.31.19656

Zhang Q, Acland GM, Wu WX, Johnson JL, Pearce-Kelling S, Tulloch B, Vervoort R, Wright AF, Aguirre GD. 2002. Different RPGR exon ORF15 mutations in Canids provide insights into photoreceptor cell degeneration. *Hum Mol Genet* **11**: 993–1003. doi:10.1093/hmg/11.9.993

* Zin EA, Ozturk BE, Dalkara D, Byrne LC. 2022. Developing new vectors for retinal gene therapy. *Cold Spring Harb Perspect Med* doi:10.1101/cshperspect.a041291

Zito I, Downes SM, Patel RJ, Cheetham ME, Ebenezer ND, Jenkins SA, Bhattacharya SS, Webster AR, Holder GE, Bird AC, et al. 2003. RPGR mutation associated with retinitis pigmentosa, impaired hearing, and sinorespiratory infections. *J Med Genet* **40**: 609–615. doi:10.1136/jmg.40.8.609

Gene Therapy for Rhodopsin Mutations

Alfred S. Lewin and W. Clay Smith

Departments of Molecular Genetics and Microbiology and Ophthalmology, University of Florida College of Medicine, Gainesville, Florida 32610, USA

Correspondence: lewin@UFL.EDU

Mutations in *RHO*, the gene for rhodopsin, account for a large fraction of autosomal-dominant retinitis pigmentosa (adRP). Patients fall into two clinical classes, those with early onset, pan retinal photoreceptor degeneration, and those who experience slowly progressive disease. The latter class of patients are candidates for photoreceptor-directed gene therapy, while former may be candidates for delivery of light-responsive proteins to interneurons or retinal ganglion cells. Gene therapy for *RHO* adRP may be targeted to the mutant gene at the DNA or RNA level, while other therapies preserve the viability of photoreceptors without addressing the underlying mutation. Correcting the *RHO* gene and replacing the mutant RNA show promise in animal models, while sustaining viable photoreceptors has the potential to delay the loss of central vision and may preserve photoreceptors for gene-directed treatments.

Rhodopsin is a prototypic G-protein-coupled receptor (GPCR) comprised of seven membrane-spanning domains that is responsible for photon capture in rod photoreceptor cells. It is the most abundant protein in the retina. Palczewski (2006) has calculated that there are approximately 5×10^9 disc membranes in the mouse retina and approximately 8×10^4 molecules per disc. Rhodopsin is densely packed in the disc membranes, where it appears to function as a dimer or multimer (Fotiadis et al. 2004; Suda et al. 2004). Therefore, rhodopsin plays a structural as well as catalytic role in the disc membranes, and mutations that cause misfolding or mistargeting of this GPCR frequently overcome cellular proteostasis systems and lead to death of rod photoreceptors (Mendes et al. 2005; Athanasiou et al. 2018). Indeed, mutations in the gene for rhodopsin (*RHO*) are a common cause of retinitis pigmentosa (RP), a disease characterized by the death first of rod photoreceptors, resulting in failure of peripheral vision and dark adaptation, and eventual death of cone photoreceptors affecting central vision and visual acuity (Fig. 1).

RP affects 1 in 3000 to 1 in 4000 people worldwide (Iannaccone et al. 2022). In the United States, this would translate into 82,500 to 110,000 people. While around half of the cases have no family history, RP is inherited in an autosomal-dominant (adRP), an autosomal-recessive (arRP), or an X-linked (xlRP) manner. Up to 30% of cases are inherited as an autosomal-dominant trait, in which only one copy of a mutated gene is responsible for the disease. Mutations in *RHO* account for a quarter of these cases, meaning that there are more than 8000 cases of *RHO*-related adRP in the United States

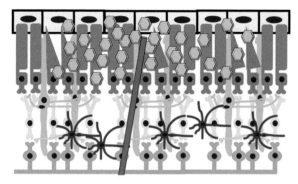

Figure 1. Overview of potential therapeutic interventions to treat retinal degeneration resulting from rhodopsin mutations.

and up to 175,000 cases worldwide. While most *RHO* mutations lead to dominantly inherited RP, some mutations lead to a recessive loss-of-function phenotype. Since loss-of-function mutations are recessive, dominance is not caused by haploinsufficiency.

More than 150 mutations in *RHO* cause adRP (Sullivan et al. 2006; Daiger et al. 2015). Studies in cell lines and in animal models indicate that *RHO* mutations impair photoreceptors by several distinct mechanisms, including increased activation of transducin (e.g., M44T), altered post-translational modification (T17M), disrupted vesicular trafficking (P347S, V345), protein misfolding, and endoplasmic reticulum (ER) retention (P23H), and constitutive activation (G90D) (Athanasiou et al. 2018).

In terms of clinical phenotype, *RHO* mutations fall into two classes: Class A mutations lead to early loss of night vision and abnormal rod function throughout the retina. Class B mutations cause more slowly progressive disease, and patients retain normal rod photoreceptors into adulthood at least in some sections of the retina (Cideciyan et al. 1998). Because of the prolonged viability of the affected cells, patients with class B mutations are better candidates for gene therapy, though slow disease progression could make it difficult to measure the efficacy of therapy. For cell-based therapies or for gene delivery to render other cell types (e.g., bipolar cells and retinal ganglion cells) photosensitive, patients with class A mutations may be better candidates, since therapy will not interfere with retained vision.

Gene therapy for recessive diseases often involves gene supplementation to deliver a normal copy of the mutant gene to the affected tissue, in this case the neural retina. For a dominant disease, however, treatment may entail suppression of the mutant allele to avoid its inhibitory impact. Another approach, gene correction, uses gene editing or base editing to simultaneously achieve gene augmentation and mutation suppression. The fact that adRP is associated with many different *RHO* mutations makes allele-specific treatment difficult, since each family may require a different treatment. As an alternative to directly treating the defect in rhodopsin, it is possible to preserve the viability and function of photoreceptors by overcoming the biochemical burden imposed by mutant rhodopsin. Such approaches include reducing ER stress, increasing turnover of misfolded rhodopsin, and improving energy metabolism in photoreceptors.

MODEL SYSTEMS FOR TESTING THERAPY

The availability of animal models has been instrumental in translating promising treatments into clinical trials. Rodent models of adRP caused by *RHO* mutations include transgenic mice and rats carrying human *RHO* transgenes containing the T17M, P23H, S334X, or P347S mutations (Olsson et al. 1992; Goto et al. 1995; Li et al. 1998a; Concepcion and Chen 2010; LaVail et al. 2018). While rodents have the advantage that they may be inbred and produced in significant numbers, larger animals such as pigs and dogs permit testing treatments in human-

Cite this article as *Cold Spring Harb Perspect Med* doi: 10.1101/cshperspect.a041283

sized eyes with a cone-rich central retina. Current porcine models include P347S and P347L transgenic lines (Petters et al. 1997; Li et al. 1998b) generated in domestic swine, and miniature pigs expressing a human P23H *RHO* (Ross et al. 2012; Fernandez de Castro et al. 2014; Scott et al. 2014). In humans, P23H is a class B mutation, but the P23H minipig model exhibits no rod electroretinographic (ERG) at birth, suggesting no rod function. Nevertheless, based on histology, rod cell bodies survive for several weeks providing a window for gene therapy. The T4R rhodopsin dog is a naturally occurring model of adRP (Kijas et al. 2002; Zhu et al. 2004). Puppies (2–3 mo old) bearing this mutation exhibit no fundus or ERG abnormalities, but in animals heterozygous for the mutant allele older than 10 mo, the ERG b-wave amplitude is attenuated, and the retina is degenerated in distinct regions. However, if young dogs are dark adapted and then exposed to flashes of light from a fundus camera, retinal degeneration begins with hours of exposure in the illuminated areas of the retina (Cideciyan et al. 2005).

As an alternative to animal models, induced pluripotent stem cells (iPSCs) may be differentiated into retinal organoids containing photoreceptor cells (Sharma et al. 2020; Eldred and Reh 2021). For DNA- or RNA-directed therapies, such as gene editing (CRISPR/Cas), RNA interference (small interfering RNA [siRNA]), or microRNA (miRNA) treatment, using human cells is essential to assess the efficacy of therapy and the nonspecific (off-target) effects of the treatment. iPSCs can be derived from patient fibroblast or other cells, but it is advisable to employ gene-editing technology to introduce the mutation of interest so that organoids with mutant rhodopsin may be compared to isogenic organoids with wild-type *RHO*. Generating retinal organoids from human iPSC is time consuming, but recent technical improvements have improved the differentiation of photoreceptors with outer segments by 4–6 mo (Capowski et al. 2019; Cowan et al. 2020; Kruczek and Swaroop 2020). Photoreceptors are displayed on the outside of retinal organoids, so that they are accessible to transduction by gene therapy vectors.

DELIVERY OF GENES TO PHOTORECEPTORS

Adeno-associated virus (AAV) is currently the most suitable viral vector for delivering genes to photoreceptor cells (Boye et al. 2013; Botto et al. 2022). Recombinant AAV (rAAV) with serotype 2 terminal repeat sequences, but pseudotyped with AAV5 or AAV8 capsids (AAV2/5 or AAV2/8), efficiently transduce photoreceptors in the area of detachment following subretinal injection. Substitution of specific surface residues leads to increased infection of photoreceptors (Petrs-Silva et al. 2009, 2011; Vandenberghe and Auricchio 2012; Kay et al. 2013). A novel serotype of AAV called AAV44.9 has the capacity to deliver genes beyond the area of retinal detachment, leading to widespread infection of photoreceptors in mouse and broader areas of transduction in macaque retinas (Boye et al. 2020). Use of this serotype or a modified version, AAV44.9(E531D) should reduce the amount of virus needed for retinal gene therapy and permit the treatment of perifoveal photoreceptors without detaching the macula.

While most preclinical gene therapy tests employ subretinal injections, several groups have tested gene delivery to photoreceptors using modified versions of AAV and intravitreal injections or suprachoroidal injections (Dalkara et al. 2013; Byrne et al. 2015, 2020; Ramachandran et al. 2017; Han et al. 2020; Pavlou et al. 2021). These approaches are theoretically safer since they avoid retinal detachment altogether. However, efficiency of transducing photoreceptors is reduced using these methods and the incidence of dose-limiting inflammation is increased by either route (Timmers et al. 2020; Yiu et al. 2020; Chung et al. 2021; Tummala et al. 2021). Induction of an inflammatory response might be avoided by selection of vector sequence to avoid unmethylated CpG sequences or inclusion of DNA sequences that antagonize activation of TLR9 (Chan et al. 2021).

There are several limitations to using AAV for gene delivery to the retina. Most humans have been infected with one or more serotypes of AAV, such that the presence of neutralizing or capsid-binding antibodies limits the efficiency of therapeutic gene delivery (Mingozzi et al.

2013; Kotterman et al. 2015; Lee et al. 2019; Bucher et al. 2021). Another disadvantage of AAV is that it can deliver a payload of no more than 4.7 kb. This size limit is not a problem for delivery of the *RHO* cDNA plus 5′ and 3′ regulatory elements, but it does limit the transfer of CRISPR/Cas gene-editing cassettes. Delivery of these larger DNA payloads may require the use of two vectors (McCullough et al. 2019; Gumerson et al. 2022; Wu et al. 2022).

OTHER DELIVERY METHODS

Adenoviral vectors (≤36 kb) and lentiviral vectors (≤8 kb) permit much larger inserts than AAV and have been tested for retinal gene therapy. Vectors derived from adenovirus lead to transient gene expression in the retina and induce a severe immune response (Trapani et al. 2014; Han et al. 2019). Lentiviral vectors derived from HIV-1 (Bainbridge et al. 2001) or EIAV (Nicoud et al. 2007) transduce the retinal pigment epithelium (RPE), but do not infect photoreceptors except in the vicinity of the injection site. Several groups have exploited nanoparticles for gene delivery to the retina (Meza-Rios et al. 2020), and this method of gene transfer is particularly attractive for gene editing tools that do not require prolonged expression of the delivered genes (Schmidt et al. 2021). For rhodopsin gene therapy, nanoparticles enable the delivery of the *RHO* genomic sequence (Han et al. 2015). The Han laboratory reported that delivering genomic DNA protected photoreceptors better than *RHO* cDNA in the P23H *Rho* model and in *Rho$^{-/-}$* mice (Mitra et al. 2018; Zheng et al. 2020).

THERAPY TARGETING *RHO*

Nearly all of the characterized *RHO* mutants are dominant and thus silencing of the mutant allele may be required to prevent blindness. A gene therapy approach would then couple knockdown of the expression of mutant rhodopsin with supplementation of a wild-type cDNA. Because of the allelic heterogeneity of adRP mutations in *RHO*, most groups have employed agents that suppress expression of all endogenous (mutant and wild-type) rhodopsin, rather than pursuing an allele-specific approach. Genome editing can be employed to block synthesis at the DNA level, or antisense oligonucleotides (ASOs) or siRNA can interrupt gene expression at the RNA stage.

Gene Editing of *RHO*

There are several technologies for gene editing, but the most commonly used technique employs clustered regularly interspaced short palindromic repeats (CRISPR) and the Cas9 nuclease or related nucleases (Mali et al. 2013; Botto et al. 2021; Fenner et al. 2022). More recent innovations, including base editing and prime editing, permit correction of point mutations or even small insertions or deletions without introducing double-stranded breaks in the genome (Komor et al. 2016; Anzalone et al. 2019; da Costa et al. 2021). CRISPR-based editing has been used to correct specific *Rho* mutations in mouse models (Bakondi et al. 2016; Li et al. 2018; Patrizi et al. 2021), but the wide variety of adRP mutations in *RHO* limit the utility of the mutation-specific approach. In contrast, an "ablate and replace" approach may be useful for all dominant *RHO* mutations. The Tsang group used dual AAV2/8 vectors to deliver the nuclease and the guide RNAs (gRNAs) in different mouse models of RHO-adRP (Tsai et al. 2018; Wu et al. 2022). The *Streptococcus pyogenes* Cas9 gene was carried by one vector, and an accompanying rAAV coded for two gRNAs for cleavage of the mutant *Rho* gene and a copy of a human *RHO* gene that did not base pair with the gRNAs. Placing the replacement gene in the same vector as the guide ensured that in photoreceptors in which *Rho* cleavage occurred, replacement with *RHO* also occurred. Using subretinal injection to treat a P23H *Rho* adRP mouse model led to improved ERG amplitudes compared to control eyes. In addition, the outer nuclear layer (ONL) thickness was greater in the treated eyes. For the C110R mutation, gene ablation and replacement preserved photoreceptors for 6 mo. Editas Medicine has announced the development of EDIT-103 for the treatment of RHO adRP. EDIT-103 also employs a dual AAV approach to ablate and switch the *RHO* gene, using the *Staphylococcus aureus* Cas9 nuclease (Editas Medicine 2022).

Cite this article as *Cold Spring Harb Perspect Med* doi: 10.1101/cshperspect.a041283

Transcriptional Repression

Zinc-finger (ZF) DNA-binding domains can be designed and tested in cells for their ability to block transcription (Liu et al. 2002). Mussolino et al. produced a series of ZF domains to bind upstream of the *RHO* gene. They fused these with the KRAB (Krüppel-associated box repressor) domain and tested them in *RHO* P347S transgenic mice using an AAV2/8 vector for delivery (Mussolino et al. 2011). This construct led to a depletion of the mutant rhodopsin and increase in the ERG response. More recently, Botta and colleagues engineered a ZF domain to obstruct a 20-base pair *cis*-regulatory element in the *RHO* promoter (Botta et al. 2016). This ZF was fused to KRAB and cloned in combination with a human *RHO* cDNA driven by another promoter (GNAT1). When delivered to pigs by subretinal injection, this combination vector suppressed expression of the endogenous *RHO* gene and replaced it with the wild-type gene delivered by the vector. The same group has shown that the ZF-DNA-binding domain that they have developed is safe when delivered to wild-type mice either via AAV or via transgenesis (Marrocco et al. 2021). Thus, this single-vector approach has considerable promise as a therapy for adRP.

Antisense Oligonucleotides (ASOs)

ASOs or antisense-ODN (oligodeoxynucleotide), can block or alter gene expression by binding to RNA and obstructing protein synthesis or RNA processing. Most often though, ASOs block gene expression by inducing mRNA degradation by RNase H, which digests the RNA in DNA:RNA hybrids. To prevent rapid turnover of antisense agents in cells or in bodily fluids, ASOs are usually linked via a phosphorothioate backbone and contain ribonucleotides with 2′-*O*-methoxyethyl or 2′-fluoro modifications at their terminal residues (Bennett and Swayze 2010). Researchers at Isis Pharmaceuticals (now Ionis) screened 20mers modified in this way. Intravitreal injection of their most potent antisense molecule caused a 70% reduction in rhodopsin mRNA over a period of 60 d (Murray et al. 2015). In P23H *Rho* transgenic rats, they observed improvement in electroretinogram a-wave and thickening of the ONL compared to eyes treated with a control ASO. A clinical trial of ASOs (QR-1123) to treat adRP associated with the P23H *RHO* mutation is in progress (ClinicalTrials.gov identifier: NCT04123626). Mutation-specific ASOs may be useful for only a small patient population, but because development of ASOs is easier than antisense techniques vectored by viruses, developing therapeutic ASOs for rare mutations is practical if a test system (animal model or organoid model) exists. In addition, in the case of adverse reaction, ASO treatment can be terminated.

RNA Replacement

RNA replacement involves depleting the levels of endogenous rhodopsin mRNA and simultaneously augmenting wild-type *RHO* mRNA. Small RNA inhibitors such as ribozymes (Wong-Staal et al. 1998; Castanotto et al. 2002), siRNAs (Grimm 2009), or artificial miRNAs (McBride et al. 2008b) may be delivered together with a resistant rhodopsin gene using plasmid or viral vectors. Several groups have tested ribozyme-based gene therapy in mouse and rat models of *RHO* adRP (Millington-Ward et al. 1997; LaVail et al. 2000; O'Neill et al. 2000; Sullivan et al. 2002; Gorbatyuk et al. 2007). More recently, siRNA has been shown to be more potent and easier to develop than ribozymes for suppressing gene expression (Reynolds et al. 2004; Boudreau et al. 2013). A group at Trinity College, Dublin, used AAV to deliver an siRNA as a small hairpin RNA (shRNA) employing the RNA polymerase III H1 promoter together with a murine *Rho* cDNA driven by the mouse *Rho* promoter (Chadderton et al. 2009; Palfi et al. 2010; Millington-Ward et al. 2011). Subretinal injection of P347S *RHO* transgenic mice with one vector expressing the shRNA and another vector expressing the replacement rhodopsin led to elevated ERG b-wave amplitudes in treated eyes for 5 mo after treatment, compared to an unchanged response in control injected eyes. In P23H *RHO* transgenic mice, Mao and coworkers used a single AAV vector to deliver both an *RHO*-shRNA and an siRNA-resistant *Rho* gene. The *Rho* gene contained silent nucleotide changes to block siRNA cleavage. The shRNA in this vector led to a 50% suppression of rhodopsin in human P23H *RHO* transgenic mice. Eyes treated with the combination vector had a twofold increase in total rhodopsin content relative to untreated eyes and protected the ERG response for 9 mo following treatment (Mao et al. 2012).

To determine whether the combination treatment would succeed in a larger animal, Cideciyan and coworkers (2018) used an RNA replacement vector as therapy for the severe retinal degeneration initiated by exposing T4R rhodopsin dogs to bright light. This vector expressed an shRNA that degrades both human and canine *RHO* mRNA. The shRNA and a *RHO* cDNA with silent mutations in the target sequence were cloned in a self-complementary AAV vector (scAAV), because such vectors result in rapid onset of gene expression (McCarty et al. 2003; Petersen-Jones et al. 2009). T4R dogs treated with this vector were protected from photoreceptor death caused by the mutation for more than 7 mo and after multiple light exposures.

Rather than supplying an siRNA as an shRNA, the siRNA sequence can be delivered as an artificial miRNA by including the flanking sequences and loop sequence of a natural miRNA (Borel et al. 2014). MiRNAs control biological processes by suppressing gene expression through binding to mRNAs (Bartel 2018). RNA polymerase II promoters can be used to drive the expression of artificial miRNAs. Unlike pol III promoters used to drive shRNA production, pol II promoters can be cell-type specific and are easier to regulate. This approach is effective in mice with dominantly inherited liver degeneration associated with the PiZ mutation in α-1-antitrypsin (Mueller et al. 2012; Mueller and Flotte 2013) and in human patients with *SOD1* mutations that cause familial amyotrophic lateral sclerosis (ALS) (Mueller et al. 2020). Artificial miRNAs appear be less inflammatory and more specific than shRNAs (Boudreau et al. 2008; McBride et al. 2008a). Greenwald and colleagues used artificial miRNAs to treat P347S *RHO* transgenic mice. They employed one AAV vector to produce an *RHO*-specific artificial miRNA and a second vector to produce an miRNA-re-

sistant *RHO* cDNA. Mice treated with either vector exhibited elevated ERG amplitudes, even though the P347S *RHO* mutation causes rapid retinal degeneration (Greenwald et al. 2013). More recently, Orlans and colleagues (2021) have used mirtrons, RNA inhibitors that are produced as short introns, as a component of a suppression and replacement therapy for adRP. A panel of mirtrons was screened in cells, and then the most potent inhibitors tested via AAV delivery. The synthesis of the mirtrons was directed by an *RHO* promoter, limiting their expression to rod photoreceptor cells. When tested by subretinal injection in P23H *Rho* knockin mice, a combination vector producing both a mirtron and a replacement rhodopsin delayed the degeneration of the retina based on OCT measurement of retinal thickness and ERG amplitudes. Development of this technology to target human rhodopsin mRNA, thus has promise for therapy of RHO-adRP.

Off-target effects are a potential complication of any antisense technology. ASOs, gRNAs, ribozymes, miRNAs, or shRNAs can bind to a non-*RHO* sequence causing its accidental destruction or editing. In addition, highly expressed hairpin RNAs or miRNAs can inhibit nuclear export of natural miRNAs by saturating RNA Exportin-5 (needed for transport from the nucleus). SiRNA, whether provided as shRNA or artificial miRNA, can block the translation of unintended genes by acting via the miRNA pathway (Birmingham et al. 2006). Although it is possible to screen for potential off-target effects using bioinformatics tools (Birmingham et al. 2007; Boudreau et al. 2013), experimental validation of specificity is ultimately required.

PRESERVING VIABILITY OF PHOTORECEPTORS

Rather than dealing directly with the rhodopsin mutations, it may be possible to prevent or delay the death of rod photoreceptors by indirect means. Since the viability of cone photoreceptors depends the preservation of rods, central vision might be maintained if rods remain viable, even with limited response to light.

Suppression of the Unfolded Protein Response (UPR)

Class II *RHO* mutations accumulate misfolded rhodopsin in the ER (Illing et al. 2002; Chiang et al. 2015; Athanasiou et al. 2017, 2018). This buildup initiates a stress pathway called the unfolded protein response (UPR) as a reaction to the imbalance between protein synthesis and protein degradation or trafficking. Three transmembrane proteins act as proximal signals for the UPR: activating transcription factor 6 (ATF6), inositol-requiring enzyme 1 (IRE1), and protein kinase R-like ER protein kinase (PERK1) (Walter and Ron 2011). Continuous stimulation of the PERK pathway in particular results in apoptosis. Activation of the UPR by T17M rhodopsin also leads to the production of inflammatory cytokines that can damage the neural retina (Rana et al. 2014). Binding of BiP/Grp78, a chaperone of the HSP70 family, keeps the transducers in an inactive state (Lin et al. 2007; Ron and Walter 2007). To prevent activation of the UPR in an adRP model, Gorbatyuk and colleagues increased the level of Grp78 by injection of AAV-Grp78 in the eyes of P23H *Rho* transgenic rats (Gorbatyuk et al. 2010). Increased levels of Grp78 reduced the death of photoreceptors and elevated the electroretinogram a-wave and b-wave responses. In other adRP models, such as the T17M-*Rho* mice and S334ter-*Rho* rats, the UPR is also elevated (Kunte et al. 2012; Shinde et al. 2012). Consequently, dampening this response is a target for preserving retinal function in *RHO* adRP (Bhootada et al. 2015; Athanasiou et al. 2017).

Neurotrophic Factors

Both GDNF (glial-derived neurotrophic factor) and CNTF (ciliary-derived neurotrophic factor) protect the retina in rodent models of RP. GDNF, a member of the TGF-β family, has receptors in Müller glia cells, but not in photoreceptors (Hauck et al. 2006). Dalkara and colleagues tested AAV-GDNF using ShH10, a capsid variant selected to specifically transduce Müller cells following injection in the vitreous. This treatment reduced the decline in ERG amplitudes and the decrease in thickness of retinal layers in S334Ter *RHO* transgenic rats (Dalkara et al. 2011). Wu and colleagues reported no impairment of retinal function in wild-type rats treated with AAV-GDNF over a year-long time course (Wu et al. 2005). Consequently, gene therapy with GDNF seems to be a safe and effective method to delay retinal degeneration caused by *RHO* adRP.

CNTF belongs to the IL-6 family and has been used for gene therapy in rat models of adRP. Intravitreal injection of AAV-CNTF in transgenic rat models of adRP diminished the loss of photoreceptors, but also dampened the ERG amplitudes (Liang et al. 2001). AAV-CNTF stimulated rhodopsin production and the viability of rod photoreceptors but reduced the expression of cone opsins (Rhee et al. 2007). In a clinical study of an implantable device secreting CNTF in the vitreous of patients with RP, Birch and colleagues concluded "ciliary neurotrophic factor released continuously from an intravitreal implant led to loss of total visual field sensitivity that was greater than the natural progression in the sham-treated eye" (Birch et al. 2016). The reduced visual field sensitivity improved upon removal of the treatment, suggesting that CNTF treatment reduced sensitivity, but did not accelerate photoreceptor degeneration. Therefore, despite promoting survival of rods, continuous delivery of CNTF is not a promising therapy for adRP.

A thioredoxin-like protein, rod-derived cone viability factor (RdCVF), supports the viability of cone photoreceptors (Léveillard et al. 2004a, b). RdCVF promotes glucose transport into photoreceptor cells using the transmembrane signaling protein basigin (Aït-Ali et al. 2015). Treatment of P23H *Rho* knockin mice with RdCVF delivered through AAV7m8 led to an increased photopic ERG response in treated eyes compared to control eyes for up to 4 mo (Byrne et al. 2015).

Modulation of Retinal Bioenergetics

The retina is one of the most energetically demanding tissues of the body (Warburg et al. 1924; Hurley et al. 2015; Kanow et al. 2017). Within the retina, rod and cone photoreceptors are some of the most metabolically active cells, using on the order of 10^5 ATP/sec/cell (Okawa et al. 2008). This high rate of energy use is driven largely by the activity of the Na^+/K^+ ATPase ion channels to maintain the appropriate ionic balance in photoreceptors, which are partially depolarized in their resting state. Recent studies to more carefully define the flow of fuel and metabolites in the retina have identified an interdependence between the layers of the retina (Hurley et al. 2015; Du et al. 2016; Kanow et al. 2017). In the outer retina, glucose is the principal fuel delivered to the RPE from the choroidal circulation. Rather than using this glucose as its main fuel source, the RPE transfers the glucose to the photoreceptors where it is metabolized primarily through aerobic glycolysis (Kanow et al. 2017). Photoreceptors secrete the lactate product of this pathway for use by the RPE and Müller glia as their principal metabolic fuel.

This high rate of metabolism and metabolic interdependence of retinal cell types is highlighted by the large number and diversity of mutations in metabolic genes that lead to retinal degeneration, which span the range of enzymes involved in glycolysis, metabolite transport, tricarboxylic acid (TCA) cycle, redox homeostasis, and fatty acid metabolism (recently, for review, see Pan et al. 2021). A number of studies have attempted to capitalize on the metabolic interdependence of the retina by modulation of retinal bioenergetics as a mechanism to slow the loss of photoreceptors in inherited retinal diseases, reasoning that improved metabolic flow would be broadly beneficial to the retina. The homeostatic plasticity of the retina has been empirically demonstrated in the *Rho*-P23H mouse, suggesting that enhancing metabolism could be of significant benefit to the retina (Leinonen et al. 2020).

Various groups have taken different approaches to enhancing retinal metabolism. One approach is to target enhanced delivery of metabolic substrate. For example, induction of Glut1, a glucose receptor, expression on the RPE with an injection of phosphatidyl serine results in transient recovery of both photopic and scotopic ERG function in *Rho*-P23H mice and in recovery of cone response in *RHO*-P23H

pigs (Wang et al. 2019). Altering glucose metabolism in rd10 and rd1 mice led to prolonged survival of cone photoreceptors (Punzo et al. 2009; Xue et al. 2021). In another substrate-targeted approach, dietary supplementation with the specific α-ketoglutarate slowed photoreceptor loss in a mouse with deficits in the PDE6α (Wert et al. 2020). Dietary supplementation has not been tested in mice with rhodopsin defects, but it is likely to retard degeneration in models of *RHO* adRP.

Another tactic for enhancing metabolism is to target enzyme activity selectively. Nelson et al. (2022) have shown that disinhibition of enolase activity using a modified arrestin1 delivered by AAV increases glycolytic output of lactate. In the *Rho*-P23H model of adRP, this increase of glycolytic output slows the loss of both rod and cone photoreceptors. Enzyme activity can also be modulated at the gene expression level. The Tsang laboratory demonstrated that knockdown of sirtuin 6, a repressor of glycolytic enzyme expression, results in enhanced production of glycolytic and TCA cycle metabolites. When these authors knocked down sirtuin 6 in mouse models of retinal degeneration with defects in *Pde6*, up-regulation of glycolysis slowed the loss of both rods and cones (Zhang et al. 2016).

Another approach for using metabolism for potential therapy is the level of mitochondrial metabolism. Photomodulation of the mitochondrial redox state shows significant benefit in *Rho*-P23H rats (Gopalakrishnan et al. 2020). In a similar manner, targeting mitochondrial biogenesis through the administration of metformin can also slow retinal degeneration as shown in the rd10-PDE6b mouse (Xu et al. 2018).

It is not surprising that the overall theme of all of these studies is that although there is a slowing of retinal degeneration with these approaches, retinal degeneration continues to progress. This observation likely reflects the fact that these therapies are not treating the underlying defect, but rather are attempting to create a more favorable metabolic environment. The expectation is that most of these metabolic types of interventions will be most effective in late-onset disease or in combination with other therapeutic interventions.

MicroRNA Gene Therapy

Dysregulation of miRNAs have been linked to some retinal diseases (Anasagasti et al. 2018; Zuzic et al. 2019). The levels of several retinal miRNAs (miR-96, -183, -1, and -133) are altered in P347S *RHO* transgenic mice (Loscher et al. 2008). In addition, a mutation in the seed region (nucleotides 2–7) of miR-204 is linked to retinal dystrophy and coloboma in humans (Conte et al. 2015). Disruption of miR-211 by knockout in mice leads to progressive cone dystrophy (Barbato et al. 2017). The Conte laboratory used an AAV2/8 vector to deliver pre-miR-204 to neonatal P247S *RHO* transgenic mice. This early-stage miRNA gene therapy caused an increase in the ERG responses, but no measurable difference in ONL thickness. When they injected mice at postnatal day 30, they observed an increase in the ERG b-wave that lasted until P60 (Karali et al. 2020). RNA sequence analysis revealed suppression of genes associated with innate immunity and elevated expression of genes related to visual transduction. Since AAV delivery also protected the retina in *Aipl1* knockout mice, gene delivery using miR-204 may be beneficial for a variety of inherited retinal diseases by stimulating common prosurvival pathways.

DELIVERING OPSIN GENES TO THE INNER RETINA

In some cases, clinical and genetic diagnosis may come too late to permit rescue of rod photoreceptors by gene therapy. However, the retinal ganglion cells and bipolar cells may not be affected in RP (Aleman et al. 2008; Bonilha et al. 2015). For this reason, transferring genes for light-responsive proteins to cells in the inner retina is a potential approach to restore some visual function. This treatment approach is reviewed in other articles in this collection.

CONCLUDING REMARKS

This review of the various approaches being developed to treat disease caused by mutations in the *RHO* gene suggests an optimistic future for developing therapies for affected patients. The success of AAV-mediated gene therapy for patients with defects in the RPE65 gene (Maguire et al. 2021; Deng et al. 2022; Sengillo et al. 2022) has provided a foundation for transferring this gene therapy to *RHO* defects. The constellation of strategies reviewed here that have demonstrated success at slowing photoreceptor loss caused by mutations in *RHO* make it likely that therapies can be developed that are either selective in their targeting of *RHO*, or may use a combination of direct and indirect approaches for preserving photoreceptor function.

ACKNOWLEDGMENTS

Shaler Richardson Professorship Endowment to the University of Florida supported both of the authors. The authors thank Dr. Michael Massengill for the graphic used in Figure 1.

REFERENCES

Aït-Ali N, Fridlich R, Millet-Puel G, Clérin E, Delalande F, Jaillard C, Blond F, Perrocheau L, Reichman S, Byrne LC, et al. 2015. Rod-derived cone viability factor promotes cone survival by stimulating aerobic glycolysis. *Cell* **161:** 817–832. doi:10.1016/j.cell.2015.03.023

Aleman TS, Cideciyan AV, Sumaroka A, Windsor EA, Herrera W, White DA, Kaushal S, Naidu A, Roman AJ, Schwartz SB, et al. 2008. Retinal laminar architecture in human retinitis pigmentosa caused by *Rhodopsin* gene mutations. *Invest Ophthalmol Vis Sci* **49:** 1580–1590. doi:10.1167/iovs.07-1110

Anasagasti A, Ezquerra-Inchausti M, Barandika O, Muñoz-Culla M, Caffarel MM, Otaegui D, López de Munain A, Ruiz-Ederra J. 2018. Expression profiling analysis reveals key microRNA-mRNA interactions in early retinal degeneration in retinitis pigmentosa. *Invest Ophthalmol Vis Sci* **59:** 2381–2392. doi:10.1167/iovs.18-24091

Anzalone AV, Randolph PB, Davis JR, Sousa AA, Koblan LW, Levy JM, Chen PJ, Wilson C, Newby GA, Raguram A, et al. 2019. Search-and-replace genome editing without double-strand breaks or donor DNA. *Nature* **576:** 149–157. doi:10.1038/s41586-019-1711-4

Athanasiou D, Aguila M, Bellingham J, Kanuga N, Adamson P, Cheetham ME. 2017. The role of the ER stress-response protein PERK in rhodopsin retinitis pigmentosa. *Hum Mol Genet* **26:** 4896–4905. doi:10.1093/hmg/ddx370

Athanasiou D, Aguila M, Bellingham J, Li W, McCulley C, Reeves PJ, Cheetham ME. 2018. The molecular and cellular basis of rhodopsin retinitis pigmentosa reveals potential strategies for therapy. *Prog Retin Eye Res* **62:** 1–23. doi:10.1016/j.preteyeres.2017.10.002

Bainbridge JW, Stephens C, Parsley K, Demaison C, Halfyard A, Thrasher AJ, Ali RR. 2001. In vivo gene transfer to the mouse eye using an HIV-based lentiviral vector; efficient long-term transduction of corneal endothelium and retinal pigment epithelium. *Gene Ther* **8:** 1665–1668. doi:10.1038/sj.gt.3301574

Bakondi B, Lv W, Lu B, Jones MK, Tsai Y, Kim KJ, Levy R, Akhtar AA, Breunig JJ, Svendsen CN, et al. 2016. In vivo CRISPR/Cas9 gene editing corrects retinal dystrophy in the S334ter-3 rat model of autosomal dominant retinitis pigmentosa. *Mol Ther* **24:** 556–563. doi:10.1038/mt.2015.220

Barbato S, Marrocco E, Intartaglia D, Pizzo M, Asteriti S, Naso F, Falanga D, Bhat RS, Meola N, Carissimo A, et al. 2017. MiR-211 is essential for adult cone photoreceptor maintenance and visual function. *Sci Rep* **7:** 17004. doi:10.1038/s41598-017-17331-z

Bartel DP. 2018. Metazoan microRNAs. *Cell* **173:** 20–51. doi:10.1016/j.cell.2018.03.006

Bennett CF, Swayze EE. 2010. RNA targeting therapeutics: molecular mechanisms of antisense oligonucleotides as a therapeutic platform. *Annu Rev Pharmacol Toxicol* **50:** 259–293. doi:10.1146/annurev.pharmtox.010909.105654

Bhootada Y, Choudhury S, Gully C, Gorbatyuk M. 2015. Targeting caspase-12 to preserve vision in mice with inherited retinal degeneration. *Invest Ophthalmol Vis Sci* **56:** 4725–4733. doi:10.1167/iovs.15-16924

Birch DG, Bennett LD, Duncan JL, Weleber RG, Pennesi ME. 2016. Long-term follow-up of patients with retinitis pigmentosa receiving intraocular ciliary neurotrophic factor implants. *Am J Ophthalmol* **170:** 10–14. doi:10.1016/j.ajo.2016.07.013

Birmingham A, Anderson EM, Reynolds A, Ilsley-Tyree D, Leake D, Fedorov Y, Baskerville S, Maksimova E, Robinson K, Karpilow J, et al. 2006. 3′ UTR seed matches, but not overall identity, are associated with RNAi off-targets. *Nat Methods* **3:** 199–204. doi:10.1038/nmeth854

Birmingham A, Anderson E, Sullivan K, Reynolds A, Boese Q, Leake D, Karpilow J, Khvorova A. 2007. A protocol for designing siRNAs with high functionality and specificity. *Nat Protocols* **2:** 2068–2078. doi:10.1038/nprot.2007.278

Bonilha VL, Rayborn ME, Bell BA, Marino MJ, Beight CD, Pauer GJ, Traboulsi EI, Hollyfield JG, Hagstrom SA. 2015. Retinal histopathology in eyes from patients with autosomal dominant retinitis pigmentosa caused by rhodopsin mutations. *Graefes Arch Clin Exp Ophthalmol* **253:** 2161–2169. doi:10.1007/s00417-015-3099-7

Borel F, Kay MA, Mueller C. 2014. Recombinant AAV as a platform for translating the therapeutic potential of RNA interference. *Mol Ther* **22:** 692–701. doi:10.1038/mt.2013.285

Botta S, Marrocco E, de Prisco N, Curion F, Renda M, Sofia M, Lupo M, Carissimo A, Bacci ML, Gesualdo C, et al. 2016. Rhodopsin targeted transcriptional silencing by DNA-binding. *eLife* **5:** e12242. doi:10.7554/eLife.12242

Botto C, Dalkara D, El-Amraoui A. 2021. Progress in gene editing tools and their potential for correcting mutations underlying hearing and vision loss. *Front Genome Ed* **3:** 737632. doi:10.3389/fgeed.2021.737632

Botto C, Rucli M, Tekinsoy MD, Pulman J, Sahel JA, Dalkara D. 2022. Early and late stage gene therapy interventions for inherited retinal degenerations. *Prog Retin Eye Res* **86:** 100975. doi:10.1016/j.preteyeres.2021.100975

Boudreau RL, Monteys AM, Davidson BL. 2008. Minimizing variables among hairpin-based RNAi vectors reveals the potency of shRNAs. *RNA* **14:** 1834–1844. doi:10.1261/rna.1062908

Boudreau RL, Spengler RM, Hylock RH, Kusenda BJ, Davis HA, Eichmann DA, Davidson BL. 2013. siSPOTR: a tool for designing highly specific and potent siRNAs for human and mouse. *Nucleic Acids Res* **41:** e9. doi:10.1093/nar/gks797

Boye SE, Boye SL, Lewin AS, Hauswirth WW. 2013. A comprehensive review of retinal gene therapy. *Mol Ther* **21:** 509–519. doi:10.1038/mt.2012.280

Boye SL, Choudhury S, Crosson S, Di Pasquale G, Afione S, Mellen R, Makal V, Calabro KR, Fajardo D, Peterson J, et al. 2020. Novel AAV44.9-based vectors display exceptional characteristics for retinal gene therapy. *Mol Ther* **28:** 1464–1478. doi:10.1016/j.ymthe.2020.04.002

Bucher K, Rodríguez-Bocanegra E, Dauletbekov D, Fischer MD. 2021. Immune responses to retinal gene therapy using adeno-associated viral vectors—implications for treatment success and safety. *Prog Retin Eye Res* **83:** 100915. doi:10.1016/j.preteyeres.2020.100915

Byrne LC, Dalkara D, Luna G, Fisher SK, Clérin E, Sahel JA, Léveillard T, Flannery JG. 2015. Viral-mediated RdCVF and RdCVFL expression protects cone and rod photoreceptors in retinal degeneration. *J Clin Invest* **125:** 105–116. doi:10.1172/JCI65654

Byrne LC, Day TP, Visel M, Strazzeri JA, Fortuny C, Dalkara D, Merigan WH, Schaffer DV, Flannery JG. 2020. In vivo–directed evolution of adeno-associated virus in the primate retina. *JCI Insight* **5:** e135112. doi:10.1172/jci.insight.135112

Capowski EE, Samimi K, Mayerl SJ, Phillips MJ, Pinilla I, Howden SE, Saha J, Jansen AD, Edwards KL, Jager LD, et al. 2019. Reproducibility and staging of 3D human retinal organoids across multiple pluripotent stem cell lines. *Development* **146:** dev171686. doi:10.1242/dev.171686

Castanotto D, Li JR, Michienzi A, Langlois MA, Lee NS, Puymirat J, Rossi JJ. 2002. Intracellular ribozyme applications. *Biochem Soc Trans* **30:** 1140–1145. doi:10.1042/bst0301140

Chadderton N, Millington-Ward S, Palfi A, O'Reilly M, Tuohy G, Humphries MM, Li T, Humphries P, Kenna PF, Farrar GJ. 2009. Improved retinal function in a mouse model of dominant retinitis pigmentosa following AAV-delivered gene therapy. *Mol Ther* **17:** 593–599. doi:10.1038/mt.2008.301

Chan YK, Wang SK, Chu CJ, Copland DA, Letizia AJ, Costa Verdera H, Chiang JJ, Sethi M, Wang MK, Neidermyer WJ Jr, et al. 2021. Engineering adeno-associated viral vectors to evade innate immune and inflammatory responses. *Sci Transl Med* **13:** eabd3438. doi:10.1126/scitranslmed.abd3438

Chiang WC, Kroeger H, Sakami S, Messah C, Yasumura D, Matthes MT, Coppinger JA, Palczewski K, LaVail MM, Lin JH. 2015. Robust endoplasmic reticulum-associated degradation of rhodopsin precedes retinal degeneration. *Mol Neurobiol* **52:** 679–695. doi:10.1007/s12035-014-8881-8

Chung SH, Mollhoff IN, Mishra A, Sin TN, Ngo T, Ciulla T, Sieving P, Thomasy SM, Yiu G. 2021. Host immune responses after suprachoroidal delivery of AAV8 in nonhuman primate eyes. *Hum Gene Ther* **32:** 682–693. doi:10.1089/hum.2020.281

Cite this article as *Cold Spring Harb Perspect Med* doi: 10.1101/cshperspect.a041283

Cideciyan AV, Hood DC, Huang Y, Banin E, Li ZY, Stone EM, Milam AH, Jacobson SG. 1998. Disease sequence from mutant *rhodopsin* allele to rod and cone photoreceptor degeneration in man. *Proc Natl Acad Sci* **95**: 7103–7108. doi:10.1073/pnas.95.12.7103

Cideciyan AV, Jacobson SG, Aleman TS, Gu D, Pearce-Kelling SE, Sumaroka A, Acland GM, Aguirre GD. 2005. In vivo dynamics of retinal injury and repair in the *rhodopsin* mutant dog model of human retinitis pigmentosa. *Proc Natl Acad Sci* **102**: 5233–5238. doi:10.1073/pnas .0408892102

Cideciyan AV, Sudharsan R, Dufour VL, Massengill MT, Iwabe S, Swider M, Lisi B, Sumaroka A, Marinho LF, Appelbaum T, et al. 2018. Mutation-independent rhodopsin gene therapy by knockdown and replacement with a single AAV vector. *Proc Natl Acad Sci* **115**: E8547–E8556. doi:10.1073/pnas.1805055115

Concepcion F, Chen J. 2010. Q344ter mutation causes mislocalization of rhodopsin molecules that are catalytically active: a mouse model of Q344ter-induced retinal degeneration. *PLoS ONE* **5**: e10904. doi:10.1371/journal.pone .0010904

Conte I, Hadfield KD, Barbato S, Carrella S, Pizzo M, Bhat RS, Carissimo A, Karali M, Porter LF, Urquhart J, et al. 2015. MiR-204 is responsible for inherited retinal dystrophy associated with ocular coloboma. *Proc Natl Acad Sci* **112**: E3236–E3245. doi:10.1073/pnas.1401464112

Cowan CS, Renner M, De Gennaro M, Gross-Scherf B, Goldblum D, Hou Y, Munz M, Rodrigues TM, Krol J, Szikra T, et al. 2020. Cell types of the human retina and its organoids at single-cell resolution. *Cell* **182**: 1623–1640.e34. doi:10.1016/j.cell.2020.08.013

da Costa BL, Levi SR, Eulau E, Tsai YT, Quinn PMJ. 2021. Prime editing for inherited retinal diseases. *Front Genome Ed* **3**: 775330. doi:10.3389/fgeed.2021.775330

Daiger SP, Bowne SJ, Sullivan LS. 2015. Genes and mutations causing autosomal dominant retinitis pigmentosa. *Cold Spring Harb Perspect Med* **5**: a017129. doi:10.1101/cshper spect.a017129

Dalkara D, Kolstad KD, Guerin KI, Hoffmann NV, Visel M, Klimczak RR, Schaffer DV, Flannery JG. 2011. AAV mediated GDNF secretion from retinal glia slows down retinal degeneration in a rat model of retinitis pigmentosa. *Mol Ther* **19**: 1602–1608. doi:10.1038/mt.2011.62

Dalkara D, Byrne LC, Klimczak RR, Visel M, Yin L, Merigan WH, Flannery JG, Schaffer DV. 2013. In vivo–directed evolution of a new adeno-associated virus for therapeutic outer retinal gene delivery from the vitreous. *Sci Transl Med* **5**: 189ra176. doi:10.1126/scitranslmed.3005708

Deng C, Zhao PY, Branham K, Schlegel D, Fahim AT, Jayasundera TK, Khan N, Besirli CG. 2022. Real-world outcomes of voretigene neparvovec treatment in pediatric patients with RPE65-associated Leber congenital amaurosis. *Graefes Arch Clin Exp Ophthalmol* **260**: 1543–1550. doi:10.1007/s00417-021-05508-2

Du J, Rountree A, Cleghorn WM, Contreras L, Lindsay KJ, Sadilek M, Gu H, Djukovic D, Raftery D, Satrústegui J, et al. 2016. Phototransduction influences metabolic flux and nucleotide metabolism in mouse retina. *J Biol Chem* **291**: 4698–4710. doi:10.1074/jbc.M115.698985

Editas Medicine. 2022. Editas Medicine announces fourth quarter and full year 2021 results and business updates.

https://ir.editasmedicine.com/news-releases/news-release-details/editas-medicine-announces-fourth-quarter-and-full-year-2021#:~:text=Fourth%20Quarter%202021&text=Collaboration%20and%20other%20research%20and,the%20same%20period%20in%202020

Eldred KC, Reh TA. 2021. Human retinal model systems: strengths, weaknesses, and future directions. *Dev Biol* **480**: 114–122. doi:10.1016/j.ydbio.2021.09.001

Fenner BJ, Tan TE, Barathi AV, Tun SBB, Yeo SW, Tsai ASH, Lee SY, Cheung CMG, Chan CM, Mehta JS, et al. 2022. Gene-based therapeutics for inherited retinal diseases. *Front Genet* **12**: 794805. doi:10.3389/fgene.2021.794805

Fernandez de Castro J, Scott PA, Fransen JW, Demas J, DeMarco PJ, Kaplan HJ, McCall MA. 2014. Cone photoreceptors develop normally in the absence of functional rod photoreceptors in a transgenic swine model of retinitis pigmentosa. *Invest Ophthalmol Vis Sci* **55**: 2460–2468. doi:10.1167/iovs.13-13724

Fotiadis D, Liang Y, Filipek S, Saperstein DA, Engel A, Palczewski K. 2004. The G protein-coupled receptor rhodopsin in the native membrane. *FEBS Lett* **564**: 281–288. doi:10.1016/S0014-5793(04)00194-2

Gopalakrishnan S, Mehrvar S, Maleki S, Schmitt H, Summerfelt P, Dubis AM, Abroe B, Connor TB, Carroll J, Huddleston W, et al. 2020. Photobiomodulation preserves mitochondrial redox state and is retinoprotective in a rodent model of retinitis pigmentosa. *Sci Rep* **10**: 20382. doi:10.1038/s41598-020-77290-w

Gorbatyuk M, Justilien V, Liu J, Hauswirth WW, Lewin AS. 2007. Preservation of photoreceptor morphology and function in P23H rats using an allele independent ribozyme. *Exp Eye Res* **84**: 44–52. doi:10.1016/j.exer.2006.08 .014

Gorbatyuk MS, Knox T, LaVail MM, Gorbatyuk OS, Noorwez SM, Hauswirth WW, Lin JH, Muzyczka N, Lewin AS. 2010. Restoration of visual function in P23H rhodopsin transgenic rats by gene delivery of BiP/Grp78. *Proc Natl Acad Sci* **107**: 5961–5966. doi:10.1073/pnas.0911991107

Goto Y, Peachey NS, Ripps H, Naash MI. 1995. Functional abnormalities in transgenic mice expressing a mutant rhodopsin gene. *Invest Ophthalmol Vis Sci* **36**: 62–71.

Greenwald DL, Cashman SM, Kumar-Singh R. 2013. Mutation-independent rescue of a novel mouse model of retinitis pigmentosa. *Gene Ther* **20**: 425–434. doi:10.1038/gt .2012.53

Grimm D. 2009. Small silencing RNAs: state-of-the-art. *Adv Drug Delivery Rev* **61**: 672–703. doi:10.1016/j.addr.2009 .05.002

Gumerson JD, Alsufyani A, Yu W, Lei J, Sun X, Dong L, Wu Z, Li T. 2022. Restoration of RPGR expression in vivo using CRISPR/Cas9 gene editing. *Gene Ther* **29**: 81–93. doi:10.1038/s41434-021-00258-6

Han Z, Banworth MJ, Makkia R, Conley SM, Al-Ubaidi MR, Cooper MJ, Naash MI. 2015. Genomic DNA nanoparticles rescue rhodopsin-associated retinitis pigmentosa phenotype. *FASEB J* **29**: 2535–2544. doi:10.1096/fj.15-270363

Han IC, Burnight ER, Ulferts MJ, Worthington KS, Russell SR, Sohn EH, Mullins RF, Stone EM, Tucker BA, Wiley LA. 2019. Helper-dependent adenovirus transduces the human and rat retina but elicits an inflammatory reaction when delivered subretinally in rats. *Hum Gene Ther* **30:** 1371–1384. doi:10.1089/hum.2019.159

Han IC, Cheng JL, Burnight ER, Ralston CL, Fick JL, Thomsen GJ, Tovar EF, Russell SR, Sohn EH, Mullins RF, et al. 2020. Retinal tropism and transduction of adeno-associated virus varies by serotype and route of delivery (intravitreal, subretinal, or suprachoroidal) in rats. *Hum Gene Ther* **31:** 1288–1299. doi:10.1089/hum.2020.043

Hauck SM, Kinkl N, Deeg CA, Swiatek-de Lange M, Schöffmann S, Ueffing M. 2006. GDNF family ligands trigger indirect neuroprotective signaling in retinal glial cells. *Mol Cell Biol* **26:** 2746–2757. doi:10.1128/MCB.26.7 .2746-2757.2006

Hurley JB, Lindsay KJ, Du J. 2015. Glucose, lactate, and shuttling of metabolites in vertebrate retinas. *J Neurosci Res* **93:** 1079–1092. doi:10.1002/jnr.23583

Iannaccone A, Alekseev O, Kraus E. 2022. Retinitis pigmentosa. In *Rare disease database*. National Organization for Rare Disorders, Danbury, CT.

Illing ME, Rajan RS, Bence NF, Kopito RR. 2002. A rhodopsin mutant linked to autosomal dominant retinitis pigmentosa is prone to aggregate and interacts with the ubiquitin proteasome system. *J Biol Chem* **277:** 34150–34160. doi:10.1074/jbc.M204955200

Kanow MA, Giarmarco MM, Jankowski CSR, Tsantilas K, Engel AL, Du J, Linton JD, Farnsworth CC, Sloat SR, Rountree A, et al. 2017. Biochemical adaptations of the retina and retinal pigment epithelium support a metabolic ecosystem in the vertebrate eye. *eLife* **6:** e28899. doi:10 .7554/eLife.28899

Karali M, Guadagnino I, Marrocco E, De Cegli R, Carissimo A, Pizzo M, Casarosa S, Conte I, Surace EM, Banfi S. 2020. AAV-miR-204 protects from retinal degeneration by attenuation of microglia activation and photoreceptor cell death. *Mol Ther Nucleic Acids* **19:** 144–156. doi:10.1016/j .omtn.2019.11.005

Kay CN, Ryals RC, Aslanidi GV, Min SH, Ruan Q, Sun J, Dyka FM, Kasuga D, Ayala AE, Van VK, et al. 2013. Targeting photoreceptors via intravitreal delivery using novel, capsid-mutated AAV vectors. *PLoS ONE* **8:** e62097. doi:10.1371/journal.pone.0062097

Kijas JW, Cideciyan AV, Aleman TS, Pianta MJ, Pearce-Kelling SE, Miller BJ, Jacobson SG, Aguirre GD, Acland GM. 2002. Naturally occurring *rhodopsin* mutation in the dog causes retinal dysfunction and degeneration mimicking human dominant retinitis pigmentosa. *Proc Natl Acad Sci* **99:** 6328–6333. doi:10.1073/pnas.082714499

Komor AC, Kim YB, Packer MS, Zuris JA, Liu DR. 2016. Programmable editing of a target base in genomic DNA without double-stranded DNA cleavage. *Nature* **533:** 420–424. doi:10.1038/nature17946

Kotterman MA, Yin L, Strazzeri JM, Flannery JG, Merigan WH, Schaffer DV. 2015. Antibody neutralization poses a barrier to intravitreal adeno-associated viral vector gene delivery to non-human primates. *Gene Ther* **22:** 116–126. doi:10.1038/gt.2014.115

Kruczek K, Swaroop A. 2020. Pluripotent stem cell-derived retinal organoids for disease modeling and development of therapies. *Stem Cells* **38:** 1206–1215. doi:10.1002/stem .3239

Kunte MM, Choudhury S, Manheim JF, Shinde VM, Miura M, Chiodo VA, Hauswirth WW, Gorbatyuk OS, Gorba-

tyuk MS. 2012. ER stress is involved in T17M rhodopsin-induced retinal degeneration. *Invest Ophthalmol Vis Sci* **53:** 3792–3800. doi:10.1167/iovs.11-9235

LaVail MM, Yasumura D, Matthes MT, Drenser KA, Flannery JG, Lewin AS, Hauswirth WW. 2000. Ribozyme rescue of photoreceptor cells in P23H transgenic rats: long-term survival and late-stage therapy. *Proc Natl Acad Sci* **97:** 11488–11493. doi:10.1073/pnas.210319397

LaVail MM, Nishikawa S, Steinberg RH, Naash MI, Duncan JL, Trautmann N, Matthes MT, Yasumura D, Lau-Villacorta C, Chen J, et al. 2018. Phenotypic characterization of P23H and S334ter rhodopsin transgenic rat models of inherited retinal degeneration. *Exp Eye Res* **167:** 56–90. doi:10.1016/j.exer.2017.10.023

Lee S, Kang IK, Kim JH, Jung BK, Park K, Chang H, Lee JY, Lee H. 2019. Relationship between neutralizing antibodies against adeno-associated virus in the vitreous and serum: effects on retinal gene therapy. *Transl Vis Sci Technol* **8:** 14. doi:10.1167/tvst.8.2.14

Leinonen H, Pham NC, Boyd T, Santoso J, Palczewski K, Vinberg F. 2020. Homeostatic plasticity in the retina is associated with maintenance of night vision during retinal degenerative disease. *eLife* **9:** e59422. doi:10.7554/eLife.59422

Léveillard T, Mohand-Saïd S, Fintz AC, Lambrou G, Sahel JA. 2004a. The search for rod-dependent cone viability factors, secreted factors promoting cone viability. *Novartis Found Symp* **255:** 117–127.

Léveillard T, Mohand-Saïd S, Lorentz O, Hicks D, Fintz AC, Clérin E, Simonutti M, Forster V, Cavusoglu N, Chalmel F, et al. 2004b. Identification and characterization of rod-derived cone viability factor. *Nat Genet* **36:** 755–759. doi:10.1038/ng1386

Li T, Sandberg MA, Pawlyk BS, Rosner B, Hayes KC, Dryja TP, Berson EL. 1998a. Effect of vitamin A supplementation on rhodopsin mutants threonine-17 → methionine and proline-347 → serine in transgenic mice and in cell cultures. *Proc Natl Acad Sci* **95:** 11933–11938. doi:10 .1073/pnas.95.20.11933

Li ZY, Wong F, Chang JH, Possin DE, Hao Y, Petters RM, Milam AH. 1998b. Rhodopsin transgenic pigs as a model for human retinitis pigmentosa. *Invest Ophthalmol Vis Sci* **39:** 808–819.

Li P, Kleinstiver BP, Leon MY, Prew MS, Navarro-Gomez D, Greenwald SH, Pierce EA, Joung JK, Liu Q. 2018. Allele-specific CRISPR-Cas9 genome editing of the single-base P23H mutation for rhodopsin-associated dominant retinitis pigmentosa. *CRISPR J* **1:** 55–64. doi:10.1089/crispr .2017.0009

Liang FQ, Aleman TS, Dejneka NS, Dudus L, Fisher KJ, Maguire AM, Jacobson SG, Bennett J. 2001. Long-term protection of retinal structure but not function using RAAV.CNTF in animal models of retinitis pigmentosa. *Mol Ther* **4:** 461–472. doi:10.1006/mthe.2001.0473

Lin JH, Li H, Yasumura D, Cohen HR, Zhang C, Panning B, Shokat KM, LaVail MM, Walter P. 2007. IRE1 signaling affects cell fate during the unfolded protein response. *Science* **318:** 944–949. doi:10.1126/science.1146361

Liu Q, Xia Z, Zhong X, Case CC. 2002. Validated zinc finger protein designs for all 16 GNN DNA triplet targets. *J Biol Chem* **277:** 3850–3856. doi:10.1074/jbc.M110669200

 Cite this article as *Cold Spring Harb Perspect Med* doi: 10.1101/cshperspect.a041283

Loscher CJ, Hokamp K, Wilson JH, Li T, Humphries P, Farrar GJ, Palfi A. 2008. A common microRNA signature in mouse models of retinal degeneration. *Exp Eye Res* **87:** 529–534. doi:10.1016/j.exer.2008.08.016

Maguire AM, Russell S, Chung DC, Yu ZF, Tillman A, Drack AV, Simonelli F, Leroy BP, Reape KZ, High KA, et al. 2021. Durability of voretigene neparvovec for biallelic RPE65-mediated inherited retinal disease: phase 3 results at 3 and 4 years. *Ophthalmology* **128:** 1460–1468. doi:10.1016/j.ophtha.2021.03.031

Mali P, Yang L, Esvelt KM, Aach J, Guell M, DiCarlo JE, Norville JE, Church GM. 2013. RNA-guided human genome engineering via Cas9. *Science* **339:** 823–826. doi:10.1126/science.1232033

Mao H, Gorbatyuk MS, Rossmiller B, Hauswirth WW, Lewin AS. 2012. Long-term rescue of retinal structure and function by rhodopsin RNA replacement with a single adeno-associated viral vector in P23H *RHO* transgenic mice. *Hum Gene Ther* **23:** 356–366. doi:10.1089/hum.2011.213

Marrocco E, Maritato R, Botta S, Esposito M, Surace EM. 2021. Challenging safety and efficacy of retinal gene therapies by retinogenesis. *Int J Mol Sci* **22:** 5767. doi:10.3390/ijms22115767

McBride JL, Boudreau RL, Harper SQ, Staber PD, Monteys AM, Martins I, Gilmore BL, Burstein H, Peluso RW, Polisky B, et al. 2008a. Artificial miRNAs mitigate shRNA-mediated toxicity in the brain: implications for the therapeutic development of RNAi. *Proc Natl Acad Sci* **105:** 5868–5873. doi:10.1073/pnas.080177510

McBride JL, Boudreau RL, Harper SQ, Staber PD, Monteys AM, Martins I, Gilmore BL, Burstein H, Peluso RW, Polisky B, et al. 2008b. Artificial miRNAs mitigate shRNA-mediated toxicity in the brain: implications for the therapeutic development of RNAi. *Proc Natl Acad Sci* **105:** 5868–5873. doi:10.1073/pnas.0801775105

McCarty DM, Fu H, Monahan PE, Toulson CE, Naik P, Samulski RJ. 2003. Adeno-associated virus terminal repeat (TR) mutant generates self-complementary vectors to overcome the rate-limiting step to transduction in vivo. *Gene Ther* **10:** 2112–2118. doi:10.1038/sj.gt.3302134

McCullough KT, Boye SL, Fajardo D, Calabro K, Peterson JJ, Strang CE, Chakraborty D, Gloskowski S, Haskett S, Samuelsson S, et al. 2019. Somatic gene editing of *GUCY2D* by AAV-CRISPR/Cas9 alters retinal structure and function in mouse and macaque. *Hum Gene Ther* **30:** 571–589. doi:10.1089/hum.2018.193

Mendes HF, van der Spuy J, Chapple JP, Cheetham ME. 2005. Mechanisms of cell death in rhodopsin retinitis pigmentosa: implications for therapy. *Trends Mol Med* **11:** 177–185. doi:10.1016/j.molmed.2005.02.007

Meza-Rios A, Navarro-Partida J, Armendariz-Borunda J, Santos A. 2020. Therapies based on nanoparticles for eye drug delivery. *Ophthalmol Ther* **9:** 1–14. doi:10.1007/s40123-020-00257-7

Millington-Ward S, O'Neill B, Tuohy G, Al-Jandal N, Kiang AS, Kenna PF, Palfi A, Hayden P, Mansergh F, Kennan A, et al. 1997. Strategems in vitro for gene therapies directed to dominant mutations. *Hum Mol Genet* **6:** 1415–1426. doi:10.1093/hmg/6.9.1415

Millington-Ward S, Chadderton N, O'Reilly M, Palfi A, Goldmann T, Kilty C, Humphries M, Wolfrum U, Bennett J, Humphries P, et al. 2011. Suppression and replacement gene therapy for autosomal dominant disease in a murine model of dominant retinitis pigmentosa. *Mol Ther* **19:** 642–649. doi:10.1038/mt.2010.293

Mingozzi F, Chen Y, Edmonson SC, Zhou S, Thurlings RM, Tak PP, High KA, Vervoordeldonk MJ. 2013. Prevalence and pharmacological modulation of humoral immunity to AAV vectors in gene transfer to synovial tissue. *Gene Ther* **20:** 417–424. doi:10.1038/gt.2012.55

Mitra RN, Zheng M, Weiss ER, Han Z. 2018. Genomic form of rhodopsin DNA nanoparticles rescued autosomal dominant retinitis pigmentosa in the P23H knock-in mouse model. *Biomaterials* **157:** 26–39. doi:10.1016/j.biomaterials.2017.12.004

Mueller C, Flotte TR. 2013. Gene-based therapy for α-1 antitrypsin deficiency. *COPD* **10:** 44–49. doi:10.3109/15412555.2013.764978

Mueller C, Tang Q, Gruntman A, Blomenkamp K, Teckman J, Song L, Zamore PD, Flotte TR. 2012. Sustained miRNA-mediated knockdown of mutant AAT with simultaneous augmentation of wild-type AAT has minimal effect on global liver miRNA profiles. *Mol Ther* **20:** 590–600. doi:10.1038/mt.2011.292

Mueller C, Berry JD, McKenna-Yasek DM, Gernoux G, Owegi MA, Pothier LM, Douthwright CL, Gelevski D, Luppino SD, Blackwood M, et al. 2020. *SOD1* suppression with adeno-associated virus and MicroRNA in familial ALS. *N Engl J Med* **383:** 151–158. doi:10.1056/NEJMoa2005056

Murray SF, Jazayeri A, Matthes MT, Yasumura D, Yang H, Peralta R, Watt A, Freier S, Hung G, Adamson PS, et al. 2015. Allele-specific inhibition of rhodopsin with an antisense oligonucleotide slows photoreceptor cell degeneration. *Invest Ophthalmol Vis Sci* **56:** 6362–6375. doi:10.1167/iovs.15-16400

Mussolino C, Sanges D, Marrocco E, Bonetti C, Di Vicino U, Marigo V, Auricchio A, Meroni G, Surace EM. 2011. Zinc-finger-based transcriptional repression of rhodopsin in a model of dominant retinitis pigmentosa. *EMBO Mol Med* **3:** 118–128. doi:10.1002/emmm.201000119

Nelson TS, Simpson C, Dyka FM, Dinculescu A, Smith WC. 2022. A modified arrestin1 increases lactate production in the retina and slows retinal degeneration. *Hum Gene Ther* doi:10.1089/hum.2021.272

Nicoud M, Kong J, Iqball S, Kan O, Naylor S, Gouras P, Allikmets R, Binley K. 2007. Development of photoreceptor-specific promoters and their utility to investigate EIAV lentiviral vector mediated gene transfer to photoreceptors. *J Gene Med* **9:** 1015–1023. doi:10.1002/jgm.1115

Okawa H, Sampath AP, Laughlin SB, Fain GL. 2008. ATP consumption by mammalian rod photoreceptors in darkness and in light. *Curr Biol* **18:** 1917–1921. doi:10.1016/j.cub.2008.10.029

Olsson JE, Gordon JW, Pawlyk BS, Roof D, Hayes A, Molday RS, Mukai S, Cowley GS, Berson EL, Dryja TP. 1992. Transgenic mice with a rhodopsin mutation (Pro23His): a mouse model of autosomal dominant retinitis pigmentosa. *Neuron* **9:** 815–830. doi:10.1016/0896-6273(92)90236-7

O'Neill B, Millington-Ward S, O'Reilly M, Tuohy G, Kiang AS, Kenna PF, Humphries P, Farrar GJ. 2000. Ribozyme-based therapeutic approaches for autosomal dominant retinitis pigmentosa. *Invest Ophthalmol Vis Sci* **41**: 2863–2869.

Orlans HO, McClements ME, Barnard AR, Martinez-Fernandez de la Camara C, MacLaren RE. 2021. Mirtron-mediated RNA knockdown/replacement therapy for the treatment of dominant retinitis pigmentosa. *Nat Commun* **12**: 4934. doi:10.1038/s41467-021-25204-3

Palczewski K. 2006. G protein-coupled receptor rhodopsin. *Annu Rev Biochem* **75**: 743–767. doi:10.1146/annurev.biochem.75.103004.142743

Palfi A, Millington-Ward S, Chadderton N, O'Reilly M, Goldmann T, Humphries MM, Li T, Wolfrum U, Humphries P, Kenna PF, et al. 2010. Adeno-associated virus-mediated rhodopsin replacement provides therapeutic benefit in mice with a targeted disruption of the rhodopsin gene. *Hum Gene Ther* **21**: 311–323. doi:10.1089/hum.2009.119

Pan WW, Wubben TJ, Besirli CG. 2021. Photoreceptor metabolic reprogramming: current understanding and therapeutic implications. *Commun Biol* **4**: 245. doi:10.1038/s42003-021-01765-3

Patrizi C, Llado M, Benati D, Iodice C, Marrocco E, Guarascio R, Surace EM, Cheetham ME, Auricchio A, Recchia A. 2021. Allele-specific editing ameliorates dominant retinitis pigmentosa in a transgenic mouse model. *Am J Hum Genet* **108**: 295–308. doi:10.1016/j.ajhg.2021.01.006

Pavlou M, Schön C, Occelli LM, Rossi A, Meumann N, Boyd RF, Bartoe JT, Siedlecki J, Gerhardt MJ, Babutzka S, et al. 2021. Novel AAV capsids for intravitreal gene therapy of photoreceptor disorders. *EMBO Mol Med* **13**: e13392. doi:10.15252/emmm.202013392

Petersen-Jones SM, Bartoe JT, Fischer AJ, Scott M, Boye SL, Chiodo V, Hauswirth WW. 2009. AAV retinal transduction in a large animal model species: comparison of a self-complementary AAV2/5 with a single-stranded AAV2/5 vector. *Mol Vis* **15**: 1835–1842.

Petrs-Silva H, Dinculescu A, Li Q, Min SH, Chiodo V, Pang JJ, Zhong L, Zolotukhin S, Srivastava A, Lewin AS, et al. 2009. High-efficiency transduction of the mouse retina by tyrosine-mutant AAV serotype vectors. *Mol Ther* **17**: 463–471. doi:10.1038/mt.2008.269

Petrs-Silva H, Dinculescu A, Li Q, Deng WT, Pang JJ, Min SH, Chiodo V, Neeley AW, Govindasamy L, Bennett A, et al. 2011. Novel properties of tyrosine-mutant AAV2 vectors in the mouse retina. *Mol Ther* **19**: 293–301. doi:10.1038/mt.2010.234

Petters RM, Alexander CA, Wells KD, Collins EB, Sommer JR, Blanton MR, Rojas G, Hao Y, Flowers WL, Banin E, et al. 1997. Genetically engineered large animal model for studying cone photoreceptor survival and degeneration in retinitis pigmentosa. *Nat Biotechnol* **15**: 965–970. doi:10.1038/nbt1097-965

Punzo C, Kornacker K, Cepko CL. 2009. Stimulation of the insulin/mTOR pathway delays cone death in a mouse model of retinitis pigmentosa. *Nat Neurosci* **12**: 44–52. doi:10.1038/nn.2234

Ramachandran PS, Lee V, Wei Z, Song JY, Casal G, Cronin T, Willett K, Huckfeldt R, Morgan JI, Aleman TS, et al. 2017. Evaluation of dose and safety of AAV7m8 and AAV8BP2 in the non-human primate retina. *Hum Gene Ther* **28**: 154–167. doi:10.1089/hum.2016.111

Rana T, Shinde VM, Starr CR, Kruglov AA, Boitet ER, Kotla P, Zolotukhin S, Gross AK, Gorbatyuk MS. 2014. An activated unfolded protein response promotes retinal degeneration and triggers an inflammatory response in the mouse retina. *Cell Death Dis* **5**: e1578. doi:10.1038/cddis.2014.539

Reynolds A, Leake D, Boese Q, Scaringe S, Marshall WS, Khvorova A. 2004. Rational siRNA design for RNA interference. *Nat Biotechnol* **22**: 326–330. doi:10.1038/nbt936

Rhee KD, Ruiz A, Duncan JL, Hauswirth WW, LaVail MM, Bok D, Yang XJ. 2007. Molecular and cellular alterations induced by sustained expression of ciliary neurotrophic factor in a mouse model of retinitis pigmentosa. *Invest Ophthalmology Vis Sci* **48**: 1389–1400. doi:10.1167/iovs.06-0677

Ron D, Walter P. 2007. Signal integration in the endoplasmic reticulum unfolded protein response. *Nat Rev Mol Cell Biol* **8**: 519–529. doi:10.1038/nrm2199

Ross JW, Fernandez de Castro JP, Zhao J, Samuel M, Walters E, Rios C, Bray-Ward P, Jones BW, Marc RE, Wang W, et al. 2012. Generation of an inbred miniature pig model of retinitis pigmentosa. *Invest Ophthalmol Vis Sci* **53**: 501–507. doi:10.1167/iovs.11-8784

Schmidt MJ, Gupta A, Bednarski C, Gehrig-Giannini S, Richter F, Pitzler C, Gamalinda M, Galonska C, Takeuchi R, Wang K, et al. 2021. Improved CRISPR genome editing using small highly active and specific engineered RNA-guided nucleases. *Nat Commun* **12**: 4219–4219. doi:10.1038/s41467-021-24454-5

Scott PA, Fernandez de Castro J, Kaplan HJ, McCall MA. 2014. A Pro23His mutation alters prenatal rod photoreceptor morphology in a transgenic swine model of retinitis pigmentosa. *Invest Ophthalmol Vis Sci* **55**: 2452–2459. doi:10.1167/iovs.13-13723

Sengillo JD, Gregori NZ, Sisk RA, Weng CY, Berrocal AM, Davis JL, Mendoza-Santiesteban CE, Zheng DD, Feuer WJ, Lam BL. 2022. Visual acuity, retinal morphology, and patients' perceptions after voretigene neparvovecrzyl therapy for RPE65-associated retinal disease. *Ophthalmol Retina* **6**: 273–283. doi:10.1016/j.oret.2021.11.005

Sharma K, Krohne TU, Busskamp V. 2020. The rise of retinal organoids for vision research. *Int J Mol Sci* **21**: 8484. doi:10.3390/ijms21228484

Shinde VM, Sizova OS, Lin JH, LaVail MM, Gorbatyuk MS. 2012. ER stress in retinal degeneration in S334ter Rho rats. *PLoS ONE* **7**: e33266. doi:10.1371/journal.pone.0033266

Suda K, Filipek S, Palczewski K, Engel A, Fotiadis D. 2004. The supramolecular structure of the GPCR rhodopsin in solution and native disc membranes. *Mol Membr Biol* **21**: 435–446. doi:10.1080/09687860400020291

Sullivan JM, Pietras KM, Shin BJ, Misasi JN. 2002. Hammerhead ribozymes designed to cleave all human rod opsin mRNAs which cause autosomal dominant retinitis pigmentosa. *Mol Vis* **8**: 102–113.

Sullivan LS, Bowne SJ, Birch DG, Hughbanks-Wheaton D, Heckenlively JR, Lewis RA, Garcia CA, Ruiz RS, Blanton SH, Northrup H, et al. 2006. Prevalence of disease-causing mutations in families with autosomal dominant retinitis pigmentosa: a screen of known genes in 200 families.

Cite this article as *Cold Spring Harb Perspect Med* doi: 10.1101/cshperspect.a041283

Invest Ophthalmol Vis Sci **47:** 3052–3064. doi:10.1167/iovs.05-1443

Timmers AM, Newmark JA, Turunen HT, Farivar T, Liu J, Song C, Ye GJ, Pennock S, Gaskin C, Knop DR, et al. 2020. Ocular inflammatory response to intravitreal injection of adeno-associated virus vector: relative contribution of genome and capsid. *Hum Gene Ther* **31:** 80–89. doi:10.1089/hum.2019.144

Trapani I, Puppo A, Auricchio A. 2014. Vector platforms for gene therapy of inherited retinopathies. *Prog Retin Eye Res* **43:** 108–128. doi:10.1016/j.preteyeres.2014.08.001

Tsai YT, Wu WH, Lee TT, Wu WP, Xu CL, Park KS, Cui X, Justus S, Lin CS, Jauregui R, et al. 2018. Clustered regularly interspaced short palindromic repeats-based genome surgery for the treatment of autosomal dominant retinitis pigmentosa. *Ophthalmology* **125:** 1421–1430. doi:10.1016/j.ophtha.2018.04.001

Tummala G, Crain A, Rowlan J, Pepple KL. 2021. Characterization of gene therapy associated uveitis following intravitreal adeno-associated virus injection in mice. *Invest Ophthalmol Vis Sci* **62:** 41. doi:10.1167/iovs.62.2.41

Vandenberghe LH, Auricchio A. 2012. Novel adeno-associated viral vectors for retinal gene therapy. *Gene Ther* **19:** 162–168. doi:10.1038/gt.2011.151

Walter P, Ron D. 2011. The unfolded protein response: from stress pathway to homeostatic regulation. *Science* **334:** 1081–1086. doi:10.1126/science.1209038

Wang W, Kini A, Wang Y, Liu T, Chen Y, Vukmanic E, Emery D, Liu Y, Lu X, Jin L, et al. 2019. Metabolic deregulation of the blood-outer retinal barrier in retinitis pigmentosa. *Cell Rep* **28:** 1323–1334.e4. doi:10.1016/j.celrep.2019.06.093

Warburg O, Posener K, Negrelein E. 1924. On the metabolism of carcinoma cells. *Bioschemische Zeitschrift* **152:** 309–344.

Wert KJ, Velez G, Kanchustambham VL, Shankar V, Evans LP, Sengillo JD, Zare RN, Bassuk AG, Tsang SH, Mahajan VB. 2020. Metabolite therapy guided by liquid biopsy proteomics delays retinal neurodegeneration. *EBioMedicine* **52:** 102636. doi:10.1016/j.ebiom.2020.102636

Wong-Staal F, Poeschla EM, Looney DJ. 1998. A controlled, phase 1 clinical trial to evaluate the safety and effects in HIV-1 infected humans of autologous lymphocytes transduced with a ribozyme that cleaves HIV-1 RNA.

Hum Gene Ther **9:** 2407–2425. doi:10.1089/hum.1998.9.16-2407

Wu WC, Lai CC, Chen SL, Sun MH, Xiao X, Chen TL, Lin KK, Kuo SW, Tsao YP. 2005. Long-term safety of GDNF gene delivery in the retina. *Curr Eye Res* **30:** 715–722. doi:10.1080/02713680591005922

Wu WH, Tsai YT, Huang IW, Cheng CH, Hsu CW, Cui X, Ryu J, Quinn PMJ, Caruso SM, Lin CS, et al. 2022. CRISPR genome surgery in a novel humanized model for autosomal dominant retinitis pigmentosa. *Mol Ther* **30:** 1407–1420. doi:10.1016/j.ymthe.2022.02.010

Xu L, Kong L, Wang J, Ash JD. 2018. Stimulation of AMPK prevents degeneration of photoreceptors and the retinal pigment epithelium. *Proc Natl Acad Sci* **115:** 10475–10480. doi:10.1073/pnas.1802724115

Xue Y, Wang SK, Rana P, West ER, Hong CM, Feng H, Wu DM, Cepko CL. 2021. AAV-Txnip prolongs cone survival and vision in mouse models of retinitis pigmentosa. *eLife* **10:** e66240. doi:10.7554/eLife.66240

Yiu G, Chung SH, Mollhoff IN, Nguyen UT, Thomasy SM, Yoo J, Taraborelli D, Noronha G. 2020. Suprachoroidal and subretinal injections of AAV using transscleral microneedles for retinal gene delivery in nonhuman primates. *Mol Ther Methods Clin Dev* **16:** 179–191. doi:10.1016/j.omtm.2020.01.002

Zhang L, Du J, Justus S, Hsu CW, Bonet-Ponce L, Wu WH, Tsai YT, Wu WP, Jia Y, Duong JK, et al. 2016. Reprogramming metabolism by targeting sirtuin 6 attenuates retinal degeneration. *J Clin Invest* **126:** 4659–4673. doi:10.1172/JCI86905

Zheng M, Mitra RN, Weiss ER, Han Z. 2020. Rhodopsin genomic loci DNA nanoparticles improve expression and rescue of retinal degeneration in a model for retinitis pigmentosa. *Mol Ther* **28:** 523–535. doi:10.1016/j.ymthe.2019.11.031

Zhu L, Jang GF, Jastrzebska B, Filipek S, Pearce-Kelling SE, Aguirre GD, Stenkamp RE, Acland GM, Palczewski K. 2004. A naturally occurring mutation of the opsin gene (T4R) in dogs affects glycosylation and stability of the G protein-coupled receptor. *J Biol Chem* **279:** 53828–53839. doi:10.1074/jbc.M408472200

Zuzic M, Rojo Arias JE, Wohl SG, Busskamp V. 2019. Retinal miRNA functions in health and disease. *Genes (Basel)* **10:** 377. doi:10.3390/genes10050377

X-Linked Retinoschisis

Cristy A. Ku,[1] Lisa W. Wei,[2] and Paul A. Sieving[1,3]

[1]Department of Ophthalmology & Vision Science, University of California Davis, Sacramento, California 95817, USA

[2]National Institutes of Health, National Institute of Allergy and Infectious Diseases, NIH Office of Biodefense, Research Resources and Translational Research/Vaccine Section, Bethesda, Maryland 20892, USA

Correspondence: pasieving@ucdavis.edu

X-linked retinoschisis (XLRS) is an inherited vitreoretinal dystrophy causing visual impairment in males starting at a young age with an estimated prevalence of 1:5000 to 1:25,000. The condition was first observed in two affected brothers by Josef Haas in 1898 and is clinically diagnosed by characteristic intraretinal cysts arranged in a petaloid "spoke-wheel" pattern centered in the macula. When clinical electroretinogram (ERG) testing began in the 1960s, XLRS was noted to have a characteristic reduction of the dark-adapted b-wave amplitude despite normal or usually nearly normal a-wave amplitudes, which became known as the "electronegative ERG response" of XLRS disease. The causative gene, *RS1*, was identified on the X-chromosome in 1997 and led to understanding the molecular and cellular basis of the condition, discerning the structure and function of the retinoschisin protein, and generating XLRS murine models. Along with parallel development of gene delivery vectors suitable for targeting retinal diseases, successful gene augmentation therapy was demonstrated by rescuing the XLRS phenotype in mouse. Two human phase I/II therapeutic XLRS gene augmentation studies were initiated; and although these did not yield definitive improvement in visual function, they gave significant new knowledge and experience, which positions the field for further near-term clinical testing with enhanced, next-generation gene therapy for XLRS patients.

XLRS CLINICAL DISEASE

Males affected by X-linked retinoschisis (XLRS) show visual impairment early in life, most frequently in childhood with visual acuities of 20/50 to less than 20/200 in some patients.[4] Estimated prevalence in the population is 1:5000 to 1:25,000 (George et al. 1995). Central vision is affected by characteristic "spoke-wheel" cystic maculopathy, with intraretinal schisis cavities arranged in a radial petaloid perifoveal pattern (Fig. 1A), as first described in two brothers by Josef Haas in 1989 (Haas 1989). Unlike cystoid macular edema of other acquired retinal conditions, XLRS cystic changes result from abnormal splitting or schisis through the retinal neurosensory layers and respond infrequently to carbonic anhydrase inhibitors (CAIs) (Pennesi et al. 2018).

Individuals with X-linked retinoschisis can manifest a spectrum of clinical severity, making

---

[3]Formerly at the National Eye Institute, National Institutes of Health (NIH), Bethesda, MD.

[4]This is an update to a previous article published in *Cold Spring Harbor Perspectives in Medicine* (Bush et al. 2015).

Cite this article as *Cold Spring Harb Perspect Med* doi: 10.1101/cshperspect.a041288

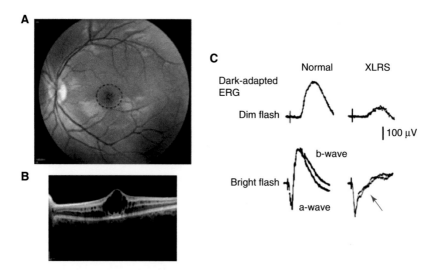

Figure 1. Fundus photograph, optical coherence tomography (OCT) scan, and electroretinogram (ERG) responses typical for an X-linked retinoschisis (XLRS) patient. (*A*) The macula (highlighted with dashed circle) has intraretinal schisis cystic cavities and some retinal pigment epithelium (RPE) pigmentary mottling. (*B*) The OCT shows a high-peaked central cystic space, and the underlying photoreceptor layer is thin and is missing many inner/outer segments. (*C*) On ERGs, responses for XLRS show an abnormally small b-wave to a dim flash under dark adapted conditions, and the b-wave to a bright flash is "absent" (red arrow), while the a-wave amplitude is preserved, giving in "electronegative" b-wave configuration.

initial diagnosis potentially challenging. Retinoschisis occurs in various and often multiple locations including foveal schisis, diffuse macular schisis, peripheral schisis, or any combination. The advent of noninvasive optical coherence tomography (OCT), particularly spectral domain OCT (SD-OCT), has provided detailed structural characterization of these retinoschisis cavities (Fig. 1B). Retinoschisis may occur in all retinal layers particularly involving the inner nuclear layer (INL) and outer plexiform layers (OPLs) (Gerth et al. 2008). Extrafoveal macular schisis may also occur in inner and outer nuclear layers, and the ganglion cell layer (Gerth et al. 2008). The electroretinogram (ERG) b-wave (bipolar cell response) amplitude is reduced in comparison to the a-wave (from photoreceptors) (Forsius et al. 1963) and may reach an "electronegative response" configuration if the b-wave does not even return to baseline amplitude (Fig 1C).

Peripheral retinoschisis occurs in 40%–75% of XLRS patients (George et al. 1996; Prenner et al. 2006) and may cause associated visual field defects. Peripheral schisis may be complicated by complex rhegmatogenous retinal detachments, which occur in areas of schisis with outer retinal wall holes. Holes in the inner retinal wall can progress to the commonly associated finding of "vitreous veils" first described in 1938 (Mann and Macrae 1938), appearing as wispy sheets of partial thickness inner retinal layers that delaminate into the vitreous along with overlying retinal vessels. These may bleed and cause vitreous hemorrhage. The frequency of complications with XLRS, such as vitreous hemorrhage, ranges from 3% to 21%, and retinal detachment ranges from 5% to 40% in the literature (Peachey 1987; Kellner et al. 1990; George et al. 1996; Roesch et al. 1998; Fahim et al. 2017; Cukras et al. 2018b; Orès et al. 2018; Pennesi et al. 2018). Over time, schisis often progresses to clinically evident RPE changes and chorioretinal scarring, with RPE atrophy in both the periphery and macula. A golden retinal sheen is frequently observed throughout the fundus in XLRS patients (Wakabayashi et al. 2022). Unusual manifestations include macular dragging and fovea ectopia (McKibbin et al. 2001), or accumulations of retinal white flecks (Hotta et al. 2001) that simulate fundus albipunctatus (van Schooneveld and Miyake 1994), although XLRS does not feature the prolonged time required for dark adaptation that occurs with fundus albipunctatus. Dark-adapted final thresholds frequently are elevated by one-half to one log unit but do not result in patient complaints.

INHERITANCE, GENE, AND CELL BIOLOGY OF XLRS

The *RS1* gene associated with XLRS was identified on the X chromosome in 1997 by positional cloning (Sauer et al. 1997). XLRS is transmitted in a classic X-linked recessive pattern, in which female carriers have a 50% chance of transmitting a disease-causing mutation in the *RS1* gene in each pregnancy. Males who inherit the causative mutation are clinically affected with high penetrance, and they transmit the mutation to all daughters and none of their sons. However, females who inherit *RS1* mutations are nearly always clinically and functionally asymptomatic. On only rare occasions, female carriers can show white flecks or areas of schisis within the peripheral retina (Kaplan et al. 1991). The absence of retinal clinical XLRS disease in carrier females indicates that full expression of the RS1 gene is not requisite for disease amelioration in affected men by gene replacement therapy.

RS1 encodes for the secreted 224–amino acid retinoschisin protein expressed by many retinal neurons but not retinal glia, as it is not expressed by either RPE or Müller glial cells. In early postnatal mouse retinal development, retinoschisin is expressed in retinal ganglion cells (RGCs), followed by expression in other inner retinal neurons throughout ocular development, and most prominently in photoreceptors by 14 days into adulthood (Fig. 2; Takada et al. 2004). Retinoschisin contains several key domains: an amino-terminal signal peptide, the RS1 domain, and a discoidin domain, which is a specialized domain found in a family of extracellular surface proteins that function in cell adhesion and signaling, and in extracellular matrix remodeling (Sauer et al. 1997; Grayson et al. 2000; Vogel et al. 2006). The protein contains 10 key structural cysteine

residues throughout the RS1 and discoidin domains that are vital to assembly of the mature protein into disulfide-linked homo-octameric complexes (Wu et al. 2005). The RS1 signaling peptide sequence allows retinoschisin to be secreted extracellularly, where it plays a critical role in retinal cell–cell adhesion and photoreceptor–bipolar cell synaptic structure and signaling (Takada et al. 2004; Molday et al. 2007), possibly through interactions with the retinal cationic channel Na/K-ATPase—SARM complex (Molday et al. 2007; Friedrich et al. 2011), and/or L-type, voltage-gated calcium channels (Shi et al. 2017), membrane lipid phosphatidylserine (Kotova et al. 2010), and vital postsynaptic signaling receptors TRPM1 channel (Ou et al. 2015).

DIAGNOSTICS

In addition to the characteristic XLRS fundus appearance, affected individuals show a distinguishing ERG waveform with subnormal dark-adapted b-wave relative to a-wave amplitudes (Fig. 1C). For reference, normal ERG responses are characterized by an initial negative polarity a-wave representing photoreceptor hyperpolarization, followed by the positive b-wave response from second-order retinal neurons, which represent bipolar cell depolarization. However, patients with XLRS demonstrate perturbed b-wave amplitudes ranging from severely electronegative waveforms in which the positive b-wave fails to rise to or above baseline, to other cases showing only a mild decrease in b/a-wave amplitude ratios. A proportion of *RS1* mutation-positive patients may even have nearly normal b-wave amplitudes (Bowles et al. 2011; Vincent et al. 2013).

These characteristic ERG findings correspond to the role of retinoschisin protein in proper synaptic functioning between photoreceptors and bipolar cells, as shown by immunohistochemistry to be consequent to a failure of intracellular proteins to properly localize in the postsynaptic structure (Takada et al. 2004). Genotype–phenotype studies have proven difficult, but work has indicated that null allele mutations or those that significantly disturb protein structure by altering cysteine residues of the hydrophobic core (Sergeev et al. 2010, 2013; Bowles

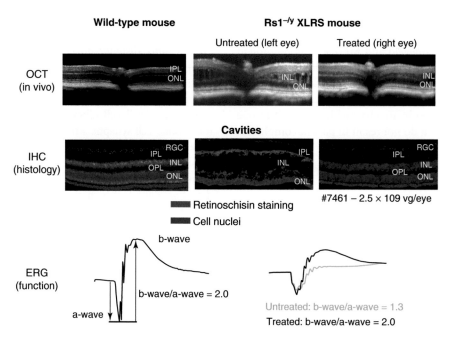

Figure 2. Retinal histopathology and electroretinogram (ERG) responses of an Rs1 knockout mouse, with images from a wild-type (WT) normal mouse for comparison. The histology *middle* panel shows retinoschisis cystic cavities in the inner retina proximal to the photoreceptors in the outer nuclear layer (ONL) of the Rs1$^{-/y}$ XLRS mouse. ERG responses of the WT mouse retina show the characteristic initial negative-going a-wave (from photoreceptors) followed by the positive-going b-wave (from depolarizing bipolar cells). The size of the ratio of (b-/a-wave) reflects transmission through the synaptic outer plexiform layer (OPL), from photoreceptors to the bipolar cells. This ratio is reduced to 1.3 in the Rs1$^{-/y}$ XLRS mouse (green waveform), indicating defective transmission from photoreceptors to the bipolar cells. The *right* panel shows the Rs1$^{-/y}$ XLRS retina after delivery of a therapeutic vector AAV8-RS1-RS1 carrying the human retinoschisin cDNA. This preserves retinal lamination and thickness of the photoreceptor ONL, and the ERG b-wave response has increased, and the (b-/a-wave) ratio grown to 2.0, indicating that transmission between photoreceptors and bipolar cells has been restored.

et al. 2011) generally result in absent or severe decrease of retinoschisin protein (Bowles et al. 2011) and are associated with worse retinal function, as measured by ERG b/a-wave ratios.

MEDICAL MANAGEMENT OF SCHISIS CAVITIES

Currently there are no approved treatments for retinal degeneration nor for the retinal schisis cavities associated with XLRS. Various experimental treatment options have been explored, including use of CAIs (e.g., dorzolamide and acetazolamide) with the mechanism of action: acidification of the subretinal space, resulting in fluid transport across the RPE and reduction of intraretinal fluid (Apushkin and Fishman

2006; Ghajarnia and Gorin 2007). While some studies report that foveal schisis may improve with CAI, acuity changes are quite variable (Ghajarnia and Gorin, 2007). Pennesi reviewed seven larger studies with four or more XLRS subjects and concluded that CAIs provided little or no gain in visual acuity (Pennesi et al. 2018). Some larger, retrospective and prospective studies do indicate that some smaller percentage of XLRS patients show reduction of central cystic cavities as measured by central foveal thickness, and to a lesser degree, they may have improvements in visual acuity, microperimetry, and ERG responses in select patients (Gurbaxani et al. 2014; Andreuzzi et al. 2017; Testa et al. 2019; Ambrosio et al. 2021), but this is generally not to be expected for most XLRS patients (Pennesi et al. 2018). Variable CAI responses could be related to differences in retinoschisin protein secretion, although no definitive genotype–phenotype correlations have been found (Walia et al. 2009; Testa et al. 2019). This may be worth pursuing for therapeutic ends once the mechanism of intraretinal fluid compartments is understood for the XLRS retina.

MOUSE MODELS

XLRS mouse models have contributed greatly to our understanding of disease pathophysiology, and they provide in vivo preclinical models for developing XLRS therapeutics. There are currently at least seven XLRS mouse models targeting the murine ortholog of the human *RS1* gene (Vijayasarathy et al. 2022) and also a rat XLRS model with *Rs1* exon 3 deletion (Zeng et al. 2021; Vijayasarathy et al. 2022). All are deficient in producing endogenous murine/rat retinoschisin, either due to effectively null alleles or by targeted knockin of known human deleterious mutations. The first mouse model was engineered with targeted disruption of exons 3 and 4 by insertion of a LacZ/ Neo^r cassette (Weber et al. 2002). A second model inserted a neomycin gene into exon 1 and most of intron 1 (Zeng et al. 2004). These two models supported preclinical studies leading to investigational new drug (IND) registration with the U.S. Food and Drug Administration (FDA) and subsequent human gene augmentation trials (ClinicalTrials.gov: NCT02317887; NCT02416622).

Murine *Rs1* knockout (KO) models generally display structural and functional retinal phenotypes similar to human XLRS, some with similarly slow progression (Zeng et al. 2004), while others progress more rapidly (Vijayasarathy et al. 2022). ERG evaluations of mouse models show characteristic reductions of the dark-adapted b-wave as observed in human XLRS. Histologically, retina structure is disorganized, with misaligned retinal lamina and splitting evident particularly within the INL and OPL, as characteristic of XLRS human disease. Figure 2 shows the retinal structure and dampened ERGs in male XLRS mice (Zeng et al. 2004). Ou et al. showed XLRS pathology of the critical synapse between photoreceptors and bipolar cells in the OPL (Ou et al. 2015).

Findings observed in mouse models supported the feasibility for gene augmentation as a useful therapeutic approach to explore for human XLRS. While retinoschisin normally is expressed during development, persistent expression in adult tissue suggests that it remains important in maintaining retinal architecture and to sustain synaptic integrity (Takada et al. 2004). Retinoschisin is expressed by almost all retinal neurons, except possibly horizontal cells, and does not require transport from the outer to the inner retina for its expression and function at the photoreceptor–bipolar cell synapse (Takada et al. 2004). Unlike most inherited retinal dystrophies, XLRS dysfunction is not limited exclusively to the outer retina and therefore may offer potential for intravitreal gene delivery.

GENE THERAPY CONSIDERATIONS

Considerations in gene augmentation therapy include selecting an appropriate gene vector and route of delivery. Current viral vectors being investigated in ocular gene therapy clinical trials include adeno-associated virus (AAV) and equine infectious anemia virus (EIAV), which have shown transduction efficacy in retinal cells. AAV vectors currently are commonly used gene vectors in ocular diseases due to their safety and efficacy (Buch et al. 2008). The AAV vector is a small, nonenveloped, single-stranded DNA virus that is nonpathogenic and shows low immunogenicity. EIAV is a non-HIV1-based, nonprimate lentivirus in the *Retroviridae* family (Trapani et al. 2014). Lentiviral vectors are used to deliver large genes that surpass the 4.8-kb size limitation of AAV, as EIAV has packaging capacity up to 8 kb (Trapani et al. 2014). Other gene vectors that are being explored in preclinical studies to extend packaging capacities include nanoparticles and dual AAV vectors.

RS1 fits within the 4.8 kb packaging limit of AAV, and AAV-*RS1* viral vectors have been used in preclinical and clinical ocular gene therapy trials (Min et al. 2005; Marangoni et al. 2014, 2016; Ou et al. 2015; Cukras et al. 2018a; Pennesi et al. 2022). Multiple available AAV serotypes, defined by variations of the viral capsid, allow for differential cell targeting or tropism (Lebherz et al. 2008). Beyond naturally occurring AAV capsid variants, developments in capsid engineering aim to generate vectors with novel or more desirable properties such as improved transduction efficiency, panretinal transduction, cell-specific tropism, or outer retinal transduction through an intravitreal administration (Dalkara et al. 2013). Currently, the most efficient method of outer retinal transduction for retinal dystrophies is achieved through a delicately performed surgical subretinal injection, which has disadvantages of relatively localized transduction in the surgical bleb and potential for surgically induced damage to the retina. In contrast, intravitreal injections are routinely performed as in-office procedures for conditions such as diabetic retinopathy and exudative age-related macular degeneration. An intravitreal route of administration would make ocular gene therapy more accessible and safer for ocular conditions with particularly fragile retinal tissue. Recently an alternative strategy using a localized subretinal injection is being developed with a "spreading vector," which disseminates more readily through the subretinal space after local application (Boye et al. 2020), and Atsena Therapeutics is developing preclinical studies toward deploying this for XLRS gene augmentation therapy.

Factors to consider with routes of delivery for ocular gene therapy include which retinal cells are targeted for gene expression, the desire for transduction of foveal and macular neurons, and the nature of disease and pathophysiology being treated. Several properties of XLRS make intravitreal injections more feasible and desirable for this condition than other inherited retinal dystrophies. Multiple retinal cells normally express the secreted retinoschisin protein, including both outer retinal photoreceptors and inner retinal bipolar cells. Further, retinoschisin is particularly necessary for function at photoreceptor–bipolar cell synapses, which bridge the outer and inner retinal layers, a site of disease that is unlike many other inherited retinal dystrophies. XLRS has an inherent impairment in retinal structural integrity that makes vitrecto-my and subretinal gene delivery challenging. However, it is conjectured that these inherent structural defects advantageously allow for greater transduction across the outer retina following an intravitreal injection of viral vector, as was observed with XLRS mice.

When administered by intravitreal injection, first-generation AAV vectors demonstrated transduction limited and localized primarily to the ganglion cells near the retinal surface. Early advances in AAV capsid engineering with tyrosine to phenylalanine substitutions (Y-F mutations) created vectors with the ability to enter the retina and transduce outer retinal cells following intravitreal injection in rodent retina (Petrs-Silva et al. 2009, 2011; Dalkara et al. 2013). Still newer capsids are in development using a strategy of "directed evolution" by repeatedly harvesting mutant capsids from the retina after intravitreal application, to enrich for capsids with this ability. It is expected these will eventually be employed for vector-based gene therapy for IRD conditions, including XLRS. Preclinical efficacy studies in XLRS mouse models demonstrated a greater extent of penetration of enhanced green fluorescent protein (EGFP) and expression in the outer retina following intravitreal injection of both first-generation and early AAV capsid mutant vectors as compared to wild-type retina (Park et al. 2009; Byrne et al. 2014). Studies further supported intravitreal delivery as a viable therapeutic option for *RS1* gene augmentation using AAV2 or AAV8 into *Rs1*-KO mice, as this reduced the schisis cavities and reversed the ERG b-wave abnormalities (Fig. 2; Zeng et al. 2004; Kjellstrom et al. 2007; Park et al. 2009; Byrne et al. 2014; Bush et al. 2015, 2016) in a dose-dependent manner (Bush et al. 2016; Zeng et al. 2021). Of interest, studies demonstrated that functional and anatomical improvement was greater when retinoschisin was expressed by photoreceptor cells as compared to targeting Müller glia for sole expression (Byrne et al. 2014) following intravitreal delivery of promoter-specific AAV vectors.

Following successful preclinical studies in mice, preclinical safety studies in larger animal/larger eyes in New Zealand white rabbits showed tolerability and safety of the AAV8-

scRS-IRBPhRS vector at two viral doses, $2e^{10}$ and $2e^{11}$ vector genomes [vg]/eye, with dose-dependent mild ocular inflammation in the retrolental, prepapillary and central vitreous spaces without anterior segment inflammation (Marangoni et al. 2014). Two larger-scale good laboratory practice (GLP) studies demonstrated safety and efficacy in the New Zealand white rabbit and *Rs1*-KO mouse (Marangoni et al. 2016).

Improved functional and structural results were also shown by AAV-*Rs1* subretinal gene augmentation in *Rs1*-KO mice (Min et al. 2005; Janssen et al. 2008). While no studies have performed head-to-head comparisons in *Rs1*-KO mice, subretinal injections generally show higher transduction of photoreceptors given the close proximity as compared to intravitreal injections. This becomes increasingly true in animal models with larger eyes than rodents. Despite promising results in rodent models, second-generation AAV vectors still showed limited outer retinal transduction via the vitreous in large animals including canine (Mowat et al. 2014) and nonhuman primate retina (Yin et al. 2011) due to barriers from the vitreous and inner limiting membrane (Takahashi et al. 2017) and overall dilution and neutralization in the vitreous.

While both delivery routes offered phenotypic improvements in XLRS mice, the first human clinical trial that entered phase I/IIa studies used the AAV8-*RS1* intravitreal vector that had demonstrated safety in GLP studies. Following IND studies required by the FDA, a prospective, nonrandomized, open-label, single-center, dose-escalation study was initiated at the National Eye Institute (NEI) in the Clinical Center of the National Institutes of Health (NIH) in Bethesda, MD (NCT02317887). Three viral vector doses ($1e^9$, $1e^{10}$, and $1e^{11}$ vg/eye) were studied, with three patients receiving each dose in the first segment of the trial (Cukras et al. 2018a). The intravitreal treatment was well-tolerated in a majority of patients. Mild vitritis and anterior segment inflammation at grade 1 or less was observed in one patient receiving $1e^{10}$ vg/eye, and two patients receiving $1e^{11}$ vg/eye exhibited the next level of ocular inflammation; all resolved promptly with topical or oral steroids.

The third patient receiving $1e^{11}$ vg/eye had a greater inflammatory response with moderate vitritis and acromioclavicular (AC) inflammation, complicated by elevated intraocular pressures, vasculitis, and postinflammatory posterior vitreous detachment leading to a retinal tear treated successfully with laser retinopexy with subsequent vitreous hemorrhage requiring vitrectomy; this subject's visual acuity returned to baseline level. Of interest, this same patient had complete closure of macular schisis cavities transiently; this closure appeared complete on OCT imaging (Cukras et al. 2018a). Other than this positive response in one of the three subjects who received the higher dose of $1e^{11}$ vg/eye, no other definite clinical improvements were observed by visual acuity, central macular thickness, microperimetry, or ERGs. This trial is continuing.

A second trial of AAV-*RS1* for XLRS was mounted as a multicenter, dose-escalation phase I/II study, sponsored by AGTC (ClinicalTrials. Gov: NCT02416622), by intravitreal administration of a second-generation tyrosine mutant vector (AAV2tYF-CB-hRS1). This study dosed 22 adult XLRS subjects and five children by intravitreal application, at vector dose levels of $1e^{11}$ to $6e^{11}$ vg/eye. Year 1 outcomes are reported as generally well tolerated but with varying levels of ocular inflammation at all dose levels, that could be medically managed with topical and oral immunosuppressive therapy (Pennesi et al. 2022). No significant overall improvement in visual function was reported. Three subjects who received the highest, $6e^{11}$ vg/eye dose developed chronic recurrent uveitis that persisted beyond a year. It is worth noting that AAV gene trials for other IRD conditions also encountered considerable inflammatory activity by $6e^{11}$ vg/eye dose level.

The minimal improvement in outcome measures in these clinical trials thus far have been attributed in part to the more limited outer retinal transduction efficiency with intravitreal application in humans than was found during small animal studies, leading to an overall subtherapeutic response (Takahashi et al. 2017). Both of the XLRS trials point out the delicate balance between elevated dose levels, which may give therapeutic improvement, but which also risk intraocular inflammation. At sustained high levels this is deleterious to ocular structure and function. Inflammation also signals an attack by the host on the therapeutic viral agent, thereby potentially limiting the benefit.

Recent efforts in the field of ocular gene augmentation therapy have been directed at improving treatment efficacy, including capsid engineering by directed evolution, whereby candidate AAV capsid mutations are selected from among a library of numerous random capsid mutations by their performance in specific advantageous properties (e.g., excellent retinal penetration of vector capsids delivered via the vitreous cavity) and reduced capsid immunogenicity. Candidate AAV vectors are in development for XLRS trials through enhanced, directed evolution studies specifically assayed for improved outer retinal transduction through intravitreal injections in the nonhuman primate retina (Byrne et al. 2020).

Among causes suspected for the lower transduction efficacy with intravitreal injections in humans and nonhuman primates are preexisting and post-treatment antibodies against the AAV capsid or transgene. Many people in the general population have had prior exposure to one or more AAV capsids and carry circulating neutralizing antibodies. Antibody cross-reactivity may still occur despite use of novel engineered AAV gene therapy viral vectors (Li et al. 2008; Kotterman et al. 2015). Intravitreal injections are at greater exposure to neutralizing antibodies due to viral shedding and extraocular biodistribution in the blood and draining lymphatic tissue, as compared to the relatively immunoprivileged subretinal compartment (Seitz et al. 2017; Reichel et al. 2018). Whether the newer enhanced AAV capsids will show immune evasion or will be efficient enough to overcome this opposing problem remains to be seen; but if overall delivery efficiency can be increased to lower the therapeutically effective required dose, this itself would be of considerable benefit.

The immune status of patients in AAV gene augmentation trials may also influence outcomes (Olivares-Gonzalez et al. 2021), and disease progression of inherited retinal dystrophies is affected by immune cell dysregulation. To understand whether the retinal microenvironment of XLRS might play into progression or inflammatory response to viral gene therapy vectors, immune cell responses have been studied in both XLRS mouse models and XLRS subjects. Analysis of the XLRS mouse retina ($Rs1^{-/y}$) using differential gene expression profiles and pathway enrichment showed massive dysregulation of immune response genes as early as postnatal day 14, with characteristics of a microglia-driven proinflammatory state coinciding with development of retinal splitting as markers for schisis cell injury (Vijayasarathy et al. 2021) Both innate and adaptive immune response genes were dysregulated. AAV8-$RS1$ delivery to XLRS mouse retina to provide wild-type $RS1$ gene function quieted the retinal immune status, which transitioned from a degenerative inflammatory phenotype and toward immune quiescence.

An immune state analysis was also performed in humans with data from 11 XLRS subjects in the AAV8-$RS1$ gene-augmentation trial (ClinicalTrials.Gov: NCT02317887). At predosing baseline, immune cell subset frequencies of the XLRS subjects differed from 12 healthy male controls, most notably by the elevated mean CD4/CD8 ratios in XLRS, and elevated serum interferon γ (IFN-γ) and tumor necrosis factor α (TNF-α). The XLRS baseline changes conformed with immune dysregulation and immune intolerance, implicating likely increased susceptibility to immune activation and enhanced cytotoxic T-cell response. This was observed across all vector doses of $1e^9$ to $3e^{11}$ vg/eye.

Systemic antibodies against AAV8 increased in a dose-related fashion following treatment, but no antibodies were observed against the $RS1$ transgene. Analysis of the six XLRS subjects who developed clinical ocular inflammation after vector application gave a modestly positive correlation of the inflammation score to their respective baseline CD4/CD8 ratios. With the caveat of a very small sample size, these findings suggest that XLRS subjects at baseline have a proinflammatory immune phenotype, and that intravitreal AAV8-$RS1$ dosing leads to systemic immune activation with an increase of activated lymphocytes, macrophages, and proinflammatory cytokines. Given this baseline XLRS inflammatory activity even before application of therapeutic AAV vector, in both XLRS mouse and XLRS human, a question arises whether an XLRS disease inflammatory activity itself may contribute to a hostile immune environment for vector placement.

With these concerns, there is new consideration for using a subretinal approach for treatment for XLRS. This expansion in treatment strategies was supported by growing experience and advancements in the surgical techniques for subretinal injections through other clinical trials for inherited retinal dystrophies (Davis 2018; Davis et al. 2019; Bertin et al. 2020), concurrent advancements in AAV vectors, and increasing concerns of gene therapy–associated uveitis particularly with intravitreal injections (Li et al. 2008; Kotterman et al. 2015; Reichel et al. 2018; Timmers et al. 2020). There is current preclinical development work toward future XLRS therapeutic clinical trials using a novel AAV44.9 capsid, generated through directed evolution and subsequent rational design by Boye et al. (2020) and produced by Atsena Therapeutics. This AAV44.9 capsid demonstrates greater transduction efficiencies with lower viral titers, and a characteristic lateral spread of transduction beyond the local subretinal injection site. In macaque monkey, this subretinal spread provided highly efficient foveal cone transduction following extrafoveal bleb placements, to the level comparable to blebs that detached the fovea (Boye et al. 2020). If successful in human trials, this capsid could well be useful for many inherited retinal dystrophies, including other conditions with fragile retinal anatomy such as choroideremia, and conditions requiring foveal and macular cone targeting, including achromatopsia or cone and cone–rod dystrophies.

CONCLUDING REMARKS

Continued developments in viral vectors, new knowledge gained from current gene therapy trials for other inherited retinal dystrophies, and the lessons learned from prior preclinical and clinical trials for XLRS provide a strong basis for mounting additional phase 1 XLRS gene augmentation trials. One pending trial uses a novel approach toward XLRS treatment through subretinal administration. If successful, its properties could be useful for other retinal dystrophies, thus compensating for current inherent limitations of subretinal gene delivery. As authors, we expect that the growing knowledge base and treatment experience in gene therapy–associated uveitis will lead to future development of intravitreal gene therapy as a treatment option. Support was provided by the UC Davis School of Medicine Dean's Fund for laboratory startup to P.A.S., and from the Department of Ophthalmology and Vision Science at UC Davis.

REFERENCES

Ambrosio L, Williams JS, Gutierrez A, Swanson EA, Munro RJ, Ferguson RD, Fulton AB, Akula JD. 2021. Carbonic anhydrase inhibition in X-linked retinoschisis: an eye on the photoreceptors. *Exp Eye Res* **202:** 108344. doi:10.1016/j.exer.2020.108344

Andreuzzi P, Fishman GA, Anderson RJ. 2017. Use of a carbonic anhydrase inhibitor in X-linked retinoschisis: effect on cystic-appearing macular lesions and visual acuity. *Retina* **37:** 1555–1561. doi:10.1097/IAE.0000000000001379

Apushkin MA, Fishman GA. 2006. Use of dorzolamide for patients with X-linked retinoschisis. *Retina* **26:** 741–745. doi:10.1097/01.iae.0000237081.80600.51

Bertin S, Brazhnikova E, Jaillard C, Sahel JA, Dalkara D. 2020. AAV-mediated gene delivery to foveal cones. *Methods Mol Biol* **2173:** 101–112. doi:10.1007/978-1-0716-0755-8_6

Bowles K, Cukras C, Turriff A, Sergeev Y, Vitale S, Bush RA, Sieving PA. 2011. X-linked retinoschisis: *RS1* mutation severity and age affect the ERG phenotype in a cohort of 68 affected male subjects. *Invest Ophthalmol Vis Sci* **52:** 9250–9256. doi:10.1167/iovs.11-8115

Boye SL, Choudhury S, Crosson S, Di Pasquale G, Afione S, Mellen R, Makal V, Calabro KR, Fajardo D, Peterson J, et al. 2020. Novel AAV44.9-based vectors display exceptional characteristics for retinal gene therapy. *Mol Ther* **28:** 1464–1478. doi:10.1016/j.ymthe.2020.04.002

Buch PK, Bainbridge JW, Ali RR. 2008. AAV-mediated gene therapy for retinal disorders: from mouse to man. *Gene Ther* **15:** 849–857. doi:10.1038/gt.2008.66

Bush RA, Wei LL, Sieving PA. 2015. Convergence of human genetics and animal studies: gene therapy for X-linked retinoschisis. *Cold Spring Harb Perspect Med* **5:** a017368. doi:10.1101/cshperspect.a017368

Bush RA, Zeng Y, Colosi P, Kjellstrom S, Hiriyanna S, Vijayasarathy C, Santos M, Li J, Wu Z, Sieving PA. 2016. Preclinical dose-escalation study of intravitreal AAV-RS1 gene therapy in a mouse model of X-linked retinoschisis: dose-dependent expression and improved retinal struc-

ture and function. *Hum Gene Ther* **27**: 376–389. doi:10
.1089/hum.2015.142

Byrne LC, Öztürk BE, Lee T, Fortuny C, Visel M, Dalkara D,
Schaffer DV, Flannery JG. 2014. Retinoschisin gene therapy in photoreceptors, Müller glia or all retinal cells in the
Rs1h$^{-/-}$ mouse. *Gene Ther* **21**: 585–592. doi:10.1038/gt
.2014.31

Byrne LC, Day TP, Visel M, Strazzeri JA, Fortuny C, Dalkara
D, Merigan WH, Schaffer DV, Flannery JG. 2020. In vivo-
directed evolution of adeno-associated virus in the primate retina. *JCI Insight* **5**: e135112. doi:10.1172/jci.insight
.135112

Cukras C, Wiley HE, Jeffrey BG, Sen HN, Turriff A, Zeng Y,
Vijayasarathy C, Marangoni D, Ziccardi L, Kjellstrom S, et
al. 2018a. Retinal AAV8-RS1 gene therapy for X-linked
retinoschisis: initial findings from a phase I/IIa trial by
intravitreal delivery. *Mol Ther* **26**: 2282–2294. doi:10
.1016/j.ymthe.2018.05.025

Cukras CA, Huryn LA, Jeffrey BP, Turriff A, Sieving PA.
2018b. Analysis of anatomic and functional measures in
X-linked retinoschisis. *Invest Ophthalmol Vis Sci* **59**:
2841–2847. doi:10.1167/iovs.17-23297

Dalkara D, Byrne LC, Klimczak RR, Visel M, Yin L, Merigan
WH, Flannery JG, Schaffer DV. 2013. In vivo-directed
evolution of a new adeno-associated virus for therapeutic
outer retinal gene delivery from the vitreous. *Sci Transl
Med* **5**: 189ra176. doi:10.1126/scitranslmed.3005708

Davis JL. 2018. The blunt end: surgical challenges of gene
therapy for inherited retinal diseases. *Am J Ophthalmol*
196: xxv–xxix. doi:10.1016/j.ajo.2018.08.038

Davis JL, Gregori NZ, MacLaren RE, Lam BL. 2019. Surgical
technique for subretinal gene therapy in humans with
inherited retinal degeneration. *Retina* **39**: S2–S8. doi:10
.1097/IAE.0000000000002609

Fahim AT, Ali N, Blachley T, Michaelides M. 2017. Peripheral fundus findings in X-linked retinoschisis. *Br J Ophthalmol* **101**: 1555–1559. doi:10.1136/bjophthalmol-
2016-310110

Forsius H, Eriksson A, Vainio-Mattila B. 1963. Sex-related
hereditary retinoschisis in 2 families in Finland. *Klin
Monbl Augenheilkd* **143**: 806–816.

Friedrich U, Stöhr H, Hilfinger D, Loenhardt T, Schachner
M, Langmann T, Weber BH. 2011. The Na/K-ATPase is
obligatory for membrane anchorage of retinoschisin, the
protein involved in the pathogenesis of X-linked juvenile
retinoschisis. *Hum Mol Genet* **20**: 1132–1142. doi:10
.1093/hmg/ddq557

George ND, Yates JR, Moore AT. 1995. X linked retinoschisis. *Br J Ophthalmol* **79**: 697–702. doi:10.1136/bjo
.79.7.697

George N, Yates J, Moore A. 1996. Clinical features in
affected males with X-linked retinoschisis. *Arch
Ophthalmol* **114**: 274–280. doi:10.1001/archopht.1996
.01100130270007

Gerth C, Zawadzki RJ, Werner JS, Heon E. 2008. Retinal
morphological changes of patients with X-linked retinoschisis evaluated by Fourier-domain optical coherence
tomography. *Arch Ophthalmol* **126**: 807–811. doi:10
.1001/archopht.126.6.807

Ghajarnia M, Gorin MB. 2007. Acetazolamide in the treatment of X-linked retinoschisis maculopathy. *Arch Ophthalmol* **125**: 571–573. doi:10.1001/archopht.125.4.571

Grayson C, Reid SN, Ellis JA, Rutherford A, Sowden JC,
Yates JR, Farber DB, Trump D. 2000. Retinoschisin, the
X-linked retinoschisis protein, is a secreted photoreceptor
protein, and is expressed and released by Weri-Rb1 cells.
Hum Mol Genet **9**: 1873–1879. doi:10.1093/hmg/9.12
.1873

Gurbaxani A, Wei M, Succar T, McCluskey PJ, Jamieson RV,
Grigg JR. 2014. Acetazolamide in retinoschisis: a prospective study. *Ophthalmology* **121**: 802–803 e803. doi:10
.1016/j.ophtha.2013.10.025

Haas J. 1989. Ueber das zusammenvorkommen von veran-
derungen der retina and choroidea. *Arch Augenheilkd* **37**:
343–348.

Hotta Y, Nakamura M, Okamoto Y, Nomura R, Terasaki H,
Miyake Y. 2001. Different mutation of the XLRS1 gene
causes juvenile retinoschisis with retinal white flecks. *Br J
Ophthalmol* **85**: 238–238. doi:10.1136/bjo.85.2.238

Janssen A, Min SH, Molday LL, Tanimoto N, Seeliger MW,
Hauswirth WW, Molday RS, Weber BH. 2008. Effect of
late-stage therapy on disease progression in AAV-mediated rescue of photoreceptor cells in the retinoschisin-
deficient mouse. *Mol Ther* **16**: 1010–1017. doi:10.1038/
mt.2008.57

Kaplan J, Pelet A, Hentati H, Jeanpierre M, Briard ML, Jour-
nel H, Munnich A, Dufier JL. 1991. Contribution to
carrier detection and genetic counselling in X linked
retinoschisis. *J Med Genet* **28**: 383–388. doi:10.1136/jmg
.28.6.383

Kellner U, Brümmer S, Foerster MH, Wessing A. 1990. X-
linked congenital retinoschisis. *Graefes Arch Clin Exp
Ophthalmol* **228**: 432–437. doi:10.1007/BF00927256

Kjellstrom S, Bush RA, Zeng Y, Takada Y, Sieving PA. 2007.
Retinoschisin gene therapy and natural history in the
Rs1h-KO mouse: long-term rescue from retinal degeneration. *Invest Ophthalmol Vis Sci* **48**: 3837–3845. doi:10
.1167/iovs.07-0203

Kotova S, Vijayasarathy C, Dimitriadis EK, Ikonomou L,
Jaffe H, Sieving PA. 2010. Retinoschisin (RS1) interacts
with negatively charged lipid bilayers in the presence of
Ca^{2+}: an atomic force microscopy study. *Biochemistry* **49**:
7023–7032. doi:10.1021/bi1007029

Kotterman MA, Yin L, Strazzeri JM, Flannery JG, Merigan
WH, Schaffer DV. 2015. Antibody neutralization poses a
barrier to intravitreal adeno-associated viral vector gene
delivery to non-human primates. *Gene Ther* **22**: 116–126.
doi:10.1038/gt.2014.115

Lebherz C, Maguire A, Tang W, Bennett J, Wilson JM. 2008.
Novel AAV serotypes for improved ocular gene transfer. *J
Gene Med* **10**: 375–382. doi:10.1002/jgm.1126

Li Q, Miller R, Han PY, Pang J, Dinculescu A, Chiodo V,
Hauswirth WW. 2008. Intraocular route of AAV2 vector
administration defines humoral immune response and
therapeutic potential. *Mol Vis* **14**: 1760–1769.

Mann I, Macrae A. 1938. Congenital vascular veils in
the vitreous. *Br J Ophthalmol* **22**: 1–10. doi:10.1136/bjo
.22.1.1

Marangoni D, Wu Z, Wiley HE, Zeiss CJ, Vijayasarathy C,
Zeng Y, Hiriyanna S, Bush RA, Wei LL, Colosi P, et al.
2014. Preclinical safety evaluation of a recombinant
AAV8 vector for X-linked retinoschisis after intravitreal
administration in rabbits. *Hum Gene Ther Clin Dev* **25**:
202–211. doi:10.1089/humc.2014.067

Marangoni D, Bush RA, Zeng Y, Wei LL, Ziccardi L, Vijaya-sarathy C, Bartoe JT, Palyada K, Santos M, Hiriyanna S, et al. 2016. Ocular and systemic safety of a recombinant AAV8 vector for X-linked retinoschisis gene therapy: GLP studies in rabbits and Rs1-KO mice. *Mol Ther Methods Clin Dev* **5:** 16011. doi:10.1038/mtm.2016.11

McKibbin M, Booth AP, George ND. 2001. Foveal ectopia in X-linked retinoschisis. *Retina* **21:** 361–366. doi:10.1097/00006982-200108000-00011

Min SH, Molday LL, Seeliger MW, Dinculescu A, Timmers AM, Janssen A, Tonagel F, Tanimoto N, Weber BH, Molday RS, et al. 2005. Prolonged recovery of retinal structure/function after gene therapy in an Rs1h-deficient mouse model of x-linked juvenile retinoschisis. *Mol Ther* **12:** 644–651. doi:10.1016/j.ymthe.2005.06.002

Molday LL, Wu WW, Molday RS. 2007. Retinoschisin (RS1), the protein encoded by the X-linked retinoschisis gene, is anchored to the surface of retinal photoreceptor and bipolar cells through its interactions with a Na/K ATPase-SARM1 complex. *J Biol Chem* **282:** 32792–32801. doi:10.1074/jbc.M706321200

Mowat FM, Gornik KR, Dinculescu A, Boye SL, Hauswirth WW, Petersen-Jones SM, Bartoe JT. 2014. Tyrosine capsid-mutant AAV vectors for gene delivery to the canine retina from a subretinal or intravitreal approach. *Gene Ther* **21:** 96–105. doi:10.1038/gt.2013.64

Olivares-Gonzalez L, Velasco S, Campillo I, Rodrigo R. 2021. Retinal inflammation, cell death and inherited retinal dystrophies. *Int J Mol Sci* **22.** doi:10.3390/ijms22042096

Orès R, Mohand-Said S, Dhaenens CM, Antonio A, Zeitz C, Augstburger E, Andrieu C, Sahel JA, Audo I. 2018. Phenotypic characteristics of a French cohort of patients with X-linked retinoschisis. *Ophthalmology* **125:** 1587–1596. doi:10.1016/j.ophtha.2018.03.057

Ou J, Vijayasarathy C, Ziccardi L, Chen S, Zeng Y, Marangoni D, Pope JG, Bush RA, Wu Z, Li W, et al. 2015. Synaptic pathology and therapeutic repair in adult retinoschisis mouse by AAV-RS1 transfer. *J Clin Invest* **125:** 2891–2903. doi:10.1172/JCI81380

Park TK, Wu Z, Kjellstrom S, Zeng Y, Bush RA, Sieving PA, Colosi P. 2009. Intravitreal delivery of AAV8 retinoschisin results in cell type-specific gene expression and retinal rescue in the Rs1-KO mouse. *Gene Ther* **16:** 916–926. doi:10.1038/gt.2009.61

Peachey NSN. 1987. Psychophysical and electroretinographic findings in X-linked juvenile retinoschisis. *Arch Ophthalmol* **105:** 513–516. doi:10.1001/archopht.1987.01060040083038

Pennesi ME, Birch DG, Jayasundera KT, Parker M, Tan O, Gurses-Ozden R, Reichley C, Beasley KN, Yang P, Weleber RG, et al. 2018. Prospective evaluation of patients with X-linked retinoschisis during 18 months. *Invest Ophthalmol Vis Sci* **59:** 5941–5956.

Pennesi ME, Yang P, Birch DG, Weng CY, Moore AT, Iannaccone A, Comander JI, Jayasundera T, Chulay J; XLRS-001 Study Group. 2022. Intravitreal delivery of rAAV2tYF-CB-hRS1 vector for gene augmentation therapy in X-linked retinoschisis—1 year clinical results. *Ophthalmol Retina* doi: 10.1016/j.oret.2022.06.013

Petrs-Silva H, Dinculescu A, Li Q, Min SH, Chiodo V, Pang JJ, Zhong L, Zolotukhin S, Srivastava A, Lewin AS, et al. 2009. High-efficiency transduction of the mouse retina by

tyrosine-mutant AAV serotype vectors. *Mol Ther* **17:** 463–471. doi:10.1038/mt.2008.269

Petrs-Silva H, Dinculescu A, Li Q, Deng WT, Pang JJ, Min SH, Chiodo V, Neeley AW, Govindasamy L, Bennett A, et al. 2011. Novel properties of tyrosine-mutant AAV2 vectors in the mouse retina. *Mol Ther* **19:** 293–301. doi:10.1038/mt.2010.234

Prenner JL, Capone A, Jr, Ciaccia S, Takada Y, Sieving PA, Trese MT. 2006. Congenital X-linked retinoschisis classification system. *Retina* **26:** S61–S64. doi:10.1097/01.iae.0000244290.09499.c1

Reichel FF, Peters T, Wilhelm B, Biel M, Ueffing M, Wissinger B, Bartz-Schmidt KU, Klein R, Michalakis S, Fischer MD, et al. 2018. Humoral immune response after intravitreal but not after subretinal AAV8 in primates and patients. *Invest Ophthalmol Vis Sci* **59:** 1910–1915. doi:10.1167/iovs.17-22494

Roesch MT, Ewing CC, Gibson AE, Weber BH. 1998. The natural history of X-linked retinoschisis. *Can J Ophthalmol* **33:** 149–158.

Sauer CG, Gehrig A, Warneke-Wittstock R, Marquardt A, Ewing CC, Gibson A, Lorenz B, Jurklies B, Weber BH. 1997. Positional cloning of the gene associated with X-linked juvenile retinoschisis. *Nat Genet* **17:** 164–170. doi:10.1038/ng1097-164

Seitz IP, Michalakis S, Wilhelm B, Reichel FF, Ochakovski GA, Zrenner E, Ueffing M, Biel M, Wissinger B, Bartz-Schmidt KU, et al. 2017. Superior retinal gene transfer and biodistribution profile of subretinal versus intravitreal delivery of AAV8 in nonhuman primates. *Invest Ophthalmol Vis Sci* **58:** 5792–5801. doi:10.1167/iovs.17-22473

Sergeev YV, Caruso RC, Meltzer MR, Smaoui N, MacDonald IM, Sieving PA. 2010. Molecular modeling of retinoschisin with functional analysis of pathogenic mutations from human X-linked retinoschisis. *Hum Mol Genet* **19:** 1302–1313. doi:10.1093/hmg/ddq006

Sergeev YV, Vitale S, Sieving PA, Vincent A, Robson AG, Moore AT, Webster AR, Holder GE. 2013. Molecular modeling indicates distinct classes of missense variants with mild and severe XLRS phenotypes. *Hum Mol Genet* **22:** 4756–4767. doi:10.1093/hmg/ddt329

Shi L, Ko ML, Ko GY. 2017. Retinoschisin facilitates the function of L-type voltage-gated calcium channels. *Front Cell Neurosci* **11:** 232. doi:10.3389/fncel.2017.00232

Takada Y, Fariss RN, Tanikawa A, Zeng Y, Carper D, Bush R, Sieving PA. 2004. A retinal neuronal developmental wave of retinoschisin expression begins in ganglion cells during layer formation. *Invest Ophthalmol Vis Sci* **45:** 3302–3312. doi:10.1167/iovs.04-0156

Takahashi K, Igarashi T, Miyake K, Kobayashi M, Yaguchi C, Iijima O, Yamazaki Y, Katakai Y, Miyake N, Kameya S, et al. 2017. Improved intravitreal AAV-mediated inner retinal gene transduction after surgical internal limiting membrane peeling in cynomolgus monkeys. *Mol Ther* **25:** 296–302. doi:10.1016/j.ymthe.2016.10.008

Testa F, Di Iorio V, Gallo B, Marchese M, Nesti A, De Rosa G, Melillo P, Simonelli F. 2019. Carbonic anhydrase inhibitors in patients with X-linked retinoschisis: effects on macular morphology and function. *Ophthalmic Genet* **40:** 207–212. doi:10.1080/13816810.2019.1616303

Timmers AM, Newmark JA, Turunen HT, Farivar T, Liu J, Song C, Ye GJ, Pennock S, Gaskin C, Knop DR, et al. 2020. Ocular inflammatory response to intravitreal injection of adeno-associated virus vector: relative contribution of genome and capsid. *Hum Gene Ther* **31:** 80–89. doi:10 .1089/hum.2019.144

Trapani I, Puppo A, Auricchio A. 2014. Vector platforms for gene therapy of inherited retinopathies. *Prog Retin Eye Res* **43:** 108–128. doi:10.1016/j.preteyeres.2014.08.001

van Schooneveld MJ, Miyake Y. 1994. Fundus albipunctatus-like lesions in juvenile retinoschisis. *Br J Ophthalmol* **78:** 659. doi:10.1136/bjo.78.8.659

Vijayasarathy C, Zeng Y, Brooks MJ, Fariss RN, Sieving PA. 2021. Genetic rescue of X-linked retinoschisis mouse (Rs1$^{-/y}$) retina induces quiescence of the retinal microglial inflammatory state following AAV8-*RS1* gene transfer and identifies gene networks underlying retinal recovery. *Hum Gene Ther* **32:** 667–681. doi:10.1089/ hum.2020.213

Vijayasarathy C, Sardar Pasha SPB, Sieving PA. 2022. Of men and mice: human X-linked retinoschisis and fidelity in mouse modeling. *Prog Retin Eye Res* **87:** 100999. doi:10 .1016/j.preteyeres.2021.100999

Vincent A, Robson AG, Neveu MM, Wright GA, Moore AT, Webster AR, Holder GE. 2013. A phenotype-genotype correlation study of X-linked retinoschisis. *Ophthalmology* **120:** 1454–1464. doi:10.1016/j.ophtha.2012.12.008

Vogel WF, Abdulhussein R, Ford CE. 2006. Sensing extracellular matrix: An update on discoidin domain receptor function. *Cell Signal* **18:** 1108–1116. doi:10.1016/j.cellsig .2006.02.012

Wakabayashi K, Sakai-Wakabayashi Y, Ishigami C. 2022. Mizuo–Nakamura phenomenon in X-linked retinoschisis. *Am J Ophthalmol Case Rep* **26:** 101529. doi:10.1016/j .ajoc.2022.101529

Walia S, Fishman GA, Molday RS, Dyka FM, Kumar NM, Ehlinger MA, Stone EM. 2009. Relation of response to treatment with dorzolamide in X-linked retinoschisis to the mechanism of functional loss in retinoschisin. *Am J Ophthalmol* **147:** 111–115 e1. doi:10.1016/j.ajo.2008 .07.041

Weber BH, Schrewe H, Molday LL, Gehrig A, White KL, Seeliger MW, Jaissle GB, Friedburg C, Tamm E, Molday RS. 2002. Inactivation of the murine X-linked juvenile retinoschisis gene, Rs1h, suggests a role of retinoschisin in retinal cell layer organization and synaptic structure. *Proc Natl Acad Sci* **99:** 6222–6227. doi:10.1073/pnas .092528599

Wu WW, Wong JP, Kast J, Molday RS. 2005. RS1, a discoidin domain-containing retinal cell adhesion protein associated with X-linked retinoschisis, exists as a novel disulfide-linked octamer. *J Biol Chem* **280:** 10721–10730. doi:10 .1074/jbc.M413117200

Yin L, Greenberg K, Hunter JJ, Dalkara D, Kolstad KD, Masella BD, Wolfe R, Visel M, Stone D, Libby RT, et al. 2011. Intravitreal injection of AAV2 transduces macaque inner retina. *Invest Ophthalmol Vis Sci* **52:** 2775–2783. doi:10.1167/iovs.10-6250

Zeng Y, Takada Y, Kjellstrom S, Hiriyanna K, Tanikawa A, Wawrousek E, Smaoui N, Caruso R, Bush RA, Sieving PA. 2004. *RS-1* gene delivery to an adult *Rs1h* knockout mouse model restores ERG b-wave with reversal of the electronegative waveform of X-linked retinoschisis. *Invest Ophthalmol Vis Sci* **45:** 3279–3285. doi:10.1167/iovs.04-0576

Zeng Y, Qian H, Campos MM, Li Y, Vijayasarathy C, Sieving PA. 2021. Rs1h$^{-/y}$ exon 3-del rat model of X-linked retinoschisis with early onset and rapid phenotype is rescued by RS1 supplementation. *Gene Ther* **29:** 431–440. doi:10 .1038/s41434-021-00290-6

From Bench to Bedside—Delivering Gene Therapy for Leber Hereditary Optic Neuropathy

Benson S. Chen[1,2,5] and Patrick Yu-Wai-Man[1,2,3,4]

[1]John van Geest Centre for Brain Repair and MRC Mitochondrial Biology Unit, Department of Clinical Neurosciences, University of Cambridge, Cambridge CB2 0PY, United Kingdom

[2]Cambridge Eye Unit, Addenbrooke's Hospital, Cambridge University Hospitals, Cambridge CB2 0QQ, United Kingdom

[3]Moorfields Eye Hospital NHS Foundation Trust, London EC1V 2PD, United Kingdom

[4]Institute of Ophthalmology, University College London, London EC1V 9EL, United Kingdom

Correspondence: py237@cam.ac.uk

Leber hereditary optic neuropathy (LHON) is a rare, maternally inherited mitochondrial disorder that presents with severe bilateral sequential vision loss, due to the selective degeneration of retinal ganglion cells (RGCs). Since the mitochondrial genetic basis for LHON was uncovered in 1988, considerable progress has been made in understanding the pathogenetic mechanisms driving RGC loss, which has enabled the development of therapeutic approaches aimed at mitigating the underlying mitochondrial dysfunction. In this review, we explore the genetics of LHON, from bench to bedside, focusing on the pathogenetic mechanisms and how these have informed the development of different gene therapy approaches, in particular the technique of allotopic expression with adeno-associated viral vectors. Finally, we provide an overview of the recent gene therapy clinical trials and consider the unanswered questions, challenges, and future prospects.

In 1871, Theodor Leber, a German ophthalmologist, published "Ueber Hereditäre und Congenital-Angelegte Sehnervenleiden" (On hereditary and congenital optic nerve diseases) in which he described four families with a distinct clinical syndrome of vision loss (Leber 1871). Affected individuals experienced bilateral sequential vision loss manifesting with central scotomas. Disease progression was rapid within the first few weeks to months, followed by slow or no progression with little improvement thereafter. Leber observed that there was evidence of maternal transmission, with predominantly young males being affected, and the syndrome almost exclusively involved the optic nerves leading to optic atrophy (Leber 1871). These observations formed the classic features of the eponymous condition, Leber hereditary optic neuropathy (LHON).

The pathogenetic mechanisms underpinning LHON remained poorly understood until 1988, when Douglas Wallace (Emory University, Atlanta, Georgia, USA), Eeva Nikoskelainen (University of Turku, Turku, Finland), and colleagues

[5]Present address: Gonville and Caius College, Trinity Street, Cambridge CB2 1TA, United Kingdom.

determined that LHON in a number of well characterized pedigrees arose from a specific point mutation specifically affecting the mitochondrial genome, an organelle with critical functions in the production of cellular adenosine triphosphate (ATP) (Wallace et al. 1988). LHON is the most common cause of inherited mitochondrial blindness, affecting ~1 in 30,000 individuals (Yu-Wai-Man et al. 2003). Three primary mitochondrial DNA (mtDNA) point mutations (m.3460G > A in *MT-ND1*, m.11778G > A in *MT-ND4*, and m.14484T > C in *MT-ND6*) have been identified and account for ~90% of LHON cases globally (Yu-Wai-Man et al. 2011). The remaining cases are due to rarer pathogenic mtDNA mutations and, in some cases, recessive mutations in nuclear genes (*NDUFS2, NDUFAF5, DNAJC30, MCAT*) that directly or indirectly compromise complex I of the mitochondrial respiratory chain (Gerber et al. 2017, 2021; Jurkute et al. 2019; Mansukhani et al. 2021; Moore and Yu-Wai-Man 2021; Stenton et al. 2021). Discovery of the genetic basis of LHON and recent advancements in gene therapy techniques have facilitated the development of gene therapy for a devastating condition that has not had any effective therapies until now.

CLINICAL FEATURES OF LHON

The clinical observations made by Leber in his seminal work on LHON have prevailed for over 150 years. Most individuals who carry a genetic mutation associated with LHON remain asymptomatic, with ~50% of males and ~10% of females at risk of experiencing visual loss (Yu-Wai-Man et al. 2009). In a national Australian cohort, the penetrance of LHON was reported to be lower at 17.5% for males and 5.4% for females (Lopez Sanchez et al. 2021). LHON typically affects men, with a male-to-female ratio of 3:1 (Poincenot et al. 2020). The peak age of onset is between 15 and 35 years, with 90% of those losing vision doing so before the age of 50 years. In most affected individuals, vision loss is the only symptom of LHON. Although it can prove difficult to establish a direct causal link with the LHON mutation, a subgroup of affected individuals can develop extraocular manifestations, with the strongest association being a multiple

sclerosis-like illnesses and movement disorders (Yu-Wai-Man et al. 2016).

LHON has been classified into three stages based on the time from disease onset: (1) subacute (0–6 mo), (2) dynamic (6–12 mo), and chronic (>12 mo) (Carelli et al. 2017). In the subacute phase of LHON (0–6 mo from onset), affected individuals experience painless visual loss, typically beginning with blurring or clouding of vision in one eye, accompanied by impaired perception of color vision (Fig. 1). Almost all patients experience bilateral vision loss, either simultaneously with the first eye (25%) or sequentially (75%), with the second eye being affected weeks to months later. The characteristic visual field defect in LHON is a dense central or cecocentral scotoma. Visual acuity may be mildly reduced initially, but declines severely to 20/200 or less, reaching a nadir ~4–6 wk after onset of visual symptoms. During the subacute phase, the optic disc may appear normal (~20%) or hyperemic, with "pseudo-edema" characterized by elevation of the optic nerve, peripapillary telangiectasias, and tortuosity of retinal arterioles, without contrast leakage on fluorescein angiography if performed. There is preferential involvement of the smaller fibers that constitute the papillomacular bundle (PMB), as evidenced by increased peripapillary retinal nerve fiber layer (RNFL) thickness, spreading initially from the temporal and inferior quadrants on optical coherence tomography (OCT), before involvement of the superior and nasal quadrants (Barboni et al. 2010). Recent studies utilizing OCT-angiography (OCT-A) have also demonstrated a reduction in peripapillary capillary vascular density (VD) in the temporal region, preceding the involvement of other regions (Balducci et al. 2018). Progressive loss of retinal ganglion cells (RGCs) results in generalized thinning of RNFL and ganglion cell–inner plexiform layer (GC-IPL) on peripapillary and macular OCT, ending 6 mo after onset of vision loss (Balducci et al. 2016). Atrophy of the optic nerves can be detected on fundoscopy as early as 6 wk after onset of visual loss.

In the dynamic phase (6–12 mo after onset), visual acuity tends to stabilize. In most cases, visual acuity is worse than 3/60 (logMAR 1.3), fulfilling the criteria for legal blindness in most

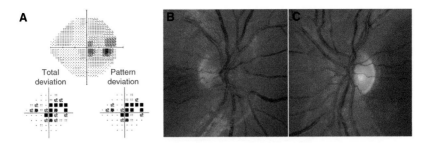

Figure 1. Ophthalmological findings in a patient with Leber hereditary optic neuropathy (LHON). A 16-year-old male developed painless blurring of vision in his left eye, without any preceding history of trauma or illness. Three months later, vision in his right eye began to deteriorate. He had no past medical history or ocular history of note. There was a family history of myopia, but no known family history of LHON or visual impairment. He was reviewed 5 mo after onset of vision loss in the left eye and found to have a visual acuity of 2/60 in the right eye and hand motion in the left eye. On assessment of color vision, he could identify 6/15 Ishihara plates with the right eye, but none with the left eye. He could only complete Humphrey visual field testing in the right eye. This revealed a cecocentral scotoma (*A*). On fundus examination, the right optic nerve appeared edematous, with hyperemia and peripapillary telangiectasia (*B*). The left optic nerve was pale temporally with resolving disc edema (*C*). Optical coherence tomography (OCT) of the optic nerve head revealed peripapillary retinal nerve fiber layer (RNFL) thickening on the right more than the left. Genetic testing confirmed the m.11778G > A mutation.

countries (Yu-Wai-Man et al. 2022). The rate of spontaneous improvement in vision ("recovery" as sometimes described in the literature) is variable but depends on the underlying mtDNA mutation and the age of onset, with the m.14484T > C mutation and childhood onset <12 yr portending a better prognosis. In a systematic review of 695 affected individuals carrying the m.11778G > A mutation, visual recovery occurred in 14%, with the important caveat that recovery was variably defined in the included studies (Newman et al. 2020). The term "recovery" is a misnomer, as the majority of patients with LHON remain significantly visually impaired with visual acuity of 6/60 (logMAR 1.0) or less.

In the chronic phase of LHON (>12 mo after onset), there is established optic atrophy with significant thinning of peripapillary RNFL and macular GC-IPL on OCT, and a global reduction in VD on OCT-A (Balducci et al. 2018).

PATHOGENETIC MECHANISMS OF LHON

LHON has been considered the classical paradigm of a mtDNA-related disease. In contrast to nuclear DNA, mtDNA is transmitted strictly through the maternal line. A cell can have over 1000 mitochondria, with each mitochondrion containing 2–10 copies of the mitochondrial genome. The mitochondrial genome has a higher mutation rate than the nuclear genome, leading to a heterogeneous population of mtDNA within the same cell, known as heteroplasmy. For a pathogenic mutation in mtDNA to manifest clinically, a heteroplasmy threshold must be reached to impair mitochondrial oxidative phosphorylation (OXPHOS) and precipitate a bioenergetic crisis. This threshold is tissue-specific and dependent on the metabolic rate of cells and organs.

To understand the pathogenetic mechanisms underpinning LHON, it is essential to understand the critical role of mitochondrial OXPHOS in generating cellular energy (Fig. 2). In OXPHOS, the mitochondrial respiratory chain complexes catalyze the oxidation of fuel molecules derived from our diet and transfers the electrons to molecular oxygen, with concomitant energy transduction into adenosine triphosphate (ATP). The mitochondrial respiratory chain consists of five distinct multisubunit respiratory complexes that transfer high-energy electrons via redox reactions that create the electrochemical gradient driving the synthesis of ATP.

The three primary mutations of LHON all involve genes encoding subunits of respiratory complex I, the first enzyme of the respiratory

Mitochondria Structural Features

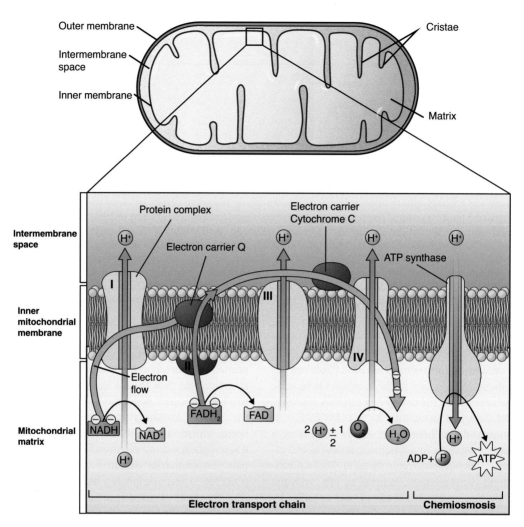

Oxidative Phosphorylation

Figure 2. Mitochondrial respiration chain and oxidative phosphorylation. Oxidative phosphorylation (OXPHOS) is the process by which the synthesis of adenosine triphosphate (ATP) is coupled to the movement of electrons through the mitochondrial respiratory chain. The respiratory chain consists of ~92 nuclear DNA- and mitochondrial DNA–encoded protein subunits, organized into a series of five protein complexes (I: NADH-coenzyme Q reductase; II: succinate-coenzyme Q reductase; III: co-enzyme QH_2 cytochrome-c reductase; IV: cytochrome-c oxidase; V: ATP synthase) embedded in the inner membrane of the mitochondria, which transfer electrons extracted from the carbon substrates of nutrients along a redox potential. In complex I, two electrons are transferred from NADH to coenzyme Q, generating ubiquinol (QH_2) and producing the translocation of four protons from the matrix to the inner membrane space. In complex II, two electrons are transferred from $FADH_2$ to coenzyme Q, by dehydrogenizing succinate to fumarate. Electrons from complexes I and II are carried by $CoQH_2$ to enter the Q cycle processed by complex III. Each Q cycle generates two reduced cytochrome c and transports two protons. The reduced cytochrome c shuttles electrons to complex IV, which mediates the final reaction in the respiratory chain. Electrons from reduced cytochrome c reduce molecular oxygen to water. For each cytochrome c that is oxidized, a proton is simultaneously translocated to the intermembrane space. The oxidized cytochrome c then returns to the pool. In the final step of OXPHOS, the proton gradient established by complexes I, II, and IV forms an electrochemical membrane potential (ΔP) that drives complex V to generate ATP, through the phosphorylation of adenosine diphosphate (ADP) to ATP.

Cite this article as *Cold Spring Harb Perspect Med* doi: 10.1101/cshperspect.a041282

chain. Complex I plays a central role in energy metabolism, as it is the major entry point for electrons to the respiratory chain. RGCs are highly energy-dependent cells that require a constant source of ATP. Animal models of LHON and patient-derived induced pluripotent stem cells (iPSCs) carrying LHON mutations show reduced complex I activity and respiratory defects (Lin et al. 2012; Wu et al. 2018). However, the pathogenesis of LHON is not simply a bioenergetic issue. Reactive oxygen species (ROS) are also produced in large amounts by complex I, in particular superoxide, with increased production of ROS evident in animal models of LHON, cybrids carrying the LHON mutation, and patient-derived iPSCs (Yang et al. 2020).

Initially considered an unwanted by-product of oxidative metabolism, there is evidence that ROS play a crucial role in regulating several cellular processes when present in low levels. At higher levels, ROS can disrupt normal cellular function resulting in oxidative damage to DNA, proteins, and lipids, including increased permeability of the mitochondrial membrane. The latter leads to increased mitochondrial genome instability, further OXPHOS dysfunction, and disrupted Ca^{2+} homeostasis; allowing for the release of many factors signaling cellular apoptosis, in particular cytochrome c, which is sequestered in the mitochondrial cristae. Dysregulation of superoxide appears to be an important cause of aberrant apoptosis signaling in RGCs, and may explain why LHON mutations preferentially affect RGC and lead to isolated loss of RGC, without involvement of other highly energy-dependent cells such as photoreceptors (Levin 2007). The unique architecture of RGCs is also likely to be an important factor that accounts for why these neuronal populations are exquisitely sensitive to mitochondrial dysfunction. Their projecting axons have a relatively long course extending from the inner retina to the lateral geniculate nucleus, with myelination only occurring after the lamina cribosa. As a result, there is a higher concentration of mitochondria in the prelaminar segment and the smaller caliber of the RGCs in the PMB result in a lower mitochondrial reserve that can be more easily overwhelmed in the setting of impaired mito-chondrial biogenesis caused by a pathogenic mtDNA mutation (Yu-Wai-Man et al. 2005).

Although the aforementioned processes are pivotal in the pathogenesis of LHON, they do not fully account for the pathophysiology of LHON. Only a proportion of LHON carriers develop vision loss, with men at most risk. This incomplete penetrance is not fully explained by mitochondrial heteroplasmy, as most LHON carriers are homoplasmic. Alterations in the balance between mitochondrial biogenesis and mitochondria-selective autophagy (mitophagy), which may be exacerbated by external metabolic stressors, have been identified as a major determinant of conversion to symptomatic disease (Mejia-Vergara et al. 2020).

As part of normal homeostasis, mitochondria contain "quality-control" pathways that monitor, degrade, repair, and eliminate damaged mitochondrial proteins and components (Tatsuta and Langer 2008). Mitochondrial biogenesis occurs in response to cellular stress or increased metabolic demands, while mitophagy is triggered in the presence of severely damaged or nonfunctioning mitochondria. Increased metabolic biogenesis in unaffected carriers of LHON mutations likely compensates for reduced complex I activity and OXPHOS dysfunction. This system can become overwhelmed in the presence of external metabolic stressors such as excessive alcohol consumption, smoke (in all forms), and certain medications and toxins. These stressors all have targets in the mitochondria that disrupt OXPHOS, leading to overproduction and accumulation of ROS, which drives mitophagy and activation of apoptosis pathways. Ultimately, loss of RGC ensues.

Hormonal influences have also been proposed for the observed male predominance in disease penetrance, including the protective effects of estrogen from oxidative stress (Pisano et al. 2015), and the role of testosterone in increasing RGC apoptosis and reduced mitophagy (Jankauskaite et al. 2020).

GENE THERAPY FOR LHON

There are limited treatment options for LHON (Hage and Vignal-Clermont 2021). Idebenone

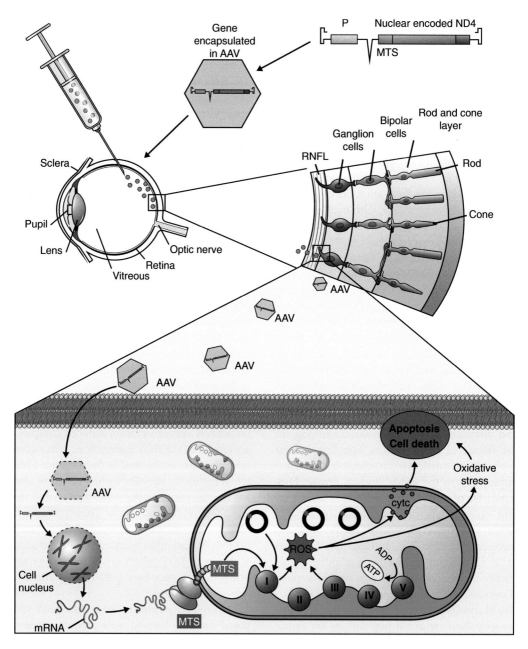

Figure 3. Mitochondrial gene therapy for Leber hereditary optic neuropathy (LHON) using the technique of allotopic expression. Viral vectors are unable to efficiently import genes into the mammalian mitochondrial genome. Instead, mitochondrial genes can be allotopically expressed, whereby the gene is modified so that it can be optimally expressed in the nuclear-cytosolic compartment and the synthesized protein is transported into the mitochondria. For successful expression of the mitochondrial gene in the nuclear-cytosolic compartment, several requirements must be met: the mitochondrial genes must be compatible with the nuclear expression system; a means of delivering the cytoplasmically synthesized protein into the mitochondria must be established; and a system to maintain and replicate the mitochondrial genes in the nucleus must be developed (Nagley and Devenish 1989). In LHON, the therapeutic gene being delivered (for example, *ND4*) is modified so that mitochondrial codons are converted to nuclear codons. (*Legend continues on following page.*)

(trade name Raxone) has been approved for use in LHON in some European countries with ~50% of treated patients experiencing a clinically relevant recovery (Klopstock et al. 2011; Catarino et al. 2020). However, the improvement in visual parameters is variable and most patients remain significantly visually impaired, indicating a clear need for more targeted efficacious therapies. Gene therapy for the treatment of vision loss in LHON has been attractive to researchers for several reasons. For most patients, a single gene defect responsible for the condition can be identified. Vision loss is acute and occurs sequentially, providing a natural time window for treatment to be initiated. Additionally, the RGCs are located on the inner surface of the retina, and they can, therefore, be easily accessed using a minimally invasive intravitreal injection. The eye also benefits from relative immune privilege and there is a long safety track record of using adeno-associated virus (AAV) for intraocular gene delivery. The scientific rationale and preclinical studies will be discussed first, before reviewing the published data for LHON gene therapy trials aimed at the most common pathogenic mutation—m.11778G > A in the *MT-ND4* gene.

Preclinical Studies

Preclinical studies have focused on using viral vectors to replace the defective mitochondrial gene or gene product in yeast and mammalian cells, with the goal of restoring mitochondrial function. Although exogenous genes can be successfully imported using viral vectors into the nuclear genome to protect the optic nerves, these methods have proven ineffective for introducing genes into mammalian mtDNA due to the relatively impervious double-membrane structure of mitochondria. Instead, the technique of allotopic expression has been adopted to overcome this physical barrier (Fig. 3).

Allotopic expression was first successfully demonstrated in yeast, in which transcription of an artificial nuclear gene (*aap1*) encoding subunit 8 of the mitochondrial ATPase complex of *Saccharomyces cerevisiae* was efficiently expressed in the nuclear-cytosolic system and imported into mitochondria (Gearing et al. 1985; Gearing and Nagley 1986). In the artificial nuclear *aap1* gene, the wild-type mitochondrial subunit 8 gene was changed to optimize expression in the nuclear-cytosolic compartment and mitochondrial codons were converted into a nuclear codon (Nagley and Devenish 1989). To achieve import into the mitochondria, the cytoplasmically synthesized subunit 8 was furnished with the amino-terminal leader from a precursor of the *Neurospora crassa* mtATPase subunit 9, which is a nuclear-encoded mitochondrial protein. Insertion of this mitochondrial targeting sequence (MTS) facilitated transportation of the synthesized protein to the mitochondria and then into the correct location in the mitochondrial compartment. When expressed in vivo from its artificial nuclear gene, the cytoplasmically synthesized subunit 8 restored the growth defects of *aap1* mutants unable to produce subunit 8 inside the mitochondria.

Subsequent studies identified two critical factors determining the import efficiency of allotopically expressed mitochondrial proteins. First, the protein being expressed had to be compatible with the MTS. A study attempting to import a

Figure 3. (*Continued*) The nuclear-encoded gene is fused to a mitochondrial targeting sequence (MTS), which will facilitate transportation of the synthesized protein to the mitochondria and into the correct location in the mitochondrial compartment, and a promotor (P) that drives constitutive expression of the gene. The therapeutic gene is encapsulated in an adeno-associated virus (AAV), which is then delivered by intravitreal injection into the eye. After transfection of the retinal ganglion cell, the therapeutic gene is delivered to the nucleus and transcribed to mRNA. The therapeutic mRNA is directed to polysomes on the mitochondrial surface, which synthesizes the therapeutic ND4 protein. The MTS assists with sorting of the protein to the inner mitochondrial membrane, where it finally integrates into complex I. Allotopic expression of *ND4* allows for the formation of functional and stable complex I units restoring mitochondrial oxidative phosphorylation and reducing the generation of reactive oxygen species, both important factors that lead to activation of cellular apoptotic pathways and death of retinal ganglion cells.

cytoplasmically synthesized version of subunit 9 of the mitochondrial ATPase complex of *S. cerevisiae* with the same MTS as before, showed less efficient import compared to the earlier experiment of the cytoplasmically synthesized version of subunit 8 (Law et al. 1988). It was thought that the MTS compromised the assembly and function of the subunit 9 protein, due to generation of additional amino-terminal residues by matrix proteases at cleavage sites defined by the MTS (Farrell et al. 1988; Law et al. 1988). Second, it was recognized that proteins encoded by the mitochondrial genome are highly hydrophobic and had difficulty crossing the mitochondrial inner membrane after cytoplasmic synthesis. In a study comparing import efficiency of cytoplasmically synthesized subunit 9 proteins of *S. cerevisiae* and *Podospora anserina*, a filamentous fungus, the production of functional ATPase was significantly restored by 30%–40% in yeast cells containing the *P. anserina* subunit 9 protein compared to *S. cerevisiae*, which had a poor rate of import into mitochondria (Bietenhader et al. 2012). The sequences of subunit 9 proteins of *S. cerevisiae* and *P. anserina* are 70% identical, but the first transmembrane segment of the *P. anserina* subunit 9 protein is less hydrophobic allowing better import across the mitochondrial inner membrane.

The success of allotopic expression in yeast led to studies in mammalian cells, including the pioneering studies of John Guy and colleagues (Bascom Palmer Eye Institute, Miami, Florida, USA), demonstrating proof-of-concept in human cybrids containing the m.11778G > A LHON mutation (Guy et al. 2002). A gene containing the nuclear-encoded *ND4* fused to an MTS specifying the amino-terminal region of ATP1 (the P1 isoform of subunit *c* of human ATP synthase [ATPc]) was constructed, and when delivered using an AAV vector into homoplasmic osteosarcoma-derived cybrids containing wild-type (m.11778G) or mutated (m.11778A) mtDNA, the MTS successfully directed the allotopically expressed ND4 polypeptide into mitochondria. A second study showed that homoplasmic cybrids derived from a patient with the m.11778G > A mutation LHON could be allotopically rescued (Guy et al. 2002). When

transfected with recombinant AAV containing the nuclear-encoded *ND4* (AAV-*ND4*), the m.11778G > A cybrids showed a threefold increase in the rate of complex I–dependent ATP synthesis compared to cybrids treated with a mock AAV vector. The degree of recovery led to levels of ATP synthesis that were virtually indistinguishable from the corresponding wild-type cell line with normal mtDNA.

Having confirmed that allotopic expression could be demonstrated in vitro, the same technique was used to develop a murine model of LHON by delivering mutant (11778G > A) human *ND4* DNA with a self-complimentary AAV2 vector also containing a *COX8* presequence MTS (Yu et al. 2012). The murine model recapitulated the hallmarks of human LHON including optic disc edema at 1-mo postinjection and optic nerve head atrophy with marked thinning of the inner retina at 1 year on spectral-domain OCT (SD-OCT). They then determined the efficacy of the *ND4* fusion gene (with MTS-specifying ATP1) that they had previously constructed, by injecting the fusion gene (packaged in AAV2 capsids) into both eyes of the murine model (Guy et al. 2009; Koilkonda et al. 2014). Visual function assessed by serial pattern electroretinogram (PERG) and retinal structure by serial SD-OCT showed a significant rescue by the fusion gene. Histology and ultrastructural analysis confirmed that loss of RGCs and demise of axons was also prevented by the fusion gene.

Approaches to allotopic expression were further optimized by researchers at the Institut de la Vision (Paris, France), with studies conducted using skin fibroblasts isolated from LHON patients (Bonnet et al. 2007, 2008). To improve import efficiency across the mitochondrial inner membrane, sorting of the *ND4* mRNA to the mitochondrial surface was maximized by generation of an expression vector, in which the engineered *ND4* gene was combined with an MTS comprising the mRNA *cis*-acting elements of the *COX10* gene, known to localize exclusively to the mitochondrial surface, and seven additional amino acids (Sylvestre et al. 2003; Bonnet et al. 2007). Compared to untreated fibroblasts, allotopic expression of *ND4* in patient-derived skin fibroblasts carrying the m.11778G > A mutation exhibited improved growth rate and survival rate on galactose medium and had almost identical complex IV/I and V/I activity ratios compared to healthy control fibroblasts (Bonnet et al. 2008). To further optimize allotopic expression, a recombinant AAV2 serotype 2 (rAAV2/2) vector was constructed, in which the mtDNA sequence was combined with the MTS in 5′ and the 3′ UTR of the nuclear *COX10* gene, which was under the control of the cytomegalovirus (CMV) immediate early promoter. The rAAV2/2 vector was selected due to its high efficiency in transducing the inner retina, primarily RGCs (Hellström et al. 2009). Allotopic expression of *ND4* in a rat model of LHON harboring the m.11778G > A mutation demonstrated prevention of RGC degeneration, preservation of complex I function in optic nerves, and preservation of visual function (Cwerman-Thibault et al. 2015).

Phase I and II Clinical Trials

Preclinical studies served as a proof-of-concept for the viability of allotopic expression of wild-type human *ND4* as a therapeutic option for patients with LHON harboring the m.11778G > A mutation. A summary of the study design and key findings of clinical trials is outlined in Table 1.

The first phase I open-label study (NCT01267422) was commenced in 2011 and conducted by Bin Li and colleagues (Huazhong University of Science and Technology, Wuhan, China) (Wan et al. 2016). Nine patients received a single unilateral intravitreal injection of rAAV2-*ND4*, consisting of the nuclear encoded *ND4*, *COX10*-MTS, and the CMV promoter. Inclusion criteria required patients to have disease duration of at least 12 mo, with visual acuity of both eyes <1.5 logMAR. Three patients received a dose of 5×10^9 viral genomes (vg) and the remaining patients received a 1×10^{10} vg dose. Gene therapy was administered to the worst affected eye with a concurrent course of oral prednisolone. Treatment was well tolerated and none of the patients experienced any side effects. Systemic physical examinations and the results of routine blood and urine, and liver, renal, and immune function tests all remained normal during the follow-up period.

Six of the nine patients improved ≥0.30 logMAR in the treated eye after 9 mo of follow-up (Table 1; Wan et al. 2016). Mean logMAR acuity (± standard deviation) was 1.69 ± 0.43 before treatment, 1.58 ± 0.44 at 1 mo, 1.38 ± 0.46 at 3 mo, 1.23 ± 0.60 at 6 mo, and 1.27 ± 0.58 at 9 mo after treatment. At 36 mo, four patients showed significant improvement of both treated and untreated eyes, with improvement in the untreated eye lagging the treated eye by 3–12 mo (Yang et al. 2016). Visual fields also improved simultaneously with visual acuity. Long-term follow-up data was reported for eight patients up to 90 mo (7.5 yr) (Yuan et al. 2020). Six patients maintained clinically significant improvement in best corrected visual acuity (BCVA) (five patients in both eyes) at 75–90 mo after treatment. There was no significant difference in the mean age of onset, duration, and baseline RNFL thickness between patients who experienced an improvement after treatment and those who did not.

A second study was conducted by Bin Li and colleagues (Huazhong University of Science and Technology, Wuhan, China), involving 149 patients with a mean disease duration of 40.56 ± 49.99 mo (Liu et al. 2020). Participants received unilateral intravitreal injection of rAAV2-*ND4*. Visual outcomes after treatment were not reported. Instead, factors identified with rapid and significant improvements within 3 d of treatment were explored. Important predictors included pretreatment BCVA, and the period between onset and treatment of LHON, suggesting that disease duration and severity may predict treatment response. Pretreatment RNFL thickness was not predictive of treatment response.

A phase I open-label dose escalation study (NCT02161380) of the self-complementary AAV2-*ND4* containing the ATPc targeting MTS ("scAAV2(Y444,500,730F)—*P1ND4v2*"), was conducted by the group at Bascom Palmer Eye Institute (Feuer et al. 2016). Five patients received a unilateral intravitreal injection of the study drug to the worst affected eye, either a "low dose" (5×10^9 vg) or a "medium dose" (2.46×10^{10} vg). For inclusion, the acuity of all

Table 1. Summary of published gene therapy clinical trials in Leber hereditary optic neuropathy for m.11778G>A mutation

NCT number Name: type of study (intervention)	Author (year)	Number of patients: disease duration at treatment[a]	Follow-up duration	Main findings
NCT01267422 Single-center, open-label, single-arm study (single IVT rAAV2-ND4 in one eye; one patient received treatment in second eye 12 mo later)	Wan et al. 2016	n = 9 ≤1 yr: two patients >1 to ≤5 yr: four patients	9 mo	At 9 mo, treated eyes in six patients improved ≥0.3 logMAR, with most improvement occurring between 3 and 6 mo after treatment. No ocular or systemic adverse events.
	Yang et al. 2016	>5 yr: two patients	Up to 36 mo	At 36 mo, in patients with disease duration <2 yr, treated eyes improved by 0.3 logMAR and untreated eyes by 0.35 logMAR; in patients with disease duration ≥2 yr, treated eyes improved by 0.4 logMAR and untreated eyes by 0.25 logMAR. In four patients, BCVA of both treated and untreated eyes improved ≥0.3 logMAR during 36 mo follow-up.
	Yuan et al. 2020		Up to 75–90 mo	Follow-up data available for eight patients; at 75–90 mo, 11/16 eyes had improved ≥0.3 logMAR, including five patients with bilateral improvement. Greater visual recovery in younger patients and those treated within 1–2 yr of disease onset. No ocular or systemic adverse events.
NCT02161380 Phase I single-center, open-label, dose-escalation study (single IVT scAAV2–P1ND4v2 in one eye [four escalating doses])	Feuer et al. 2016	n = 5 ≤1 yr: one patient >1–≤5 yr: three patients >5 yr: one patient	90–180 d	At 90 d, two patients improved ≥0.3 logMAR: one patient improved from hand movements acuity to seven ETDRS letters; the other patient improved by 15 ETDRS letters; three patients remained unchanged. No serious ocular or systemic adverse events.
	Guy et al. 2017	n = 14 ≤1 yr: eight patients (including two with unilateral vision loss only) >1–≤5 yr: four patients >5 yr: two patients	Up to 24 mo	At 12 mo, in patients with bilateral visual loss (groups 1 and 2—see text for description), treated eyes improved by 0.24 logMAR and untreated eyes improved by 0.09 logMAR (compared to baseline). At 18 mo, in patients with bilateral visual loss (groups 1 and 2—see text for description), treated eyes improved by 0.45 logMAR and untreated eyes improved by 0.13 logMAR (compared to baseline). Only 1/6 patients with chronic visual loss (group 1) improved by ≥0.3 logMAR. At 12 and 18 mo, difference in improvement between treated eyes and untreated eyes in group 2 patients (bilateral vision

Study	Reference	n	Follow-up	Comments
	Lam et al. 2022	n = 28 ≤1 yr: 17 participants (including eight with unilateral vision loss only) >1 yr: 11 patients	Up to 36 mo	loss <1 yr), significantly more than that observed in an unmatched prior acute natural history cohort. In group 3 (acute unilateral visual loss), treatment of the better seeing eye did not prevent visual loss in one patient; the other patient maintained visual function in the treated eye. No noteworthy changes in visual acuity were observed in patients with chronic bilateral visual loss (group 1) over time, comparable to a natural history cohort; among group 1 patients, the largest percent improvements occurred with the "high" and "higher" doses. Improvement in treated and untreated eyes of patients with acute bilateral visual loss (group 2) was not significant when compared to improvement in visual acuity observed in the natural history cohort. Baseline BCVA in the treated eye was a crude predictor of the final BCVA: treated eyes that improved remarkably had baseline BCVA ≥20/800; treated eyes that improved but had baseline BCVA <20/800 never improved to better than 20/200; amount and timing of improvement highly variable. In group 3 (acute unilateral visual loss), all treated eyes lost ≥0.3 logMAR within the first year despite treatment. Incident uveitis occurred in 8/28 patients, and was related to vector dose; uveitis did not result in any vision sequelae.
NCT02064569 REVEAL: phase I/IIa single-center, open-label, dose-escalation study (single IVT GS010 in one eye [four escalating doses])	Vignal et al. 2018	n = 15 ≤1 yr: five patients >1–≤5 yr: five patients	96 wk	The most frequent ocular adverse events were intraocular inflammation and elevation of intraocular pressure (all mild). At week 96, 6/14 patients had improved ≥0.3 logMAR.
	Vignal-Clermont et al. 2021	>5 yr: five patients	Up to 5 yr	Follow-up data at 5 yr was available for 12 treated eyes and 10 untreated eyes; mean improvement from baseline in treated eyes was 0.44 logMAR, and in untreated eyes was 0.49 logMAR. Patients receiving the optimal dose of 9×10^{10} vg had a mean disease duration of 4.6 ± 8.7 yr (median 1.1 yr). Despite the delay in receiving treatment, BCVA improved in 4/6

Continued

Table 1. *Continued*

NCT number Name: type of study (intervention)	Author (year)	Number of patients: disease duration at treatment[a]	Follow-up duration	Main findings
				patients: two had experienced visual loss within 1 yr and two had experienced visual loss between 1 and 2 yr before treatment; improvement was observed beginning at 24 wk and remaining stable to 5 yr. At 5 yr, mean improvement from baseline in treated eyes was 0.68 logMAR, and in untreated eyes was 0.64 logMAR; however, final BCVA was still off-chart: mean acuity 1.77 and 1.78 logMAR in treated and untreated eyes, respectively.
NCT03153293 Phase II/III single-center, open-label, single-arm study (single IVT rAAV2-ND4 in one eye)	Liu et al. 2020	$n = 149$ 40.56 ± 49.99 (1– 312) mo	Up to 12 mo	54 (36.2%) patients exhibited rapid and significant improvement (≥0.3 logMAR) in visual acuity within 3 d of treatment: 26 patients in treated eye only, 11 patients in untreated eye only, and 17 patients in both eyes. For treated eyes, bivariate logistic regression modeling revealed that patient age, the period between onset and treatment, and pretreatment baseline BCVA of the treated eye were important predictors of rapid and significant improvement after gene therapy; pretreatment baseline visual field index and RNFL not predictive. For untreated eyes, the period between onset and treatment (of the fellow eye) and pretreatment baseline BCVA of the untreated eye were important predictors of rapid and significant improvement after gene therapy; patient age, pretreatment baseline visual field index, and RNFL not predictive.
NCT02652780 REVERSE: phase III multicenter, randomized, double-masked, sham-controlled (single IVT GS010 in one eye and sham in fellow eye in patients 6–12 mo after onset of visual loss)	Yu-Wai-Man, et al. 2020	$n = 37$ Treated eyes: 263.1 ± 53.9 (181– 362) d Sham-treated eyes: 278.8 ± 64.5 (181– 364) d	96 wk	At baseline, mean BCVA for treated and sham-treated eyes was 1.67 and 1.55 logMAR, respectively. At week 48, mean improvement in BCVA from baseline for treated and sham-treated eyes was −0.218 and −0.211 logMAR, respectively. At week 96, mean improvement in BCVA from baseline for treated and sham-treated eyes was −0.308 and −0.259 logMAR, respectively. The proportion of eyes with a CRR[b] was significantly higher in treated eyes (62%) compared to the sham-treated eyes (43%).

| NCT02652767 | Newman et al. 2021b | n = 38 | 96 wk | |

RESCUE: phase III multicenter, randomized, double-masked, sham-controlled (single IVT GS010 in one eye and sham in fellow eye in patients up to 6 mo after onset of visual loss)

Treated eyes: 108.5 ± 43.0 (40–179) d
Sham-treated eyes: 115.8 ± 42.9 (24–179) d

At week 96, 25 (68%) patients showed CRR[b] in at least one eye (14 patients in both eyes, nine patients in treated eye only, and two patients in sham-treated eye only). Contrast sensitivity and mean deviation on automated perimetry also showed improvement in treated and sham-treated eyes at week 96; no difference in OCT parameters.

At week 96, mean NEI-VFQ-25 composite score increased by 9.5 points compared to baseline.

At baseline, mean BCVA for treated and sham-treated eyes was 1.31 and 1.26 logMAR, respectively.

At week 48, mean change in BCVA from baseline for treated and sham-treated eyes was a deterioration of 0.38 and 0.39 logMAR, respectively.

At week 96, mean change in BCVA from baseline for treated and sham-treated eyes was a deterioration of 0.18 and 0.21 logMAR, respectively. Change in BCVA from baseline showed a parallel evolution for both treated and sham-treated eyes; BCVA deteriorated over initial weeks, reaching the worse levels at week 24, followed by a plateau phase at week 48, then improved by week 96.

A nadir BCVA was identified for each eye; average nadir BCVA was 1.9 logMAR (20/1600) in both eyes; mean time to nadir from baseline was 153.5 d and 164.1 d for treated and sham-treated eyes, respectively.

At week 96, mean change in BCVA from nadir for treated and sham-treated eyes was an improvement of 0.53 and 0.46 logMAR, respectively. Proportion of eyes that improved ≥0.3 logMAR from nadir to 96 wk was 63% treated eyes and 55% sham-treated eyes.

At week 96, mean NEI-VFQ-25 composite score decreased by 2.2 points compared to baseline.

| NCT03406104 | Biousse et al. 2021 | n = 61 | 3 yr | |

RESTORE: prospective, long-term follow-up of participants from REVERSE and

6.5 (2.3–12.8) mo

Due to differences in the timing of when patients received treatment in REVERSE and RESCUE, analysis of changes in BCVA were started at 12 mo after onset of vision loss.

Continued

Table 1. *Continued*

NCT number Name: type of study (intervention)	Author (year)	Number of patients: disease duration at treatment[a]	Follow-up duration	Main findings
RESCUE, including comparison with a natural history cohort (no additional intervention)	Newman et al. 2021a	$n = 76$ (treated with GS010) 6.5 (2.3–12.8) mo $n = 208$ (controls from natural history cohort; not treated)	Up to 48 mo from onset of vision loss	LOESS regression model showed a progressive and sustained BCVA improvement from 12 to 51.5 mo after onset of vision loss; mean BCVA steadily improved from 1.57 logMAR at 12 mo to 1.26 logMAR at 48 mo after onset of vision loss; mean BCVA remained on-chart (i.e., <1.6 logMAR) throughout the follow-up period. Absolute difference in change from baseline between treated and sham-treated eyes was 0.006 logMAR at 2 yr after treatment, and 0.018 logMAR at 3 yr after treatment. At week 96 after treatment, mean NEI-VFQ-25 composite score improved by 4 points compared to baseline. At 3 yr after treatment, mean NEI-VFQ-25 composite score improved by 7 points compared to baseline. BCVA from REVERSE, RESCUE, and RESTORE up to 4.3 yr after vision loss was compared to the visual acuity of 208 natural history subjects matched for age and *ND4* genotype; natural history subjects were from a LHON registry and from 10 previously published natural history studies; both treated and sham-treated eyes in REVERSE, RESCUE, and RESTORE were considered as "treated" due to bilateral improvement. Data for 150 "treated" eyes and 76 natural history eyes were available at month 12, and for 62 "treated" eyes and 27 natural history eyes at month 48. LOESS curves showed that BCVA of treated patients progressively improved from month 12 to 52 after onset of vision loss. At month 48, there was a statistically significant difference in BCVA of 0.33 logMAR in favor of treated eyes compared to natural history eyes. At month 48, most treated eyes (88.7%) were on-chart (i.e., <1.6 logMAR) compared to 48.1% of natural history eyes. The proportion of eyes at month 48 showing a meaningful improvement from nadir of ≥0.3 logMAR was 35/62

Cite this article as *Cold Spring Harb Perspect Med* doi: 10.1101/cshperspect.a041282

				(56.5%) treated eyes compared to 4/25 (16%) natural history eyes. When adjusted for age and duration of follow-up, the treatment effect at last observation (0.32 logMAR improvement in favor of treated eyes) remained statistically and clinically significant.
NCT03293524 REFLECT: phase III multicenter, randomized, double-masked, placebo-controlled (single IVT GS010 in first affected eye; second affected eye randomized to IVT GS010 or IVT placebo in patients up to 12 mo after onset of vision loss)	GenSight Biologics (2021)	$n = 98$ (48 treated bilaterally and 50 treated unilaterally) Disease duration not stated; but only those within 12 mo of onset of vision loss eligible	2 yr	At year 2, mean improvement in BCVA from baseline for bilaterally treated patients was −0.25 and −0.18 logMAR for the first and second treated eyes, respectively; and for unilaterally treated patients was −0.16 and −0.10 logMAR for the treated and placebo-treated eyes, respectively. At year 2, mean improvement in BCVA from nadir for bilaterally treated patients was −0.39 and −0.34 logMAR for the first and second treated eyes, respectively; and for unilaterally treated patients was −0.38 and −0.27 logMAR for the treated and placebo-treated eyes, respectively. The proportion of patients at year 2 who had improved ≥0.3 logMAR compared to nadir, was 35/48 (73%) of bilaterally treated patients and 33/50 (66%) of unilaterally treated patients. The mean BCVA for bilaterally and unilaterally treated patients reached 1.32 and 1.44 logMAR, respectively, with an absolute difference of +6 ETDRS letters in favor of bilaterally treated patients. The proportion of patients at year 2 who achieved CRR[b] in at least one eye, was 36/48 (75%) of bilaterally treated patients and 30/50 (60%) of unilaterally treated patients.

(BCVA) Best corrected visual acuity, (CRR) clinically relevant response, (ETDRS) Early Treatment Diabetic Retinopathy Study, (GS010) lenadogene nolparvovec, (IVT) intravitreal injection, (LOESS) locally estimated scatterplot smoothing, (logMAR) logarithm of the minimum angle of resolution, (NEI-VFQ-25) 25-item version of the National Eye Institute Visual Function Questionnaire, (OCT) optical coherence tomography, (RNFL) retinal nerve fiber layer.

[a] All disease duration at treatment values are reported as mean ± standard deviation (range), except values for RESTORE study, which are reported as median (range).

[b] Clinically relevant response (CRR) is defined as an improvement of at least 10 ETDRS letters from nadir (for on-chart eyes at nadir), or an improvement from an off-chart level of visual acuity at nadir to being able to read at least five ETDRS letters.

affected eyes had to be reduced to ≤35 ETDRS letters. Oral corticosteroids were not administered. Off-chart acuities were assigned logMAR values of 2.0 logMAR for counting fingers, 2.3 logMAR for hand motion, and 2.6 logMAR for light perception. None of the patients experienced serious ocular or systemic adverse effects. Only two patients (one with visual loss <12 mo receiving the low dose, and one with visual loss >12 mo receiving the medium dose) showed ≥0.3 logMAR improvement in BCVA (equivalent to three lines of ETDRS letters) at 3 mo.

Additional patients were treated in an extension of the initial study (Guy et al. 2017). Fourteen patients (including the original five) were organized into three groups: (group 1) chronic bilateral visual loss ≥12 mo in one eye and ≥6 mo in the fellow eye; (group 2) bilateral visual loss <12 mo both eyes; and (group 3) unilateral visual loss. Although primarily a safety study, the authors found that both treated and untreated eyes in groups 1 and 2 improved. Compared to baseline, treated eyes improved 0.45 logMAR at 18 mo postinjection, while untreated fellow eyes improved 0.13 logMAR. On OCT, treated eyes demonstrated stable average temporal RNFL thickness at 12 mo compared to baseline, while untreated eyes demonstrated significant temporal RNFL thinning.

The group at Bascom Palmer Eye Institute then assessed the safety of unilateral intravitreal injection of a "high" (2.4×10^9 vg) and "higher" (1.0×10^{10} vg) dose of scAAV2(Y444,500,730F) —$P1ND4v2$ (Lam et al. 2022). Confusingly the doses designated "low," "medium," "high," and "higher" were relabeled at the recommendation of the Food and Drug Administration (FDA), due to a change in the manufacturer of the gene therapy product. The outcomes of 28 patients were analyzed, including the previous 14 patients, and organized into the three previously stated groups. The only drug-related adverse event was incident uveitis, which was significantly correlated to vector dose. The study authors found variable improvement in treated and untreated eyes in groups 1 and 2, but a consistent relationship between acuity improvement and dose could not be established. In group 3, who received treatment to the better seeing eye, there was worsening of BCVA of treated eyes.

The final phase I/IIa study ("REVEAL") was an open-label, single-center, dose-escalation study (NCT02064569) conducted at Centre Hospitalier National d'Ophtalmologie des Quinze-Vingts (Paris, France) (Vignal et al. 2018; Vignal-Clermont et al. 2021). Fifteen patients with baseline acuity ≤20/200 in both eyes (except three patients with acuity ≤20/63) received a unilateral intravitreal injection of rAAV2/2-ND4 (also known as GS010, lenadogene nolparvovec, and trade name LUMEVOQ). Patients received injection of either a 9×10^9, 3×10^{10}, 9×10^{10}, or 1.8×10^{11} vg dose. The highest dose of 1.8×10^{11} vg was not sufficiently tolerated and was associated with more marked intraocular inflammation compared to lower doses. The dose of 9×10^{10} vg was selected as the maximum tolerated dose to be taken into phase III studies. Both treated and untreated eyes showed significant improvements in acuity at 5 yr compared with baseline, with mean improvements of −0.44 and −0.49 logMAR for treated and untreated eyes, respectively.

Phase III Clinical Trials

The early phase studies confirmed the safety of allotopic $ND4$ gene therapy for the treatment of LHON caused by the m.11778G > A mutation. Although not specifically designed to demonstrate efficacy, early phase studies found that gene therapy appeared to be more efficacious for those treated within 12 mo onset of visual loss and sustained response in long-term follow-up. Unexpectedly, untreated eyes also demonstrated improved visual acuity.

The results of the first phase III clinical trial to be reported was "REVERSE" (NCT02652 780), a randomized, double-masked, sham-controlled, multicenter clinical trial (Yu-Wai-Man et al. 2020). Thirty-seven patients with bilateral vision loss duration of 6–12 mo received an intravitreal injection of GS010 (9×10^9 vg dose) in one eye and sham treatment to the fellow eye, without concurrent corticosteroids. Off-chart acuities were assigned logMAR values of 2.0 for counting fingers, 2.3 for hand motion, 4.0 for light perception, and 4.5 for no light perception. Mean logMAR acuity at baseline was 1.67 ± 0.50 in treated eyes and 1.55 ± 0.42 in sham-

Cite this article as *Cold Spring Harb Perspect Med* doi: 10.1101/cshperspect.a041282

treated eyes. At week 96, the mean change in logMAR acuity from baseline was −0.308 ± 0.068 (equivalent to +15 ETDRS letters) in treated eyes and −0.259 ± 0.068 (+13 ETDRS letters) in sham-treated eyes. Bilateral improvements were also detected in contrast sensitivity and on automated perimetry. To investigate the bilateral improvement detected in the REVERSE trial, a study was conducted using nonhuman primates to probe possible underlying mechanisms. Three months after unilateral intravitreal injection of rAAV2/2-ND4 in the right eye, rAAV2/2-ND4 DNA was detected in all the tissue and fluid samples tested in animals receiving treatment, including the anterior segment of the eye, retina, optic nerve, optic tract, optic chiasm, and lateral geniculate nucleus. The authors hypothesized that inter-eye transfer of the rAAV2/2-ND4 viral vector could be the result of transneuronal spread of VVF, possibly through synaptic transfer mechanisms.

A second phase III clinical trial, "RESCUE" (NCT02652767), was designed concurrently with the REVERSE trial, using similar assessment protocols and outcome measures (Newman et al. 2021b). The RESCUE study included 38 participants with bilateral vision loss where the duration of vision loss for each eye was ≤6 mo, enabling a study of earlier treatment in the subacute phase of LHON. The mean BCVA for both treated and untreated eyes deteriorated over initial weeks, reaching the worse levels at week 24, followed by a plateau phase until week 48. Mean logMAR acuity at 96 wk was 1.47 ± 0.77 for treated eyes and 1.49 ± 0.74 for sham-treated eyes. This represented a mean worsening of +0.18 (−9 ETDRS letters) and +0.21 (−10 ETDRS letters) in treated and sham-treated eyes, respectively, compared to baseline, or an improvement of −0.53 (+26 ETDRS letters) and −0.46 (+23 ETDRS letters) in treated and sham-treated eyes, respectively, compared to the nadir. Despite earlier treatment and better baseline BCVA in RESCUE, visual outcomes at 96 wk were actually inferior to those seen in REVERSE. The difference in mean BCVA between the two trials was statistically significant from week 63.5 after disease onset. The trial investigators speculated that the greater RNFL thickness due to axonal swelling in the initial stages of disease could play a role by imposing a physical barrier to the diffusion of GS010 to RGCs and potentially impede the distribution of the viral vector throughout the RNFL after viral transduction (Newman et al. 2021b).

A long-term follow-up study ("RESTORE") was conducted as an extension of REVERSE and RESCUE, with participants of both studies being followed for an additional 3 yr, corresponding to 5 yr post-treatment administration (Biousse et al. 2021). Analysis of BCVA was conducted from 12 mo after onset of vision loss, when 92.7% of eyes (139/150) had received treatment, using a locally estimated scatterplot smoothing (LOESS) nonparametric local regression model, in which each patient's eyes were considered independently. The LOESS regression model showed a progressive and sustained BCVA improvement from 12 to 51.5 mo after onset of vision loss, with the mean BCVA of treated patients remaining on-chart (better than 1.6 logMAR) throughout the follow-up period.

The most recent phase III clinical trial of GS010, "REFLECT" (NCT03293524), was a randomized, double-masked, placebo-controlled trial (GenSight Biologics 2021). REFLECT included 98 patients with bilateral vision loss ≤1 yr from onset, each receiving an intravitreal injection of GS010 in their first affected eye, and intravitreal injection of either GS010 or a placebo in their second affected eye. An oral corticosteroid regimen was administered concurrently to reduce intraocular inflammation, which was mild and comparable in unilaterally and bilaterally treated patients. Preliminary data analysis indicates a trend toward slightly better visual improvement with bilateral treatment. At 2 yr, the mean improvement in logMAR acuity of bilaterally treated eyes was −0.25 (+13 ETDRS letters) and −0.18 (+9 ETDRS letters) in the first and second treated eyes, respectively, compared to baseline; or −0.39 (+20 ETDRS letters) and −0.34 (+17 ETDRS letters) in the first and second treated eyes, respectively, compared to nadir. Both eyes in unilaterally treated patients also improved significantly compared to nadir, with a −0.38 (+19 ETDRS letters) and −0.27 (+14

ETDRS letters) improvement observed in treated and placebo-treated eyes, respectively. The proportion of patients experiencing a ≥0.3 logMAR (+15 ETDRS letters) improvement relative to their observed nadir was 63% and 73% for unilaterally and bilaterally treated participants, respectively.

UNANSWERED QUESTIONS AND FUTURE AREAS FOR RESEARCH

To accurately assess the therapeutic efficacy of any treatment, regulatory agencies such as the FDA and European Medicines Agency (EMA) require well-controlled trials that use a valid comparison, typically an internal control. It is known that a proportion of patients with LHON experience spontaneous improvement in vision (Newman et al. 2020; Yu-Wai-Man et al. 2022). However, none of the phase III clinical trials were conducted with an internal control to determine if the observed improvement was a treatment effect or due to spontaneous improvement. A recent literature review and meta-analysis combined visual function information from 695 patients with the m.11778G > A mutation from 15 studies and found that 100 (14.4%) patients were reported to have "recovered" some vision (Newman et al. 2020). However, definitions of "recovery" varied among studies and there was inconsistent reporting of use of idebenone, an EMA-authorized medication for LHON. Meaningful visual recovery from the nadir likely occurred in <20% of patients aged ≥15 yr, with ultimate visual acuity of better than 20/200 rare.

Data from this review was combined with data from the REALITY LHON registry (NCT03295071), an international observational retrospective registry of LHON patients, and used as an external control for the REVERSE, RESCUE, and RESTORE trials (Newman et al. 2021a). Using a LOESS regression model, the BCVA of treated patients was found to progressively improve from month 12–52 after vision loss. At month 48, there was a statistically and clinically relevant difference in visual acuity of −0.33 logMAR (16.5 ETDRS equivalent) in favor of treated eyes compared to matched natural history eyes (P < 0.01). Nearly 90% of treated eyes were on-chart at month 48 compared to nearly 50% of natural history eyes (P < 0.01). Although this external control was helpful in understanding the efficacy of rAAV2/2-ND4 gene therapy, future clinical trials for LHON will require more standardized reporting of the natural history of this disorder to serve as an external control. Regulatory agencies do permit the use of external controls, including data derived from natural history studies, when it is not feasible or ethical to use an internal control, such as in studies of rare disorders.

The efficacy of gene therapy for chronic LHON has only been investigated in early phase studies with mixed results. These studies have been limited by lack of masking and small patient numbers. It remains unclear whether gene therapy for chronic LHON has the same efficacy as for patients treated within a year of disease onset.

An unexpected finding of all the clinical trials of gene therapy for ND4 has been visual improvement in both the treated and untreated eyes of study participants. To probe the underlying mechanisms leading to bilateral improvement, a study was conducted using nonhuman primates (Yu-Wai-Man et al. 2020). Three months after unilateral intravitreal injection of rAAV2/2-ND4, viral vector DNA was detected in all the tissue and fluid samples including the anterior segment, retina, and optic nerve of the contralateral untreated eye. Viral vector DNA was also found in the optic chiasm, optic tract, and lateral geniculate nucleus. The authors hypothesized that inter-eye transfer of the rAAV2/2-ND4 viral vector could be the result of transneuronal spread via the optic nerve and chiasm. This is supported by evidence of transneuronal spread of adenovirus vector through synaptic transfer mechanisms (Zingg et al. 2017). Systemic transfer was thought to be less likely, as bio-dissemination studies have shown limited transfer of rAAV2/2-ND4 in blood (Vignal-Clermont et al. 2021). Other explanations include transfer of mitochondrial material into the contralateral eye, increased expression of coactivators and transcription factors that regulate mitochondrial biogenesis in the contralateral eye, and improved visual function in the contralateral eye as a result of brain plasticity (Yu-Wai-Man et al. 2020; Vignal-Clermont et al. 2021).

Last, it is uncertain whether the technique used in the allotopic expression of *ND4* also apply to the other primary mutations of LHON. There is increased interest in studying allotopic expression of *ND1* and *ND6*, corresponding to the m.3460G > A and m.11484T > C mutations, respectively. Allotopic rescue of respiratory chain dysfunction in fibroblasts harboring the m.3460G > A mutation has been demonstrated already by the group at Institut de la Vision (Bonnet et al. 2007, 2008). In patient-derived fibroblasts carrying the m.3460G > A mutation, allotopic expression of *ND1* was associated with an 80% increase in overall ATP production rate compared to untreated fibroblasts and an ~1.8-fold increase in the overall amount of ND1 protein. However, on spectrometric assessment of complex I enzymatic activity, there was only a partial but significant rescue of complex I defect (60% for the V/I activity ratio), which was attributed to the central role *ND1* plays in the first step of complex I biogenesis (Bonnet et al. 2008). Currently, there are no gene therapy trials for *ND1* or *ND6* registered on the clinicaltrials.gov database. Further preclinical studies are required, aided by the learnings from the studies that lead to the development of AAV2-*ND4*.

OTHER APPROACHES TO GENE THERAPY

There is interest in therapies that prevent or delay conversion to symptomatic LHON, in particular neuroprotective approaches that reduce mitochondrial stress, inhibit RGC apoptosis, and promote RGC survival. Current strategies under investigation include AAV vectors encoding *SOD2*, *NDI1*, *NRF2*, and *BDNF*. Alternative gene therapy strategies that are nonspecific for the type of LHON mutation that individuals carry can potentially be used in all patients.

In m.11778G > A LHON cybrids transfected with an AAV vector encoding the *SOD2* gene, increased expression of superoxide dismutase results in increased cell survival (Qi et al. 2007). Superoxide dismutase, encoded by the *SOD2* gene, catalyzes the dismutation of superoxide

radicals in mitochondria and is a key mediator of the cell's antioxidant defense mechanism.

In a rotenone-induced murine model of LHON, rescue of optic nerve degeneration was achieved using an AAV vector to deliver yeast *NDI1* (Marella et al. 2010; Chadderton et al. 2013). Ndi1 (encoded by the *NDI1* gene), is an alternative NADH dehydrogenase expressed in yeast (*S. cerevisiae*) mitochondria (equivalent to mammalian complex I), and acts as functional replacement for defective complex I, restoring downstream electron transfer while at the same time suppressing ROS overproduction. However, safety issues will need to be studied further given the cross-species nature of this gene therapy approach.

In HEK293T cybrids subjected to oxidative stress, overexpression of Nrf2 by transfecting cybrids with AAV-*NRF2* resulted in reduction of ROS levels (Liang et al. 2017). Nrf2 (encoded by the *NRF2* gene) is a transcription factor involved mitochondrial biogenesis and a major regulator of antioxidant and cellular protective genes including *SOD2*.

The brain-derived neurotrophic factor (BDNF)/tropomycin receptor kinase B (TrkB) signaling pathway has also been the focus of several studies of because of its role in regulating the survival, development, function, and plasticity of neurons (Osborne et al. 2018). In in vivo and in vitro animal studies, AAV vectors encoding BDNF have demonstrated consistent and considerable neuroprotection of RGC. Based on these promising preclinical studies, neuroprotective BDNF gene therapy trials are under consideration for glaucoma, and could also prove relevant for mitochondrial optic neuropathies, including LHON.

Gene editing using CRISPR/Cas 9 is a promising technique that allows the in vivo correction of the underlying genetic defect and this approach is being considered for various inherited retinal degenerations (Suzuki et al. 2016; Kim et al. 2017; Tsai et al. 2018; Cai et al. 2019; Maeder et al. 2019; Sladen et al. 2021). Genetic modification of mtDNA has for a long time not been feasible, but recent major breakthroughs in mitochondrial genome engineering are now making this a reality (Mok et al. 2020; Silva-Pinheiro and Minczuk 2022). The efficiency and safety of in vivo mitochondrial base editing delivered using

AAV delivery methods are being further optimized, and the translational benefit for primary mtDNA diseases is likely to be explored first for the mitochondrial optic neuropathies given the obvious advantages of intraocular gene therapy.

CONCLUDING REMARKS

One hundred and fifty years ago, Theodor Leber described four families in which a number of young men suffered abrupt bilateral vision loss. In the last 30 yr, considerable progress has been made in understanding the genetic basis of LHON and the underpinning pathological mechanisms, enabling the development of targeted treatments. The unique challenge of developing gene therapy for mitochondrial disease is the inability of viral vectors to efficiently introduce genes directly into the mitochondrial genome. This has been overcome to some extent with the technique of allotopic gene expression using AAV vectors with carefully selected MTSs, facilitating transportation of the synthesized protein to the mitochondria and into the correct location within the mitochondrial compartment. Phase II and III clinical trials have confirmed the safety and efficacy of allotopically expressed *ND4* for the treatment of LHON due to the m.11778G > A mutation within 12 mo of vision loss onset, with the unexpected finding of sustained bilateral visual improvement despite unilateral intravitreal injection. Although recent clinical trials have not been designed with an internal control group, the improvement in visual outcomes is to a degree not demonstrated when natural history data is used as an external comparator. The efficacy of allotopically expressed *ND4* for chronic LHON and the viability of other gene therapies, including mutation-specific therapies for *ND1* and *ND6* and mutation-independent neuroprotective approaches, have yet to be established. However, these unanswered questions present further opportunities for investigation and give hope to patients and their families affected by LHON.

ACKNOWLEDGMENTS

B.S.C. is recipient of the Cambridge-Rutherford Memorial Scholarship awarded by the Royal Society Te Apārangi – Rutherford Foundation and the Cambridge Commonwealth, European & International Trust. P.Y.W.M. is supported by an Advanced Fellowship Award (NIHR301696) from the UK National Institute of Health Research (NIHR) and a Clinician Scientist Fellowship Award (G1002570) from the UK Medical Research Council (MRC). P.Y.W.M. also receives funding from Fight for Sight (UK), the Isaac Newton Trust (UK), Moorfields Eye Charity (GR001376), the Addenbrooke's Charitable Trust, the National Eye Research Centre (UK), the International Foundation for Optic Nerve Disease (IFOND), the NIHR as part of the Rare Diseases Translational Research Collaboration, the NIHR Cambridge Biomedical Research Centre (BRC-1215-20014), and the NIHR Biomedical Research Centre based at Moorfields Eye Hospital NHS Foundation Trust and UCL Institute of Ophthalmology. The views expressed are those of the author(s) and not necessarily those of the NHS, the NIHR, or the Department of Health.

REFERENCES

Balducci N, Savini G, Cascavilla ML, La Morgia C, Triolo G, Giglio R, Carbonelli M, Parisi V, Sadun AA, Bandello F, et al. 2016. Macular nerve fibre and ganglion cell layer changes in acute Leber's hereditary optic neuropathy. *Br J Ophthalmol* **100:** 1232–1237. doi:10.1136/bjophthalmol-2015-307326

Balducci N, Cascavilla ML, Ciardella A, La Morgia C, Triolo G, Parisi V, Bandello F, Sadun AA, Carelli V, Barboni P. 2018. Peripapillary vessel density changes in Leber's hereditary optic neuropathy: a new biomarker. *Clin Exp Ophthalmol* **46:** 1055–1062. doi:10.1111/ceo.13326

Barboni P, Carbonelli M, Savini G, Ramos Carolina do V, Carta A, Berezovsky A, Salomao SR, Carelli V, Sadun AA. 2010. Natural history of Leber's hereditary optic neuropathy: longitudinal analysis of the retinal nerve fiber layer by optical coherence tomography. *Ophthalmology* **117:** 623–627. doi:10.1016/j.ophtha.2009.07.026

Bietenhader M, Martos A, Tetaud E, Aiyar RS, Sellem CH, Kucharczyk R, Clauder-Münster S, Giraud MF, Godard F, Salin B, et al. 2012. Experimental relocation of the mitochondrial ATP9 gene to the nucleus reveals forces underlying mitochondrial genome evolution. *PLoS Genet* **8:** e1002876. doi:10.1371/journal.pgen.1002876

Biousse V, Newman NJ, Yu-Wai-Man P, Carelli V, Moster ML, Vignal-Clermont C, Klopstock T, Sadun AA, Sergott RC, Hage R, et al. 2021. Long-term follow-up after unilateral intravitreal gene therapy for Leber hereditary optic neuropathy: the RESTORE study. *J Neuroophthalmol* **41:** 309–315. doi:10.1097/WNO.0000000000001367

Cite this article as *Cold Spring Harb Perspect Med* doi: 10.1101/cshperspect.a041282

Bonnet C, Kaltimbacher V, Ellouze S, Augustin S, Bénit P, Forster V, Rustin P, Sahel JA, Corral-Debrinski M. 2007. Allotopic mRNA localization to the mitochondrial surface rescues respiratory chain defects in fibroblasts harboring mitochondrial DNA mutations affecting complex I or v subunits. *Rejuvenation Res* **10:** 127–144. doi:10.1089/rej.2006.0526

Bonnet C, Augustin S, Ellouze S, Bénit P, Bouaita A, Rustin P, Sahel JA, Corral-Debrinski M. 2008. The optimized allotopic expression of ND1 or ND4 genes restores respiratory chain complex I activity in fibroblasts harboring mutations in these genes. *Biochim Biophys Acta* **1783:** 1707–1717. doi:10.1016/j.bbamcr.2008.04.018

Cai Y, Cheng T, Yao Y, Li X, Ma Y, Li L, Zhao H, Bao J, Zhang M, Qiu Z, et al. 2019. In vivo genome editing rescues photoreceptor degeneration via a Cas9/RecA-mediated homology-directed repair pathway. *Sci Adv* **5:** eaav3335. doi:10.1126/sciadv.aav3335

Carelli V, Carbonelli M, de Coo IF, Kawasaki A, Klopstock T, Lagrèze WA, La Morgia C, Newman NJ, Orssaud C, Pott JWR, et al. 2017. International consensus statement on the clinical and therapeutic management of Leber hereditary optic neuropathy. *J Neuroophthalmol* **37:** 371–381. doi:10.1097/WNO.0000000000000570

Catarino CB, von Livonius B, Priglinger C, Banik R, Matloob S, Tamhankar MA, Castillo L, Friedburg C, Halfpenny CA, Lincoln JA, et al. 2020. Real-world clinical experience with idebenone in the treatment of Leber hereditary optic neuropathy. *J Neuroophthalmol* **40:** 558–565. doi:10.1097/WNO.0000000000001023

Chadderton N, Palfi A, Millington-Ward S, Gobbo O, Overlack N, Carrigan M, O'Reilly M, Campbell M, Ehrhardt C, Wolfrum U, et al. 2013. Intravitreal delivery of AAV-NDI1 provides functional benefit in a murine model of Leber hereditary optic neuropathy. *Eur J Hum Genet* **21:** 62–68. doi:10.1038/ejhg.2012.112

Cwerman-Thibault H, Augustin S, Lechauve C, Ayache J, Ellouze S, Sahel JA, Corral-Debrinski M. 2015. Nuclear expression of mitochondrial ND4 leads to the protein assembling in complex I and prevents optic atrophy and visual loss. *Mol Ther Methods Clin Dev* **2:** 15003. doi:10.1038/mtm.2015.3

Farrell LB, Gearing DP, Nagley P. 1988. Reprogrammed expression of subunit 9 of the mitochondrial ATPase complex of *Saccharomyces cerevisiae*. Expression in vitro from a chemically synthesized gene and import into isolated mitochondria. *Eur J Biochem* **173:** 131–137. doi:10.1111/j.1432-1033.1988.tb13976.x

Feuer WJ, Schiffman JC, Davis JL, Porciatti V, Gonzalez P, Koilkonda RD, Yuan H, Lalwani A, Lam BL, Guy J. 2016. Gene therapy for Leber hereditary optic neuropathy: initial results. *Ophthalmology* **123:** 558–570. doi:10.1016/j.ophtha.2015.10.025

Gearing DP, Nagley P. 1986. Yeast mitochondrial ATPase subunit 8, normally a mitochondrial gene product, expressed in vitro and imported back into the organelle. *EMBO J* **5:** 3651–3655. doi:10.1002/j.1460-2075.1986.tb04695.x

Gearing DP, McMullen GL, Nagley P. 1985. Chemical synthesis of a mitochondrial gene designed for expression in the yeast nucleus. *Biochem Int* **10:** 907–915.

GenSight Biologics. 2021. GenSight Biologics confirms sustained efficacy and safety of bilateral LUMEVOQ injections at 2-year follow-up of REFLECT Phase III Trial. Paris, France. https://www.gensight-biologics.com/2021/12/14/gensight-biologics-confirms-sustained-efficacy-and-safety-of-bilateral-lumevoq-injections-at-2-year-follow-up-of-reflect-phase-iii-trial

Gerber S, Ding MG, Gérard X, Zwicker K, Zanlonghi X, Rio M, Serre V, Hanein S, Munnich A, Rotig A, et al. 2017. Compound heterozygosity for severe and hypomorphic *NDUFS2* mutations cause non-syndromic LHON-like optic neuropathy. *J Med Genet* **54:** 346–356. doi:10.1136/jmedgenet-2016-104212

Gerber S, Orssaud C, Kaplan J, Johansson C, Rozet JM. 2021. *MCAT* mutations cause nuclear LHON-like optic neuropathy. *Genes (Basel)* **12:** 521. doi: 10.3390/genes12040521

Guy J, Qi X, Pallotti F, Schon EA, Manfredi G, Carelli V, Martinuzzi A, Hauswirth WW, Lewin AS. 2002. Rescue of a mitochondrial deficiency causing Leber hereditary optic neuropathy. *Ann Neurol* **52:** 534–542. doi:10.1002/ana.10354

Guy J, Qi X, Koilkonda RD, Arguello T, Chou TH, Ruggeri M, Porciatti V, Lewin AS, Hauswirth WW. 2009. Efficiency and safety of AAV-mediated gene delivery of the human ND4 complex I subunit in the mouse visual system. *Invest Ophthalmol Vis Sci* **50:** 4205–4214. doi:10.1167/iovs.08-3214

Guy J, Feuer WJ, Davis JL, Porciatti V, Gonzalez PJ, Koilkonda RD, Yuan H, Hauswirth WW, Lam BL. 2017. Gene therapy for Leber hereditary optic neuropathy: low- and medium-dose visual results. *Ophthalmology* **124:** 1621–1634. doi:10.1016/j.ophtha.2017.05.016

Hage R, Vignal-Clermont C. 2021. Leber hereditary optic neuropathy: review of treatment and management. *Front Neurol* **12:** 651639. doi:10.3389/fneur.2021.651639

Hellström M, Ruitenberg MJ, Pollett MA, Ehlert EM, Twisk J, Verhaagen J, Harvey AR. 2009. Cellular tropism and transduction properties of seven adeno-associated viral vector serotypes in adult retina after intravitreal injection. *Gene Ther* **16:** 521–532. doi:10.1038/gt.2008.178

Jankauskaite E, Ambroziak AM, Hajieva P, Ołdak M, Tońska K, Korwin M, Bartnik E, Kodroń A. 2020. Testosterone increases apoptotic cell death and decreases mitophagy in Leber's hereditary optic neuropathy cells. *J Appl Genet* **61:** 195–203. doi:10.1007/s13353-020-00550-y

Jurkute N, Majander A, Bowman R, Votruba M, Abbs S, Acheson J, Lenaers G, Amati-Bonneau P, Moosajee M, Arno G, et al. 2019. Clinical utility gene card for: inherited optic neuropathies including next-generation sequencing-based approaches. *Eur J Hum Genet* **27:** 494–502. doi:10.1038/s41431-018-0235-y

Kim E, Koo T, Park SW, Kim D, Kim K, Cho HY, Song DW, Lee KJ, Jung MH, Kim S, et al. 2017. In vivo genome editing with a small Cas9 orthologue derived from *Campylobacter jejuni*. *Nat Commun* **8:** 14500. doi:10.1038/ncomms14500

Klopstock T, Yu-Wai-Man P, Dimitriadis K, Rouleau J, Heck S, Bailie M, Atawan A, Chattopadhyay S, Schubert M, Garip A, et al. 2011. A randomized placebo-controlled trial of idebenone in Leber's hereditary optic neuropathy. *Brain* **134:** 2677–2686. doi:10.1093/brain/awr170

Koilkonda R, Yu H, Talla V, Porciatti V, Feuer WJ, Hauswirth WW, Chiodo V, Erger KE, Boye SL, Lewin AS, et al. 2014. LHON gene therapy vector prevents visual loss and optic neuropathy induced by G11778A mutant mitochondrial DNA: biodistribution and toxicology profile. *Invest Ophthalmol Vis Sci* **55:** 7739–7753. doi:10.1167/iovs.14-15388

Lam BL, Feuer WJ, Davis JL, Porciatti V, Yu H, Levy RB, Vanner E, Guy J. 2022. Leber hereditary optic neuropathy gene therapy: adverse events and visual acuity results of all patient groups. *Am J Ophthalmol* doi:10.1016/j.ajo.2022.02.023

Law RH, Farrell LB, Nero D, Devenish RJ, Nagley P. 1988. Studies on the import into mitochondria of yeast ATP synthase subunits 8 and 9 encoded by artificial nuclear genes. *FEBS Lett* **236:** 501–505. doi:10.1016/0014-5793(88)80086-3

Leber T. 1871. Ueber hereditäre und congenital-angelegte sehnervenleiden [On hereditary and congenital optic nerve diseases]. *Albrecht von Graefes Archiv für Ophthalmologie* **17:** 249–291. doi:10.1007/BF01694557

Levin LA. 2007. Mechanisms of retinal ganglion specific-cell death in Leber hereditary optic neuropathy. *Trans Am Ophthalmol Soc* **105:** 379–391.

Liang KJ, Woodard KT, Weaver MA, Gaylor JP, Weiss ER, Samulski RJ. 2017. AAV- Nrf2 promotes protection and recovery in animal models of oxidative stress. *Mol Ther* **25:** 765–779. doi:10.1016/j.ymthe.2016.12.016

Lin CS, Sharpley MS, Fan W, Waymire KG, Sadun AA, Carelli V, Ross-Cisneros FN, Baciu P, Sung E, McManus MJ, et al. 2012. Mouse mtDNA mutant model of Leber hereditary optic neuropathy. *Proc Natl Acad Sci* **109:** 20065–20070. doi:10.1073/pnas.1217113109

Liu HL, Yuan JJ, Zhang Y, Tian Z, Li X, Wang D, Du YY, Song L, Li B. 2020. Factors associated with rapid improvement in visual acuity in patients with Leber's hereditary optic neuropathy after gene therapy. *Acta Ophthalmol* **98:** e730–e733.

Lopez Sanchez MIG, Kearns LS, Staffieri SE, Clarke L, McGuinness MB, Meteoukki W, Samuel S, Ruddle JB, Chen C, Fraser CL, et al. 2021. Establishing risk of vision loss in Leber hereditary optic neuropathy. *Am J Hum Genet* **108:** 2159–2170. doi:10.1016/j.ajhg.2021.09.015

Maeder ML, Stefanidakis M, Wilson CJ, Baral R, Barrera LA, Bounoutas GS, Bumcrot D, Chao H, Ciulla DM, DaSilva JA, et al. 2019. Development of a gene-editing approach to restore vision loss in Leber congenital amaurosis type 10. *Nat Med* **25:** 229–233. doi:10.1038/s41591-018-0327-9

Mansukhani SA, Mehta DG, Renaud DL, Whealy MA, Chen JJ, Bhatti MT. 2021. Nuclear DNA mutation causing a phenotypic Leber hereditary optic neuropathy plus. *Ophthalmology* **128:** 628–631. doi:10.1016/j.ophtha.2020.09.011

Marella M, Seo BB, Thomas BB, Matsuno-Yagi A, Yagi T. 2010. Successful amelioration of mitochondrial optic neuropathy using the yeast NDI1 gene in a rat animal model. *PLoS ONE* **5:** e11472. doi:10.1371/journal.pone.0011472

Mejia-Vergara AJ, Seleme N, Sadun AA, Karanjia R. 2020. Pathophysiology of conversion to symptomatic Leber hereditary optic neuropathy and therapeutic implications: a review. *Curr Neurol Neurosci Rep* **20:** 11. doi:10.1007/s11910-020-01032-8

Mok BY, de Moraes MH, Zeng J, Bosch DE, Kotrys AV, Raguram A, Hsu F, Radey MC, Peterson SB, Mootha VK, et al. 2020. A bacterial cytidine deaminase toxin enables CRISPR-free mitochondrial base editing. *Nature* **583:** 631–637. doi:10.1038/s41586-020-2477-4

Moore AT, Yu-Wai-Man P. 2021. Mitochondrial disorders and the eye: a new era for diagnosis. *Ophthalmology* **128:** 632–633. doi:10.1016/j.ophtha.2020.12.032

Nagley P, Devenish RJ. 1989. Leading organellar proteins along new pathways: the relocation of mitochondrial and chloroplast genes to the nucleus. *Trends Biochem Sci* **14:** 31–35. doi:10.1016/0968-0004(89)90087-X

Newman NJ, Carelli V, Taiel M, Yu-Wai-Man P. 2020. Visual outcomes in Leber hereditary optic neuropathy patients with the m.11778G>A (MTND4) mitochondrial DNA mutation. *J Neuroophthalmol* **40:** 547–557. doi:10.1097/WNO.0000000000001045

Newman NJ, Yu-Wai-Man P, Carelli V, Biousse V, Moster ML, Vignal-Clermont C, Sergott RC, Klopstock T, Sadun AA, Girmens JF, et al. 2021a. Intravitreal gene therapy vs. natural history in patients with Leber hereditary optic neuropathy carrying the m.11778G>A ND4 mutation: systematic review and indirect comparison. *Front Neurol* **12:** 662838. doi:10.3389/fneur.2021.662838

Newman NJ, Yu-Wai-Man P, Carelli V, Moster ML, Biousse V, Vignal-Clermont C, Sergott RC, Klopstock T, Sadun AA, Barboni P, et al. 2021b. Efficacy and safety of intravitreal gene therapy for Leber hereditary optic neuropathy treated within 6 months of disease onset. *Ophthalmology* **128:** 649–660. doi:10.1016/j.ophtha.2020.12.012

Osborne A, Khatib TZ, Songra L, Barber AC, Hall K, Kong GYX, Widdowson PS, Martin KR. 2018. Neuroprotection of retinal ganglion cells by a novel gene therapy construct that achieves sustained enhancement of brain-derived neurotrophic factor/tropomyosin-related kinase receptor-B signaling. *Cell Death Dis* **9:** 1007. doi:10.1038/s41419-018-1041-8

Pisano A, Preziuso C, Iommarini L, Perli E, Grazioli P, Campese AF, Maresca A, Montopoli M, Masuelli L, Sadun AA, et al. 2015. Targeting estrogen receptor beta as preventive therapeutic strategy for Leber's hereditary optic neuropathy. *Hum Mol Genet* **24:** 6921–6931.

Poincenot L, Pearson AL, Karanjia R. 2020. Demographics of a large international population of patients affected by Leber's hereditary optic neuropathy. *Ophthalmology* **127:** 679–688. doi:10.1016/j.ophtha.2019.11.014

Qi X, Sun L, Hauswirth WW, Lewin AS, Guy J. 2007. Use of mitochondrial antioxidant defenses for rescue of cells with a Leber hereditary optic neuropathy-causing mutation. *Arch Ophthalmol* **125:** 268–272. doi:10.1001/archopht.125.2.268

Silva-Pinheiro P, Minczuk M. 2022. The potential of mitochondrial genome engineering. *Nat Rev Genet* **23:** 199–214. doi:10.1038/s41576-021-00432-x

Sladen PE, Perdigão PRL, Salsbury G, Novoselova T, van der Spuy J, Chapple JP, Yu-Wai-Man P, Cheetham ME. 2021. CRISPR-Cas9 correction of OPA1 c.1334G>A: p.R445H restores mitochondrial homeostasis in dominant optic atrophy patient-derived iPSCs. *Mol Ther Nucleic Acids* **26:** 432–443. doi:10.1016/j.omtn.2021.08.015

Cite this article as *Cold Spring Harb Perspect Med* doi: 10.1101/cshperspect.a041282

Stenton SL, Sheremet NL, Catarino CB, Andreeva NA, Assouline Z, Barboni P, Barel O, Berutti R, Bychkov I, Caporali L, et al. 2021. Impaired complex I repair causes recessive Leber's hereditary optic neuropathy. *J Clin Invest* **131:** e138267. doi:10.1172/JCI138267

Suzuki K, Tsunekawa Y, Hernandez-Benitez R, Wu J, Zhu J, Kim EJ, Hatanaka F, Yamamoto M, Araoka T, Li Z, et al. 2016. In vivo genome editing via CRISPR/Cas9 mediated homology-independent targeted integration. *Nature* **540:** 144–149. doi:10.1038/nature20565

Sylvestre J, Margeot A, Jacq C, Dujardin G, Corral-Debrinski M. 2003. The role of the 3′ untranslated region in mRNA sorting to the vicinity of mitochondria is conserved from yeast to human cells. *Mol Biol Cell* **14:** 3848–3856. doi:10.1091/mbc.e03-02-0074

Tatsuta T, Langer T. 2008. Quality control of mitochondria: protection against neurodegeneration and ageing. *EMBO J* **27:** 306–314. doi:10.1038/sj.emboj.7601972

Tsai YT, Wu WH, Lee TT, Wu WP, Xu CL, Park KS, Cui X, Justus S, Lin CS, Jauregui R, et al. 2018. Clustered regularly interspaced short palindromic repeats-based genome surgery for the treatment of autosomal dominant retinitis pigmentosa. *Ophthalmology* **125:** 1421–1430. doi:10.1016/j.ophtha.2018.04.001

Vignal C, Uretsky S, Fitoussi S, Galy A, Blouin L, Girmens JF, Bidot S, Thomasson N, Bouquet C, Valero S, et al. 2018. Safety of rAAV2/2- ND4 gene therapy for Leber hereditary optic neuropathy. *Ophthalmology* **125:** 945–947. doi:10.1016/j.ophtha.2017.12.036

Vignal-Clermont C, Girmens JF, Audo I, Said SM, Errera MH, Plaine L, O'Shaughnessy D, Taiel M, Sahel JA. 2021. Safety of intravitreal gene therapy for treatment of subjects with Leber hereditary optic neuropathy due to mutations in the mitochondrial ND4 gene: the REVEAL study. *BioDrugs* **35:** 201–214. doi:10.1007/s40259-021-00468-9

Wallace DC, Singh G, Lott MT, Hodge JA, Schurr TG, Lezza AM, Elsas LJ II, Nikoskelainen EK. 1988. Mitochondrial DNA mutation associated with Leber's hereditary optic neuropathy. *Science* **242:** 1427–1430. doi:10.1126/science.3201231

Wan X, Pei H, Zhao MJ, Yang S, Hu WK, He H, Ma SQ, Zhang G, Dong XY, Chen C, et al. 2016. Efficacy and safety of rAAV2-ND4 treatment for Leber's hereditary optic neuropathy. *Sci Rep* **6:** 21587. doi:10.1038/srep 21587

Wu YR, Wang AG, Chen YT, Yarmishyn AA, Buddhakosai W, Yang TC, Hwang DK, Yang YP, Shen CN, Lee HC, et al. 2018. Bioactivity and gene expression profiles of hiPSC-generated retinal ganglion cells in MT-ND4 mutated Leber's hereditary optic neuropathy. *Exp Cell Res* **363:** 299–309. doi:10.1016/j.yexcr.2018.01.020

Yang S, Ma SQ, Wan X, He H, Pei H, Zhao MJ, Chen C, Wang DW, Dong XY, Yuan JJ, et al. 2016. Long-term outcomes of gene therapy for the treatment of Leber's hereditary optic neuropathy. *EBioMedicine* **10:** 258–268. doi:10.1016/j.ebiom.2016.07.002

Yang TC, Yarmishyn AA, Yang YP, Lu PC, Chou SJ, Wang ML, Lin TC, Hwang DK, Chou YB, Chen SJ, et al. 2020. Mitochondrial transport mediates survival of retinal ganglion cells in affected LHON patients. *Hum Mol Genet* **29:** 1454–1464. doi:10.1093/hmg/ddaa063

Yu H, Ozdemir SS, Koilkonda RD, Chou TH, Porciatti V, Chiodo V, Boye SL, Hauswirth WW, Lewin AS, Guy J. 2012. Mutant NADH dehydrogenase subunit 4 gene delivery to mitochondria by targeting sequence-modified adeno-associated virus induces visual loss and optic atrophy in mice. *Mol Vis* **18:** 1668–e11683.

Yuan J, Zhang Y, Liu H, Wang D, Du Y, Tian Z, Li X, Yang S, Pei H, Wan X, et al. 2020. Seven-year follow-up of gene therapy for Leber's hereditary optic neuropathy. *Ophthalmology* **127:** 1125–1127. doi:10.1016/j.ophtha.2020.02.023

Yu-Wai-Man P, Griffiths PG, Brown DT, Howell N, Turnbull DM, Chinnery PF. 2003. The epidemiology of Leber hereditary optic neuropathy in the north east of England. *Am J Hum Genet* **72:** 333–339. doi:10.1086/346066

Yu-Wai-Man CY, Chinnery PF, Griffiths PG. 2005. Optic neuropathies—importance of spatial distribution of mitochondria as well as function. *Med Hypotheses* **65:** 1038–1042. doi:10.1016/j.mehy.2004.10.021

Yu-Wai-Man P, Griffiths PG, Hudson G, Chinnery PF. 2009. Inherited mitochondrial optic neuropathies. *J Med Genet* **46:** 145–158. doi:10.1136/jmg.2007.054270

Yu-Wai-Man P, Griffiths PG, Chinnery PF. 2011. Mitochondrial optic neuropathies—disease mechanisms and therapeutic strategies. *Prog Retin Eye Res* **30:** 81–114. doi:10.1016/j.preteyeres.2010.11.002

Yu-Wai-Man P, Votruba M, Burté F, La Morgia C, Barboni P, Carelli V. 2016. A neurodegenerative perspective on mitochondrial optic neuropathies. *Acta Neuropathol* **132:** 789–806. doi:10.1007/s00401-016-1625-2

Yu-Wai-Man P, Newman NJ, Carelli V, Moster ML, Biousse V, Sadun AA, Klopstock T, Vignal-Clermont C, Sergott RC, Rudolph G, et al. 2020. Bilateral visual improvement with unilateral gene therapy injection for Leber hereditary optic neuropathy. *Sci Transl Med* **12:** eaaz7423. doi:10.1126/scitranslmed.aaz7423

Yu-Wai-Man P, Newman NJ, Carelli V, La Morgia C, Biousse V, Bandello FM, Clermont CV, Campillo LC, Leruez S, Moster ML, et al. 2022. Natural history of patients with Leber hereditary optic neuropathy—results from the REALITY study. *Eye (Lond)* **36:** 818–826. doi:10.1038/s41433-021-01535-9

Zingg B, Chou XL, Zhang ZG, Mesik L, Liang F, Tao HW, Zhang LI. 2017. AAV-mediated anterograde transsynaptic tagging: mapping corticocollicular input-defined neural pathways for defense behaviors. *Neuron* **93:** 33–47. doi:10.1016/j.neuron.2016.11.045

A Systematic Review of Optogenetic Vision Restoration: History, Challenges, and New Inventions from Bench to Bedside

Antonia Stefanov[1] and John G. Flannery[1,2]

[1]Helen Wills Neuroscience Institute, University of California, Berkeley, California 94720, USA

[2]Department of Molecular and Cell Biology, University of California, Berkeley, California 94720, USA

Corresponding author: flannery@berkeley.edu

Blindness due to rod-cone dystrophies is a significant comorbidity and cause of reduced quality of life worldwide. Optogenetics uses adeno-associated viral (AAV) vectors to bypass lost photoreceptors and transfect remnant cell populations of the degenerated retina aiming to restore vision via the ectopic expression of opsins. The optogenetic targeting of retinal ganglion cells (RGCs) has been remarkably successful and several studies have advanced to clinical trials over the recent years. The inner retina and specifically ON bipolar cells represent even more appealing targets due to their intrinsically coded tasks in parallel processing and fine-tuning of visual signals before reaching the output: RGCs. However, present success with pursuing inner and outer retinal cells for optogenetic vision restoration is limited by multiple factors, including AAV tropism, promoter specificity, and retinal morphofunctional remodeling. Here we provide a review of the evolution of optogenetics, its greatest challenges, and solutions from bench to bedside.

In the broadest possible sense, optogenetic technology combines optics, genetics, and bioengineering to study intact, living neural circuits by introducing new genetic information to the target cells and artificially expressing light-sensitive proteins with the purpose of stimulating them by light (Deisseroth et al. 2006; Simunovic et al. 2019).

Evolution refined nature's apparatus for translating light stimuli into electrical signaling —with the aid of photoreceptive neurons expressing light-sensitive proteins—from simple phototaxis into image-forming vision. Mammalian vision is triggered by light entering the eye and activating opsins naturally occurring in the photoreceptors of the retina (i.e., rhodopsin and cone opsins), which bind a retinoid chromophore that changes conformation and thus initiates a chain of molecular events initially in the photoreceptor, later processed in three cellular and two plexiform layers of the neural retina to eventually be conveyed by the optic nerve into the brain. Therefore, a very obvious field that is continuously developing and benefiting from optogenetics today is vision science with a very straightforward aim: vision restoration.

The concept underpinning optogenetic vision restoration in inherited retinal degenera-

Cite this article as *Cold Spring Harb Perspect Med* doi: 10.1101/cshperspect.a041304

tions (IRDs) is to use virus vectors (most commonly at present—adeno-associated virus [AAV]) to deliver opsins into surviving retinal neurons, which normally respond to synaptic transmitter molecules, not photons. Expression of the ectopic, light-sensitive transgene is driven and restricted by cell-specific promoters with the purpose of turning second- and/or third-order neurons into light sensors or rarely to resensitize degenerated, "dormant" photoreceptors.

Here we provide a systematic review of the history and evolution of optogenetics, its greatest challenges, and solutions from preclinical to clinical studies.

OPSINS

There are two broad types of opsins suitable for vision restoration: type 1 or bacterial opsins and type 2 or animal opsins. In addition, there are chemical photoswitches termed PORTLs (photoswitchable orthogonal remotely tethered ligands) that combine a photochromic ligand (typically azobenzene) with a tether, a glutamate molecule, and a covalent attachment "tag" such as SNAP-tag to impart light sensitivity to a G-protein-coupled receptor (GPCR). In this respect, azobenzene-based photoswitches are promising nanoscale tools for neuronal photo stimulation (Broichhagen et al. 2015).

Examples of type 1 opsins are channelrhodopsins (ChRs), halorhodopsins (NpHRs), and archeorhodopsins (Archs). NpHRs are chloride pumps most effectively activated by absorbing light in the yellow spectrum resulting in hyperpolarization of the cell caused by the increased influx of chloride ions. Archs, on the other hand, are light-activated, intra-, or extracellular proton pumps with highest sensitivity to yellow-to-green wavelengths, again resulting in cellular hyperpolarization (Duebel et al. 2015). Finally, ChRs are the only known light-gated ion channels (Lin 2011). The most appealing feature that makes ChRs widely used in optogenetic vision restoration is resistance to photobleaching. Bleaching desensitization refers to the temporary inhibition of phototransduction initiation in rod photoreceptors following exposure to bright light (photolysis) due to the photoisomerization

of the chromophore 11-*cis* retinal into all-*trans* retinal (bleaching product) that remains bound to the apoprotein, opsin. Rod regeneration from bleaching depends on the removal of all-*trans* retinal and the delivery of 11-*cis* retinal to rhodopsin's chromophore binding site (Pepperberg 2003). In ChRs, the covalently bound all-*trans* retinal isomerizes to 13-*cis* retinal hence preventing bleaching, which is a well-known issue with type 2 opsins. ChRs employed in optogenetic vision restoration typically have peak light sensitivities in short wavelength illumination limiting their potential uses in natural environmental settings, where blue light is less abundant than longer wavelength light (Wyszecki and Stiles 1982). Additionally, ocular surfaces and especially ocular media exhibit significant absorbance properties in the blue, short wavelength spectrum (Norren and Vos 1974). Another challenge in using naturally occurring ChRs—and in fact all type 1 opsins—for optogenetic vision restoration is that their light sensitivities are not sufficient for activation in environments with typical ambient light levels. One might think that this challenge is easy to overcome by artificial means, incorporating amplifying or intensifying the light that enters the eye with goggles; however, this solution could pose another threat to the surviving photoreceptors in a patient: phototoxicity. Phototoxicity (type I and II) happens when the eye gets exposed to bright, short-to-medium wavelength light. The difference between the two types lies within exposure time and light intensity: type I phototoxicity is triggered by prolonged exposure, whereas type II phototoxicity is known to affect the retina after a shorter irradiation to more intense light (Ham et al. 1984). Therefore, using high-intensity light of the short wavelength spectrum to activate wild-type ChRs in retinal cells is a cause of significant concern. Today's ChR variants are modern designer proteins with modifications that are shifting their peak sensitivities to longer wavelength light, decreasing the risk of phototoxicity as well as better complementing the distribution of visible light spectra in naturally lit environments. The perfect optogenetic molecule would in fact be able to deliver operational limits that more faithfully mimic human cone vision in commonly encountered light conditions that can range from 10^{-4} (moonless night) to 10^{5} (direct sunlight). Currently though, type 1 opsins provide an operational range that is completely outpaced by the physiological human visual system. However, modern red-shifted designer molecules have allowed the development of devices including light-intensifying goggles, that with minimal risk of phototoxicity are able to modify and adjust the incoming light intensity to match the sensitivity of type 1 opsins (Yue et al. 2016). These devices are also able to modify other stimulus properties like wavelength, as well as spatial and temporal properties. Regarding temporal response characteristics, the ideal optogenetic molecule will function at response kinetics of at least the same order as retinal neurons.

Type 2 or mammalian opsins also have the potential to be used in optogenetic vision restoration. They do in general have higher light sensitivities than type 1 opsins, although high-reaction kinetics is a feature of bacterial opsins that is hard to beat. Quite intriguingly, all type 1 opsins exhibit faster response kinetics than photoreceptors (Busskamp et al. 2010), ~35 msec for dark adapted cones (Hood and Birch 1993a) and ~190 msec for dark adapted rods (Hood and Birch 1993b). Human opsins—melanopsin, rhodopsin, and cone opsins—may also be ectopically expressed in cells surviving photoreceptor loss in IRDs. Human opsins are G-protein-coupled receptors that are presumed to naturally enhance sensitivity by signal amplification. Besides having excellent light sensitivity, these opsins have another major advantage from a therapeutic viewpoint. These proteins are naturally expressed by human tissues and are less likely to be recognized as foreign antigens by the patients' immune system; therefore, these are not anticipated to elicit a significant inflammatory (uveitis) response. Reaction kinetics—especially in melanopsin, which is the slowest known animal opsin (De Silva et al. 2017)—is in fact a painful tradeoff when it comes to choosing from type 1 and 2 opsins in optogenetics. A further issue with type 2 opsins—as mentioned above—is bleaching and recovery happening at a particularly slow rate in rhodopsin, which is a process fundamentally dependent on the retinal pigment epithelium (RPE). It remains unclear whether the RPE will continue to deliver the 11-*cis* retinal chromophore to the retina after the photoreceptors have degenerated. It remains possible that the RPE will down-regulate this function as the photoreceptors are lost. However, the complement of intact photoreceptor outer segments in a healthy retina represents a huge "sink" for 11-*cis* retinal, and in the absence of these cells, the amount of 11-*cis* required for "charging" the optogenetic opsin when expressed in inner retinal neurons should only be a small portion of that required for supplying an intact outer nuclear layer. In addition, a Müller glia–driven cone photopigment recycling pathway (Wang and Kefalov 2011) may be sufficient when it comes to employing cone opsins in optogenetic vision restoration.

VECTORS

AAV vectors are the best studied and most often used gene delivery vectors in optogenetics because of their lack of pathogenicity, extremely low incidence of host genome integration, and long-term episomal persistence in the target tissue/cell.

Current AAV production methods generate titers (>10e13) high enough to be used in human subjects with the small volumes required for intraocular administration (Ferreira et al. 2014). AAV was accidentally discovered in 1965 as a contaminant in an adenovirus preparation and by the 1980s it was recognized and repurposed "from defective virus to effective vector" (Gonçalves 2005). AAV is a dependovirus and without the presence of a helper virus like adenovirus (hence the name) it is unable to replicate, which is another reassurance of its safe application as a vector in human gene therapy. In addition to its natural role as a "helper" virus that requires coinfection with adenovirus for replication, the deletion of the "rep" and "cap" genes from the therapeutic construct further cripple its replication capabilities.

Of the nine naturally occurring AAV serotypes, 12 human and >100 animal AAV capsid variants have been identified to date. While all AAV serotypes are able to infect the RPE, some show tropism toward different retinal cell types (e.g., AAV2, 5, 7–9 are capable of transfecting photoreceptors) (Day et al. 2014), while AAV2 shows a propensity to transfect inner retinal cells (Yin et al. 2011). The RPE may be particularly permissive to AAV transduction from its apical (subretinal) face as these are highly phagocytic epithelia with elaborate apical microvilli and lamellipodia.

Fortunately, opsins are encoded by genes short enough to be packaged into AAV vectors, including the required promoter elements and inverted terminal repeats (ITRs). AAV vectors are known to have a maximum gene packaging capacity of 4.7–5 kb without compromised transduction efficiency and truncated or fragmented genomes (Wu et al. 2010). It has been shown that when a cargo of larger than 5.3 kb was packaged into AAVs, their capacity to transduce targets was significantly reduced, due to a preferential degradation process of oversized vector particles (Grieger and Samulski 2005). Although the same study by Grieger and Samulski found evidence that successful protein expression from overpackaged AAVs with fragmented genomes was possible after the reconstitution of overlapping fragments, this is not an acceptable option for clinical application with strict FDA requirements for complete sequence validation in the clinical grade good manufacturing practice (GMP) vector product. Due to this inconvenient limit in encapsidated genome size, however, it is nearly impossible to apply AAV-based gene therapy to treat a variety of diseases like congenital stationery night blindness type 2A caused by mutations in the *CACNA1F* gene (Carr 1974), which is longer than 35 kb and thus impossible to fit into an AAV capsid. Understandably, there is a great deal of interest in increasing the size of therapeutic transgenes while at the same time benefiting from the numerous advantages of AAV transduction. As a result, a so-called dual AAV vector system has been and is to date under development to address the aforementioned issue (Chamberlain et al. 2016).

ADMINISTRATION

Administration routes of optogenetic therapy carry challenges as well. The neural retina, like any nervous tissue, is extremely compact with small extracellular spaces and outer (OLMs) and inner limiting "membranes" (ILMs) on each side. It should be noted that neither of these structures are true cell membranes, as the ILM is formed by the "end feet" of Müller cells. The ILM is an interface between the retina and the vitreous composed of collagen fibers, glycosaminoglycans, laminin, and fibronectin. The OLM is similarly not a true cell membrane, but a row of junctional complexes formed of Crb1 and Crb2—linking the photoreceptor inner segments and Müller glia and demarking the inner border of the subretinal space. Despite not being "true" cell lipid-bilayer membranes, these structures both constitute barriers restricting viral penetration between retinal cells (Dalkara et al. 2009). Although photoreceptor degeneration significantly reduces retinal thickness, Müller glial hypertrophy creating the so-called "glial seal" only makes permeability more challenging (De Silva et al. 2017).

Two delivery routes have been applied in the eye: intravitreal and subretinal. Intravitreal injection of AAV vectors is the easiest and least invasive way of administration that most ophthalmologists are very competent at performing (Ochakovski et al. 2017). Although intravitreal injection represents the most efficient method of transducing the widest possible retinal area in small laboratory animals, a major limitation in larger animals and human subjects is that achieving a similar transduction efficiency may require AAV injections volumes and titers high enough to induce intraocular inflammation (Simunovic et al. 2019), whereas safe AAV dosing has never been able to produce panretinal transgene expression and was, until recently, still struggling to reach deeper layers of the tissue to access inner retinal neurons, photoreceptors, or the RPE from the vitreous cavity. The latter issue may be addressed by pars plana vitrectomy and surgical peeling of the ILM before AAV injection; however, these procedures require the expertise of vitreoretinal surgeons and may jeopardize surgical outcomes by serious side effects like cataracts (Do et al. 2008), or retinal detachment with a case study reporting a full-thickness macular hole in one patient (Maguire et al. 2008).

Cite this article as *Cold Spring Harb Perspect Med* doi: 10.1101/cshperspect.a041304

Advances in vector design and directed evolution largely contribute to the development of AAV capsid variants that are able to penetrate full retinal depth and reach all layers as well as the RPE via intravitreal administration (Dalkara et al. 2013; Byrne et al. 2020).

Subretinal injection is a feasible alternative to intravitreal administration to access photoreceptors and the RPE. Indeed, it has been the gene delivery route of choice in clinical trials (Ochakovski et al. 2017). The major setback of the procedure is the necessity of a pars plana vitrectomy as well as piercing through the retina with a needle and dispensing the AAV into an artificially detached subretinal space, often described as a bleb. This approach results in retinal damage at the piercing and detachment sites and transgene expression is often restricted to the bleb area. Although iatrogenic retinal detachment is agreed to have a devastating effect on retinal function, it has been shown that spatial vision is swiftly recovered following the procedure. Other visual functions, for example, color matching, were found to be temporarily disturbed as well, which in combination with outer retinal thinning confirmed via optical coherence tomographic (OCT) findings, suggest photoreceptor loss or outer segment shortening in some patients after surgery (Simunovic et al. 2017). Therefore, engineering capsid modifications enabling enhanced retinal penetration of the AAVs from the vitreous cavity would be more favorable. The most effective recombinant AAV serotypes to date deployed in nonhuman primate (NHP) preclinical and human clinical trials are AAV2/2(4YF) (Petrs-Silva et al. 2011) and AAV2.7m8 (Dalkara et al. 2013). However, in vivo–directed evolution of AAVs in NHP retina recently revealed promising, more efficient alternatives (Byrne et al. 2020).

PROMOTERS

The choice of vector serotype, viral capsid modifications exhibiting different tissue and cell tropisms, and the vector delivery routes—with intravitreal injections preferentially targeting ganglion cells, whereas subretinal injections target outer retinal cells and the RPE—are meant to specify therapeutic targets to a certain extent.

Promoters driving ectopic transgene expression can potentially enhance cell-type specificity, although a major advantage of ubiquitous promoters is that they might be able to withstand retinal morphofunctional remodeling caused by retinal degeneration, which is known to largely alter endogenous promoter activity and gene expression (Hackam et al. 2004). Hence, the most straightforward way to transfect the retina is via ubiquitous promoters like the cytomegalovirus (CMV) enhancer/chicken β actin/rabbit β globulin (CAG) promoter, with or without a downstream woodchuck hepatitis virus post-translational regulatory element (WPRE), which is known to improve and increase expression in retinal cells (Patrício et al. 2017).

Photoreceptor degeneration in most IRDs typically progresses in a rod-to-cone pattern, where cone demise is a bystander effect of rod death. However, degenerated cone cells not only remain for almost a year following the complete loss of rods in the rd1 mouse model of early onset, recessive retinitis pigmentosa, but they were also shown to maintain active gene expression, although at altered levels (Narayan et al. 2019). Also, imaging of human patients with advanced IRD revealed degenerated but remnant cone photoreceptors often referenced as dormant cone cells (Wong and Kwok 2016). In theory, cone dormancy enables therapeutic intervention with the optogenetic reactivation of cone photosensitivity using specific promoters like cone arrestin (mCAR and hCAR) or a more efficient chimeric promoter consisting of an enhancer element of inter-photoreceptor retinoid-binding protein promoter and a minimal sequence of the human transducin α-subunit promoter (IRBPe/GNAT2) (Dyka et al. 2014). However, additional treatment might be necessary to improve their viability as cones represent a gradually degenerating cell population.

Retinal ganglion cells (RGCs) are the easiest targets for optogenetics partially because their proximity to the retinal surface makes them intravitreally accessible for most vectors and also because their long-term persistence leaves them unaffected despite retinal degeneration. However, RGCs are third-order neurons, and the majority of visual signal processing is completed prior to them; thus, the extent of vision restoration targeting these cells over second-order neurons is currently being debated and remains unclear. The only deployed and effective RGC-specific promoter to date is represented by the nonselective, panneuronal human synapsin 1 (hSyn1) promoter (Simunovic et al. 2019), stimulating discussions over the necessity of ON-selective promoters.

Visual signal processing first occurs at the level of second-order neurons, including the bipolar cells, referred to as the retina's switchboard by Thomas Euler (Euler et al. 2014). Each of the more than 10 types of bipolar cells plays a distinct role in transforming the photoreceptor input in a unique way, thus creating individual channels that encode stimulus properties including polarity, contrast, temporal profile, and chromatic composition. Finally, the axonal endings of each bipolar cell type systematically stratify at different inner plexiform layer (IPL) strata and by this means provide synaptic input to specific groups of RGCs and amacrine cells. Parallel processing and signal refinement abilities make bipolar cells the most desired targets in optogenetic vision restoration strategies to date. However, present success in bipolar cell targeting is limited by multiple factors including promoter specificity. At present, the most widely used ON bipolar cell-specific promoter is represented by the mGluR6 promoter and its modified, enhanced variants.

Numerous optogenetic preclinical trials have been and are being conducted in murine, canine, and NHP models to date. These may be divided into categories based on the targeted cell population (ubiquitous, photoreceptors, bipolar cells, ganglion cells), the expressed optogenetic proteins (type 1 or 2 opsins), the delivery route, and the capsid variant used. Major studies until 2017 are summarized in Table 1 (Simunovic et al. 2019). Studies and clinical trials published between 2017 and 2022 are listed and summarized in Table 1.

NEW PROMOTERS

Toward the end of 2017, a report was published from the Dalkara laboratory on a new promoter with great potential for optogenetic vision resto-
ration. The new promoter sequence was identified based on the regulatory region of the human γ-synuclein gene (SNCG) granting strong transgene expression in RGCs across species. Intravitreal injections of SNCG-driven channelrhodopsin-Ca^{2+}-permeable channelrhodopsin (CatCh) with green fluorescent protein (GFP) packaged into AAV2 vectors showed panretinal expression and obvious CatCh responses in the retina and cortex of rd1 mice. When injected into NHPs, the same construct resulted in strong expression in perifoveolar ganglion cells that responded strongly to light levels safe for the human eye, even 6 months after injection. With the same vector and plasmid construct, the new SNCG promoter was compared to the ubiquitous CMV promoter with the latter requiring higher activation thresholds and leaving much more unresponsive cells based on multielectrode array (MEA) recordings, suggesting that cell-type-specific promoters are key for the clinical translation of optogenetics (Chaffiol et al. 2017).

Ferrari and colleagues administered intravitreal injections of AAV2-hSyn-ReaChR-mCitrine to target RGCs in rd1 mice as well as AAV2-SNCG-CatCh-GFP in NHPs. Since transgene expression is also present in axons, it is unclear whether RGCs will be responding only to a stimulation area covering their somas and dendrites, or to any stimulation reaching their axons, severely impairing spatial resolution. Using MEAs, they recorded responses of mouse and macaque retinas to random checkerboard patterns after optogenetic treatment and found that transduced RGCs were only sensitive to a small region of the visual space. They then created a simplified model based on this small receptive field, which predicted RGC responses to complex stimuli accurately. From this model, in a simulation, they estimated how the entire light-sensing RGC population would respond to letters of different sizes, similar to a human visual acuity test. Then the maximal acuity expected by a patient could be estimated and the obtained acuity was found to be above the limit of legal blindness (Ferrari et al. 2020).

Developing methods for noninvasive cone targeting led to the identification of a strongly cone-specific promoter—PR1.7—in both

Table 1. A summary of major studies of optogenetic approaches to vision restoration in animal models

Study	Model	Vector	Mode of delivery	Promoter/enhancer	Opsin	Functional estimates	Comments
Ubiquitous promotors							
Bi et al. 2006	Murine rd1	AAV2	Intravitreal (P1 or P60–360)	CAG/WPRE	ChR2	1. Patch clamp 2. MEA 3. VEP	• Light sensitivity estimated from patch clamp recordings • 9/13 eyes demonstrated VEPs • Sensitivity maintained at up to 6 mo
Zhang et al. 2009	Murine rd1	AAV2	Intravitreal (P80)	CMV/WPRE	ChR2 and NpHR	1. Patch clamp 2. MEA	• Light sensitivity estimated from patch clamp recordings • NpHR-expressing cells 20 times less sensitive than ChR2-expressing cells • Sensitivity maintained at up to 4 mo
Tomita et al. 2007	Murine RCS	AAV2	Intravitreal (P300)	CAG	ChR2	1. Electroretinogram 2. Visually evoked cortical potentials	• Chr2 expressed in 28% of RGCs • Expression also seen in the inner plexiform and inner nuclear layers
Tomita et al. 2010	Murine RCS	AAV2	Intravitreal (P180)	CAG	ChR2	1. Visually evoked cortical potentials 2. Behavioral response (optomotor)	• Recovery of visually evoked cortical potentials commencing 2 wk following injection and peaking at 6 wk • Evidence of functional rescue behaviorally at high photopic levels (2.25×10^{15} photon cm^{-2})
Tomita et al. 2014	Murine RCS	AAV2	Intravitreal (age not specified)	CAG	mVChR1	1. Visually evoked cortical potentials at 4 and 12 mo 2. Behavioral response (optomotor)	• Recovery of VEP observed up to 12 mo postinjection
Sato et al. 2017	Murine ChR2-expressing/MNU-induced degeneration	AAV2	Intravitreal (age not specified)	CAG	mVChR1 (+ChR2)	1. Patch clamp recordings 2. ERG 3. VEP	• Coexpression of mVChR1 and Chr2 in 12% of RGCs • Lack of response to longer wavelengths proposed to be due to lack of chromophore in mVChR1/ChR2 coexpressing cells
Lin et al. 2008	Murine rd1	AAV2	Intravitreal (P30)	CMV	OPN4	1. Patch clamping 2. PLR 3. Light avoidance 4. Two AFC visual discrimination	• Light sensitivity estimated from PLR • Sensitivity retained at 11 mo
Liu et al. 2016	Murine rd1	AAV2/8	Subretinal (P30)	CMV	OPN4	1. ERG 2. VEP 3. Light avoidance	• Functional rescue at day 30; none at day 45

Continued

Table 1. *Continued*

Study	Model	Vector	Mode of delivery	Promoter/enhancer	Opsin	Functional estimates	Comments
De Silva et al. 2017	Murine rd1	AAV2/8(Y773F)	Subretinal (P42–45)	CAG/WPRE	OPN4	1. MEA 2. LASER cortical imaging 3. PLR 4. Light avoidance 5. Object recognition test	• Threshold for light sensitivity estimated by MEA • Function retained at up to 13 mo following injection
Photoreceptor-specific promoters							
Busskamp et al. 2010	Murine 1. rd1 2. CNGA3$^{-/-}$/Rho$^{-/-}$ double-knockout	AAV2.1	Subretinal (P53–264)	1. hRHO 2. hRO 3. mCAR	eNpHR	1. Patch clamp 2. MEA 3. VEP 4. Behavior ("dark light box") 5. Optomotor response	• ON, OFF, and ON–OFF RGC responses were demonstrated • Transient and sustained RGC responses preserved • Lateral inhibition and directional selectivity demonstrated • Cortical activity and optomotor responses evident in rd1, but not CNGA3$^{-/-}$/Rho$^{-/-}$ double-knockout mice
Bipolar cell-specific promoters							
Lagali et al. 2008	Murine rd1	Electroporation	Subretinal (P0–1)	mGRM6/SV40	ChR2	1. Patch clamp 2. MEA 3. VEP 4. Behavior ("light-induced locomotion") 5. Optomotor response	• About 7% of ON bipolar cells expressed ChR2 • Threshold estimated by MEA
Doroudchi et al. 2011	Murine 1. rd 2. rd10 3. rd16	AAV8 (capsid mutation Y733F)	Subretinal (P ≅ 56)	mGRM6/SV40	ChR2	1. MEA (P290) 2. Behavior ("water maze task")	• Sustained benefit evident at up to 10 mo • No evidence of a significant local or system immune response • Threshold for light sensitivity estimated by MEA
Cronin et al. 2014	Murine 1. rd1	AAV2/8 or AAV2/8BP2	Subretinal (P = 70)	"4X" mGRM6 (4 enhancer elements)	ChR2	1. MEA (P84–98)	• Transduction efficiency 59% • Electrophysiological responses suggest responses from ON, OFF, and ON–OFF ganglion cells
Macé et al. 2015	Murine rd1	AAV2 (7m8 mutant)	Intravitreal (P = 28–56)	mGRM6/SV40	ChR2	1. MEA (P = 132–324 d) 2. Extracellular cortical recordings (P = 245–346 d) 3. Light-induced locomotory behavior (P > 105 d)	• Threshold estimated by MEA • ON and OFF responses demonstrated • Cortical activity and improvements in visually guided behavior demonstrated
van Wyk et al. 2015	Murine rd1	AAV2 (tyrosine mutant)	Intravitreal and subretinal (P > 168)	mGRM6/SV40/WPRE	mGluR6/OPN4 chimera	1. Patch clamped human embryonic kidney cells 2. Cell-attached recordings from RGCs 3. Whole-cell patch clamp recordings from bipolar cells 4. Intrinsic signal imaging from visual cortex 5. Behavioral assessment (optomotor reflex and water maze)	• Similar efficacy demonstrated for intravitreal and subretinal routes • Expression demonstrated at up to 8 mo • 12% transduction of target ON bipolar cells • Reported sensitivity of transgenic rd1 mice expressing mGluR6/OPN4 similar to transfected mice • Response kinetics similar to native bipolar cells • Responses are "sign inverting"

Reference	Model	Vector	Route	Promoter	Opsin	Assessment	Findings
Cehajic-Kapetanovic et al. 2015	Murine rd1	AAV2/2	Intravitreal (P56–70)	mGRM6 or CAG (i.e., selective and nonselective)	Rho	1. MEA (P112–154) 2. Multielectrode probe recording from LGN 3. Behavioral (light-induced locomotion, simulated predator-induced locomotion)	• Threshold estimated from MEA • Behavioral responses elicited under low photopic illumination levels • Selective expression in bipolar cells results in increased responses at behavioral tests compared to nonselective expression
Gaub et al. 2015	Murine rd1	AAV2/2, 4 YF	Intravitreal (P21–42)	mGRM6	Rho and ChR2 (H134R)	1. MEA (P63–112) 2. VEPs 3. Behavior (light avoidance, modified water maze, and temporal light pattern discrimination)	• Only direct comparison of type 1 and type 2 opsin • Rhodopsin at least 1000 times more sensitive than ChR2 • Firing rate in treated retinas similar to wild-type • ON and OFF RGC responses demonstrated
Ganglion cell-specific promoters							
Thyagarajan et al. 2010	Murine rd1	Chr2 × rd1 cross	NA (cross-bred)	NA (cross-bred)	ChR2	1. MEA 2. Cortical imaging (optical) 3. Behavior (optomotor response, water maze)	• ChR2 expressed in 30%–40% of RGCs • No evidence of functional rescue at behavioral tasks
Sengupta et al. 2016	Murine rd1	AAV2	Intravitreal (P28–35)	hSyn1	ReaChR	1. Patch clamp recordings from RGCs 2. MEA ($P \geq 60$) 3. Cortical responses (extracellular) 4. Behavior (light avoidance)	• Thresholds 1000× below threshold for photochemical damage • Functional responses also recorded from macaque and human RGCs—their temporal response characteristics were preserved (i.e., transient vs. sustained)
Ameline et al. 2017	Canine RPE65	AAV2	Intravitreal following vitrectomy	hSyn1	Chr2 or OPN4	1. MEA (21 mo postinjection)	• No evidence of injection-induced thinning on optical coherence tomography

Table adapted from Simunovic et al. 2019, with permission, from Elsevier © 2019.
(rd) Retinal degeneration, (RCS) Royal College of Surgeons, (MNU) *N*-methyl-*N*-nitrosourea, (CNGA3) α-subunit of the cone cGMP-gated cation channel, (Rho) rhodopsin, (AAV) adeno-associated virus, (P) days postnatal, (CAG) CMV enhancer/chicken β actin/rabbit β globulin, (CMV) cytomegalovirus, (WPRE) Woodchuck hepatitis virus post-translational regulatory element, (hRHO) human rod opsin, (hRO) human red opsin, (mCAR) mouse cone arrestin, (mGRM6) metabotropic glutamate receptor 6, (SV40) simian virus 40, (hSyn1) human synactin 1, (ChR2) channel rhodopsin 2, (OPN4) melanopsin, (eNpHR) halorhodopsin, (ChR2/H134R) humanized channelrhodopsin 2, (OPN4/mGluR6) melanopsin/glutamate receptor chimera, (Rho) rhodopsin, (MEA) multielectrode array, (VEP) visual evoked potential.

healthy and degenerating retinas across species: wild-type and rd10 mice as well as NHPs in vivo and human retinas in vitro (Khabou et al. 2018). Khabou and colleagues used Jaws, a hyperpolarizing microbial opsin (Chuong et al. 2014), to evaluate its potential for optogenetic vision restoration. The intravitreal injection of AAV2-7m8-PR1.7-Jaws-GFP in macaques produced robust and highly cone-specific GFP expression in the foveola and resulted in measurable optogenetic reactivation of cones (Khabou et al. 2018).

Jüttner et al. created a library of 230 AAV-promoter constructs, with synthetic promoters created using four innovative and independent design strategies. They also demonstrated that some of the identified promoters specifically target neuronal and glial cell types in the murine and NHP retina in vivo and in the human retina in vitro, applications for recording and stimulation, as well as the intersectional and combinatorial labeling of cell types (Jüttner et al. 2019).

Hulliger and colleagues are "Empowering retinal gene therapy with a specific promoter for human rod and cone ON bipolar cells." They describe the design and functional assessment of 770En_454P(hGRM6), a human GRM6 gene-derived, short promoter that drives strong and specific expression in the ON bipolar cells of the human retina. 770En_454P(hGRM6)-driven medium wavelength cone opsin (MW-opsin) expression in ON bipolar cells resulted in lasting restoration of the optomotor reflex in rd1 mice (Hulliger et al. 2020).

VECTOR DEVELOPMENT

Maddalena and colleagues addressed another issue in AAV-based gene therapy: packaging capacity. The known 5 kb limit in transfer capacity can be expanded to about 9 kb using dual AAV vectors, although this strategy would still not enable effective treatment of certain types of Usher or Alström syndromes caused by mutations in very large genes. To overcome this limitation, they have generated a triple AAV vector system with a maximal transfer capacity of about 14 kb (Maddalena et al. 2018).

Dias and colleagues compared intravitreally administered AAV transfection and penetration efficacy in mice versus rats when adjuvant pharmacological agents are applied to enhance the preservation and penetration of viral particles. They used wild-type AAV2 and recombinant AAV2 with a quadruple Y-F mutation carrying the ubiquitous CBA promoter driving GFP expression and applied tyrosine kinase inhibitors like imatinib and genistein, which were highly effective and promoted even outer retinal transgene expression in mice, but not in rats. They conclude that eye size and ILM differences in mice versus rats are too large to achieve similar results in the two species and thus further vector and administration strategy development is needed (Dias et al. 2019).

AAV variant development via in vivo–directed evolution created a replication-incompetent AAV library, guided by deep sequencing and controlled by GFP barcoded capsids that went through six rounds of in vivo secondary selection in primates (Byrne et al. 2020). The selection process involved intravitreal administration of the library and recovery of genomes from the outer retina followed by next-generation sequencing of each round. Directed evolution resulted in vectors with redirected tropism to the outer retina and increased gene delivery to retinal cells expanding the pool of effective AAV vectors for primate retina and potentially enabling less invasive administration of gene therapy in human patients (Byrne et al. 2020).

NEW OPTOGENETIC PROTEINS

Retinitis pigmentosa causes degeneration of photoreceptors, whereas other retinal cells survive. It has been shown that the expression of light-activated signaling proteins in those surviving cells could restore vision. Berry et al. used a retinal G-protein-coupled receptor, mGluR2, which was chemically engineered to respond to light. In RGCs of rd1 mice, photoswitch-charged mGluR2 ("SNAG-mGluR2") evoked robust OFF responses to light, but not in wild-type retinas, suggesting selectivity for RGCs that have lost photoreceptor input. SNAG-mGluR2 enabled animals to discriminate between high-contrast patterns. Simultaneous viral delivery of the inhibitory SNAG-mGluR2 and excitatory light-activated ionotropic glutamate receptor LiGluR restored ON, OFF, and ON–OFF light responses and improved visual acuity (Berry et al. 2017).

Wright and colleagues have developed the so-called multicharacteristic opsin (MCO) to restore visually guided behavior as shown via the radial water maze test in rd10 mice using intravitreal AAV delivery and the mGluR6 promoter (Wright et al. 2017). Batabyal et al. used the same AAV2-mGluR6-MCO-mCherry construct to intravitreally inject rd10 mice and reported that MCO was highly sensitive and functional in ambient light, reporter expression was detectable 6 mo after injection, and water maze and optomotor assays showed significant changes 8 wk postinjection (Batabyal et al. 2021). Intravitreal injections of the construct in wild-type dogs produced transgene expression in the inner nuclear layer with no detectable inflammatory response in the dog retina. The virus vector was secreted and cleared from the body via urine and feces in about 3–13 wk postinjection. Moreover, intravitreal injection of AAV-MCO resulted in a few off-target expressions in the mesenteric lymph node, liver, spleen, and testis. The group concluded that AAV2-mGluR6-MCO-mCherry gene therapy is safe (Tchedre et al. 2021). MCO is currently being tested in two first-in-human clinical trials.

Ganjawala et al. reported that the optimization of the kinetics of a recently described ChR variant resulted in the identification of two highly light-sensitive *Chloromonas oogama* ChR mutants: CoChR-L112C and CoChR-H94E/L112C/K264T. C57Bl6 and TKO (Opn4$^{-/-}$Gnat1$^{-/-}$Cnga3$^{-/-}$ triple-knockout) mice received intraocular injections of AAV2 carrying the CoChR mutants under control of the CAG promoter. The improved light sensitivity was confirmed by ex vivo electrophysiological recordings of the AAV transfected retina. Also, the CoChR mutants were found to restore the optomotor reflex in ambient light conditions, eliminating a major setback in ChR-based optogenetic vision restoration (Ganjawala et al. 2019).

Lu and coworkers compared the CAG promoter to an improved mGluR6 promoter (In4s-In3-200En-mGluR500P [Lu et al. 2016]) by driving CoChR-GFP expression using the AAV2.7m8-Y444F vector in a mouse model of retinal degeneration. They reported that, based on MEA recordings, pupillary light response, and optomotor tests, CAG promoter-driven CoChR expression restored higher light and contrast sensitivity to the degenerated mouse retina (Lu et al. 2020).

Optogenetic strategies are restricted by either low light sensitivity or slow kinetics and lack adaptation to changes in ambient light. Berry et al. found that the mammalian MW-opsin under control of the RGC-specific hSyn promoter delivered intravitreally via AAV2/2(4YF) conquers these limitations and is able to grant visually guided behavior in dim light conditions. MW-opsin allows rd1 mice to discriminate temporal and spatial light patterns displayed on an LCD screen, exhibits adaptation to increments and decrements in ambient light, and restores novel object exploration in an open field arena providing the kinetics, sensitivity, and adaptation needed to restore patterned vision (Berry et al. 2019).

McClements et al. reported successful expression of rod and cone opsin in ON bipolar cells of the rd1 retina via both subretinal and intravitreal delivery routes when using the well-known 4xGrm6 promoter and various AAV capsid variants: AAV2.4YF, AAV8.BP2, and AAV2.7m8 (McClements et al. 2021).

ChrimsonR

Gauvain and colleagues describe the selection of an optogenetic construct in NHPs as groundwork for an ongoing clinical trial (reference number was not mentioned) testing AAV2.7m8-ChR-tdTomato in retinitis pigmentosa patients. They showed that the AAV2.7m8 vector had a higher transfection efficacy than AAV2 in RGCs and that ChrimsonR fused to tdTomato was expressed more powerfully than ChrimsonR alone. The tested vector doses transfected robust numbers of RGCs in the perifovea, with no significant inflammation. After recording RGC responses, they estimated a visual acuity of 20/249, above the level of legal blindness (20/400) (Gauvain et al. 2021).

Chaffiol et al. demonstrated that a single intravitreal injection of AAV2.7m8-CAG-ChrimsonR-tdTomato can efficiently target perifoveal RGCs and, 20 mo after injection, optogene expression and cortical visually evoked potentials were still detectable and sufficient in macaques (Chaffiol et al. 2022). ChrimsonR is currently being tested in a clinical trial.

NEW METHODS

McGregor et al. reported that AAV2-CAG-tdTomato-ChrimsonR and AAV2-CAG-GCaMP6s coinfection enables the combination of adaptive optics ophthalmoscopy with calcium imaging to optically record optogenetically restored RGC activity in the fovea of the living primate. This in vivo imaging method could be combined with any gene therapy to reduce the number of primates needed to evaluate restored retinal activity, while maximizing translational benefit by using an appropriate preclinical model of the human visual system (McGregor et al. 2020).

Gilhooley and colleagues compared two optogenetic tools: mammalian melanopsin (hOPN4) and microbial red-shifted channelrhodopsin (ReaChR) expressed within RGCs versus (mainly) bipolar cells in the degenerating retina. Constructs packaged into AAV2/2(quadY-F) were administered intravitreally into Cre/lox transgenic mice where expression was restricted only to cells expressing the Cre recombinase enzyme—target cell populations dominated by ON bipolar cells via floxed hOPN4 gene in L7-Cre mice or RGCs via floxed hOPN4 in Grik4-Cre mice—and was compared with nontargeted delivery using the CBA promoter. In summary, they found that bipolar-targeted optogenetic tools produced faster kinetics and flatter intensity-response curves compared with nontargeted or RGC-targeted tools. They concluded that both mammalian and microbial opsins granted better results when targeted to bipolar cells and thus bipolar cell targeting for vision restoration in IRDs has obvious advantages over RGC targeting (Gilhooley et al. 2022).

DOG MODEL

Nikonov and coworkers demonstrated restoration of retinal responses and partial restoration of vision in the rod-cone dystrophy 1 (Rcd1) dog model of retinitis pigmentosa after unilateral subretinal injection of the AAV9 vector, ensuring cone-specific expression by including the chimeric antigen receptor (CAR) promoter to drive the enhanced version of the optogenetic gene eNpHR, a light-gated hyperpolarizing chloride pump belonging to the halorhodopsin family (Nikonov et al. 2022).

ETHICS

Harris and Gilbert (2022) emphasize the importance of fair treatment and informed consent of patient volunteers and raise ethical issues to be resolved in high-profile, first-in-human clinical trials.

CLINICAL TRIALS

Clinical trials of optogenetics are underway.

Nanoscope Therapeutics' product-vMCO-010, also known as AAV-delivered multicharacteristic opsin, is being tested in a phase 1 and 2 dose escalation study and a phase 2 efficacy and safety study: NCT04945772, NCT04919473.

In September 2021, GenSight announced positive results regarding safety of GS030 in human patients with retinitis pigmentosa. GS030 was delivered intravitreally using AAV2 carrying ChrimsonR targeting RGCs (NCT03326336).

A phase 1/2 trial for advanced retinitis pigmentosa is testing ChR as product RST-001 by RetroSense Therapeutics with an estimated completion date of April 2035.

MEASURES OF VISUAL ACUITY IN PRECLINICAL OPTOGENETIC STUDIES

The optomotor reflex test (OptoMotry) is commonly used for behavioral visual acuity assessment in the field of optogenetic vision restoration. Visual acuity by definition is a measure of ability to differentiate and recognize shapes and details of environmental objects at a given distance. It has multiple components, including contrast sensitivity (stationary and dynamic), color vision, image vision, depth perception, and visual memory. The optomotor reflex is the involuntary movement of the eyes and head in the direction of horizontally moving environmental object(s). In testing mice, the phenomenon relies on the proper functioning of horizontal cells (contrast sensitivity) and direction selective ganglion cells (horizontal motion), satisfying only one component of visual acuity as a collective term. Therefore, OptoMotry should not be the only means of visual acuity testing. Instead, we suggest the use of the following series of behavioral assays:

1. Light-dark paradigm or photophobia test to confirm light perception (Bourin and Hascoët 2003),

2. OptoMotry to confirm dynamic contrast sensitivity (using colored background lighting can provide information on color contrast sensitivity) (Abdeljalil et al. 2005),

3. Open field and object exploration test for image vision (Berry et al. 2019),

4. Visual cliff test for depth perception (binocular vision) (Fox 1965), and

5. Water maze test or the two-chamber active avoidance test for contrast sensitivity and visual memory (Frick et al. 2000; Berry et al. 2019).

The summarized data from these five tests should be used to interpret the extent of restored (or missing) visual acuity and be used as a standard for all laboratories to adhere to in the future allowing the comparison of results originating from laboratories around the world.

CONCLUDING REMARKS

IRDs are the leading cause of blindness and visual impairment, affecting between 1 in 3000–5000 individuals worldwide. Gene therapy might be a solution for some patients; however, it is not applicable to all known genotypes or to patients with advanced disease and unknown genotypes. Optogenetics proposes genotype-independent

vision restoration, and unlike electronic retinal implants, it offers advantages in sensitivity, retinal area, and precision. Experiments in animal models confirm that the choice between type 1 versus type 2 opsins comes with a tradeoff of sensitivity versus reaction kinetics. Targeting interneurons might restore higher acuity vision than output neurons and using cell-specific promoters may be more advantageous than generic ones. Furthermore, many outstanding questions remain, including the optimal vector and surgical approach of delivery. Nevertheless, preclinical trials of optogenetics for vision restoration are promising and the results of the first phase 1/2 trials in humans are awaited.

REFERENCES

Abdeljalil J, Hamid M, Abdel-Mouttalib O, Stéphane R, Raymond R, Johan A, José S, Pierre C, Serge P. 2005. The optomotor response: a robust first-line visual screening method for mice. *Vision Res* **45:** 1439–1446. doi:10.1016/j.visres.2004.12.015

Ameline B, Tshilenge KT, Weber M, Biget M, Libeau L, Caplette R, Mendes-Madeira A, Provost N, Guihal C, Picaud S, et al. 2017. Long-term expression of melanopsin and channelrhodopsin causes no gross alterations in the dystrophic dog retina. *Gene Ther* **24:** 735–741. doi:10.1038/gt.2017.63

Batabyal S, Gajjeraman S, Pradhan S, Bhattacharya S, Wright W, Mohanty S. 2021. Sensitization of ON-bipolar cells with ambient light activatable multi-characteristic opsin rescues vision in mice. *Gene Ther* **28:** 162–176. doi:10.1038/s41434-020-00200-2

Berry MH, Holt A, Levitz J, Broichhagen J, Gaub BM, Visel M, Stanley C, Aghi K, Kim YJ, Cao K, et al. 2017. Restoration of patterned vision with an engineered photoactivatable G protein-coupled receptor. *Nat Commun* **8:** 1–12. doi:10.1038/s41467-017-01990-7

Berry MH, Holt A, Salari A, Veit J, Visel M, Levitz J, Aghi K, Gaub BM, Sivyer B, Flannery JG, et al. 2019. Restoration of high-sensitivity and adapting vision with a cone opsin. *Nat Commun* **10:** 1221. doi:10.1038/s41467-019-09124-x

Bi A, Cui J, Ma YP, Olshevskaya E, Pu M, Dizhoor AM, Pan ZH. 2006. Ectopic expression of a microbial-type rhodopsin restores visual responses in mice with photoreceptor degeneration. *Neuron* **50:** 23–33. doi:10.1016/j.neuron.2006.02.026

Bourin M, Hascoët M. 2003. The mouse light/dark box test. *Eur J Pharmacol* **463:** 55–65. doi:10.1016/S0014-2999(03)01274-3

Broichhagen J, Damijonaitis A, Levitz J, Sokol KR, Leippe P, Konrad D, Isacoff EY, Trauner D. 2015. Orthogonal optical control of a G protein-coupled receptor with a SNAP-tethered photochromic ligand. *ACS Cent Sci* **1:** 383–393. doi:10.1021/acscentsci.5b00260

Busskamp V, Duebel J, Balya D, Fradot M, Viney TJ, Siegert S, Groner AC, Cabuy E, Forster V, Seeliger M, et al. 2010. Genetic reactivation of cone photoreceptors restores visual responses in retinitis pigmentosa. *Science* **329:** 413–417. doi:10.1126/science.1190897

Byrne LC, Day TP, Visel M, Strazzeri JA, Fortuny C, Dalkara D, Merigan WH, Schaffer DV, Flannery JG. 2020. In vivo-directed evolution of adeno-associated virus in the primate retina. *JCI Insight* **5:** e134112. doi:10.1172/jci.insight.135112

Carr RE. 1974. Congenital stationary nightblindness. *Trans Am Ophthalmol Soc* **72:** 448–487.

Cehajic-Kapetanovic J, Eleftheriou C, Allen AE, Milosavljevic N, Pienaar A, Bedford R, Davis KE, Bishop PN, Lucas RJ. 2015. Restoration of vision with ectopic expression of human rod opsin. *Curr Biol* **25:** 2111–2122. doi:10.1016/j.cub.2015.07.029

Chaffiol A, Caplette R, Jaillard C, Brazhnikova E, Desrosiers M, Dubus E, Duhamel L, Macé E, Marré O, Benoit P, et al. 2017. A new promoter allows optogenetic vision restoration with enhanced sensitivity in macaque retina. *Mol Ther* **25:** 2546–2560. doi:10.1016/j.ymthe.2017.07.011

Chaffiol A, Provansal M, Joffrois C, Blaize K, Labernede G, Goulet R, Burban E, Brazhnikova E, Duebel J, Pouget P, et al. 2022. In vivo optogenetic stimulation of the primate retina activates the visual cortex after long-term transduction. *Mol Ther Methods Clin Dev* **24:** 1–10. doi:10.1016/j.omtm.2021.11.009

Chamberlain K, Riyad JM, Weber T. 2016. Expressing transgenes that exceed the packaging capacity of adeno-associated virus capsids. *Hum Gene Ther Methods* **27:** 1–12. doi:10.1089/hgtb.2015.140

Chuong AS, Miri ML, Busskamp V, Matthews GAC, Acker LC, Sørensen AT, Young A, Klapoetke NC, Henninger MA, Kodandaramaiah SB, et al. 2014. Noninvasive optical inhibition with a red-shifted microbial rhodopsin. *Nat Neurosci* **17:** 1123–1129. doi:10.1038/nn.3752

Cronin T, Vandenberghe LH, Hantz P, Juttner J, Reimann A, Kacsó AE, Huckfeldt RM, Busskamp V, Kohler H, Lagali PS, et al. 2014. Efficient transduction and optogenetic stimulation of retinal bipolar cells by a synthetic adeno-associated virus capsid and promoter. *EMBO Mol Med* **6:** 1175–1190. doi:10.15252/emmm.201404077

Dalkara D, Kolstad KD, Caporale N, Visel M, Klimczak RR, Schaffer DV, Flannery JG. 2009. Inner limiting membrane barriers to AAV-mediated retinal transduction from the vitreous. *Mol Ther* **17:** 2096–2102. doi:10.1038/mt.2009.181

Dalkara D, Byrne LC, Klimczak RR, Visel M, Yin L, Merigan WH, Flannery JG, Schaffer DV. 2013. In vivo-directed evolution of a new adeno-associated virus for therapeutic outer retinal gene delivery from the vitreous. *Sci Transl Med* **5:** 189ra76. doi:10.1126/scitranslmed.3005708

Day TP, Byrne LC, Schaffer DV, Flannery JG. 2014. Advances in AAV vector development for gene therapy in the retina. *Adv Exp Med Biol* **801:** 687–693. doi:10.1007/978-1-4614-3209-8_86

De Silva SR, Barnard AR, Hughes S, Tam SKE, Martin C, Singh MS, Barnea-Cramer AO, McClements ME, During MJ, Peirson SN, et al. 2017. Long-term restoration of visual function in end-stage retinal degeneration using subretinal human melanopsin gene therapy. *Proc Natl Acad Sci* **114:** 11211–11216. doi:10.1073/pnas.1701589114

Dias MS, Araujo VG, Vasconcelos T, Li Q, Hauswirth WW, Linden R, Petrs-Silva H. 2019. Retina transduction by rAAV2 after intravitreal injection: comparison between mouse and rat. *Gene Ther* **26:** 479–490. doi:10.1038/s41434-019-0100-9

Deisseroth K, Feng G, Majewska AK, Miesenböck G, Ting A, Schnitzer MJ. 2006. Next-generation optical technologies for illuminating genetically targeted brain circuits. *J Neurosci* **26:** 10380–10386. doi:10.1523/JNEUROSCI.3863-06.2006

Do DV, Hawkins B, Gichuhi S, Vedula SS. 2008. Surgery for post-vitrectomy cataract. *Cochrane Database Syst Rev* **3:** CD006366. doi:10.1002/14651858.CD006366.pub2

Doroudchi MM, Greenberg KP, Liu J, Silka KA, Boyden ES, Lockridge JA, Arman AC, Janani R, Boye SE, Boye SL, et al. 2011. Virally delivered channelrhodopsin-2 safely and effectively restores visual function in multiple mouse models of blindness. *Mol Ther* **19:** 1220–1229. doi:10.1038/mt.2011.69

Duebel J, Marazova K, Sahel J-A. 2015. Optogenetics. *Curr Opin Ophthalmol* **26:** 226–232. doi:10.1097/ICU.0000000000000140

Dyka FM, Boye SL, Ryals RC, Chiodo VA, Boye SE, Hauswirth WW. 2014. Cone specific promoter for use in gene therapy of retinal degenerative diseases. *Adv Exp Med Biol* **801:** 695–701. doi:10.1007/978-1-4614-3209-8_87

Euler T, Haverkamp S, Schubert T, Baden T. 2014. Retinal bipolar cells: elementary building blocks of vision. *Nat Rev Neurosci* **15:** 507–519. doi:10.1038/nrn3783

Ferrari U, Deny S, Sengupta A, Caplette R, Trapani F, Sahel JA, Dalkara D, Picaud S, Duebel J, Marre O. 2020. Towards optogenetic vision restoration with high resolution. *PLoS Comput Biol* **16:** e1007857. doi:10.1371/journal.pcbi.1007857

Ferreira V, Petry H, Salmon F. 2014. Immune responses to AAV-vectors, the Glybera example from bench to bedside. *Front Immunol* **5:** 82. doi:10.3389/fimmu.2014.00082

Fox MW. 1965. The visual cliff test for the study of visual depth perception in the mouse. *Anim Behav* **13:** 232–233. doi:10.1016/0003-3472(65)90040-0

Frick KM, Stillner ET, Berger-Sweeney J. 2000. Mice are not little rats: Species differences in a one-day water maze task. *Neuroreport* **11:** 3461–3465. doi:10.1097/00001756-200011090-00013

Ganjawala TH, Lu Q, Fenner MD, Abrams GW, Pan ZH. 2019. Improved CoChR variants restore visual acuity and contrast sensitivity in a mouse model of blindness under ambient light conditions. *Mol Ther* **27:** 1195–1205. doi:10.1016/j.ymthe.2019.04.002

Gaub BM, Berry MH, Holt AE, Isacoff EY, Flannery JG. 2015. Optogenetic vision restoration using rhodopsin for enhanced sensitivity. *Mol Ther* **23:** 1562–1571. doi:10.1038/mt.2015.121

Gauvain G, Akolkar H, Chaffiol A, Arcizet F, Khoei MA, Desrosiers M, Jaillard C, Caplette R, Marre O, Bertin S, et al. 2021. Optogenetic therapy: high spatiotemporal resolution and pattern discrimination compatible with vision restoration in non-human primates. *Commun Biol* **4:** 125. doi:10.1038/s42003-020-01594-w

Cite this article as *Cold Spring Harb Perspect Med* doi: 10.1101/cshperspect.a041304

Gilhooley MJ, Lindner M, Palumaa T, Hughes S, Peirson SN, Hankins MW. 2022. A systematic comparison of optogenetic approaches to visual restoration. *Mol Ther Methods Clin Dev* 25: 111–123. doi:10.1016/j.omtm.2022.03.003

Gonçalves MAFV. 2005. Adeno-associated virus: from defective virus to effective vector. *Virol J* 2: 43. doi:10.1186/1743-422X-2-43

Grieger JC, Samulski RJ. 2005. Packaging capacity of adeno-associated virus serotypes: impact of larger genomes on infectivity and postentry steps. *J Virol* 79: 9933–9944. doi:10.1128/JVI.79.15.9933-9944.2005

Hackam AS, Strom R, Liu D, Qian J, Wang C, Otteson D, Gunatilaka T, Farkas RH, Chowers I, Kageyama M, et al. 2004. Identification of gene expression changes associated with the progression of retinal degeneration in the rd1 mouse. *Invest Ophthalmol Vis Sci* 45: 2929–2942. doi:10.1167/iovs.03-1184

Ham WTJ, Mueller HA, Ruffolo JJJ, Millen JE, Cleary SF, Guerry RK, Guerry D 3rd. 1984. Basic mechanisms underlying the production of photochemical lesions in the mammalian retina. *Curr Eye Res* 3: 165–174. doi:10.3109/02713688408997198

Harris AR, Gilbert F. 2022. Restoring vision using optogenetics without being blind to the risks. *Graefes Arch Clin Exp Ophthalmol* 260: 41–45. doi:10.1007/s00417-021-05477-6

Hood DC, Birch DG. 1993a. Human cone receptor activity: the leading edge of the a-wave and models of receptor activity. *Vis Neurosci* 10: 857–871. doi:10.1017/s0952523800006076

Hood DC, Birch DG. 1993b. Light adaptation of human rod receptors: the leading edge of the human a-wave and models of rod receptor activity. *Vision Res* 33: 1605–1618. doi:10.1016/0042-6989(93)90027-t

Hulliger EC, Hostettler SM, Kleinlogel S. 2020. Empowering retinal gene therapy with a specific promoter for human rod and cone ON-bipolar cells. *Mol Ther Methods Clin Dev* 17: 505–519. doi:10.1016/j.omtm.2020.03.003

Jüttner J, Szabo A, Gross-Scherf B, Morikawa RK, Rompani SB, Hantz P, Szikra T, Esposti F, Cowan CS, Bharioke A, et al. 2019. Targeting neuronal and glial cell types with synthetic promoter AAVs in mice, non-human primates and humans. *Nat Neurosci* 22: 1345–1356. doi:10.1038/s41593-019-0431-2

Khabou H, Garita-Hernandez M, Chaffiol A, Reichman S, Jaillard C, Brazhnikova E, Bertin S, Forster V, Desrosiers M, Winckler C, et al. 2018. Noninvasive gene delivery to foveal cones for vision restoration. *JCI Insight* 3: e96029. doi:10.1172/jci.insight.96029

Lagali PS, Balya D, Awatramani GB, Münch TA, Kim DS, Busskamp V, Cepko CL, Roska B. 2008. Light-activated channels targeted to ON bipolar cells restore visual function in retinal degeneration. *Nat Neurosci* 11: 667–675. doi:10.1038/nn.2117

Lin JY. 2011. A user's guide to channelrhodopsin variants: features, limitations and future developments. *Exp Physiol* 96: 19–25. doi:10.1113/expphysiol.2009.051961

Lin B, Koizumi A, Tanaka N, Panda S, Masland RH. 2008. Restoration of visual function in retinal degeneration mice by ectopic expression of melanopsin. *Proc Natl Acad Sci* 105: 16009–16014. doi:10.1073/pnas.0806114105

Liu MM, Dai JM, Liu WY, Zhao CJ, Lin B, Yin ZQ. 2016. Human melanopsin-AAV2/8 transfection to retina transiently restores visual function in rd1 mice. *Int J Ophthalmol* 9: 655–661.

Lu Q, Ganjawala TH, Ivanova E, Cheng JG, Troilo D, Pan ZH. 2016. AAV-mediated transduction and targeting of retinal bipolar cells with improved mGluR6 promoters in rodents and primates. *Gene Ther* 23: 680–689. doi:10.1038/gt.2016.42

Lu Q, Ganjawala TH, Krstevski A, Abrams GW, Pan ZH. 2020. Comparison of AAV-mediated optogenetic vision restoration between retinal ganglion cell expression and ON bipolar cell targeting. *Mol Ther Methods Clin Dev* 18: 15–23. doi:10.1016/j.omtm.2020.05.009

Macé E, Caplette R, Marre O, Sengupta A, Chaffiol A, Barbe P, Desrosiers M, Bamberg E, Sahel JA, Picaud S, et al. 2015. Targeting channelrhodopsin-2 to ON-bipolar cells with vitreally administered AAV restores ON and OFF visual responses in blind mice. *Mol Ther* 23: 7–16. doi:10.1038/mt.2014.154

Maddalena A, Tornabene P, Tiberi P, Minopoli R, Manfredi A, Mutarelli M, Rossi S, Simonelli F, Naggert JK, Cacchiarelli D, et al. 2018. Triple vectors expand AAV transfer capacity in the retina. *Mol Ther* 26: 524–541. doi:10.1016/j.ymthe.2017.11.019

Maguire AM, Simonelli F, Pierce EA, Pugh EN Jr, Mingozzi F, Bennicelli J, Banfi S, Marshall KA, Testa F, Surace EM, et al. 2008. Safety and efficacy of gene transfer for Leber's congenital amaurosis. *New Engl J Med* 358: 2240–2248. doi:10.1056/NEJMoa0802315

McClements ME, Staurenghi F, Visel M, Flannery JG, MacLaren RE, Cehajic-Kapetanovic J. 2021. AAV induced expression of human rod and cone opsin in bipolar cells of a mouse model of retinal degeneration. *Biomed Res Int* 2021: 1–8. doi:10.1155/2021/4014797

McGregor JE, Godat T, Dhakal KR, Parkins K, Strazzeri JM, Bateman BA, Fisher WS, Williams DR, Merigan WH. 2020. Optogenetic restoration of retinal ganglion cell activity in the living primate. *Nat Commun* 11: 1703. doi:10.1038/s41467-020-15317-6

Narayan DS, Ao J, Wood JPM, Casson RJ, Chidlow G. 2019. Spatio-temporal characterization of S- and M/L-cone degeneration in the Rd1 mouse model of retinitis pigmentosa. *BMC Neurosci* 20: 46. doi:10.1186/s12868-019-0528-2

Nikonov S, Aravand P, Lyubarsky A, Nikonov R, Luo AJ, Wei Z, Maguire AM, Phelps NT, Shpylchak I, Willet K, et al. 2022. Restoration of vision and retinal responses after adeno-associated virus–mediated optogenetic therapy in blind dogs. *Trans Vis Sci Technol* 11: 24. doi:10.1167/tvst.11.5.24

Norren DV, Vos JJ. 1974. Spectral transmission of the human ocular media. *Vision Res* 14: 1237–1244. doi:10.1016/0042-6989(74)90222-3

Ochakovski GA, Bartz-Schmidt KU, Fischer MD. 2017. Retinal gene therapy: surgical vector delivery in the translation to clinical trials. *Front Neurosci* 11: 174. doi:10.3389/fnins.2017.00174

Patrício MI, Barnard AR, Orlans HO, McClements ME, MacLaren RE. 2017. Inclusion of the woodchuck hepatitis virus posttranscriptional regulatory element enhances AAV$_2$-driven transduction of mouse and human retina.

Mol Ther Nucleic Acids **6**: 198–208. doi:10.1016/j.omtn .2016.12.006

Pepperberg DR. 2003. Bleaching desensitization: background and current challenges. *Vision Res* **43**: 3011–3019. doi:10.1016/S0042-6989(03)00484-X

Petrs-Silva H, Dinculescu A, Li Q, Deng WT, Pang JJ, Min SH, Chiodo V, Neeley AW, Govindasamy L, Bennett A, et al. 2011. Novel properties of tyrosine-mutant AAV2 vectors in the mouse retina. *Mol Ther* **19**: 293–301. doi:10 .1038/mt.2010.234

Sato M, Sugano E, Tabata K, Sannohe K, Watanabe Y, Ozaki T, Tamai M, Tomita H. 2017. Visual responses of photoreceptor-degenerated rats expressing two different types of channelrhodopsin genes. *Sci Rep* **7**: 41210. doi:10.1038/ srep41210

Sengupta A, Chaffiol A, Macé E, Caplette R, Desrosiers M, Lampič M, Forster V, Marre O, Lin JY, Sahel JA, et al. 2016. Red-shifted channelrhodopsin stimulation restores light responses in blind mice, macaque retina, and human retina. *EMBO Mol Med* **8**: 1248–1264. doi:10.15252/ emmm.201505699

Simunovic MP, Xue K, Jolly JK, MacLaren RE. 2017. Structural and functional recovery following limited iatrogenic macular detachment for retinal gene therapy. *JAMA Ophthalmol* **135**: 234–241. doi:10.1001/jamaophthalmol .2016.5630

Simunovic MP, Shen W, Lin JY, Protti DA, Lisowski L, Gillies MC. 2019. Optogenetic approaches to vision restoration. *Exp Eye Res* **178**: 15–26. doi:10.1016/j.exer.2018.09.003

Tchedre KT, Batabyal S, Galicia M, Narcisse D, Mustafi SM, Ayyagari A, Chavala S, Mohanty SK. 2021. Biodistribution of adeno-associated virus type 2 carrying multi-characteristic opsin in dogs following intravitreal injection. *J Cell Mol Med* **25**: 8676–8686. doi:10.1111/jcmm.16823

Thyagarajan S, van Wyk M, Lehmann K, Lowel S, Feng G, Wassle H. 2010. Visual function in mice with photoreceptor degeneration and transgenic expression of channelrhodopsin 2 in ganglion cells. *J Neurosci* **30**: 8745–8758. doi:10.1523/JNEUROSCI.4417-09.2010

Tomita H, Sugano E, Yawo H, Ishizuka T, Isago H, Narikawa S, Kügler S, Tamai M. 2007. Restoration of visual response in aged dystrophic RCS rats using AAV-mediated channelopsin-2 gene transfer. *Invest Ophthalmol Vis Sci* **48**: 3821–3826. doi:10.1167/iovs.06-1501

Tomita H, Sugano E, Isago H, Hiroi T, Wang Z, Ohta E, Tamai M. 2010. Channelrhodopsin-2 gene transduced into retinal ganglion cells restores functional vision in genetically blind rats. *Exp Eye Res* **90**: 429–436. doi:10 .1016/j.exer.2009.12.006

Tomita H, Sugano E, Murayama N, Ozaki T, Nishiyama F, Tabata K, Takahashi M, Saito T, Tamai M. 2014. Restoration of the majority of the visual spectrum by using modified volvox channelrhodopsin-1. *Mol Ther* **22**: 1434–1440. doi:10.1038/mt.2014.81

van Wyk M, Pielecka-Fortuna J, Löwel S, Kleinlogel S. 2015. Restoring the ON switch in blind retinas: opto-mGluR6, a next-generation, cell-tailored optogenetic tool. *PLoS Biol* **13**: e1002143. doi:10.1371/journal.pbio.1002143

Wang J-S, Kefalov VJ. 2011. The cone-specific visual cycle. *Prog Retin Eye Res* **30**: 115–128. doi:10.1016/j.preteyeres .2010.11.001

Wong F, Kwok SY. 2016. The survival of cone photoreceptors in retinitis pigmentosa. *JAMA Ophthalmol* **134**: 249–250. doi:10.1001/jamaophthalmol.2015.5490

Wright W, Gajjeraman S, Batabyal S, Pradhan S, Bhattacharya S, Mahapatra V, Tripathy A, Mohanty S. 2017. Restoring vision in mice with retinal degeneration using multicharacteristic opsin. *Neurophotonics* **4**: 041505.

Wu Z, Yang H, Colosi P. 2010. Effect of genome size on AAV vector packaging. *Mol Ther* **18**: 80–86. doi:10.1038/mt .2009.255

Wyszecki G, Stiles WS. 1982. *Color science: concepts and methods, quantitative data and formulae*, 2nd ed. Wiley, New York.

Yin L, Greenberg K, Hunter JJ, Dalkara D, Kolstad KD, Masella BD, Wolfe R, Visel M, Stone D, Libby RT, et al. 2011. Intravitreal injection of AAV2 transduces macaque inner retina. *Invest Ophthalmol Vis Sci* **52**: 2775–2783. doi:10.1167/iovs.10-6250

Yue L, Weiland JD, Roska B, Humayun MS. 2016. Retinal stimulation strategies to restore vision: fundamentals and systems. *Prog Retin Eye Res* **53**: 21–47. doi:10.1016/j .preteyeres.2016.05.002

Zhang Y, Ivanova E, Bi A, Pan ZH. 2009. Ectopic expression of multiple microbial rhodopsins restores ON and OFF light responses in retinas with photoreceptor degeneration. *J Neurosci* **29**: 9186–9196. doi:10.1523/JNEUROSCI .0184-09.2009

Optogenetic Vision Restoration

Volker Busskamp,[1] Botond Roska,[2,3] and José-Alain Sahel[4,5]

[1]Degenerative Retinal Diseases, University Hospital Bonn, 53127 Bonn, Germany

[2]Institute of Molecular and Clinical Ophthalmology Basel, 4031 Basel, Switzerland

[3]Department of Ophthalmology, University of Basel, 4001 Basel, Switzerland

[4]Department of Ophthalmology, UPMC Vision Institute, University of Pittsburgh School of Medicine, Pittsburgh, Pennsylvania 15213, USA

[5]Institut Hospitalo-Universitaire FOReSIGHT, Sorbonne Universite, Inserm, Quinze-Vingts Hopital de la Vision, 75012 Paris, France

Correspondence: sahelja@upmc.edu

Optogenetics has emerged over the past 20 years as a powerful tool to investigate the various circuits underlying numerous functions, especially in neuroscience. The ability to control by light the activity of neurons has enabled the development of therapeutic strategies aimed at restoring some level of vision in blinding retinal conditions. Promising preclinical and initial clinical data support such expectations. Numerous challenges remain to be tackled (e.g., confirmation of safety, cell and circuit specificity, patterns, intensity and mode of stimulation, rehabilitation programs) on the path toward useful vision restoration.

THE RETINA

The retinal is a layered tissue at the back of the eyeball. It consists of three nuclear and two plexiform layers. The outer nuclear layer (ONL) consists of nuclei of photoreceptors, rods for night vision, and cones for high acuity, color, and daylight vision. The light-sensitive compartments of photoreceptors are surrounded by microvilli from retinal pigment epithelium (RPE) cells. The inner nuclear layer (INL) includes the nuclei of horizontal (HC), bipolar (BC), and amacrine cells (AC). Retinal ganglion cell (RGC) nuclei form the ganglion cell layer (GCL), and their axons are bundled within the optic nerve relaying the retinal output information to higher brain areas. Retinal neurons are interconnected within the plexiform layers, namely, photoreceptors, HCs, and BCs in the outer plexiform layer (OPL) as well as BCs, ACs, and RGCs in the inner plexiform layer (IPL). Müller glia (MG) cells span all retinal layers while their cell bodies are also located in the INL. The retina is a transparent tissue, and the light passes all layers before the photons are converted into electrical signals within the outer segments (OSs) of photoreceptors (Masland 2001).

The conversion of photons to electrical signals is mediated via the phototransduction cascade, a complex interplay of many enzymatic reactions involving sets of proteins, which leads to the closure of cyclic nucleotide-gated channels.

Thereby, the photoreceptor cell becomes hyperpolarized. As in every neuron, photoreceptors release neurotransmitters via their synapses when depolarized. Hence, light-mediated hyperpolarization blocks the steady dark currents, which HCs and BCs detect downstream. BCs consist of two classes: OFF-BCs are activated by light contrast decrements and ON-BCs are activated by contrast increments. Vertically, BCs relay the activity to corresponding postsynaptic OFF, ON, and ON–OFF RGCs. HCs and ACs provide inhibitory input to the retinal pathways, further refining the light information before it is sent via the optic nerve to higher visual brain areas. The RGCs fire action potentials to encode the neuronal activity. RGCs are very diverse in morphology and function. Individual RGC types form a mosaic across the retina and each type can be considered as a specific channel transmitting a specific visual feature. Of note, primate vision is further refined by the formation of the macula, a cone-enriched central spot that is used for color and high acuity vision such as reading and recognizing faces. Overall, the retina is a sophisticated biological computer and our window to the outside world.

RETINAL DEGENERATION

Vision requires a large energy and oxygen supply, as well as precise neural circuit development and maintenance at the molecular level to function properly. Environmental disturbances or genetic mutations can perturb visual processing within the retina and may also trigger progressive photoreceptor degeneration, as in forms of retinitis pigmentosa (RP). In RP, first the rod photoreceptors die, leading to reduced night vision and tunnel vision. At late stages, the cone photoreceptors in the macula lose their light sensitivity, resulting in overall blindness.

RP presents with much variability in genetic mutations, forms of progression, and severity of vision loss. Basic and clinical research has investigated many different therapeutic interventions; however, only one is approved for clinical use at this stage. Due to the complexities of the individual mutations, pathologies, and clinical manifestations, a one-size-fits-all solution does not exist. To preserve the natural vision, early interventions

are needed to stop the progressing loss of photoreceptors. There is a successful gene therapy, voretigene neparvovec rzyl, that substitutes the *RPE65* gene to prevent Leber congenital amaurosis (LCA) (Russell et al. 2017). However, developing gene therapies for every mutation would be cumbersome. Notably, the human retina has no intrinsic regenerative capacity. Cell-replacement therapies for RPE and photoreceptor cells are promising, but also require further advancement before becoming a standard treatment to overcome blindness.

In this review, we focus on optogenetic vision restoration therapy, which is independent of the cause of blindness as long as the optic nerve is preserved. Optogenetic therapy is making use of DNA-encoded, light-sensitive proteins that are delivered to remaining retinal cells and thereby rendering the target cells light sensitive. Technically, optogenetic therapy uses the same procedure that has already been established and approved for other types of retinal gene therapy.

OPTOGENETIC TOOLS

Optogenetic sensors refer to proteins that trigger or inhibit biological processes within living cells upon light exposure. These proteins are typically ion channels, ion pumps, or intracellular enzymes within signaling cascades. The most well-known optogenetic sensor is an ion channel, Channelrhodopsin-2 (ChR2), which has a seven-transmembrane helix motif. One helix binds the chromophore retinal via a Schiff base. Upon chromophore activation by a photon, conformational changes of the transmembrane helices result in the influx of cations from the extracellular membrane into the cell, thereby leading to depolarization (Nagel et al. 2003; Bamann et al. 2008). Electrically active cells are thereby excited. ChR2 was discovered in the eyespot of green algae and is used for phototaxis. ChR2 is permeable for Na^+, K^+, and Ca^{2+} and biophysically also a leaky outwardly directed proton pump (Feldbauer et al. 2009). However, under physiological conditions, the channel properties are dominating. The peak activity is at 470 nm, meaning it absorbs blue light. The channel kinetics are determined by the biophysical properties of the photocycle including the isomerization of the chromophore. Wild-type ChR2 was described to reliably trigger action potentials in neurons up to 30 Hz (Boyden et al. 2005). Targeted mutagenesis of ChR2 was performed by many groups to enhance its kinetic properties and additional optogenetic sensors from different species were discovered (Gunaydin et al. 2010; Berndt et al. 2011; Kleinlogel et al. 2011; Klapoetke et al. 2014). Importantly, kinetics and sensitivity are inversely correlated: fast ChR2 mutants require higher light levels, whereas slow ChR2 variants with long channel opening times require less light and fewer photons (Klapper et al. 2016).

The dependence on blue light for in vivo applications is also not preferable as 470 nm photons have a higher energy level. Extensive blue light illumination can cause photochemical damage to cells. Especially for retinal applications, blue light also activates the melanopsin-containing RGCs important for triggering the pupillary reflex. Thereby, blue light leads to pupillary contraction limiting the amount of light arriving at the retina to activate ChR2-expressing cells. Therefore, red-shifted ChR species such as volvox ChR (Zhang et al. 2008), ReaChR (Lin et al. 2013), and Chrimson (Klapoetke et al. 2014) provide safer light stimulation with less pupil constriction.

Another type of optogenetic sensor is halorhodopsins, which are inward chloride or outward proton pumps. These pumps also have seven transmembrane helices and require the chromophore retinal. Here, one photocycle results in transfer of one chloride ion or proton translocation over the cell membrane. The halorhodopsin from *Natronomonas pharaonis* (NpHR) was first applied as an optogenetic tool (Han and Boyden 2007; Zhang et al. 2007). Physiologically, this pump hyperpolarizes archaebacteria up to −200 mV for ATP synthesis and for the activation of secondary transporters in the cell membrane (Duschl et al. 1988; Bamberg et al. 1993). Ectopically expressed in other cell types, they become hyperpolarized upon light activation. Thereby, neuronal activity gets inhibited. In the retina, halorhodopsin could mimic OFF responses as well as light responses of photoreceptors. The peak activity of NpHR is red-shifted at 580 nm. There exist also light-sensitive

proton pumps such as Arch from *Halorubrum sodomense* with a peak activity at 566 nm and Mac from the fungus *Leptosphaeria maculans* at 540 nm (Chow et al. 2010). Another light-sensitive chloride pump from *Haloarcula salinarum* called Jaws was discovered with red-shifted peak activity at 632 nm and higher photocurrents compared to other halorhodopsin species (Chuong et al. 2014).

The rhodopsin protein in rod photoreceptors, the cone opsins in cone photoreceptors, and the melanopsin protein in light-sensitive ganglion cells are all G-protein-coupled receptors (GPCRs) that require a downstream signaling cascade to convert photons into electrical signals. These GPCRs also have seven transmembrane domains like the microbial optogenetic sensors; however, due to the signaling cascade, they are more sensitive to light. The chromophore retinal requires re-isomerization by RPE and MG cells while melanopsin has intrinsic re-isomerization properties. While sensitivity is superior over microbial optogenes, the GPCR kinetics are tuned by other proteins and sufficient for photoreceptors and melanopsin-expressing ganglion cells but very slow for other retinal cell types. Of note, for ON BCs, a chimeric protein consisting of the intracellular domains of the ON-BC-specific metabotropic glutamate receptor mGluR6 and the light-sensing domains of melanopsin, called Opto-mGluR6, has been engineered (van Wyk et al. 2015).

EXPRESSION CONTROL

Ectopic gene expression requires promoter elements that initiate transcription. Promoter elements can be ubiquitous or cell-type specific. The expression levels of optogenetic sensors can be indirectly visualized live using fluorescent reporter proteins. These fluorescent reporters such as enhanced green fluorescent protein (EGFP) are fused to the carboxyl terminus of the optogene, resulting in fluorescent labeling of the host cell's membrane. There exist also cleaving signals, such as 2A elements, in which the fluorescent protein is separated during protein translation, resulting in cytoplasmic labeling. Optogenetic sensors require high expression levels to cause sufficient neuronal depolarization or hyperpolarization for changes in neuronal function. Therefore, optimal optogene expression requires promoter elements that drive transcription at sufficient levels. For biomedical applications, the choice of promoter elements must be adjusted and adapted for preclinical model systems and finally optimized for adequate expression in the human target cells (Jüttner et al. 2019). For example, promoter systems that work well in rodent cell types can underperform in human cell types and vice versa.

The ectopic expression of optogenes in mammalian cell types may require further modifications to facilitate optimal expression levels. In the case of nonhuman genes, changing the codon usage to the default human codons has been shown to be beneficial.

Optogenes are membrane proteins that require specific intracellular processing steps to be properly integrated into the cell membrane. In this light, intrinsic membrane proteins have specific protein domains that enhance the release from the endoplasmic reticulum (ER). Initially, optogenes, especially NpHR, have been found to aggregate within the ER around the nucleus when highly expressed in neurons. The addition of an ER-releasing tag from the inward-rectifier potassium channel Kir2.1 enhanced the segregation of the optogenetic proteins from the ER. The combination with another modification, the membrane-trafficking signal peptide from the β subunit of the nAChR, further improved membrane localization. This modified optogene was called eNpHR2.0 (Gradinaru et al. 2008) and further modified to eNpHR3.0 (Gradinaru et al. 2010). Protein engineering by adding trafficking signal domains from Kir2.1 and ER export domains led to improved membrane targeting. In some cases, clustering optogene expression in the soma within the dendrites or to the axonal initial segment was also explored (Greenberg et al. 2011; Wu et al. 2013; Zhang et al. 2015). Here, additional protein tags for the anticipated expression location were fused to the optogene.

GENE TRANSFER

Adeno-associated viruses (AAVs) are currently the most frequent gene transfer tool for retinal transduction. AAVs can deliver about 4.8 kb of single-stranded DNA (Grieger and Samulski 2005a). These viral particles are about 20 nm in diameter and are potent to diffuse through tissues until they bind to matching cell surface receptors. The AAV genomes are encapsulated in capsids defining their serotype. Serotypes have different affinities to cell surface receptors and, therefore, AAV vector serotype choice can enhance the transduction of specific cell types (Grieger and Samulski 2005b; Ojala et al. 2015; Salganik et al. 2015). The genetic elements within the recombinant AAV genome are flanked by inverted terminal repeats (ITRs), which form hairpins at the ends of the single-stranded viral DNA genome (Bohenzky et al. 1988). These secondary structures are important as primers for the secondary strand synthesis, which is important for stability in the nucleus as episomal concatemers and gene expression. The first approved ocular AAV gene therapy, voretigene neparvovec rzyl, for humans transferred the human RPE65 cDNA to RPE cells of LCA patients (Russell et al. 2017).

AAV capsids have also been improved by in vivo–directed evolution (Dalkara et al. 2013; Pavlou et al. 2021) or targeted protein engineering (Dalkara et al. 2012; Cronin et al. 2014; Hickey et al. 2017) for retinal gene transfer (Zolotukhin and Vandenberghe 2022). These AAV particles can be injected into the vitreous where the inner limiting membrane may inhibit diffusion and transduction of RGCs (Dalkara et al. 2009). For targeting RPE cells and photoreceptors, subretinal injections, although more challenging from a surgical aspect, are the default administration to target high cell numbers.

OPTOGENETIC ACTIVATION OF RGCs

The first evidence for optogenetic vision restoration was provided in rodents in 2006 (Bi et al. 2006). ChR2 was fused to EGFP and was driven from a ubiquitous promoter, the CMV enhancer/ chicken β-actin (CAG) promoter. Gene transfer was achieved with AAV serotype 2 that was injected into the intravitreal space in mice and rats. Thereby, RGCs were efficiently transduced, as shown by EGFP expression. ChR2-expressing RGCs were sensitive to 460-nm light. Blind *rd1* mice were treated and showed light responses in RGCs with average action potential frequencies up to 150 Hz as well as visual-evoked potentials in the visual cortex. Behavior responses were not reported. Of note, targeting all RGCs changed OFF responses to ON so that the entire retinal output consisted of ON responses. This approach was also successfully tested in blind rats (Tomita et al. 2007) and also showed, to some extent, optomotor behavioral responses (Tomita et al. 2009, 2010).

The relatively low light sensitivity compared to normal vision requires high light levels for stimulation. Instead of using flashes of light, holographic stimulation was successfully tested to drive ChR2-expressing RGCs in blind mice (Reutsky-Gefen et al. 2013). Thereby, single cells can be precisely controlled, and the overall light intensities were reduced. The nonhuman origin of ChR2 or the fluorescent proteins was considered to induce immunogenicity and to be problematic for clinical applications. In rats, optogenes did not induce immune responses (Sugano et al. 2016) and the light levels used did not induce phototoxicity (Tabata et al. 2021). To overcome the limitation to optogenetic-induced ON responses of RGCs, the coexpression of NpHR and ChR2 was shown to induce OFF, ON–OFF, and ON responses, depending on the wavelengths used (Zhang et al. 2009). However, the gene expression targeted random RGCs irrespectively of their intrinsic response features.

To overcome the sensitivity problem and exogenous origin of the microbial optogenetic tools, the GPCR melanopsin normally expressed in intrinsically light-sensitive RGCs was driven from a ubiquitous CMV promoter element, and RGCs in *rd1* mice were transduced by AAV transfer (Lin et al. 2008). Upon light activation, a G-protein cascade was triggered and the melanopsin-expressing RGCs fired action potentials on average at ~40 Hz. However, the long latency of action potential onset and the continuous responses after the termination of the light stimulus were not optimal for precise temporal vision. Nevertheless, the light responses robustly triggered the pupillary reflex and the treated former blind mice performed well in the dark–light box light-avoidance behavioral assay. Mutations to naturally occurring

melanopsin mutations are performed to overcome the kinetic drawbacks of applying melanopsin for vision restoration (Rodgers et al. 2018). The GPCRs from rod and cone photoreceptors rhodopsin and medium-wavelength cone opsin also restored light sensitivity in blind mice upon ectopic expression in RGCs (Berry et al. 2019). Of note, the cone opsin was active at ambient light levels and the treated mice were able to discriminate temporal and spatial light patterns.

While GPCRs require a downstream signaling cascade to work, microbial optogenes are simpler and work as a single unit. These tools have also been further improved by targeted mutagenesis (Pan et al. 2014), and novel tools with advanced biophysical properties such as having a red-shifted action spectrum, faster kinetics, and higher sensitivity have been discovered. In this line, a chimera of Volvox channelrhodopsin-1 and Chlamydomonas channelrhodopsin-1, called (mVChR1), was engineered and successfully applied to ganglion cells of rats (Tomita et al. 2014). The activity range was broad, spanning wavelengths between 468 nm and 640 nm. MVChR1 was also tested in combination with ChR2 (Sato et al. 2017). A more sensitive ChR2 derivative called CatCh was successfully applied to RGCs in the peri-foveolar region of macaque retinas (Chaffiol et al. 2017). Another red-shifted channelrhodopsin called ReaChR drove RGC activity in former blind mouse retinas as well as in macaque retinas and human retinal explants (Sengupta et al. 2016). The optogene bReaChES also reactivated RGCs in blind mice (Too et al. 2022). A more red-shifted tool, called ChrimsonR, drove RGC responses in macaque retinas (McGregor et al. 2020). Another study showed that ChrimsonR when fused to tdTomato (ChR-tdT) induced robust light responses in macaque RGCs using safe light levels. No significant immune response following ChR-tdT expression was detected (Gauvain et al. 2021). When removing the fluorescent protein tdTomato, optogenetic responses were significantly reduced suggesting that the fluorescent protein was beneficial for the functional performance. That study also provided dose-ranging information relevant for clinical trials.

In 2021, the first evidence for partial vision restoration in a blind patient from end-stage RP following optogenetic activation of RGCs was published (Sahel et al. 2021). The trial used AAV-2-mediated expression of ChrimsonR in RGCs following an intravitreal injection. Goggles emitting light in the relevant amber wavelength corresponding to visual patterns generated from a camera activated visual responses as demonstrated by the ability to locate and quantify elementary objects and the demonstration of cortical activation using multielectrode electroencephalogram (EEG). The safety of the use of a red-shifted optogene was demonstrated in that study. Several other patients have been treated using the same protocol.

OPTOGENETIC ACTIVATION OF ON BIPOLAR CELLS

As aforementioned, the retina performs visual signal processing upstream of RGSs. To maintain these functional features upon optogenetic intervention in retinal degenerative diseases, rendering BCs into artificial photoreceptors was attempted. Targeting ChR2 to ON BCs would restore the retinal ON pathways. To this end, an ON BC-specific promoter element from the metabotropic glutamate receptor 6 (Grm6) gene was used to drive ChR2 fused to EYFP (Lagali et al. 2008). At that time, there did not exist AAV capsids that efficiently targeted retinal BCs. Therefore, in vivo electroporation was used and, in combination with the ON BC-specific promoter element, resulted in robust ChR2 transduction of ON BCs in the *rd1* mouse model. Illumination with light induced robust action potentials in RGCs of treated animals. The center-surround organization of ON RGCs' receptive fields was restored and feedforward inhibition was measured, highlighting the restoration of some visual signal processing. In addition, visual-evoked potentials were recorded in the visual cortex of treated animals. These former blind mice also successfully passed visual behavior tests including the optomotor response test for two spatial frequencies.

For translating this approach, changing the gene-delivery methodology to AAV was essential (Macé et al. 2015; Lu et al. 2016). Using a modified AAV capsid and the generation of a tandem array of the Grm6 enhancer sequence further improved

ON BC targeting and optogenetic reactivation (Cronin et al. 2014). Like for the RGC approach, more sensitive optogenetic tools were tested. For example, a chimeric protein was engineered and applied to ON BCs, showing advanced light sensitivity. This tool consisted of the light-sensing domains of melanopsin and of the intracellular GRM6 domains (van Wyk et al. 2015). Melanopsin was also successfully tested to sensitize ON BCs as well as other inner retinal cell types for extended time periods (De Silva et al. 2017). The sensitivity was further improved by applying rhodopsin (Cehajic-Kapetanovic et al. 2015; Gaub et al. 2015) and cone opsins to ON BCs (McClements et al. 2021). However, to determine whether human opsins ectopically expressed in other retinal cell types and recruiting host cell G-protein cascades can overcome the light adaptation features of the retina requires further testing. Normal photoreceptors respond through adaptation to light intensities spanning more than 8 log units. Of note, microbial rhodopsins are only functional over about 2 log units.

To date, the field still lacks an efficient promoter element for OFF BCs, useful for adding an optogene to reactivate the OFF pathway. By using spectrally shifted tools to target ON and OFF BCs, both major signal-processing pathways might be reactivated. Still, optogenetic reactivation of ON BCs is promising.

REACTIVATING DORMANT CONE PHOTORECEPTORS

In RP, the mutations of rod-expressed genes lead to rod degeneration, whereas the cone photoreceptors function normally, at first. However, at later stages, the cones are also affected and lose their light-sensitive OS first, resulting in overall blindness. This is accompanied with changes in cone morphology and protein expression. Therefore, it was thought that cone photoreceptors degenerate fast upon OS loss but evidence from animal and human studies indicated longer cone cell body survival (Li et al. 1995; Milam et al. 1998; Lin et al. 2009). However, it was not known whether these cone cell bodies were still synaptically connected to downstream retinal BCs. Resensitizing dormant cone photoreceptors has the potential to activate all downstream cone processing including the ON and OFF pathways. As photoreceptors react with hyperpolarization to light, the light-sensitive chloride pump eNpHR was tested (Busskamp et al. 2010). The mouse cone arrestin (mCAR) promoter element driving this halorhodopsin showed the best expression levels upon subretinal AAV delivery into fast and slow RP mouse models. Robust photocurrents upon light activity with a peak of activity at 580 nm were recorded in cones. These reactivated cones were still connected to BCs, and light-induced responses of RGCs with action potential frequencies over 200 Hz were measured. Importantly, both the ON and the OFF pathways, as well as signal-processing features including direction selectivity were reactivated. Former blind animals performed visually guided behavior including the optomotor response test. In addition, the halorhodopsin was also able to drive human cones in retinal explants from organ donors highlighting the potential of this approach for clinical applications.

Over time, the number of cones declined; however, at postnatal day 500, treated animals still had eNpHR-expressing cones that induced robust light responses in RGCs (Zuzic et al. 2022). This also showed that a single AAV administration resulted in efficient and long-term transduction efficiency in mice. Additional hyperpolarizing optogenes with better biophysical characteristics were also tested in cones (Chuong et al. 2014). The safety and efficacy of reactivating dormant cone photoreceptors was also tested in a dog model highlighting its clinical potential (Nikonov et al. 2022). In addition, combining photoreceptor cell-replacement therapies with optogenetic reactivation was shown (Garita-Hernandez et al. 2019). This approach was also found useful to reactivate light responses in human explants showing that halorhodopsin-expressing human cones drive activity in human ganglion cells (Kamar et al. 2020), thereby facilitating functional studies when intrinsic light responses are lost in human retinas.

As in many human blindness diseases, such as age-related macular degeneration (AMD), the loss of photoreceptor function is incomplete; optogenetic approaches may interfere with remaining intrinsic light perceptions such as in the peripheral areas of the retina. To overcome this, a near-infrared (NIR) light, >900 nm, was tested in cone photoreceptors (Nelidova et al. 2020). Thereby, dormant cones would be sensitive to light outside the intrinsic visual range enabling intrinsic and optogenetic vision to functionally coexist. To this end, mammalian or snake temperature-sensitive engineered transient receptor potential (TRP) channels were expressed in dormant cones upon AAV delivery. Gold nanorods were coinjected and bound to the TRP channels. Thereby, the dormant cones were sensitive to NIR light and drove robust activity in RGSs and the visual cortex as well as behavioral responses in former blind mice. The nanorods were well tolerated in the retina. This approach was also successfully translated to postmortem retinal explants in which cones were resensitized. Of note, TRP channels led to a depolarization of the cone photoreceptors upon light activation, which led to functional restoration of light activity. Although this approach requires two components to be injected into the subretinal space, NIR optogenetic tools do not impede remaining vision and thereby offer treatments to larger patient groups that are not completely blind. In summary, targeting dormant cone photoreceptors reactivated all downstream cone pathways and retinal-processing features.

SUMMARY AND OUTLOOK

Optogenetic vision restoration is a good example of how new biomedical approaches are developed based on fundamental research on retinal cell types and circuits as well as biophysical characterization of light-sensitive proteins. First, this required the discovery of microbial optogenetic tools to drive robust neuronal activity before mammalian opsins were also successfully tested. Existing and growing knowledge of retinal function and signal processing will contribute to the quality of regained vision. It also guided the hierarchical targeting of retinal cell types for optogenetic activation, first testing in RGCs, ON BCs, and dormant cones. The discovery of cell-type-specific promoter elements and vectors, and progress in transducing inner retinal cell types with AAVs, will further boost this approach. Research to improve optogenetic tools such as cell localization, sensitivity, and kinetics is ongoing. With the first clinical human data at hand, clinicians now have the opportunity to thoroughly test treated patients to understand the quality of regained vision and current limitations. Many groups are working on eliminating the need for goggles but the need to adapt to various levels of lighting (10 log units in natural conditions), the need for retinal preprocessing, and the prevention of photophobia when using highly light-sensitive proteins, may represent significant issues that must be addressed. It is likely that optogenetic therapy will not restore normal vision including adaptation to many light levels; however, the goal is to restore vision to a degree that is useful for patients in their daily lives.

REFERENCES

Bamann C, Kirsch T, Nagel G, Bamberg E. 2008. Spectral characteristics of the photocycle of channelrhodopsin-2 and its implication for channel function. *J Mol Biol* **375:** 686–694. doi:10.1016/j.jmb.2007.10.072

Bamberg E, Tittor J, Oesterhelt D. 1993. Light-driven proton or chloride pumping by halorhodopsin. *Proc Natl Acad Sci* **90:** 639–643. doi:10.1073/pnas.90.2.639

Berndt A, Schoenenberger P, Mattis J, Tye KM, Deisseroth K, Hegemann P, Oertner TG. 2011. High-efficiency channelrhodopsins for fast neuronal stimulation at low light levels. *Proc Natl Acad Sci* **108:** 7595–7600. doi:10.1073/pnas.1017210108

Berry MH, Holt A, Salari A, Veit J, Visel M, Levitz J, Aghi K, Gaub BM, Sivyer B, Flannery JG, et al. 2019. Restoration of high-sensitivity and adapting vision with a cone opsin. *Nat Commun* **10:** 1221. doi:10.1038/s41467-019-09124-x

Bi A, Cui J, Ma YP, Olshevskaya E, Pu M, Dizhoor AM, Pan ZH. 2006. Ectopic expression of a microbial-type rhodopsin restores visual responses in mice with photoreceptor degeneration. *Neuron* **50:** 23–33. doi:10.1016/j.neuron.2006.02.026

Bohenzky RA, LeFebvre RB, Berns KI. 1988. Sequence and symmetry requirements within the internal palindromic sequences of the adeno-associated virus terminal repeat. *Virology* **166:** 316–327. doi:10.1016/0042-6822(88)90502-8

Boyden ES, Zhang F, Bamberg E, Nagel G, Deisseroth K. 2005. Millisecond-timescale, genetically targeted optical control of neural activity. *Nat Neurosci* **8:** 1263–1268. doi:10.1038/nn1525

Busskamp V, Duebel J, Balya D, Fradot M, Viney TJ, Siegert S, Groner AC, Cabuy E, Forster V, Seeliger M, et al. 2010. Genetic reactivation of cone photoreceptors restores visual responses in retinitis pigmentosa. *Science* **329:** 413–417. doi:10.1126/science.1190897

Cehajic-Kapetanovic J, Eleftheriou C, Allen AE, Milosavljevic N, Pienaar A, Bedford R, Davis KE, Bishop PN, Lucas RJ. 2015. Restoration of vision with ectopic expression of human rod opsin. *Curr Biol* **25:** 2111–2122. doi:10.1016/j.cub.2015.07.029

Chaffiol A, Caplette R, Jaillard C, Brazhnikova E, Desrosiers M, Dubus E, Duhamel L, Macé E, Marre O, Benoit P, et al. 2017. A new promoter allows optogenetic vision restoration with enhanced sensitivity in macaque retina. *Mol Ther* **25:** 2546–2560. doi:10.1016/j.ymthe.2017.07.011

Chow BY, Han X, Dobry AS, Qian X, Chuong AS, Li M, Henninger MA, Belfort GM, Lin Y, Monahan PE, et al. 2010. High-performance genetically targetable optical neural silencing by light-driven proton pumps. *Nature* **463:** 98–102. doi:10.1038/nature08652

Chuong AS, Miri ML, Busskamp V, Matthews GA, Acker LC, Sørensen AT, Young A, Klapoetke NC, Henninger MA, Kodandaramaiah SB, et al. 2014. Noninvasive optical inhibition with a red-shifted microbial rhodopsin. *Nat Neurosci* **17:** 1123–1129. doi:10.1038/nn.3752

Cronin T, Vandenberghe LH, Hantz P, Juttner J, Reimann A, Kacsó AE, Huckfeldt RM, Busskamp V, Kohler H, Lagali PS, et al. 2014. Efficient transduction and optogenetic stimulation of retinal bipolar cells by a synthetic adeno-associated virus capsid and promoter. *EMBO Mol Med* **6:** 1175–1190. doi:10.15252/emmm.201404077

Dalkara D, Kolstad KD, Caporale N, Visel M, Klimczak RR, Schaffer DV, Flannery JG. 2009. Inner limiting membrane barriers to AAV-mediated retinal transduction from the vitreous. *Mol Ther* **17:** 2096–2102. doi:10.1038/mt.2009.181

Dalkara D, Byrne LC, Lee T, Hoffmann NV, Schaffer DV, Flannery JG. 2012. Enhanced gene delivery to the neonatal retina through systemic administration of tyrosine-mutated AAV9. *Gene Ther* **19:** 176–181. doi:10.1038/gt.2011.163

Dalkara D, Byrne LC, Klimczak RR, Visel M, Yin L, Merigan WH, Flannery JG, Schaffer DV. 2013. In vivo–directed evolution of a new adeno-associated virus for therapeutic outer retinal gene delivery from the vitreous. *Sci Transl Med* **5:** 189ra76. doi:10.1126/scitranslmed.3005708

De Silva SR, Barnard AR, Hughes S, Tam SKE, Martin C, Singh MS, Barnea-Cramer AO, McClements ME, During MJ, Peirson SN, et al. 2017. Long-term restoration of visual function in end-stage retinal degeneration using subretinal human melanopsin gene therapy. *Proc Natl Acad Sci* **114:** 11211–11216. doi:10.1073/pnas.1701589114

Duschl A, McCloskey MA, Lanyi JK. 1988. Functional reconstitution of halorhodopsin. Properties of halorhodopsin-containing proteoliposomes. *J Biol Chem* **263:** 17016–17022. doi:10.1016/S0021-9258(18)37491-X

Feldbauer K, Zimmermann D, Pintschovius V, Spitz J, Bamann C, Bamberg E. 2009. Channelrhodopsin-2 is a leaky proton pump. *Proc Natl Acad Sci* **106:** 12317–12322. doi:10.1073/pnas.0905852106

Garita-Hernandez M, Lampič M, Chaffiol A, Guibbal L, Routet F, Santos-Ferreira T, Gasparini S, Borsch O, Gagliardi G, Reichman S, et al. 2019. Restoration of visual function by transplantation of optogenetically engineered photoreceptors. *Nat Commun* **10:** 4524. doi:10.1038/s41467-019-12330-2

Gaub BM, Berry MH, Holt AE, Isacoff EY, Flannery JG. 2015. Optogenetic vision restoration using rhodopsin for enhanced sensitivity. *Mol Ther* **23:** 1562–1571. doi:10.1038/mt.2015.121

Gauvain G, Akolkar H, Chaffiol A, Arcizet F, Khoei MA, Desrosiers M, Jaillard C, Caplette R, Marre O, Bertin S, et al. 2021. Optogenetic therapy: high spatiotemporal resolution and pattern discrimination compatible with vision restoration in non-human primates. *Commun Biol* **4:** 125. doi:10.1038/s42003-020-01594-w

Gradinaru V, Thompson KR, Deisseroth K. 2008. eNpHR: a natronomonas halorhodopsin enhanced for optogenetic applications. *Brain Cell Biol* **36:** 129–139. doi:10.1007/s11068-008-9027-6

Gradinaru V, Zhang F, Ramakrishnan C, Mattis J, Prakash R, Diester I, Goshen I, Thompson KR, Deisseroth K. 2010. Molecular and cellular approaches for diversifying and extending optogenetics. *Cell* **141:** 154–165. doi:10.1016/j.cell.2010.02.037

Greenberg KP, Pham A, Werblin FS. 2011. Differential targeting of optical neuromodulators to ganglion cell soma and dendrites allows dynamic control of center-surround antagonism. *Neuron* **69:** 713–720. doi:10.1016/j.neuron.2011.01.024

Grieger JC, Samulski RJ. 2005a. Packaging capacity of adeno-associated virus serotypes: impact of larger genomes on infectivity and postentry steps. *J Virol* **79:** 9933–9944. doi:10.1128/JVI.79.15.9933-9944.2005

Grieger JC, Samulski RJ. 2005b. Adeno-associated virus as a gene therapy vector: vector development, production and clinical applications. *Adv Biochem Eng Biotechnol* **99:** 119–145.

Gunaydin LA, Yizhar O, Berndt A, Sohal VS, Deisseroth K, Hegemann P. 2010. Ultrafast optogenetic control. *Nat Neurosci* **13:** 387–392. doi:10.1038/nn.2495

Han X, Boyden ES. 2007. Multiple-color optical activation, silencing, and desynchronization of neural activity, with single-spike temporal resolution. *PLoS ONE* **2:** e299. doi:10.1371/journal.pone.0000299

Hickey DG, Edwards TL, Barnard AR, Singh MS, de Silva SR, McClements ME, Flannery JG, Hankins MW, MacLaren RE. 2017. Tropism of engineered and evolved recombinant AAV serotypes in the rd1 mouse and ex vivo primate retina. *Gene Ther* **24:** 787–800. doi:10.1038/gt.2017.85

Jüttner J, Szabo A, Gross-Scherf B, Morikawa RK, Rompani SB, Hantz P, Szikra T, Esposti F, Cowan CS, Bharioke A, et al. 2019. Targeting neuronal and glial cell types with synthetic promoter AAVs in mice, non-human primates and humans. *Nat Neurosci* **22:** 1345–1356. doi:10.1038/s41593-019-0431-2

Kamar S, Howlett MHC, Klooster J, Graaff W, Csikós T, Rabelink MJWE, Hoeben RC, Kamermans M. 2020. Degenerated cones in cultured human retinas can successfully be optogenetically reactivated. *Int J Mol Sci* **21:** 522. doi:10.3390/ijms21020522

Klapoetke NC, Murata Y, Kim SS, Pulver SR, Birdsey-Benson A, Cho YK, Morimoto TK, Chuong AS, Carpenter EJ, Tian Z, et al. 2014. Independent optical excitation of distinct neural populations. *Nat Methods* **11:** 338–346. doi:10.1038/nmeth.2836

Klapper SD, Swiersy A, Bamberg E, Busskamp V. 2016. Biophysical properties of optogenetic tools and their application for vision restoration approaches. *Front Syst Neurosci* **10:** 74. doi:10.3389/fnsys.2016.00074

Kleinlogel S, Feldbauer K, Dempski RE, Fotis H, Wood PG, Bamann C, Bamberg E. 2011. Ultra light-sensitive and fast neuronal activation with the Ca²⁺-permeable channelrhodopsin CatCh. *Nat Neurosci* **14:** 513–518. doi:10.1038/nn.2776

Lagali PS, Balya D, Awatramani GB, Münch TA, Kim DS, Busskamp V, Cepko CL, Roska B. 2008. Light-activated channels targeted to ON bipolar cells restore visual function in retinal degeneration. *Nat Neurosci* **11:** 667–675. doi:10.1038/nn.2117

Li ZY, Kljavin IJ, Milam AH. 1995. Rod photoreceptor neurite sprouting in retinitis pigmentosa. *J Neurosci* **15:** 5429–5438. doi:10.1523/JNEUROSCI.15-08-05429.1995

Lin B, Koizumi A, Tanaka N, Panda S, Masland RH. 2008. Restoration of visual function in retinal degeneration mice by ectopic expression of melanopsin. *Proc Natl Acad Sci* **105:** 16009–16014. doi:10.1073/pnas.0806114105

Lin B, Masland RH, Strettoi E. 2009. Remodeling of cone photoreceptor cells after rod degeneration in *rd* mice. *Exp Eye Res* **88:** 589–599. doi:10.1016/j.exer.2008.11.022

Lin JY, Knutsen PM, Muller A, Kleinfeld D, Tsien RY. 2013. Reachr: a red-shifted variant of channelrhodopsin enables deep transcranial optogenetic excitation. *Nat Neurosci* **16:** 1499–1508. doi:10.1038/nn.3502

Lu Q, Ganjawala TH, Ivanova E, Cheng JG, Troilo D, Pan ZH. 2016. AAV-mediated transduction and targeting of retinal bipolar cells with improved mGluR6 promoters in rodents and primates. *Gene Ther* **23:** 680–689. doi:10.1038/gt.2016.42

Macé E, Caplette R, Marre O, Sengupta A, Chaffiol A, Barbe P, Desrosiers M, Bamberg E, Sahel JA, Picaud S, et al. 2015. Targeting channelrhodopsin-2 to ON-bipolar cells with vitreally administered AAV restores ON and OFF visual responses in blind mice. *Mol Ther* **23:** 7–16. doi:10.1038/mt.2014.154

Masland RH. 2001. The fundamental plan of the retina. *Nat Neurosci* **4:** 877–886. doi:10.1038/nn0901-877

McClements ME, Staurenghi F, Visel M, Flannery JG, MacLaren RE, Cehajic-Kapetanovic J. 2021. AAV induced expression of human rod and cone opsin in bipolar cells of a mouse model of retinal degeneration. *Biomed Res Int* **2021:** 1–8. doi:10.1155/2021/4014797

McGregor JE, Godat T, Dhakal KR, Parkins K, Strazzeri JM, Bateman BA, Fischer WS, Williams DR, Merigan WH. 2020. Optogenetic restoration of retinal ganglion cell activity in the living primate. *Nat Commun* **11:** 1703. doi:10.1038/s41467-020-15317-6

Milam AH, Li ZY, Fariss RN. 1998. Histopathology of the human retina in retinitis pigmentosa. *Prog Retin Eye Res* **17:** 175–205. doi:10.1016/s1350-9462(97)00012-8

Nagel G, Szellas T, Huhn W, Kateriya S, Adeishvili N, Berthold P, Ollig D, Hegemann P, Bamberg E. 2003. Channelrhodopsin-2, a directly light-gated cation-selective membrane channel. *Proc Natl Acad Sci* **100:** 13940–13945. doi:10.1073/pnas.1936192100

Nelidova D, Morikawa RK, Cowan CS, Raics Z, Goldblum D, Scholl HPN, Szikra T, Szabo A, Hillier D, Roska B. 2020. Restoring light sensitivity using tunable near-infrared sensors. *Science* **368:** 1108–1113. doi:10.1126/science.aaz5887

Nikonov S, Aravand P, Lyubarsky A, Nikonov R, Luo AJ, Wei Z, Maguire AM, Phelps NT, Shpylchak I, Willett K, et al. 2022. Restoration of vision and retinal responses after adeno-associated virus-mediated optogenetic therapy in blind dogs. *Transl Vis Sci Technol* **11:** 24. doi:10.1167/tvst.11.5.24

Ojala DS, Amara DP, Schaffer DV. 2015. Adeno-associated virus vectors and neurological gene therapy. *Neuroscientist* **21:** 84–98. doi:10.1177/1073858414521870

Pan ZH, Ganjawala TH, Lu Q, Ivanova E, Zhang Z. 2014. Chr2 mutants at L132 and T159 with improved operational light sensitivity for vision restoration. *PLoS ONE* **9:** e98924. doi:10.1371/journal.pone.0098924

Pavlou M, Schön C, Occelli LM, Rossi A, Meumann N, Boyd RF, Bartoe JT, Siedlecki J, Gerhardt MJ, Babutzka S, et al. 2021. Novel AAV capsids for intravitreal gene therapy of photoreceptor disorders. *EMBO Mol Med* **13:** e13392. doi:10.15252/emmm.202013392

Reutsky-Gefen I, Golan L, Farah N, Schejter A, Tsur L, Brosh I, Shoham S. 2013. Holographic optogenetic stimulation of patterned neuronal activity for vision restoration. *Nat Commun* **4:** 1509. doi:10.1038/ncomms2500

Rodgers J, Peirson SN, Hughes S, Hankins MW. 2018. Functional characterisation of naturally occurring mutations in human melanopsin. *Cell Mol Life Sci* **75:** 3609–3624. doi:10.1007/s00018-018-2813-0

Russell S, Bennett J, Wellman JA, Chung DC, Yu ZF, Tillman A, Wittes J, Pappas J, Elci O, McCague S, et al. 2017. Efficacy and safety of voretigene neparvovec (AAV2-hRPE65v2) in patients with RPE65-mediated inherited retinal dystrophy: a randomised, controlled, open-label, phase 3 trial. *Lancet* **390:** 849–860. doi:10.1016/S0140-6736(17)31868-8

Sahel JA, Boulanger-Scemama E, Pagot C, Arleo A, Galluppi F, Martel JN, Esposti SD, Delaux A, de Saint Aubert JB, de Montleau C, et al. 2021. Partial recovery of visual function in a blind patient after optogenetic therapy. *Nat Med* **27:** 1223–1229. doi:10.1038/s41591-021-01351-4

Salganik M, Hirsch ML, Samulski RJ. 2015. Adeno-associated virus as a mammalian DNA vector. *Microbiol Spectr* **3:** 10.1128/microbiolspec.MDNA3-0052-2014. doi:10.1128/microbiolspec.MDNA3-0052-2014

Sato M, Sugano E, Tabata K, Sannohe K, Watanabe Y, Ozaki T, Tamai M, Tomita H. 2017. Visual responses of photoreceptor-degenerated rats expressing two different types of channelrhodopsin genes. *Sci Rep* **7:** 41210. doi:10.1038/srep41210

Sengupta A, Chaffiol A, Macé E, Caplette R, Desrosiers M, Lampič M, Forster V, Marre O, Lin JY, Sahel JA, et al. 2016. Red-shifted channelrhodopsin stimulation restores light responses in blind mice, macaque retina, and human retina. *EMBO Mol Med* **8:** 1248–1264. doi:10.15252/emmm.201505699

Sugano E, Tabata K, Takahashi M, Nishiyama F, Shimizu H, Sato M, Tamai M, Tomita H. 2016. Local and systemic responses following intravitreous injection of AAV2-encoded modified volvox channelrhodopsin-1 in a genetically blind rat model. *Gene Ther* **23:** 158–166. doi:10.1038/gt.2015.99

Tabata K, Sugano E, Hatakeyama A, Watanabe Y, Suzuki T, Ozaki T, Fukuda T, Tomita H. 2021. Phototoxicities caused by continuous light exposure were not induced in retinal ganglion cells transduced by an optogenetic gene. *Int J Mol Sci* **22:** 6732. doi:10.3390/ijms22136732

Tomita H, Sugano E, Yawo H, Ishizuka T, Isago H, Narikawa S, Kügler S, Tamai M. 2007. Restoration of visual response in aged dystrophic RCS rats using AAV-mediated channelopsin-2 gene transfer. *Invest Ophthalmol Vis Sci* **48:** 3821–3826. doi:10.1167/iovs.06-1501

Tomita H, Sugano E, Fukazawa Y, Isago H, Sugiyama Y, Hiroi T, Ishizuka T, Mushiake H, Kato M, Hirabayashi M, et al. 2009. Visual properties of transgenic rats harboring the channelrhodopsin-2 gene regulated by the thy-1.2 promoter. *PLoS ONE* **4:** e7679. doi:10.1371/journal.pone.0007679

Tomita H, Sugano E, Isago H, Hiroi T, Wang Z, Ohta E, Tamai M. 2010. Channelrhodopsin-2 gene transduced into retinal ganglion cells restores functional vision in genetically blind rats. *Exp Eye Res* **90:** 429–436. doi:10.1016/j.exer.2009.12.006

Tomita H, Sugano E, Murayama N, Ozaki T, Nishiyama F, Tabata K, Takahashi M, Saito T, Tamai M. 2014. Restoration of the majority of the visual spectrum by using modified volvox channelrhodopsin-1. *Mol Ther* **22:** 1434–1440. doi:10.1038/mt.2014.81

Too LK, Shen W, Protti DA, Sawatari A, A Black D, Leamey CA, Y Huang J, Lee SR, E Mathai A, Lisowski L, et al. 2022. Optogenetic restoration of high sensitivity vision with bReaChES, a red-shifted channelrhodopsin. *Sci Rep* **12:** 19312. doi:10.1038/s41598-022-23572-4

van Wyk M, Pielecka-Fortuna J, Löwel S, Kleinlogel S. 2015. Restoring the ON switch in blind retinas: opto-mGluR6, a next-generation, cell-tailored optogenetic tool. *PLoS Biol* **13:** e1002143. doi:10.1371/journal.pbio.1002143

Wu C, Ivanova E, Zhang Y, Pan ZH. 2013. rAAV-mediated subcellular targeting of optogenetic tools in retinal ganglion cells in vivo. *PLoS ONE* **8:** e66332. doi:10.1371/journal.pone.0066332

Zhang F, Wang LP, Brauner M, Liewald JF, Kay K, Watzke N, Wood PG, Bamberg E, Nagel G, Gottschalk A, et al. 2007. Multimodal fast optical interrogation of neural circuitry. *Nature* **446:** 633–639. doi:10.1038/nature05744

Zhang F, Prigge M, Beyrière F, Tsunoda SP, Mattis J, Yizhar O, Hegemann P, Deisseroth K. 2008. Red-shifted optogenetic excitation: a tool for fast neural control derived from *Volvox carteri. Nat Neurosci* **11:** 631–633. doi:10.1038/nn.2120

Zhang Y, Ivanova E, Bi A, Pan ZH. 2009. Ectopic expression of multiple microbial rhodopsins restores ON and OFF light responses in retinas with photoreceptor degeneration. *J Neurosci* **29:** 9186–9196. doi:10.1523/JNEUROSCI.0184-09.2009

Zhang Z, Feng J, Wu C, Lu Q, Pan ZH. 2015. Targeted expression of channelrhodopsin-2 to the axon initial segment alters the temporal firing properties of retinal ganglion cells. *PLoS ONE* **10:** e0142052. doi:10.1371/journal.pone.0142052

Zolotukhin S, Vandenberghe LH. 2022. AAV capsid design: a Goldilocks challenge. *Trends Mol Med* **28:** 183–193. doi:10.1016/j.molmed.2022.01.003

Zuzic M, Striebel J, Pawlick JS, Sharma K, Holz FG, Busskamp V. 2022. Gene-independent therapeutic interventions to maintain and restore light sensitivity in degenerating photoreceptors. *Prog Retin Eye Res* **90:** 101065. doi:10.1016/j.preteyeres.2022.101065

Therapeutic Gene Editing in Inherited Retinal Disorders

Jinjie Ling,[1] Laura A. Jenny,[2] Ashley Zhou,[1] and Stephen H. Tsang[2,3,4,5]

[1]Columbia University Vagelos College of Physicians and Surgeons, New York, New York 10032, USA

[2]Jonas Children's Vision Care, and Bernard and Shirley Brown Glaucoma Laboratory, Edward Harkness Eye Institute, Department of Ophthalmology, New York-Presbyterian Hospital, New York, New York 10032, USA

[3]Department of Biomedical Engineering, Columbia University, New York, New York 10032, USA

[4]Columbia Stem Cell Initiative, and Institute of Human Nutrition, Columbia University, New York, New York 10032, USA

[5]Department of Pathology and Cell Biology, Columbia University, New York, New York 10032, USA

Correspondence: sht2@columbia.edu

Since the development of CRISPR/Cas9 gene editing in 2012, therapeutic editing research has produced several phase 1-2a trials. Here we provide an overview of the mechanisms and applications of various gene-editing technologies including adeno-associated virus vectors, lentiviruses, CRISPR/Cas9 systems, base and prime editing, antisense oligonucleotides, short-hairpin RNAs, Cas13, and adenosine deaminase acting on RNA for the treatment of various inherited retinal diseases (IRDs). We outline the various stages of clinical trials using these technologies and the impacts they have made in advancing the practice of medicine.

The eye is an extraordinary organ that harbors several characteristics conducive for the implementation of gene therapy. The retinal–blood barrier, which excludes ocular immune cell penetration, and the presence of cytokines and signaling molecules, which promotes regulatory T-cell activation and immunosuppression, confer a unique immune-privileged state to the eye (Medawar 1948; Stein-Streilein and Taylor 2007; Caspi 2010). Anatomically, the eye consists of a limited volume of cells, and the organization of these cells into their functional layers is amenable to the delivery of gene therapy vectors. The bilateral nature of human eyes is of particular interest for clinical trials as it enables one eye to serve as the treatment recipient and the other to serve as the control. Here we provide an overview of the current applications of gene editing in the treatment of retinal diseases and include an update on promising developments in recent clinical trials and cutting-edge technologies.

STRATEGIES IN GENE THERAPY AND EDITING

Adeno-Associated Virus

Historically, the adeno-associated virus (AAV) vector has served as the delivery modality of choice for the treatment of ocular disease as it exhibits low immunogenicity and high transduction efficiency in retinal cells (Timmers et al. 2020). Although AAV-based therapies have found success in the treatment of some retinal diseases (i.e., *RPE65*-associated Leber congenital amaurosis [LCA] summarized in Table 1; Bainbridge et al. 2008, 2015; Maguire et al. 2008; Cideciyan et al. 2013; Russell et al. 2017; Duncan et al. 2018), the genetic payloads delivered by AAV-based therapies are restricted to ~4.5 kb due to the small size of the AAV genome (Bainbridge et al. 2008, 2015). Thus, retinal disease-causing alterations in larger genes such as *ABCA4*, *USH2A*, and *CEP290*, have been difficult to correct using conventional AAV-based methods. In addition, AAV-based strategies rely on the supplementation of a wild-type (WT) copy of the mutant gene, which is not conducive to the treatment of autosomal-dominant retinal diseases. Finally, gene therapy applications of AAV vectors often require removal of the *rep* open reading frame (ORF) to prevent vector integration into the host genome. Thus, AAV vectors are conventionally expressed as episomes with waning therapeutic efficacy over time (Trapani and Auricchio 2018). Some groups have circumvented these obstacles by engineering dual AAV systems that carry segmented transgenes or by constructing a truncated, yet functional form of the gene of interest that is operable within the size constraints of the AAV vector (Lai et al. 2009).

Lentiviruses

Lentiviruses are retroviruses with the ability to accommodate delivery of larger genetic payloads of up to ~9 kb and have been viewed as attractive alternatives for the treatment of retinal diseases mediated by mutations in large causative genes (Coffin et al. 1997). However, lentiviral transduction results in integration of foreign DNA into the host, which can lead to unwanted insertional mutations (Trapani et al. 2014). The development of integration-deficient lentiviral vectors (IDLVs) enables expression of the lentiviral vector as a stable episome and has been successfully applied to the treatment of retinal dystrophy in a murine model (Yáñez-Muñoz et al. 2006).

DNA EDITING

CRISPR/Cas9

The CRISPR/Cas9 system is the current state-of-the-art technique for genomic surgery. Conventional applications center on a Cas9 endonuclease that is directed across the genome by a single-guide RNA (sgRNA) (Jinek et al. 2012). The sgRNA hybridizes with a complementary target DNA strand, and the Cas9 endonuclease delivers a precise molecular incision. This Cas9-mediated DNA cleavage relies on positioning near a spacer sequence or protospacer-adjacent motif (PAM), which must be directly downstream of the incision site. These DNA double-strand breaks (DSBs) subsequently activate one of two DNA repair pathways, the homology-directed repair (HDR) or nonhomologous end joining (NHEJ), which are exploited to generate a desired genetic alteration.

Cas 12

Cas12a (previously known as Cpf1) and its orthologs possess unique properties that expand on the repertoire of CRISPR/Cas applications. Compared to Cas9, they are more compact in size, generate staggered double-stranded DNA (dsDNA) breaks instead of blunt-ended dsDNA breaks, and reportedly have lower overall off-target effects (Anzalone et al. 2020). In addition, Cas12 can also cleave single-stranded DNA (ssDNA). Recent studies demonstrate that following recognition of a complementary DNA sequence, Cas12 can indiscriminately cleave surrounding ssDNA molecules, a property that has been exploited for the development of novel diagnostic technologies (Broughton et al. 2020). One key limitation of Cas9 and its orthologs is their heavy reliance on G-rich PAM sequences for localization. In contrast, Cas12a and its variants primarily recognize T-rich PAM sequences. Thus, a combination of Cas9 and Cas12 applications may expand the areas of the genome that are amenable to gene editing in retinal diseases.

CasX, also known as Cas12e, harbors many of the same features as the other Cas12 proteins in its family (Liu et al. 2019). However, it has an even lighter molecular weight with a size of only

Table 1. Description of various gene-editing strategies that have been developed in recent years along with any associated ongoing clinical trials

Gene-editing strategy	Diseases	Clinical trial status	Notes
Adeno-associated virus (AAV) vector	*RPE65*-associated Leber congenital amaurosis (LCA) (FDA approved; NCT00999609) CEP290-associated LCA (phase 2; NCT03872479)	CMS and FDA approved	Low immunogenicity and high transduction efficiency in retinal pigmented epithelium Therapeutic gene is limited to ~4.5 kb in size Difficult to apply to autosomal-dominant retinal diseases Waning therapeutic efficacy over time
Lentiviruses	Stargardt patients (NCT01367444)	Phase 1-2a; terminated as sponsor decided to stop development of product	Larger genetic payloads of up to ~9 kb Unwanted insertional mutations in host
CRISPR/Cas system	*RHO*-adRP (preclinical) Stargardt macular degeneration LCA	Preclinical	Off-target effects Inability to cleave single-stranded DNA (ssDNA) (Cas9) Requires specific G-rich protospacer-adjacent motif (PAM) sequence localization (Cas9) Inefficient in mitotically inactive cells (Cas9)
Base editing	Muscular atrophy; inherited liver and skin diseases; *RPE65*-associated LCA; sickle cell disease; ALL; α1 antitrypsin deficiency; Stargardt disease	Preclinical	Independent of double-strand break (DSB) formation and homology-directed repair (HDR)-dependent DNA repair High fidelity and efficiency Minimal off-target mutations and indel events
Prime editing			Facilitates reverse transcriptase (RT) hybridization and mutation correction on the opposing strand Does not require HDR-mediated DNA repair or DSB formation Limited to transition mutations Dependent on PAM position near the desired incision site

Continued

Table 1. *Continued*

Gene-editing strategy	Diseases	Clinical trial status	Notes
Antisense oligonucleotides	*RHO*-adRP (preclinical, phase 1/2; NCT04855045) *CEP290*-associated LCA (preclinical) Usher syndrome type 2 (phase 1/2; NCT03780257) SCA7 (preclinical murine model)	Preclinical, phase 1/2	May be used in treatment of inherited retinal diseases (IRDs) Unscalable to all mutated genes causing disease
Short-hairpin RNAs	*RHO*-adRP (preclinical canine model)	Preclinical	Require delivery via a viral vector
Cas13 and ADAR	Usher syndrome type 2 (preclinical)	Preclinical	Improved specificity and off-target effects compared to previous RNAi approaches

~980 amino acids (aa), which may facilitate efficient delivery. Furthermore, the mechanism by which the CasX protein processes and cleaves DNA differs from its predecessors. Scribe Therapeutics is optimizing this novel editor toward the treatment of several ophthalmologic diseases including retinitis pigmentosa, Stargardt macular degeneration, and LCA.

Cas14

Cas14 is a remarkably compact endonuclease identified from uncultivated archaea bacteria with a size ranging from 400 to 700 aa. In contrast to prior Cas proteins, it is guided by an RNA molecule and selectively binds and cleaves ssDNA. Strikingly, its function and localization are not dependent on the proximity of a PAM sequence, and like Cas12a, harbors potential to be used in the future for exquisite diagnostic applications.

Base Editing

CRISPR/Cas9 approaches for the correction of point mutations initially centered on the delivery of a WT Cas9 and an sgRNA directed toward the site of the point mutation followed by HDR using a functional donor sequence (Chapman et al. 2012). Unfortunately, HDR-mediated repair is highly inefficient, particularly in mitotically inactive cells. In addition, Cas9-mediated DSB for-

mation is susceptible to widespread, inadvertent indels that may produce unwanted deleterious effects (Lin et al. 2014; Zhang et al. 2015).

Recent advancements have revealed a new class of gene-editing tools that are capable of editing ssDNA independent of DSB formation and HDR-dependent DNA repair. Termed base editors, they include cytosine base editors (CBEs), which consist of a catalytically inactivated Cas9 protein (dCas9) linked to a cytosine deaminase (rAPOBEC1), and adenine base editors (ABEs), which consist of a dCas9 linked to an adenine deaminase (Komor et al. 2016; Gaudelli et al. 2017). CBEs and ABEs perform point changes of C•G to T•A and vice versa, respectively, with high fidelity and efficiency and have been successfully applied to a variety of genetic diseases including muscular atrophy and inherited liver and skin diseases in preclinical studies (Rossidis et al. 2018; Villiger et al. 2018; Osborn et al. 2020).

Suh et al. demonstrated the utility of base editors in the treatment of *RPE65*-associated LCA caused by an underlying point mutation. Specifically, the group engineered a lentiviral vector containing a codon-optimized ABE variant (ABEmax) and an sgRNA directed toward a point mutation in exon 3 (c.130C > T; p.R44X) of the *Rpe65* gene. In *rd12* mice, lentiviral transduction via subretinal injection corrected the de novo nonsense mutation with a maximum 29% efficiency, recovered visual chromophore production, and restored retinal function as assessed by scotopic electroretinography (ERG), optomotor responses (OMRs), and visually evoked potentials (VEPs) (Suh et al. 2021). Strikingly, these improvements were achieved with minimal off-target mutations and indel events. Recently, base editing was demonstrated to be efficacious in long-lasting restoration of cone functionality and survival in mice, building on the success of AAV-mediated treatment of retinal pigment epithelium (RPE)-LCA. The patients with LCA who were treated with the AAV-mediated therapy often developed continued retinal degeneration after treatment (Cideciyan et al. 2013; Bainbridge et al. 2015). Base editing offers promising development of treatment for a variety of retinal diseases on a long-term basis (Caruso et al. 2022; Choi et al. 2022).

BEAM Therapeutics is leveraging base-editing techniques in the treatment of a variety of genetic diseases including sickle cell disease, acute lymphoblastic leukemia (ALL), α1 antitrypsin deficiency, and Stargardt disease, an inherited retinal disease caused by a wide array of mutations in the *ABC4A* gene (Tanna et al. 2017).

Prime Editing

While base editing is able to overcome a critical obstacle in its avoidance of DSB formation and HDR-dependent repair, its applications are limited to transition mutations and are dependent on PAM position near the desired incision site. Prime editing (PE) relies on reverse transcriptase (RT)-mediated repair to expand on the repertoire of desired mutational corrections including deletions, insertions, and all types of transitions and transversions, and, like base editing, PE does not require HDR-mediated DNA repair or DSB formation. PE consists of an RT, a pegRNA, and an SpCas9 nickase modified with an H840A mutation that causes the nickase to preferentially generate a single-strand break (SSB) along the PAM-containing strand (da Costa et al. 2021). The pegRNA contains an sgRNA directed toward the mutation site and an extension segment containing a spacer sequence, an sgRNA scaffold, a primer-binding sequence (PBS), and a reverse transcription template (RTT). The spacer sequence extends the 3′ end of the sgRNA, facilitating RT hybridization and mutation correction on the opposing strand (Fig. 1).

Recently, Zhi et al. (2022) engineered a dual AAV8 split-PE system, which consists of Split-ABE- and Split-CBE-containing vectors. Split-ABE was then generated by two distinct mechanisms of splicing either by mRNA *trans*-splicing or intern-mediated protein slicing, the latter of which produces a Split-ABE that is more efficient in genome editing in vivo. Using this approach, the group delivered the dual AAV8 split-PE system into adult mouse retina via subretinal injection and successfully generated a G•A transversion in the *Dnmt1* gene at the p.P55Q, c.G164T position. The transversion efficiency of the dual system was only 1.71%.

RNA Editing

CRISPR/Cas9 and other relevant genome surgery approaches result in permanent alterations to the patient's genomic DNA. Many patients often opt for strategies that ensure the integrity of the genome and limit permanent modifications to their underlying DNA. Thus, approaches that modulate disease processes at the RNA level are highly desirable and can address these patient-centered concerns. RNA-editing strategies include degradation of pathological mRNA molecules, modulation of pre-mRNA splicing, and, more recently, individual base editing of mRNA transcripts.

Antisense Oligonucleotides

Antisense oligonucleotides (ASOs) are synthetic small RNA molecules or nucleotide analogs that bind to complementary pre-mRNA sequences. Depending on the chemical modification made to these molecules, ASOs can initiate a variety of biochemical activities following pre-mRNA hybridization including mRNA degradation, translational obstruction, and exon exclusion/inclusion (Hammond and Wood 2011).

ASOs with the ability to degrade mRNA are of particular interest in the treatment of autosomal-dominant inherited retinal diseases (IRDs), which have been unamenable to gene replace-

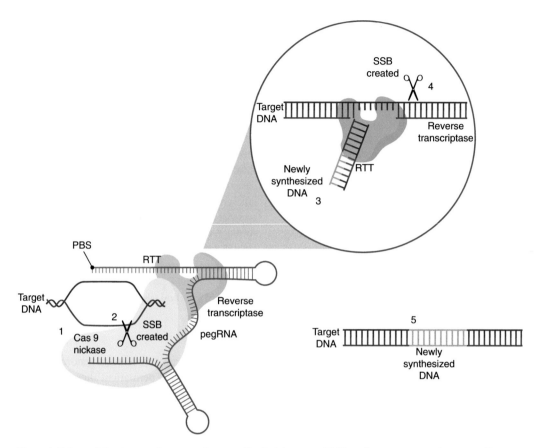

Figure 1. Prime editing is a novel strategy that uses Cas 9 nickase, pegRNA, and reverse transcriptase to edit target DNA. (1) The target DNA binds to the prime editing complex via protospacer-adjacent motif (PAM), and (2) the Cas 9 nickase creates a single-strand break (SSB) in the target DNA. (3) The reverse transcriptase reads the RNA and synthesizes new DNA to the edited strand. (4) The edited strand and unedited strand now have a base pair mismatch, and then a guide RNA (gRNA) directs the prime editor complex to create another SSB in the unedited strand. (5) The cell remakes the nicked strand using the edited strand as a template, creating a double-stranded section of edited DNA (in yellow). (RTT) Reverse transcription template, (PBS) primer-binding sequence.

ment strategies in mouse models of retinal dystrophies (Wu et al. 2022). These ASO moieties hybridize to complementary pre-mRNA molecules and recruit ribonuclease H (RNase H1) to cleave the bound pre-mRNA molecule. Several ASO therapies centered on an mRNA degradation strategy have been developed for various diseases, and one such therapy is currently in phase 2 of clinical trials testing for the treatment of rhodopsin-mediated autosomal-dominant retinitis pigmentosa (*RHO*-adRP) (NCT04123626).

Other ASO moieties can facilitate skipping of pathological exon or pseudoexon containing stop codon mutations. By avoiding these harmful segments, an appropriate reading frame can be reestablished, and the production of functional protein with the required domains can be restored. ProQR Therapeutics is employing this strategy in the treatment of LCA caused by an underlying c.2991 + 1655 > G intronic mutation in the *CEP290* gene and in the treatment of Usher syndrome type 2 with underlying exon 13 mutation.

Short-Hairpin RNAs

Short-hairpin RNAs (shRNAs) are small RNA molecules that initiate the intracellular RNA interference (RNAi) pathway. Specifically, the RNase III Dicer complex is recruited to process the shRNAs into small-interfering RNAs (siRNAs). These RNA molecules can then hybridize to complementary mRNA molecules and recruit the RNA-induced silencing complex (RISC) for mRNA degradation. Importantly, while siRNAs can be delivered as discrete RNA molecules, shRNAs require delivery via a lentiviral DNA vector (Lambeth and Smith 2013).

Cas13 and ADARs

Recent advances in CRISPR/Cas therapies have yielded unique Cas proteins with the capacity to precisely target and degrade RNA transcripts. Abudayyeh et al. isolated an RNA-guided, RNA endonuclease from the *Leptotrichia shahii* bacterium (Abudayyeh et al. 2017; Cabral et al. 2017; Sengillo et al. 2017). Previously termed C2c2, Cas13a relies on an sgRNA to localize to and target mRNA transcripts for degradation, achieving the same efficacy as previous RNAi approaches but with improved specificity and off-target effects.

While the aforementioned RNA-based therapies center on transcript degradation, recent advances in Cas13 systems have yielded the possibility of base editing at the mRNA level. These approaches employ a catalytically inactive dCas13 and an adenosine deaminase acting on RNA (ADAR). dCas13 guides the ADAR to the desired editing site to facilitate A·I *trans* conversions. As of now, however, ADARs are only able to facilitate A·I conversions and therefore can only correct A > G mutations.

DISEASE-SPECIFIC ADVANCEMENTS

RPE65-Associated LCA

The *RPE65* gene encodes a crucial retinoid isomerase that regenerates 11-*cis*-retinal for rod and cone photoreceptors in the classical RPE visual cycle. Mutations in the *RPE65* gene among several other genes have been extensively linked to LCA, a recessively inherited retinal disease characterized by severe vision impairment, nystagmus, and diminished ERG responses by the first year of life (Gu et al. 1997; Perrault et al. 1999).

In 2017, Voretigene neparvovec-rzyl (Luxturna) was approved by the U.S. Food and Drug Administration (FDA) as the first gene-replacement therapy for the treatment of RPE-associated LCA. Luxturna is an AAV serotype 2 (AAV2) vector that contains a WT copy of the *RPE65* gene and is delivered via subretinal injection to restore RPE65 production by RPE cells (Bainbridge et al. 2008). The AAV2 vector is expressed intracellularly as a stable episome in nonmitotic RPE cells. Thus, the therapy could conceivably serve as a one-time treatment solution for patients with *RPE*-associated LCA. In clinical trials, Luxturna-treated patients demonstrated dramatic improvements in bilateral multi-luminance mobility testing (MLMT) compared to control patients following 1 year of treatment. Moreover, patients also reported improvements in visual field testing, best corrected visual acuity (BCVA), and overall navigational ability in both light and dark conditions (Maguire et al. 2019). These exciting clinical developments in the landmark case of Luxturna provide compelling support for future investigation and the use of gene therapy strategies in the treatment of retinal diseases.

CEP290-Associated LCA

The *CEP290* gene encodes a critical regulator protein that directs ciliary trafficking and synthesis. These processes are vital to the function of the photoreceptor outer segment, which is dependent on effective transport of proteins and lipids synthesized in the photoreceptor inner segment. Mutations in *CEP290* lead to a form of LCA, LCA10, which is highlighted by nystagmus, compromised ERG response, and severe vision loss by the first year of life (Perrault et al. 2007). Mutations in the *CEP290* primarily exhibit an autosomal-recessive pattern of inheritance and have been implicated in ~30% of all LCA patients. The c.2991 + 1655A > G mutation in the intervening sequence in intron 26 (IVS26) represents the most frequent underlying mutation for LCA10 and produces an mRNA with a premature stop codon (p.Cys998*). Subsequently, both a nonfunctional truncated CEP290 protein and a full length-WT CEP290 protein are produced, resulting in haploinsufficiency (Ruan et al. 2017).

Gene augmentation approaches in the treatment of CEP290-mediated LCA have been hindered by the size of the *CEP290* gene (~8 kb), which is not able to be accommodated by the size restrictions of the AAV vector. However, one group circumvented this size limitation by developing a truncated, yet fully functional version of the gene, termed miniCEP290. The truncated gene was successfully packaged and delivered by an AAV vector with demonstrable improvement in photoreceptor viability in a murine model (Zhang et al. 2018).

In the realm of gene editing, Maeder et al. (2019) developed an AAV5 vector containing a *Staphylococcus aureus* Cas9 (saCas9) and two sgRNAs flanking the IVS26 mutation in the *CEP290* gene. This construct, termed EDIT-101, removes the IVS26-containing segment in the *CEP290* gene to restore mRNA splicing and functional CEP290 protein expression. The group demonstrated that EDIT-101 was able to recover *CEP290* mRNA splicing and protein function in an ex vivo, postmortem human retinal model with a productive edit rate of ~17%. These results were recapitulated in HuCEP290 mice, a human *CEP290* IVS26 knock-in mouse model. Because mouse retina harbors lower proportions of cones (~3%), the group further evaluated the efficacy of EDIT-101 in a cynomolgus monkey nonhuman primate (NHP) model, which better recapitulates the human eye (Carter-Dawson and LaVail 1979; Curcio et al. 1987). In this NHP model, administration of EDIT-101 via subretinal injection in the perifoveal region achieved a maximum 28% productive edit rate with a vector concentration of 1×10^{12} vgml^{-1}.

In 2019, Editas Medicine spearheaded the phase 1/2 Brilliance clinical trial (NCT03872479) to assess the safety, tolerability, and efficacy of EDIT-101 (Fig. 2) in LCA patients aged 3 and older with at least one mutation in the *CEP290* gene (including c.2991 + 1655A > G) and a visual acuity no better than 0.4 LogMAR (NCT03872479). Primary outcome measures include drug toxicity and adverse effects assessed every 3 months for up to 1 year. Secondary measures including BCVA, color vision, full-field stimulus

testing (FST), microperimetry, and quality of life scores, among other metrics. The efficacy component of the study consists of five subjects, three of which received a single dose of EDIT-101 at the moderate-level dose and two at the low-level dose (1.1×10^{12} vg/mL and 6×10^{11} vg/mL, respectively). Unfortunately, initial results have been inconclusive with only two patients demonstrating improvement in outcome measures at 6 months following treatment. Furthermore, only one patient achieved clinically meaningful improvement, an increase of 0.7logMAR in BCVA. Reported adverse effects include retinal tears and hemorrhages.

Toward an RNA-editing approach, Dulla et al. (2018) developed an optimized ASO capable of restoring normal RNA splicing in LCA10 with an underlying *CEP290* c.2991 + 1655A > G mutation. Also known as QR-110 and sepofarsen, this construct does not require AAV packaging but can be delivered directly via intravitreal injection (IVT). In preclinical studies, QR-110 treatment successfully corrected *CEP290* c.2991 + 1655A > G mutations in human retinal organoids and demonstrated robust bioavailability in WT mice and rabbit retinas and excellent tolerability in an NHP model.

ProQR Therapeutics is currently conducting the phase 2/3 Illuminate clinical trial (NCT03913143) to assess the safety, tolerability, and efficacy of sepofarsen in the treatment of LCA10 caused by underlying *CEP290* p.Cys998X mutation (Fig. 2). Thirty-six patients aged 8 and older received one treatment dose of sepofarsen at 0 mo and 3 mo and every 6 mo thereafter, up to 24 mo. The primary outcome measure is the mean change in BCVA following 12 mo of treatment, and secondary outcome measures include navigational ability, FST, ERG, ocular adverse events, and changes in photoreceptor outer/inner layer, among others. While an initial case study reported sustained visual improvement in one enrolled patient 15 mo following treatment, the Illuminate trial ultimately failed to meet primary outcome measure (Cideciyan et al. 2019). In addition, differences in secondary outcome measures between the treatment and control groups were not statistically significant. Although sepofarsen was

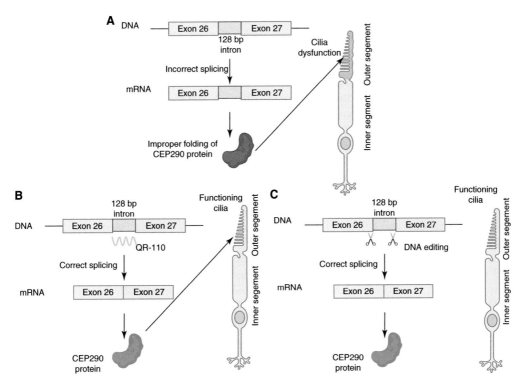

Figure 2. Mechanisms of two therapies for *CEP290*. (*A*) Mutations in *CEP290* cause incorrect splicing, which results in a truncated CEP290 protein. The CEP290 protein is a crucial component of protein trafficking in cilia and results in vision loss due to the malfunction of the outer segment of the photoreceptors. (*B*) QR-110 is an RNA therapeutic designed by ProQR, which binds to the mutated intronic sequence in *CEP290* to prevent improper splicing and allow for correct protein formation. (*C*) EDIT-101 is a gene-editing therapy developed by Editas Medicine, which removes the disease-causing mutation, allowing for correct splicing and full-length CEP290 formation.

overall well-tolerated, adverse events included retinal thinning and cystoid macular edema (CME), which were consistent with findings from phase 1/2 of the trial.

RHO-adRP

Retinitis pigmentosa (RP) is a group of rare inherited retinal disorders initiated by rod photoreceptor degeneration with progression to a wide range of disease phenotypes from mild night blindness to severe reductions in visual acuity (Verbakel et al. 2018). In the early stages of RP, patients report diminishing night vision that then progresses to deterioration of peripheral vision, termed "tunnel vision." In later stages, significant rod photoreceptor loss subsequently leads to secondary cone photoreceptor death, which may compromise daytime visual acuity

and result in complete blindness (Narayan et al. 2016).

RP can be precipitated by a compendium of defects in the photoreceptors and RPE. In particular, the rhodopsin (*RHO*) gene encodes a G-protein coupled receptor that serves as the primary visual pigment for rod photoreceptors (Nathans et al. 1986). Mutations in the *RHO* gene exhibit an autosomal-dominant hereditary pattern of retinitis pigmentosa and were the first to be associated with the development of RP. Rhodopsin-mediated autosomal-dominant retinitis pigmentosa (*RHO*-adRP) accounts for almost 25% of all autosomal-dominant retinitis pigmentosa (adRP) cases (Jacobson et al. 1991).

Conventional gene therapy approaches for the treatment of *RHO*-adRP centered on attenuating expression of the mutant *RHO* gene, which is directly implicated in the retinal degeneration process. QR-1123 is an ASO therapy designed to treat *RHO*-adRP with underlying P23H mutation in the *RHO* gene by targeting P23H mutant RHO transcripts for degradation (Murray et al. 2015). In preclinical studies, intravitreal injection of QR-1123 effectively attenuated P23H mutant *RHO* expression while preserving WT *RHO* expression, restored ERG response, and augmented outer nuclear layer (ONL) thickness in a P23H mutant murine model. In 2018, ProQR Therapeutics acquired QR-1123 from Ionis Pharmaceuticals and initiated a phase 1/2 Aurora clinical trial (NCT04123626) to assess the safety, tolerability, and efficacy of QR-1123 in the treatment of patients with P23H mutated *RHO*-adRP. Phase 1 results indicate that QR-1123 is well tolerated with an excellent overall safety profile.

One critical limitation for therapies such as QR-1123 is that they are not scalable to the over 150 reported mutations in the *RHO* gene that have been shown to cause *RHO*-adRP. Thus, a more conventional paradigm involves eliminating expression of both the patient WT and mutant *RHO* genes followed by gene replacement with an exogenous WT *RHO* gene (Meng et al. 2020). Such a strategy can be expanded to treat all forms of *RHO*-adRP without designing individually tailored therapies for each underlying mutation.

Cideciyan et al. (2018) developed a single AAV system containing both a WT copy of the human *RHO* gene and a component encoding an shRNA that targets the human *RHO* gene. Importantly, the group engineered the codon-modified *RHO* gene to be resistant to degradation by the vector-carrying shRNA (Gorbatyuk et al. 2007; O'Reilly et al. 2007; Palfi et al. 2012).

A single subretinal injection of the shRNA$_{820}$ candidate in a canine model for light-induced *RHO*-adRP degeneration model dramatically attenuated *RHO* mRNA and protein expression in mutant *RHO* retinas. Next, the group delivered the AAV system containing the shRNA$_{820}$ and the codon-modified human *RHO* gene and showed that the rescue *RHO* gene could be expressed at maximum 132% and 33%, at the mRNA and protein level, respectively, in comparison to control retinas. The group also demonstrated that vector administration could preserve retinal ONL thickness, photoreceptor cells, and the outer segment layers in treated retinas (Cideciyan et al. 2018). In 2018, IVERIC Bio acquired the rights to the therapy, now named IC-100, with plans to initiate a phase 1/2 clinical trial. However, subsequent preclinical studies in NHPs were unable to recapitulate the safety profiles previously reported in canine models and have stalled clinical trial proposals. IVERIC Bio is seeking potential collaborations as it turns its attention to other products in its portfolio. Natural history studies and IND-enabling activities for IC-100 are ongoing (Meng et al. 2020).

Using a CRISPR/Cas9-based approach in the treatment of *RHO*-adRP, Editas Medicine developed a dual AAV5 system to knock out and replace the mutant *RHO* gene. The dual system consists of a vector encoding an *S. aureus* Cas9 (SaCas) cRNA and a second encoding several gRNAs and a codon-optimized copy of the *RHO* cRNA. Widespread frameshift deletions generated by this dual system dramatically diminished *RHO* expression in human retinal explants, and a rescue *RHO* vector was sufficient to restore *RHO* expression similar to physiological levels (Diner et al. 2020).

USH2A

Biallelic mutations in the *USH2A* gene result in Usher syndrome type 2, an autosomal-recessive syndrome characterized by congenital hearing deficits and late-onset retinitis pigmentosa with late-onset, or nonsyndromic retinitis pigmentosa (nsRP) (van Wijk et al. 2004). *USH2A* encodes usherin, a transmembrane protein that is critical for photoreceptor outer layer and periciliary region structure (Géléoc and El-Amraoui 2020). ~35% of *USH2A* mutations occur in exon 13, which can cause premature termination and inappropriate splicing resulting in dysfunctional usherin protein. Like *CEP290*-mediated LCA, Usher syndrome type 2 has been difficult to approach using AAV-based gene augmentation strategies due to the size of the *USH2A* gene.

Dulla et al. developed the novel ASO QR-421a, which promotes exon 13 skipping in the mutant *USH2A* gene, thereby restoring normal pre-mRNA splicing (Dulla et al. 2021). QR-421a treatment selectively induced exon 13 skipping in an induced pluripotent stem cell model derived from the photoreceptors of a patient with homozygous c.2299delG mutation in the *USH2A* gene. In addition, the group showed that QR-421a had high bioavailability in the photoreceptor outer layer of WT mice. Based on these promising results, ProQR Therapeutics initiated phase 1/2 Stellar clinical trial (NCT03780257) to assess the safety, tolerability, and efficacy of QR-421a (also termed ultevursen) in patients with exon 13 mutations in the *USH2A* gene. Results from phase 1/2 have been moderately positive. Ultevursen is well tolerated and is without significant adverse effects, and the 16 subjects that received a single dose of the therapy reported a mean 6.0 letter improvement in BCVA. ProQR has since initiated two phase 2/3 clinical trials, Sirius (NCT05158296) and Celeste (NCT05176717), with results expected in 2024.

Currently, Locanabio is developing a Cas13d-centered RNA-editing approach to promote exon 13 skipping in the *USH2A* gene. In preliminary studies, a single AAV vector containing a catalytically inactive Cas13d (dCas13d) and a gRNA targeting a portion of exon 13 augmented the proportion of truncated usherin protein with exon 13 exclusion in HEK293T cells (Lardelli et al. 2021).

Spinocerebellar Ataxia

Polyglutamine spinocerebellar ataxias (SCAs) represent a heterogeneous group of six autosomal-dominant, neurodegenerative diseases characterized by a constellation of symptoms including ataxia, speech difficulties, impaired gait, and motor dysfunction (Duenas et al. 2006). The six disease groups, SCA1, SCA2, SCA3, SCA6, SCA7, and SCA17, are defined by CAG (glutamate) repeat expansions in the coding region of their associated genes, *ATXN1, ATXN2, ATXN3, CACNA1A, ATXN7,* and *TBP,* respectively (Paulson et al. 2017; Buijsen et al. 2019).

In particular, SCA7 distinctively presents with pigmentary regional dystrophy and progressive visual loss beginning in the macular region and spreading to the retinal periphery

(Lebre and Brice 2003). These pathological changes can be clinically monitored via optical coherence tomography (OCT), ERG, and full-field ERG (ffERG), which demonstrate retinal thinning of the retinal nerve fiber layer, diminished amplitudes, and diminished 30 Hz cone flicker amplitudes, respectively (Campos-Romo et al. 2018; Park et al. 2020).

Niu et al. (2018) successfully developed an ASO against *Ataxin-7*, and delivery of the ASO in a SCA7 266Q knockin mouse model via intravitreal injection dramatically attenuated *Ataxin-7* expression. In addition, mice receiving the ASO therapy recovered rod and cone function. Ramachandran developed short double-stranded RNA (dsRNA) molecules to target repeat expansion of SCA7 (Ramachandran et al. 2014). In preclinical studies, this RNAi strategy significantly reduced WT and mutant *Ataxin-7* expression, improved disease phenotype in a murine model of SCA7, and demonstrated minimal toxic effects.

CONCLUSION

The past decade has seen an explosion in gene therapy and editing techniques with major improvements to existing technologies. While Luxturna remains the only FDA-approved AAV2 therapy for the treatment of RPE65-mediated LCA, editing tools including CRISPR/Cas9 and its emerging novel variants have expanded the ways that we may approach the treatment of IRDs. These technologies have opened the possibility for researchers to treat IRDs with varying inheritance patterns and disease pathologies, IRDs with underlying mutations in previously inoperable genes due to size constraints, and IRDs with aberrations at the DNA and/or RNA levels. Meanwhile, existing RNA-editing techniques such as RNAi continue to be refined and optimized, and several trials assessing the efficacy of ASOs and RNA-based therapies have since been initiated with promising results. While the majority of clinical trials have failed to translate preclinical findings in patients and the recent results from ProQR's Brilliance trial for the treatment of *CEP290*-mediated LCA represents one such trial, gene therapy and editing techniques are still in the early stages of development. Undoubtedly, gene therapy and editing will continue to encounter challenges and several rounds of refinement in clinical trials before it is shown to be safe and effective in the treatment of many IRDs. Simultaneously, gene therapy has garnered overwhelming public support and financial backing. Cas14a-Scribe Therapeutics recently closed a 100-million-dollar series B round, and other top gene therapy companies carry robust market caps. There are more gene therapy–based clinical trials than ever before with more than 20 recruiting, enrolling by invitation, and active (not recruiting) trials designated on Clinicaltrials.gov as of July 2022. Finally, the success story of Luxturna and the profound impact that it has had on patients with RPE65-mediated LCA indicate that gene therapy and editing are viable strategies in the treatment of IRDs and will inevitably become mainstays in the way we manage patient IRDs in the future.

COMPETING INTEREST STATEMENT

S.H.T. receives financial support from Abeona Therapeutics and Emendo. He is also the founder of Rejuvitas and is on the scientific and clinical advisory board for Nanoscope Therapeutics and Medical Excellence Capital.

ACKNOWLEDGMENTS

Jonas Children's Vision Care receives support from the National Institutes of Health (grant numbers: 5P30CA013696, U01EY030580, U54OD020351, R24EY028758, R24EY027285, 5P30EY019007, R01EY018213, R01EY024698, R01EY033770, R21AG05043; the Schneeweiss Stem Cell Fund; New York State (grant number SDHDOH01-C32590GG-3450000); the Foundation Fighting Blindness New York Regional Research Center Grant (grant numbers PPA-1218-0751-COLU and TA-NMT-0116-0692-COLU); Nancy & Kobi Karp; the Crowley Family Funds; The Rosenbaum Family Foundation; Alcon Research Institute; the Gebroe Family Foundation; and unrestricted funds from Research to Prevent Blindness, New York, NY, USA.

REFERENCES

Abudayyeh OO, Gootenberg JS, Essletzbichler P, Han S, Joung J, Belanto JJ, Verdine V, Cox DBT, Kellner MJ, Regev A, et al. 2017. RNA targeting with CRISPR-Cas13. *Nature* **550**: 280–284. doi:10.1038/nature24049

Anzalone AV, Koblan LW, Liu DR. 2020. Genome editing with CRISPR-Cas nucleases, base editors, transposases and prime editors. *Nat Biotechnol* **38**: 824–844. doi:10.1038/s41587-020-0561-9

Bainbridge JW, Smith AJ, Barker SS, Robbie S, Henderson R, Balaggan K, Viswanathan A, Holder GE, Stockman A, Tyler N, et al. 2008. Effect of gene therapy on visual function in Leber's congenital amaurosis. *N Engl J Med* **358**: 2231–2239. doi:10.1056/NEJMoa0802268

Bainbridge JW, Mehat MS, Sundaram V, Robbie SJ, Barker SE, Ripamonti C, Georgiadis A, Mowat FM, Beattie SG, Gardner PJ, et al. 2015. Long-term effect of gene therapy on Leber's congenital amaurosis. *N Engl J Med* **372**: 1887–1897. doi:10.1056/NEJMoa1414221

Broughton JP, Deng X, Yu G, Fasching CL, Servellita V, Singh J, Miao X, Streithorst JA, Granados A, Sotomayor-Gonzalez A, et al. 2020. CRISPR-Cas12-based detection of SARS-CoV-2. *Nat Biotechnol* **38**: 870–874. doi:10.1038/s41587-020-0513-4

Buijsen RAM, Toonen LJA, Gardiner SL, van Roon-Mom WMC. 2019. Genetics, mechanisms, and therapeutic progress in polyglutamine spinocerebellar ataxias. *Neurotherapeutics* **16**: 263–286. doi:10.1007/s13311-018-00696-y

Cabral T, DiCarlo JE, Justus S, Sengillo JD, Xu Y, Tsang SH. 2017. CRISPR applications in ophthalmologic genome surgery. *Curr Opin Ophthalmol* **28**: 252–259. doi:10.1097/ICU.0000000000000359

Campos-Romo A, Graue-Hernandez EO, Pedro-Aguilar L, Hernandez-Camarena JC, Rivera-De la Parra D, Galvez V, Diaz R, Jimenez-Corona A, Fernandez-Ruiz J. 2018. Ophthalmic features of spinocerebellar ataxia type 7. *Eye (Lond)* **32**: 120–127. doi:10.1038/eye.2017.135

Carter-Dawson LD, LaVail MM. 1979. Rods and cones in the mouse retina. I: Structural analysis using light and electron microscopy. *J Comp Neurol* **188**: 245–262. doi:10.1002/cne.901880204

Caruso SM, Quinn PM, da Costa BL, Tsang SH. 2022. CRISPR/Cas therapeutic strategies for autosomal dominant disorders. *J Clin Invest* **132**: e158287. doi:10.1172/JCI158287

Caspi RR. 2010. A look at autoimmunity and inflammation in the eye. *J Clin Invest* **120**: 3073–3083. doi:10.1172/JCI42440

Chapman JR, Taylor MR, Boulton SJ. 2012. Playing the end game: DNA double-strand break repair pathway choice. *Mol Cell* **47**: 497–510. doi:10.1016/j.molcel.2012.07.029

Choi EH, Suh S, Foik AT, Leinonen H, Newby GA, Gao XD, Banskota S, Hoang T, Du SW, Dong Z, et al. 2022. In vivo base editing rescues cone photoreceptors in a mouse model of early-onset inherited retinal degeneration. *Nat Commun* **13**: 1830. doi:10.1038/s41467-022-29490-3

Cideciyan AV, Jacobson SG, Beltran WA, Sumaroka A, Swider M, Iwabe S, Roman AJ, Olivares MB, Schwartz

SB, Komaromy AM, et al. 2013. Human retinal gene therapy for Leber congenital amaurosis shows advancing retinal degeneration despite enduring visual improvement. *Proc Natl Acad Sci* **110**: E517–E525.

Cideciyan AV, Sudharsan R, Dufour VL, Massengill MT, Iwabe S, Swider M, Lisi B, Sumaroka A, Marinho LF, Appelbaum T, et al. 2018. Mutation-independent rhodopsin gene therapy by knockdown and replacement with a single AAV vector. *Proc Natl Acad Sci* **115**: E8547–E8556. doi:10.1073/pnas.1805055115

Cideciyan AV, Jacobson SG, Drack AV, Ho AC, Charng J, Garafalo AV, Roman AJ, Sumaroka A, Han IC, Hochstedler MD, et al. 2019. Effect of an intravitreal antisense oligonucleotide on vision in Leber congenital amaurosis due to a photoreceptor cilium defect. *Nat Med* **25**: 225–228. doi:10.1038/s41591-018-0295-0

Coffin JM, Hughes SH, Varmus HE. 1997. *Retroviruses.* Cold Spring Harbor Laboratory Press, Cold Spring Harbor, NY.

Curcio CA, Sloan KR Jr, Packer O, Hendrickson AE, Kalina RE. 1987. Distribution of cones in human and monkey retina: individual variability and radial asymmetry. *Science* **236**: 579–582. doi:10.1126/science.3576186

da Costa BL, Levi SR, Eulau E, Tsai YT, Quinn PMJ. 2021. Prime editing for inherited retinal diseases. *Front Genome Ed* **3**: 775330. doi:10.3389/fgeed.2021.775330

Diner BA, Dass A, Nayak R, Flinkstrom Z, Tallo T, Miller M, DaSilva J, Gotta G, Wang T, Marco E, et al. 2020. Dual AAV-based "knock-out-and-replace" of RHO as a therapeutic approach to treat RHO-associated autosomal dominant retinitis pigmentosa (RHO adRP). Editas Medicine, Cambridge MA.

Duenas AM, Goold R, Giunti P. 2006. Molecular pathogenesis of spinocerebellar ataxias. *Brain* **129**: 1357–1370. doi:10.1093/brain/awl081

Dulla K, Aguila M, Lane A, Jovanovic K, Parfitt DA, Schulkens I, Chan HL, Schmidt I, Beumer W, Vorthoren L, et al. 2018. Splice-modulating oligonucleotide QR-110 restores CEP290 mRNA and function in human c.2991+ 1655A>G LCA10 models. *Mol Ther Nucleic Acids* **12**: 730–740. doi:10.1016/j.omtn.2018.07.010

Dulla K, Slijkerman R, van Diepen HC, Albert S, Dona M, Beumer W, Turunen JJ, Chan HL, Schulkens IA, Vorthoren L, et al. 2021. Antisense oligonucleotide-based treatment of retinitis pigmentosa caused by USH2A exon 13 mutations. *Mol Ther* **29**: 2441–2455. doi:10.1016/j.ymthe .2021.04.024

Duncan JL, Pierce EA, Laster AM, Daiger SP, Birch DG, Ash JD, Iannaccone A, Flannery JG, Sahel JA, Zack DJ, et al. 2018. Inherited retinal degenerations: current landscape and knowledge gaps. *Transl Vis Sci Technol* **7**: 6. doi:10 .1167/tvst.7.4.6

Gaudelli NM, Komor AC, Rees HA, Packer MS, Badran AH, Bryson DI, Liu DR. 2017. Programmable base editing of A•T to G•C in genomic DNA without DNA cleavage. *Nature* **551**: 464–471. doi:10.1038/nature24644

Géléoc GGS, El-Amraoui A. 2020. Disease mechanisms and gene therapy for Usher syndrome. *Hear Res* **394**: 107932. doi:10.1016/j.heares.2020.107932

Gorbatyuk M, Justilien V, Liu J, Hauswirth WW, Lewin AS. 2007. Suppression of mouse rhodopsin expression in vivo by AAV mediated siRNA delivery. *Vision Res* **47**: 1202–1208. doi:10.1016/j.visres.2006.11.026

Gu SM, Thompson DA, Srikumari CR, Lorenz B, Finckh U, Nicoletti A, Murthy KR, Rathmann M, Kumaramanickavel G, Denton MJ, Gal A. 1997. Mutations in RPE65 cause autosomal recessive childhood-onset severe retinal dystrophy. *Nat Genet* **17**: 194–197. doi:10.1038/ ng1097-194

Hammond SM, Wood MJ. 2011. Genetic therapies for RNA mis-splicing diseases. *Trends Genet* **27**: 196–205. doi:10 .1016/j.tig.2011.02.004

Jacobson SG, Kemp CM, Sung CH, Nathans J. 1991. Retinal function and rhodopsin levels in autosomal dominant retinitis pigmentosa with rhodopsin mutations. *Am J Ophthalmol* **112**: 256–271. doi:10.1016/S0002-9394(14) 76726-1

Jinek M, Chylinski K, Fonfara I, Hauer M, Doudna JA, Charpentier E. 2012. A programmable dual-RNA-guided DNA endonuclease in adaptive bacterial immunity. *Science* **337**: 816–821. doi:10.1126/science.1225829

Komor AC, Kim YB, Packer MS, Zuris JA, Liu DR. 2016. Programmable editing of a target base in genomic DNA without double-stranded DNA cleavage. *Nature* **533**: 420–424. doi:10.1038/nature17946

Lai Y, Thomas GD, Yue Y, Yang HT, Li D, Long C, Judge L, Bostick B, Chamberlain JS, Terjung RL, et al. 2009. Dystrophins carrying spectrin-like repeats 16 and 17 anchor nNOS to the sarcolemma and enhance exercise performance in a mouse model of muscular dystrophy. *J Clin Invest* **119**: 624–635. doi:10.1172/JCI36612

Lambeth LS, Smith CA. 2013. Short hairpin RNA-mediated gene silencing. *Methods Mol Biol* **942**: 205–232. doi:10 .1007/978-1-62703-119-6_12

Lardelli R, Roth DM, Nachtrab G, Geddes C, Wilson A, Narayan N, Villegas G, Adams R, Gibbs D, Batra R. 2021. RNA-targeting gene therapy exon-skipping strategy to treat genetic diseases. Locanabio, San Diego, CA.

Lebre AS, Brice A. 2003. Spinocerebellar ataxia 7 (SCA7). *Cytogenet Genome Res* **100**: 154–163. doi:10.1159/ 000073850

Lin S, Staahl BT, Alla RK, Doudna JA. 2014. Enhanced homology-directed human genome engineering by controlled timing of CRISPR/Cas9 delivery. *eLife* **3**: e04766. doi:10.7554/eLife.04766

Liu JJ, Orlova N, Oakes BL, Ma E, Spinner HB, Baney KLM, Chuck J, Tan D, Knott GJ, Harrington LB, et al. 2019. Author correction: CasX enzymes comprise a distinct family of RNA-guided genome editors. *Nature* **568**: E8–E10. doi:10.1038/s41586-019-1084-8

Maeder ML, Stefanidakis M, Wilson CJ, Baral R, Barrera LA, Bounoutas GS, Bumcrot D, Chao H, Ciulla DM, DaSilva JA, et al. 2019. Development of a gene-editing approach to restore vision loss in Leber congenital amaurosis type 10. *Nat Med* **25**: 229–233. doi:10.1038/s41591-018-0327-9

Maguire AM, Simonelli F, Pierce EA, Pugh EN Jr, Mingozzi F, Bennicelli J, Banfi S, Marshall KA, Testa F, Surace EM, et al. 2008. Safety and efficacy of gene transfer for Leber's congenital amaurosis. *N Engl J Med* **358**: 2240–2248. doi:10.1056/NEJMoa0802315

Maguire AM, Russell S, Wellman JA, Chung DC, Yu ZF, Tillman A, Wittes J, Pappas J, Elci O, Marshall KA, et al. 2019. Efficacy, safety, and durability of voretigene neparvovec-rzyl in RPE65 mutation-associated inherited retinal dystrophy: results of phase 1 and 3 trials. *Ophthalmology* **126:** 1273–1285. doi:10.1016/j.ophtha.2019.06.017

Medawar PB. 1948. Immunity to homologous grafted skin; the fate of skin homografts transplanted to the brain, to subcutaneous tissue, and to the anterior chamber of the eye. *Br J Exp Pathol* **29:** 58–69.

Meng D, Ragi SD, Tsang SH. 2020. Therapy in rhodopsin-mediated autosomal dominant retinitis pigmentosa. *Mol Ther* **28:** 2139–2149. doi:10.1016/j.ymthe.2020.08.012

Murray SF, Jazayeri A, Matthes MT, Yasumura D, Yang H, Peralta R, Watt A, Freier S, Hung G, Adamson PS, et al. 2015. Allele-specific inhibition of rhodopsin with an antisense oligonucleotide slows photoreceptor cell degeneration. *Invest Ophthalmol Vis Sci* **56:** 6362–6375. doi:10.1167/iovs.15-16400

Narayan DS, Wood JP, Chidlow G, Casson RJ. 2016. A review of the mechanisms of cone degeneration in retinitis pigmentosa. *Acta Ophthalmol* **94:** 748–754. doi:10.1111/aos.13141

Nathans J, Piantanida TP, Eddy RL, Shows TB, Hogness DS. 1986. Molecular genetics of inherited variation in human color vision. *Science* **232:** 203–210. doi:10.1126/science.3485310

Niu C, Prakash TP, Kim A, Quach JL, Huryn LA, Yang Y, Lopez E, Jazayeri A, Hung G, Sopher BL, et al. 2018. Antisense oligonucleotides targeting mutant Ataxin-7 restore visual function in a mouse model of spinocerebellar ataxia type 7. *Sci Transl Med* **10:** eaap8677. doi:10.1126/scitranslmed.aap8677

O'Reilly M, Palfi A, Chadderton N, Millington-Ward S, Ader M, Cronin T, Tuohy T, Auricchio A, Hildinger M, Tivnan A, et al. 2007. RNA interference–mediated suppression and replacement of human rhodopsin in vivo. *Am J Hum Genet* **81:** 127–135. doi:10.1086/519025

Osborn MJ, Newby GA, McElroy AN, Knipping F, Nielsen SC, Riddle MJ, Xia L, Chen W, Eide CR, Webber BR, et al. 2020. Base editor correction of COL7A1 in recessive dystrophic epidermolysis bullosa patient-derived fibroblasts and iPSCs. *J Invest Dermatol* **140:** 338–347.e5. doi:10.1016/j.jid.2019.07.701

Palfi A, Chadderton N, McKee AG, Blanco Fernandez A, Humphries P, Kenna PF, Farrar GJ. 2012. Efficacy of co-delivery of dual AAV2/5 vectors in the murine retina and hippocampus. *Hum Gene Ther* **23:** 847–858. doi:10.1089/hum.2011.142

Park JY, Joo K, Woo SJ. 2020. Ophthalmic manifestations and genetics of the polyglutamine autosomal dominant spinocerebellar ataxias: a review. *Front Neurosci* **14:** 892. doi:10.3389/fnins.2020.00892

Paulson HL, Shakkottai VG, Clark HB, Orr HT. 2017. Polyglutamine spinocerebellar ataxias—from genes to potential treatments. *Nat Rev Neurosci* **18:** 613–626. doi:10.1038/nrn.2017.92

Perrault I, Delphin N, Hanein S, Gerber S, Dufier JL, Roche O, Defoort-Dhellemmes S, Dollfus H, Fazzi E, Munnich A, et al. 2007. Spectrum of NPHP6/CEP290 mutations in Leber congenital amaurosis and delineation of the associated phenotype. *Hum Mutat* **28:** 416. doi:10.1002/humu.9485

Perrault I, Rozet JM, Gerber S, Ghazi C, Leowski C, Ducroq D, Souied E, Dufier JL, Munnich A, Kaplan J. 1999. Leber congenital amaurosis. *Mol Genet Metab* **68:** 200–208. doi:10.1006/mgme.1999.2906

Ramachandran PS, Boudreau RL, Schaefer KA, La Spada AR, Davidson BL. 2014. Nonallele specific silencing of ataxin-7 improves disease phenotypes in a mouse model of SCA7. *Mol Ther* **22:** 1635–1642. doi:10.1038/mt.2014.108

Rossidis AC, Stratigis JD, Chadwick AC, Hartman HA, Ahn NJ, Li H, Singh K, Coons BE, Li L, Lv W, et al. 2018. In utero CRISPR-mediated therapeutic editing of metabolic genes. *Nat Med* **24:** 1513–1518. doi:10.1038/s41591-018-0184-6

Ruan GX, Barry E, Yu D, Lukason M, Cheng SH, Scaria A. 2017. CRISPR/Cas9-mediated genome editing as a therapeutic approach for Leber congenital amaurosis 10. *Mol Ther* **25:** 331–341. doi:10.1016/j.ymthe.2016.12.006

Russell S, Bennett J, Wellman JA, Chung DC, Yu ZF, Tillman A, Wittes J, Pappas J, Elci O, McCague S, et al. 2017. Efficacy and safety of voretigene neparvovec (AAV2-hRPE65v2) in patients with RPE65-mediated inherited retinal dystrophy: a randomised, controlled, open-label, phase 3 trial. *Lancet* **390:** 849–860. doi:10.1016/S0140-6736(17)31868-8

Sengillo JD, Justus S, Cabral T, Tsang SH. 2017. Correction of monogenic and common retinal disorders with gene therapy. *Genes (Basel)* **8:** 53. doi:10.3390/genes8020053

Stein-Streilein J, Taylor AW. 2007. An eye's view of T regulatory cells. *J Leukoc Biol* **81:** 593–598. doi:10.1189/jlb.0606383

Suh S, Choi EH, Leinonen H, Foik AT, Newby GA, Yeh WH, Dong Z, Kiser PD, Lyon DC, Liu DR, et al. 2021. Restoration of visual function in adult mice with an inherited retinal disease via adenine base editing. *Nat Biomed Eng* **5:** 169–178. doi:10.1038/s41551-020-00632-6

Tanna P, Strauss RW, Fujinami K, Michaelides M. 2017. Stargardt disease: clinical features, molecular genetics, animal models and therapeutic options. *Br J Ophthalmol* **101:** 25–30. doi:10.1136/bjophthalmol-2016-308823

Timmers AM, Newmark JA, Turunen HT, Farivar T, Liu J, Song C, Ye GJ, Pennock S, Gaskin C, Knop DR, et al. 2020. Ocular inflammatory response to intravitreal injection of adeno-associated virus vector: relative contribution of genome and capsid. *Hum Gene Ther* **31:** 80–89. doi:10.1089/hum.2019.144

Trapani I, Auricchio A. 2018. Seeing the light after 25 years of retinal gene therapy. *Trends Mol Med* **24:** 669–681. doi:10.1016/j.molmed.2018.06.006

Trapani I, Puppo A, Auricchio A. 2014. Vector platforms for gene therapy of inherited retinopathies. *Prog Retin Eye Res* **43:** 108–128. doi:10.1016/j.preteyeres.2014.08.001

van Wijk E, Pennings RJ, te Brinke H, Claassen A, Yntema HG, Hoefsloot LH, Cremers FP, Cremers CW, Kremer H. 2004. Identification of 51 novel exons of the Usher syndrome type 2A (USH2A) gene that encode multiple conserved functional domains and that are mutated in patients with Usher syndrome type II. *Am J Hum Genet* **74:** 738–744. doi:10.1086/383096

Verbakel SK, van Huet RAC, Boon CJF, den Hollander AI, Collin RWJ, Klaver CCW, Hoyng CB, Roepman R, Klevering BJ. 2018. Non-syndromic retinitis pigmentosa. *Prog Retin Eye Res* **66:** 157–186. doi:10.1016/j.preteyeres.2018.03.005

Villiger L, Grisch-Chan HM, Lindsay H, Ringnalda F, Pogliano CB, Allegri G, Fingerhut R, Häberle J, Matos J, Robinson MD, et al. 2018. Treatment of a metabolic liver disease by in vivo genome base editing in adult mice. *Nat Med* **24:** 1519–1525. doi:10.1038/s41591-018-0209-1

Wu W, Tsai YT, Huang IW, Cheng CH, Hsu CW, Cui X, Ryu J, Quinn PM, Caruso S, Lin CS, et al. 2022. CRISPR genome surgery in a novel humanized model for autosomal dominant retinitis pigmentosa. *Mol Ther* **30:** 1407–1420. doi:10.1016/j.ymthe.2022.02.010

Yáñez-Muñoz RJ, Balaggan KS, MacNeil A, Howe SJ, Schmidt M, Smith AJ, Buch P, MacLaren RE, Anderson PN, Barker SE, et al. 2006. Effective gene therapy with nonintegrating lentiviral vectors. *Nat Med* **12:** 348–353. doi:10.1038/nm1365

Zhang XH, Tee LY, Wang XG, Huang QS, Yang SH. 2015. Off-target effects in CRISPR/Cas9-mediated genome engineering. *Mol Ther Nucleic Acids* **4:** e264. doi:10.1038/mtna.2015.37

Zhang W, Li L, Su Q, Gao G, Khanna H. 2018. Gene therapy using a miniCEP290 fragment delays photoreceptor degeneration in a mouse model of Leber congenital amaurosis. *Hum Gene Ther* **29:** 42–50. doi:10.1089/hum.2017.049

Zhi S, Chen Y, Wu G, Wen J, Wu J, Liu Q, Li Y, Kang R, Hu S, Wang J, et al. 2022. Dual-AAV delivering split prime editor system for in vivo genome editing. *Mol Ther* **30:** 283–294. doi:10.1016/j.ymthe.2021.07.011

Alternative RNA Splicing in the Retina: Insights and Perspectives

Casey J. Keuthan,[1] Sadik Karma,[1] and Donald J. Zack[2]

[1]Department of Ophthalmology, Wilmer Eye Institute, Johns Hopkins University School of Medicine, Baltimore, Maryland 21231, USA

[2]Departments of Ophthalmology, Wilmer Eye Institute, Neuroscience, Molecular Biology and Genetics, and Genetic Medicine, Johns Hopkins University School of Medicine, Baltimore, Maryland 21231, USA

Correspondence: donzack@gmail.com

Alternative splicing is a fundamental and highly regulated post-transcriptional process that enhances transcriptome and proteome diversity. This process is particularly important in neuronal tissues, such as the retina, which exhibit some of the highest levels of differentially spliced genes in the body. Alternative splicing is regulated both temporally and spatially during neuronal development, can be cell-type-specific, and when altered can cause a number of pathologies, including retinal degeneration. Advancements in high-throughput sequencing technologies have facilitated investigations of the alternative splicing landscape of the retina in both healthy and disease states. Additionally, innovations in human stem cell engineering, specifically in the generation of 3D retinal organoids, which recapitulate many aspects of the in vivo retinal microenvironment, have aided studies of the role of alternative splicing in human retinal development and degeneration. Here we review these advances and discuss the ongoing development of strategies for the treatment of alternative splicing-related retinal disease.

Electron microscopy experiments of RNA–DNA hybrids with human adenovirus 2, as well as other studies, in the 1960s and 1970s led to the dogma-breaking publications in 1977 by Berget and colleagues and Chow and colleagues that described the discovery of RNA splicing (Berget et al. 1977; Chow et al. 1977). Soon after the initial finding of spliced adenoviral RNA transcripts, the phenomena was observed for genes of other viruses and was also shown to occur in eukaryotic organisms (Early et al. 1980). Decades of insights into RNA splicing have continued to show the central importance of this process in human health and disease (Marasco and Kornblihtt 2022).

In conjunction with the finding of RNA splicing, Berget et al.'s original study also discovered the process of alternative splicing, the differential use of mRNA splice sites to yield multiple, functional mRNAs. Today, we understand that alternative splicing is an important regulatory mechanism that helps eukaryotes generate the enormous diversity of proteins needed for their many cellular and physiological processes. Studies have estimated that as many as 95% of human genes undergo alternative splicing (Pan et al. 2008; Wang et al. 2008). Particularly high levels of alternative splicing are found in nervous system tissues, including the retina (Modrek et al. 2001; Yeo et al. 2004; Cao et al. 2011). Retinal development is largely dependent upon finely controlled, cell-type-specific patterns of gene expression, and alternative splicing contributes to this complex developmental program. Additionally, given the importance of this process in the retina, it should come as no surprise that aberrant splicing events can greatly impact retinal cell survival and function.

Retinal tissue exhibits tightly regulated splicing patterns that contribute to retinal cells' cellular and subcellular diversity (Aísa-Marín et al. 2021), and the retina is particularly sensitive to splicing dysregulation, with numerous inherited retinal dystrophies (IRDs) and diseases arising from splicing dysregulations (Liu and Zack 2013). The IRDs, a group of heterogeneous genetic disorders affecting approximately one in 3000 individuals, are characterized by the progressive degeneration of rod and/or cone photoreceptors (Garanto and Collin 2018). Examples of IRDs include retinitis pigmentosa (RP), cone-rod dystrophy, and Usher syndrome (USH). In this article, we summarize the different types of splicing mutations linked to retinal disease, as well as review various high-throughput methodologies available and the value of human retinal organoid models for studying alternative splicing in the retina. Finally, we discuss current therapeutic strategies being developed for correcting splicing-related diseases.

TYPES OF SPLICING EVENTS AND THEIR CONNECTION TO IRD

RNA splicing occurs as a two-step *trans*-esterification reaction (Lee and Rio 2015). In the first step, introns are cleaved at a consensus sequence found at the 5′ end of the intron, or 5′ splice site. The cleaved end then attaches to a second splice site on the 3′ end of the intron, forming what is called an intron lariat. This reaction is followed by positioning the 5′ and 3′ spliced ends together for fusion of the exons and excision of the intron lariat. With constitutive splicing, introns are removed and exons are retained in the same order of appearance as the pre-mRNA transcript (Fig. 1A). Alternative splicing occurs when alternative splice forms are processed, which results in the exclusion of particular exons and/or the in-

clusion of additional exons (Fig. 1B–F). Alternative splicing is a crucial mechanism in generating the diversity of the transcriptome and proteome.

Cassette Exon Inclusion or Skipping

Exon skipping/inclusion (or cassette exon splicing) is a common alternative splicing event in which a particular exon, the cassette exon, can either be included or skipped to result in two distinct, mature mRNAs (Fig. 1B). Cassette exon alternative splicing is extremely prevalent during retinal development (Wan et al. 2011). Cell-type-specific exon skipping/inclusion can also contribute to retinal disease. Mutations in *COL2A1* exon 2, which is skipped in most tissues but included in the eye, result in the largely ocular phenotypes associated with Stickler syndrome (Ryan and Sandell 1990; Bishop et al. 1994; Richards et al. 2000). Multiple alternatively spliced *CRB1* isoforms are expressed in a cell-type-specific manner in the retina (Ray et al. 2020). These isoforms have different functions, some of which are functionally relevant to *CRB1*-related retinal disease (Ray et al. 2020). Exon skipping may also explain, at least partially, the diversity of phenotypes observed in patients with *CEP290* mutations (Drivas et al. 2015).

Alternative Splice Sites

Alternative 5′ and 3′ splice site events can render more subtle changes to the mRNA, since only a portion of an exon is spliced in or out of the transcript (Fig. 1C,D). Over 300 different splice site mutations in 83 genes/loci have been documented as retinal disease–causing variants in the NCBI ClinVar database (Table 1). Progress has been made to understand the biological role splice site mutations play in IRD pathogenesis. For example, investigation of families with the autosomal-dominant erosive vitreoretinopathy and Wagner disease suggests pathogenesis is a result of an imbalance in the ratio of *CSPG2/Versican* splice site variants (Mukhopadhyay et al. 2006). Moreover, Sangermano et al. (2018) generated a midigene library of all *ABCA4* splice var-

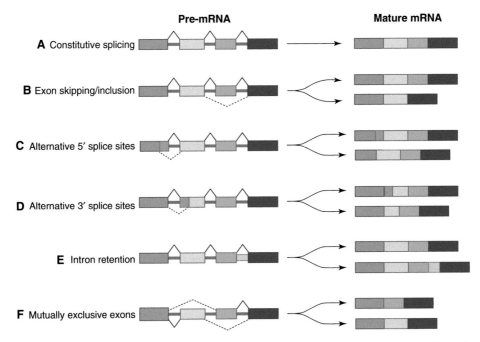

Figure 1. Types of alternative splicing events. (*A*) Constitutive RNA splicing removes introns from the pre-mRNA in sequential order, resulting in a mature mRNA transcript that includes all exons. (*B*) Exon skipping/inclusion (or cassette exon splicing) is a common alternative splicing event in which a particular exon, the cassette exon, can either be included or skipped to result in two distinct, mature mRNAs. (*C,D*) Alternative 5′ and 3′ splice sites can occur where only part of an exon is preferentially included or excluded in the mature mRNA transcript. (*E*) Alternative splicing events can also result in the retention of intronic sequences in the final mRNA. (*F*) For mutually exclusive exon events, one of two exons (or exon groups) is preferentially spliced in while the other is spliced out of the mature mRNA. (Adapted from the "mRNA Splicing Types" template with permission from BioRender.com [2022].)

iants reported in Stargardt disease patients for deeper analysis of aberrant splice site events.

Intron Retention

Splicing events where intronic regions are included in the mature mRNA can occur when intron sequences with high similarity to canonical splice acceptor or donor sites, known as cryptic splice sites, are activated (Fig. 1E). When the reading frame remains intact, these intron sequences can be translated, resulting in mutant protein that can affect its normal function. Intron-retaining splicing events have been linked to several forms of retinal disease. A 65-kDa cryptic splice site mutation in a patient's *RPE65* gene was reported as the causative variant for the patient's Leber's congenital amaurosis (LCA) (Tucker et al. 2015). The most common disease-causing vari-

ant in *CEP290* LCA is the intronic splicing mutation c.2991 + 1655A>G (den Hollander et al. 2006; Coppieters et al. 2010). This intron-retention event introduces a pseudoexon (also known as a cryptic exon) into the mRNA that creates a premature stop codon. Interestingly, a significant amount of the normal *CEP290* transcript is correctly spliced in these patients, emphasizing the unique threshold for splicing defects that seem to affect the retina compared to other nonimpacted tissues.

Intron retention is frequently observed in USH type 2 (*USH2A*) patients. Like other intronic mutations, intron retention in c.7595-2144A>G patients creates a pseudoexon that causes premature termination of the translated protein (Vaché et al. 2012; Slijkerman et al. 2016). The c.82 + 5G variant of *ATF6*, an unfolded protein response gene linked to achroma-

Table 1. Summary of splice site mutations that cause retinal disease

Gene(s)	No. of variants	Gene(s)	No. of variants
ABCA4	43	LOC112806037/MERTK	1
ACBD5	1	MERTK	12
ACO2	1	NR2E3	1
ADGRV1	2	OFD1	1
AHR	1	OPA1	1
ALMS1	1	PANK2	1
ARL2BP	4	PDE6A	11
ARL6	1	PDE6B/PDE6B-AS1	5
BBS1/ZDHHC24	1	PDE6B	3
BBS2	1	PDE6G	1
BBS5	1	PHYH	1
CDH23	2	POMGNT1/TSPAN1	1
CDHR1	1	PROM1	8
CDKL5/RS1	1	PRPF3	1
CEP290	6	PRPF31	4
CERKL	6	PRPF31/PRPF31-AS1	6
CFAP410	1	PRPF31-AS1/PRPF31	2
CFAP418	1	PRPH2	1
CHM	5	RBP4	1
CLN3	1	REEP6	1
CNGB1	8	RHO	3
CNGB3	4	RP1	3
COL18A1	1	RP2	4
COL2A1	2	RPE65	11
CRB1	11	RPGR	13
CYGB/PRCD	2	RPGRIP1	1
EYS	11	RS1	1
FAM161A	1	SAG	2
FRMD7	1	SCAPER	1
GPHN/RDH12/ZFYVE26	1	STX3	1
GPHN/RDH12	1	TRPM1	1
GUCY2D	1	TTC8	3
HGSNAT	9	TTLL5	2
IFT140/LOC105371046	1	TUB/RIC3	1
IFT140	1	TULP1	2
IFT172	1	USH2A	35
IGFBP7	1	USH2A/USH2A-AS1	5
IMPG1	1	USH2A/USH2A-AS2	3
IMPG2	8	VCAN/VCAN-AS1	1
KIZ/KIZ-AS1	1	VPS13B	1
KIZ	1	ZNF408	1
LOC105371046/IFT140	1		

Genes with splice site mutations with pathogenic clinical significance for retinal degeneration in NCBI's ClinVar database (Landrum et al. 2018). Last accessed August 4, 2022.

Cite this article as *Cold Spring Harb Perspect Med* doi: 10.1101/cshperspect.a041313

topsia, also results in usage of a cryptic splice site that produces a mutant transcript that can evade nonsense-mediated decay (NMD) (Kohl et al. 2015). An additional *ATF6* achromatopsia variant, c.1533 + 1G-C, results in a mutant protein with an 83 bp retention of intron 12 (Kohl et al. 2015). This particular variant also yields a second, aberrantly spliced *ATF6* transcript that causes skipping of exon 12, resulting in premature termination (Kohl et al. 2015). Several intron retention mutations in *CNGB3*, another achromatopsia-causing gene, create cryptic splice sites that lead to inclusion and subsequent activation of pseudoexons (Weisschuh et al. 2020). *Nr2e3* mutant mouse models have been generated to investigate the significance of alternative isoforms, including an intron-retaining transcript, to RP and enhanced S-cone syndrome phenotypes (Aísa-Marín et al. 2020).

Mutually Exclusive Exons

Mutually exclusive exon splicing involves coordination of multiple splicing events, where one of two exons, or one group of two exon groups, is skipped and the other retained in the mature mRNA transcript (Fig. 1F). This type of splicing event occurs at significantly high levels during human retinal development as the retina transitions from a fetal to adult state, particularly for exons in genes involved in the maintenance of photoreceptors (Mellough et al. 2019).

MUTATIONS IN SPLICING FACTORS THAT CAUSE RD

Spliceosome

The spliceosome is a complex assembly of ribonucleoproteins, including small nuclear RNPs (snRNPs) (U1, U2, U4, U5, and U6) and various cofactors that execute splicing reactions within a cell. While these splicing factors are ubiquitously expressed, by a mechanism that is incompletely understood, mutations in a number of spliceosome components uniquely (or primarily) affect the retina. For example, mutations in the premRNA processing factors *PRPF3*, *PRPF4*, *PRPF6*, *PRPF8*, and *PRPF31* all cause autoso-

mal-dominant RP (Heng et al. 1998; McKie et al. 2001; Vithana et al. 2001, 2003; Chakarova et al. 2002; Sullivan et al. 2006; Cao et al. 2011; Tanackovic et al. 2011; Venturini et al. 2012; Chen et al. 2014; Linder et al. 2014). Mutations in other factors involved in pre-mRNA splicing have also been identified with IRDs (e.g., RNA helicases encoded by *SNRNP200* and *DHX38* have been identified as dominant and recessive RP genes, respectively) (Zhao et al. 2009; Li et al. 2010; Benaglio et al. 2011; Ajmal et al. 2014). *CWC27*, a factor associated with the U2-type spliceosome, is also associated with retinal diseases that manifest an array of phenotypes ranging from nonsyndromic RP to retinal degeneration with additional skeletal abnormalities (Xu et al. 2017). Moreover, the widely expressed PIM1-kinase-associated protein 1 (*PAP1*) that also interacts with the U2 spliceosome complex may be connected to the RP 9 form of disease (Keen et al. 2002; Maita et al. 2004).

RNA-Binding Proteins

RNA-binding proteins include *trans*-acting splicing factors that can modulate the inclusion or exclusion of alternatively spliced exons through either recruitment or repression of the splicing machinery. Dysregulation through RNA-binding factors can also contribute to retinal disease. For example, *SFRS10* is up-regulated in age-related macular degeneration (AMD) patients and believed to be involved in the splicing regulation of stress response genes during disease pathogenesis (Karunakaran et al. 2013). Additionally, mutations in the gene encoding the RNA-binding protein *CERKL* have been reported to cause RP and cone-rod dystrophy (Bayes et al. 1998; Tuson et al. 2004; Auslender et al. 2007; Garanto et al. 2011; Fathinajafabadi et al. 2014).

SPLICING IN THE AGE OF HIGH-THROUGHPUT SEQUENCING

Isoform Identification/Quantification with Short-Read RNA-Sequencing (RNA-seq)

High-throughput sequencing has transformed the field of RNA biology, allowing us to garner detailed transcriptome information at a single-cell resolution. Typical RNA next-generation sequencing (NGS) generates reads from short fragments of amplified cDNA, which are later computationally assembled and quantified. However, alternatively spliced isoforms of the same gene are often quite similar and may have significantly overlapping regions of the short reads, making it challenging to accurately identify splicing events with this methodology. To overcome these challenges, a multitude of computational tools have been developed for isoform quantification from short-read RNA-seq data. Cufflinks is a well-known program for transcript assembly and quantification (Trapnell et al. 2010, 2013). Similarly, tools such as RSEM, TIGAR2, and eXpress can be used for quantifying known transcripts (Li and Dewey 2011; Roberts and Pachter 2013; Nariai et al. 2014). Alignment-free methods have also been developed, including Sailfish, Salmon, and Kallisto, for more rapid and flexible read mapping (Patro et al. 2014, 2017; Bray et al. 2016). Alternatively, programs like iReckon, SLIDE, and StringTie all support novel transcript discovery to uncover previously unknown transcripts (Wang et al. 2008; Mezlini et al. 2013; Pertea et al. 2015). These methods, and others, have been reviewed extensively (Wang et al. 2015; Zhang et al. 2017; Mehmood et al. 2020; Halperin et al. 2021). Grant et al. have also compared several algorithms for evaluating splicing, including TopHat, SpliceMap, and their newly developed pipeline, the RNA-seq unified mapper (RUM), using RNA-seq data from the mouse retina (Grant et al. 2011).

Large-scale transcriptome analysis by RNA-seq has been performed mostly on healthy human retina tissue, and this work has identified almost 80,000 retinal alternative splicing events (Farkas et al. 2013). This study found a sizeable portion of novel splice events that maintained an open reading frame, suggesting previously unknown protein isoforms expressed in the retina. ASCOT, a recently developed resource for the analysis of splice variants across a variety of transcriptome datasets, used publicly archived RNA-seq data from mouse and human tissue to identify the synergistic regulation of *MSI1* and *PTBP1* in modulating photoreceptor-specific splicing (Ling

et al. 2020). Hence, NGS has and will continue to be a powerful tool to broaden our understanding of RNA splicing in retinal disease.

Long-Read Sequencing for Isoform Detection

Long-read sequencing (LRS) is an alternative and powerful technique to obtain sequence information of splice variants that cannot be resolved using short-read sequencing methods. In general, LRS methods acquire real-time sequence information of full-length molecules, allowing more contiguous isoform assembly. PacBio Single-Molecule Real-Time (SMRT) is a widely used LRS platform that uses a sequencing-by-synthesis strategy to capture sequence information of single DNA molecules (Eid et al. 2009). In this method, flow cells are equipped with zero-mode waveguides that act as the sequencing units to emit light as nucleotides are added by the DNA polymerase (Korlach et al. 2010). A long-read optimized de novo transcriptome pipeline has been developed using PacBio sequencing to identify novel isoforms in the eye and assess their significance to ocular development and disease (Swamy et al. 2020). A modified version of PacBio LRS, lrCaptureSeq, successfully uncovered a previously unknown *CRB1* variant specific to photoreceptors (Ray et al. 2020). Nanopore sequencing (Oxford Nanopore Technologies [ONT]) is another single-molecule LRS platform that takes advantage of the unique sizes and electrical properties of distinct nucleotides (Deamer et al. 2016). Single strands of DNA or RNA are fed through the nanopores of the flow cell, where changes in electrical current are measured and used to deduce the identity of each nucleotide (Laver et al. 2015). ONT's PromethION sequencer can run up to 48 flow cells, each containing almost 3000 individual channels, in parallel, to generate upward of 290 Gb of data per flow cell (ONT, unpubl.). Long-read nanopore sequencing was recently used to identify novel structural variants of *CEP78* that cause cone-rod dystrophy and hearing loss (Ascari et al. 2021).

Single-Cell Resolution of Isoforms

While advancements in LRS technology continue to be made, the technology is not yet optimal for single-cell studies. The relatively low read accuracy of LRS methods, compared to NGS methods, makes it difficult to demultiplex reads based on short indexes like those used in typical single-cell RNA-seq protocols. Most of the single-cell methods rely on unique molecular identifiers (UMIs) associated with a fragment of an RNA molecule. RNA counts are generated by sequencing one end, resulting in limited coverage to suitably identify splice variants. SMART-seq2/3 is a plate-based, single-cell RNA-seq method that combines full-length transcriptome coverage with UMIs to detect isoform-specific RNA on a per-cell basis (Hagemann-Jensen et al. 2020). Single-molecule fluorescent in situ hybridization (smFISH) is another technique to detect unique isoform sequences in single cells (Femino et al. 1998; Raj et al. 2008). One powerful advantage to using smFISH is the ability to glean spatial information, as well as sequence data, from individual cells. Similarly, 10x Genomics' newly developed Xenium In Situ platform labels cells with circularizable DNA probes, rather than poly(A) capture, making it possible to build spatial transcriptome maps with isoform-level detection in single cells (10x Genomics, unpubl.) Although powerful, these methods have limited throughput.

RETINAL ORGANOIDS AS A HUMAN MODEL FOR SPLICING-RELATED RETINAL DISEASE

Animal models, particularly rodents, have been the gold standard for studying splicing and the effects of specific splicing mutations on mammalian tissues and organ systems. However, animal models do not always exhibit comparable biology and clinical retinal phenotypes to those observed in humans. Recent advances in stem cell engineering have led to the development of three-dimensional (3D) retinal organoids as an alternative system for modeling the human retina and retinal disease. Stem cell–derived retinal organoids form the major cell types of the mammalian neuroretina with 3D organization that mimics the connectivity and microenvironment of the in vivo retina. Generation of retinal organoids typically involves aggregation of either embryonic

or induced pluripotent stem cells (iPSCs) into embryoid bodies, followed by treatment with small molecules to mimic the signaling events that occur during in vivo development (Fig. 2). A multitude of retinal organoid differentiation protocols have been developed (Zhong et al. 2014; Wahlin et al. 2017; Capowski et al. 2019; Cowan et al. 2020; Fligor et al. 2020; Kallman et al. 2020), and detailed use of these 3D cell cultures have been comprehensively reviewed (Bell et al. 2020; O'Hara-Wright and Gonzalez-Cordero 2020; Fathi et al. 2021; Vielle et al. 2021).

Recently, RNA-sequencing of retinal organoids has been used to explore the temporal relationship of photoreceptor-specific splicing events during retinal development (Ottaviani et al. 2019). Retinal organoids generated from stem cell lines in which retinal disease–associated mutations have been engineered or from retinal degeneration patient-derived iPSC lines have also provided powerful models for studying the mechanisms of disease-causing mutations, including those caused by aberrations in the normal splicing program. As one example, *PRPF31* RP retinal organoids have been used to comprehensively characterize the ciliary abnormalities and transcriptomic changes associated with the RP variant (Buskin et al. 2018). Differentiation of retinal organoids has also verified retina-specific expression of a particular *REEP1* splice variant implicated in autosomal-recessive RP (Arno et al. 2016). Wild-type (WT) retinal organoids have even been used to identify the cilia gene that appears to explain the nonsyndromic nature of *DYNC2H1* RP (Vig et al. 2020). Furthermore, retinal organoids differentiated from iPSCs of a *CEP290* LCA patient have revealed that tissue-specific differences in splicing could drive the pleiotropic phenotypes that arise from different *CEP290* mutations (Parfitt et al. 2016).

THERAPIES FOR THE MODULATION OF SPLICING

Given the important role that splicing abnormalities can play in disease pathogenesis, increasing efforts are being made to develop splicing modulation-based therapeutic approaches, particularly for cancer treatment (Urbanski et al. 2018;

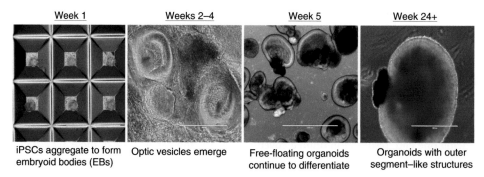

| Week 1 | Weeks 2–4 | Week 5 | Week 24+ |

iPSCs aggregate to form embryoid bodies (EBs) | Optic vesicles emerge | Free-floating organoids continue to differentiate | Organoids with outer segment–like structures

Figure 2. Stem cell–derived organoids recapitulate human retinal development. Generally, three-dimensional aggregates, or embryoid bodies (EBs), of induced pluripotent stem cells (iPSCs) or embryonic stem cells are first formed in suspension (week 1). Scale bar, 1000 µm. The EBs are composed of all three embryonic germ layers. Next, the EBs are transferred to Matrigel wells where they are cultured for several weeks while optic vesicles emerge (weeks 2–4). Scale bar, 400 µm. These vesicles are eventually lifted from the adherent plate and maintained as free-floating organoids that ultimately form all of the major cell types of the human retina (week 5). Scale bar, 1000 µm. The cellular organization and timeline of cell development mimics that of human retinal development. For example, retinal ganglion cells (RGCs) are one of the first cell types to arise and self-localize to the innermost portions of the organoid (week 5; red = tdTomato-expressing RGCs). Retinal organoids eventually give rise to terminally differentiated photoreceptors, which can continue to mature to form outer segment–like protrusions along the surface (week 24+). Scale bar, 400 µm.

Wang and Aifantis 2020). Progress has also been made in developing splicing-based strategies for some neurological conditions (Jaudon et al. 2020; Hill and Meisler 2021). Interestingly, the first drug approved for the treatment of spinal muscular atrophy was an antisense oligonucleotide (ASO) splicing modulator (Schorling et al. 2020). Here, we will review some of the molecular strategies that are being developed for therapeutic splicing modulation and will discuss some of the ongoing, early efforts to apply these strategies to retinal diseases.

CRISPR-Based Splicing Therapeutics

The discovery and use of the clustered regularly interspaced short palindromic repeat (CRISPR)/ Cas system has revolutionized how we approach genetic engineering. Cas9 is an endonuclease that uses guide RNA (gRNA) to generate a double-stranded break (DSB) at a specific site in the genome (Zhang et al. 2014). This break is then repaired by either non-homologous end joining (NHEJ) in the absence of a homologous DNA template, an error-prone process that usually leads to gene knockout, or homology-directed repair (HDR) in the presence of a synthetic

DNA strand to lead to specifically engineered genomic alterations (Savić and Schwank 2016).

CRISPR has been adapted for use as a splicing modulator (Fig. 3A). CRISPR-SKIP exploits the fact that most intronic acceptor sites end with a guanosine; it uses C > T single-base repair to target the complementary sequence to mutate cytosine to thymine, leading to intronic acceptor sites ending with two consecutive adenosines and thus skipping the exon (Gapinske et al. 2018). This system, although dependent on the presence of proto-spaced adjacent motifs (PAMs) ~16 nucleotides away from the cytosine of the intronic acceptor site, provides a potential therapy for diseases that result from erroneous inclusion of a pseudo-exon, such as specific variants of LCA (Gerard et al. 2012; Barny et al. 2019).

Beyond genomic engineering, CRISPR can also be used to directly modify RNA to modulate splicing. One promising strategy uses the CRISPR/Cas13 system to edit full-length transcripts through RNA editing for programmable A to I replacement (REPAIR), a single-base RNA-editing technique (Cox et al. 2017). REPAIR has shown favorable results in modifying splicing with few side effects. The base conver-

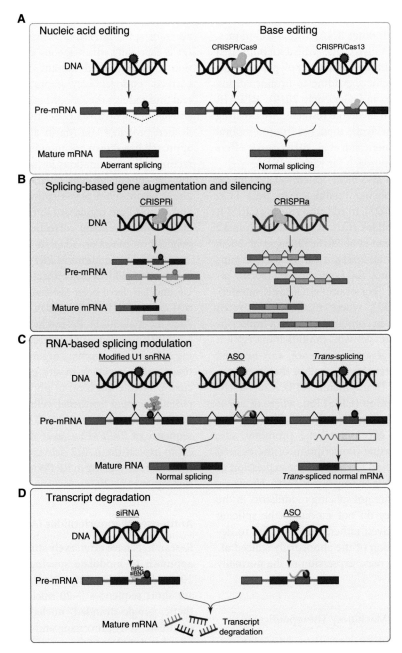

Figure 3. Therapies to target splicing-related defects. (*A*) Base editing using a modified clustered regularly interspaced short palindromic repeat (CRISPR)/Cas system can correct splicing mutations at both the DNA and pre-mRNA level to restore normal RNA splicing of the gene. (*B*) CRISPRa/i has the potential to either deplete aberrantly spliced mRNA transcripts or increase transcription of the mRNA from a normal allele, respectively. (*C*) RNA-based splicing modulation can be accomplished by either (1) a modified U1 snRNA that recognizes a mutated splice donor site (SDS) to reestablish normal splicing, (2) antisense oligonucleotides (ASOs), short nucleotide sequences to restore normal splicing levels, or (3) *trans*-splicing, which hijacks a naturally occurring mechanism to increase the ratio of normal to mutated transcript. (*D*) siRNA and ASO therapies can be designed to target the splicing defect within the pre-mRNA molecule for degradation of the mutant transcripts. (Figure created with BioRender.com.)

sion of REPAIR can be further broadened by infusing it with other RNA-editing techniques, such as combining REPAIR with apolipoprotein B mRNA editing catalytic polypeptide–like APOBEC to achieve cytidine-to-uridine editing (Pickar-Oliver and Gersbach 2019). REPAIR has also shown favorable results in modulating splicing in a neuronal model of frontotemporal dementia (Konermann et al. 2018), and it offers a promising approach for various IRDs.

CRISPR is also being tested in IRD clinical trials as a splicing modulator to treat LCA (Quinn et al. 2021). In addition to using CRISPR to edit nucleotides (Cox et al. 2017; Gapinske et al. 2018; Yuan et al. 2018; Zhang et al. 2020; Aísa-Marín et al. 2021), it can be used to suppress or enhance the expression of specific alleles (Fig. 3B). For example, CRISPR interference (CRISPRi), where nuclease-deactivated Cas9 (dCas9), in combination with a transcriptional repressor domain, inhibits transcription of a specific genomic sequence, can be used to inhibit expression of an allele that is erroneously spliced (Kampmann 2018). Conversely, CRISPR activation (CRISPRa), where dCas9 is fused with an activation domain that recruits transcription effectors to the promoter site, thereby increasing transcription of the desired gene, can be used to augment the expression of the desired allele (Kampmann 2018). However, both systems are not splicing modulators in the sense that they do not modulate the splicing events themselves; rather, they are used to decrease expression of the abnormally spliced allele and/or increase expression of the normally spliced allele.

Spliceosome Machinery Therapeutics

Since the spliceosome is responsible for the removal of introns and carrying out the splicing process, it offers a therapeutic target to explore. As aforementioned, U1 binds to the 5′ intronic splice site by recognizing the splice donor site (SDS) and initiates the splicing process (Yang et al. 2019). Splicing dysregulation in IRDs often involves U1 binding to a mutated SDS. With recent advancements in genetic engineering, a mutation-adapted U1 can be designed to match

a specific patient with a particular SDS to correct aberrant splicing (Fig. 3C). Mutation-adapted U1 is especially advantageous for gain-of-function mutations of dominant diseases since it corrects endogenously expressed transcripts and thus reduces the amount of mutated protein and simultaneously increases the amount of the desired protein (Aísa-Marín et al. 2021). This approach has shown encouraging results in correcting splicing mutations in the retina, including the rhodopsin gene (*RHO*) (Tanner et al. 2009), where ~95% of WT splicing was restored, and RP GTPase regulator (*RPGR*) (Glaus et al. 2011), where splicing correction was dose-dependent on mutation-adapted U1.

Similarly, mutations in *PRPF31*, an essential component to form the connection between U4/U6 and U5, have been associated with autosomal-dominant RP (Azizzadeh Pormehr et al. 2020; Li et al. 2021). Researchers have used the CRISPR/Cas9 system to correct aberrant splicing in both human retinal organoids and mouse tissue cultures, where in situ gene editing rescued protein expression in photoreceptors and retinal pigment epithelial cells (Buskin et al. 2018; Rodrigues et al. 2022). The small coding sequence of *PRPF31* has also allowed researchers to exploit the AAV2 delivery system to correct aberrant splicing in RP (Wheway et al. 2020; Rodrigues et al. 2022).

Antisense Oligonucleotides (ASOs)

Researchers have extensively studied ASOs as an approach to modulate splicing (Gerard et al. 2016; Vázquez-Domínguez et al. 2019). ASOs are short sequences (~20 nucleotides) of synthetic, single-stranded nucleotides that can modulate RNA processing and translation (Gemayel et al. 2021). ASOs can be used to either (1) silence an allele or inhibit a specific mutation at the DNA level, or (2) skip a mutated sequence (pseudoexon) normally skipped, or retain a sequence normally included (circumvent erroneous exon skipping), at the pre-mRNA level (Fig. 3C,D; Garanto 2019). The silencing of a genomic allele is especially advantageous in the case of an autosomal-dominant mutation (e.g., with Nuclear Receptor Subfamily 2 Group E Member

3 [*NR2E3*]), an ASO designed against the mutated allele rescues the mutation by decreasing expression of mutated *NR2E3* at the RNA and protein levels, while WT-*NR2E3* RNA and protein levels remain unaffected (Naessens et al. 2019).

Several studies have been done in the context of the IRDs to modulate splicing at the pre-mRNA level using ASOs. One example is a recurrent intronic mutation that causes the insertion of a pseudoexon and a premature stop codon in *CEP290*, representing 15% of all LCA cases in the United States and Europe (Mellough et al. 2019). An ASO that targets the *CEP290* pseudoexon biases the exclusion of the exon and restores normal levels of the protein (Collin et al. 2012; Gerard et al. 2012; Cideciyan et al. 2019). ASOs have also been used to induce inclusion of sequences that are skipped in certain mutations, such as using an ASO to rescue a recurrent mutation in the *USH1C* gene that activates a cryptic splice donor site prematurely in the exon, leading to a shortened mature mRNA and decreased protein level underlying USH (Lentz et al. 2013). Similarly, ASOs can be used to modulate pre-mRNA splicing (Lentz et al. 2013; Naessens et al. 2019); examples include *OPA1* (Bonifert et al. 2016), *OFD1* (Webb et al. 2012), *CHM* (Garanto et al. 2018), *USH2A* (Slijkerman et al. 2016; Dulla et al. 2021), *ABCA4* (Albert et al. 2018; Bauwens et al. 2019; Garanto et al. 2019; Sangermano et al. 2019), *RHO* (Murray et al. 2015; Gemayel et al. 2021), and *PRPF31* (Wheway et al. 2020).

Trans-Splicing-Mediated Therapeutics

In humans, most pre-mRNA splicing occurs in a *cis* fashion, meaning the mature mRNA has the 5′ end and the 3′ end of the same pre-mRNA transcript. However, that is not the case for all organisms. Scientists first discovered *trans*-splicing in trypanosomes, where the mature mRNA has the 5′ end of one pre-mRNA transcript and the 3′ end of another, and more recently found that some human and rat transcripts also undergo this process (Berger et al. 2015). *Trans*-splicing has been used to target several diseases, especially ones that (1) have a

gain-of-function mutation, (2) endogenous expression levels are tightly regulated, and/or (3) there are a large number of mutations, so a "generic" (rather than personalized) treatment is needed (Puttaraju et al. 1999; Berger et al. 2015). Spliceosome-mediated RNA *trans*-splicing (SMaRT) exploits endogenous *trans*-splicing machinery and engineers molecules that can *trans*-splice with endogenous, mutated, pre-mRNA transcripts, increasing the desired transcript and protein while simultaneously decreasing the mutated transcript and protein (Fig. 3C; Puttaraju et al. 1999; Berger et al. 2015). SMaRT is conducted through the introduction of a pre-mRNA *trans*-splicing molecule (PTM) that consists of (1) a binding domain for specific targeting of the endogenous pre-mRNA, (2) an artificial intron sequence containing all the elements required for splicing, and (3) the cDNA "replacement sequence" (Berger et al. 2015). Additionally, the PTM lacks the first exon and therefore it does not have an initiation codon (AUG), rendering it inert in the cell unless it gets spliced in in the presence of its target pre-mRNA (Berger et al. 2015). SMaRT has been used to correct aberrant splicing in the *RHO* gene in both in vitro and in vivo models (Berger et al. 2015). Recently, Ascidian Therapeutics was launched with a lead program to develop *trans*-splicing therapies for *ABCA4*-causing retinal disease (Ascidian Therapeutics, press release, 2022).

Mature mRNAs and Proteins Therapeutics

RNA interference (RNAi), an endogenous mechanism for transcriptional and post-transcriptional gene silencing (Hannon 2002), is a prominent example of a therapeutic method that targets the RNA through exogenous small interfering RNA (siRNA) (Fig. 3D). First, Dicer, an endonuclease, cleaves long, double-stranded RNA into siRNA. Next, the siRNA is loaded into an RISC complex, unwound by a helicase, and then binds to mRNA with a complementary sequence, marking it for degradation (Gavrilov and Saltzman 2012; Nikam and Gore 2018). siRNA has been studied and used in clinical trials as a potential therapeutic agent for ocular diseases, such as targeting *VEGF* or PF-655 to treat AMD and diabetic macular edema (Singerman 2009; Kaiser et al. 2010; Lares et al. 2010; Vaishnaw et al. 2010), targeting caspase-2 to treat optic neuropathies like non-arteritic anterior ischemic optic neuropathy (Solano et al. 2014), targeting *TRPV1* for ocular pain (Benitez-Del-Castillo et al. 2016), or β2-adrenergic receptors to treat ocular hypertension (Martínez et al. 2014). Although siRNAs can be used therapeutically to target splicing events or specific and mature mRNAs to down-regulate the expression of distinct protein isoforms, they are generally used as RNA therapeutics rather than splicing modulators (Hombach and Kretz 2016).

Protein kinases are also being targeted to modulate splicing, examples being the use of CLK inhibitors in breast cancer, amyotrophic lateral sclerosis (ALS), and colorectal cancer (Muraki et al. 2004; Araki et al. 2015). While kinase inhibitors present a possible avenue to explore for IRDs, research in this area has so far been limited.

CONCLUDING REMARKS

Clearly, there have been major advances in understanding the role alternative splicing plays in retinal development and defining many of the splicing-related mutations that can cause retinal degeneration and other forms of retinal disease. The retina demonstrates an unusually high degree of alternative splicing and many retina-specific splice isoforms have been identified. Less clear are the reasons why mutations in ubiquitously expressed splicing-related factors can lead to diseases in which the clinical phenotype is largely, or completely, limited to the retina. A variety of hypotheses have been proposed to explain this relative specificity, but none of them seem to fully explain the specificity and further research will be needed to more fully understand this interesting phenomenon. Another exciting area of ongoing research is directed at developing splicing modulation-based therapies for the splicing-related IRDs, and these approaches are showing great promise and hopefully will lead to safe and effective ways to reduce vision loss.

REFERENCES

Aísa-Marín I, López-Iniesta MJ, Milla S, Lillo J, Navarro G, de la Villa P, Marfany G. 2020. Nr2e3 functional domain ablation by CRISPR-Cas9D10A identifies a new isoform and generates retinitis pigmentosa and enhanced S-cone syndrome models. *Neurobiol Dis* **146:** 105122. doi:10.1016/j.nbd.2020.105122

Aísa-Marín I, García-Arroyo R, Mirra S, Marfany G. 2021. The alter retina: alternative splicing of retinal genes in health and disease. *Int J Mol Sci* **22:** 1855. doi:10.3390/ijms22041855

Ajmal M, Khan MI, Neveling K, Khan YM, Azam M, Waheed NK, Hamel CP, Ben-Yosef T, De Baere E, Koenekoop RK, et al. 2014. A missense mutation in the splicing factor gene *DHX38* is associated with early-onset retinitis pigmentosa with macular coloboma. *J Med Genet* **51:** 444–448. doi:10.1136/jmedgenet-2014-102316

Albert S, Garanto A, Sangermano R, Khan M, Bax NM, Hoyng CB, Zernant J, Lee W, Allikmets R, Collin RWJ, et al. 2018. Identification and rescue of splice defects caused by two neighboring deep-intronic ABCA4 mutations underlying Stargardt disease. *Am J Hum Genet* **102:** 517–527. doi:10.1016/j.ajhg.2018.02.008

Araki S, Dairiki R, Nakayama Y, Murai A, Miyashita R, Iwatani M, Nomura T, Nakanishi O. 2015. Inhibitors of CLK protein kinases suppress cell growth and induce apoptosis by modulating pre-mRNA splicing. *PLoS ONE* **10:** e0116929. doi:10.1371/journal.pone.0116929

Arno G, Agrawal SA, Eblimit A, Bellingham J, Xu M, Wang F, Chakarova C, Parfitt DA, Lane A, Burgoyne T, et al. 2016. Mutations in REEP6 cause autosomal-recessive retinitis pigmentosa. *Am J Hum Genet* **99:** 1305–1315. doi:10.1016/j.ajhg.2016.10.008

Ascari G, Rendtorff ND, De Bruyne M, De Zaeytijd J, Van Lint M, Bauwens M, Van Heetvelde M, Arno G, Jacob J, Creytens D, et al. 2021. Long-read sequencing to unravel complex structural variants of CEP78 leading to cone-rod dystrophy and hearing loss. *Front Cell Dev Biol* **9:** 664317. doi:10.3389/fcell.2021.664317

Ascidian Therapeutics. 2022. Ascidian Therapeutics launches to rewrite RNA. https://www.ascidian-tx.com/media/Ascidian%20Therapeutics%20PR_12%20October%202022.pdf

Auslender N, Sharon D, Abbasi AH, Garzozi HJ, Banin E, Ben-Yosef T. 2007. A common founder mutation of *CERKL* underlies autosomal recessive retinal degeneration with early macular involvement among Yemenite Jews. *Invest Ophthalmol Vis Sci* **48:** 5431–5438. doi:10.1167/iovs.07-0736

Azizzadeh Pormehr L, Ahmadian S, Daftarian N, Mousavi SA, Shafiezadeh M. 2020. PRPF31 reduction causes missplicing of the phototransduction genes in human organotypic retinal culture. *Eur J Hum Genet* **28:** 491–498. doi:10.1038/s41431-019-0531-1

Barny I, Perrault I, Michel C, Goudin N, Defoort-Dhellemmes S, Ghazi I, Kaplan J, Rozet JM, Gerard X. 2019. AON-mediated exon skipping to bypass protein truncation in retinal dystrophies due to the recurrent CEP290 c.4723A>T mutation. Fact or fiction? *Genes (Basel)* **10:** 368. doi:10.3390/genes10050368

Bauwens M, Garanto A, Sangermano R, Naessens S, Weisschuh N, De Zaeytijd J, Khan M, Sadler F, Balikova I, Van Cauwenbergh C, et al. 2019. ABCA4-associated disease as a model for missing heritability in autosomal recessive disorders: novel noncoding splice, *cis*-regulatory, structural, and recurrent hypomorphic variants. *Genet Med* **21:** 1761–1771. doi:10.1038/s41436-018-0420-y

Bayes M, Goldaracena B, Martinez-Mir A, Iragui-Madoz MI, Solans T, Chivelet P, Bussaglia E, Ramos-Arroyo MA, Baiget M, Vilageliu L, et al. 1998. A new autosomal recessive retinitis pigmentosa locus maps on chromosome 2q31-q33. *J Med Genet* **35:** 141–145. doi:10.1136/jmg.35.2.141

Bell CM, Zack DJ, Berlinicke CA. 2020. Human organoids for the study of retinal development and disease. *Annu Rev Vis Sci* **6:** 91–114. doi:10.1146/annurev-vision-121219-081855

Benaglio P, McGee TL, Capelli LP, Harper S, Berson EL, Rivolta C. 2011. Next generation sequencing of pooled samples reveals new SNRNP200 mutations associated with retinitis pigmentosa. *Hum Mutat* **32:** E2246–E2258. doi:10.1002/humu.21485

Benitez-Del-Castillo JM, Moreno-Montañés J, Jiménez-Alfaro I, Muñoz-Negrete FJ, Turman K, Palumaa K, Sádaba B, González MV, Ruz V, Vargas B, et al. 2016. Safety and efficacy clinical trials for SYL1001, a novel short interfering RNA for the treatment of dry eye disease. *Invest Ophthalmol Vis Sci* **57:** 6447–6454. doi:10.1167/iovs.16-20303

Berger A, Lorain S, Joséphine C, Desrosiers M, Peccate C, Voit T, Garcia L, Sahel JA, Bemelmans AP. 2015. Repair of rhodopsin mRNA by spliceosome-mediated RNA *trans*-splicing: a new approach for autosomal dominant retinitis pigmentosa. *Mol Ther* **23:** 918–930. doi:10.1038/mt.2015.11

Berget SM, Moore C, Sharp PA. 1977. Spliced segments at the 5′ terminus of adenovirus 2 late mRNA. *Proc Natl Acad Sci* **74:** 3171–3175. doi:10.1073/pnas.74.8.3171

Bishop PN, Reardon AJ, McLeod D, Ayad S. 1994. Identification of alternatively spliced variants of type II procollagen in vitreous. *Biochem Biophys Res Commun* **203:** 289–295. doi:10.1006/bbrc.1994.2180

Bonifert T, Gonzalez Menendez I, Battke F, Theurer Y, Synofzik M, Schöls L, Wissinger B. 2016. Antisense oligonucleotide mediated splice correction of a deep intronic mutation in OPA1. *Mol Ther Nucleic Acids* **5:** e390. doi:10.1038/mtna.2016.93

Bray NL, Pimentel H, Melsted P, Pachter L. 2016. Near-optimal probabilistic RNA-seq quantification. *Nat Biotechnol* **34:** 525–527. doi:10.1038/nbt.3519

Buskin A, Zhu L, Chichagova V, Basu B, Mozaffari-Jovin S, Dolan D, Droop A, Collin J, Bronstein R, Mehrotra S, et al. 2018. Disrupted alternative splicing for genes implicated in splicing and ciliogenesis causes PRPF31 retinitis pigmentosa. *Nat Commun* **9:** 4234. doi:10.1038/s41467-018-06448-y

Cao H, Wu J, Lam S, Duan R, Newnham C, Molday RS, Graziotto JJ, Pierce EA, Hu J. 2011. Temporal and tissue specific regulation of RP-associated splicing factor genes PRPF3, PRPF31 and PRPC8—implications in the pathogenesis of RP. *PLoS ONE* **6:** e15860. doi:10.1371/journal.pone.0015860

Capowski EE, Samimi K, Mayerl SJ, Phillips MJ, Pinilla I, Howden SE, Saha J, Jansen AD, Edwards KL, Jager LD, et al. 2019. Reproducibility and staging of 3D human retinal organoids across multiple pluripotent stem cell lines. *Development* **146:** dev171686. doi:10.1242/dev.171686

Chakarova CF, Hims MM, Bolz H, Abu-Safieh L, Patel RJ, Papaioannou MG, Inglehearn CF, Keen TJ, Willis C, Moore AT, et al. 2002. Mutations in HPRP3, a third member of pre-mRNA splicing factor genes, implicated in autosomal dominant retinitis pigmentosa. *Hum Mol Genet* **11:** 87–92. doi:10.1093/hmg/11.1.87

Chen X, Liu Y, Sheng X, Tam PO, Zhao K, Chen X, Rong W, Liu Y, Liu X, Pan X, et al. 2014. PRPF4 mutations cause autosomal dominant retinitis pigmentosa. *Hum Mol Genet* **23:** 2926–2939. doi:10.1093/hmg/ddu005

Chow LT, Gelinas RE, Broker TR, Roberts RJ. 1977. An amazing sequence arrangement at the 5′ ends of adenovirus 2 messenger RNA. *Cell* **12:** 1–8. doi:10.1016/0092-8674(77)90180-5

Cideciyan AV, Jacobson SG, Drack AV, Ho AC, Charng J, Garafalo AV, Roman AJ, Sumaroka A, Han IC, Hochstedler MD, et al. 2019. Effect of an intravitreal antisense oligonucleotide on vision in Leber congenital amaurosis due to a photoreceptor cilium defect. *Nat Med* **25:** 225–228. doi:10.1038/s41591-018-0295-0

Collin RW, den Hollander AI, van der Velde-Visser SD, Bennicelli J, Bennett J, Cremers FP. 2012. Antisense oligonucleotide (AON)-based therapy for Leber congenital amaurosis caused by a frequent mutation in CEP290. *Mol Ther Nucleic Acids* **1:** e14. doi:10.1038/mtna.2012.3

Coppieters F, Casteels I, Meire F, De Jaegere S, Hooghe S, van Regemorter N, Van Esch H, Matulevičienė A, Nunes L, Meersschaut V, et al. 2010. Genetic screening of LCA in Belgium: predominance of CEP290 and identification of potential modifier alleles in AHI1 of CEP290-related phenotypes. *Hum Mutat* **31:** E1709–E1766. doi:10.1002/humu.21336

Cowan CS, Renner M, De Gennaro M, Gross-Scherf B, Goldblum D, Hou Y, Munz M, Rodrigues TM, Krol J, Szikra T, et al. 2020. Cell types of the human retina and its organoids at single-cell resolution. *Cell* **182:** 1623–1640.e34. doi:10.1016/j.cell.2020.08.013

Cox DBT, Gootenberg JS, Abudayyeh OO, Franklin B, Kellner MJ, Joung J, Zhang F. 2017. RNA editing with CRISPR-Cas13. *Science* **358:** 1019–1027. doi:10.1126/science.aaq0180

Deamer D, Akeson M, Branton D. 2016. Three decades of nanopore sequencing. *Nat Biotechnol* **34:** 518–524. doi:10.1038/nbt.3423

den Hollander AI, Koenekoop RK, Yzer S, Lopez I, Arends ML, Voesenek KE, Zonneveld MN, Strom TM, Meitinger T, Brunner HG, et al. 2006. Mutations in the CEP290 (NPHP6) gene are a frequent cause of Leber congenital amaurosis. *Am J Hum Genet* **79:** 556–561. doi:10.1086/507318

Drivas TG, Wojno AP, Tucker BA, Stone EM, Bennett J. 2015. Basal exon skipping and genetic pleiotropy: a predictive model of disease pathogenesis. *Sci Transl Med* **7:** 291ra297. doi:10.1126/scitranslmed.aaa5370

Dullaʼ K, Slijkerman R, van Diepen HC, Albert S, Dona M, Beumer W, Turunen JJ, Chan HL, Schulkens IA, Vorthoren L, et al. 2021. Antisense oligonucleotide-based treatment of retinitis pigmentosa caused by USH2A exon 13 mutations. *Mol Ther* **29**: 2441–2455. doi:10.1016/j.ymthe.2021.04.024

Early P, Rogers J, Davis M, Calame K, Bond M, Wall R, Hood L. 1980. Two mRNAs can be produced from a single immunoglobulin μ gene by alternative RNA processing pathways. *Cell* **20**: 313–319. doi:10.1016/0092-8674(80)90617-0

Eid J, Fehr A, Gray J, Luong K, Lyle J, Otto G, Peluso P, Rank D, Baybayan P, Bettman B, et al. 2009. Real-time DNA sequencing from single polymerase molecules. *Science* **323**: 133–138. doi:10.1126/science.1162986

Farkas MH, Grant GR, White JA, Sousa ME, Consugar MB, Pierce EA. 2013. Transcriptome analyses of the human retina identify unprecedented transcript diversity and 3.5 Mb of novel transcribed sequence via significant alternative splicing and novel genes. *BMC Genomics* **14**: 486. doi:10.1186/1471-2164-14-486

Fathi M, Ross CT, Hosseinzadeh Z. 2021. Functional 3-dimensional retinal organoids: technological progress and existing challenges. *Front Neurosci* **15**: 668857. doi:10.3389/fnins.2021.668857

Fathinajafabadi A, Pérez-Jiménez E, Riera M, Knecht E, Gonzàlez-Duarte R. 2014. CERKL, a retinal disease gene, encodes an mRNA-binding protein that localizes in compact and untranslated mRNPs associated with microtubules. *PLoS ONE* **9**: e87898. doi:10.1371/journal.pone.0087898

Femino AM, Fay FS, Fogarty K, Singer RH. 1998. Visualization of single RNA transcripts in situ. *Science* **280**: 585–590. doi:10.1126/science.280.5363.585

Fligor CM, Huang KC, Lavekar SS, VanderWall KB, Meyer JS. 2020. Differentiation of retinal organoids from human pluripotent stem cells. *Methods Cell Biol* **159**: 279–302. doi:10.1016/bs.mcb.2020.02.005

Gapinske M, Luu A, Winter J, Woods WS, Kostan KA, Shiva N, Song JS, Perez-Pinera P. 2018. CRISPR-SKIP: programmable gene splicing with single base editors. *Genome Biol* **19**: 107. doi:10.1186/s13059-018-1482-5

Garanto A. 2019. RNA-based therapeutic strategies for inherited retinal dystrophies. *Adv Exp Med Biol* **1185**: 71–77. doi:10.1007/978-3-030-27378-1_12

Garanto A, Collin RWJ. 2018. Design and in vitro use of antisense oligonucleotides to correct pre-mRNA splicing defects in inherited retinal dystrophies. *Methods Mol Biol* **1715**: 61–78. doi:10.1007/978-1-4939-7522-8_5

Garanto A, Riera M, Pomares E, Permanyer J, de Castro-Miró M, Sava F, Abril JF, Marfany G, Gonzàlez-Duarte R. 2011. High transcriptional complexity of the retinitis pigmentosa *CERKL* gene in human and mouse. *Invest Ophthalmol Vis Sci* **52**: 5202–5214. doi:10.1167/iovs.10-7101

Garanto A, van der Velde-Visser SD, Cremers FPM, Collin RWJ. 2018. Antisense oligonucleotide-based splice correction of a deep-intronic mutation in CHM underlying choroideremia. *Adv Exp Med Biol* **1074**: 83–89. doi:10.1007/978-3-319-75402-4_11

Garanto A, Duijkers L, Tomkiewicz TZ, Collin RWJ. 2019. Antisense oligonucleotide screening to optimize the rescue of the splicing defect caused by the recurrent deep-intronic ABCA4 variant c.4539+2001G>A in Stargardt

disease. *Genes (Basel)* **10**: 452. doi:10.3390/genes10060452

Gavrilov K, Saltzman WM. 2012. Therapeutic siRNA: principles, challenges, and strategies. *Yale J Biol Med* **85**: 187–200.

Gemayel MC, Bhatwadekar AD, Ciulla T. 2021. RNA therapeutics for retinal diseases. *Expert Opin Biol Ther* **21**: 603–613. doi:10.1080/14712598.2021.1856365

Gerard X, Perrault I, Hanein S, Silva E, Bigot K, Defoort-Delhemmes S, Rio M, Munnich A, Scherman D, Kaplan J, et al. 2012. AON-mediated exon skipping restores ciliation in fibroblasts harboring the common Leber congenital amaurosis CEP290 mutation. *Mol Ther Nucleic Acids* **1**: e29. doi:10.1038/mtna.2012.21

Gerard X, Garanto A, Rozet JM, Collin RW. 2016. Antisense oligonucleotide therapy for inherited retinal dystrophies. *Adv Exp Med Biol* **854**: 517–524. doi:10.1007/978-3-319-17121-0_69

Glaus E, Schmid F, Da Costa R, Berger W, Neidhardt J. 2011. Gene therapeutic approach using mutation-adapted U1 snRNA to correct a RPGR splice defect in patient-derived cells. *Mol Ther* **19**: 936–941. doi:10.1038/mt.2011.7

Grant GR, Farkas MH, Pizarro AD, Lahens NF, Schug J, Brunk BP, Stoeckert CJ, Hogenesch JB, Pierce EA. 2011. Comparative analysis of RNA-seq alignment algorithms and the RNA-seq unified mapper (RUM). *Bioinformatics* **27**: 2518–2528. doi:10.1093/bioinformatics/btr427

Hagemann-Jensen M, Ziegenhain C, Chen P, Ramsköld D, Hendriks GJ, Larsson AJM, Faridani OR, Sandberg R. 2020. Single-cell RNA counting at allele and isoform resolution using Smart-seq3. *Nat Biotechnol* **38**: 708–714. doi:10.1038/s41587-020-0497-0

Halperin RF, Hegde A, Lang JD, Raupach EA, Group CRR, Legendre C, Liang WS, LoRusso PM, Sekulic A, Sosman JA, et al. 2021. Improved methods for RNAseq-based alternative splicing analysis. *Sci Rep* **11**: 10740. doi:10.1038/s41598-021-89938-2

Hannon GJ. 2002. RNA interference. *Nature* **418**: 244–251. doi:10.1038/418244a

Heng HH, Wang A, Hu J. 1998. Mapping of the human HPRP3 and HPRP4 genes encoding U4/U6-associated splicing factors to chromosomes 1q21.1 and 9q31–q33. *Genomics* **48**: 273–275. doi:10.1006/geno.1997.5181

Hill SF, Meisler MH. 2021. Antisense oligonucleotide therapy for neurodevelopmental disorders. *Dev Neurosci* **43**: 247–252. doi:10.1159/000517686

Hombach S, Kretz M. 2016. Non-coding RNAs: classification, biology and functioning. *Adv Exp Med Biol* **937**: 3–17. doi:10.1007/978-3-319-42059-2_1

Jaudon F, Baldassari S, Musante I, Thalhammer A, Zara F, Cingolani LA. 2020. Targeting alternative splicing as a potential therapy for episodic ataxia type 2. *Biomedicines* **8**: 332. doi:10.3390/biomedicines8090332

Kaiser PK, Symons RC, Shah SM, Quinlan EJ, Tabandeh H, Do DV, Reisen G, Lockridge JA, Short B, Guerciolini R, et al. 2010. RNAi-based treatment for neovascular age-related macular degeneration by Sirna-027. *Am J Ophthalmol* **150**: 33–39.e2. doi:10.1016/j.ajo.2010.02.006

Kallman A, Capowski EE, Wang J, Kaushik AM, Jansen AD, Edwards KL, Chen L, Berlinicke CA, Joseph Phillips M, Pierce EA, et al. 2020. Investigating cone photoreceptor development using patient-derived NRL null retinal organoids. *Commun Biol* **3**: 82. doi:10.1038/s42003-020-0808-5

Kampmann M. 2018. CRISPRi and CRISPRa screens in mammalian cells for precision biology and medicine. *ACS Chem Biol* **13**: 406–416. doi:10.1021/acschembio.7b00657

Karunakaran DK, Banday AR, Wu Q, Kanadia R. 2013. Expression analysis of an evolutionarily conserved alternative splicing factor, Sfrs10, in age-related macular degeneration. *PLoS ONE* **8**: e75964. doi:10.1371/journal.pone.0075964

Keen TJ, Hims MM, McKie AB, Moore AT, Doran RM, Mackey DA, Mansfield DC, Mueller RF, Bhattacharya SS, Bird AC, et al. 2002. Mutations in a protein target of the Pim-1 kinase associated with the RP9 form of autosomal dominant retinitis pigmentosa. *Eur J Hum Genet* **10**: 245–249. doi:10.1038/sj.ejhg.5200797

Kohl S, Zobor D, Chiang WC, Weisschuh N, Staller J, Gonzalez Menendez I, Chang S, Beck SC, Garcia Garrido M, Sothilingam V, et al. 2015. Mutations in the unfolded protein response regulator ATF6 cause the cone dysfunction disorder achromatopsia. *Nat Genet* **47**: 757–765. doi:10.1038/ng.3319

Konermann S, Lotfy P, Brideau NJ, Oki J, Shokhirev MN, Hsu PD. 2018. Transcriptome engineering with RNA-targeting type VI-D CRISPR effectors. *Cell* **173**: 665–676.e14. doi:10.1016/j.cell.2018.02.033

Korlach J, Bjornson KP, Chaudhuri BP, Cicero RL, Flusberg BA, Gray JJ, Holden D, Saxena R, Wegener J, Turner SW. 2010. Real-time DNA sequencing from single polymerase molecules. *Methods Enzymol* **472**: 431–455. doi:10.1016/S0076-6879(10)72001-2

Landrum MJ, Lee JM, Benson M, Brown GR, Chao C, Chitipiralla S, Gu B, Hart J, Hoffman D, Jang W, et al. 2018. ClinVar: improving access to variant interpretations and supporting evidence. *Nucleic Acids Res* **46**: D1062–D1067. doi:10.1093/nar/gkx1153

Lares MR, Rossi JJ, Ouellet DL. 2010. RNAi and small interfering RNAs in human disease therapeutic applications. *Trends Biotechnol* **28**: 570–579. doi:10.1016/j.tibtech.2010.07.009

Laver T, Harrison J, O'Neill PA, Moore K, Farbos A, Paszkiewicz K, Studholme DJ. 2015. Assessing the performance of the Oxford nanopore technologies MinION. *Biomol Detect Quantif* **3**: 1–8. doi:10.1016/j.bdq.2015.02.001

Lee Y, Rio DC. 2015. Mechanisms and regulation of alternative pre-mRNA splicing. *Annu Rev Biochem* **84**: 291–323. doi:10.1146/annurev-biochem-060614-034316

Lentz JJ, Jodelka FM, Hinrich AJ, McCaffrey KE, Farris HE, Spalitta MJ, Bazan NG, Duelli DM, Rigo F, Hastings ML. 2013. Rescue of hearing and vestibular function by antisense oligonucleotides in a mouse model of human deafness. *Nat Med* **19**: 345–350. doi:10.1038/nm.3106

Li B, Dewey CN. 2011. RSEM: accurate transcript quantification from RNA-seq data with or without a reference genome. *BMC Bioinformatics* **12**: 323. doi:10.1186/1471-2105-12-323

Li N, Mei H, MacDonald IM, Jiao X, Hejtmancik JF. 2010. Mutations in ASCC3L1 on 2q11.2 are associated with autosomal dominant retinitis pigmentosa in a Chinese

family. *Invest Ophthalmol Vis Sci* **51**: 1036–1043. doi:10.1167/iovs.09-3725

Li J, Liu F, Lv Y, Sun K, Zhao Y, Reilly J, Zhang Y, Tu J, Yu S, Liu X, et al. 2021. Prpf31 is essential for the survival and differentiation of retinal progenitor cells by modulating alternative splicing. *Nucleic Acids Res* **49**: 2027–2043. doi:10.1093/nar/gkab003

Linder B, Hirmer A, Gal A, Rüther K, Bolz HJ, Winkler C, Laggerbauer B, Fischer U. 2014. Identification of a PRPF4 loss-of-function variant that abrogates U4/U6.U5 tri-snRNP integration and is associated with retinitis pigmentosa. *PLoS ONE* **9**: e111754. doi:10.1371/journal.pone.0111754

Ling JP, Wilks C, Charles R, Leavey PJ, Ghosh D, Jiang L, Santiago CP, Pang B, Venkataraman A, Clark BS, et al. 2020. ASCOT identifies key regulators of neuronal subtype-specific splicing. *Nat Commun* **11**: 137. doi:10.1038/s41467-019-14020-5

Liu MM, Zack DJ. 2013. Alternative splicing and retinal degeneration. *Clin Genet* **84**: 142–149. doi:10.1111/cge.12181

Maita H, Kitaura H, Keen TJ, Inglehearn CF, Ariga H, Iguchi-Ariga SM. 2004. PAP-1, the mutated gene underlying the RP9 form of dominant retinitis pigmentosa, is a splicing factor. *Exp Cell Res* **300**: 283–296. doi:10.1016/j.yexcr.2004.07.029

Marasco LE, Kornblihtt AR. 2022. The physiology of alternative splicing. *Nat Rev Mol Cell Biol* doi:10.1038/s41580-022-00545-z

Martínez T, Gonzalez MV, Roehl I, Wright N, Paneda C, Jimenez AI. 2014. In vitro and in vivo efficacy of SYL040012, a novel siRNA compound for treatment of glaucoma. *Mol Ther* **22**: 81–91. doi:10.1038/mt.2013.216

McKie AB, McHale JC, Keen TJ, Tarttelin EE, Goliath R, van Lith-Verhoeven JJ, Greenberg J, Ramesar RS, Hoyng CB, Cremers FP, et al. 2001. Mutations in the pre-mRNA splicing factor gene PRPC8 in autosomal dominant retinitis pigmentosa (RP13). *Hum Mol Genet* **10**: 1555–1562. doi:10.1093/hmg/10.15.1555

Mehmood A, Laiho A, Venäläinen MS, McGlinchey AJ, Wang N, Elo LL. 2020. Systematic evaluation of differential splicing tools for RNA-seq studies. *Brief Bioinform* **21**: 2052–2065. doi:10.1093/bib/bbz126

Mellough CB, Bauer R, Collin J, Dorgau B, Zerti D, Dolan DWP, Jones CM, Izuogu OG, Yu M, Hallam D, et al. 2019. An integrated transcriptional analysis of the developing human retina. *Development* **146**: dev169474. doi:10.1242/dev.169474

Mezlini AM, Smith EJ, Fiume M, Buske O, Savich GL, Shah S, Aparicio S, Chiang DY, Goldenberg A, Brudno M. 2013. iReckon: simultaneous isoform discovery and abundance estimation from RNA-seq data. *Genome Res* **23**: 519–529. doi:10.1101/gr.142232.112

Modrek B, Resch A, Grasso C, Lee C. 2001. Genome-wide detection of alternative splicing in expressed sequences of human genes. *Nucleic Acids Res* **29**: 2850–2859. doi:10.1093/nar/29.13.2850

Mukhopadhyay A, Nikopoulos K, Maugeri A, de Brouwer AP, van Nouhuys CE, Boon CJ, Perveen R, Zegers HA, Wittebol-Post D, van den Biesen PR, et al. 2006. Erosive vitreoretinopathy and Wagner disease are caused by intronic mutations in *CSPG2/Versican* that result in an imbalance of splice variants. *Invest Ophthalmol Vis Sci* **47:** 3565–3572. doi:10.1167/iovs.06-0141

Muraki M, Ohkawara B, Hosoya T, Onogi H, Koizumi J, Koizumi T, Sumi K, Yomoda J, Murray MV, Kimura H, et al. 2004. Manipulation of alternative splicing by a newly developed inhibitor of Clks. *J Biol Chem* **279:** 24246–24254. doi:10.1074/jbc.M314298200

Murray SF, Jazayeri A, Matthes MT, Yasumura D, Yang H, Peralta R, Watt A, Freier S, Hung G, Adamson PS, et al. 2015. Allele-specific inhibition of rhodopsin with an antisense oligonucleotide slows photoreceptor cell degeneration. *Invest Ophthalmol Vis Sci* **56:** 6362–6375. doi:10.1167/iovs.15-16400

Naessens S, Ruysschaert L, Lefever S, Coppieters F, De Baere E. 2019. Antisense oligonucleotide-based downregulation of the G56R pathogenic variant causing NR2E3-associated autosomal dominant retinitis pigmentosa. *Genes (Basel)* **10:** 363. doi:10.3390/genes10050363

Nariai N, Kojima K, Mimori T, Sato Y, Kawai Y, Yamaguchi-Kabata Y, Nagasaki M. 2014. TIGAR2: sensitive and accurate estimation of transcript isoform expression with longer RNA-seq reads. *BMC Genomics* **15**(Suppl 10): S5. doi:10.1186/1471-2164-15-S10-S5

Nikam RR, Gore KR. 2018. Journey of siRNA: clinical developments and targeted delivery. *Nucleic Acid Ther* **28:** 209–224. doi:10.1089/nat.2017.0715

O'Hara-Wright M, Gonzalez-Cordero A. 2020. Retinal organoids: a window into human retinal development. *Development* **147:** dev189746. doi:10.1242/dev.189746

Ottaviani D, Lane A, Parfitt DA, Jovanovic K, Sladen PE, Gardner JC, Hardcastle AJ, Cheetham ME. 2019. Temporal resolution of alternative splicing in the developing human retina using 3D retinal organoids. *Invest Ophthalmol Vis Sci* **60:** 3333.

Pan Q, Shai O, Lee LJ, Frey BJ, Blencowe BJ. 2008. Deep surveying of alternative splicing complexity in the human transcriptome by high-throughput sequencing. *Nat Genet* **40:** 1413–1415. doi:10.1038/ng.259

Parfitt DA, Lane A, Ramsden CM, Carr AF, Munro PM, Jovanovic K, Schwarz N, Kanuga N, Muthiah MN, Hull S, et al. 2016. Identification and correction of mechanisms underlying inherited blindness in human iPSC-derived optic cups. *Cell Stem Cell* **18:** 769–781. doi:10.1016/j.stem.2016.03.021

Patro R, Mount SM, Kingsford C. 2014. Sailfish enables alignment-free isoform quantification from RNA-seq reads using lightweight algorithms. *Nat Biotechnol* **32:** 462–464. doi:10.1038/nbt.2862

Patro R, Duggal G, Love MI, Irizarry RA, Kingsford C. 2017. Salmon provides fast and bias-aware quantification of transcript expression. *Nat Methods* **14:** 417–419. doi:10.1038/nmeth.4197

Pertea M, Pertea GM, Antonescu CM, Chang TC, Mendell JT, Salzberg SL. 2015. StringTie enables improved reconstruction of a transcriptome from RNA-seq reads. *Nat Biotechnol* **33:** 290–295. doi:10.1038/nbt.3122

Pickar-Oliver A, Gersbach CA. 2019. The next generation of CRISPR-Cas technologies and applications. *Nat Rev Mol Cell Biol* **20:** 490–507. doi:10.1038/s41580-019-0131-5

Puttaraju M, Jamison SF, Mansfield SG, Garcia-Blanco MA, Mitchell LG. 1999. Spliceosome-mediated RNA trans-splicing as a tool for gene therapy. *Nat Biotechnol* **17:** 246–252. doi:10.1038/6986

Quinn J, Musa A, Kantor A, McClements ME, Cehajic-Kapetanovic J, MacLaren RE, Xue K. 2021. Genome-editing strategies for treating human retinal degenerations. *Hum Gene Ther* **32:** 247–259. doi:10.1089/hum.2020.231

Raj A, van den Bogaard P, Rifkin SA, van Oudenaarden A, Tyagi S. 2008. Imaging individual mRNA molecules using multiple singly labeled probes. *Nat Methods* **5:** 877–879. doi:10.1038/nmeth.1253

Ray TA, Cochran K, Kozlowski C, Wang J, Alexander G, Cady MA, Spencer WJ, Ruzycki PA, Clark BS, Laeremans A, et al. 2020. Comprehensive identification of mRNA isoforms reveals the diversity of neural cell-surface molecules with roles in retinal development and disease. *Nat Commun* **11:** 3328. doi:10.1038/s41467-020-17009-7

Richards AJ, Martin S, Yates JR, Scott JD, Baguley DM, Pope FM, Snead MP. 2000. COL2A1 exon 2 mutations: relevance to the Stickler and Wagner syndromes. *Br J Ophthalmol* **84:** 364–371. doi:10.1136/bjo.84.4.364

Roberts A, Pachter L. 2013. Streaming fragment assignment for real-time analysis of sequencing experiments. *Nat Methods* **10:** 71–73. doi:10.1038/nmeth.2251

Rodrigues A, Slembrouck-Brec A, Nanteau C, Terray A, Tymoshenko Y, Zagar Y, Reichman S, Xi Z, Sahel JA, Fouquet S, et al. 2022. Modeling PRPF31 retinitis pigmentosa using retinal pigment epithelium and organoids combined with gene augmentation rescue. *NPJ Regen Med* **7:** 39. doi:10.1038/s41536-022-00235-6

Ryan MC, Sandell LJ. 1990. Differential expression of a cysteine-rich domain in the amino-terminal propeptide of type II (cartilage) procollagen by alternative splicing of mRNA. *J Biol Chem* **265:** 10334–10339. doi:10.1016/S0021-9258(18)86950-2

Sangermano R, Khan M, Cornelis SS, Richelle V, Albert S, Garanto A, Elmelik D, Qamar R, Lugtenberg D, van den Born LI, et al. 2018. *ABCA4* midigenes reveal the full splice spectrum of all reported noncanonical splice site variants in Stargardt disease. *Genome Res* **28:** 100–110. doi:10.1101/gr.226621.117

Sangermano R, Garanto A, Khan M, Runhart EH, Bauwens M, Bax NM, van den Born LI, Khan MI, Cornelis SS, Verheij J, et al. 2019. Deep-intronic ABCA4 variants explain missing heritability in Stargardt disease and allow correction of splice defects by antisense oligonucleotides. *Genet Med* **21:** 1751–1760. doi:10.1038/s41436-018-0414-9

Savić N, Schwank G. 2016. Advances in therapeutic CRISPR/Cas9 genome editing. *Transl Res* **168:** 15–21. doi:10.1016/j.trsl.2015.09.008

Schorling DC, Pechmann A, Kirschner J. 2020. Advances in treatment of spinal muscular atrophy—new phenotypes, new challenges, new implications for care. *J Neuromuscul Dis* **7:** 1–13. doi:10.3233/JND-190424

Singerman L. 2009. Combination therapy using the small interfering RNA bevasiranib. *Retina* **29:** S49–S50. doi:10.1097/IAE.0b013e3181ad2341

Slijkerman RW, Vaché C, Dona M, García-García G, Claustres M, Hetterschijt L, Peters TA, Hartel BP, Pennings RJ, Millan JM, et al. 2016. Antisense oligonucleotide-based splice correction for USH2A-associated retinal degeneration caused by a frequent deep-intronic mutation. *Mol Ther Nucleic Acids* **5**: e381. doi:10.1038/mtna .2016.89

Solano EC, Kornbrust DJ, Beaudry A, Foy JW, Schneider DJ, Thompson JD. 2014. Toxicological and pharmacokinetic properties of QPI-1007, a chemically modified synthetic siRNA targeting caspase 2 mRNA, following intravitreal injection. *Nucleic Acid Ther* **24**: 258–266. doi:10.1089/nat .2014.0489

Sullivan LS, Bowne SJ, Seaman CR, Blanton SH, Lewis RA, Heckenlively JR, Birch DG, Hughbanks-Wheaton D, Daiger SP. 2006. Genomic rearrangements of the *PRPF31* gene account for 2.5% of autosomal dominant retinitis pigmentosa. *Invest Ophthalmol Vis Sci* **47**: 4579–4588. doi:10.1167/iovs.06-0440

Swamy VS, Fufa TD, Hufnagel RB, McGaughey DM. 2020. A long read optimized de novo transcriptome pipeline reveals novel ocular developmentally regulated gene isoforms and disease targets. bioRxiv doi:10.1101/2020.08 .21.261644

Tanackovic G, Ransijn A, Ayuso C, Harper S, Berson EL, Rivolta C. 2011. A missense mutation in PRPF6 causes impairment of pre-mRNA splicing and autosomal-dominant retinitis pigmentosa. *Am J Hum Genet* **88**: 643–649. doi:10.1016/j.ajhg.2011.04.008

Tanner G, Glaus E, Barthelmes D, Ader M, Fleischhauer J, Pagani F, Berger W, Neidhardt J. 2009. Therapeutic strategy to rescue mutation-induced exon skipping in rhodopsin by adaptation of U1 snRNA. *Hum Mutat* **30**: 255–263. doi:10.1002/humu.20861

Trapnell C, Williams BA, Pertea G, Mortazavi A, Kwan G, van Baren MJ, Salzberg SL, Wold BJ, Pachter L. 2010. Transcript assembly and quantification by RNA-seq reveals unannotated transcripts and isoform switching during cell differentiation. *Nat Biotechnol* **28**: 511–515. doi:10.1038/nbt.1621

Trapnell C, Hendrickson DG, Sauvageau M, Goff L, Rinn JL, Pachter L. 2013. Differential analysis of gene regulation at transcript resolution with RNA-seq. *Nat Biotechnol* **31**: 46–53. doi:10.1038/nbt.2450

Tucker BA, Cranston CM, Anfinson KA, Shrestha S, Streb LM, Leon A, Mullins RF, Stone EM. 2015. Using patient-specific induced pluripotent stem cells to interrogate the pathogenicity of a novel retinal pigment epithelium-specific 65 kDa cryptic splice site mutation and confirm eligibility for enrollment into a clinical gene augmentation trial. *Transl Res* **166**: 740–749.e1. doi:10.1016/j.trsl.2015 .08.007

Tuson M, Marfany G, Gonzàlez-Duarte R. 2004. Mutation of CERKL, a novel human ceramide kinase gene, causes autosomal recessive retinitis pigmentosa (RP26). *Am J Hum Genet* **74**: 128–138. doi:10.1086/381055

Urbanski LM, Leclair N, Anczuków O. 2018. Alternative-splicing defects in cancer: splicing regulators and their downstream targets, guiding the way to novel cancer therapeutics. *Wiley Interdiscip Rev RNA* **9**: e1476. doi:10 .1002/wrna.1476

Vaché C, Besnard T, le Berre P, García-García G, Baux D, Larrieu L, Abadie C, Blanchet C, Bolz HJ, Millan J, et al. 2012. Usher syndrome type 2 caused by activation of an USH2A pseudoexon: implications for diagnosis and therapy. *Hum Mutat* **33**: 104–108. doi:10.1002/humu.21634

Vaishnaw AK, Gollob J, Gamba-Vitalo C, Hutabarat R, Sah D, Meyers R, de Fougerolles T, Maraganore J. 2010. A status report on RNAi therapeutics. *Silence* **1**: 14. doi:10 .1186/1758-907X-1-14

Vázquez-Domínguez I, Garanto A, Collin RWJ. 2019. Molecular therapies for inherited retinal diseases—current standing, opportunities and challenges. *Genes (Basel)* **10**: 654. doi:10.3390/genes10090654

Venturini G, Rose AM, Shah AZ, Bhattacharya SS, Rivolta C. 2012. CNOT3 is a modifier of PRPF31 mutations in retinitis pigmentosa with incomplete penetrance. *PLoS Genet* **8**: e1003040. doi:10.1371/journal.pgen.1003040

Vielle A, Park YK, Secora C, Vergara MN. 2021. Organoids for the study of retinal development and developmental abnormalities. *Front Cell Neurosci* **15**: 667880. doi:10 .3389/fncel.2021.667880

Vig A, Poulter JA, Ottaviani D, Tavares E, Toropova K, Tracewska AM, Mollica A, Kang J, Kehelwathugoda O, Paton T, et al. 2020. DYNC2H1 hypomorphic or retina-predominant variants cause nonsyndromic retinal degeneration. *Genet Med* **22**: 2041–2051. doi:10.1038/s41436-020-0915-1

Vithana EN, Abu-Safieh L, Allen MJ, Carey A, Papaioannou M, Chakarova C, Al-Maghtheh M, Ebenezer ND, Willis C, Moore AT, et al. 2001. A human homolog of yeast pre-mRNA splicing gene, PRP31, underlies autosomal dominant retinitis pigmentosa on chromosome 19q13.4 (RP11). *Mol Cell* **8**: 375–381. doi:10.1016/S1097-2765 (01)00305-7

Vithana EN, Abu-Safieh L, Pelosini L, Winchester E, Hornan D, Bird AC, Hunt DM, Bustin SA, Bhattacharya SS. 2003. Expression of *PRPF31* mRNA in patients with autosomal dominant retinitis pigmentosa: a molecular clue for incomplete penetrance. *Invest Ophthalmol Vis Sci* **44**: 4204–4209. doi:10.1167/iovs.03-0253

Wahlin KJ, Maruotti JA, Sripathi SR, Ball J, Angueyra JM, Kim C, Grebe R, Li W, Jones BW, Zack DJ. 2017. Photoreceptor outer segment-like structures in long-term 3d retinas from human pluripotent stem cells. *Sci Rep* **7**: 766. doi:10.1038/s41598-017-00774-9

Wan J, Masuda T, Hackler L Jr, Torres KM, Merbs SL, Zack DJ, Qian J. 2011. Dynamic usage of alternative splicing exons during mouse retina development. *Nucleic Acids Res* **39**: 7920–7930. doi:10.1093/nar/gkr545

Wang J, Aifantis I. 2020. RNA splicing and cancer. *Trends Cancer* **6**: 631–644. doi:10.1016/j.trecan.2020.04.011

Wang ET, Sandberg R, Luo S, Khrebtukova I, Zhang L, Mayr C, Kingsmore SF, Schroth GP, Burge CB. 2008. Alternative isoform regulation in human tissue transcriptomes. *Nature* **456**: 470–476. doi:10.1038/nature07509

Wang J, Ye Z, Huang TH, Shi H, Jin V. 2015. A survey of computational methods in transcriptome-wide alternative splicing analysis. *Biomol Concepts* **6**: 59–66. doi:10 .1515/bmc-2014-0040

Webb TR, Parfitt DA, Gardner JC, Martinez A, Bevilacqua D, Davidson AE, Zito I, Thiselton DL, Ressa JH, Apergi M, et al. 2012. Deep intronic mutation in OFD1, identified by targeted genomic next-generation sequencing, causes a severe form of X-linked retinitis pigmentosa (RP23). *Hum Mol Genet* **21**: 3647–3654. doi:10.1093/ hmg/dds194

Weisschuh N, Sturm M, Baumann B, Audo I, Ayuso C, Bocquet B, Branham K, Brooks BP, Catalá-Mora J, Giorda R, et al. 2020. Deep-intronic variants in *CNGB3* cause achromatopsia by pseudoexon activation. *Hum Mutat* **41:** 255–264. doi:10.1002/humu.23920

Wheway G, Douglas A, Baralle D, Guillot E. 2020. Mutation spectrum of PRPF31, genotype–phenotype correlation in retinitis pigmentosa, and opportunities for therapy. *Exp Eye Res* **192:** 107950. doi:10.1016/j.exer.2020.107950

Xu M, Xie YA, Abouzeid H, Gordon CT, Fiorentino A, Sun Z, Lehman A, Osman IS, Dharmat R, Riveiro-Alvarez R, et al. 2017. Mutations in the spliceosome component CWC27 cause retinal degeneration with or without additional developmental anomalies. *Am J Hum Genet* **100:** 592–604. doi:10.1016/j.ajhg.2017.02.008

Yang Q, Zhao J, Zhang W, Chen D, Wang Y. 2019. Aberrant alternative splicing in breast cancer. *J Mol Cell Biol* **11:** 920–929. doi:10.1093/jmcb/mjz033

Yeo G, Holste D, Kreiman G, Burge CB. 2004. Variation in alternative splicing across human tissues. *Genome Biol* **5:** R74. doi:10.1186/gb-2004-5-10-r74

Yuan J, Ma Y, Huang T, Chen Y, Peng Y, Li B, Li J, Zhang Y, Song B, Sun X, et al. 2018. Genetic modulation of RNA splicing with a CRISPR-guided cytidine deaminase.

Mol Cell **72:** 380–394.e7. doi:10.1016/j.molcel.2018.09.002

Zhang F, Wen Y, Guo X. 2014. CRISPR/Cas9 for genome editing: progress, implications and challenges. *Hum Mol Genet* **23:** R40–R46. doi:10.1093/hmg/ddu125

Zhang C, Zhang B, Lin LL, Zhao S. 2017. Evaluation and comparison of computational tools for RNA-seq isoform quantification. *BMC Genomics* **18:** 583. doi:10.1186/s12864-017-4002-1

Zhang Q, Fu Y, Thakur C, Bi Z, Wadgaonkar P, Qiu Y, Xu L, Rice M, Zhang W, Almutairy B, et al. 2020. CRISPR-Cas9 gene editing causes alternative splicing of the targeting mRNA. *Biochem Biophys Res Commun* **528:** 54–61. doi:10.1016/j.bbrc.2020.04.145

Zhao C, Bellur DL, Lu S, Zhao F, Grassi MA, Bowne SJ, Sullivan LS, Daiger SP, Chen LJ, Pang CP, et al. 2009. Autosomal-dominant retinitis pigmentosa caused by a mutation in SNRNP200, a gene required for unwinding of U4/U6 snRNAs. *Am J Hum Genet* **85:** 617–627. doi:10.1016/j.ajhg.2009.09.020

Zhong X, Gutierrez C, Xue T, Hampton C, Vergara MN, Cao LH, Peters A, Park TS, Zambidis ET, Meyer JS, et al. 2014. Generation of three-dimensional retinal tissue with functional photoreceptors from human iPSCs. *Nat Commun* **5:** 4047. doi:10.1038/ncomms5047

Pathomechanisms of Inherited Retinal Degeneration and Perspectives for Neuroprotection

Arianna Tolone,[1] Merve Sen,[1] Yiyi Chen, Marius Ueffing, Blanca Arango-Gonzalez, and François Paquet-Durand

Institute for Ophthalmic Research, Eberhard-Karls-Universität Tübingen, Tübingen 72076, Germany

Correspondence: marius.ueffing@uni-tuebingen.de; blanca.arango-gonzalez@klinikum.uni-tuebingen.de

The precise processes causing photoreceptor cell death in retinal degeneration (RD) are still largely unknown but are likely to follow a variety of degenerative mechanisms. While different genetic insults can trigger distinct molecular pathways, eventually these may converge into a limited number of common cell death mechanisms. These mechanisms often involve deregulation of cyclic guanosine monophosphate (cGMP)-signaling and proteostasis, which both may increase photoreceptor energy expenditure. Comprehensive information on these mechanisms may allow for targeted interventions to delay or prevent photoreceptor loss. Here, we review the current knowledge on photoreceptor degenerative mechanisms, focusing on processes triggered by aberrant cGMP-signaling, proteostasis, and energy metabolism. Afterward, we discuss how these pathways could potentially be used to treat photoreceptor degeneration, highlighting data from a number of recent studies on inhibitory cGMP analogs, proteostasis blockers, and interventions aimed at fortifying energetic status. Finally, we provide perspectives on how such experimental approaches could be translated into future clinical applications.

PATHOPHYSIOLOGY OF RD: FROM NECROSIS AND APOPTOSIS TO ALTERNATIVE CELL DEATH MECHANISMS

Cell death was traditionally seen as a biological accident triggered by overwhelming physical stress (e.g., trauma, intoxication, oxidation), leading to unordered, chaotic destruction of the cellular machinery. For this phenomenon, the term "necrosis" was coined (Glücksmann 1951). However, in the past decades, especially through the works of Kerr, Wyllie, and Currie, who introduced the term "apoptosis" (Kerr et al. 1972), it has become increasingly clear that in multicellular organisms cell death is often a well-orchestrated and program-driven process, which has little to no resemblance to the original definition of necrosis. Since its introduction, the term apoptosis has in many ways become a synonym for cell death. However, it is important to understand that apoptosis is only one of several possible cell death mechanisms that a cell may

---

[1]Co–first authors.

Cite this article as *Cold Spring Harb Perspect Med* doi: 10.1101/cshperspect.a041310

employ (Galluzzi et al. 2018). Notably, apoptosis is typically associated with developmental processes (Ghose and Shaham 2020; Montero et al. 2022) while pathological cell death associated with inherited retinal degeneration (RD) is likely to be nonapoptotic (Arango-Gonzalez et al. 2014; Power et al. 2020).

In RD, but also in essentially all other neurodegenerative diseases, the execution of cell death may employ a variety of very different metabolic processes, depending on the type of trigger, developmental stage, energetic status, pathogen load, etc. (Leist and Jäättelä 2001). Consequently, many alternative cell death mechanisms could potentially be exploited for therapeutic purposes (Kepp et al. 2011). However, the targeting of these mechanisms is complicated by our current lack of knowledge and the possibility that this variety of cell death mechanisms may not be clearly delineated pathways but a continuum of processes and metabolic subroutines, with considerable ambiguity and flexibility in between (Galluzzi et al. 2018).

In preclinical RD research on animal models, another confounding factor arises from the fact that early mutation-induced degeneration often coincides with retinal development and may overlap with secondary and tertiary degenerative processes and retinal remodeling (Sancho-Pelluz et al. 2008; Strettoi 2015). Therefore, the cell death mechanisms seen in animal models must be thoroughly analyzed and related to developmental stages to assess to what extent they may reproduce the human disease condition.

As diverse as cell death mechanisms may be, they likely have at least a few things in common. Cell death may be caused either via an uncompensated loss-of-function or via a toxic gain-of-function mechanism. Loss-of-function may include hypomorphic or total loss of specific gene function that affects processes central to cellular integrity, such as intracellular ciliary transport between inner (IS) and outer segments (OS), or recycling of critical visual components like retinal between photoreceptor and retinal pigment epithelium (RPE) cells. Gain-of-function may include overactivity of certain signal transducers, such as cyclic guanosine monophosphate (cGMP), the aggregation and inclusion forma-

tion of critical gene products with subsequent activation of the unfolded protein response (UPR), mis-sorting and interference with the trafficking machinery, constitutive or dysregulated activation, or structural destabilization of the OS.

For the purposes of this review, we focus on degenerative mechanisms of photoreceptors that are related to pathologic changes in cGMP signaling, proteostasis, and energy metabolism. It is plausible to think that once the underlying mechanisms are sufficiently well understood, targeted interventions can be designed to prevent or delay photoreceptor degeneration. Accordingly, we provide an overview of recent studies on inhibitory cGMP analogs, proteostasis blockers, and interventions aimed at boosting energy production. Finally, we provide perspectives on how such experimental approaches could be translated into future clinical applications.

cGMP-SIGNALING IN PHOTORECEPTOR PHYSIOLOGY AND PATHOPHYSIOLOGY

The second messenger, cGMP, plays a key role in photoreceptor function. In the absence of light, cGMP is present at high levels in the photoreceptor OS where it maintains the cyclic nucleotide-gated channel (CNGC) in the open state, leading to an influx of Na^+ and Ca^{2+} ions. Two main exchangers regulate the outflow of these ions: The $Na^+/Ca^{2+}/K^+$ exchanger (NCKX) in the OS and the ATP-driven Na^+/K^+ exchanger (NKX) located in the IS (Tolone et al. 2019; Yan et al. 2021). The influx of positive ions through CNGC into the OS creates a depolarizing current, which is ultimately driven by the Na^+ and K^+ gradients produced by NKX in the IS (Vinberg et al. 2018). The constant flux of ions across the OS and IS membranes during darkness is referred to as the dark current, which likely is the most energy-intensive task in a photoreceptor (Wong-Riley 2010). Notably, NKX activity alone is responsible for at least 50% of the ATP consumption of a photoreceptor (Ames 1992).

cGMP is synthesized by retinal guanylyl cyclases (GCs), which are encoded by the *GUCY2D* and *GUCY2F* genes in human (*Gucy2e* in mouse), the activity of which is controlled indirectly by

Ca^{2+} via GC-activating protein (GCAP) (Lim et al. 2018). High intracellular Ca^{2+} levels in the dark inhibit GCAP and limit cGMP production, thereby establishing a negative feedback loop that holds the photoreceptor cGMP level in its physiological range (Pugh and Lamb 1990; Burns et al. 2002; Dell'Orco et al. 2009). In light, cGMP levels are decreased by the activity of phosphodiesterase 6 (PDE6) and, consequently, the CNGC closes. While the influx of Na^+ through CNGC is drastically reduced, NKX continues to pump Na^+ out of the IS. This causes photoreceptor hyperpolarization (Vinberg et al. 2018), which spreads along the cell membrane to the synaptic terminal. Here, the change in membrane potential closes the voltage-gated Ca^{2+} channel (VGCC), consequently reducing intracellular Ca^{2+} (Waldner et al. 2018). In addition, hyperpolarization in bright light induces the opening of hyperpolarization-activated cyclic nucleotide-gated channel-1 (HCN1) expressed in the IS. HCN1 opening generates an inward current of Na^+ and K^+ ions that depolarize the cell, decreasing the refractory period and increasing the temporal resolution of photoreceptors (Tanimoto et al. 2012). Overall, photoreceptor physiology rests on the balance between cGMP and Ca^{2+}, linked via the Ca^{2+}-GCAP negative feedback loop and whose disruption appears to be a feature common to several forms of RD (Olshevskaya et al. 2002).

Although, in the past decades, research on RD focused on the presumed damaging role of excessive intracellular Ca^{2+} levels and apoptosis (Orrenius et al. 2003; Zeiss et al. 2004), in recent years, the focus has shifted toward nonapoptotic and Ca^{2+}-independent mechanisms of cell death. These mechanisms are characterized by an abnormal accumulation of cGMP in photoreceptors (Power et al. 2020). This phenomenon has been observed in mouse models with loss-of-function mutations in the *Aipl1, Prph2, Cngb1, Cnga3, Pde6a, Pde6b, Pde6c, and Rho* genes and excessive photoreceptor cGMP levels are likely found in additional RD-disease genes (Arango-Gonzalez et al. 2014; Power et al. 2020).

Excessive cGMP signaling may increase the activity of one or more of its three known photoreceptor targets: CNGC, HCN1 (Biel and Michalakis 2009), and protein kinase G (PKG). While CNGC overactivation has been associated with increased Ca^{2+} levels in the cell (Paquet-Durand et al. 2011; Kulkarni et al. 2016), the direct effects of PKG overactivation have yet to be elucidated. Indeed, as a protein kinase, PKG has many potential phosphorylation targets. To date, we know that downstream of excessive cGMP and PKG signaling, there is an increase in the enzymatic activities of histone deacetylase (HDAC), poly (ADP-ribose) polymerase (PARP), and Ca^{2+}-dependent calpain-type proteases, even though for HDAC and PARP there is still no evidence linking them directly to PKG or elevated Ca^{2+} levels (Arango-Gonzalez et al. 2014; Das et al. 2021).

Recent studies identified several PKG targets with a potential role in cell death in RD (Roy et al. 2022). These include 6-phosphofructo-2-kinase/fructose-2,6-biphosphatase-3 (PFKFB3) and voltage-dependent potassium channels belonging to the Kv1 family. Both targets were found to be expressed in the retina and were more strongly phosphorylated in the *rd1* situation (Roy et al. 2022). Increased phosphorylation of Kv1 channels implies an abnormal increase in potassium leakage from the cell, which would raise energy consumption to bring the equilibrium potential of K^+ back to a physiological range. PFKFB3 converts fructose-6-phosphate to fructose-2,6-bisP (F2,6BP). F2,6BP is a potent allosteric activator of 6-phosphofructokinase-1 (PFK-1), stimulating glycolysis (Clem et al. 2008; Shi et al. 2017). A PKG-dependent change of PFKFB3 activity thus has the potential to strongly impact retinal energy metabolism, by shifting ATP-production away from the efficient Krebs cycle and oxidative phosphorylation toward the highly inefficient glycolysis (Chen et al. 2022). Thus, excessive activation of PKG by high photoreceptor cGMP-levels could, on the one hand, increase energy expenditure and at the same time reduce the efficiency of ATP-production. Overall, this has the potential of causing a serious "energy crisis" in photoreceptor cells.

PROTEOSTASIS, PROTEASOMAL DEGRADATION, AND AUTOPHAGY

Proteostasis comprises the folding, assembly, and degradation pathways that maintain a balance of functional proteins within cells. The retina can be exposed to a variety of detrimental factors, including light-induced damage, oxidative stress, or inherited mutations, each of which can lead to perturbations of proteostasis (Athanasiou et al. 2013; Zhang et al. 2014). Photoreceptors seem especially vulnerable to disruptions in protein homeostasis, notably due to the massive opsin production and high metabolic activity. This production of large quantities of the visual pigment rhodopsin in photoreceptors places a substantial strain on the protein-folding machinery, resulting in misfolded/unfolded protein accumulation and protein aggregation. Indeed, misfolded protein aggregates are a central pathological phenotype in several neurodegenerative diseases (Moreno-Gonzalez and Soto 2011), including in RD (Griciuc et al. 2010, 2011; Tzekov et al. 2011).

Cellular proteostasis is regulated by a complex network of interacting and competitive biological modules (Jayaraj et al. 2020). An imbalance between these modules will activate integrated response pathways such as the UPR, endoplasmic reticulum–associated degradation (ERAD), and autophagy, likely in an attempt to induce signaling and transcriptional changes to adapt to the stressor(s). However, if the imbalance is prolonged or too excessive, the activation of death pathways will reduce photoreceptor cell viability and function (Athanasiou et al. 2013).

The endoplasmic reticulum (ER) is the site of extensive protein synthesis, folding, maturation, and export, and it has been equipped with highly specialized systems that detect and correct abnormal protein-folding states to prevent pathology. Accumulation of misfolded proteins in the ER membrane and lumen provokes UPR (Walter and Ron 2011). The unfolded proteins are sensed by a signaling pathway that includes inositol requiring enzyme 1 (IRE1), protein kinase RNA-like ER kinase (PERK), and activating transcription factor 6 (ATF6) transmembrane receptors, which transmit signals aiming to (1) increase ER protein-folding capacity, (2) decrease ER protein-folding load, and (3) promote the clearance and degradation of misfolded proteins. To cope with misfolded or unfolded proteins, cells have evolved discrete mechanisms, which comprise

two major proteostasis networks: (1) ERAD, and (2) the autophagy pathway (Griciuc et al. 2011; Smith et al. 2011).

ERAD

In this process, the unfolded or misfolded protein in the ER is recognized by molecular chaperones and targeted to the retrotranslocation machinery (retrotranslocon) (Wu and Rapoport 2018). Subsequently, the protein is ubiquitinated by one of two ER membrane–localized ubiquitin ligases and finally extruded through the retrotranslocation channel to the cytosol. This process depends on ATP hydrolysis by the ATPase associated with diverse cellular activities (AAA) known as valosin-containing protein (VCP) or p97 (Ye et al. 2001). Once released into the cytosol, the protein is delivered to the proteasome for degradation (Griciuc et al. 2010, 2011). Failure of this degradation pathway will lead to the accumulation of polyubiquitinated protein in the cytosol.

Autophagy

An alternative and possibly complementary protein degradation route in photoreceptors is autophagy (Mizushima 2007). This pathway might benefit proteins with a high propensity to aggregate within the ER, such as rhodopsin. Autophagy is a tightly regulated process in cell growth and development that creates and maintains a balance between the synthesis, degradation, and recycling of cellular products (Griciuc et al. 2011). There are three main autophagic processes: macroautophagy, microautophagy, and chaperone-mediated autophagy (Kroemer and Levine 2008). They all degrade intracellular components via the lysosome. The most well-known mechanism of autophagy is macroautophagy, which mediates the degradation of damaged organelles or proteins, and involves forming a double-membrane structure (phagophore), which becomes an autophagosome through lipid acquisition (Baba et al. 1994). The autophagosome then fuses with the lysosome, forming autolysosomes, degrading, and recycling the cargo (Lamb et al. 2013). The initiation of macroautophagy is

Cite this article as *Cold Spring Harb Perspect Med* doi: 10.1101/cshperspect.a041310

tightly regulated by AMP-activated protein kinase (AMPK) and the mammalian target of rapamycin complex 1 (mTORC1) (Wong et al. 2013). Incidentally, AMPK is also a key regulator of cellular energy metabolism (Xu and Ash 2016).

In addition, an imbalance in proteostasis may also lead to a Ca^{2+} imbalance and mitochondrial dysfunction through excessive ER stress (Cao and Kaufman 2014). Production of reactive oxygen species (ROS) and release of cytochrome *c* from dysfunctional mitochondria to the cytosol may initiate mitochondria-mediated cell death (Shore et al. 2011). Ultimately, such mitochondrial dysfunction will compromise the energy metabolism to the extent that key cellular functions can no longer be maintained.

THE ROLE OF ENERGY METABOLISM FOR PHOTORECEPTOR CELL DEATH AND SURVIVAL

The retina is one of the most metabolically active tissues in the body (Trick and Berkowitz 2005) and the majority of its large energy demand is likely caused by the photoreceptor dark current (Okawa et al. 2008). Yet even today very little is known about how photoreceptors satisfy their energetic needs, what fuels they use, and how they obtain these. A recent hypothesis proposed that photoreceptors use predominantly glucose and aerobic glycolysis, with the resultant lactate used by the RPE and Müller glial cells for mitochondrial respiration (Kanow et al. 2017; Viegas and Neuhauss 2021). However, this hypothesis is contradicted by the inefficiency of aerobic glycolysis and the high density of mitochondria in photoreceptor IS (Giarmarco et al. 2020).

In principle, a cell may generate energy-containing substrates such as ATP via two main pathways: (1) the very rapid glycolysis in the cytoplasm, and (2) the comparatively slow mitochondrial Krebs cycle coupled to oxidative phosphorylation. Retinal cells that have access to a large supply of lipids, such as RPE cells, can also use β-oxidation for their energy production via oxidative phosphorylation. The energetic advantage of oxidative metabolism in the mitochondria far outweighs that of glycolytic metabolism in the cytosol, as one molecule of glucose yields only two molecules of ATP via the glycolytic pathway but up to 36 molecules of ATP via oxidative phosphorylation. Paradoxically, the retina has long been suggested to prefer aerobic glycolysis (Warburg 1925) (i.e., the conversion of glucose to lactate, even when O_2 is abundant, a phenomenon called the "Warburg effect") (Diaz-Ruiz et al. 2011). The incomplete glucose oxidation is suggested to promote anabolic activity, such as synthesis of nucleic acids, proteins, and lipids (Lunt and Heiden 2011). Since photoreceptor disk shedding, subsequent OS growth, and the corresponding lipid and protein synthesis follow the dark–light cycle (LaVail 1980), it is tempting to speculate that the switch from oxidative metabolism to aerobic glycolysis could be driven by cGMP- and PKG-dependent regulation of PFKFB3 activity.

AMPK is another key regulator of cell metabolism (Herzig and Shaw 2018). AMPK is triggered through an allosteric mechanism that stimulates its kinase activity in response to variations in energy availability, notably changes in the ATP-to-AMP ratio. Once activated, AMPK redirects metabolism toward increased catabolism and decreased anabolism through the phosphorylation of key proteins in multiple pathways, including mTORC1, lipid homeostasis, and glycolysis (Bando et al. 2005; Gwinn et al. 2008; Ahmadian et al. 2011). In addition, the insulin/mTOR pathway promotes anabolic processes such as protein synthesis and ribosome biogenesis under conditions of high cellular energy (Iadevaia et al. 2012). In RD, high levels of cGMP keep CNGC open, resulting in a continuous ion influx to photoreceptors (Das et al. 2021) and resembling a situation of constant darkness. To counterbalance the resultant constant dark current, ATP must be consumed (Okawa et al. 2008), leading to a net increase in energy expenditure.

Moreover, photoreceptor degeneration in 10 different animal models was found to be connected to the overactivation of PARP (Arango-Gonzalez et al. 2014), an enzyme that consumes nicotinamide dinucleotide (NAD^+) to mediate DNA repair (Bai 2015). Excessive consumption of NAD^+ by overactivated PARP-1 results in a reduced redox capacity of cells, decreasing ATP-production. Furthermore, the production of poly (ADP-ribose) polymers may compromise mitochondrial function also directly (Baek et al. 2013). Eventually, an imbalance between energy consumption and production, perhaps aggravated by an unwarranted switch from mitochondrial respiration to aerobic glycolysis, will lead to the breakdown of a cell's membrane potential and subsequently to cell death. Therefore, retinal energy metabolism and its regulation probably have direct consequences for RD disease pathogenesis.

TARGETS FOR THERAPEUTIC INTERVENTIONS AND THERAPY DEVELOPMENT

An improved understanding of the cellular mechanisms governing photoreceptor degeneration will likely enable the development of novel therapies targeting these mechanisms. Here, we detail three possible avenues for exploiting mechanistic knowledge to improve photoreceptor viability. These approaches concern intervening with cGMP-signaling, protein homeostasis, and photoreceptor energy metabolism.

Targeting CNGC and/or PKG

Rising cGMP levels appear to be an early event in photoreceptor cell death (Farber and Lolley 1974) and therefore neuroprotective strategies targeting excessive cGMP signaling may be well suited to prevent or delay the progression of RD. Downstream targets of cGMP signaling include CNGC and PKG, which could hence be addressed for therapeutic purposes.

Knockout studies on double-mutant animals carrying genetic defects that disable both CNGC and PDE6 function (i.e., $Cngb1^{-/-} \times rd1$ and $Cngb1^{-/-} \times rd10$) hinted at an important role of CNGC in RD (Paquet-Durand et al. 2011; Waldner et al. 2018). Nevertheless, targeting CNGC for therapeutic purposes faces important challenges. First, cones and rods express different isoforms of CNGC (Das et al. 2021), and the potential inhibitor should be specific for a given isoform. For example, in retinitis pigmentosa (RP), only rod-

specific channels should be inhibited to avoid impairing cone-mediated vision. Furthermore, as CNGCs are involved in visual signal transduction, their inhibition could cause detrimental effects on vision in the long run. However, pharmacological inhibition of CNGC is possible via, for example, the L-cis enantiomer of the antihypertensive drug diltiazem (Das et al. 2022). An alternative approach may be the use of antisense oligonucleotides, which would allow selective knockdown of the CNGC isoform of interest (e.g., Cngb1).

In contrast to CNGCs, PKG appears not to be expressed differently in cones and rods, and its inhibition should not affect phototransduction (Ekstrom et al. 2014; Vighi et al. 2018). These two aspects make PKG an attractive candidate for targeting excessive cGMP signaling. There are several types of PKG inhibitors on the market. The first group of inhibitors includes KT5823 and the derivative of the fungal metabolite balanol N46, which block PKG activity by targeting the ATP-binding site (Olivares-González et al. 2016; Qin et al. 2018). Another type of peptide-based PKG inhibitors can bind to the kinasés substrate recognition site (Nickl et al. 2010). Finally, an additional class of PKG inhibitors are cGMP analogs that target the cGMP-binding domains (Lohmann et al. 1997) present in no other kinase type. Such cGMP analogs are particularly effective in slowing photoreceptor degeneration in vitro and in vivo in rd1, rd2, and rd10 mouse models (Vighi et al. 2018), boding well for the development of pharmacological therapies.

Recent studies showed that pharmacological inhibition of CNGCs alone is not sufficient to prevent RD and can, in fact, accelerate photoreceptor loss (Das et al. 2022). On the other hand, cGMP analogs that inhibit PKG and are effective in vitro and in vivo are also mild inhibitors of CNGCs (Tolone et al. 2021). This suggests that a synergistic action on the different events downstream of excessive cGMP signaling might be an appropriate strategy for the development of new treatments for RD.

Rebalancing Photoreceptor Proteostasis

As mentioned above, RD can disturb the folding capacity of cellular proteins and lead to the accumulation of misfolded proteins in the ER, causing ER stress and subsequent photoreceptor cell death. Specifically, in RP, misfolded proteins, as triggered, for instance, by the P23H mutation in the rhodopsin gene, disrupt cellular proteostasis and lead to photoreceptor cell degeneration. Since dysbalanced proteostasis is a common feature of RD, strategies to manipulate its network, like targeting ERAD, autophagy, or UPR, are particularly interesting as a neuroprotective approach.

Regulation of proper protein integrity and folding is crucial for cellular processes to maintain proteostasis (Díaz-Villanueva et al. 2015). In fact, inhibition of the HSP90 protein, responsible for proper protein folding in the ER, protects photoreceptor cells in models for autosomal-dominant RP (Aguilà et al. 2014). Targeting upstream ER stress sensors via pharmacological chaperones can improve protein folding and promote misfolded P23H rod opsin trafficking (Athanasiou et al. 2018). The AMPK activator metformin improved P23H folding and trafficking and reduced cell death in cell culture models; however, metformin accelerated the progression of RD in the P23H-1 transgenic rat model and in P23H knockin (KI) mice (Athanasiou et al. 2017). Chemical chaperones, also known as Kosmotropes (Wiggins 2001), can bind to proteins nonspecifically and improve the stability in their native conformation, reducing aggregation caused by misfolded rhodopsin (Athanasiou et al. 2018). For example, in vitro studies have shown that sodium 4-phenylbutyrate (4-PBA) could decrease P23H rod opsin aggregation (Mendes and Cheetham 2008) and reduce UPR-signaling and ER stress associated with the T17M rod opsin mutation (Mendes and Cheetham 2008). Importantly, administration of 4-PBA in the $Rpe65^{R91W/R91W}$ mouse model of Leber's congenital amaurosis (LCA) improved cone survival and vision (Li et al. 2016). However, 4-PBA did not protect against photoreceptor degeneration in the P23H rat model (Athanasiou et al. 2018). Another molecule, curcumin, a polyphenolic agent derived from the *Curcuma longa* plant, was reported to improve photoreceptor function and morphology in P23H rats, reduce P23H aggregation, and enhance rhodopsin localization to the rod OS

(Vasireddy et al. 2011). The chemical chaperone tauroursodeoxycholic acid (TUDCA), which inhibits apoptosis by preventing the proapoptotic protein Bax from being transported to the mitochondria (Boatright et al. 2009), preserved photoreceptor structure and function in an LCA animal model (Fu and Zhang 2014), in the *rd1* (Lawson et al. 2016) and *rd10* mouse models of RP (Oveson et al. 2011; Drack et al. 2012), and preserved photoreceptor function and survival in the P23H-1 rat model (Athanasiou et al. 2018).

Treatment with arimoclomol, which amplifies the natural response to cellular stress by inducing the heat-shock response, also slowed down the progression of RD in P23H rats (Parfitt et al. 2014). Inhibition of the PERK branch of the UPR accelerated RD in P23H rats, suggesting that PERK activation in this model for autosomal-dominant RP was protective (Athanasiou et al. 2018). On the other hand, intravitreal administration of KIRA6, an IRE1-dependent mRNA decay inhibitor, appeared to preserve photoreceptor numbers in P23H-1 rats (Ghosh et al. 2014), suggesting that activation of the UPR was detrimental.

Overexpression of the ER-resident chaperone network between ER degradation–enhancing α-mannosidase-like 1 (EDEM1), the ER-resident protein-containing DNAJ domain (ERdj5; also known as DnaJ homolog subfamily C member 10 [DNAJC10]), and the UPR regulator-binding immunoglobulin-protein (BiP) has been shown to reduce P23H aggregation in vitro (Kosmaoglou et al. 2009; Athanasiou et al. 2012, 2014). BiP overexpression also reduced photoreceptor cell death by reducing ER stress in P23H rats (Gorbatyuk et al. 2010). Additionally, modulation of the proteostasis by VCP or proteasome inhibitors rescued photoreceptor cell degeneration in P23H rats and P23H KI mice (Arango-Gonzalez et al. 2020; Sen et al. 2021a,c). Moreover, inhibition or down-regulation of VCP promoted the correct localization of rhodopsin to the OS upon treatment in vitro as well as in vivo (Arango-Gonzalez et al. 2020; Sen et al. 2021b,c). Further studies have shown that inhibition of VCP can exert neuroprotection in animal models for other retinal pathologies, for example, autosomal recessive RP (Ikeda et al. 2014), glaucoma (Nakano et al. 2016), and retinal ischemia (Hata et al. 2017).

In RP, the autophagy pathway also appears to be involved in the degradation of misfolded rhodopsin (Wen et al. 2019), and the inactivation of autophagy leads to accumulation of rhodopsin and RD (Yao et al. 2016). Treatment with the autophagy-inducing drug rapamycin reduced P23H aggregation in vitro (Mendes and Cheetham 2008), while systemic administration of rapamycin to P23H rats slowed down rod cell degeneration (Sizova et al. 2014). In contrast, normalization of the autophagic flux in the retina of P23H KI mice relative to proteasome activity may support photoreceptor cell homeostasis, resulting in increased photoreceptor cell survival (Qiu et al. 2019).

Improving Energy Metabolism

The crucial role of retinal energy metabolism could potentially make it a target for therapeutic interventions. Such interventions could, for instance, address defects in nutrient supply, alleviate the effects of high oxidative metabolism, or redirect cellular metabolism toward increased energy production. For instance, elevated insulin levels increased glucose uptake in cones, activated cone mTOR signaling, and delayed the secondary loss of cones in four different models for RP (Punzo et al. 2009). Potentially, the regulation of glycolysis via PFKFB3 could be used to similar effect (Shi et al. 2017).

An alternative way of influencing photoreceptor energy metabolism is through the use of both antioxidants and amino acids, some of which are already used in dietary supplements to help prevent RD or age-related macular degeneration (AMD) (Grover and Samson 2014; Gastaldello et al. 2022). Notably, antioxidants may help the detoxification of ROS thought to be generated as byproducts of metabolic processes. Excess generation of ROS may lead to oxidative damage to different targets, including lipids and enzymes involved in ATP synthesis (Quijano et al. 2016). Lutein is an antioxidant belonging to the carotenoid group of compounds with antioxidative and anti-inflammatory properties. Its beneficial effects have been

studied in many diseases, such as AMD and diabetic retinopathy (Li et al. 2020). Apart from carotenoids, nutraceuticals such as polyphenols, saponins, and other compounds have revealed protective effects in retinal disorders (Rossino and Casini 2019). Fatty acids, such as omega-3, are also reported for their protective roles in the retina (Querques et al. 2011). An additional (exogenous) supply of fatty acids could be applicable to cells with access to a large supply of lipids, such as RPE cells, which can then use β-oxidation for their energy production via oxidative phosphorylation (Adijanto et al. 2014). Therefore, the use of these compounds may represent a natural alternative method to conventional retina disease treatments (Fig. 1).

Moreover, genetic alterations modifying photoreceptor metabolism so as to improve resistance to stress have been investigated in animal models (Caruso et al. 2020). Such approaches include overexpression of transforming growth factor β (TGF-β), rod-derived cone viability factor (RdCVF), ablation of sirtuin-6, pyruvate kinase M2 (PKM2), and the phosphatase and tensin homolog (PTEN) (Byrne et al. 2015; Venkatesh et al. 2015; Zhang et al. 2016, 2020; Wang et al. 2020).

Taken together, balancing the energy metabolism of photoreceptors, as well as reducing their overall energy consumption caused by high metabolic and proteostatic activity, may constitute a mutation-independent method for the treatment of RD. While relatively coarse systemic approaches, such as the addition of antioxidants in the diet, may show some effectiveness, more sophisticated and targeted approaches designed to improve energy production specifically in photoreceptors or the RPE may have significant potential in the future.

CONCLUSION: PERSPECTIVES FOR FUTURE CLINICAL DEVELOPMENT

Alterations of cGMP-signaling, ion currents, proteostasis, or lack of energy equivalents can cause photoreceptor cell death (Power et al. 2020; Yan et al. 2021; McLaughlin et al. 2022). Different pathological mechanisms may require

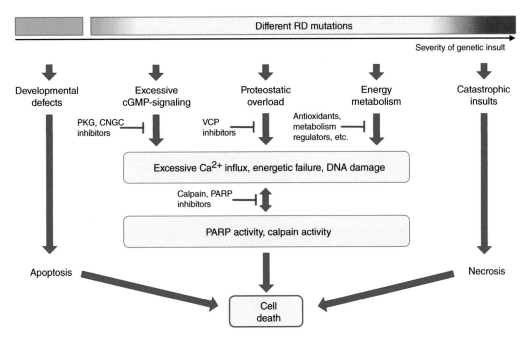

Figure 1. Degenerative mechanisms in retinal degeneration (RD) and therapeutic approaches. The ensemble of cell death mechanisms leading to photoreceptor degeneration likely forms a continuum that may be structured according to the severity of the causative genetic insult. While apoptotic cell death is typically associated with retinal development, RD-causing mutations may initially affect cyclic guanosine monophosphate (cGMP)-signaling and proteostasis. Eventually, different genetic triggers may converge on excessive photoreceptor energy consumption, ultimately resulting in cell death. (PKG) Protein kinase G, (CNGC) cyclic nucleotide-gated channel, (VCP) valosin-containing protein, (PARP) poly(ADP-ribose) polymerase.

different treatment approaches, yet there is a demand for mutation-independent treatment given the high number of distinct mutations affecting retinal function. Moreover, there is an advantage in having larger cohorts of well-stratified patients for clinical studies, especially when compared to gene-specific treatment for rare forms of RD, where the number of patients that can be recruited for a study may be very small (Schneider et al. 2022). Given the multitude of causative genetic defects in RD, gene therapy is unlikely to be available for most patients within this decade. Here, the development of mutation-independent interventions in cGMP-signaling, proteostasis, and energy metabolism may provide an alternative option to preserve a patient's vision until gene-specific treatments become available. Nevertheless, it will be of major importance to carefully select only those patients that are likely to benefit from a particular treat-

ment to reach statistically meaningful clinical end points.

Another major concern in any therapy for retinal diseases is the route of administration and the delivery of the treatment to the affected photoreceptors or RPE cells (Himawan et al. 2019). While recent years have seen the development of relatively targeted adeno-associated viruses (AAV) for gene therapy (Botto et al. 2022), the targeted delivery of pharmacological agents still faces important problems. When delivered systemically, drugs need to be able to cross the blood–retinal barrier and achieve a sufficient and long-lasting concentration in the target cell. This also applies when a local administration to the eye (e.g., intravitreal injection, topical administration) is chosen, as the administration intervals will need to be as long as possible to allow for adequate patient compliance. Smart drug delivery systems are needed for long-term sustained release, such as targeted liposomes, lipid nano-capsules, poly(lactic-co-glycolic acid)-based, methoxy-poly (ethylene glycol) 5 kDa-cholane (mPEG 5 kDa-cholane)-based, or cyclodextrin-based (Yang et al. 2020; Christensen et al. 2021; Prajapati et al. 2021; Sen et al. 2021a). Local delivery to the eye will also limit systemic side effects and improve the overall safety profile for a given treatment.

In conclusion, profound insight into the cell death mechanisms that govern photoreceptor loss in RD is needed to advance current strategies toward mutation-independent clinical treatments. As disease mechanisms may be diverse, in-depth knowledge on disease etiology is key to define the right targets as well as to ascertain appropriate patient selection for clinical trials.

REFERENCES

Adijanto J, Du J, Moffat C, Seifert EL, Hurle JB, Philp NJ. 2014. The retinal pigment epithelium utilizes fatty acids for ketogenesis. *J Biol Chem* 289: 20570–20582. doi:10.1074/jbc.M114.565457

Aguilà M, Bevilacqua D, McCulley C, Schwarz N, Athanasiou D, Kanuga N, Novoselov SS, Lange CA, Ali RR, Bainbridge JW, et al. 2014. Hsp90 inhibition protects against inherited retinal degeneration. *Hum Mol Genet* 23: 2164–2175. doi:10.1093/hmg/ddt613

Ahmadian M, Abbott MJ, Tang T, Hudak CS, Kim Y, Bruss M, Hellerstein MK, Lee HY, Samuel VT, Shulman GI. 2011. Desnutrin/ATGL is regulated by AMPK and is required for a brown adipose phenotype. *Cell Metab* 13: 739–748. doi:10.1016/j.cmet.2011.05.002

Ames A III. 1992. Energy requirements of CNS cells as related to their function and to their vulnerability to ischemia: a commentary based on studies on retina. *Can J Physiol Pharmacol* 70: S158–S164. doi:10.1139/y92-257

Arango-Gonzalez B, Trifunović D, Sahaboglu A, Kranz K, Michalakis S, Farinelli P, Koch S, Koch F, Cottet S, Janssen-Bienhold U, et al. 2014. Identification of a common non-apoptotic cell death mechanism in hereditary retinal degeneration. *PLoS ONE* 9: e112142. doi:10.1371/journal.pone.0112142

Arango-Gonzalez B, Sen M, Guarascio R, Ziaka K, del Amo EM, Hau K, Poultney H, Asfahani R, Urtti A, Chou TF, et al. 2020. Inhibition of VCP preserves retinal structure and function in autosomal dominant retinal degeneration. bioRxiv doi:10.1101/2020.11.17.384669

Athanasiou D, Kosmaoglou M, Kanuga N, Novoselov SS, Paton AW, Paton JC, Chapple JP, Cheetham ME. 2012. Bip prevents rod opsin aggregation. *Mol Biol Cell* 23: 3522–3531. doi:10.1091/mbc.e12-02-0168

Athanasiou D, Aguilà M, Bevilacqua D, Novoselov SS, Parfitt DA, Cheetham ME. 2013. The cell stress machinery and retinal degeneration. *FEBS Lett* 587: 2008–2017. doi:10.1016/j.febslet.2013.05.020

Athanasiou D, Bevilacqua D, Aguila M, McCulley C, Kanuga N, Iwawaki T, Chapple JP, Cheetham ME. 2014. The cochaperone and reductase ERdj5 facilitates rod opsin biogenesis and quality control. *Hum Mol Genet* 23: 6594–6606. doi:10.1093/hmg/ddu385

Athanasiou D, Aguila M, Opefi CA, South K, Bellingham J, Bevilacqua D, Munro PM, Kanuga N, Mackenzie FE, Dubis AM, et al. 2017. Rescue of mutant rhodopsin traffic by metformin-induced AMPK activation accelerates photoreceptor degeneration. *Hum Mol Genet* 26: 305–319. doi:10.1093/hmg/ddx370

Athanasiou D, Aguila M, Bellingham J, Li W, McCulley C, Reeves PJ, Cheetham ME. 2018. The molecular and cellular basis of rhodopsin retinitis pigmentosa reveals potential strategies for therapy. *Prog Retin Eye Res* 62: 1–23. doi:10.1016/j.preteyeres.2017.10.002

Baba M, Takeshige K, Baba N, Ohsumi Y. 1994. Ultrastructural analysis of the autophagic process in yeast: detection of autophagosomes and their characterization. *J Cell Biol* 124: 903–913. doi:10.1083/jcb.124.6.903

Baek SH, Bae ON, Kim EK, Yu SW. 2013. Induction of mitochondrial dysfunction by poly(ADP-ribose) polymer: implication for neuronal cell death. *Mol Cells* 36: 258–266. doi:10.1007/s10059-013-0172-0

Bai P. 2015. Biology of poly(ADP-ribose) polymerases: the factotums of cell maintenance. *Mol Cell* 58: 947–958. doi:10.1016/j.molcel.2015.01.034

Bando H, Atsumi T, Nishio T, Niwa H, Mishima S, Shimizu C, Yoshioka N, Bucala R, Koike T. 2005. Phosphorylation of the 6-phosphofructo-2-kinase/fructose 2,6-bisphosphatase/PFKFB3 family of glycolytic regulators in human cancer. *Clin Cancer Res* 11: 5784–5792. doi:10.1158/1078-0432.CCR-05-0149

Biel M, Michalakis S. 2009. Cyclic nucleotide-gated channels. *Handb Exp Pharmacol* 191: 111–136.

Boatright JH, Nickerson JM, Moring AG, Pardue MT. 2009. Bile acids in treatment of ocular disease. *J Ocul Biol Dis Infor* 2: 149–159. doi:10.1007/s12177-009-9030-x

Botto C, Rucli M, Tekinsoy MD, Pulman J, Sahel JA, Dalkara D. 2022. Early and late stage gene therapy interventions for inherited retinal degenerations. *Prog Retin Eye Res* 86: 100975. doi:10.1016/j.preteyeres.2021.100975

Burns ME, Mendez A, Chen J, Baylor DA. 2002. Dynamics of cyclic GMP synthesis in retinal rods. *Neuron* 36: 81–91. doi:10.1016/S0896-6273(02)00911-X

Byrne LC, Dalkara D, Luna G, Fisher SK, Clérin E, Sahel JA, Léveillard T, Flannery JG. 2015. Viral-mediated RdCVF and RdCVFL expression protects cone and rod photoreceptors in retinal degeneration. *J Clin Invest* 125: 105–116. doi:10.1172/JCI65654

Cao SS, Kaufman RJ. 2014. Endoplasmic reticulum stress and oxidative stress in cell fate decision and human disease. *Antioxid Redox Signal* 21: 396–413. doi:10.1089/ars.2014.5851

Caruso S, Ryu J, Quinn PM, Tsang SH. 2020. Precision metabolome reprogramming for imprecision therapeutics in retinitis pigmentosa. *J Clin Invest* 130: 3971–3973.

Chen Y, Zizmare L, Calbiague V, Yu S, Herberg FW, Schmachtenberg O, Paquet-Durand F, Trautwein C.

2022. Retinal energy metabolism: photoreceptors switch between Cori, Cahill, and mini-Krebs cycles to uncouple glycolysis from mitochondrial respiration. bioRxiv doi:10.1101/2022.06.20.496788

Christensen G, Barut L, Urimi D, Schipper N, Paquet-Durand F. 2021. Investigating ex vivo animal models to test the performance of intravitreal liposomal drug delivery systems. *Pharmaceutics* **13**: 1013. doi:10.3390/pharmaceutics13071013

Clem B, Telang S, Clem A, Yalcin A, Meier J, Simmons A, Rasku MA, Arumugam S, Dean WL, Eaton J, et al. 2008. Small-molecule inhibition of 6-phosphofructo-2-kinase activity suppresses glycolytic flux and tumor growth. *Mol Cancer Ther* **7**: 110–120. doi:10.1158/1535-7163.MCT-07-0482

Das S, Chen Y, Yan J, Christensen G, Belhadj S, Tolone A, Paquet-Durand F. 2021. The role of cGMP-signalling and calcium-signalling in photoreceptor cell death: perspectives for therapy development. *Pflugers Arch* **473**: 1411–1421. doi:10.1007/s00424-021-02556-9

Das S, Popp V, Power M, Groeneveld K, Yan J, Melle C, Rogerson L, Achury M, Schwede F, Strasser T, et al. 2022. Redefining the role of Ca^{2+}-permeable channels in photoreceptor degeneration using diltiazem. *Cell Death Dis* **13**: 47. doi:10.1038/s41419-021-04482-1

Dell'Orco D, Schmidt H, Mariani S, Fanelli F. 2009. Network-level analysis of light adaptation in rod cells under normal and altered conditions. *Mol Biosyst* **5**: 1232–1246. doi:10.1039/b908123b

Diaz-Ruiz R, Rigoulet M, Devin A. 2011. The warburg and crabtree effects: on the origin of cancer cell energy metabolism and of yeast glucose repression. *Biochim Biophys Acta* **1807**: 568–576. doi:10.1016/j.bbabio.2010.08.010

Díaz-Villanueva JF, Díaz-Molina R, García-González V. 2015. Protein folding and mechanisms of proteostasis. *Int J Mol Sci* **16**: 17193–17230. doi:10.3390/ijms160817193

Drack AV, Dumitrescu AV, Bhattarai S, Gratie D, Stone EM, Mullins R, Sheffield VC. 2012. TUDCA slows retinal degeneration in two different mouse models of retinitis pigmentosa and prevents obesity in Bardet–Biedl syndrome type 1 mice. *Invest Ophthalmol Vis Sci* **53**: 100–106. doi:10.1167/iovs.11-8544

Ekstrom PA, Ueffing M, Zrenner E, Paquet-Durand F. 2014. Novel in situ activity assays for the quantitative molecular analysis of neurodegenerative processes in the retina. *Curr Med Chem* **21**: 3478–3493. doi:10.2174/0929867321666140601201337

Farber DB, Lolley RN. 1974. Cyclic guanosine monophosphate: elevation in degenerating photoreceptor cells of the C3H mouse retina. *Science* **186**: 449–451. doi:10.1126/science.186.4162.449

Fu Y, Zhang T. 2014. Pathophysiological mechanism and treatment strategies for Leber congenital amaurosis. *Adv Exp Med Biol* **801**: 791–796. doi:10.1007/978-1-4614-3209-8_99

Galluzzi L, Vitale I, Aaronson SA, Abrams JM, Adam D, Agostinis P, Alnemri ES, Altucci L, Amelio I, Andrews DW, et al. 2018. Molecular mechanisms of cell death: recommendations of the nomenclature committee on cell death 2018. *Cell Death Differ* **25**: 486–541. doi:10.1038/s41418-017-0012-4

Gastaldello A, Giampieri F, Quiles JL, Navarro-Hortal MD, Aparicio S, García Villena E, Tutusaus Pifarre K, De Giuseppe R, Grosso G, Cianciosi D, et al. 2022. Adherence to the Mediterranean-style eating pattern and macular degeneration: a systematic review of observational studies. *Nutrients* **14**: 2028. doi:10.3390/nu14102028

Ghose P, Shaham S. 2020. Cell death in animal development. *Development* **147**: dev191882. doi:10.1242/dev.191882

Ghosh R, Wang L, Wang ES, Perera BG, Igbaria A, Morita S, Prado K, Thamsen M, Caswell D, Macias H, et al. 2014. Allosteric inhibition of the IRE1α RNase preserves cell viability and function during endoplasmic reticulum stress. *Cell* **158**: 534–548. doi:10.1016/j.cell.2014.07.002

Giarmarco MM, Brock DC, Robbings BM, Cleghorn WM, Tsantilas KA, Kuch KC, Ge W, Rutter KM, Parker ED, Hurley JB, et al. 2020. Daily mitochondrial dynamics in cone photoreceptors. *Proc Natl Acad Sci* **117**: 28816–28827. doi:10.1073/pnas.2007827117

Glücksmann A. 1951. Cell deaths in normal vertebrate ontogeny. *Biol Rev Camb Philos Soc* **26**: 59–86. doi:10.1111/j.1469-185X.1951.tb00774.x

Gorbatyuk MS, Knox T, LaVail MM, Gorbatyuk OS, Noorwez SM, Hauswirth WW, Lin JH, Muzyczka N, Lewin AS. 2010. Restoration of visual function in P23H rhodopsin transgenic rats by gene delivery of BiP/Grp78. *Proc Natl Acad Sci* **107**: 5961–5966. doi:10.1073/pnas.0911991107

Griciuc A, Aron L, Piccoli G, Ueffing M. 2010. Clearance of Rhodopsin[P23H] aggregates requires the ERAD effector VCP. *Biochim Biophys Acta* **1803**: 424–434. doi:10.1016/j.bbamcr.2010.01.008

Griciuc A, Aron L, Ueffing M. 2011. ER stress in retinal degeneration: a target for rational therapy? *Trends Mol Med* **17**: 442–451. doi:10.1016/j.molmed.2011.04.002

Grover AK, Samson SE. 2014. Antioxidants and vision health: facts and fiction. *Mol Cell Biochem* **388**: 173–183. doi:10.1007/s11010-013-1908-z

Gwinn DM, Shackelford DB, Egan DF, Mihaylova MM, Mery A, Vasquez DS, Turk BE, Shaw RJ. 2008. AMPK phosphorylation of raptor mediates a metabolic checkpoint. *Mol Cell* **30**: 214–226. doi:10.1016/j.molcel.2008.03.003

Herzig S, Shaw RJ. 2018. AMPK: guardian of metabolism and mitochondrial homeostasis. *Nat Rev Mol Cell Biol* **19**: 121–135. doi:10.1038/nrm.2017.95

Himawan E, Ekström P, Buzgo M, Gaillard P, Stefánsson E, Marigo V, Loftsson T, Paquet-Durand F. 2019. Drug delivery to retinal photoreceptors. *Drug Discov Today* **24**: 1637–1643. doi:10.1016/j.drudis.2019.03.004

Iadevaia V, Huo Y, Zhang Z, Foster LJ, Proud CG. 2012. Roles of the mammalian target of rapamycin, mTOR, in controlling ribosome biogenesis and protein synthesis. *Biochem Soc Trans* **40**: 168–172. doi:10.1042/BST20110682

Ikeda HO, Sasaoka N, Koike M, Nakano N, Muraoka Y, Toda Y, Fuchigami T, Shudo T, Iwata A, Hori S, et al. 2014. Novel VCP modulators mitigate major pathologies of rd10, a mouse model of retinitis pigmentosa. *Sci Rep* **4:** 5970. doi:10.1038/srep05970

Jayaraj GG, Hipp MS, Hartl FU. 2020. Functional modules of the proteostasis network. *Cold Spring Harb Perspect Biol* **12:** a033951. doi:10.1101/cshperspect.a033951

Kanow MA, Giarmarco MM, Jankowski CS, Tsantilas K, Engel AL, Du J, Linton JD, Farnsworth CC, Sloat SR, Rountree A, et al. 2017. Biochemical adaptations of the retina and retinal pigment epithelium support a metabolic ecosystem in the vertebrate eye. *eLife* **6:** e28899. doi:10.7554/eLife.28899

Kepp O, Galluzzi L, Lipinski M, Yuan J, Kroemer G. 2011. Cell death assays for drug discovery. *Nat Rev Drug Discov* **10:** 221–237. doi:10.1038/nrd3373

Kerr JF, Wyllie AH, Currie AR. 1972. Apoptosis: a basic biological phenomenon with wide-ranging implications in tissue kinetics. *Br J Cancer* **26:** 239–257. doi:10.1038/bjc.1972.33

Kosmaoglou M, Kanuga N, Aguilà M, Garriga P, Cheetham ME. 2009. A dual role for EDEM1 in the processing of rod opsin. *J Cell Sci* **122:** 4465–4472. doi:10.1242/jcs.055228

Kroemer G, Levine B. 2008. Autophagic cell death: the story of a misnomer. *Nat Rev Mol Cell Biol* **9:** 1004–1010. doi:10.1038/nrm2529

Kulkarni M, Trifunović D, Schubert T, Euler T, Paquet-Durand F. 2016. Calcium dynamics change in degenerating cone photoreceptors. *Hum Mol Genet* **25:** 3729–3740. doi:10.1093/hmg/ddw219

Lamb CA, Yoshimori T, Tooze SA. 2013. The autophagosome: origins unknown, biogenesis complex. *Nat Rev Mol Cell Biol* **14:** 759–774. doi:10.1038/nrm3696

LaVail MM. 1980. Circadian nature of rod outer segment disc shedding in the rat. *Invest Ophthalmol Vis Sci* **19:** 407–411.

Lawson EC, Bhatia SK, Han MK, Aung MH, Ciavatta V, Boatright JH, Pardue MT. 2016. Tauroursodeoxycholic acid protects retinal function and structure in rd1 mice. *Adv Exp Med Biol* **854:** 431–436. doi:10.1007/978-3-319-17121-0_57

Leist M, Jäättelä M. 2001. Four deaths and a funeral: from caspases to alternative mechanisms. *Nat Rev Mol Cell Biol* **2:** 589–598. doi:10.1038/35085008

Li S, Samardzija M, Yang Z, Grimm C, Jin M. 2016. Pharmacological amelioration of cone survival and vision in a mouse model for Leber congenital amaurosis. *J Neurosci* **36:** 5808–5819. doi:10.1523/JNEUROSCI.3857-15.2016

Li LH, Lee JC, Leung HH, Lam WC, Fu Z, Lo ACY. 2020. Lutein supplementation for eye diseases. *Nutrients* **12:** 1721. doi:10.3390/nu12061721

Lim S, Roseman G, Peshenko I, Manchala G, Cudia D, Dizhoor AM, Millhauser G, Ames JB. 2018. Retinal guanylyl cyclase activating protein 1 forms a functional dimer. *PLoS ONE* **13:** e0193947. doi:10.1371/journal.pone.0193947

Lohmann SM, Vaandrager AB, Smolenski A, Walter U, De Jonge HR. 1997. Distinct and specific functions of cGMP-dependent protein kinases. *Trends Biochem Sci* **22:** 307–312. doi:10.1016/S0968-0004(97)01086-4

Lunt SY, Heiden MGV. 2011. Aerobic glycolysis: meeting the metabolic requirements of cell proliferation. *Annu Rev Cell Dev Biol* **27:** 441–464. doi:10.1146/annurev-cellbio-092910-154237

McLaughlin T, Medina A, Perkins J, Yera M, Wang JJ, Zhang SX. 2022. Cellular stress signaling and the unfolded protein response in retinal degeneration: mechanisms and therapeutic implications. *Mol Neurodegener* **17:** 25. doi:10.1186/s13024-022-00528-w

Mendes HF, Cheetham ME. 2008. Pharmacological manipulation of gain-of-function and dominant-negative mechanisms in rhodopsin retinitis pigmentosa. *Hum Mol Genet* **17:** 3043–3054. doi:10.1093/hmg/ddn202

Mizushima N. 2007. Autophagy: process and function. *Genes Dev* **21:** 2861–2873. doi:10.1101/gad.1599207

Montero JA, Lorda-Diez CI, Hurle JM. 2022. Regulation of developmental cell death in the animal kingdom: a critical analysis of epigenetic versus genetic factors. *Int J Mol Sci* **23:** 1154. doi:10.3390/ijms23031154

Moreno-Gonzalez I, Soto C. 2011. Misfolded protein aggregates: mechanisms, structures and potential for disease transmission. *Semin Cell Dev Biol* **22:** 482–487. doi:10.1016/j.semcdb.2011.04.002

Nakano N, Ikeda HO, Hasegawa T, Muraoka Y, Iwai S, Tsuruyama T, Nakano M, Fuchigami T, Shudo T, Kakizuka A, et al. 2016. Neuroprotective effects of VCP modulators in mouse models of glaucoma. *Heliyon* **2:** e00096. doi:10.1016/j.heliyon.2016.e00096

Nickl CK, Raidas SK, Zhao H, Sausbier M, Ruth P, Tegge W, Brayden JE, Dostmann WR. 2010. (D)-Amino acid analogues of DT-2 as highly selective and superior inhibitors of cGMP-dependent protein kinase Iα. *Biochim Biophys Acta* **1804:** 524–532. doi:10.1016/j.bbapap.2009.12.004

Okawa H, Sampath AP, Laughlin SB, Fain GL. 2008. ATP consumption by mammalian rod photoreceptors in darkness and in light. *Curr Biol* **18:** 1917–1921. doi:10.1016/j.cub.2008.10.029

Olivares-González L, Martínez-Fernández de la Cámara C, Hervás D, Marín MP, Lahoz A, Millán JM, Rodrigo R. 2016. cGMP-phosphodiesterase inhibition prevents hypoxia-induced cell death activation in porcine retinal explants. *PLoS ONE* **11:** e0166717. doi:10.1371/journal.pone.0166717

Olshevskaya EV, Ermilov AN, Dizhoor AM. 2002. Factors that affect regulation of cGMP synthesis in vertebrate photoreceptors and their genetic link to human retinal degeneration. *Mol Cell Biochem* **230:** 139–147. doi:10.1023/A:1014248208584

Orrenius S, Zhivotovsky B, Nicotera P. 2003. Regulation of cell death: the calcium-apoptosis link. *Nat Rev Mol Cell Biol* **4:** 552–565. doi:10.1038/nrm1150

Oveson BC, Iwase T, Hackett SF, Lee SY, Usui S, Sedlak TW, Snyder SH, Campochiaro PA, Sung JU. 2011. Constituents of bile, bilirubin and TUDCA, protect against oxidative stress-induced retinal degeneration. *J Neurochem* **116:** 144–153. doi:10.1111/j.1471-4159.2010.07092.x

Paquet-Durand F, Beck S, Michalakis S, Goldmann T, Huber G, Mühlfriedel R, Trifunović D, Fischer MD, Fahl E, Duetsch G, et al. 2011. A key role for cyclic nucleotide gated (CNG) channels in cGMP-related retinitis pigmentosa. *Hum Mol Genet* **20:** 941–947. doi:10.1093/hmg/ddq539

Parfitt DA, Aguila M, McCulley CH, Bevilacqua D, Mendes HF, Athanasiou D, Novoselov SS, Kanuga N, Munro PM,

Coffey PJ, et al. 2014. The heat-shock response co-inducer arimoclomol protects against retinal degeneration in rhodopsin retinitis pigmentosa. *Cell Death Dis* **5:** e1236. doi:10.1038/cddis.2014.214

Power M, Das S, Schütze K, Marigo V, Ekström P, Paquet-Durand F. 2020. Cellular mechanisms of hereditary photoreceptor degeneration—focus on cGMP. *Prog Retin Eye Res* **74:** 100772. doi:10.1016/j.preteyeres.2019.07.005

Prajapati M, Christensen G, Paquet-Durand F, Loftsson T. 2021. Cytotoxicity of β-cyclodextrins in retinal explants for intravitreal drug formulations. *Molecules* **26:** 1492. doi:10.3390/molecules26051492

Pugh EN Jr, Lamb TD. 1990. Cyclic GMP and calcium: the internal messengers of excitation and adaptation in vertebrate photoreceptors. *Vision Res* **30:** 1923–1948. doi:10.1016/0042-6989(90)90013-B

Punzo C, Kornacker K, Cepko CL. 2009. Stimulation of the insulin/mTOR pathway delays cone death in a mouse model of retinitis pigmentosa. *Nat Neurosci* **12:** 44–52. doi:10.1038/nn.2234

Qin L, Sankaran B, Aminzai S, Casteel DE, Kim C. 2018. Structural basis for selective inhibition of human PKG Iα by the balanol-like compound N46. *J Biol Chem* **293:** 10985–10992. doi:10.1074/jbc.RA118.002427

Qiu Y, Yao J, Jia L, Thompson DA, Zacks DN. 2019. Shifting the balance of autophagy and proteasome activation reduces proteotoxic cell death: a novel therapeutic approach for restoring photoreceptor homeostasis. *Cell Death Dis* **10:** 547. doi:10.1038/s41419-019-1780-1

Querques G, Forte R, Souied EH. 2011. Retina and omega-3. *J Nutr Metab* **2011:** 748361. doi:10.1155/2011/748361

Quijano C, Trujillo M, Castro L, Trostchansky A. 2016. Interplay between oxidant species and energy metabolism. *Redox Biol* **8:** 28–42. doi:10.1016/j.redox.2015.11.010

Rossino MG, Casini G. 2019. Nutraceuticals for the treatment of diabetic retinopathy. *Nutrients* **11:** 771. doi:10.3390/nu11040771

Roy A, Tolone A, Hilhorst R, Groten J, Tomar T, Paquet-Durand F. 2022. Kinase activity profiling identifies putative downstream targets of cGMP/PKG signaling in inherited retinal neurodegeneration. *Cell Death Discov* **8:** 93. doi:10.1038/s41420-022-00897-7

Sancho-Pelluz J, Arango-Gonzalez B, Kustermann S, Romero FJ, van Veen T, Zrenner E, Ekström P, Paquet-Durand F. 2008. Photoreceptor cell death mechanisms in inherited retinal degeneration. *Mol Neurobiol* **38:** 253–269. doi:10.1007/s12035-008-8045-9

Schneider N, Sundaresan Y, Gopalakrishnan P, Beryozkin A, Hanany M, Levanon EY, Banin E, Ben-Aroya S, Sharon D. 2022. Inherited retinal diseases: linking genes, disease-causing variants, and relevant therapeutic modalities. *Prog Retin Eye Res* **89:** 101029. doi:10.1016/j.preteyeres.2021.101029

Sen M, Al-Amin M, Kicková E, Sadeghi A, Puranen J, Urtti A, Caliceti P, Salmaso S, Arango-Gonzalez B, Ueffing M. 2021a. Retinal neuroprotection by controlled release of a VCP inhibitor from self-assembled nanoparticles. *J Control Release* **339:** 307–320. doi:10.1016/j.jconrel.2021.09.039

Sen M, Bassetto M, Poulhes F, Zelphati O, Ueffing M, Arango-Gonzalez B. 2021b. Efficient ocular delivery of VCP siRNA via reverse magnetofection in RHO P23H

rodent retina explants. *Pharmaceutics* **13:** 225. doi:10.3390/pharmaceutics13020225

Sen M, Kutsyr O, Cao B, Bolz S, Arango-Gonzalez B, Ueffing M. 2021c. Pharmacological inhibition of the VCP/proteasome axis rescues photoreceptor degeneration in RHO (P23H) rat retinal explants. *Biomolecules* **11:** 1528. doi:10.3390/biom11101528

Shi L, Pan H, Liu Z, Xie J, Han W. 2017. Roles of PFKFB3 in cancer. *Signal Transduct Target Ther* **2:** 17044. doi:10.1038/sigtrans.2017.44

Shore GC, Papa FR, Oakes SA. 2011. Signaling cell death from the endoplasmic reticulum stress response. *Curr Opin Cell Biol* **23:** 143–149. doi:10.1016/j.ceb.2010.11.003

Sizova OS, Shinde VM, Lenox AR, Gorbatyuk MS. 2014. Modulation of cellular signaling pathways in P23H rhodopsin photoreceptors. *Cell Signal* **26:** 665–672. doi:10.1016/j.cellsig.2013.12.008

Smith MH, Ploegh HL, Weissman JS. 2011. Road to ruin: targeting proteins for degradation in the endoplasmic reticulum. *Science* **334:** 1086–1090. doi:10.1126/science.1209235

Strettoi E. 2015. A survey of retinal remodeling. *Front Cell Neurosci* **9:** 494. doi:10.3389/fncel.2015.00494

Tanimoto N, Brombas A, Müller F, Seeliger MW. 2012. HCN1 channels significantly shape retinal photoresponses. *Adv Exp Med Biol* **723:** 807–812. doi:10.1007/978-1-4614-0631-0_103

Tolone A, Belhadj S, Rentsch A, Schwede F, Paquet-Durand F. 2019. The cGMP pathway and inherited photoreceptor degeneration: targets, compounds, and biomarkers. *Genes (Basel)* **10:** 453. doi:10.3390/genes10060453

Tolone A, Haq W, Fachinger A, Rentsch A, Herberg FW, Schwede F, Paquet-Durand F. 2021. Retinal degeneration: multilevel protection of photoreceptor and ganglion cell viability and function with the novel PKG inhibitor CN238. bioRxiv doi:10.1101/2021.08.05.455191

Trick GL, Berkowitz BA. 2005. Retinal oxygenation response and retinopathy. *Prog Retin Eye Res* **24:** 259–274. doi:10.1016/j.preteyeres.2004.08.001

Tzekov R, Stein L, Kaushal S. 2011. Protein misfolding and retinal degeneration. *Cold Spring Harb Perspect Biol* **3:** a007492. doi:10.1101/cshperspect.a007492

Vasireddy V, Chavali VR, Joseph VT, Kadam R, Lin JH, Jamison JA, Kompella UB, Reddy GB, Ayyagari R. 2011. Rescue of photoreceptor degeneration by curcumin in transgenic rats with P23H rhodopsin mutation. *PLoS ONE* **6:** e21193. doi:10.1371/journal.pone.0021193

Venkatesh A, Ma S, Le YZ, Hall MN, Rüegg MA, Punzo C. 2015. Activated mTORC1 promotes long-term cone survival in retinitis pigmentosa mice. *J Clin Invest* **125:** 1446–1458. doi:10.1172/JCI79766

Viegas FO, Neuhauss SCF. 2021. A metabolic landscape for maintaining retina integrity and function. *Front Mol Neurosci* **14:** 656000. doi:10.3389/fnmol.2021.656000

Vighi E, Trifunović D, Veiga-Crespo P, Rentsch A, Hoffmann D, Sahaboglu A, Strasser T, Kulkarni M, Bertolotti E, van den Heuvel A, et al. 2018. Combination of cGMP analogue and drug delivery system provides functional protection in hereditary retinal degeneration. *Proc Natl Acad Sci* **115:** E2997–E3006. doi:10.1073/pnas.1718792115

Vinberg F, Chen J, Kefalov VJ. 2018. Regulation of calcium homeostasis in the outer segments of rod and cone photoreceptors. *Prog Retin Eye Res* **67:** 87–101. doi:10.1016/j.preteyeres.2018.06.001

Waldner DM, Bech-Hansen NT, Stell WK. 2018. Channeling vision: Ca(V)1.4—a critical link in retinal signal transmission. *Biomed Res Int* **2018:** 7272630. doi:10.1155/2018/7272630

Walter P, Ron D. 2011. The unfolded protein response: from stress pathway to homeostatic regulation. *Science* **334:** 1081–1086. doi:10.1126/science.1209038

Wang SK, Xue Y, Cepko CL. 2020. Microglia modulation by TGF-β1 protects cones in mouse models of retinal degeneration. *J Clin Invest* **130:** 4360–4369.

Warburg O. 1925. The metabolism of carcinoma cells. *J Cancer Res* **9:** 148–163. doi:10.1158/jcr.1925.148

Wen RH, Stanar P, Tam B, Moritz OL. 2019. Autophagy in *Xenopus laevis* rod photoreceptors is independently regulated by phototransduction and misfolded RHO[P23H]. *Autophagy* **15:** 1970–1989. doi:10.1080/15548627.2019.1596487

Wiggins PM. 2001. High and low density intracellular water. *Cell Mol Biol (Noisy-le-grand)* **47:** 735–744.

Wong PM, Puente C, Ganley IG, Jiang X. 2013. The ULK1 complex: sensing nutrient signals for autophagy activation. *Autophagy* **9:** 124–137. doi:10.4161/auto.23323

Wong-Riley MT. 2010. Energy metabolism of the visual system. *Eye Brain* **2:** 99–116. doi:10.2147/EB.S9078

Wu X, Rapoport TA. 2018. Mechanistic insights into ER-associated protein degradation. *Curr Opin Cell Biol* **53:** 22–28. doi:10.1016/j.ceb.2018.04.004

Xu L, Ash JD. 2016. The role of AMPK pathway in neuroprotection. *Adv Exp Med Biol* **854:** 425–430. doi:10.1007/978-3-319-17121-0_56

Yan J, Chen Y, Zhu Y, Paquet-Durand F. 2021. Programmed non-apoptotic cell death in hereditary retinal degeneration: crosstalk between cGMP-dependent pathways and PARthanatos? *Int J Mol Sci* **22:** 10567. doi:10.3390/ijms221910567

Yang J, Luo L, Oh Y, Meng T, Chai G, Xia S, Emmert D, Wang B, Eberhart CG, Lee S, et al. 2020. Sunitinib malate-loaded biodegradable microspheres for the prevention of corneal neovascularization in rats. *J Control Release* **327:** 456–466. doi:10.1016/j.jconrel.2020.08.019

Yao J, Jia L, Feathers K, Lin C, Khan NW, Klionsky DJ, Ferguson TA, Zacks DN. 2016. Autophagy-mediated catabolism of visual transduction proteins prevents retinal degeneration. *Autophagy* **12:** 2439–2450. doi:10.1080/15548627.2016.1238553

Ye Y, Meyer HH, Rapoport TA. 2001. The AAA ATPase Cdc48/p97 and its partners transport proteins from the ER into the cytosol. *Nature* **414:** 652–656. doi:10.1038/414652a

Zeiss CJ, Neal J, Johnson EA. 2004. Caspase-3 in postnatal retinal development and degeneration. *Invest Ophthalmol Vis Sci* **45:** 964–970. doi:10.1167/iovs.03-0439

Zhang SX, Sanders E, Fliesler SJ, Wang JJ. 2014. Endoplasmic reticulum stress and the unfolded protein responses in retinal degeneration. *Exp Eye Res* **125:** 30–40. doi:10.1016/j.exer.2014.04.015

Zhang L, Du J, Justus S, Hsu CW, Bonet-Ponce L, Wu WH, Tsai YT, Wu WP, Jia Y, Duong JK. 2016. Reprogramming metabolism by targeting sirtuin 6 attenuates retinal degeneration. *J Clin Invest* **126:** 4659–4673. doi:10.1172/JCI86905

Zhang E, Ryu J, Levi SR, Oh JK, Hsu CW, Cui X, Lee TT, Wang NK, de Carvalho JRL, Tsang SH. 2020. PKM2 ablation enhanced retinal function and survival in a preclinical model of retinitis pigmentosa. *Mamm Genome* **31:** 77–85. doi:10.1007/s00335-020-09837-1

Cite this article as *Cold Spring Harb Perspect Med* doi: 10.1101/cshperspect.a041310

Neurotrophic Factors in the Treatment of Inherited Retinal Diseases

Laure Blouin,[1] José-Alain Sahel,[2] and Daniel C. Chung[3]

[1]Director of Clinical Science & Medical Communications, SparingVision, 75008 Paris, France

[2]Department of Ophthalmology, University of Pittsburgh Medical Center, Pittsburgh, Pennsylvania 15219, USA

[3]Chief Medical Officer, SparingVision, Philadelphia, Pennsylvania 19103, USA

Correspondence: Daniel.chung@sparingvision.com

Inherited retinal diseases (IRDs) are the leading cause of blindness in working-age individuals worldwide. Their genetic etiology is especially heterogenous, so the development of gene-specific therapies is unlikely to meet the medical needs of the entire patient community. Considering these challenges, a complementary strategy could be to develop therapies independent of the underlying gene variant causing retinal degeneration. As the retina is a neural tissue, it is in theory amenable to neuroprotective therapies that could help prolong cell survival or promote retinal function. Many neurotrophic factors have shown favorable results in preclinical animal models of neurodegenerative diseases, but unfortunately these findings have not yet translated into successful human clinical trials. The clinical development of these new therapies is mostly impeded by selection of pertinent clinical end points and time-to-readout, as the majority of IRDs show a relatively slow disease progression rate. Despite these challenges, several strategies have moved forward into clinical development.

Inherited retinal diseases (IRDs) are a predominant focus for investigative therapeutic interventions, with modalities such as gene augmentation and gene editing having made significant strides in the past few decades. These strategies mostly target specific genes or variants within the gene of interest, as seen with the gene therapy for *RPE65*-associated IRD, Luxturna (voretigene neparvovec). However, even though voretigene neparvovec has proven effective and is now commercialized worldwide, its application remains limited to <5% of patients with rod-cone dystrophies (RCDs). With more than 300 different genes responsible for IRD, and many more retinal diseases with nonmonogenic etiologies, the development of individual gene-specific therapies will not be able to meet the medical needs of all patients with IRDs.

As a neural tissue, the retina could be amenable to neuroprotective therapies aiming to slow or prevent visual function loss caused by the degeneration of retinal cells like photoreceptors. Photoreceptors are responsible for the process of phototransduction (i.e., the transformation of a light stimulus into an electrical impulse that is then propagated through a neural network to the occipital lobe of the brain, where it is integrated). These photosensitive cells are able to detect light stimuli across a wide range of wavelengths and luminance levels critical for human vision. Any dysfunction or degeneration of photoreceptors will lead to visual impairment, as exemplified in retinitis pigmentosa (RP).

RP is the most common form of RCD and comprises a group of heterogeneous, progressively degenerative retinal pathologies that contribute to the majority of adult blindness worldwide with a prevalence of 1:4000 individuals (Hamel 2006). Although considered a rare disease, RP constitutes a large field of research and investigative clinical development, as it continues to be an area of high unmet medical need. With more than 70 different causative genes, its genetic transmission spans all modes of inheritance (RetNet, web.sph.uth.edu/RetNet/sumdis.htm).

RP is a monogenic disease that causes deficiencies in rod photoreceptors or retinal pigment epithelial (RPE) cells, leading to their slow degeneration. Secondary degeneration of cone photoreceptors ensues, due to the lack of neurotrophic support normally produced by rods. Regardless of genetic etiology, patients experience the initial degeneration of rod photoreceptors as a loss of visual perception in dim light (known as night blindness or nyctalopia), which then progresses to concentric visual field loss in daylight, ultimately affecting the central cone photoreceptors, leading to the loss of color perception and eventually visual acuity. In a minority of patients, it can ultimately deteriorate to total loss of light perception.

Neurotrophic factors are usually produced endogenously and can have different functions based on their corresponding cell receptors, such as promoting proliferation, survival, or regeneration of the targeted cell. Once they bind to their targeted cells, neurotrophic factors generally initiate a metabolic cascade responsible for a physiologic response or downstream biologic effect.

Factors specific to neurons are comprised of neurotrophins and glial-derived neurotrophic factors (GDNFs). Neurotrophins include factors such as neurotrophin 3, neurotrophin 4, nerve growth factor (NGF), and brain-derived growth factor (BDNF) (Skaper 2012). The GDNF ligand family includes artemin, neurturin, and the most investigated, GDNF (Runeberg-Roos et al. 2020). Other categories of trophic factors include fibroblast growth factor (FGF), ciliary nerve trophic factor (CNTF), insulin-like growth factor (IGF), and transforming growth factors (TGFs). An important source of growth factors are glial cells, such as retinal astrocytes and Müller cells, but other cells such as photoreceptors can also produce or secrete neurotrophic factors (Léveillard et al. 2004; Linker et al. 2009).

Many neurotrophic factors have shown favorable results in preclinical animal models of neurodegenerative diseases, but unfortunately these findings did not translate in human clinical trials, as seen with GDNF used to treat Parkinson's disease (Gash et al. 2020), or CNTF for amyotrophic lateral sclerosis (Miller et al. 1996). In ophthalmology, research has focused on agents that will slow or prevent the degeneration of photoreceptors in animal models.

A large number of different neurotrophic or survival factors were initially tested by LaVail and Steinberg in two models of photoreceptor degeneration, the light-damaged albino rat model and the Royal College of Surgeons (RCS). Their findings suggested a protective effect of neurotrophic factors against photoreceptor cell death, following direct protein injections of basic fibroblast growth factor (bFGF, or FGF-2), ciliary neurotrophic factor (CNTF), or brain-derived neurotrophic factor (BDNF) (Faktorovich et al. 1992; LaVail et al. 1992). Additional studies by other investigators have shown that bFGF, BDNF, cardiotrophin-1, NGF, FGF, and CNTF can slow the progression of photoreceptor and/or RGC degeneration in animal models (Schuettauf et al. 2005; Sahni et al. 2011). To date, none of these factors has shown efficacy in placebo-controlled human clinical trials.

This review focuses on the clinical development of FGF, GDNF, and CNTF for ophthalmic disorders, and on the discovery and preclinical development of rod-derived cone viability factor (RdCVF) that has proven integral for an endogenous pathway of cone survival.

FGF

FGF includes a family of multifunctional growth factors that have primarily been investigated for their ability to develop and maintain tissues, by promoting cell proliferation and differentiation. In the early 1990s, basic FGF was shown to induce extensive rescue of photoreceptors following subretinal injection in RCS rat models of retinal degeneration (Faktorovich et al. 1990). When injected intravitreally, the neurotrophic factor could rescue a wider area of the retina, including other cell types.

FGF is also known to promote corneal epithelial cell growth and migration. Currently, FGF-1 is assessed for the treatment of corneal diseases such as Fuchs endothelial cell dystrophy. Considering the unstable 3D structure of FGF-1 and its tendency to lose function, the protein sequence was engineered to increase its half-life. The drug candidate TTHX1114 was administered four times weekly via intracameral injections to 17 patients with corneal endothelial dystrophy (NCT04520321). The phase I/II trial has not reported any safety concerns up to 90 d of follow-up (ClinicalTrials: clinicaltrials.gov/ct2/history/NCT04520321?V_8&embedded = true).

GDNF

In the eye, GDNF is primarily expressed in the retina (Akurathi et al. 2022). Subretinal injections of GDNF were found to rescue the function and promote the survival of rod photoreceptors in *rd/rd* mice (Frasson et al. 1999), when a unique intravitreal administration was able to rescue retinal ganglion cells after optic nerve severing in Sprague–Dawley rats (Koeberle and Ball 1998).

Furthermore, a proof of concept for GDNF gene therapy was carried out in a model of RP (S334-4ter rats), using an adeno-associated viral (AAV) vector engineered to specifically transduce Müller glial cells (ShH10.Y445F) (Dalkara et al. 2011). Sustained functional rescue of photoreceptors, as measured by ERG, was reported up to 5 mo after intravitreal administration.

Sustained intraocular delivery of GDNF was investigated more recently using poly(lactic-co-glycolic acid)-coated microspheres (García-Ca-

ballero et al. 2018). Twelve weeks after administration to *rho*$^{-/-}$ mice, partial functional and structural rescue of photoreceptors was reported, compared to controls. Interestingly, no significant intraocular inflammatory reaction was observed despite the presence of foreign particles in the eye.

CNTF

CNTF is highly expressed in the brain, spinal cord, and ciliary ganglion of the eye. CNTF belongs to the family of CNTF proteins, which include interleukin 6 (IL-6) and leukemia inhibitory factor (LIF). The trophic factor is expressed by the *CNTF* gene located on chromosome 11 that encodes a 22.7-kDa polypeptide. CNTF binds to a heterotrimeric complex of receptors—comprised of CNTF receptor α (CNTFRα), gp130, and LIF receptor β (LIFRβ)—and activates a JAK kinase. The JAK kinase then phosphorylates the tyrosine residues of the intracellular domain of gp130 and LIF, which triggers the docking of STAT3 to the complex. STAT3 then undergoes phosphorylation, dimerizes, and moves to the nucleus where gene transcription is conducted.

CNTF has demonstrated remyelinating properties following sciatic nerve crush in a mouse model deficient in CNTF. The trophic factor also appears to delay cell loss in neurodegenerative diseases of the central nervous system (CNS). In a rat model of amyotrophic lateral sclerosis, a decrease in the progression of motor nerve destruction was demonstrated, maintaining motor operation and cell survival. The neuroprotective effect of CNTF has also been shown in other CNS models, like the eye. Its neuroprotective effect on neural tissue, especially on photoreceptors, has been well documented in preclinical models. The use of CNTF as a neuroprotective agent has been postulated for several ocular conditions, including diabetic retinopathy (Wu and Mo 2023), primary open-angle glaucoma (Shpak et al. 2017; Goldberg et al. 2023), age-related macular degeneration (AMD) (Zhang et al. 2011), and retinal detachment (Wen et al. 2012).

The most common area of investigation for CNTF remains its use in IRDs, especially in RP. In 1992, LaVail and colleagues reported a protective effect of intravitreal injections of CNTF protein following light-induced retinal degeneration in a rat model (LaVail et al. 1992). These results were repeated in murine models, showing similar protective effects on the photoreceptors. In the late 1990s, CNTF gene therapy proved promising in IRD models, first using adenoviral vectors, then switching to safer AAV vectors. Both vectors demonstrated a long-term protective effect in maintaining photoreceptor survival and overall retinal health. These preclinical and research results have led to the investigation of CNTF in human clinical trials.

In the new millennium, a novel approach of intraocular implants using encapsulated cell technology (ECT) was developed to facilitate sustained dosing of the CNTF protein in the retina. In a dog model of retinal degeneration, the ECT implant showed a significant improvement in protecting the retina compared to a single-bolus intravitreal injection (Tao et al. 2002).

Four clinical studies were launched based on these preclinical findings: three targeting RP and one centering on geographic atrophy related to dry AMD. Data collected in RP patients up to 96 mo postimplantation did not demonstrate efficacy on visual acuity, visual field sensitivity, or retinal anatomy as seen on optical coherence tomography (Birch et al. 2013, 2016). In dry AMD and geographic atrophy, only moderate efficacy was documented (Zhang et al. 2011).

Despite disappointing results in RP and dry AMD, CNTF was assessed for the treatment of macular telangiectasia type 2. Following a promising phase I safety trial, a phase II randomized control trial reported a greater progression of neurodegeneration in the eyes that received a sham treatment compared to the CNTF-treated eyes, 2 yr after implantation (Chew et al. 2015, 2019). Moreover, changes in area of photoreceptor loss correlated highly with changes in the retinal sensitivity measured on microperimetry, and reading speed was stabilized only in the eyes receiving the implant. The efficacy of the implant has recently been confirmed in two phase III trials that met their respective primary end points (NCT03316300 and NCT03319849) (Neurotech Pharmaceuticals 2022).

RdCVF

The sequential degeneration of rods and cones observed in RCD was initially described in a mouse model of retinal degeneration (Carter-Dawson et al. 1978). The *rd1* mouse is an extremely rapid degenerative model of rod-cone degeneration. A recessive mutation carried by the gene encoding the β-subunit of the rod-phosphodiesterase (*PDE6B*) leads to the rapid degeneration of rods through apoptosis, followed by a secondary degeneration of cones, even though they do not express the pathogenic gene variant and are not directly affected by the enzymatic deficit. This model mimics the sequence of events reported in patients affected with RCD (i.e., a primary loss of dark-adapted vision followed by loss of central and light-adapted vision).

Subretinal transplantation of a layer of wild-type rod photoreceptors was shown to slow down the secondary degeneration of cones in the *rd1* mouse (Mohand-Said et al. 1997). Further investigations revealed that the mechanism of action allowing rods to protect cone cells was linked to one or several proteins secreted by rods (Mohand-Said et al. 1998; Fintz et al. 2003). A specific trophic factor was identified by high-content screening of a retinal cDNA library in cone-enriched chicken embryo cell cultures: RdCVF.

RdCVF was shown to be expressed specifically by rod photoreceptors. In addition, the preferential localization of RdCVF on the cone extracellular matrix suggested that it bound a receptor present on the membrane of cone cells (Léveillard et al. 2004). Once secreted by rods in the retinal intercellular matrix, RdCVF binds to a receptor on the membrane of cone photoreceptors, Basigin 1, forming a complex with glucose transporter GLUT1, thereby increasing glucose uptake by the cones and promoting outer segment renewal (Aït-Ali et al. 2015). This stimulation of aerobic glycolysis is similarly used by fast-dividing cancer cells and is known as the Warburg effect.

The protective action of RdCVF on cone function and survival was robustly established in several preclinical studies using *rd1* and *rd10* mice, two models of recessive RCD (Léveillard et al. 2004), and P23H-rhodopsin mutant rats, a model of autosomal dominant RCD (Yang et al. 2009; Sahel et al. 2013).

Interestingly, the nucleoredoxin-like 1 (*NXN-L1*) gene encoding RdCVF also encodes a thioredoxin called RdCVF-Long (RdCVFL) (Léveillard et al. 2004). *NXNL1* is comprised of two exons spaced by one intron, and its alternative splicing generates two mRNA isoforms. RdCVF mRNA retains the gene intron, and RdCVFL mRNA is the product of intron splicing. The intron of *NXNL1* contains an in-frame stop codon that truncates the protein in its enzymatically active domain; therefore, RdCVF does not exhibit any redox activity, unlike RdCVFL.

Although RdCVF is expressed by rod photoreceptors only, RdCVFL is expressed by both rods and cones. RdCVFL acts as a potent antioxidant to mitigate the effects of oxidative stress produced by the high metabolism of photoreceptors. Indeed, as phototransduction is very demanding in energy, the retina is one of the organs that consumes the most oxygen, relative to its weight.

AAV-*RdCVFL* gene therapy showed a protective effect on photoreceptors of *Nxnl1*$^{-/-}$ mice exposed to photooxidative stress (Elachouri et al. 2015). RdCVFL was shown to act mainly as an antioxidant, and its protective activity was confirmed in *rd10* mice showing increased ERG responses and cone density (Mei et al. 2016).

Together, the mechanisms of action of RdCVF and RdCVFL appear to have a synergistic effect to protect cone photoreceptor function and structure. This was demonstrated by coinjecting both AAV-*RdCVF* and AAV-*RdCVFL* in *rd10* mice, resulting in a more effective protection of cones than the injection of each vector alone (Byrne et al. 2015).

This therapeutic approach is about to be investigated in a first-in-human trial due to launch in 2023 (NCT05748873). Given the large number of genetic variants leading to an impaired phototransduction response in rods, the strategic preservation of cones is a sensible approach for patients suffering from RCD, since (1) the pathogenic variants do not affect the proteins expressed by cones; (2) the secondary degeneration of cones is the main event leading to profound visual impairment; and (3) even a small proportion of functional cones is sufficient to sustain major visual functions.

DISCUSSION

Variant-specific gene therapies have predominated in the past two decades, but their success has been limited. Currently, Luxturna is the only gene therapy available for an ophthalmic disease, being intended for individuals with IRD due to variants in the *RPE65* gene. Recently, several pivotal trials for gene-specific gene therapy have not met their primary end point, specifically in the clinical development for choroideremia and X-linked RP. Drug development for ocular gene therapy has seen challenges in clinical design, indication, and end point selection, leading to delays in regulatory approval. Considering the difficulties in getting gene-specific therapies to patients, a complementary strategy could be to develop neuroprotective therapies independently of the underlying gene variant causing retinal degeneration.

The field has long sought a gene-independent approach to reverse, stop, or slow down the visual deficits brought on by retinal degeneration. However, the clinical development of these new therapies has its own challenges, mainly time-to-readout and selection of pertinent clinical end points. As the majority of IRDs show a relatively slow disease progression rate, the challenge is to capture the difference between intervention and control groups within the scope of most funding resource timelines. Commonly reported clinical end points, such as best-corrected visual acuity (BCVA) or visual field, may not in reality be the most optimal criteria for the assessment of changes in clinical trials for IRDs. Other end points of visual function and anatomy should be considered, such as the analysis of hill of vision, parameters measured by microperimetry and chromatic full-field light stimulation threshold testing (FST), as well as structural parameters measured by fundus autofluorescence, spectral-domain optical coherence tomography (SD-OCT) (such as the ellipsoid zone), and adaptive optics imaging.

In 2021, regulatory approval was granted for a complement factor C3 inhibitor in the treatment of nonproliferative AMD, based on the assessment of fundus autofluorescence. The primary end point demonstrated a reduction in the rate of geographic atrophy growth following treatment administration, allowing for a successful clinical trial based on the curbing of disease progression. This achievement gives some inference to the approvability of new treatments whose approach is to slow down the degenerative process in IRD.

CNTF has been under investigation for decades, as it was assessed in multiple preclinical models, and ultimately in human clinical trials, with minimal success. However, promising clinical results have recently been reported in trials for macular telangiectasis, indicating that the neurotrophic factor may eventually prove beneficial to patients.

Other treatments continue to be investigated, in search of a therapy that will slow down retinal degeneration, regardless of the patient's genetic etiology. RdCVF has recently entered into a clinic trial in the hope of slowing down cone degeneration in RCD. Its dual mechanism of action, leveraging innate neuroprotective and antioxidant properties, may allow to slow or potentially stop the progression of cone degeneration. Clinical development for many other gene therapy programs is underway, with the aim to demonstrate the safety and efficacy of new investigational treatments. Neuroprotective agents may one day represent a gene-independent therapeutic strategy able to address both inherited and noninherited retinal diseases.

REFERENCES

Aït-Ali N, Fridlich R, Millet-Puel G, Clérin E, Delalande F, Jaillard C, Blond F, Perrocheau L, Reichman S, Byrne LC, et al. 2015. Rod-derived cone viability factor promotes cone survival by stimulating aerobic glycolysis. *Cell* **161:** 817–832. doi:10.1016/j.cell.2015.03.023

Akurathi A, Boese EA, Kardon RH, Ledolter J, Kuehn MH, Harper MM. 2022. Decreased expression of glial-derived neurotrophic factor receptors in glaucomatous human retinas. *Curr Eye Res* **47:** 597–605. doi:10.1080/02713683.2021.2002907

Birch DG, Weleber RG, Duncan JL, Jaffe GJ, Tao W, Ciliary Neurotrophic Factor Retinitis Pigmentosa Study Groups. 2013. Randomized trial of ciliary neurotrophic factor delivered by encapsulated cell intraocular implants for retinitis pigmentosa. *Am J Ophthalmol* **156:** 283–292.e1. doi:10.1016/j.ajo.2013.03.021

Birch DG, Bennett LD, Duncan JL, Weleber RG, Pennesi ME. 2016. Long-term follow-up of patients with retinitis pigmentosa receiving intraocular ciliary neurotrophic

factor implants. *Am J Ophthalmol* **170:** 10–14. doi:10.1016/j.ajo.2016.07.013

Byrne LC, Dalkara D, Luna G, Fisher SK, Clérin E, Sahel JA, Léveillard T, Flannery JG. 2015. Viral-mediated RdCVF and RdCVFL expression protects cone and rod photoreceptors in retinal degeneration. *J Clin Invest* **125:** 105–116. doi:10.1172/JCI65654

Carter-Dawson LD, LaVail MM, Sidman RL. 1978. Differential effect of the *rd* mutation on rods and cones in the mouse retina. *Invest Ophthalmol Vis Sci* **17:** 489–498.

Chew EY, Clemons TE, Peto T, Sallo FB, Ingerman A, Tao W, Singerman L, Schwartz SD, Peachey NS, Bird AC, Mac-Tel-CNTF Research Group. 2015. Ciliary neurotrophic factor for macular telangiectasia type 2: results from a phase 1 safety trial. *Am J Ophthalmol* **159:** 659–666.e1. doi:10.1016/j.ajo.2014.12.013

Chew EY, Clemons TE, Jaffe GJ, Johnson CA, Farsiu S, Lad EM, Guymer R, Rosenfeld P, Hubschman JP, Constable I, et al. 2019. Effect of ciliary neurotrophic factor on retinal neurodegeneration in patients with macular telangiectasia type 2: a randomized clinical trial. *Ophthalmology* **126:** 540–549. doi:10.1016/j.ophtha.2018.09.041

Dalkara D, Kolstad KD, Guerin KI, Hoffmann NV, Visel M, Klimczak RR, Schaffer DV, Flannery JG. 2011. AAV mediated GDNF secretion from retinal glia slows down retinal degeneration in a rat model of retinitis pigmentosa. *Mol Ther* **19:** 1602–1608. doi:10.1038/mt.2011.62

Elachouri G, Lee-Rivera I, Clérin E, Argentini M, Fridlich R, Blond F, Ferracane V, Yang Y, Raffelsberger W, Wan J, et al. 2015. Thioredoxin rod-derived cone viability factor protects against photooxidative retinal damage. *Free Radic Biol Med* **81:** 22–29. doi:10.1016/j.freeradbiomed.2015.01.003

Faktorovich EG, Steinberg RH, Yasumura D, Matthes MT, LaVail MM. 1990. Photoreceptor degeneration in inherited retinal dystrophy delayed by basic fibroblast growth factor. *Nature* **347:** 83–86. doi:10.1038/347083a0

Faktorovich EG, Steinberg RH, Yasumura D, Matthes MT, LaVail MM. 1992. Basic fibroblast growth factor and local injury protect photoreceptors from light damage in the rat. *J Neurosci* **12:** 3554–3567. doi:10.1523/JNEUROSCI.12-09-03554.1992

Fintz AC, Audo I, Hicks D, Mohand-Said S, Léveillard T, Sahel J. 2003. Partial characterization of retina-derived cone neuroprotection in two culture models of photoreceptor degeneration. *Invest Ophthalmol Vis Sci* **44:** 818–825. doi:10.1167/iovs.01-1144

Frasson M, Picaud S, Léveillard T, Simonutti M, Mohand-Said S, Dreyfus H, Hicks D, Sabel J. 1999. Glial cell line-derived neurotrophic factor induces histologic and functional protection of rod photoreceptors in the *rd/rd* mouse. *Invest Ophthalmol Vis Sci* **40:** 2724–2734.

García-Caballero C, Lieppman B, Arranz-Romera A, Molina-Martínez IT, Bravo-Osuna I, Young M, Baranov P, Herrero-Vanrell R. 2018. Photoreceptor preservation induced by intravitreal controlled delivery of GDNF and GDNF/melatonin in rhodopsin knockout mice. *Mol Vis* **24:** 733–745.

Gash DM, Gerhardt GA, Bradley LH, Wagner R, Slevin JT. 2020. GDNF clinical trials for Parkinson's disease: a critical human dimension. *Cell Tissue Res* **382:** 65–70. doi:10.1007/s00441-020-03269-8

Goldberg JL, Beykin G, Satterfield KR, Nuñez M, Lam BL, Albini TA. 2023. Phase I NT-501 ciliary neurotrophic factor implant trial for primary open-angle glaucoma: safety, neuroprotection, and neuroenhancement. *Ophthalmol Sci* **3**: 100298. doi:10.1016/j.xops.2023.100298

Hamel C. 2006. Retinitis pigmentosa. *Orphanet J Rare Dis* **1**: 40. doi:10.1186/1750-1172-1-40

Koeberle PD, Ball AK. 1998. Effects of GDNF on retinal ganglion cell survival following axotomy. *Vision Res* **38**: 1505–1515. doi:10.1016/s0042-6989(97)00364-7

LaVail MM, Unoki K, Yasumura D, Matthes MT, Yancopoulos GD, Steinberg RH. 1992. Multiple growth factors, cytokines, and neurotrophins rescue photoreceptors from the damaging effects of constant light. *Proc Natl Acad Sci* **89**: 11249–11253. doi:10.1073/pnas.89.23.11249

Léveillard T, Mohand-Saïd S, Lorentz O, Hicks D, Fintz AC, Clérin E, Simonutti M, Forster V, Cavusoglu N, Chalmel F, et al. 2004. Identification and characterization of rod-derived cone viability factor. *Nat Genet* **36**: 755–759. doi:10.1038/ng1386

Linker R, Gold R, Luhder F. 2009. Function of neurotrophic factors beyond the nervous system: inflammation and autoimmune demyelination. *Crit Rev Immunol* **29**: 43–68. doi:10.1615/critrevimmunol.v29.i1.20

Mei X, Chaffiol A, Kole C, Yang Y, Millet-Puel G, Clérin E, Aït-Ali N, Bennett J, Dalkara D, Sahel JA, et al. 2016. The thioredoxin encoded by the rod-derived cone viability factor gene protects cone photoreceptors against oxidative stress. *Antioxid Redox Signal* **24**: 909–923. doi:10.1089/ars.2015.6509

Miller RG, Petajan JH, Bryan WW, Armon C, Barohn RJ, Goodpasture JC, Hoagland RJ, Parry GJ, Ross MA, Stromatt SC. 1996. A placebo-controlled trial of recombinant human ciliary neurotrophic (rhCNTF) factor in amyotrophic lateral sclerosis: rhCNTF ALS study group. *Ann Neurol* **39**: 256–260. doi:10.1002/ana.410390215

Mohand-Said S, Hicks D, Simonutti M, Tran-Minh D, Deudon-Combe A, Dreyfus H, Silverman MS, Ogilvie JM, Tenkova T, Sahel J. 1997. Photoreceptor transplants increase host cone survival in the retinal degeneration (*rd*) mouse. *Ophthalmic Res* **29**: 290–297. doi:10.1159/000268027

Mohand-Said S, Deudon-Combe A, Hicks D, Simonutti M, Forster V, Fintz AC, Léveillard T, Dreyfus H, Sahel JA. 1998. Normal retina releases a diffusible factor stimulating cone survival in the retinal degeneration mouse. *Proc Natl Acad Sci* **95**: 8357–8362. doi:10.1073/pnas.95.14.8357

Neurotech Pharmaceuticals. 2022. Neurotech pharmaceuticals announces positive phase 3 topline results for NT-501 implant in MacTel. Press Release, Nov. 2. https://www.neurotechpharmaceuticals.com/neurotech-pharmaceuticals-announces-positive-phase-3-topline-results-for-nt-501-implant-in-mactel

Runeberg-Roos P, Penn RD. 2020. Improving therapeutic potential of GDNF family ligands. *Cell Tissue Res* **382**: 173–183. doi:10.1007/s00441-020-03256-z

Sahel JA, Léveillard T, Picaud S, Dalkara D, Marazova K, Safran A, Paques M, Duebel J, Roska B, Mohand-Said S. 2013. Functional rescue of cone photoreceptors in retinitis pigmentosa. *Graefes Arch Clin Exp Ophthalmol* **251**: 1669–1677. doi:10.1007/s00417-013-2314-7

Sahni JN, Angi M, Irigoyen C, Semeraro F, Romano MR, Parmeggiani F. 2011. Therapeutic challenges to retinitis pigmentosa: from neuroprotection to gene therapy. *Curr Genomics* **12**: 276–284. doi:10.2174/138920211795860062

Schuettauf F, Zurakowski D, Quinto K, Varde MA, Besch D, Laties A, Anderson R, Wen R. 2005. Neuroprotective effects of cardiotrophin-like cytokine on retinal ganglion cells. *Graefes Arch Clin Exp Ophthalmol* **243**: 1036–1042. doi:10.1007/s00417-005-1152-7

Shpak AA, Guekht AB, Druzhkova TA, Kozlova KI, Gulyaeva NV. 2017. Ciliary neurotrophic factor in patients with primary open-angle glaucoma and age-related cataract. *Mol Vis* **23**: 799–809.

Skaper SD. 2012. The neurotrophin family of neurotrophic factors: an overview. In *Neurotrophic factors. Methods in molecular biology* (ed. Skaper S), Vol. 846. Humana Press, Totowa, NJ.

Tao W, Wen R, Goddard MB, Sherman SD, O'Rourke PJ, Stabila PF, Bell WJ, Dean BJ, Kauper KA, Budz VA, et al. 2002. Encapsulated cell-based delivery of CNTF reduces photoreceptor degeneration in animal models of retinitis pigmentosa. *Invest Ophthalmol Vis Sci* **43**: 3292–3298.

Wen R, Tao W, Li Y, Sieving PA. 2012. CNTF and retina. *Prog Retin Eye Res* **31**: 136–151. doi:10.1016/j.preteyeres.2011.11.005

Wu S, Mo X. 2023. Optic nerve regeneration in diabetic retinopathy: potentials and challenges ahead. *Int J Mol Sci* **24**: 1447. doi:10.3390/ijms24021447

Yang Y, Mohand-Said S, Danan A, Simonutti M, Fontaine V, Clerin E, Picaud S, Léveillard T, Sahel JA. 2009. Functional cone rescue by RdCVF protein in a dominant model of retinitis pigmentosa. *Mol Ther* **17**: 787–795. doi:10.1038/mt.2009.28

Zhang K, Hopkins JJ, Heier JS, Birch DG, Halperin LS, Albini TA, Brown DM, Jaffe GJ, Tao W, Williams GA. 2011. Ciliary neurotrophic factor delivered by encapsulated cell intraocular implants for treatment of geographic atrophy in age-related macular degeneration. *Proc Natl Acad Sci* **108**: 6241–6245. doi:10.1073/pnas.1018987108

Restoration of Rod-Derived Metabolic and Redox Signaling to Prevent Blindness

Emmanuelle Clérin,[1] Najate Aït-Ali,[1] José-Alain Sahel,[1,2,3,4] and Thierry Léveillard[1]

[1]Department of Genetics, Sorbonne Université, INSERM, CNRS, Institut de la Vision, F-75012 Paris, France

[2]CHNO des Quinze-Vingts, DHU Sight Restore, INSERM-DGOS CIC 1423, F-75012 Paris, France

[3]Department of OphthalmoloUPMC Vision Institute, University of Pittsburgh School of Medicine, Pittsburgh, Pennsylvania 15213, USA

Correspondence: emmanuelle.clerin@inserm.fr; sahelja@pitt.edu

Vision is initiated by capturing photons in highly specialized sensory cilia known as the photoreceptor outer segment. Because of its lipid and protein composition, the outer segments are prone to photo-oxidation, requiring photoreceptors to have robust antioxidant defenses and high metabolic synthesis rates to regenerate the outer segments every 10 days. Both processes required high levels of glucose uptake and utilization. Retinitis pigmentosa is a prevalent form of inherited retinal degeneration characterized by initial loss of low-light vision caused by the death of rod photoreceptors. In this disease, rods die as a direct effect of an inherited mutation. Following the loss of rods, cones eventually degenerate, resulting in complete blindness. The progression of vision loss in retinitis pigmentosa suggested that rod photoreceptors were necessary to maintain healthy cones. We identified a protein secreted by rods that functions to promote cone survival, and we named it rod-derived cone viability factor (RdCVF). RdCVF is encoded by an alternative splice product of the nucleoredoxin-like 1 (*NXNL1*) gene, and RdCVF was found to accelerate the uptake of glucose by cones. Without RdCVF, cones eventually die because of compromised glucose uptake and utilization. The *NXNL1* gene also encodes for the thioredoxin RdCVFL, which reduces cysteines in photoreceptor proteins that are oxidized, providing a defense against radical oxygen species. We will review here the main steps of discovering this novel intercellular signaling currently under translation as a broad-spectrum treatment for retinitis pigmentosa.

Patients suffering from retinitis pigmentosa (RP), the most common form of inherited retinal degeneration, lose vision in two successive steps. Early in their adult life, they lose the ability to see in dim light conditions, known as night vision loss, which corresponds to loss of function and degeneration of rod photoreceptors. This is a minor handicap in our current well-illuminated environment, and these people have an almost normal lifestyle. However, as the disease progresses, patients experience the loss of function and degeneration of cones. This

---

[4]Present address: Department of Ophthalmology, The University of Pittsburgh School of Medicine, Pittsburgh, PA 15213.

leads to blindness because cones, although representing only 3%–5% of all photoreceptors in most mammals, are essential for daylight peripheral and central vision and color discrimination and visual acuity. Cones dominate the center of the primate retina, the fovea. Because cones underlie all visual functions in a lighted environment, their protection is a medically relevant objective. In the first series of experiments, José-Alain Sahel and Saddek Mohand-Saïd showed that the transplantation of the mouse outer retina in the subretinal space of the *rd1* mouse retarded the secondary degeneration of cones in this model of recessive RP that carries a loss of function of the *Pde6b* gene (Mohand-Saïd et al. 1997). Interestingly, the protective effect is independent of the RP causing mutation because transplanted *rd1* retinas are also protective until their rods are lost (Mohand-Saïd et al. 2000). In these experiments, the graft did not make synaptic connections with the host retina, but the protective effect came from a diffusible molecule (Mohand-Saïd et al. 1998). A partial purification of the conditioned medium of neural retinal explants from the mouse retina established that the molecular weight and the thermal stability of the active compound were compatible with that of a secreted protein (Fintz et al. 2003). The same fraction prevents the death of cones from a cone-enriched culture from the retina of chicken embryos, a model established originally by Ruben Adler and Michael Hatlee (Adler and Hatlee 1989). The cone-enriched culture assay was used by this same group to partially purify a protective activity originating from the interphotoreceptor matrix (IPM) (Hewitt et al. 1990). Extracts of IPM support cone photoreceptor survival in a specific manner, but the purification of the active molecules to homogeneity was never reported. In retrospect, this failure is certainly due to the very low concentration of such signaling molecules in the IPM.

IDENTIFICATION OF ROD-DERIVED CONE VIABILITY FACTOR

We, therefore, developed an expression cloning strategy using an adapted version of the cone-enriched culture system. Following transplantation in the *rd1* retina, the active molecule can be liberated by the transplanted cells or in reaction to that transplantation through, for example, the reactivity of retinal Müller glial cells (Carwile et al. 1998; Frasson et al. 1999). To take into account this possible indirect mode of action of the protective molecules, we screened an expression library constructed with the entire neural retina (Fig. 1A). This library was not amplified to ensure that less abundant complementary DNAs (cDNAs) were not lost. To generate expression libraries, cDNAs were cloned into plasmids containing a mammalian expression cassette and an SV40 origin of replication. Plasmids were transfected into COS1 cells by pools of 100 unique clones. The COS-1 cell line has been obtained by the transformation with SV40 large T-antigen, which permits the replication of the transfected plasmids (Fig. 1B; Chen and Okayama 1987). One of the risks of such an approach is that if the expected activity is carried by a heterodimer, the probability of having the two distinct cDNAs in a single pool is very low. On the other hand, contrarily to a protein purification approach, each cDNA is a clone and not a protein fraction and so can be amplified. Using this protocol, the cDNA encoding the protective factor was transcribed and translated, and the protein was secreted by COS-1 cells. For practical reasons, the cone-enriched culture system was simplified so that the conditioned medium was produced in a serum-free medium (Millet-Puel et al. 2021). Because those primary cultures of retinal precursors adopt a cone photoreceptor cell fate in vitro, a standard protocol with two seeding densities of 96-well plates with four replicate pools of 100 plasmids was rigorously applied to test 2100 clone pools. Cone survival was measured using a live-cell esterase activity and cell death using membrane permeability of ethidium dyes and their DNA binding in the nucleus (Fig. 1C). After the primary screening, we diluted the selected pools into subpools of 10 clones, then single clones, which allowed the identification of the cDNA encoding rod-derived cone viability factor (RdCVF) in the third screening round (Léveillard et al. 2004).

Cite this article as *Cold Spring Harb Perspect Med* doi: 10.1101/cshperspect.a041284

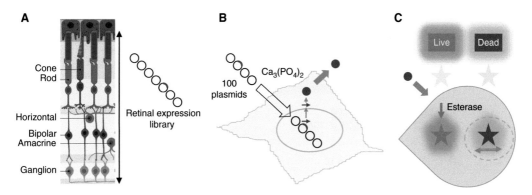

Figure 1. Expression cloning strategy. (*A*) The tissue origin of the expression library used for screening. (*B*) Transfection of pools of 100 plasmids from the unamplified neural retina cDNA library into COS-1 cells with an enhanced calcium-phosphate protocol. (*C*) We used two fluorescent probes, one that stains (in green) living cells throughout the cell's endogenous esterase activity and the second (in red) to label the dead cells by the permeability of their membranes to a dimer of the DNA intercalant, ethidium bromide.

CHARACTERIZATION OF THE NUCLEOREDOXIN-LIKE 1 GENE

To ascertain that the protective activity RdCVF was not the result of its association with any secreted COS-1 proteins, we tested a purified recombinant RdCVF protein on the cone-enriched culture as well as on retinal explants of the *rd1* mouse (Léveillard and Aït-Ali 2017). We demonstrated that RdCVF protein protects the cones in the *rd1* mouse and in the RHO^{P23H} transgenic rat (Yang et al. 2009). Immunodepletion of RdCVF from the conditioned medium of wild-type retinas shows that the protective activity is at least partially attributable to RdCVF (Léveillard et al. 2004; Yang et al. 2010). Sequence analysis suggests that RdCVF is a truncated-thioredoxin-related protein of 109 amino acids encoded by the nucleoredoxin-like 1 (*NXNL1*) gene and secreted by a leaderless secretory pathway, as other thioredoxin proteins (Rubartelli et al. 1992). The secretion of thioredoxins is induced by oxidative stress and is inhibited by serum (Sahaf and Rosén 2000; Tanudji et al. 2003). Luckily enough, serum was not present during expression cloning. The *NXNL1* gene is expressed specifically by photoreceptor cells. Its expression is rod-dependent for the mouse and human retina (Delyfer et al. 2011). In RP, rod death results in the loss of expression of RdCVF. Interestingly, the lower expression of *Nxnl1* by retinal bipolar cells is also rod-depen-

dent (Reichman et al. 2010). The *Nxnl1* expression (RdCVF and RdCVFL) is higher during daylight, which suggests a circadian rhythm (Wolloscheck et al. 2015; Camacho et al. 2019). The daily regulation of *Nxnl1* is potentially mediated by *Pax4*, which was shown to regulate the *Nxnl1* promoter (Rath et al. 2009; Reichman et al. 2010). The inactivation of the *Nxnl1* gene in the mouse triggers an age-dependent loss of cones even in the presence of a potential compensation from its paralog, *Nxnl2*, demonstrating that *Nxnl1*/RdCVF expression in rods is essential for cone survival (Cronin et al. 2010; Jaillard et al. 2012). RdCVF is the translation of an alternatively spliced mRNA encoding the exon 1 with the retention of the following intron that contains an in-frame stop codon (Fig. 2A). The other product, RdCVFL, is made by splicing intron 1 of the *Nxnl1* gene and corresponds to thioredoxin-like protein with a complete thioredoxin fold (Fig. 2C). The exclusion of the sequence of exon 2 results in the presence of a large hydrophobic pocket, incompatible with the structural model of the thioredoxin fold (Chalmel et al. 2007). Except for RdCVF2L, the only other example of truncated thioredoxin is TRX80, a proteolytic cleavage corresponding to the amino-terminal 80 residues of the thioredoxin TXN1 that acts as a pro-inflammatory cytokine, but no receptor has yet been identified (Pekkari et al. 2000). The serum concentration of TRX80

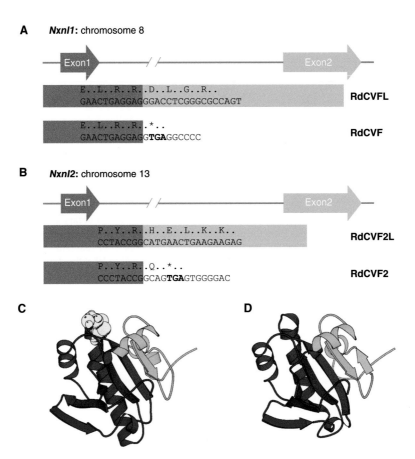

Figure 2. Genic organization of the two nucleoredoxin-like genes. (*A*) The *Nxnl1* gene and its two splicing products, rod-derived cone viability factor (RdCVF) and RdCVFL. (*B*) The *Nxnl2* gene and its two splicing products, RdCVF2 and RdCVF2L. (*C*) Structural model of RdCVF. (*D*) Structural model of RdCVF. The red ribbon corresponds to residues matching the *Crithidia fasciculata* tryparedoxin I X-ray structure (1EWX). Blue ribbons correspond to insertions in that structure. Green ribbons are the sequence arising from exon 2 of the genes and yellow ribbons represent the catalytic site of RdCVFL.

is elevated in patients suffering from Alzheimer's disease (Goikolea et al. 2022). The RdCVF protein is puzzling because thioredoxins have the capacity to lower the level of reactive oxygen species (ROS) and to reduce oxidized cysteine residues of proteins (Ren et al. 2017). Nevertheless, RdCVF has no thiol-oxidoreductase activity and is not, consequently, an active thioredoxin (Léveillard et al. 2004).

THE THIOREDOXIN PROTEIN ROD-DERIVED CONE VIABILITY FACTOR LONG

The thioredoxin RdCVFL protects rods against photo-oxidative damage (Elachouri et al. 2015).

Using proteomics, we established the interactome of RdCVFL, identifying proteins whose redox status could be regulated by RdCVFL. We showed that RdCVFL interacts with the microtubule-associated protein T (TAU) and prevents its oxidation (Fridlich et al. 2009). In the *Nxnl1*$^{-/-}$ retina, TAU is phosphorylated at a position similar to that of TAU in the brain of patients with Alzheimer's disease. The inactivation of the *Nxnl1* gene leads to photoreceptor dysfunction and death. Rod and cone function is normal in young *Nxnl1*$^{-/-}$ mice but deteriorates month by month, indicating that the gene is involved in preventing photoreceptor damage that accumulates with age. Loss of *Nxnl1* activity pos-

Cite this article as *Cold Spring Harb Perspect Med* doi: 10.1101/cshperspect.a041284

sibly contributes to the imbalance between ROS-mediated protein oxidation and its reduction by thioredoxins and glutaredoxin systems (Stadtman 2006). Transgenic expression of RdCVFL or RdCVF2L in $NXNL1^{-/-}$ mice, both prevented phosphorylation of TAU, but only RdCVFL prevented the death of rods (Elachouri et al. 2015). This observation indicates that other targets besides TAU are involved in the death of rods in $NXNL1^{-/-}$ mice (Fridlich et al. 2009) and is not related specifically to thioredoxin activity (Fig. 2D). Thioredoxins, such as TXN1, perform thiol–disulfide exchange reactions via the catalytic active site cysteine pair, the -CXXC- motif (Léveillard and Sahel 2017). This catalytic site is conserved in early vertebrate RdCVF2L proteins but was changed to -CXXS- in all placental mammals (Elachouri et al. 2015). The active site of RdCVF2L has the sequence of a monothiol glutaredoxin, such as the two monothiol glutaredoxins, GLRX3 and GLRX5 (Lillig et al. 2008; Hanschmann et al. 2013). Under oxidative stress conditions, glutathione reacts spontaneously with the thiol radical of cysteines leading to their glutathionylation. This is a defense mechanism against further oxidations that could be irreversible, such as sulfonation ($-SO_3H$). GLRXs are versatile proteins that not only reduce disulfide and protein glutathionylation but also play an important role in iron metabolism by coordinating iron–sulfur clusters ([Fe-S]) (Ogata et al. 2021). The thioredoxin (TXN) and glutaredoxin (GLRX) systems are the two antioxidant systems evolutionarily conserved from bacteria to humans (Fig. 3; Ren et al. 2017). In the mouse, GLRX3 inactivation is associated with increased expression of transferrin receptor and decreased expression of ferritin. Transferrin is an endogenous iron chelator and has therapeutic effects on RP (Bigot et al. 2020). Ferroptosis is a novel form of programmed cell death, with characteristic iron overload and lipid peroxidation (Yang et al. 2021). We observed an increase in lipid peroxidation in the $Nxnl1^{-/-}$ retina (Cronin et al. 2010). The endogenous level of peroxidation of the $rd10$ retina is reduced by the administration of RdCVFL, but not by that of RdCVF (Byrne et al. 2015). Lipid hyperoxides are re-

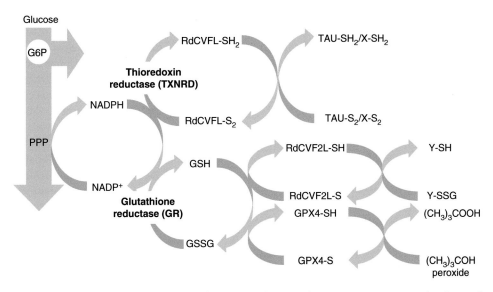

Figure 3. The thioredoxin (TXN) and glutaredoxin (GLRX) antioxidant systems. Nicotinamide adenine dinucleotide phosphate (NADPH), produced by the metabolism of glucose through the pentose phosphate pathway (PPP), serves as a cofactor for thioredoxin reductase (TXNRD) and glutathione reductase (GR). TXNRD reduces oxidized rod-derived cone viability factor (RdCVFL) that reduces TAU. GR reduces oxidized glutathione (GSSG > GSH), which reduces RdCVF2L and deglutathionylates unknown proteins (Y). Glutathione also reduces glutathione peroxidase 4 (GPX4), which reduces lipid hyperoxides [($CH_3)_3COH$]. (G6P) Glucose-6-phosphate.

duced by glutathione peroxidase 4 (GPX4), and the inactivation of the *Gpx4* gene in mouse rods and cones causes lipid peroxidation and cell death at the early stage of retinal development (Ueta et al. 2012). It seems that the change in the catalytic site of RdCVF2L allows the nucleoredoxin-like genes *NXNL1* and *NXNL2* to occupy both branches of the antioxidant system.

METABOLIC AND REDOX SIGNALING OF THE NUCLEOREDOXIN-LIKE 1 GENE

We discovered that iodinated-RdCVF binds to cells of the cone-enriched cultures, but not to COS-1 or RPE cells. This result is consistent with the expression of an RdCVF receptor by cells targeted by RdCVF, such as cones. We used a far-western blotting approach to visualize the binding protein and observed that the signal was more important in the membrane fraction of the cone-dominant chicken retina. A proteomic analysis of the signal revealed many candidate membranal proteins of appropriate migration in the gel. One important candidate protein was basigin-1 (BSG1), which was a splice variant of the basigin gene known to be expressed by chicken cones (Ochrietor et al. 2003). Mice in which the gene for *Bsg* has been deleted have several abnormalities, including blindness (Ochrietor et al. 2002). Additional studies demonstrated that BSG1 is essential to the biological activity of RdCVF on cones and that BSG1 coimmunoprecipitates with the glucose transporter GLUT1 within the periplasmic membrane of the cones (Aït-Ali et al. 2015). By binding to this complex, RdCVF accelerates the entry of glucose into the cones. We also demonstrated that the protective effect of RdCVF implies that glucose is metabolized by aerobic glycolysis (Fig. 4A). Claudio Punzo and Constance Cepko had observed previously the role of GLUT1 in the secondary degeneration of the cones in RP models (Punzo et al. 2009; Cepko and Punzo 2015). Our data showing that the truncated thioredoxin, RdCVF, is an allosteric regulator of glucose uptake is in agreement with additional data showing the role of glucose transport in secondary cone loss in RP (Camacho et al. 2016, 2019). Aerobic glycolysis favors the diversification of the carbon flux of

glycolysis to the production of glycerol-3-phosphate (G3P), the headgroup in phospholipids of the cone outer segments. Rods secrete RdCVF stimulating the renewal of cone outer segments. This model is in agreement with the clinical observations, showing that the outer segments of the cones are lost well before cones die (Busskamp et al. 2010). The essential role of aerobic glycolysis in photoreceptor outer segment renewal is consistent with work from the Cepko laboratory (Chinchore et al. 2017). These discoveries contributed to the accelerated research of metabolism in retinal biology and retinal degeneration. A series of studies addressed the role of glucose metabolism in rod and cone survival. The expression of the glycolytic enzymes was examined in the mouse retina (Rueda et al. 2016). The ablation of GLUT1 in photoreceptors in the mouse confirmed its role in rod outer segment regrowth (Daniele et al. 2022); this is the same for hexokinase 2 (HK2), which is involved in aerobic glycolysis and expressed by photoreceptor instead of HK1 (Aït-Ali et al. 2015; Petit et al. 2018; Weh et al. 2020). Conflicting results were obtained for pyruvate kinase isoform 2 (PKM2), another isoenzyme expressed by photoreceptors, and functions in aerobic glycolysis (Rajala et al. 2016, 2018a,b; Wubben et al. 2017; Zhang et al. 2020). Lactate dehydrogenase A (LDHA) deletion in the rods inhibits rod outer segment growth (Chinchore et al. 2017). Rod-specific inactivation of the *Bsg* gene that encodes for the BSG1, the RdCVF receptor, and BSG2, a chaperone for lactate transporters, leads to rod dysfunction, but cone-specific knockout has no effect on the cones (Han et al. 2020). The ablation of the sirtuin 6 (*Sirt6*) gene in rods provides electrophysiological and anatomic rescue of rods, but also of cones of a preclinical model of RP (Zhang et al. 2016). SIRT6, an NAD^+-dependent histone deacetylase is a master regulator of cellular metabolism that represses glycolysis (Zhong et al. 2010). The fact that the cones are protected when the rods are targeted fits well with the fact that RdCVF is produced by the rods to sustain the function and the viability of the cones. Similar observations have recently been reported (Reed et al. 2022). Gene inactivation studies have strongly linked glucose metabolism to rod sur-

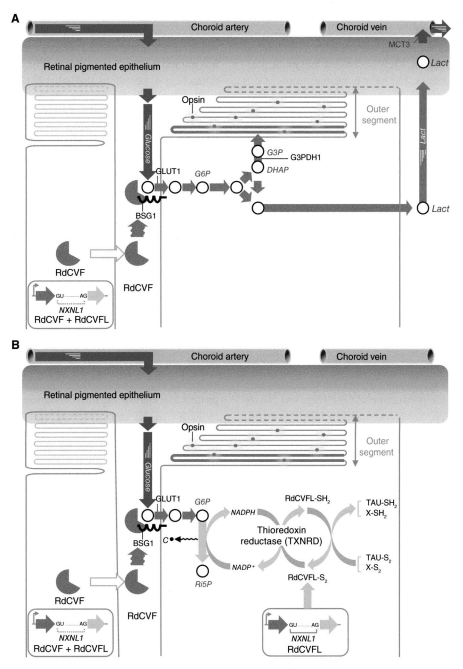

Figure 4. Metabolic and redox signaling of the nucleoredoxin-like 1 gene. (*A*) Metabolic signaling of rod-derived cone viability factor (RdCVF). The uptake of glucose, transported from the choroid arterioles to the outer retina is stimulated by RdCVF, secreted by rods, by binding to the BSG1/GLUT1 complex at the surface of the cones. Glucose is metabolized by aerobic glycolysis, which diverts to lipid synthesis at the level of dihydroxyacetone phosphate (DHAP) to participate in cone outer segment renewal. Aerobic glycolysis produces lactate that is transported out of the retina throughout the retinal pigmented epithelium (RPE) toward choroid venules by the lactate transporters MCT1 and MCT3, localized respectively on the apical and basal side of the RPE. (*B*) Redox signaling of RdCVF and RdCVFL. Glucose uptaken by cones is metabolized to glucose-6-phosphate (G6P) and then further by the pentose phosphate pathway (PPP) resulting in the reduction of $NADP^+$ to NADPH, the cofactor of thioredoxin reductase (TXNRD). TXNRD reduces oxidized RdCVFL that is produced by cones. RdCVFL reduces TAU as well as other proteins (X). (C) Carbon, (G3P) glycerol-3-phosphate, (G3PDH1) G3P-dehydrogense 1, (Ri5P) ribose-5-phosphate.

vival, but cones are less sensitive to individual gene knockout, likely because of metabolic plasticity in cones. The most famous example of this phenomenon is the protective effect of the thioredoxin interacting protein (TXNIP) on cones in mouse models of RP (Xue et al. 2021). TXNIP promotes internalization of the glucose transporter GLUT1, which reduces glucose uptake (Wu et al. 2013; Sullivan et al. 2018). TXNIP and RdCVF have antagonistic activities on glucose uptake in cones. To exert its protection on cones, TXNIP reduces glucose uptake but also requires the activity of LDHB to convert lactate into pyruvate for utilization in mitochondrial respiration, thus switching carbon sources from glucose to lactate. In contrast, RdCVF stimulates glucose uptake for biosynthetic processes and aerobic glycolysis. Increased glycolysis leads to pyruvate and lactate production. Because the renewal of cone outer segments is essential to maintain the function of the cones, one open question is how the metabolism of lactate could lead to the production of G3P (Fig. 4A). Theoretically, pyruvate, produced by LDHB from lactate, would have to be metabolized by the Krebs cycle to produce oxaloacetate (OAA) that is then converted to phosphoenolpyruvate (PEP) by mitochondrial phosphoenolpyruvate carboxykinase 2 (PCK2); PEP would then be converted to G3P by glyceroneogenesis (Fig. 5A; Yu et al. 2021). PCK2 is widely expressed and can be induced by diverse stress. Interestingly, we observed that *Pck2* mRNA is induced in the retina of the *rd1* mouse, from the onset of rod degeneration (Fig. 5B; Blond and Léveillard 2019).

Cones are vulnerable to oxidative agents (Komeima et al. 2006). By using single-cell reverse-transcription polymerase chain reaction (RT-PCR), we found that rather than expressing RdCVF, cones express the thioredoxin RdCVFL (Mei et al. 2016). The administration of RdCVFL under a cone-specific promoter protects the cones from oxidative damage that occurs when the *Nxnl1* gene is specifically inactivated in the cones. So, both products of the *NXNL1* gene are involved in the protection of the cones; the non-cell-autonomous action of RdCVF and the cell-autonomous activity of RdCVFL. Because the redox power of the thioredoxin RdCVFL depends on the metabolism of glucose, this model was named metabolic and redox signaling of the retina (Fig. 4; Léveillard and Sahel 2017).

THE EMERGENCE OF ROD–CONE CELLULAR INTERACTION DURING EVOLUTION

Conceptually, a thioredoxin gene that encodes two alternative gene products that stimulate glucose uptake or thioredoxin activity represents an interesting evolutionary step because both activities are essential for cones (Léveillard and Aït-Ali 2017). Altogether, the metabolic and redox signaling of the *NXNL* genes relies on two protein products made by alternative splicing. The evolutionary origin of this splicing event that created RdCVF protein by intron retention dates from 580 million years ago (mya), prior to the appearance of the camera-like eye in the cnidarian *Hydra vulgaris*. In *H. vulgaris*, two tandemly repeated *NXNL* genes encode for ubiquitously expressed and active RdCVFL thioredoxins that protect the organism against the damages caused by ROS (Aït-Ali and Léveillard 2022). Surprisingly, both *NXNLa* and *NXNLb* also encode for truncated thioredoxins, similar to mammalian RdCVF. *H. vulgaris* has no eye but possesses photosensitive cells located on its tentacles (Passano and McCullough 1962; Guertin and Kass-Simon 2015). These photosensitive neurons share with vertebrates the use of the mode of signal transduction of ciliary photoreceptors, as in humans (Plachetzki et al. 2012). The most abundant of these truncated proteins, RdCVFa, is expressed specifically by cells of the tentacles suggesting that those cells express a ligand of a cell-surface receptor (Fig. 6). RdCVFa interacts with a membrane protein of 25 kDa, which could have an amino-terminal immunoglobulin domain resembling that of BSG1 because RdCVFa binds BSG1. The function of this ligand–receptor interaction is an open question. We speculate that because *Cnidarians*, as *H. vulgaris*, invest a large fraction of their energy in the maintenance of their cnidocyst repertoire, which has to be constantly renewed, like the outer segments of photoreceptors, RdCVFa would be involved in the metabolic support for cnidae renewal (Beckmann and Özbek 2012). RdCVFa would be the

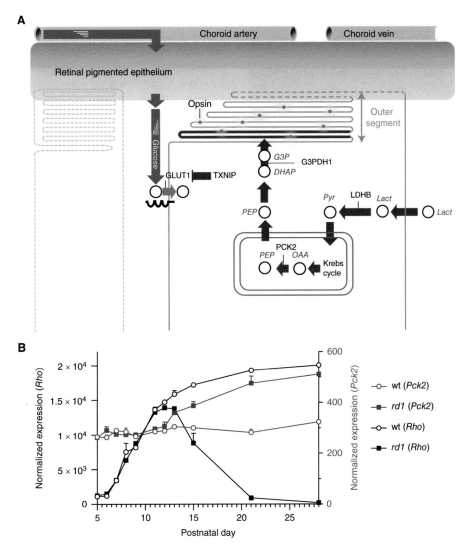

Figure 5. Metabolism of lactate by glyceroneogenesis. (*A*) To produce glycerol-3-phosphate (G3P), the precursor of phospholipids of the cone outer segment, lactate (Lact) is metabolized by lactate dehydrogenase B (LDHB) into pyruvate (Pyr). The Krebs cycle then produces oxaloacetate (OAA) that is converted to phosphoenolpyruvate (PEP) by mitochondrial phosphoenolpyruvate carboxykinase 2 (PCK2). PEP is transported to the cytoplasm and metabolized to G3P by glyceroneogenesis. (GPDH1) Glycerol-3-phosphate dehydrogenase 1, (DHAP) dihydroxyacetone phosphate. (*B*) Increasing expression of *Pck2* mRNA starts when the rods degenerate as visualized by the loss of expression of rhodopsin (*Rho*) in the *rd1* retina. (wt) Wild-type (C3H$^{wt/wt}$), *rd1* (C3H$^{rd1/rd1}$).

first functional truncated thioredoxin appearing (*terminus ad quem*) during evolution. The take-home message is that RdCVF signaling predates the appearance of the eye during evolution (Picciani et al. 2021). Lamprey represents the most ancient group of vertebrates existing for more than 360 million years. It is at this point during evolution when rods evolved from cones, even

before the emergence of rod outer segments (Morshedian and Fain 2015). The evolution of a rod with higher sensitivity may have allowed early vertebrates to inhabit deeper waters. But because cones have elevated energy requirements, this event has reduced the energy cost of the retina and perhaps permitted cephalization (Feinberg and Mallatt 2013; Ingram et al. 2020).

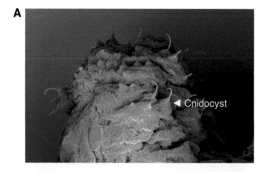

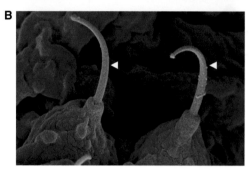

Figure 6. Speculation on the role of *Hydra vulgaris* RdCVFa in the renewal of cnidea. (*A*) The cnidocysts at the surface of a tentacle. (*B*) Higher magnification of the cnidea (arrowheads) that are ejected during cnidocyst discharge.

The unique *NXNL* gene of the lamprey genome is an ortholog of vertebrate *NXNL1* genes, with a unique intron that is partially retained by rods but not cone photoreceptors (Aït-Ali et al. 2022). Rods produce RdCVF and RdCVFL proteins and cones only RdCVFL, as in the mouse (Mei et al. 2016). This RdCVF protein binds to BSG1 of the lamprey. RdCVF, RdCVFL, and BSG1 expression are restricted to the retina, whereas the chaperone BSG2 is expressed by the RPE and other tissues. This timing agrees with the emergence of metabolic signaling between rods and cones, synchronized to the separation of ancestral cones into rods and cones. So, contrary to what we could expect, it is not the dominance of rods in the mammalian retina that resulted in the emergence of the rod to cone metabolic interaction because it was already in place in a species with an equivalent number of rods and cones. A competition between rods and cones for a survival signal was proposed by our mathematical mod-

eling of photoreceptor interaction (Camacho et al. 2016). In this model, rods have a metabolic advantage over cones in that they compensate by providing a signal that accelerates glucose uptake by cones. Considering the importance of color vision in animal life, natural selection and the advantages of cone survival in the presence of rods led to the development of a compensatory mechanism that provides cones a competitive advantage (Perini et al. 2009; Léveillard et al. 2015). The nature of this hypothetic metabolic advantage is presently unknown, but the metabolic and redox signaling of the *NXNL1* gene is likely to date from that time.

THE NUCLEOREDOXIN-LIKE SIGNALING OUTSIDE THE EYE

The nucleoredoxin-like 2 gene (*NXNL2*) has the same genic organization of *NXNL1* and encodes by alternative splicing for a trophic factor, RdCVF2, and a thioredoxin-like protein, RdCVF2L (Fig. 2B). One of the major differences between the two genes is that NXNL2 expression is not restricted to the retina (Chalmel et al. 2007; Jaillard et al. 2012). Very interestingly, the metabolic signaling of the *Nxnl2* gene supports brain function (Jaillard et al. 2021). In nonpathological conditions, blood-borne satiety hormones whose concentration increases after feeding in parallel to glucose directly transfer this information to a subset of neurons of the *area postrema*, a nonfenestrated circumventricular organ (Price et al. 2008). Somehow, this signal triggers the production and/ or release of RdCVF2 within the cerebrospinal fluid that circulates toward the pyramidal cells of the hippocampus (Fultz et al. 2019). By binding to its receptor at the surface of pyramidal neurons, RdCVF2 stimulates glucose uptake, which results in increased glycolysis for the extension of lipid membrane surface at the dendritic spines during memory acquisition or consolidation (Fig. 4A). In pathological conditions, such as those created by removing the *Nxnl2* gene in the mouse, the shortage of glucose in pyramidal neurons reduces the repair activity of the two NADPH-dependent redox pathways, the thioredoxin and glutaredoxin systems, and probably that of RdCVF2L. The metabolic resilience of pyramidal neurons allows them to deal with this redox power dysfunction for some time, but aging adds to the burden, which results in a tauopathy that may come from the lost control of the redox status of TAU by RdCVF2L. The failure of all clinical trials carried out to date on Alzheimer's disease with devastating consequences leads the scientific community to look at new avenues (Herrup 2021). As glucose is the major energy source for neurons, the regulation of its metabolism is central in this reevaluation. The therapeutic activity of the two products of the *NXNL2* gene is of special interest toward this goal (Corsi et al. 2023).

THE PATH OF THE NUCLEOREDOXIN-LIKE 1 GENE TO THE CLINIC

The administration of RdCVF protein supplements or replaces rod-to-cone signaling and prevents secondary degeneration of cones (Yang et al. 2009). The administration of RdCVF by gene therapy also prevents the secondary loss of cone function in several genetic models of RP, recessive and dominant mutations (Byrne et al. 2015). These studies suggest that an RdCVF gene therapy may have gene-independent protective activity because RdCVF protects against secondary cone loss. Preventing secondary loss of cone by the administration of RdCVF is medically rational because most patients that consult an ophthalmologist have already lost most of their rods, whereas visual acuity is only reduced when 50% of the cones become nonfunctional (Léveillard and Sahel 2010). The cones are maintained alive but nonfunctional for many years (Busskamp et al. 2010). Finally, only when the equilibrium between damage by ROS and repair by RdCVFL is broken will cones die. The combined administration of the two proteins encoded by the *NXNL1* gene as an effective treatment of all genetic forms of RP was presented at ARVO (Léveillard et al. 2017; Aït-Ali et al. 2018; Clérin et al. 2018; Léveillard 2018), and then transferred to the company SparingVision that we created on June 2016. The phase Ib clinical trial has started in 2023 (Clérin et al. 2020; Marussig et al. 2020; Chung et al. 2021; Marie et al. 2021; Noel et al. 2021a,b; Lorget et al. 2022). Because the treatment will be administrated after rod loss, the pro-

duction of RdCVF will rely on the transduction of RdCVF by RPE cells and that of RdCVFL by the cones themselves. One can ask why we are transducing the cones because they degenerate only after rods. First of all, we found this to be therapeutically effective in the *rd10* mouse (Mei et al. 2016), and in addition, even if this remains to be established, it is quite possible that the expression of RdCVFL by cones is dependent on rods, as we have shown for the expression of the *Nxnl1* gene by bipolar cells (Reichman et al. 2010).

The therapeutic strategy may also be effective for a more frequent blinding disease because *NXNL1* retinal cell signaling may be involved in age-related macular degeneration (AMD) (Léveillard et al. 2019). It is within the frame of a large international consortium on the genetics of AMD that we have identified risk alleles in the *SLC16A8* gene that encode for the lactate transporter MCT3, which is essential for the efflux of lactate produced by aerobic glycolysis in photoreceptors through the retinal pigment epithelium (RPE) (Fig. 4A; Fritsche et al. 2013, 2016). We showed in that ecosystem, RPE cells derived from induced pluripotent cells of AMD patients carrying an *SCL16A8* risk allele have a deficit in lactate transport (Klipfel et al. 2021). By maintaining the differentiation status of the RPE and the expression of *SLC16A8*, OTX2 prevents blindness in the Royal College of Surgeons (RCS) rat, a Mendelian model of dysfunction of this epithelium (Kole et al. 2018). Among 1120 AMD patients from the cohort of Quinze-Vingts hospital in Paris, 38% of them carry the *SLC16A8* major risk allele and 33% are heterozygous for this allele. So, for 33% of AMD patients, an increase in the expression of the non-risk allele by any means could have a therapeutic value.

CONCLUDING REMARKS

The ancestral nucleoredoxin-like genes, 580 mya, encode for ubiquitously expressed thioredoxin-like proteins involved in the redox control. At that time, intron retention produced a secreted protein with an unknown function. Then, 400 mya, rods diverged from cones resulting in a glucose competition between these cells (Okawa et al. 2008). We speculate that the competition most likely resulted in an advantage of rods over cones in terms of glucose uptake. The dependence on cone vision exerted selective pressure to maintain cone function, which led to the evolution of rod-derived signaling to enhance cone competition for glucose uptake to maintain daylight color vision. More than 70 mya, mammals emerged as a class with rod-dominated retinas because of the pressure of the predation by dinosaurs, the ancestors of birds, that were forcing the ancestral mammals to adopt a nocturnal lifestyle (Gerkema et al. 2013). Fifty million years ago, in primate evolution, cones became concentrated into the fovea for high-acuity central daylight vision (Williams et al. 2010). As a result of these evolutionary steps, patients suffering from RP lose central vision as a result of the interruption of the *NXNL* metabolic and redox signaling between rods and cones.

ACKNOWLEDGMENTS

We thank John Han, who pointed to glyceroneogenesis. The writing was supported by Inserm and Sorbonne Université.

REFERENCES

Adler R, Hatlee M. 1989. Plasticity and differentiation of embryonic retinal cells after terminal mitosis. *Science* **243:** 391–393. doi:10.1126/science.2911751

Aït-Ali N, Léveillard T. 2022. The emergence of rod–cone cellular interaction. *Front Genet* **13:** 900849. doi:10.3389/fgene.2022.900849

Aït-Ali N, Fridlich R, Millet-Puel G, Clérin E, Delalande F, Jaillard C, Blond F, Perrocheau L, Reichman S, Byrne LC, et al. 2015. Rod-derived cone viability factor promotes cone survival by stimulating aerobic glycolysis. *Cell* **161:** 817–832. doi:10.1016/j.cell.2015.03.023

Aït-Ali N, Delalande F, Van Dorsselaer A, Leveillard TD. 2018. Expression of RdCVF and RdCVL in non human primate retina: a credible animal model for the development of a clinical trial. *Invest Ophthalmol Vis Sci* **59:** 3066.

Aït-Ali N, Blond F, Clérin E, Morshedian A, Cesar Q, Delalande F, Koyanagi M, Birck C, Han J, Ren X. 2022. The emergence of the metabolic signaling of the nucleoredoxin-like genes during evolution. bioRxiv doi:10.1101/2022.01.06.475223

Beckmann A, Özbek S. 2012. The nematocyst: a molecular map of the cnidarian stinging organelle. *Int J Dev Biol* **56:** 577–582. doi:10.1387/ijdb.113472ab

Bigot K, Gondouin P, Bénard R, Montagne P, Youale J, Piazza M, Picard E, Bordet T, Behar-Cohen F. 2020.

Transferrin non-viral gene therapy for treatment of retinal degeneration. *Pharmaceutics* **12:** 836. doi:10.3390/pharmaceutics12090836

Blond F, Léveillard T. 2019. Functional genomics of the retina to elucidate its construction and deconstruction. *Int J Mol Sci* **20:** 4922. doi:10.3390/ijms20194922

Busskamp V, Duebel J, Balya D, Fradot M, Viney TJ, Siegert S, Groner AC, Cabuy E, Forster V, Seeliger M, et al. 2010. Genetic reactivation of cone photoreceptors restores visual responses in retinitis pigmentosa. *Science* **329:** 413–417. doi:10.1126/science.1190897

Byrne LC, Dalkara D, Luna G, Fisher SK, Clérin E, Sahel JA, Léveillard T, Flannery JG. 2015. Viral-mediated RdCVF and RdCVFL expression protects cone and rod photoreceptors in retinal degeneration. *J Clin Invest* **125:** 105–116. doi:10.1172/JCI65654

Camacho ET, Léveillard T, Sahel JA, Wirkus S. 2016. Mathematical model of the role of RdCVF in the coexistence of rods and cones in a healthy eye. *Bull Math Biol* **78:** 1394–1409. doi:10.1007/s11538-016-0185-x

Camacho ET, Brager D, Elachouri G, Korneyeva T, Millet-Puel G, Sahel JA, Léveillard T. 2019. A mathematical analysis of aerobic glycolysis triggered by glucose uptake in cones. *Sci Rep* **9:** 4162. doi:10.1038/s41598-019-39901-z

Carwile ME, Culbert RB, Sturdivant RL, Kraft TW. 1998. Rod outer segment maintenance is enhanced in the presence of bFGF, CNTF and GDNF. *Exp Eye Res* **66:** 791–805. doi:10.1006/exer.1998.0488

Cepko C, Punzo C. 2015. Cell metabolism: sugar for sight. *Nature* **522:** 428–429. doi:10.1038/522428a

Chalmel F, Léveillard T, Jaillard C, Lardenois A, Berdugo N, Morel E, Koehl P, Lambrou G, Holmgren A, Sahel JA, et al. 2007. Rod-derived cone viability factor-2 is a novel bifunctional-thioredoxin-like protein with therapeutic potential. *BMC Mol Biol* **8:** 74. doi:10.1186/1471-2199-8-74

Chen C, Okayama H. 1987. High-efficiency transformation of mammalian cells by plasmid DNA. *Mol Cell Biol* **7:** 2745–2752. doi:10.1128/mcb.7.8.2745-2752.1987

Chinchore Y, Begaj T, Wu D, Drokhlyansky E, Cepko CL. 2017. Glycolytic reliance promotes anabolism in photoreceptors. *eLife* **6:** e25946. doi:10.7554/eLife.25946

Chung DC, Vinot P-A, Marussig M, Thiébault L, Pom B, Andrieu C, Zeitz C, Léveillard TD, Boissel S, Mohand-Saïd S. 2021. Correlations between progression markers in rod- cone dystrophy due to mutations in RHO, PDE6A, or PDE6B. *Invest Ophthalmol Vis Sci* **62:** 3539–3539.

Clérin E, Yang Y, Pagan D, Achiedo S, Degardin J, Cesar Q, Simonutti M, Millet-Puel G, Blond F, Ait-Ali N, et al. 2018. The development of a therapy for retinitis pigmentosa based on the combined administration of the two products encoded by the nucleoredoxin like-1 gene. *Invest Ophthalmol Vis Sci* **59:** 3963.

Clérin E, Marussig M, Sahel JA, Léveillard T. 2020. Metabolic and redox signaling of the nucleoredoxin-like-1 gene for the treatment of genetic retinal diseases. *Int J Mol Sci* **21:** 1625. doi:10.3390/ijms21051625

Corsi M, Jaillard C, Leveillard T, Jaillard C, Léveillard T. 2023. Nucleoredoxin-like 2 metabolic signaling impairs its potential contribution to neurodegenerative diseases.

Neural Regen Res **18:** 529–530. doi:10.4103/1673-5374
.346476

Cronin T, Raffelsberger W, Lee-Rivera I, Jaillard C, Niepon
ML, Kinzel B, Clérin E, Petrosian A, Picaud S, Poch O, et
al. 2010. The disruption of the rod-derived cone viability
gene leads to photoreceptor dysfunction and susceptibility to oxidative stress. *Cell Death Differ* **17:** 1199–1210.
doi:10.1038/cdd.2010.2

Daniele LL, Han JYS, Samuels IS, Komirisetty R, Mehta N,
McCord JL, Yu M, Wang Y, Boesze-Battaglia K, Bell BA,
et al. 2022. Glucose uptake by GLUT1 in photoreceptors
is essential for outer segment renewal and rod photoreceptor survival. *FASEB J* **36:** e22428. doi:10.1096/fj.2022
00369R

Delyfer MN, Raffelsberger W, Mercier D, Korobelnik JF,
Gaudric A, Charteris DG, Tadayoni R, Metge F, Caputo
G, Barale PO, et al. 2011. Transcriptomic analysis of human retinal detachment reveals both inflammatory response and photoreceptor death. *PLoS ONE* **6:** e28791.
doi:10.1371/journal.pone.0028791

Elachouri G, Lee-Rivera I, Clérin E, Argentini M, Fridlich R,
Blond F, Ferracane V, Yang Y, Raffelsberger W, Wan J, et
al. 2015. Thioredoxin rod-derived cone viability factor
protects against photooxidative retinal damage. *Free
Radic Biol Med* **81:** 22–29. doi:10.1016/j.freeradbiomed
.2015.01.003

Feinberg TE, Mallatt J. 2013. The evolutionary and genetic
origins of consciousness in the Cambrian Period over 500
million years ago. *Front Psychol* **4:** 667. doi:10.3389/fpsyg
.2013.00667

Fintz AC, Audo I, Hicks D, Mohand-Saïd S, Léveillard T,
Sahel J. 2003. Partial characterization of retina-derived
cone neuroprotection in two culture models of photoreceptor degeneration. *Invest Ophthalmol Vis Sci* **44:** 818–
825. doi:10.1167/iovs.01-1144

Frasson M, Picaud S, Leveillard T, Simonutti M, Mohand-
Saïd S, Dreyfus H, Hicks D, Sabel J. 1999. Glial cell line-
derived neurotrophic factor induces histologic and functional protection of rod photoreceptors in the rd/rd
mouse. *Invest Ophthalmol Vis Sci* **40:** 2724–2734.

Fridlich R, Delalande F, Jaillard C, Lu J, Poidevin L, Cronin
T, Perrocheau L, Millet-Puel G, Niepon ML, Poch O, et
al. 2009. The thioredoxin-like protein rod-derived cone
viability factor (RdCVFL) interacts with TAU and inhibits its phosphorylation in the retina. *Mol Cell Proteomics* **8:** 1206–1218. doi:10.1074/mcp.M800406-MCP
200

Fritsche LG, Chen W, Schu M, Yaspan BL, Yu Y, Thorleifs-
son G, Zack DJ, Arakawa S, Cipriani V, Ripke S, et al.
2013. Seven new loci associated with age-related macular
degeneration. *Nat Genet* **45:** 433–439. doi:10.1038/ng
.2578

Fritsche LG, Igl W, Bailey JN, Grassmann F, Sengupta S,
Bragg-Gresham JL, Burdon KP, Hebbring SJ, Wen C,
Gorski M, et al. 2016. A large genome-wide association
study of age-related macular degeneration highlights contributions of rare and common variants. *Nat Genet* **48:**
134–143. doi:10.1038/ng.3448

Fultz NE, Bonmassar G, Setsompop K, Stickgold RA, Rosen
BR, Polimeni JR, Lewis LD. 2019. Coupled electrophysiological, hemodynamic, and cerebrospinal fluid oscilla-

tions in human sleep. *Science* **366:** 628–631. doi:10.1126/
science.aax5440

Gerkema MP, Davies WI, Foster RG, Menaker M, Hut RA.
2013. The nocturnal bottleneck and the evolution of activity patterns in mammals. *Proc Biol Sci* **280:** 20130508.
doi:10.1098/rspb.2013.0508

Goikolea J, Gerenu G, Daniilidou M, Mangialasche F, Me-
cocci P, Ngandu T, Rinne J, Solomon A, Kivipelto M,
Cedazo-Minguez A, et al. 2022. Serum thioredoxin-80 is
associated with age, ApoE4, and neuropathological biomarkers in Alzheimer's disease: a potential early sign of
AD. *Alzheimers Res Ther* **14:** 37. doi:10.1186/s13195-022-
00979-9

Guertin S, Kass-Simon G. 2015. Extraocular spectral photosensitivity in the tentacles of *Hydra vulgaris*. *Comp Biochem Physiol A Mol Integr Physiol* **184:** 163–170. doi:10
.1016/j.cbpa.2015.02.016

Han JYS, Kinoshita J, Bisetto S, Bell BA, Nowak RA, Peachey
NS, Philp NJ. 2020. Role of monocarboxylate transporters
in regulating metabolic homeostasis in the outer retina:
insight gained from cell-specific *Bsg* deletion. *FASEB J* **34:**
5401–5419. doi:10.1096/fj.201902961R

Hanschmann EM, Godoy JR, Berndt C, Hudemann C, Lillig
CH. 2013. Thioredoxins, glutaredoxins, and peroxire-
doxins—molecular mechanisms and health significance:
from cofactors to antioxidants to redox signaling. *Antioxid Redox Signal* **19:** 1539–1605. doi:10.1089/ars.2012
.4599

Herrup K. 2021. *How not to study a disease: the story of
Alzheimer's*. MIT Press, Cambridge, MA.

Hewitt AT, Lindsey JD, Carbott D, Adler R. 1990. Photoreceptor survival-promoting activity in interphotoreceptor
matrix preparations: characterization and partial purification. *Exp Eye Res* **50:** 79–88. doi:10.1016/0014-4835(90)
90013-K

Ingram NT, Fain GL, Sampath AP. 2020. Elevated energy
requirement of cone photoreceptors. *Proc Natl Acad Sci*
117: 19599–19603. doi:10.1073/pnas.2001776117

Jaillard C, Mouret A, Niepon ML, Clérin E, Yang Y, Lee-
Rivera I, Aït-Ali N, Millet-Puel G, Cronin T, Sedmak T, et
al. 2012. Nxnl2 splicing results in dual functions in neuronal cell survival and maintenance of cell integrity. *Hum
Mol Genet* **21:** 2298–2311. doi:10.1093/hmg/dds050

Jaillard C, Ouechtati F, Clérin E, Millet-Puel G, Corsi M, Aït-
Ali N, Blond F, Chevy Q, Gales L, Farinelli M, et al. 2021.
The metabolic signaling of the nucleoredoxin-like 2 gene
supports brain function. *Redox Biol* **48:** 102198. doi:10
.1016/j.redox.2021.102198

Klipfel L, Cordonnier M, Thiébault L, Clérin E, Blond F,
Millet-Puel G, Mohand-Saïd S, Goureau O, Sahel JA,
Nandrot EF, et al. 2021. A splice variant in *SLC16A8*
gene leads to lactate transport deficit in human iPS cell-
derived retinal pigment epithelial cells. *Cells* **10:** 179.
doi:10.3390/cells10010179

Kole C, Klipfel L, Yang Y, Ferracane V, Blond F, Reichman S,
Millet-Puel G, Clérin E, Aït-Ali N, Pagan D, et al. 2018.
Otx2-genetically modified retinal pigment epithelial cells
rescue photoreceptors after transplantation. *Mol Ther* **26:**
219–237. doi:10.1016/j.ymthe.2017.09.007

Komeima K, Rogers BS, Lu L, Campochiaro PA. 2006. Antioxidants reduce cone cell death in a model of retinitis

pigmentosa. *Proc Natl Acad Sci* **103**: 11300–11305. doi:10.1073/pnas.0604056103

Léveillard TD. 2018. Photoreceptor metabolic and redox signaling in health and disease. *Invest Ophthalmol Vis Sci* **59**: 5999.

Léveillard T, Aït-Ali N. 2017. Cell signaling with extracellular thioredoxin and thioredoxin- like proteins: insight into their mechanisms of action. *Oxid Med Cell Longev* **2017**: 8475125. doi:10.1155/2017/8475125

Léveillard T, Sahel JA. 2010. Rod-derived cone viability factor for treating blinding diseases: from clinic to redox signaling. *Sci Transl Med* **2**: 26ps16. doi:10.1126/scitranslmed.3000866

Léveillard T, Sahel JA. 2017. Metabolic and redox signaling in the retina. *Cell Mol Life Sci* **74**: 3649–3665. doi:10.1007/s00018-016-2318-7

Léveillard T, Mohand-Saïd S, Lorentz O, Hicks D, Fintz AC, Clérin E, Simonutti M, Forster V, Cavusoglu N, Chalmel F, et al. 2004. Identification and characterization of rod-derived cone viability factor. *Nat Genet* **36**: 755–759. doi:10.1038/ng1386

Léveillard T, Van Dorsselaer A, Sahel JA. 2015. Altruism in the retina: sticks feed cones. *Med Sci (Paris)* **31**: 828–830. doi:10.1051/medsci/20153110005

Léveillard TD, Clérin E, Maamri NM, Millet-Puel G, Blond F, Dalkara D, Van Dorsselaer A. 2017. The combined administration of the two products encoded by the nucleoredoxin-like-I gene stabilizes vision in a mouse model of retinitis pigmentosa. *Invest Ophthalmol Vis Sci* **58**: 1576–1576.

Léveillard T, Philp NJ, Sennlaub F. 2019. Is retinal metabolic dysfunction at the center of the pathogenesis of age-related macular degeneration? *Int J Mol Sci* **20**: 762. doi:10.3390/ijms20030762

Lillig CH, Berndt C, Holmgren A. 2008. Glutaredoxin systems. *Biochim Biophys Acta* **1780**: 1304–1317. doi:10.1016/j.bbagen.2008.06.003

Lorget F, Marie M, Khabou H, Simon C, Nuno D, Vanlandingham P, Quiambao A, Farjo R, Dalkara D, Sahel JA. 2022. SPVN06, a novel mutation-independent AAV-based gene therapy, dramatically reduces vision loss in the rd10 mouse model of rod–cone dystrophy. *Invest Ophthalmol Vis Sci* **63**: 56–A0029.

Marie M, Marussig M, Vinot PA, Vihtelic T, Boyd RF, Knupp L, Lamoureux J, Leveillard TD, Sahel JA, Lorget F. 2021. A 1-month toxicology and biodistribution NHP pilot study evaluating a single subretinal bilateral administration of SPVN06-a novel AAV-based gene therapy for the treatment of rod-cone dystrophies agnostic of the causative mutation. *Invest Ophthalmol Vis Sci* **62**: 194.

Marussig M, Thiebault L, Vinot PA, Pom B, Andrieu C, Zeitz C, Leveillard TD, Allouche F, Mohand-Saïd S, Audo IS, et al. 2020. Natural history of retinitis pigmentosa due to RHO, PDE6A OR PDE6B mutations. *Invest Ophthalmol Vis Sci* **61**: 3035.

Mei X, Chaffiol A, Kole C, Yang Y, Millet-Puel G, Clérin E, Aït-Ali N, Bennett J, Dalkara D, Sahel JA, et al. 2016. The thioredoxin encoded by the rod-derived cone viability factor gene protects cone photoreceptors against oxidative stress. *Antioxid Redox Signal* **24**: 909–923. doi:10.1089/ars.2015.6509

Millet-Puel G, Pinault M, Cordonnier M, Fontaine V, Sahel JA, Léveillard T. 2021. Cone-enriched cultures from the retina of chicken embryos to study rod to cone cellular interactions. *J Vis Exp* doi: 10.3791/61998

Mohand-Saïd S, Hicks D, Simonutti M, Tran-Minh D, Deudon-Combe A, Dreyfus H, Silverman MS, Ogilvie JM, Tenkova T, Sahel J. 1997. Photoreceptor transplants increase host cone survival in the retinal degeneration (*rd*) mouse. *Ophthalmic Res* **29**: 290–297. doi:10.1159/000268027

Mohand-Saïd S, Deudon-Combe A, Hicks D, Simonutti M, Forster V, Fintz AC, Léveillard T, Dreyfus H, Sahel JA. 1998. Normal retina releases a diffusible factor stimulating cone survival in the retinal degeneration mouse. *Proc Natl Acad Sci* **95**: 8357–8362. doi:10.1073/pnas.95.14.8357

Mohand-Saïd S, Hicks D, Dreyfus H, Sahel JA. 2000. Selective transplantation of rods delays cone loss in a retinitis pigmentosa model. *Arch Ophthalmol* **118**: 807–811. doi:10.1001/archopht.118.6.807

Morshedian A, Fain GL. 2015. Single-photon sensitivity of lamprey rods with cone-like outer segments. *Curr Biol* **25**: 484–487. doi:10.1016/j.cub.2014.12.031

Noel J, Jalligampala A, Marussig M, Vinot PA, Marie M, Butler M, Lorget F, Boissel S, Leveillard TD, Sahel JA, et al. 2021a. SPVN06, a novel mutation-independent AAV-based gene therapy, protects cone degeneration in a pig model of retinitis pigmentosa. *Invest Ophthalmol Vis Sci* **62**.

Noel JM, Jalligampala A, Marussig M, Vinot PA, Marie M, Butler M, Lorget F, Boissel S, Leveillard TD, Sahel JA, et al. 2021b. Rod-derived cone viability factor provides trophic support for cone photoreceptors in a pig model of retinitis pigmentosa. *Mol Ther* **29**: 269–269.

Ochrietor JD, Moroz TP, Clamp MF, Timmers AM, Muramatsu T, Linser PJ. 2002. Inactivation of the Basigin gene impairs normal retinal development and maturation. *Vis Res* **42**: 447–453. doi:10.1016/S0042-6989(01)00236-X

Ochrietor JD, Moroz TP, van Ekeris L, Clamp MF, Jefferson SC, deCarvalho AC, Fadool JM, Wistow G, Muramatsu T, Linser PJ. 2003. Retina-specific expression of 5A11/Basigin-2, a member of the immunoglobulin gene superfamily. *Invest Ophthalmol Vis Sci* **44**: 4086–4096. doi:10.1167/iovs.02-0995

Ogata FT, Branco V, Vale FF, Coppo L. 2021. Glutaredoxin: discovery, redox defense and much more. *Redox Biol* **43**: 101975. doi:10.1016/j.redox.2021.101975

Okawa H, Sampath AP, Laughlin SB, Fain GL. 2008. ATP consumption by mammalian rod photoreceptors in darkness and in light. *Curr Biol* **18**: 1917–1921. doi:10.1016/j.cub.2008.10.029

Passano LM, McCullough CB. 1962. The light response and the rhythmic potentials of hydra. *Proc Natl Acad Sci* **48**: 1376–1382. doi:10.1073/pnas.48.8.1376

Pekkari K, Gurunath R, Arner ES, Holmgren A. 2000. Truncated thioredoxin is a mitogenic cytokine for resting human peripheral blood mononuclear cells and is present in human plasma. *The J Biol Chem* **275**: 37474–37480. doi:10.1074/jbc.M001012200

Perini ES, Pessoa VF, Pessoa DM. 2009. Detection of fruit by the *Cerrado*'s marmoset (*Callithrix penicillata*): modeling color signals for different background scenarios and ambient light intensities. *J Exp Zoology A Ecol Genet Physiol* **311:** 289–302. doi:10.1002/jez.531

Petit L, Ma S, Cipi J, Cheng SY, Zieger M, Hay N, Punzo C. 2018. Aerobic glycolysis is essential for normal rod function and controls secondary cone death in retinitis pigmentosa. *Cell Rep* **23:** 2629–2642. doi:10.1016/j.celrep.2018.04.111

Picciani N, Kerlin JR, Jindrich K, Hensley NM, Gold DA, Oakley TH. 2021. Light modulated cnidocyte discharge predates the origins of eyes in Cnidaria. *Ecol Evol* **11:** 3933–3940. doi:10.1002/ece3.7280

Plachetzki DC, Fong CR, Oakley TH. 2012. Cnidocyte discharge is regulated by light and opsin-mediated phototransduction. *BMC Biol* **10:** 17. doi:10.1186/1741-7007-10-17

Price CJ, Hoyda TD, Ferguson AV. 2008. The area postrema: a brain monitor and integrator of systemic autonomic state. *Neuroscientist* **14:** 182–194. doi:10.1177/1073858407311100

Punzo C, Kornacker K, Cepko CL. 2009. Stimulation of the insulin/mTOR pathway delays cone death in a mouse model of retinitis pigmentosa. *Nat Neurosci* **12:** 44–52. doi:10.1038/nn.2234

Rajala RV, Rajala A, Kooker C, Wang Y, Anderson RE. 2016. The Warburg effect mediator pyruvate kinase M2 expression and regulation in the retina. *Sci Rep* **6:** 37727. doi:10.1038/srep37727

Rajala A, Wang Y, Brush RS, Tsantilas K, Jankowski CSR, Lindsay KJ, Linton JD, Hurley JB, Anderson RE, Rajala RVS. 2018a. Pyruvate kinase M2 regulates photoreceptor structure, function, and viability. *Cell Death Dis* **9:** 240. doi:10.1038/s41419-018-0296-4

Rajala A, Wang Y, Soni K, Rajala RVS. 2018b. Pyruvate kinase M2 isoform deletion in cone photoreceptors results in age-related cone degeneration. *Cell Death Dis* **9:** 737. doi:10.1038/s41419-018-0712-9

Rath MF, Bailey MJ, Kim JS, Coon SL, Klein DC, Moller M. 2009. Developmental and daily expression of the Pax4 and Pax6 homeobox genes in the rat retina: localization of Pax4 in photoreceptor cells. *J Neurochem* **108:** 285–294. doi:10.1111/j.1471-4159.2008.05765.x

Reed M, Takemaru KI, Ying G, Frederick JM, Baehr W. 2022. Deletion of CEP164 in mouse photoreceptors post-ciliogenesis interrupts ciliary intraflagellar transport (IFT). *PLoS Genet* **18:** e1010154. doi:10.1371/journal.pgen.1010154

Reichman S, Kalathur RK, Lambard S, Aït-Ali N, Yang Y, Lardenois A, Ripp R, Poch O, Zack DJ, Sahel JA, et al. 2010. The homeobox gene CHX10/VSX2 regulates RdCVF promoter activity in the inner retina. *Hum Mol Genet* **19:** 250–261. doi:10.1093/hmg/ddp484

Ren X, Zou L, Zhang X, Branco V, Wang J, Carvalho C, Holmgren A, Lu J. 2017. Redox signaling mediated by thioredoxin and glutathione systems in the central nervous system. *Antioxid Redox Signal* **27:** 989–1010. doi:10.1089/ars.2016.6925

Rubartelli A, Bajetto A, Allavena G, Wollman E, Sitia R. 1992. Secretion of thioredoxin by normal and neoplastic-cells through a leaderless secretory pathway. *J Biol Chem* **267:** 24161–24164. doi:10.1016/S0021-9258(18)35742-9

Rueda EM, Johnson JE Jr, Giddabasappa A, Swaroop A, Brooks MJ, Sigel I, Chaney SY, Fox DA. 2016. The cellular and compartmental profile of mouse retinal glycolysis, tricarboxylic acid cycle, oxidative phosphorylation, and ~P transferring kinases. *Mol Vis* **22:** 847–885.

Sahaf B, Rosén A. 2000. Secretion of 10-kDa and 12-kDa thioredoxin species from blood monocytes and transformed leukocytes. *Antioxid Redox Signal* **2:** 717–726. doi:10.1089/ars.2000.2.4-717

Stadtman ER. 2006. Protein oxidation and aging. *Free Radic Res* **40:** 1250–1258. doi:10.1080/10715760600918142

Sullivan WJ, Mullen PJ, Schmid EW, Flores A, Momcilovic M, Sharpley MS, Jelinek D, Whiteley AE, Maxwell MB, Wilde BR, et al. 2018. Extracellular matrix remodeling regulates glucose metabolism through TXNIP destabilization. *Cell* **175:** 117–132.e21. doi:10.1016/j.cell.2018.08.017

Tanudji M, Hevi S, Chuck SL. 2003. The nonclassic secretion of thioredoxin is not sensitive to redox state. *Am J Physiol Cell Physiol* **284:** C1272–C1279. doi:10.1152/ajpcell.00521.2002

Ueta T, Inoue T, Furukawa T, Tamaki Y, Nakagawa Y, Imai H, Yanagi Y. 2012. Glutathione peroxidase 4 is required for maturation of photoreceptor cells. *J Biol Chem* **287:** 7675–7682. doi:10.1074/jbc.M111.335174

Weh E, Lutrzykowska Z, Smith A, Hager H, Pawar M, Wubben TJ, Besirli CG. 2020. Hexokinase 2 is dispensable for photoreceptor development but is required for survival during aging and outer retinal stress. *Cell Death Dis* **11:** 422. doi:10.1038/s41419-020-2638-2

Williams BA, Kay RF, Kirk EC. 2010. New perspectives on anthropoid origins. *Proc Natl Acad Sci* **107:** 4797–4804. doi:10.1073/pnas.0908320107

Wolloscheck T, Kunst S, Kelleher DK, Spessert R. 2015. Transcriptional regulation of nucleoredoxin-like genes takes place on a daily basis in the retina and pineal gland of rats. *Vis Neurosci* **32:** E002. doi:10.1017/S0952523814000352

Wu N, Zheng B, Shaywitz A, Dagon Y, Tower C, Bellinger G, Shen CH, Wen J, Asara J, McGraw TE, et al. 2013. AMPK-dependent degradation of TXNIP upon energy stress leads to enhanced glucose uptake via GLUT1. *Mol Cell* **49:** 1167–1175. doi:10.1016/j.molcel.2013.01.035

Wubben TJ, Pawar M, Smith A, Toolan K, Hager H, Besirli CG. 2017. Photoreceptor metabolic reprogramming provides survival advantage in acute stress while causing chronic degeneration. *Sci Rep* **7:** 17863. doi:10.1038/s41598-017-18098-z

Xue Y, Wang SK, Rana P, West ER, Hong CM, Feng H, Wu DM, Cepko CL. 2021. AAV-Txnip prolongs cone survival and vision in mouse models of retinitis pigmentosa. *eLife* **10:** e66240. doi:10.7554/eLife.66240

Yang Y, Mohand-Saïd S, Danan A, Simonutti M, Fontaine V, Clérin E, Picaud S, Léveillard T, Sahel JA. 2009. Functional cone rescue by RdCVF protein in a dominant model of retinitis pigmentosa. *Mol Ther* **17:** 787–795. doi:10.1038/mt.2009.28

Yang Y, Mohand-Saïd S, Léveillard T, Fontaine V, Simonutti M, Sahel JA. 2010. Transplantation of photoreceptor and total neural retina preserves cone function in P23H rhodopsin transgenic rat. *PLoS ONE* **5:** e13469. doi:10.1371/journal.pone.0013469

Yang M, So KF, Lam WC, Lo ACY. 2021. Cell ferroptosis: new mechanism and new hope for retinitis pigmentosa. *Cells* **10**. doi:10.3390/cells10082153

Yu S, Meng S, Xiang M, Ma H. 2021. Phosphoenolpyruvate carboxykinase in cell metabolism: roles and mechanisms beyond gluconeogenesis. *Mol Metab* **53:** 101257. doi:10.1016/j.molmet.2021.101257

Zhang L, Du J, Justus S, Hsu C-W, Bonet-Ponce L, Wu W-H, Tsai Y-T, Wu W-P, Jia Y, Duong JK, et al. 2016. Reprogramming metabolism by targeting sirtuin 6 attenuates

retinal degeneration. *The J Clin Invest* **126:** 4659–4673. doi:10.1172/JCI86905

Zhang E, Ryu J, Levi SR, Oh JK, Hsu CW, Cui X, Lee TT, Wang NK, de Carvalho JRL, Tsang SH. 2020. PKM2 ablation enhanced retinal function and survival in a preclinical model of retinitis pigmentosa. *Mamm Genome* **31:** 77–85. doi:10.1007/s00335-020-09837-1

Zhong L, D'Urso A, Toiber D, Sebastian C, Henry RE, Vadysirisack DD, Guimaraes A, Marinelli B, Wikstrom JD, Nir T, et al. 2010. The histone deacetylase Sirt6 regulates glucose homeostasis via Hif1α. *Cell* **140:** 280–293. doi:10.1016/j.cell.2009.12.041

Gene Therapies for Retinitis Pigmentosa that Target Glucose Metabolism

Yunlu Xue[1] and Constance L. Cepko[2]

[1]Lingang Laboratory, Shanghai 200031, China

[2]Departments of Genetics and Ophthalmology, Howard Hughes Medical Institute, Harvard Medical School, Boston, Massachusetts 02115, USA

Correspondence: ylxue@lglab.ac.cn; cepko@genetics.med.harvard.edu

Retinitis pigmentosa is a blinding disease wherein rod photoreceptors are affected first, due to the expression of a disease gene, leading to the loss of dim light vision. In many cases, cones do not express the disease gene, yet they are also affected and eventually die, typically after most of the rods in their neighborhood have died. The cause of secondary cone death is unclear. Photoreceptors are one of the most energy-demanding cell types in the body and consume a high amount of glucose. At an early stage of degeneration, the cones appear to have a shortage of glucose to fuel their metabolism. This review focuses on gene therapy approaches that address this potential metabolic shortcoming.

About 100 years ago, Warburg observed that the mammalian retina consumed vast amounts of glucose, and quickly turned it into lactate, even in the presence of oxygen (Warburg 1925). This phenomenon is known as the "Warburg effect" or aerobic glycolysis. Cohen and Noell (1960) ran metabolic assays using neonatal versus adult rabbit retinas and discovered that glucose metabolism was higher in adult retinas than in neonatal retinas. Interestingly, the neonatal retinas were not yet active in phototransduction, leading to the hypothesis that the high glucose metabolism is related to the function of the retina. Subsequently, Winkler (1981) studied the relationship between metabolism and electrical activity of photoreceptors with drugs that inhibit phototransduction, and found that the lactate production was reduced with a Na/K-ATPase inhibitor. Using short hairpin RNA (shRNA) knockdown of key enzymes of glucose metabolism in rod photoreceptors, we found that the photoreceptors were the cell type that drove the high glycolytic demand (Chinchore et al. 2017). The Warburg effect is thought to support the high anabolic needs of photoreceptors, which need to build a portion of their membrane-rich outer segments each day, and consume ATP to run the ion pumps that maintain their membrane potential and their synaptic function. Studies of the interplay between the support cells of the photoreceptors, the retinal pigmented epithelial (RPE) cells, and photoreceptors have also been carried out, leading to the model where glucose and lactate are exchanged between these two cell types (Fig. 1; Kanow et al. 2017; Bisbach et al. 2020).

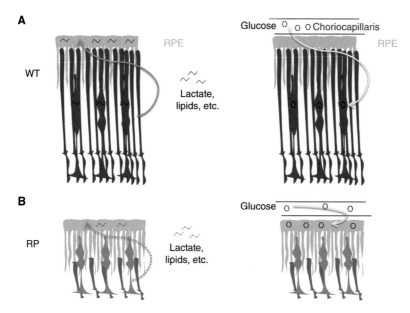

Figure 1. Schematics showing the metabolic relationship between photoreceptors and retinal pigmented epithelial (RPE) cells. (*A*) Glucose and lactate might be the main fuel sources for photoreceptors and RPE cells in the wild-type (WT) eye, respectively (Kanow et al. 2017). (*B*) There may be a shortage of glucose for cones in retinitis pigmentosa (RP) due to a reduction in the supply of lactate made by rods as well as their outer segments. This may cause the RPE cells to retain more glucose in the RP eye than in the wild-type eye.

INSUFFICIENT GLUCOSE FOR RP CONES?

Retinitis pigmentosa (RP) rods die due to inherited genetic mutations, many of which are expressed specifically in rods. RP cones, which usually do not express the disease genes, die secondarily after rod death, due to reasons that are not entirely clear. There are likely multiple mechanisms for this, possibly involving oxidative stress, metabolic imbalance, inflammation, and/or insufficient trophic factor(s) (Mohand-Said et al. 1998; Komeima et al. 2006; Punzo et al. 2009; Wang et al. 2019a).

A study by Punzo et al. (2009) from our laboratory led to the first suggestion that there was a glucose shortage for RP cones. By quantifying RNA changes during degeneration in four RP mouse strains, a common signature across the strains included many genes involved in metabolism. To follow this up, an immunohistochemical analysis of RP retinal tissue showed that the loss of phosphorylated mTOR was one of the earliest signs of cone degeneration. This was true across all four strains that were exam-

ined. The loss of phosphorylated mTOR was recapitulated in short-term explant cultures in glucose-free medium, suggesting the RP cones might suffer from a glucose shortage. In a follow-up study, the Punzo laboratory found that the mTORC1 complex, which is a central regulator of metabolism, was important for RP cone survival (Venkatesh et al. 2015). Recently, photoreceptor metabolic problems have also been linked to age-related macular degeneration (AMD)-like pathology in mouse models (Cheng et al. 2020).

An independent line of experiments involving rod-derived cone viability factor (RdCVF) arrived at a potential glucose transport issue for RP cones. RdCVF was found to interact with Basigin1, a chaperone needed to fold glucose transporter 1 (GLUT1), the major glucose transporter of photoreceptors and the RPE. Addition of RdCVF to cone-enriched cultures from chicks facilitated glucose uptake and glycolysis (Aït-Ali et al. 2015). These studies also pointed to a potentially insufficient glucose supply for RP cones (Fig. 2A).

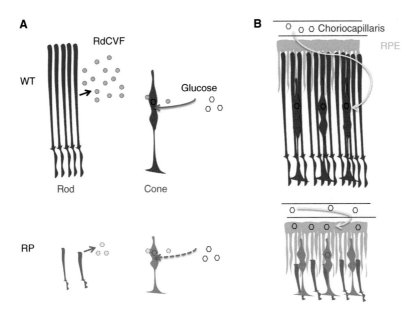

Figure 2. Schematics showing two possible reasons that cones may not have sufficient glucose. (*A*) Glucose uptake might be insufficient in retinitis pigmentosa (RP), with rod-derived cone viability factor (RdCVF) improving glucose uptake via glucose transporter 1 (GLUT1), as it facilitates the folding of GLUT1 via its interaction with Basigin1 (Aït-Ali et al. 2015). (*B*) Glucose supply might be insufficient as the retinal pigmented epithelial (RPE) cells may retain glucose due to a lactate and outer segment reduction when rods die (Wang et al. 2016). (WT) Wild-type.

The transport of glucose from the choriocapillaris to the photoreceptors is via glucose transporters in the RPE. Systemic delivery of 2-NBDG, a fluorescent analog of glucose, into RP mice showed fluorescence concentrated along the apical side of the RPE (Wang et al. 2016). In contrast, in wild-type mice, the fluorescence was enriched in the photoreceptor inner segments. The investigators proposed that glucose was trapped in the RPE during degeneration, causing a shortage of glucose for the RP cones (Fig. 2B). In a follow-up study, loss of GLUT1 from the RPE was proposed to lead to this transportation issue, at least in the Rho^{P23H} RP strain (Wang et al. 2019b). However, there are issues with 2-NBDG being an accurate indicator of glucose localization (Dunn et al. 2021; Keller et al. 2021), and verification in other strains has not been reported.

Hurley and colleagues made an analogy of the relationship between the RPE and the retina as an ecosystem (Kanow et al. 2017). In wild-type animals, glucose enters the RPE via GLUT1 and travels through the RPE to the photoreceptors with little retention. Glucose is then taken up by the photoreceptors and used primarily for glycolysis. Lactate is the end product, which is released from the photoreceptors via monocarboxylate transporters (MCTs). The RPE, and almost no other cell type in the body, expresses a high level of MCT3 (Philp et al. 1998; Halestrap and Price 1999), which can take up the lactate. Lactate is then thought to fuel RPE metabolism, enabling the RPE to release glucose to the photoreceptors (Fig. 1A). In RP, due to the massive loss of rods, which are the dominant photoreceptor type in mouse and human, the lactate supply to the RPE would drop. In addition to a reduction in lactate, the RPE may also miss the supply of outer segments, which they take up following daily shedding by photoreceptors. The outer segments could be a source of anabolic building blocks and energy for the RPE (Bazan et al. 1990; Curcio et al. 2009). Even before they die, RP rods lack outer segments, so that their daily shedding would be greatly reduced. To make up for the loss of adequate lactate and/or outer segment–derived nutrients, the RPE might retain glucose that is normally destined for the photoreceptors, creating a shortage of glucose for cones (Fig. 1B).

GENE THERAPIES TO PROLONG RP CONE SURVIVAL

mTOR

The initial observation of RNA changes in genes involved with metabolism, and lack of mTOR phosphorylation, suggested that the stimulation of mTOR via the systemic injection of insulin might prolong cone survival. Punzo et al. found that systemic insulin injection improved RP cone survival in mice, while streptozotocin, a drug that kills the pancreatic β-cells, accelerated RP cone death (Punzo et al. 2009). To determine whether these effects were direct on cones, and to achieve better targeting of the mTOR pathway, multiple genetically modified animals were tested for effects on cone survival. It was found that mTORC1 pathway activation specifically in cones could enhance RP cone survival (Venkatesh et al. 2015).

RdCVF

RdCVF was discovered in a cDNA screen on embryonic chick cone cultures, with the readout of increased cone survival. As mentioned above, it was later discovered to enhance glucose uptake and glycolysis in chick cone cultures via its binding to Basigin1, which improved the folding of GLUT1 (Fig. 2A; Aït-Ali et al. 2015). Initially, RdCVF therapy was designed to be delivered as a protein to RP eyes (Yang et al. 2009). To achieve better delivery with only a single or few injections, an AAV-based gene therapy was designed. AAV transduction to RP mouse models led to increased cone survival (Aït-Ali et al. 2015; Byrne et al. 2015). In a rat RP model, addition of RdCVF improved cone function as well as outer segments (Yang et al. 2009). A study in RP pigs is ongoing (Noel et al. 2021).

Gluconeogenesis

Another strategy to enable cones to have more glucose, in the case where uptake or supply might be limiting, was to have cones make their own. This approach was carried out by Chinchore et al. where improved RP cone survival was observed (Chinchore et al. 2019). The broadly active cytomegalovirus (CMV) promoter was used in this study, so it is not clear whether this was due to cones making their own glucose, or the benefit derived from glucose made by the cones and/or the RPE.

Txnip

By surveying 20 genes involved in metabolism and targeting only cones, using cone-specific promoters, we identified that thioredoxin interacting protein (Txnip) prolongs cone survival (Xue et al. 2021). Txnip is an α-arrestin protein that interacts with several proteins (Forred et al. 2016). One of its binding partners is thioredoxin, an antioxidation protein, wherein binding nullifies the activity of thioredoxin (Nishiyama et al. 1999; Junn et al. 2000). A mutant of Txnip, C247S, which abolishes its interaction with thioredoxins (Patwari et al. 2006), showed better RP cone rescue than the wild-type allele. Potentially, this mutation frees thioredoxin to help reduce oxidative damage, and/or frees Txnip to interact with other partners that benefit cones. The Txnip rescue is dependent on LDHB, a subunit of lactate dehydrogenase that facilitates lactate catabolism. Txnip was also shown to improve RP cone mitochondrial structure and function. We have suggested that Txnip prolongs RP cone survival by switching the fuel choice from glucose to lactate, with the pyruvate produced by LDHB fueling mitochondrial metabolism. Lactate may be more available to RP cones (e.g., from the systemic circulation via the RPE and/or Müller glia) (Fig. 3).

Alterations in Rod Metabolism

The hypothesis of a glucose shortage for RP cones concerns nonautonomous cone death. Nonetheless, any treatment to maintain rods,

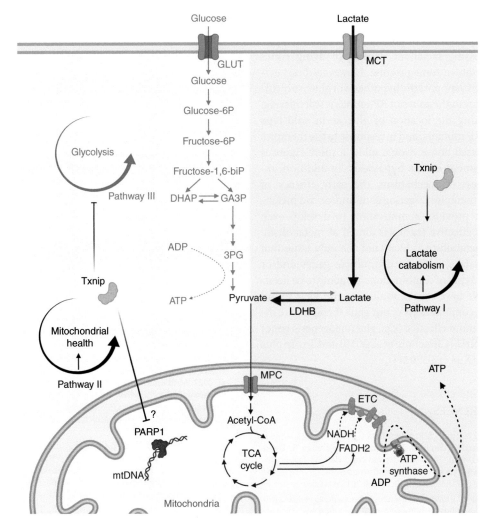

Figure 3. Model for the mechanism of thioredoxin interacting protein (Txnip)-mediated cone rescue. The data suggest that at least two pathways are required for Txnip rescue. Pathway I: enhancement of lactate catabolism, which requires the function of LDHB; and pathway II: improved mitochondrial health, possibly through mitochondrial Parp1 inhibition. An additional pathway, pathway III: inhibiting glycolysis by removing glucose transporter 1 (GLUT1) from the cell surface may partially contribute to rescue by working with improved lactate metabolism and improved mitochondrial health and/or unidentified pathways. (Diagram and figure legend adapted from Xue et al. 2021, © 2021.) (MCT) Monocarboxylate transporter.

even if they are not functional in phototransduction, might also benefit cones (Zhang et al. 2016). Sirt6, an inhibitor of glycolytic flux, was inhibited specifically in the rods of PDE6β mutant mice. This strain has elevated cGMP and calcium in rods, and responded to the Sirt6 reduction with greater rod survival and function. Interestingly, cones also benefitted, as would be hoped due to the effect of rod death on cones. This method has not been extended to other models, but could be a generic approach. Efforts also have been made toward characterizing the metabolomics of entire retinas, and changes of metabolites have been noted (Jiang et al. 2022). Interpretation of these changes awaits studies aimed at the function of the implicated pathways.

CONCLUDING REMARKS

In animal models, gene-independent therapies addressing metabolic aspects of dying cones have shown some promise. However, direct evidence to support the hypothesis of glucose insufficiency in the cones of RP retinas is still missing. Tracking the location of glucose in wild-type and RP mutants, and in response to the therapies discussed above, would allow a more rigorous assessment of this hypothesis. In addition, regardless of mechanism, the early efficacy of gene therapies targeting cone and/or rod metabolism provides a motivation to develop even more effective therapies aimed at metabolism. As metabolism is likely not the only issue that cones face, addition of multiple genes and/or other types of combinations are going to be needed. We have started to do this and have found some combinations of our gene therapies are indeed more effective (e.g., gluconeogenesis genes plus Nrf2 [Chinchore et al. 2019] and Txnip plus Nrf2 [Xue et al. 2021]).

REFERENCES

Aït-Ali N, Fridlich R, Millet-Puel G, Clérin E, Delalande F, Jaillard C, Blond F, Perrocheau L, Reichman S, Byrne LCC, et al. 2015. Rod-derived cone viability factor promotes cone survival by stimulating aerobic glycolysis. *Cell* **161:** 817–832. doi:10.1016/j.cell.2015.03.023

Bazan HE, Bazan NG, Feeney-Burns L, Berman ER. 1990. Lipids in human lipofuscin-enriched subcellular fractions of two age populations. Comparison with rod outer segments and neural retina. *Invest Ophthalmol Vis Sci* **31:** 1433–1443.

Bisbach CM, Hass DT, Robbings BM, Rountree AM, Sadilek M, Sweet IR, Hurley JB. 2020. Succinate can shuttle reducing power from the hypoxic retina to the O_2-rich pigment epithelium. *Cell Rep* **31:** 107606. doi:10.1016/j.celrep.2020.107606

Byrne LC, Dalkara D, Luna G, Fisher SK, Clérin E, Sahel JA, Léveillard T, Flannery JG. 2015. Viral-mediated RdCVF and RdCVFL expression protects cone and rod photoreceptors in retinal degeneration. *J Clin Invest* **125:** 105–116. doi:10.1172/JCI65654

Cheng SY, Cipi J, Ma S, Hafler BP, Kanadia RN, Brush RS, Agbaga MP, Punzo C. 2020. Altered photoreceptor metabolism in mouse causes late stage age-related macular degeneration-like pathologies. *Proc Natl Acad Sci* **117:** 13094–13104. doi:10.1073/pnas.2000339117

Chinchore Y, Begaj T, Wu D, Drokhlyansky E, Cepko CL. 2017. Glycolytic reliance promotes anabolism in photoreceptors. *eLife* **6:** e25946. doi:10.7554/eLife.25946

Chinchore Y, Begaj T, Guillermeir C, Steinhauser M, Punzo C, Cepko C. 2019. Transduction of gluconeogenic enzymes prolongs cone photoreceptor survival and function in models of retinitis pigmentosa. bioRxiv doi:10.1101/569665

Cohen LH, Noell WK. 1960. Glucose catabolism of rabbit retina before and after development of visual function. *J Neurochem* **5:** 253–276. doi:10.1111/j.1471-4159.1960.tb13363.x

Curcio CA, Johnson M, Huang JD, Rudolf M. 2009. Aging, age-related macular degeneration, and the response-to-retention of apolipoprotein B-containing lipoproteins. *Prog Retin Eye Res* **28:** 393–422. doi:10.1016/j.preteyeres.2009.08.001

Dunn AF, Catterton MA, Dixon DD, Pompano RR. 2021. Spatially resolved measurement of dynamic glucose uptake in live ex vivo tissues. *Anal Chim Acta* **1141:** 47–56. doi:10.1016/j.aca.2020.10.027

Forred BJ, Neuharth S, Kim DI, Amolins MW, Motamedchaboki K, Roux KJ, Vitiello PF. 2016. Identification of redox and glucose-dependent Txnip protein interactions. *Oxid Med Cell Longev* **2016:** 1–10. doi:10.1155/2016/5829063

Halestrap AP, Price NT. 1999. The proton-linked monocarboxylate transporter (MCT) family: structure, function and regulation. *Biochem J* **343:** 281–299. doi:10.1042/bj3430281

Jiang K, Mondal AK, Adlakha YK, Gumerson J, Aponte A, Gieser L, Kim J-W, Boleda A, Brooks MJ, Nellissery J, et al. 2022. Multiomics analyses reveal early metabolic imbalance and mitochondrial stress in neonatal photoreceptors leading to cell death in *Pde6brd1/rd1* mouse model of retinal degeneration. *Hum Mol Genet* **31:** 2137–2154. doi:10.1093/hmg/ddac013

Junn E, Han SH, Im JY, Yang Y, Cho EW, Um HD, Kim DK, Lee KW, Han PL, Rhee SG, et al. 2000. Vitamin D3 upregulated protein 1 mediates oxidative stress via suppressing the thioredoxin function. *J Immunol* **164:** 6287–6295. doi:10.4049/jimmunol.164.12.6287

Kanow MA, Giarmarco MM, Jankowski CS, Tsantilas K, Engel AL, Du J, Linton JD, Farnsworth CC, Sloat SR, Rountree A, et al. 2017. Biochemical adaptations of the retina and retinal pigment epithelium support a metabolic ecosystem in the vertebrate eye. *eLife* **6:** e28899. doi:10.7554/eLife.28899

Keller JP, Marvin JS, Lacin H, Lemon WC, Shea J, Kim S, Lee RT, Koyama M, Keller PJ, Looger LL. 2021. In vivo glucose imaging in multiple model organisms with an engineered single-wavelength sensor. *Cell Rep* **35:** 109284. doi:10.1016/j.celrep.2021.109284

Komeima K, Rogers BS, Lu L, Campochiaro PA. 2006. Antioxidants reduce cone cell death in a model of retinitis pigmentosa. *Proc Natl Acad Sci* **103:** 11300–11305. doi:10.1073/pnas.0604056103

Mohand-Said S, Deudon-Combe A, Hicks D, Simonutti M, Forster V, Fintz AC, Léveillard T, Dreyfus H, Sahel JA. 1998. Normal retina releases a diffusible factor stimulating cone survival in the retinal degeneration mouse. *Proc Natl Acad Sci* **95:** 8357–8362. doi:10.1073/pnas.95.14.8357

Nishiyama A, Matsui M, Iwata S, Hirota K, Masutani H, Nakamura H, Takagi Y, Sono H, Gon Y, Yodoi J. 1999.

Cite this article as *Cold Spring Harb Perspect Med* doi: 10.1101/cshperspect.a041289

Identification of thioredoxin-binding protein-2/vitamin D_3 up-regulated protein 1 as a negative regulator of thioredoxin function and expression. *J Biol Chem* **274:** 21645–21650. doi:10.1074/jbc.274.31.21645

Noel J, Jalligampala A, Marussig M, Vinot PA, Marie M, Butler M, Lorget F, Boissel S, Leveillard TD, Sahel JA, et al. 2021. SPVN06, a novel mutation-independent AAV-based gene therapy, protects cone degeneration in a pig model of retinitis pigmentosa. *Invest Ophthalmol Vis Sci* **62:** 1189–1189.

Patwari P, Higgins LJ, Chutkow WA, Yoshioka J, Lee RT. 2006. The interaction of thioredoxin with Txnip: evidence for formation of a mixed disulfide by disulfide exchange. *J Biol Chem* **281:** 21884–21891. doi:10.1074/jbc.M600427200

Philp NJ, Yoon H, Grollman EF. 1998. Monocarboxylate transporter MCT1 is located in the apical membrane and MCT3 in the basal membrane of rat RPE. *Am J Physiol* **274:** R1824–R1828. doi:10.1152/ajpregu.1998.274.6.R1824

Punzo C, Kornacker K, Cepko CL. 2009. Stimulation of the insulin/mTOR pathway delays cone death in a mouse model of retinitis pigmentosa. *Nat Neurosci* **12:** 44–52. doi:10.1038/nn.2234

Venkatesh A, Ma S, Le YZ, Hall MN, Rüegg MA, Punzo C. 2015. Activated mTORC1 promotes long-term cone survival in retinitis pigmentosa mice. *J Clin Invest* **125:** 1446–1458. doi:10.1172/JCI79766

Wang W, Lee SJ, Scott PA, Lu X, Emery D, Liu Y, Ezashi T, Roberts MR, Ross JW, Kaplan HJ, et al. 2016. Two-step reactivation of dormant cones in retinitis pigmentosa. *Cell Rep* **15:** 372–385. doi:10.1016/j.celrep.2016.03.022

Wang SK, Xue Y, Rana P, Hong CM, Cepko CL. 2019a. Soluble CX3CL1 gene therapy improves cone survival and function in mouse models of retinitis pigmentosa. *Proc Natl Acad Sci* **116:** 10140–10149. doi:10.1073/pnas.1901787116

Wang W, Kini A, Wang Y, Liu T, Chen Y, Vukmanic E, Emery D, Liu Y, Lu X, Jin L, et al. 2019b. Metabolic deregulation of the blood-outer retinal barrier in retinitis pigmentosa. *Cell Rep* **28:** 1323–1334.e4. doi:10.1016/j.celrep.2019.06.093

Warburg O. 1925. The metabolism of carcinoma cells. *J Cancer Res* **9:** 148–163. doi:10.1158/jcr.1925.148

Winkler BS. 1981. Glycolytic and oxidative metabolism in relation to retinal function. *J Gen Physiol* **77:** 667–692. doi:10.1085/jgp.77.6.667

Xue Y, Wang SK, Rana P, West ER, Hong CM, Feng H, Wu DM, Cepko CL. 2021. AAV-Txnip prolongs cone survival and vision in mouse models of retinitis pigmentosa. *eLife* **10:** e66240. doi:10.7554/eLife.66240

Yang Y, Mohand-Said S, Danan A, Simonutti M, Fontaine V, Clerin E, Picaud S, Léveillard T, Sahel JA. 2009. Functional cone rescue by RdCVF protein in a dominant model of retinitis pigmentosa. *Mol Ther* **17:** 787–795. doi:10.1038/mt.2009.28

Zhang L, Du J, Justus S, Hsu CW, Bonet-Ponce L, Wu WH, Tsai YT, Wu WP, Jia Y, Duong JK, et al. 2016. Reprogramming metabolism by targeting sirtuin 6 attenuates retinal degeneration. *J Clin Invest* **126:** 4659–4673. doi:10.1172/JCI86905

Electronic Retinal Prostheses

Daniel Palanker

Department of Ophthalmology and Hansen Experimental Physics Laboratory, Stanford University, Stanford, California 94305, USA

Correspondence: palanker@stanford.edu

Retinal prostheses are a promising means for restoring sight to patients blinded by photoreceptor atrophy. They introduce visual information by electrical stimulation of the surviving inner retinal neurons. Subretinal implants target the graded-response secondary neurons, primarily the bipolar cells, which then transfer the information to the ganglion cells via the retinal neural network. Therefore, many features of natural retinal signal processing can be preserved in this approach if the inner retinal network is retained. Epiretinal implants stimulate primarily the ganglion cells, and hence should encode the visual information in spiking patterns, which, ideally, should match the target cell types. Currently, subretinal arrays are being developed primarily for restoration of central vision in patients impaired by age-related macular degeneration (AMD), while epiretinal implants—for patients blinded by retinitis pigmentosa, where the inner retina is less preserved. This review describes the concepts and technologies, preclinical characterization of prosthetic vision and clinical outcomes, and provides a glimpse into future developments.

Retinal degenerative diseases are among the leading causes of incurable blindness today (Smith et al. 2001). While photoreceptors are lost in retinal degeneration, the inner retinal neurons survive to a large extent (Humayun et al. 1999; Kim et al. 2002; Mazzoni et al. 2008), providing an opportunity to reintroduce visual information into the neural system by electrical stimulation of the remaining neurons.

Photoreceptors (about 100 million in a human eye) hyperpolarize upon illumination, which, in turn, reduces the glutamate release rate in synapses with about a dozen types of bipolar cells (BCs). Two types of horizontal cells modulate these synapses, providing edge enhancement and some aspects of the contrast adaptation. BCs (about 10 million in total) are also graded-response neurons, which integrate visual information from multiple photoreceptors and relay it to about two dozen types of retinal ganglion cells (RGCs, about one million), which generate the action potentials propagating to the brain (Fig. 1A,B). About 30 types of amacrine cells (Masland 2001; Wässle 2004) regulate the synapses between BCs and ganglion cells, providing various aspects of spatiotemporal filtering. Different types of RGCs encode various aspects of the visual information in a plurality of ways, including increments or decrements of light (ON and OFF cells), color opponency (blue-yellow, red-green) (Field et al. 2007), various sizes of receptive fields (midget and parasol), segregation of the object motion from that of a background (Olveczky et al. 2003), and many others.

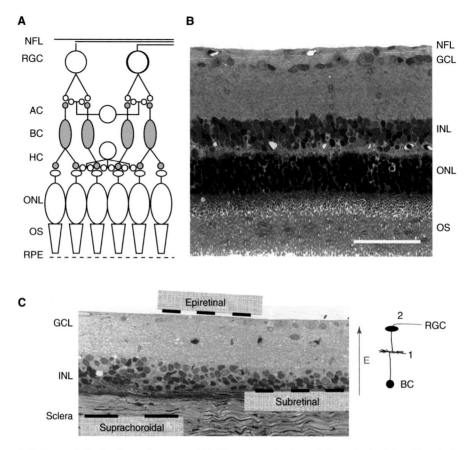

Figure 1. Retina and the implant placement. (*A*) Diagrammatic view of the retinal wiring. Signals from the photoreceptors (including the nuclei in the outer nuclear layer [ONL] and the outer segments [OS]) are processed by the second-order neurons (horizontal [HCs] and bipolar cells [BCs], located in the inner nuclear layer [INL]) and relayed to the third-order neurons—the retinal ganglion cells (RGCs) regulated by the amacrine cells (ACs). The RGC axons in the nerve fiber layer (NFL) transmit the visual signals to the brain. Photoreceptor OS are in contact with the retinal pigment epithelium (RPE). (*B*) Histology of a healthy rat retina. Scale bar, 50 μm. (*C*) Histology of a degenerate rat retina (RCS). Epiretinal implants are placed above the nerve fiber layer. Subretinal implants are placed below the INL instead of the missing photoreceptors. Suprachoroidal implants are inserted into the sclera below the choroid. (GCL) Ganglion cell layer.

Age-related macular degeneration (AMD) is a leading cause of untreatable vision loss, affecting over 8.7% of the population worldwide (Wong et al. 2014). Advanced forms of AMD are associated with severe visual impairment, and their prevalence dramatically increases with age: from 1.5% above 40 yr to more than 15% in populations older than 80 in the United States (Friedman et al. 2004). The dry form of advanced AMD, called geographic atrophy (GA), is associated with a loss of photoreceptors in the center of the macula. Since human visual

acuity decreases with eccentricity (Wandell 1995), loss of high-resolution central vision severely impairs reading and face recognition, while the low-resolution peripheral vision still allows for normal ambulation. Therefore, restoration of central vision in such conditions should provide sufficiently high acuity for reading and face recognition, without jeopardizing the surrounding peripheral retina.

Retinitis pigmentosa (RP) is a broad class of genetic disorders, which typically affects relatively young patients (in their twenties or thirties), with an incidence rate of approximately 1:4000 (Haim 2002). This inherited disease typically begins with a loss of rod photoreceptors in the mid-periphery, that gradually expands toward the peripheral retina and toward the fovea, eventually leading to blindness due to loss of the cone photoreceptors in the central retina. For these patients, independent ambulation would already be a great benefit, even if resolution of prosthetic vision would not suffice for reading.

While retinal degenerations leave the number of the inner retinal neurons (inner nuclear layers [INLs] and ganglion cell layers [GCLs]) relatively intact for an extended period of time (Humayun et al. 1999; Kim et al. 2002), significant changes in wiring of the retinal network can take place at the end phases of the disease, when the vast majority of the photoreceptors are lost (Marc and Jones 2003; Marc et al. 2003; Jones and Marc 2005). During retinal remodeling, amacrine and BCs can migrate either to the distal retina or to the GCL. In the final stages of the retinal remodeling, neuronal death can also significantly deplete the INL and GCL, with glial cells partially filling the space left by deceased neurons (Marc and Jones 2003; Marc et al. 2003). Spontaneous firing patterns of RGCs change significantly with degeneration (Margolis et al. 2008; Menzler and Zeck 2011; Sekirnjak et al. 2011), and electrical stimulation thresholds of certain types of RGCs can increase (Cho et al. 2016).

AMD patients are less likely to suffer from extensive retinal remodeling compared to RP since (1) the peripheral retina is preserved, which helps in maintaining more normal neural activity in the center via lateral connectivity in the retinal network, and (2) the onset of the disease is much later in life and hence its duration is shorter. However, even in such a local retinal degeneration, the RGC spiking rate may increase significantly (Tochitsky et al. 2014).

ELECTRICAL STIMULATION OF NEURONS

Neural activity can be affected by modulating the cell potential with electric current. Extracellular stimulation works by polarizing the cells in an electric field: since the cell membrane is highly resistive while its cytoplasm is very conductive, electric fields in extracellular medium redistribute the charges along the cell membrane such that the cytoplasm rapidly (sub-µs in cell soma) becomes equipotential (Boinagrov et al. 2010). As a result, the transmembrane potential step increases (i.e., the membrane is hyperpolarized) on the side of the cell facing the anode and decreases (the membrane is depolarized) on the opposite side. When the membrane potential exceeds a certain threshold (typically around 10 mV [Boinagrov et al. 2010]) on a depolarized side, the voltage-gated ion channels open, increasing the influx of positive ions (Na^+ in ganglion cells, Ca^{2+} in BCs), resulting in cellular depolarization as a whole. This, in turn, may lead to generation of the action potential in spiking cells (RGCs), or just increase in the neurotransmitter release rate from axonal terminals in the graded-response cells (BCs).

Since the distribution of ion channels over neurons is typically anisotropic, orientation of the electric field significantly affects the stimulation threshold. It is lower when the side of a cell with the highest concentration of the responding ion channels is depolarized. Therefore, the pulse polarity (anodic or cathodic), as well as placement of the stimulating electrode (above or below the retina—epiretinal or subretinal), affects the stimulation threshold. For epiretinal stimulation of RGCs, cathodic-first pulses have a lower stimulation threshold than anodic (Jensen et al. 2005; Fried et al. 2006; Boinagrov et al. 2014) due to a higher concentration of Na voltage-sensitive ion channels near the axon initial segment (Fried et al. 2006). For subretinal stimulation of RGCs, anodic-first pulses have lower stimulation thresholds for the same reason (Jensen and Rizzo 2006; Boinagrov et al. 2014). Similarly, for subretinal stimulation of the BCs in the INL, anodic pulses have a lower threshold (Boinagrov et al. 2014) because of higher concentration of the voltage-sensitive Ca channels in BC's axonal terminals (Werginz et al. 2015). For small electrodes, proximity to the target neuron is another factor that significantly affects the stimulation threshold, since in this case the electric potential rapidly decreases with distance. A combination of a good placement of the stimulating electrode and a proper choice of the stimulation parameters can help achieve selective activation of various retinal neurons (Boinagrov et al. 2014).

Epiretinal prostheses aim at eliciting RGC response directly. Since the Na ion channels underlying the RGC stimulation are much faster than the Ca channels responsible for BC response, RGCs have shorter chronaxie (around 1 msec) than BCs (around 3–4 msec), so the stimulation threshold continues to decrease with increasing pulse duration at least to 20 msec. The strength–duration relationships of the stimulation thresholds for direct and network-mediated responses demonstrated that short (<1 msec) cathodic-first pulses from an epiretinal electrode provide the best RGC/BC selectivity of about a factor of 3 (Boinagrov et al. 2014). Conversely, subretinal anodic-first pulses provide higher selectivity for BCs using longer stimuli, exceeding a factor of 6 for 20 msec pulses (Boinagrov et al. 2014).

Relative position of the active and return electrodes in the implant affects the cross talk between neighboring pixels, and thereby can also affect the contrast, selectivity, and attainable resolution (Palanker et al. 2005; Loudin et al. 2007; Flores et al. 2016). Many implants operate with a remote return electrode in the so-called monopolar configuration. Cross talk between the neighboring pixels increases with a larger number of simultaneously activated electrodes. To overcome this limitation, local return electrodes can be placed around each stimulating electrode (Loudin et al. 2007; Mathieson et al. 2012). However, local returns decrease the electric field penetration depth, compared to a monopolar configuration, and thus impose more stringent limits on distance between the stimulating electrodes and the target neurons. This has led to development of three-dimensional implants (Ho et al. 2019) and current steering approaches (Chen et al. 2020) to optimize the field shaping.

In cell somas, membrane polarization is defined largely by the voltage step across the cell boundaries (i.e., by the integral of the electric field along the cell length). Axons are modeled as leaky cables, where the activating function is defined by the derivative of the electric field along the axon (Malmivuo and Plonsey 1995). Unfortunately, RGC stimulation with epiretinal electrodes is primarily axonal, making the selective and local activation of RGCs rather difficult to achieve (Nanduri et al. 2012; Grosberg et al. 2017).

APPROACHES TO RETINAL PROSTHETICS

Anatomical Placement and the Target Cells

Depending on their location in patient's eye, retinal implants are categorized as epiretinal, subretinal, or suprachoroidal (Fig. 1C).

Epiretinal Implants

In the "epiretinal" approach, electrodes are placed on top of the inner limiting membrane, targeting primarily the RGCs (Fig. 1C; Ahuja et al. 2011; Humayun et al. 2012). Epiretinal stimulation is less dependent on the health of the inner retinal neurons and can operate as long as the RGCs are alive. Since the action potential is a binary response, modulating the stimulus amplitude, or duration above the threshold does not affect the amplitude of the elicited spike, and hence a more appropriate modulation strategy for RGCs is by controlling the stimulation timing, frequency, and burst duration. RGCs can generally respond to stimuli at frequencies of at least 100 Hz (Sekirnjak et al. 2006; Cai et al. 2011), thus enabling generation of naturalistic spike trains by direct electrical activation (Jepson et al. 2014).

A major issue with epiretinal activation of RGCs is axonal stimulation (Weitz et al. 2015; Grosberg et al. 2017). Even though the RGC stimulation threshold at the axon initial segment can be three times lower than the axonal threshold (Werginz et al. 2020), axons from distant cells in the nerve fiber layer, passing between the stimulating electrodes and the ganglion cells, may get activated, resulting in arcuate visual percepts (Nanduri et al. 2012). This effect, leading to distortion of the retinotopic map, remains a major hurdle for epiretinal implants. One approach for circumventing the problem of axonal stimulation is based on the use of much longer (>20 msec) pulses to stimulate the bipolar rather than ganglion cells (Weitz et al. 2015). Doing so significantly improved the localization of phosphenes in patients; however, it precludes encoding the retinal output by direct stimulation of RGCs at high frequencies. Another approach is based on careful measurements of the local stimulation threshold under each electrode using a bidirectional implant and avoiding the electrodes that activate remote cells (Shah et al. 2019). Epiretinal implants that aim at restoring the natural visual code in specific types of RGCs (Fried et al. 2006; Jepson et al. 2014) should activate individual neurons without affecting the surrounding cells. Different RGC types were found to have somewhat different activation thresholds (Fried et al. 2009), likely due to differences in the Na channels and other anatomical or physiological properties. However, selective activation of RGCs is quite challenging: only ~7% of cells could be activated selectively even in the peripheral primate retina (Grosberg et al. 2017), while in the central macula it is even harder due to multilayered RGCs and denser axonal bundles.

Another challenge with direct encoding of the proper spiking patterns in various RGCs is identification of the cell types in the degenerate retina (Chichilnisky and Kalmar 2002). Instead of light responses, proposed cell classification is based on electrical signatures of the RGC spontaneous activity, including their electrophysiological images and autocorrelation functions (Richard et al. 2015). Applicability of this method to a degenerate retina, where spontaneous firing patterns become abnormal, remains to be tested. Another issue with an abnormally high spontaneous firing rate of RGCs frequently observed in animal models of retinal degeneration (Sekirnjak et al. 2011) is that it may diminish the corresponding perception or impede the ability of the implant to encode a desired spikes sequence.

Typically, implantation of the epiretinal devices involves vitrectomy and attachment of the implant to the retina using retinal tacks. In some epiretinal implants, such as Argus, antennae and data processors are placed outside the eyeball, under the conjunctiva, connected to the intra-

ocular part by a transscleral cable (da Cruz et al. 2013).

Subretinal Implants

In the "subretinal" approach, arrays of electrodes placed between the pigment epithelium and the INL replace the degenerated photoreceptors and target primarily the surviving BCs (Fig. 1C; Zrenner et al. 2011; Lorach et al. 2015). In nonspiking neurons, stronger stimuli can be encoded with higher amplitude or longer pulses. Output signals from BCs are then transmitted via synapses to RGCs, which convert them into the action potential trains. This approach retains some of the remaining signal-processing properties of the retinal network, and hence the spiking patterns elicited in RGCs resemble those observed in normal retina. However, changes in the retinal network during degeneration may impact the retinal signal processing, and therefore alter the encoding of the visual information. To elicit a steady percept using pulsatile stimulation, its frequency should exceed that of flicker fusion (Lorach et al. 2015; Ho et al. 2019; Palanker et al. 2020). In BCs, this occurs at frequencies exceeding ~30–60 Hz due to accumulation of Ca in the axonal terminals and due to temporal filtering properties of the glutamate vesicles release (Werginz et al. 2020).

Implantation of the subretinal arrays in human patients involves formation of a local retinal detachment induced by subretinal injection of fluid, followed by a small retinal incision through which the device is inserted into the subretinal space, ending with the retinal reattachment (Palanker et al. 2020). In the case of wired subretinal implants, large areas of the retina are typically detached during implantation, which is a significant challenge with fragile diseased retinas. Excessively traumatic implantations can lead to fibrosis and scarring.

In a "suprachoroidal" approach, the device is inserted into the sclera below the choroid (Fig. 1C). While this approach is assumed to be surgically less risky than the epi- and subretinal prostheses (Fujikado et al. 2011; Ayton et al. 2014), the larger distance between the stimulating electrodes and the target neurons greatly limits the attainable selectivity of retinal stimulation and the spatial resolution. Therefore, such implants have large (~1 mm) electrodes and are placed in the periphery of the visual field to help with low-resolution tasks, primarily for ambulation (Kolic et al. 2020).

Delivery of Power and Data to the Implant

Transmission of power and data to the implant is an engineering challenge since direct transcutaneous wiring of an implant to external electronics is prone to infections and severe scarring (Knutson et al. 2002). Therefore, transfer of power and information to modern implants is done wirelessly, using the following approaches: (1) delivery of data and power through radiofrequency (RF) coils, (2) optical delivery of data with power transmission through RF coils, or (3) optical transmission of data and power to the implant.

Several retinal implant systems use serial telemetry for data transmission: the Argus II (Second Sight Medical Systems, Sylmar, CA), shown in Figure 2, IRIS II (Hornig et al. 2017), a suprachoroidal device (Ayton et al. 2014), and the Boston Retinal Implant (Rizzo et al. 2011). Increasing the number of electrodes to thousands in the coil-based designs is rather difficult since (1) it requires a very wide bandwidth, and (2) wiring of a large number of electrodes makes the feedthrough connector rather bulky and the cable quite rigid. Multiplexing the signals on the retinal implant itself would reduce the required number of wires, but it adds electronics to the implant, which affects its heating, weight, size, and flexibility.

Another option is transmission of power via RF coils, and the data—via a serial optical link from the glasses to the implant—as was done in the IRIS II system (Pixium Vision, Paris, France)

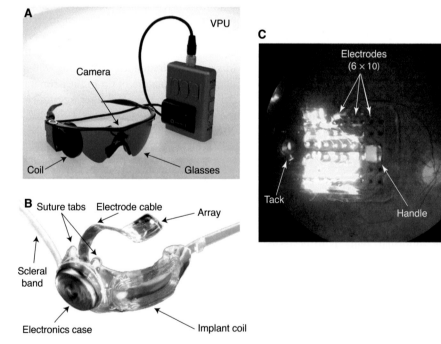

Figure 2. The Argus II epiretinal system. (*A*) External portion of the Argus II, including glasses with a video camera, radiofrequency (RF) coil, and a video processing unit (VPU). (*B*) The implantable portion of Argus II, including the implant RF coil, the electronics case, and the electrode array. (*C*) Fundus photo of an Argus II implant in the macula. A retinal tack attaches the electrode array to the sclera. A white handle is used for positioning the device in the eye. (All figure panels are reprinted from Humayun et al. 2012, with permission from Elsevier © 2012.)

(Hornig et al. 2017). Since the optical data-transmission rate is typically much higher than with RF, more information can be delivered to the implant.

In both approaches, the visual information is transmitted to the implant via serial telemetry, and hence it does not depend on eye movements. Since the brain expects images to shift on the retina with eye movements, static patterns with such retinal implants are perceived as moving objects. Similar phenomena have been reported with cortical visual prostheses (Naumann 2012). To avoid this effect, patients are asked to keep their gaze steady and scan the visual field with the head-mounted cameras—a very unnatural paradigm. Such problems can be alleviated by incorporating an eye tracking, which can shift the images on the implant according to the direction of gaze (Caspi et al. 2018).

A few designs have been proposed for power delivery through RF coupling and transmission of the visual information through the eye optics (Woodburn et al. 2002; Loudin et al. 2007; Zrenner et al. 2011; Ha et al. 2016). The best known was the Alpha IMS/AMS (Retina Implant AG, Reutlingen, Germany) shown in Figure 3. The subretinal implant includes photodiodes with amplifiers and stimulating electrodes in each pixel, which convert the incident images into electrical current flowing through the retina. Such optical implants naturally couple the eye movements to the stimulation pattern on the implant. The subdermal power-receiving coil with electronics placed behind the ear was connected to the subretinal implant via a transscleral cable (Stingl et al. 2017), which makes the implantation procedure difficult and prone to complications, and the feedthrough connector to the moving implant remains a challenging engineering problem (Daschner et al. 2017).

The third category of retinal implants receives both the power and data by light, via natural eye optics (Fig. 4; Mathieson et al. 2012; Ghezzi et al. 2013). Such photovoltaic implants directly convert incident light into electric current to stimulate the nearby neurons (Palanker et al. 2005; Mathieson et al. 2012; Lorach et al. 2015). To provide sufficient current for retinal stimulation, intense illumination is projected from a near-the-eye display (Goetz et al. 2013). To avoid the photophobic and phototoxic effects of bright light, invisible near-infrared (880–915 nm) wavelengths are used. Instead of silicon photodiodes, photovoltaic elements based on light-sensitive polymers have also been proposed (Ghezzi et al. 2013). Since photovoltaic systems do not require cables (Mathieson et al. 2012; Lorach et al. 2015), the implantation procedure is greatly simplified. Implants can be composed of several modules to tile the visual field. These modules can be inserted into the subretinal space via a smaller incision and follow the eye curvature, making the surgery less traumatic than with a single larger implant (Lee et al. 2016).

PRECLINICAL EVALUATION OF PROSTHETIC VISION

Retinal Response to Electric Stimulation

Electric Receptive Fields

RGC receptive fields characterize the spatial extent sampled by individual ganglion cells. With prosthetic stimulation, it characterizes the combined point spread function of the implant and of the retinal neural network (Sim et al. 2014; Lorach et al. 2015). Spatiotemporal properties of RGCs can be assessed from the spike-triggered average responses to various stimuli in healthy and degenerate retina using a multielectrode array ex vivo (Ho et al. 2018a). The average photovoltaic receptive field size with 70 μm pixels was found to be similar to that of the natural visual responses: 191 μm versus 228 μm, respectively (Fig. 5A,B). Both the natural and photovoltaic receptive fields in healthy retina had an antagonistic center-surround organization (Ho et al. 2018a). In healthy retina, ON RGCs exhibited photovoltaic OFF responses, and vice versa (Fig. 5A,B). This reversal is consistent with depolarization of the photoreceptor terminals by subretinal anodic stimuli, as opposed to their hyperpolarization under light. In the degenerate rat retina, both ON and OFF photovoltaic responses were also observed: ON—primarily in RGCs with low spontaneous firing rate and OFF—in

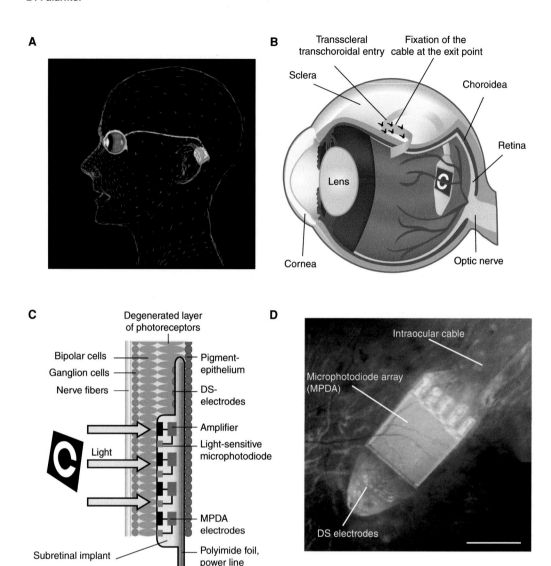

Figure 3. The Alpha IMS subretinal system. (*A*) A cable from the radiofrequency (RF) receiver implanted behind the ear runs under the temporal muscle, through the sclera, to the implanted chip under the retina. (*B*) A power cable from the implant exits the eye 3 mm behind the limbus. (*C*) Pixels with photodiodes, amplifiers, and electrodes are located between the pigment epithelium and the inner nuclear layer. (*D*) View of the subretinal implant through a pupil. Scale bar, 3 mm, corresponding to 10° of the visual angle. (Panels *B*, *C*, and *D* reprinted from Zrenner et al. 2011 under the terms of the Creative Commons Attribution License.)

cells with high spontaneous firing (Ho et al. 2018b). Despite the disconnected horizontal cells, the degenerate retina maintained the antagonistic center-surround organization of the receptive fields under electrical stimulation, most likely due to lateral inhibition by amacrine cells, as in healthy retina (Fig. 5C,D).

Lateral Resolution

One of the most important characteristics of vision in general and of prosthetic sight, in particular, is the visual acuity. In healthy rats, visual acuity is approximately 1 cpd (cycle per degree), which corresponds to about 28 μm on the retina

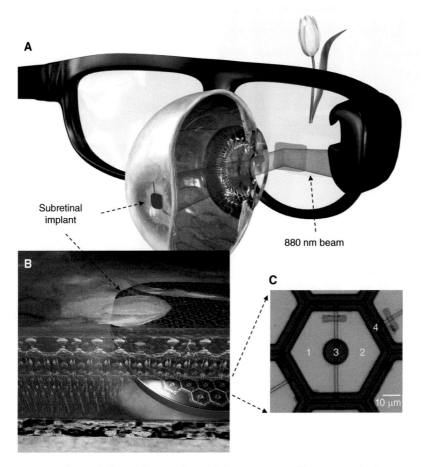

Figure 4. PRIMA: a subretinal photovoltaic implant. (*A*) Images captured by a camera in the augmented-reality glasses are processed and projected into the eye using pulsed near infrared (880 nm) light. (*B*) Pixels in the 30-μm-thick subretinal implant convert incident light into electric current flowing through the retina to stimulate the bipolar cells. (*C*) A 55 μm pixel is composed of two diodes (1 and 2) connected in a series between the active (3) and return (4) electrodes. Scale bar, 10 μm.

(Harnois et al. 1984). This is much smaller than the average size of the RGC receptive fields in rats (~200 μm) (Lorach et al. 2015). The difference might be due to nonlinear spatial integration of BC subunits connected to the same ganglion cell RGCs, which allows detecting much finer structures over their receptive fields (Caldwell and Daw 1978; Thibos and Levick 1983; Demb et al. 1999; Brown et al. 2000; Passaglia et al. 2002; Petrusca et al. 2007; Heine and Passaglia 2011; Schwartz et al. 2012). This feature is preserved with subretinal electrical stimulation (Lorach et al. 2015). Spatial resolution measured with alternating gratings projected onto the sub-

retinal photovoltaic pixels of 75 μm and 55 μm in size matched the row pitch of the hexagonal array: 65 μm (Lorach et al. 2015) and 48 μm (Ho et al. 2019), respectively.

Contrast Sensitivity

Similar multiple electrode array (MEA) measurements of the retinal response to steps in irradiance demonstrated the contrast threshold of ±12% with photovoltaic stimulation in the degenerate retinas, as opposed to ±2.3% with visible light in healthy retinas (Ho et al. 2018b). Interestingly, observed decrease of the

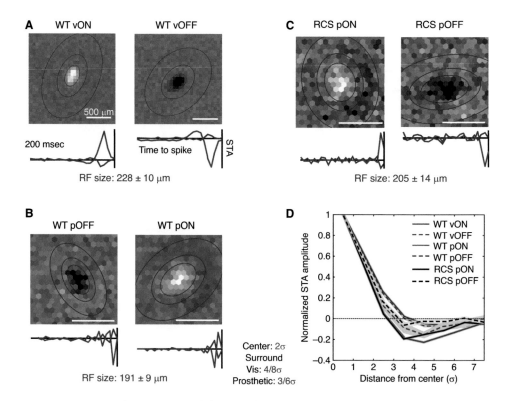

Figure 5. Center-surround organization of the natural and prosthetic receptive fields. (*A*) The visual spike-triggered average (STA) receptive fields of the ON and OFF retinal ganglion cell (RGC) in the healthy rat retina. The time courses for center and for surround are shown at the *bottom*. (*B*) Receptive fields and the time courses for photovoltaic response in the healthy rat retina. The vON cells become pOFF, and vOFF cells—pON. (*C*) Similar receptive field maps and the center and surround time courses for pON and pOFF RGCs in a degenerate rat retina (RCS). (*D*) The average STA response amplitude, normalized to the deflection in the most central bin versus distance from the center of the receptive field, measured in standard deviations of the 2D Gaussian fit to the STA receptive field. Visual and photovoltaic OFF responses were inverted for ease of comparison.

contrast sensitivity by a factor of 5 in prosthetic vision is similar in magnitude to the natural contrast enhancement between the photoreceptors and BCs (Burkhardt and Fahey 1998), which is absent in the degenerate retina. Loss of this contrast enhancement can be compensated by image processing prior to its delivery to a subretinal implant.

In Vivo Characterization of Prosthetic Vision

Common characteristics of vision, such as resolution, contrast sensitivity, and dynamic range, have been studied extensively with retinal implants (Behrend et al. 2011; Lorach et al. 2015; Ho et al. 2018a,b, 2019). Perception of motion, thought to be transmitted to the brain by the

magnocellular-projecting parasol cells in the primate visual system (Newsome et al. 1985; Merigan and Maunsell 1993), has also been explored with epiretinal implants. Promising results were reported with elicitation of naturalistic motion stimuli in the primate retina (Jepson et al. 2014).

Studies in vivo begin with implantation of the devices in an adequate animal model, such as a subretinal photovoltaic prosthesis in rats (Mandel et al. 2013) for example. In this case, surgery begins with a scleral incision, followed by a retinal detachment using injection of saline. The implant is then slid into the gap, which is subsequently sutured. Integration of the device into the subretinal space can be evaluated by retinal imaging, including optical coherence tomography (OCT), fundus imaging, and fluorescein angiography.

To characterize prosthetic vision, visually evoked potentials (VEPs), can be measured via transcranial screw electrodes implanted over the visual cortex. Corneal signals can help evaluate the electric current produced by individual pixels (Lorach et al. 2015). Behavioral measurements have also been used in assessment of the stimulation thresholds, contrast sensitivity, ON and OFF responses, and other characteristics of vision (Prevot et al. 2017; Ho et al. 2018b).

Lateral Resolution

Natural and prosthetic visual acuity was studied in rats by recording the VEPs in response to alternating gratings (Fig. 6). This method matches well the visual acuity measured in behavioral tests of natural vision (Dean 1981; Silveira et al. 1987). Grating acuity measured with subretinal photovoltaic pixels of 75 μm (Lorach et al. 2015), 55 μm (Ho et al. 2019), and 40 μm (Wang et al. 2022) in size matched the row pitch of the hexagonal arrays. However, with 20 μm

pixels, prosthetic acuity did not exceed their natural level of 28 μm, indicating that the limiting factor became the retinal signal integration (Wang et al. 2022).

Behavioral tests of subretinal photovoltaic implants PRIMA (Pixium Vision, Paris, France), based on saccadic response to stimulation with 140 μm pixels in nonhuman primates, demonstrated perceptual thresholds of 0.2 mW/mm^2 with 10 msec pulses (Prevot et al. 2017), similar to the earlier observations in RCS rats (Ho et al. 2018b). These measurements also demonstrated visual response with a spot size down to a single pixel.

Contrast Sensitivity

For behavioral measurements of contrast sensitivity, RCS rats with photovoltaic subretinal implants were placed in cages surrounded by near infrared (NIR) displays. Bursts of pulses at various irradiance levels and durations were applied at 20 Hz frequency for 2 sec. Rats' startling response to changes in lighting revealed the average contrast threshold of 12%, as compared to

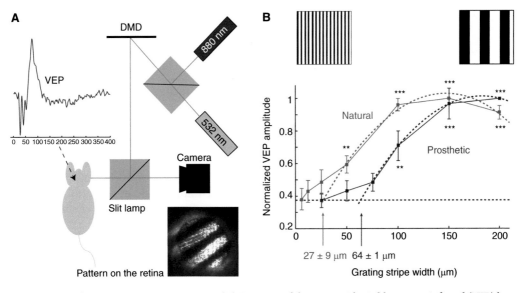

Figure 6. Visual acuity measurements in vivo. (*A*) Diagram of the setup with visible or near infrared (NIR) laser illumination of a digital micromirror device (DMD) imaged onto the retina. Visual evoked potential (VEP) signals are recorded from three transcranial electrodes. (*B*) Amplitude of the VEP in response to alternating gratings decreases with the decreasing stripe width, and acuity is defined as an intersection of the extrapolated fit with the noise level.

2.3% with visible light stimulation in healthy controls (Long–Evans rats) matching the ex vivo results described above (Ho et al. 2018b).

Frequency Dependence

Amplitude of the rat VEP in response to pulsatile stimulation decreased with frequency for both the subretinal prosthetic and natural vision in a similar manner: it decreased by half at 10 Hz, compared to 2 Hz, and became practically undetectable at 60 Hz (Ho et al. 2019). Human tests of prosthetic vision with subretinal photovoltaic array, described below, confirmed the flicker fusion between 30 and 60 Hz (Palanker et al. 2020).

CLINICAL EVALUATION

Prosthetic vision in human patients is assessed by a wide variety of psychophysical methods. Several companies and research consortia have reached the clinical phase, thereby providing invaluable evidence that implants can elicit meaningful visual percepts in patients blinded by retinal degenerations. In this section, we review the current status and clinical outcomes with several retinal prostheses.

Criteria for Evaluating Prosthetic Vision

The nonbinding FDA recommendations for assessment of the visual function were issued as a part of their investigational device exemption (IDE) guidance for retinal prostheses (Cohen and Lepri 2013). The suggested tests include the following: (1) low vision letter acuity with limited response time; (2) grating acuity using a forced-choice paradigm and fixed presentation time; (3) mapping of stimulated visual phosphene fields, including two-point discrimination; and (4) assessment of form vision and functional vision in real-world situations, including orientation and mobility. The Second Sight Medical Implants (Sylmar, CA) introduced a set of low vision tests, called FLORA (Functional Low-Vision Observer Rated Assessment), for their Argus II retinal prosthesis trial (Ho et al. 2015). More recently, another set of tests and

measurement methodologies was suggested by a group of investigators working on prosthetic vision (Ayton et al. 2020).

Reports on prosthetic light perception in the other clinical trials describe the perceived brightness, shape, and color of the elicited phosphenes (Ayton et al. 2014; Stingl et al. 2015). In addition to the grating visual acuity, some patients could distinguish Landolt C optotypes and letters. Some reports include temporal characteristics of prosthetic vision and detection of motion.

The Argus II Epiretinal Prosthesis

The only retinal prosthesis approved for commercial use by the FDA (as a humanitarian use device) was the Argus II epiretinal prosthetic system (Second Sight Medical Products, Sylmar, CA). Its head-mounted unit includes a video camera and an RF antenna, which transmits the data and power to the intraocular receiver via serial telemetry (Fig. 2). The signals are then decoded and processed inside the implant, before being distributed via a transscleral cable to the 60 stimulating electrodes on a flexible epiretinal array. Electrodes are 200 μm in diameter, arranged in a square grid with a 575 μm pitch (da Cruz et al. 2016). The array was floating, on average, at 180 μm above the retina (Ahuja et al. 2013). The Argus II has been implanted in more than 200 RP patients, with the best reported grating visual acuity of 20/1260 (Ho et al. 2015). Serious adverse events (SAEs) reported over the course of the clinical trial affected ~30% of the patients, the majority (82%) of which occurred within the first 6 mo. The most common occurrences included conjunctival erosion and dehiscence over the extraocular implant (Ho et al. 2015). No device failures were reported within 3 yr after implantation (Ho et al. 2015).

All patients in the Argus II trial perceived light with the implant turned ON, and almost all subjects performed better at the square localization test with the implant ON than without it. Only 57% of the patients improved in detection of the direction of motion with the system ON versus OFF. Improvements in orientation and mobility with the system was also reported by the clinical trial, but in other studies, a significantly worse performance at spatial orientation tasks with the implant was observed (Garcia et al. 2014). One reason for this discrepancy could be that prosthetic visual percepts interfered with patient's natural orientation habits, including tactile and auditory perception. Alternatively, Argus II could complicate the spatial orientation since its visual percepts are unrelated to the direction of gaze. Adding the eye tracking with the corresponding shift of the images on the implant indeed improved the object localization (Caspi et al. 2018).

A significant problem with the Argus II epiretinal implant is the stimulation of axons passing near the electrodes from remote RGCs. Percepts induced by axonal stimulation have arcuate rather than punctate shapes (Behrend et al. 2011; Nanduri et al. 2012), which severely distorts a retinotopic map of the visual field. One solution to this problem can be in application of much longer pulses (>25 msec instead of the typical 0.5–1 msec) to activate the BCs rather than ganglion cells, thereby evoking the network-mediated retinal responses without an axonal stimulation (Weitz et al. 2015).

None of the RP patients with Argus II gained vision to the extent that would allow ambulation without a white cane or a guide dog. In March 2019, Second Sight closed the Argus II project, and turned its focus to the cortical visual prosthesis, called Orion (Beauchamp et al. 2020).

The Subretinal Implant Alpha IMS/AMS

The subretinal approach has been spearheaded by the Retina Implant AG (Reutlingen, Germany) with their Alpha IMS system (Zrenner et al. 2011), which received CE mark in 2013. In this device, a subretinal chip with light-sensitive pixels and amplifiers converts images projected naturally by ambient light onto the retina into electrical currents that flow through the retina and stimulate the inner retinal neurons (Fig. 3).

This implant includes 1600 (40×40) pixels of $70 \times 70 \ \mu m^2$ in size, each having a photodiode, an amplifier, and a 30 μm diameter TiN or SIROF electrode arranged into an array of 2.8×2.8 mm in size, corresponding to a visual field of 9.3° (Fig. 3). Biphasic pulses (cathodic phase first) ranging from 0.1 to 2.0 msec in duration are applied at frequencies of 0.5–500 Hz to all electrodes. Patients could adjust the photodiode sensitivity and the maximum current according to the ambient lighting conditions and the individual retinal response (Stingl et al. 2017; Daschner et al. 2018). The return electrode, common to all the pixels, is located at the power supply behind the ear. Power is delivered to the implant via a cable that runs under the retina, crossing the sclera pars-plana, and then subdermally to an implant located behind the ear, where power is transmitted via an RF coil (Fig. 3), as in the cochlear implants.

The detection, localization, and counting of objects was significantly better with the implant ON than OFF in 13 out of 15 RP patients in a trial. With foveal placement of the implant ($n = 8$), functional outcomes were significantly better than with parafoveal ($n = 12$): 75% of the patients with foveal location of the chip distinguished a direction of motion, while none of the patients with nonfoveal placement could accomplish this task (Stingl et al. 2013). Two patients could detect Landolt C at 20/546 acuity, which is about half of the Nyquist sampling limit for 70 μm pixels (20/280). Twelve patients demonstrated a grating acuity ranging from between 0.1 and 3.3 cpd (Stingl et al. 2017), and 4.6 ± 0.8 gray levels could be distinguished, on average.

The eye movements of RP patients without stimulation were large and scanning. However, with the implant ON, they significantly improved: patients could fixate well and they exhibited the classic fixational movement patterns, such as ocular tremor, drift, and microsaccades (Hafed et al. 2016).

The majority of the Alpha IMS implants failed within a year postimplantation, while half of the Alpha AMS devices failed within 30 mo (Daschner et al. 2018). In March 2019, Retina Implant AG closed.

A Photovoltaic Subretinal Implant PRIMA

The photovoltaic PRIMA implant (Pixium Vision, Paris) is designed for restoration of central vision in patients impaired by GA in AMD.

Photodiodes in each pixel convert light into biphasic (anodic first) pulses of electric current (Lorach et al. 2015). The implant used in the first feasibility trial was 2 × 2 mm in width (corresponding to about 7° of the visual field), 30 μm thick, with 378 pixels of 100 μm in size (Palanker et al. 2020). Images captured by the camera are processed and projected from the augmented-reality (AR) glasses into an 18° wide field on the retina. To avoid photophobic and phototoxic effects of bright illumination, NIR (880 nm) light is applied (Fig. 4; Goetz et al. 2013). For a steady perception under pulsed illumination, frequencies exceeding the flicker fusion are applied (30–60 Hz). Perceptual brightness is adjusted by modulating the pulse duration in a DMD display of the AR glasses from 0.7 to 10 msec.

The first feasibility study was conducted in five patients with GA of at least three optic disc diameters and a visual acuity 20/400–20/1000 in the worse-seeing "study" eye. Residual natural acuity due to preserved peripheral vision and eccentric fixation did not decrease after the implantation in any of the patients, demonstrating the safety and stability of the submacular chip, with a follow-up period now exceeding 36 mo. Prosthetic vision was initially tested using the virtual-reality glasses (PRIMA-1), and then with augmented-reality glasses (PRIMA-2).

All five patients perceived monochromatic (white-yellowish "sun color") patterns with the brightness adjustable by pulse duration in the range of 0.7–10 msec in retinotopically correct locations within the previous scotomata. All four patients with a subretinal placement of the chip demonstrated Landolt C acuity of 1.17 ± 0.13 pixels, corresponding to the Snellen range of 20/438–20/564 (Palanker et al. 2020, 2022). Such a close match of prosthetic acuity to the pixel size indicates that smaller pixels may provide even higher resolution and hence offer real benefits to a larger number of patients. Remarkably, patients perceive simultaneously the prosthetic central vision and peripheral natural vision in the treated and in the fellow eye (Palanker et al. 2022).

Interestingly, despite the lack of selectivity in stimulation of the ON and OFF BCs, patients perceive the displayed images in a correct contrast: for example, as light patterns on a dark background, and not as a mixture of the bright and dark spots. One reason could be that the rod BCs have only the ON pathway, split into ON and OFF RGCs via amacrine cells, so there should be no polarity reversal upon electrical stimulation here. Similarly, the ON-cone pathway should preserve the polarity of the RGC response under electrical stimulation. The OFF-cone pathway is expected to be reversed in electrical stimulation, but its input into the visual system may be attenuated by the low signal-to-noise ratio since spontaneous firing in OFF-RGCs greatly increases in retinal degeneration (Sekirnjak et al. 2011; Denlinger et al. 2020). Another potential difference is the fact that ON BCs have longer axons than the OFF BCs (Euler et al. 2014) and therefore should experience a larger voltage step across the cell in a similar electric field, yielding a stronger response than the OFF BCs.

A noticeable difference between the prosthetic and natural vision is a slower than normal image recognition, even when resolution is not a limiting factor. This might be due to a lower number of BCs activated electrically than naturally due to the limited penetration depth of electric field into the INL. Reduced flow of the visual information may be compensated by longer integration (Ho et al. 2020).

Suprachoroidal Systems

A suprachoroidal placement of the electrode array has been tested by Bionic Vision Australia (three patients) (Ayton et al. 2014) and by a group in Osaka University (two patients) (Fujikado et al. 2011). Phosphene perception in RP patients was reported over the 12-month Bionic Vision trial, but the equivalent visual acuity was in the realm of ultralow vision, ranging from 20/4000 to 20/20,000. Its utility for ambulation and object localization remains to be explored (Kolic et al. 2020).

Other Clinical Results

Optobionics Inc. conducted a clinical trial of their subretinal array of photodiodes (artificial silicon retina [ASR]). They reported improvements in central vision following implantation of the ASR in the periphery, possibly due to neurotrophic effects of surgery or of the implant (Chow et al. 2004). The company closed in 2007. The EPIRET3—an epiretinal array of 25 electrodes of 100 μm in diameter spaced 500 μm apart (Klauke et al. 2011), implanted in six patients for a period of 4 wk, successfully elicited visual percepts. However, the studies did not continue beyond 2010. Clinical trials of the IRIS II epiretinal implant with 150 electrodes have been conducted by Pixium Vision (Muqit et al. 2019). Patients reported some visual percepts, but the trial was discontinued in 2017.

In early 2020, Nano Retina started a clinical trial of their NR600 epiretinal implant in patients with advanced RP. Wireless implant includes a camera, image processor, and an array of 600 electrodes spaced by 100 μm and penetrating by about 100 μm into the retina. Implant is powered by NIR light emitted from the glasses (Nano Retina [Yanovitch et al. 2022]). First reports of the clinical outcomes include localization of a square of light on a screen, and the ability to follow a white line on the floor.

SUMMARY AND OUTLOOK

The first two companies that tested an idea of electronic restoration of sight in patients blinded by inherited retinal degeneration (RP) using epiretinal (Second Sight) and subretinal (Retina Implant AG) implants have proven the concept. However, since they failed to reach satisfactory performance, both products were discontinued in 2019, after about 20 yr of development. Commercialization of such a complex technology for a relatively small market is one of the challenges, and therefore such projects are usually undertaken by consortiums of academic research groups and commercial companies. The next generation of implants and stimulation protocols is designed to address some of the shortcomings of the first systems.

On a subretinal side, the wireless nature of the photovoltaic implant PRIMA enables its application to AMD patients, where retinal network is better preserved than in the end-stage RP. In addition, local return electrodes in PRIMA pixels provide much better confinement of electric field than with a remote return, thereby improving contrast, selectivity, and resolution of retinal stimulation (Palanker et al. 2022). The next challenge is to reduce the pixel size down to 25 μm and achieve acuity of 20/100, which would provide real benefit to many AMD patients. Iridium Medical Technology (www.irmedtech.com/Advantage/index_en.html) is developing a flexible retinal implant to cover a wide visual field, essential for ambulation of RP patients.

On the epiretinal side, an implant for selective activation of the many classes of RGCs with the appropriate retinal code is being developed for the end-stage RP patients (Shah and Chichilnisky 2020). A group of D. Ghezzy at EPFL is developing a flexible epiretinal implant to cover a wide visual field, essential for ambulation of RP patients (Woodburn et al. 2002; Chenais et al. 2021), as described below.

Electric Field Shaping for High Resolution in Subretinal Approach

Distance between the implant and the target neurons becomes a limiting factor when it exceeds the electrode size or a separation between the active and return electrodes (Fig. 7A; Palanker et al. 2005; Loudin et al. 2007; Flores et al. 2019). Since the INL thickness is ~30–40 μm, planar bipolar implants with local return electrodes and pixel pitch smaller than 60 μm (30 μm radius) are unlikely to stimulate all the neurons in the INL within the safe charge injection limits (Flores et al. 2019).

One way to improve the proximity to the target neurons is to use three-dimensional electrodes, such as pillars and honeycombs, using retinal migration into the voids (Fig. 7B,C). Recent measurements with 40 and 55 μm pixels in rats demonstrated that 10 μm tall pillar electrodes reduce the stimulation threshold by half (Ho et al. 2019). Honeycombs are expected to provide even bigger benefit since the insulating walls between the pixels direct the electric field vertically, along the BCs in the retina, and thereby decreasing the stimulation threshold (Flores et al. 2019). These walls also decouple the field penetration depth from the pixel width, making

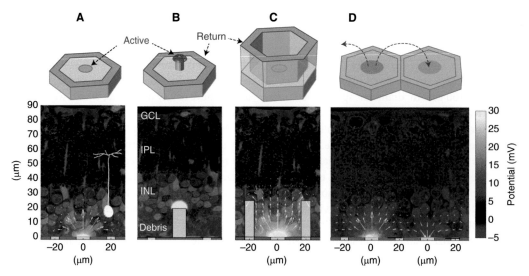

Figure 7. Electric field shaping strategies. (*A*) As flat bipolar pixels decrease in size, penetration of electric field into the retina becomes insufficient for stimulation of the bipolar cells (diagrammatically shown in white on *top* of the retinal histology). (*B,C*) Within a few weeks postimplantation, cells in the inner nuclear layer (INL) migrate into the voids between the pillars or walls in the subretinal implant, thereby getting closer to the active electrodes. (*C*) With a return electrode on top of the walls, an electric field is aligned vertically, along the bipolar cells. Since the field penetration depth is decoupled from the pixel width, stimulation threshold does not change with the pixel size. (*D*) Current steering, with some pixels serving as anodes and some as cathodes intermittently, enables field shaping for optimal lateral and axial confinement. (GCL) Ganglion cell layer, (IPL) inner plexiform layer.

the stimulation threshold independent of pixel width.

Yet another possibility for the optimal field confinement is a current steering, where active electrodes can be used as anodes and as cathodes intermittently (Fig. 7D). Such a strategy may allow optimizing the electric field penetration depth and lateral confinement for every patient, depending on the retinal thickness and its proximity to the implant (Wang et al. 2022).

Selective Stimulation of RGCs

A group called "Artificial Retina," led by Dr. Chichilnisky at Stanford, is working on a device for selective activation of RGCs to mimic the natural retinal code for proper restoration of sight (Shah and Chichilnisky 2020). During the initial calibration, the epiretinal implant will record and identify the many distinct RGC types based on characteristics of their spontaneous firing. The implant will then activate the appropriate ganglion cells at the appropriate times, effectively trans-

forming the captured visual scene into the proper spiking sequence of the various cells.

Flexible Implants for a Wide Visual Field

For a comfortable ambulation of the patients blinded by RP, the prosthetic visual field should exceed 20°, which corresponds to 6 mm length on the retina. To ensure proximity to the retina over such a large area, implants should follow the eye curvature. Two groups are working on wide flexible implants to address this need: an epiretinal array based on organic photodiodes (Polyretina) (Chenais et al. 2021), and a subretinal device based on flexible CMOS electronics (Iridium Medical) (Woodburn et al. 2002).

Image Processing

In addition to improvements in esthetic appearance and in optical performance of the virtual and augmented reality glasses, prosthetic vision may advance with applications of advanced image processing. Besides the obvious functions, such as optical or electronic zoom, contrast enhancement, and autofocus of the camera, visual scenes could be simplified prior to projection onto the implant, which would help better match its resolution and contrast and make the visual percepts easier to understand. Computer algorithms rapidly advance at visual categorization (e.g., segregation of the visual content by distance and displaying only the closer objects [Jung et al. 2015]) or by encoding the depth instead of luminance to facilitate navigation (Hicks et al. 2014) have been recently demonstrated. Other improvements may include simplified or symbolic representation of common objects, such as banknotes, as well as integration of the other assistive technologies, such as text-to-voice conversion, face recognition, etc.

REFERENCES

Ahuja AK, Dorn JD, Caspi A, McMahon MJ, Dagnelie G, Dacruz L, Stanga P, Humayun MS, Greenberg RJ. 2011. Blind subjects implanted with the Argus II retinal prosthesis are able to improve performance in a spatial-motor task. *Br J Ophthalmol* **95:** 539–543. doi:10.1136/bjo.2010 .179622

Ahuja AK, Yeoh J, Dorn JD, Caspi A, Wuyyuru V, McMahon MJ, Humayun MS, Greenberg RJ, Dacruz L. 2013. Factors affecting perceptual threshold in Argus II retinal prosthesis subjects. *Transl Vis Sci Technol* **2:** 1. doi:10 .1167/tvst.2.4.1

Ayton LN, Blamey PJ, Guymer RH, Luu CD, Nayagam DA, Sinclair NC, Shivdasani MN, Yeoh J, McCombe MF, Briggs RJ, et al. 2014. First-in-human trial of a novel suprachoroidal retinal prosthesis. *PLoS ONE* **9:** e115239. doi:10.1371/journal.pone.0115239

Ayton LN, Rizzo JF, Bailey IL, Colenbrander A, Dagnelie G, Geruschat DR, Hessburg PC, McCarthy CD, Petoe MA, Rubin GS, et al. 2020. Harmonization of outcomes and vision endpoints in vision restoration trials: recommendations from the International HOVER Taskforce. *Transl Vis Sci Technol* **9:** 25. doi:10.1167/tvst.9.8.25

Beauchamp MS, Oswalt D, Sun P, Foster BL, Magnotti JF, Niketeghad S, Pouratian N, Bosking WH, Yoshor D. 2020. Dynamic stimulation of visual cortex produces form vision in sighted and blind humans. *Cell* **181:** 774–783.e5. doi:10.1016/j.cell.2020.04.033

Behrend MR, Ahuja AK, Humayun MS, Chow RH, Weiland JD. 2011. Resolution of the epiretinal prosthesis is not limited by electrode size. *IEEE Trans Neural Syst Rehabil Eng* **19:** 436–442. doi:10.1109/TNSRE.2011.2140132

Boinagrov D, Loudin J, Palanker D. 2010. Strength-duration relationship for extracellular neural stimulation: numerical and analytical models. *J Neurophysiol* **104:** 2236–2248. doi:10.1152/jn.00343.2010

Boinagrov D, Pangratz-Fuehrer S, Goetz G, Palanker D. 2014. Selectivity of direct and network-mediated stimulation of the retinal ganglion cells with epi-, sub- and intraretinal electrodes. *J Neural Eng* **11:** 026008. doi:10 .1088/1741-2560/11/2/026008

Brown SP, He S, Masland RH. 2000. Receptive field microstructure and dendritic geometry of retinal ganglion cells. *Neuron* **27:** 371–383. doi:10.1016/S0896-6273(00) 00044-1

Burkhardt DA, Fahey PK. 1998. Contrast enhancement and distributed encoding by bipolar cells in the retina. *J Neurophysiol* **80:** 1070–1081. doi:10.1152/jn.1998.80.3.1070

Cai C, Ren Q, Desai NJ, Rizzo JF III, Fried SI. 2011. Response variability to high rates of electric stimulation in retinal ganglion cells. *J Neurophysiol* **106:** 153–162. doi:10.1152/ jn.00956.2010

Caldwell JH, Daw NW. 1978. New properties of rabbit retinal ganglion cells. *J Physiol* **276:** 257–276. doi:10.1113/jphy siol.1978.sp012232

Caspi A, Roy A, Wuyyuru V, Rosendall PE, Harper JW, Katyal KD, Barry MP, Dagnelie G, Greenberg RJ. 2018. Eye movement control in the Argus II retinal-prosthesis enables reduced head movement and better localization precision. *Invest Ophthalmol Vis Sci* **59:** 792–802. doi:10 .1167/iovs.17-22377

Chen ZC, Wang BY, Palanker D. 2020. Real-time optimization of the current steering for visual prosthesis. In *Proceedings of the 10th International IEEE/EMBS Conference on Neural Engineering (NER)*. Virtual Event, May 4–6.

Chenais NAL, Leccardi MJIA, Ghezzi D. 2021. Photovoltaic retinal prosthesis restores high-resolution responses to single-pixel stimulation in blind retinas. *Commun Mater* **2:** 28. doi:10.1038/s43246-021-00133-2

Chichilnisky EJ, Kalmar RS. 2002. Functional asymmetries in ON and OFF ganglion cells of primate retina. *J Neurosci* **22:** 2737–2747. doi:10.1523/JNEUROSCI.22-07-02737.2002

Cho A, Ratliff C, Sampath A, Weiland J. 2016. Changes in ganglion cell physiology during retinal degeneration influence excitability by prosthetic electrodes. *J Neural Eng* **13:** 025001. doi:10.1088/1741-2560/13/2/025001

Chow AY, Chow VY, Packo KH, Pollack JS, Peyman GA, Schuchard R. 2004. The artificial silicon retina microchip for the treatment of vision loss from retinitis pigmentosa. *Arch Ophthalmol-Chic* **122:** 460–469. doi:10.1001/arch opht.122.4.460

Cohen E, Lepri B. 2013. Investigational device exemption guidance for retinal prostheses. In *The senses: a comprehensive reference*, 2nd ed. Center for Devices and Radiological Health-FDA, Elsevier, Amsterdam.

da Cruz L, Coley BF, Dorn J, Merlini F, Filley E, Christopher P, Chen FK, Wuyyuru V, Sahel J, Stanga P, et al. 2013. The Argus II epiretinal prosthesis system allows letter and word reading and long-term function in patients with profound vision loss. *Br J Ophthalmol* **97:** 632–636. doi:10.1136/bjophthalmol-2012-301525

da Cruz L, Dorn JD, Humayun MS, Dagnelie G, Handa J, Barale PO, Sahel JA, Stanga PE, Hafezi F, Safran AB, et al. 2016. Five-year safety and performance results from the Argus II retinal prosthesis system clinical trial. *Ophthalmology* **123:** 2248–2254. doi:10.1016/j.ophtha.2016.06 .049

Daschner R, Greppmaier U, Kokelmann M, Rudorf S, Rudorf R, Schleehauf S, Wrobel WG. 2017. Laboratory and clinical reliability of conformally coated subretinal implants. *Biomed Microdevices* **19:** 7. doi:10.1007/s10544-017-0147-6

Daschner R, Rothermel A, Rudorf R, Rudorf S, Stett A. 2018. Functionality and performance of the subretinal implant chip Alpha AMS. *Sensor Mater* **30:** 179–192. doi:10.18494/SAM.2018.1726

Dean P. 1981. Visual pathways and acuity hooded rats. *Behav Brain Res* **3:** 239–271. doi:10.1016/0166-4328(81)90050-4

Demb JB, Haarsma L, Freed MA, Sterling P. 1999. Functional circuitry of the retinal ganglion cell's nonlinear receptive field. *J Neurosci* **19:** 9756–9767. doi:10.1523/JNEUROSCI.19-22-09756.1999

Denlinger B, Helft Z, Telias M, Lorach H, Palanker D, Kramer RH. 2020. Local photoreceptor degeneration causes local pathophysiological remodeling of retinal neurons. *JCI Insight* **5:** e132114. doi:10.1172/jci.insight.132114

Euler T, Haverkamp S, Schubert T, Baden T. 2014. Retinal bipolar cells: elementary building blocks of vision. *Nat Rev Neurosci* **15:** 507–519. doi:10.1038/nrn3783

Field GD, Sher A, Gauthier JL, Greschner M, Shlens J, Litke AM, Chichilnisky EJ. 2007. Spatial properties and functional organization of small bistratified ganglion cells in primate retina. *J Neurosci* **27:** 13261–13272.

Flores T, Goetz G, Lei X, Palanker D. 2016. Optimization of return electrodes in neurostimulating arrays. *J Neural Eng* **13:** 036010. doi:10.1088/1741-2560/13/3/036010

Flores T, Huang T, Bhuckory M, Ho E, Chen Z, Dalal R, Galambos L, Kamins T, Mathieson K, Palanker D. 2019. Honeycomb-shaped electro-neural interface enables cellular-scale pixels in subretinal prosthesis. *Sci Rep* **9:** 10657. doi:10.1038/s41598-019-47082-y

Fried SI, Hsueh HA, Werblin FS. 2006. A method for generating precise temporal patterns of retinal spiking using prosthetic stimulation. *J Neurophysiol* **95:** 970–978. doi:10.1152/jn.00849.2005

Fried SI, Lasker ACW, Desai NJ, Eddington DK, Rizzo JF. 2009. Axonal sodium-channel bands shape the response to electric stimulation in retinal ganglion cells. *J Neurophysiol* **101:** 1972–1987.

Friedman DS, O'Colmain BJ, Munoz B, Tomany SC, McCarty C, de Jong PT, Nemesure B, Mitchell P, Kempen J; Eye Diseases Prevalence Research Group. 2004. Prevalence of age-related macular degeneration in the United States. *Arch Ophthalmol* **122:** 564–572.

Fujikado T, Kamei M, Sakaguchi H, Kanda H, Morimoto T, Ikuno Y, Nishida H, Kishima H, Maruo T, Konoma K. 2011. Testing of semichronically implanted retinal prosthesis by suprachoroidal-transretinal stimulation in patients with retinitis pigmentosa. *Invest Ophthalmol Vis Sci* **52:** 4726–4733. doi:10.1167/iovs.10-6836

Garcia S, Petrini K, Da Cruz L, Rubin GS, Nardini M. 2014. Assessing improvements in perception afforded by retinal prostheses in multisensory tasks. *Invest Ophthalmol Vis Sci* **55:** 5962.

Ghezzi D, Antognazza MR, Maccarone R, Bellani S, Lanzarini E, Martino N, Mete M, Pertile G, Bisti S, Lanzani G, et al. 2013. A polymer optoelectronic interface restores light

sensitivity in blind rat retinas. *Nat Photonics* **7:** 400–406. doi:10.1038/nphoton.2013.34

Goetz GA, Mandel Y, Manivanh R, Palanker DV, Čižmár T. 2013. Holographic display system for restoration of sight to the blind. *J Neural Eng* **10:** 056021. doi:10.1088/1741-2560/10/5/056021

Grosberg LE, Ganesan K, Goetz GA, Madugula SS, Bhaskhar N, Fan V, Li P, Hottowy P, Dabrowski W, Sher A, et al. 2017. Activation of ganglion cells and axon bundles using epiretinal electrical stimulation. *J Neurophysiol* **118:** 1457–1471. doi:10.1152/jn.00750.2016

Ha S, Khraiche ML, Akinin A, Jing Y, Damle S, Kuang Y, Bauchner S, Lo YH, Freeman WR, Silva GA, et al. 2016. Towards high-resolution retinal prostheses with direct optical addressing and inductive telemetry. *J Neural Eng* **13:** 056008. doi:10.1088/1741-2560/13/5/056008

Hafed ZM, Stingl K, Bartz-Schmidt KU, Gekeler F, Zrenner E. 2016. Oculomotor behavior of blind patients seeing with a subretinal visual implant. *Vision Res* **118:** 119–131.

Haim M. 2022. Epidemiology of retinitis pigmentosa in Denmark. *Acta Ophthalmol Scand Suppl* **233:** 1–34.

Harnois C, Bodis-Wollner I, Onofrj M. 1984. The effect of contrast and spatial frequency on the visual evoked potential of the hooded rat. *Exp Brain Res* **57:** 1–8.

Heine WF, Passaglia CL. 2011. Spatial receptive field properties of rat retinal ganglion cells. *Vis Neurosci* **28:** 403–417. doi:10.1017/S0952523811000307

Hicks SL, Wilson I, van Rheede JJ, MacLaren RE, Downes SM, Kennard C. 2014. Improved mobility with depth-based residual vision glasses. *Invest Ophthalmol Vis Sci* **55:** 2153.

Ho AC, Humayun MS, Dorn JD, da Cruz L, Dagnelie G, Handa J, Barale PO, Sahel JA, Stanga PE, Hafezi F, et al. 2015. Long-term results from an epiretinal prosthesis to restore sight to the blind. *Ophthalmology* **122:** 1547–1554.

Ho E, Smith R, Goetz G, Lei X, Galambos L, Kamins TI, Harris J, Mathieson K, Palanker D, Sher A. 2018a. Spatiotemporal characteristics of retinal response to network-mediated photovoltaic stimulation. *J Neurophysiol* **119:** 389–400. doi:10.1152/jn.00872.2016

Ho E, Lorach H, Goetz G, Laszlo F, Lei X, Kamins T, Mariani JC, Sher A, Palanker D. 2018b. Temporal structure in spiking patterns of ganglion cells defines perceptual thresholds in rodents with subretinal prosthesis. *Sci Rep* **8:** 3145. doi:10.1038/s41598-018-21447-1

Ho E, Lei X, Flores T, Lorach H, Huang T, Galambos L, Kamins T, Harris J, Mathieson K, Palanker D. 2019. Characteristics of prosthetic vision in rats with subretinal flat and pillar electrode arrays. *J Neural Eng* **16:** 066027. doi:10.1088/1741-2552/ab34b3

Ho E, Shmakov A, Palanker D. 2020. Decoding network-mediated retinal response to electrical stimulation: implications for fidelity of prosthetic vision. *J Neural Eng* **17:** 1–24.

Hornig R, Dapper M, Le Joliff E, Hill R, Ishaque K, Posch C, Benosman R, LeMer Y, Sahel J-A, Picaud S. 2017. Pixium vision: first clinical results and innovative developments. In *Artificial vision: a clinical guide* (ed. Gabel VP), pp. 99–113. Springer, Amsterdam.

Humayun MS, Prince M, de Juan E, Barron Y, Moskowitz M, Klock IB, Milam AH. 1999. Morphometric analysis of the extramacular retina from postmortem eyes with retinitis pigmentosa. *Invest Ophth Vis Sci* **40**: 143–148.

Humayun MS, Dorn JD, da Cruz L, Dagnelie G, Sahel JA, Stanga PE, Cideciyan AV, Duncan JL, Eliott D, Filley E, et al. 2012. Interim results from the international trial of second sight's visual prosthesis. *Ophthalmology* **119**: 779–788. doi:10.1016/j.ophtha.2011.09.028

Jensen RJ, Rizzo JF III. 2006. Thresholds for activation of rabbit retinal ganglion cells with a subretinal electrode. *Exp Eye Res* **83**: 367–373. doi:10.1016/j.exer.2006.01.012

Jensen RJ, Ziv OR, Rizzo JF III. 2005. Thresholds for activation of rabbit retinal ganglion cells with relatively large, extracellular microelectrodes. *Invest Ophthalmol Vis Sci* **46**: 1486–1496. doi:10.1167/iovs.04-1018

Jepson LH, Hottowy P, Weiner GA, Dabrowski W, Litke AM, Chichilnisky EJ. 2014. High-fidelity reproduction of spatiotemporal visual signals for retinal prosthesis. *Neuron* **83**: 87–92. doi:10.1016/j.neuron.2014.04.044

Jones BW, Marc RE. 2005. Retinal remodeling during retinal degeneration. *Exp Eye Res* **81**: 123–137. doi:10.1016/j.exer.2005.03.006

Jung JH, Aloni D, Yitzhaky Y, Peli E. 2015. Active confocal imaging for visual prostheses. *Vision Res* **111** (Part B): 182–196.

Kim SY, Sadda S, Pearlman J, Humayun MS, de Juan E Jr, Melia BM, Green WR. 2002. Morphometric analysis of the macula in eyes with disciform age-related macular degeneration. *Retina* **22**: 471–477. doi:10.1097/00006982-200208000-00012

Klauke S, Goetz M, Rein S, Hoehl D, Thomas U, Eckhorn R, Bremmer F, Wachtler T. 2011. Stimulation with a wireless intraocular epiretinal implant elicits visual percepts in blind humans. *Invest Ophthalmol Vis Sci* **52**: 449–455.

Knutson JS, Naples GG, Peckham PH, Keith MW. 2002. Electrode fracture rates and occurrences of infection and granuloma associated with percutaneous intramuscular electrodes in upper-limb functional electrical stimulation applications. *J Rehab Res Devel* **39**: 671–683.

Kolic M, Baglin EK, Titchener S, Kvansakul J, Abbott CJ, Barnes N, McGuinness M, Kentler W, Young K, Walker J, et al. 2020. A 44 channel suprachoroidal retinal prosthesis: interim functional vision results. *Invest Ophth Vis Sci* **61**: 2199.

Lee DY, Lorach H, Huie P, Palanker D. 2016. Implantation of modular photovoltaic subretinal prosthesis. *Ophthalmic Surg Lasers Imaging Retina* **47**: 171–174.

Lorach H, Goetz G, Smith R, Lei X, Mandel Y, Kamins T, Mathieson K, Huie P, Harris J, Sher A, et al. 2015. Photovoltaic restoration of sight with high visual acuity. *Nat Med* **21**: 476–482. doi:10.1038/nm.3851

Loudin JD, Simanovskii DM, Vijayraghavan K, Sramek CK, Butterwick AF, Huie P, McLean GY, Palanker DV. 2007. Optoelectronic retinal prosthesis: system design and performance. *J Neural Eng* **4**: S72–S84. doi:10.1088/1741-2560/4/1/S09

Malmivuo J, Plonsey R. 1995. Functional electric stimulation. In *Bioelectromagnetism* (pp. 363–375). Oxford University Press, New York.

Mandel Y, Goetz G, Lavinsky D, Huie P, Mathieson K, Wang L, Kamins T, Galambos L, Manivanh R, Harris J, et al. 2013. Cortical responses elicited by photovoltaic subreti-

nal prostheses exhibit similarities to visually evoked potentials. *Nat Commun* **4**: 1980.

Marc RE, Jones BW. 2003. Retinal remodeling in inherited photoreceptor degenerations. *Mol Neurobiol* **28**: 139–147. doi:10.1385/MN:28:2:139

Marc RE, Jones BW, Watt CB, Strettoi E. 2003. Neural remodeling in retinal degeneration. *Prog Retin Eye Res* **22**: 607–655. doi:10.1016/S1350-9462(03)00039-9

Margolis DJ, Newkirk G, Euler T, Detwiler PB. 2008. Functional stability of retinal ganglion cells after degeneration-induced changes in synaptic input. *J Neurosci* **28**: 6526–6536. doi:10.1523/JNEUROSCI.1533-08.2008

Masland RH. 2001. The fundamental plan of the retina. *Nat Neurosci* **4**: 877–886. doi:10.1038/nn0901-877

Mathieson K, Loudin J, Goetz G, Huie P, Wang L, Kamins TI, Galambos L, Smith R, Harris JS, Sher A, et al. 2012. Photovoltaic retinal prosthesis with high pixel density. *Nat Photon* **6**: 391–397. doi:10.1038/nphoton.2012.104

Mazzoni F, Novelli E, Strettoi E. 2008. Retinal ganglion cells survive and maintain normal dendritic morphology in a mouse model of inherited photoreceptor degeneration. *J Neurosci* **28**: 14282–14292. doi:10.1523/JNEUROSCI.4968-08.2008

Menzler J, Zeck G. 2011. Network oscillations in rod-degenerated mouse retinas. *J Neurosci* **31**: 2280–2291. doi:10.1523/JNEUROSCI.4238-10.2011

Merigan WH, Maunsell JH. 1993. How parallel are the primate visual pathways? *Annu Rev Neurosci* **16**: 369–402. doi:10.1146/annurev.ne.16.030193.002101

Muqit MMK, Velikay-Parel M, Weber M, Dupeyron G, Audemard D, Corcostegui B, Sahel J, Le Mer Y. 2019. Six-month safety and efficacy of the intelligent retinal implant system II device in retinitis pigmentosa. *Ophthalmology* **126**: 637–639.

Nanduri D, Fine I, Horsager A, Boynton GM, Humayun MS, Greenberg RJ, Weiland JD. 2012. Frequency and amplitude modulation have different effects on the percepts elicited by retinal stimulation. *Invest Ophth Vis Sci* **53**: 205–214. doi:10.1167/iovs.11-8401

Naumann J. 2012. *Search for paradise: a patient's account of the artificial vision experiment.* Xlibris, Bloomington, IN.

Newsome WT, Wurtz RH, Dursteler MR, Mikami A. 1985. Deficits in visual-motion processing following ibotenic acid lesions of the middle temporal visual area of the Macaque monkey. *J Neurosci* **5**: 825–840. doi:10.1523/JNEUROSCI.05-03-00825.1985

Olveczky BP, Baccus SA, Meister M. 2003. Segregation of object and background motion in the retina. *Nature* **423**: 401–408.

Palanker D, Blumenkranz MS, Weiter JJ. 2005. Retinal laser therapy: biophysical basis and applications. In *Retina*, Vol 1, 4th ed. (ed. Ryan SJ), pp. 539-553. Mosby, St Louis.

Palanker D, Le Mer Y, Mohand-Said S, Muqit M, Sahel JA. 2020. Photovoltaic restoration of central vision in atrophic age-related macular degeneration. *Ophthalmology* **127**: 1097–1104. doi:10.1016/j.ophtha.2020.02.024

Palanker D, Le Mer Y, Mohand-Said S, Sahel JA. 2022. Simultaneous perception of prosthetic and natural vision in AMD patients. *Nat Commun* **13**: 513.

Passaglia CL, Troy JB, Rüttiger L, Lee BB. 2002. Orientation sensitivity of ganglion cells in primate retina. *Vision Res* **42:** 683–694. doi:10.1016/S0042-6989(01)00312-1

Petrusca D, Grivich MI, Sher A, Field GD, Gauthier JL, Greschner M, Shlens J, Chichilnisky EJ, Litke AM. 2007. Identification and characterization of a Y-like primate retinal ganglion cell type. *J Neurosci* **27:** 11019–11027. doi:10.1523/JNEUROSCI.2836-07.2007

Prevot PH, Lanoë M, Dalouz S, Blaize K, Oubari O, Gehere K, Akolkar H, Buc G, Picaud SA, Sahel JA. 2017. Behavioral and electrophysiological characterization of photovoltaic subretinal implants in non-human primates. *Invest Ophth Vis Sci* **58:** 4270–4270.

Richard E, Goetz G, Chichilnisky EJ. 2015. Recognizing retinal ganglion cells in the dark. *Adv Neural Inf Proc Syst* **28:** 1–9.

Rizzo JF 3rd, Shire DB, Kelly SK, Troyk P, Gingerich M, McKee B, Priplata A, Chen J, Drohan W, Doyle P, et al. 2011. Overview of the Boston retinal prosthesis: challenges and opportunities to restore useful vision to the blind. In *Conference proceedings: Annual International Conference of the IEEE Engineering in Medicine and Biology Society IEEE Engineering in Medicine and Biology Society Conference 2011*, pp. 7492–7495.

Schwartz GW, Okawa H, Dunn FA, Morgan JL, Kerschensteiner D, Wong RO, Rieke F. 2012. The spatial structure of a nonlinear receptive field. *Nat Neurosci* **15:** 1572–1580. doi:10.1038/nn.3225

Sekirnjak C, Hottowy P, Sher A, Dabrowski W, Litke AM, Chichilnisky EJ. 2006. Electrical stimulation of mammalian retinal ganglion cells with multielectrode arrays. *J Neurophysiol* **95:** 3311–3327. doi:10.1152/jn.01168.2005

Sekirnjak C, Jepson LH, Hottowy P, Sher A, Dabrowski W, Litke AM, Chichilnisky EJ. 2011. Changes in physiological properties of rat ganglion cells during retinal degeneration. *J Neurophysiol* **105:** 2560–2571. doi:10.1152/jn.01061.2010

Shah NP, Chichilnisky EJ. 2020. Computational challenges and opportunities for a bi-directional artificial retina. *J Neural Eng* **17:** 055002.

Shah NP, Madugula S, Grosberg L, Mena G, Tandon P, Hottowy P, Sher A, Litke A, Mitra S, Chichilnisky EJ. 2019. Optimization of electrical stimulation for a high-fidelity artificial retina. In *9th International IEEE/EMBS Conference on Neural Engineering (NER)*, pp. 714–718. March 20–23.

Silveira LCL, Heywood CA, Cowey A. 1987. Contrast sensitivity and visual-acuity of the pigmented rat determined electrophysiologically. *Vision Res* **27:** 1719–1731. doi:10.1016/0042-6989(87)90101-5

Sim SL, Szalewski RJ, Johnson LJ, Akah LE, Shoemaker LE, Thoreson WB, Margalit E. 2014. Simultaneous recording of mouse retinal ganglion cells during epiretinal or subretinal stimulation. *Vision Res* **101:** 41–50. doi:10.1016/j.visres.2014.05.005

Smith W, Assink J, Klein R, Mitchell P, Klaver CC, Klein BE, Hofman A, Jensen S, Wang JJ, de Jong PT. 2001. Risk factors for age-related macular degeneration: pooled findings from three continents. *Ophthalmology* **108:** 697–704.

Stingl K, Bartz-Schmidt KU, Gekeler F, Kusnyerik A, Sachs H, Zrenner E. 2013. Functional outcome in subretinal electronic implants depends on foveal eccentricity. *Invest Ophthalmol Vis Sci* **54:** 7658–7665.

Stingl K, Bartz-Schmidt KU, Besch D, Chee CK, Cottriall CL, Gekeler F, Groppe M, Jackson TL, MacLaren RE, Koitschev A, et al. 2015. Subretinal visual implant Alpha IMS—clinical trial interim report. *Vision Res* **111:** 149–160. doi:10.1016/j.visres.2015.03.001

Stingl K, Schippert R, Bartz-Schmidt KU, Besch D, Cottriall CL, Edwards TL, Gekeler F, Greppmaier U, Kiel K, Koitschev A, et al. 2017. Interim results of a multicenter trial with the new electronic subretinal implant Alpha AMS in 15 patients blind from inherited retinal degenerations. *Front Neurosci* **11:** 445. doi:10.3389/fnins.2017.00445

Thibos LN, Levick WR. 1983. Bimodal receptive fields of cat retinal ganglion cells. *Vision Res* **23:** 1561–1572. doi:10.1016/0042-6989(83)90170-0

Tochitsky I, Polosukhina A, Degtyar VE, Gallerani N, Smith CM, Friedman A, Van Gelder RN, Trauner D, Kaufer D, Kramer RH. 2014. Restoring visual function to blind mice with a photoswitch that exploits electrophysiological remodeling of retinal ganglion cells. *Neuron* **81:** 800–813.

Wandell B. 1995. *Foundations of vision*. Sinauer Associates, Sunderland, MA.

Wang BY, Chen ZC, Bhuckory M, Huang T, Shin A, Zuckerman V, Ho E, Rosenfeld E, Galambos L, Kamins T, et al. 2022. Electronic photoreceptors enable prosthetic visual acuity matching the natural resolution in rats. *Nat Commun* **13:** 6627.

Wässle H. 2004. Parallel processing in the mammalian retina. *Nat Rev Neurosci* **5:** 747–757. doi:10.1038/nrn1497

Weitz AC, Nanduri D, Behrend MR, Gonzalez-Calle A, Greenberg RJ, Humayun MS, Chow RH, Weiland JD. 2015. Improving the spatial resolution of epiretinal implants by increasing stimulus pulse duration. *Sci Transl Med* **7:** 318ra203. doi:10.1126/scitranslmed.aac4877

Werginz P, Benav H, Zrenner E, Rattay F. 2015. Modeling the response of ON and OFF retinal bipolar cells during electric stimulation. *Vision Res* **111:** 170–181.

Werginz P, Wang B-Y, Chen ZC, Palanker D. 2020. On optimal coupling of the "electronic photoreceptors" into the degenerate retina. *J Neural Eng* **17:** 045008.

Wong WL, Su XY, Li X, Cheung CMG, Klein R, Cheng CY, Wong TY. 2014. Global prevalence of age-related macular degeneration and disease burden projection for 2020 and 2040: a systematic review and meta-analysis. *Lancet Glob Health* **2:** E106–E116.

Woodburn KW, Engelman CJ, Blumenkranz MS. 2002. Photodynamic therapy for choroidal neovascularization: A review. *Retina* **22:** 391–405. doi:10.1097/00006982-200208000-00001

Yanovitch L, Raz-Prag D, Hanein Y. 2022. A new high-resolution three-dimensional retinal implant: system design and preliminary human results. bioRxiv doi:10.1101/2022.09.14.507901

Zrenner E, Bartz-Schmidt KU, Benav H, Besch D, Bruckmann A, Gabel VP, Gekeler F, Greppmaier U, Harscher A, Kibbel S, et al. 2011. Subretinal electronic chips allow blind patients to read letters and combine them to words. *Proc Biol Sci* **278:** 1489–1497. doi:10.1098/rspb.2010.1747

iPSC-RPE in Retinal Degeneration: Recent Advancements and Future Perspectives

Tadao Maeda[1,2,3] and Masayo Takahashi[1,2,3]

[1]Research Center, Kobe City Eye Hospital, Kobe 6500-047, Japan

[2]Department of Ophthalmology, Kobe City Eye Hospital, Kobe 6500-047, Japan

[3]Vision Care Cell Therapy, Kobe 650-0047, Japan

Correspondence: takahashisec@vision-care.jp

Regenerative medicine is a great hope for patients suffering from diseases for which no effective treatment is available. With the creation of induced pluripotent stem cells (iPSCs) in 2006, research and development has accelerated expeditiously, reaching a practical stage worldwide. The iPSC-regenerative medicine in ophthalmology is one of the pioneers, which has kicked off clinical application ahead of other fields owing to its advantages. The clinical safety issues of iPSC-derived retinal pigment epithelial (iPSC-RPE) transplantation for exudative age-related macular degeneration have been addressed to a certain extent. Preparations are being made for the next clinical study based on the improvement of its therapeutic effects and expansion of indications globally. Steady progress toward the practical applications of regenerative medicine for the treatment of retinal disorders is expected in the future while strengthening global cooperation amid various research areas, clinical fields, and regulations.

Regenerative medicine, which overcomes intractable and serious diseases by replacing tissues and organs using stem cells to regain lost physical function, is a promising treatment to be used worldwide. Since the mid-1990s, following the dramatic progress of neural stem cells, embryonic stem (ES) cells, and induced pluripotent stem cells (iPSCs) in basic science, regenerative treatment of several diseases by cell transplantation of various tissues has recently commenced, including the diseases of the central nervous system. In the last 10 years, there has been a remarkable progress in research related to regenerative medicine of the eye, including clinical studies on bullous keratopathy using cultured human corneal endothelial cells, age-related macular degeneration, retinitis pigmentosa, and corneal stem cell deficiency using iPSCs. This has been possible because the world's first iPSC-RPE transplantation has obtained promising results well within safety limits. In Japan alone, a total of 11 clinical studies using iPSCs were started. Furthermore, until recently, gene therapy for retinitis pigmentosa and related diseases, for which there existed no cure, has been started in Japan and some other countries of the world. In this study, we describe future prospects, issues, and limitations from the viewpoint of practical treatment with a focus on iPSC-based retinal regenerative medicine.

iPSCs AS A RESOURCE IN REGENERATIVE MEDICINE

Stem cells such as ES cells, iPSCs, and somatic stem cells are characterized by self-renewability and multipotency. ES cells are stem cells that are separated and established from the cell mass inside the blastocyst after fertilization and are capable of differentiating into almost all types of cells/tissues. In 2006, iPSCs designed as ES cell–like pluripotent stem cells were induced from mouse fibroblasts by Professor Shinya Yamanaka at Kyoto University using four transcription factors (Oct3/4, Flk1, Sox2, and c-Myc). Further on, in 2007, the same group succeeded in creating human iPSCs for applications in regenerative medicine, drug discovery support, and in basic research for elucidating the mechanisms of cell differentiation, rejuvenation, and aging processes. Adult somatic stem cells are present in niches in living tissues that maintain a special local microenvironment. They are thought to be responsible for tissue regeneration by replenishing cells lost, owing to developmental processes and tissue damage.

iPSCs used in regenerative medicine can be broadly divided into autologous and allogeneic cells (Fig. 1). Autologous transplantation is a treatment method in which cells are collected from a patient, cultured, processed, and returned to the patient. The risk of immune rejection and infection due to incompatibility of donor cells is reduced, as the patient's own cells are reintroduced into his/her body. Since cells need to be cultured and processed from somatic cells, the time and cost required for such treatment per patient is quite high. In addition, it requires a high level of skill/high efficiency to maintain the same quality of the final product due to differences in cell properties among individuals. On the other hand, in allogeneic transplantation cells collected from selected healthy donors, that meet certain quality standards are used as raw materials, but there is always a risk of immune rejection. In many cases, it is possible to store the cultured and processed cells as intermediates (cell stock) for a long period using methods such as cryopreservation. By such techniques, it is possible to decrease the time and cost

required for allogeneic treatment compared to autologous treatment, and also to suppress variations in the quality of the cultured cells making them more suitable for practical use. The pioneer in preparing this material for allogeneic transplantation is the iPS Cell Stock Project for Regenerative Medicine, which has been underway since 2013 at the Center for iPS Cell Research and Application, Kyoto University, Japan (www.cira.kyoto-u.ac.jp/e/research/stock.html). In this project, it was estimated that more than 80% of the Japanese people can be treated with less immune rejection by collecting 75 types of iPSCs using healthy volunteers' cells with human leukocyte antigens (HLAs) in a homozygous combination at 6 loci. Most recently, to further improve its practical application, the group has started to provide research-grade iPSCs by knocking out the part of *HLA* that caused rejection, by using gene editing. If this technology is put into practical use, it is expected that only seven types of HLA class C-KO cell lines will be able to cover 95% of the Japanese population in the future (Xu et al. 2019). In addition, several other iPSC lines that can be used in clinical trials are being prepared globally for practical applications in regenerative medicine (commonfund.nih.gov/stemcells/lines; ct.catapult.org.uk/clinical-grade-iPS-cell-line).

CONCEPT OF STEM CELL–BASED THERAPIES FOR RETINAL DEGENERATION

According to some recent reports, the prevalence of retinal degeneration, such as age-related macular degeneration (AMD) and retinitis pigmentosa (RP), is the leading cause of blindness in the working age group of 15–64 yr, especially in developed countries (Buch et al. 2001; Al-Merjan et al. 2005; Morizane et al. 2019; GBD 2019 Blindness and Vision Impairment Collaborators 2021). However, there is no established treatment for patients with RP or AMD with photoreceptor cell and/or RPE degeneration to date (Scholl et al. 2016; Fleckenstein et al. 2018; Maeda et al. 2021). Stem cell–based therapies are drawing worldwide attention as ES/iPSC-RPE cell studies have evaluated safety and effica-

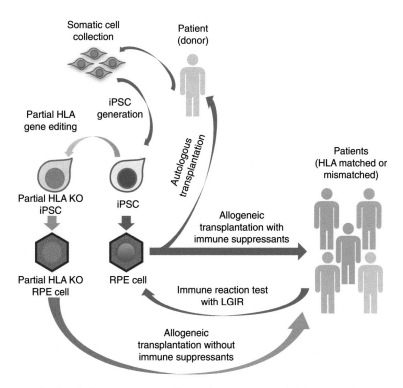

Figure 1. Concept of induced pluripotent stem cell retinal pigment epithelial (iPSC-RPE) preparation as regenerative medicine. Transfection of somatic cells with the four Yamanaka factors, including *OCT4, SOX2, KLF4,* and *CMYC* (OSKM), results in iPSCs. iPSCs differentiate into RPE cells and are used for autologous or allogeneic transplantation. In the case of allogeneic transplantation, human leucocyte antigen (HLA) matching between donor and host is assessed to determine the protocols of immunosuppressant administration and monitoring of immune rejection against transplanted iPSC-RPE cells. Allogeneic iPSCs with partial HLA gene editing were tested to avoid unfavorable immune rejection against transplanted RPE cells and to minimize immunosuppressant administration. (KO) Knockout, (LGIR) lymphocyte graft immune reaction.

cy to a certain extent (Scholl et al. 2016; Maeda et al. 2019, 2021).

Retinal degeneration is an ideal target for stem cell–based therapies because fewer stem cells are required for the human eye compared to other organs owing to its anatomical characteristics (Fig. 2A). Furthermore, high-resolution in vivo retinal imaging systems, such as spectral domain optical coherence tomography (SD-OCT), and adaptive optics scanning laser ophthalmoscopy (AO-SLO) (Fig. 2A), enable precise clinical observation of the retina and allow for close follow-up of stem cell–based therapies. Currently, these therapies are being applied for retinal diseases affecting the outer retinal layers including photoreceptors and RPE, such as AMD (Maeda et al. 2021) and RP with RPE-

related gene mutation (Fig. 3). RPE cell products have been used for AMD to halt disease progression via reconstruction of the RPE layer and to restore partial visual function in RP with RPE-related gene mutations (Fig. 1B). Two types of formulations have been in use for the administration of iPSC-RPE at our institute: cell sheets without scaffolds and cell suspensions for patients with wet AMD (Mandai et al. 2017; Sugita et al. 2020). Due to the greater extent of surgical invasiveness involving a wider incision site and occasional removal of choroidal neovascularization (CNV) before RPE sheet transplantation, the risk of surgical complications following RPE sheet transplantation is generally higher than that following RPE cell suspension. Several adverse events associated with surgery such as

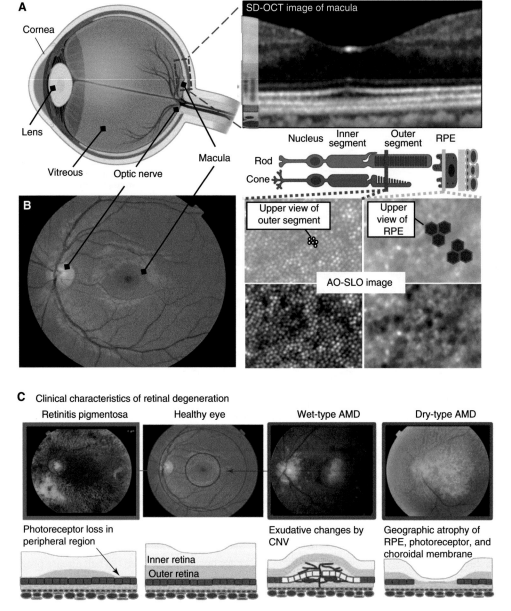

Figure 2. Characteristics of the human eye as a target of regenerative medicine: Anatomical structure of the human eye. The anatomical structures of the human eye can be observed using spectral domain optical coherence tomography (SD-OCT) (*A*) and a fundus camera (*B*). SD-OCT provides a cross-sectional image of retinal laminar structures consisting of different types of neural structures at micrometer resolution (*A, right* panel). The positions of the photoreceptor cells and the retinal pigment epithelium (RPE) are indicated in the OCT images. The fundus camera provides an en face image of the retina at various magnifications; for example, a color fundus image shows a wide-angled macro image, and an adaptive optics scanning laser ophthalmoscopy (AO-SLO) image shows the cellular structure of the outer segment of a photoreceptor and RPE at high resolution. (*C*) Clinical characteristics of retinal degeneration: Retinal degeneration is characterized by various clinical features, which can be observed in ophthalmological examinations and fundus images of retinitis pigmentosa (RP), healthy eyes, wet-type age-related macular degeneration (AMD), and dry-type AMD. In cases of RP with RPE-related gene mutations, degeneration of the outer retina starts from the peripheral retinal region and the macular region is relatively secure. In AMD with either wet- or dry-type features, the macular region is damaged by exudative changes caused by choroidal neovascularization (CNV) formation or geographic atrophy (GA) of the outer retina.

Cite this article as *Cold Spring Harb Perspect Med* doi: 10.1101/cshperspect.a041308

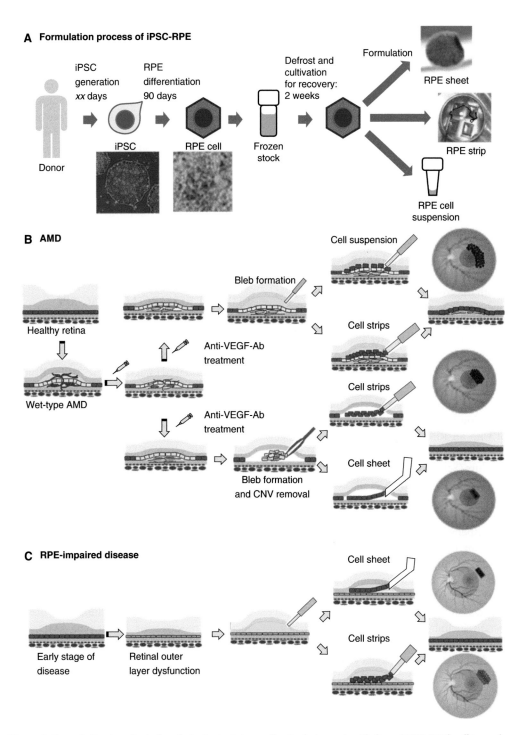

Figure 3. Formulation type for induced pluripotent stem cell retinal pigment epithelium (iPSC-RPE) cell transplantation for retinal degeneration. Formulation of iPSC-RPE cells (*A*). iPSC-RPE cells prepared from iPSCs were stored as a frozen stock/intermediate product. The frozen stock was defrosted, and RPE cells were cultivated for 2 weeks to recover their functions. iPSC-RPE cells can be formulated into three different types: cell sheets, strips, or suspensions. These formulations can be used for wet-type age-related macular degeneration (AMD) according to the pathological condition and size of exudative lesions to maximize the advantage of each formulation (*B*). In the case of RPE-impaired disease, including dry-type AMD, RPE cell suspension or cell strips could be used to cover pathological lesions enough to predict the efficacy of RPE cell therapy (*C*). (VEGF) Vascular endothelial growth factor, (CNV) choroidal neovascularization.

retinal hemorrhage and edema have been reported in some clinical trials of ES-RPE cell transplantation (da Cruz et al. 2018; Kashani et al. 2018, 2021). However, survival and integration of grafted RPE cells can be improved significantly compared to cell suspension. In fact, in a promising approach, clinical trials of autologous iPSC-RPE on a biodegradable scaffold have been initiated (NCT04627428). It has been reported that long-term outcomes may be affected by the use of non-biodegradable scaffolds in RPE sheet formulation (da Cruz et al. 2018; Kashani et al. 2018, 2021). Although there are several reports on both improvement as well as maintenance of visual acuity to various extents after RPE cell sheet transplantation, several cases of adverse events related to surgery have also been reported (Mandai et al. 2017; da Cruz et al. 2018; Kashani et al. 2018, 2021; Takagi et al. 2019).

On the other hand, clinical trials that used ES or iPSC-RPE cells have reported that RPE cell suspension transplantation is less invasive than that with an RPE sheet because a small-gauge cannula with a soft tip (38G) is used in the former procedure (Schwartz et al. 2015; Song et al. 2015; Mehat et al. 2018; Sugita et al. 2020). Similar reports exist on adverse events in the epiretinal membrane both for ES and iPSC-RPE associated with suspension, most likely due to leakage of cells from the transplanted lesions (Schwartz et al. 2015; Song et al. 2015; Mehat et al. 2018; Sugita et al. 2020). Although some cases showed retinal sensitivity improvement in these areas, there was no significant improvement in visual function, including visual acuity, or quality-of-life assessment (Schwartz et al. 2015; Song et al. 2015; Mehat et al. 2018; Sugita et al. 2020).

To improve the efficacy and safety of RPE cell transplantation, a new formulation using RPE strips has been reported (Nishida et al. 2021) and preparation for clinical research is underway (jRCTa050210178). RPE strips have the advantage of both cell sheets and cell suspensions and can be prepared in 2 d. RPE strips are expected to be a useful alternative to the other two formulations because of their ability to expand into a monolayer sheet in the subretinal space after transplantation from a small retinal hole (Fig. 3A,B).

Furthermore, clinical research on iPSC retinal sheets for RP with photoreceptor degeneration has just begun to find ways to restore the functional and anatomical integrity of the neural retina (jRCTa050200027). In the future, a combination of cell products with RPE and retinal sheets might be a viable option for the treatment of advanced AMD with both photoreceptor and RPE degeneration, as well as for RP with similar pathology (jRCTa050190084). The clinical studies on iPSC-RPE cell transplantation are summarized in Table 1.

CLINICAL RESEARCH ON iPSC-RPE TRANSPLANTATION FOR AMD

AMD is a leading cause of severe central vision loss in the elderly worldwide. AMD is induced via sequential damage to the RPE, Bruch's membrane, the choroidal membrane, and photoreceptors due to pathological changes with age. The global prevalence of AMD is 8.7%, and it is estimated to affect approximately 288 million individuals globally by 2040 (Wong et al. 2014). Advanced stages of AMD are categorized into two forms: non-neovascular (dry, nonexudative, or geographic atrophy [GA]), and neovascular (wet or exudative). Dry AMD is characterized by GA of the outer retina, including the RPE, photoreceptors, and choriocapillaris, which results in gradual retinal cell loss and decreased visual acuity. In wet-type AMD, CNV causes exudative changes involving subretinal leakage of blood, lipids, and fluids, and the formation of fibrous scars. In wet-type AMD, anti-vascular endothelial growth factor (VEGF) antibodies are used as a standard treatment to improve visual function in many cases. However, some patients are resistant to anti-VEGF antibody treatment. In addition, cases of RPE atrophy or RPE tear due to the long-term administration of anti-VEGF antibody treatment have been reported (Nagiel et al. 2013; Young et al. 2014; Kuroda et al. 2015, 2016; Daniel et al. 2020). Furthermore, they only suppressed the proliferation of CNV and did not ameliorate RPE atrophy. Since no cure for RPE degeneration exists to date, reconstruction and functional recovery of RPE by cell transplanta-

Table 1. Clinical studies on stem cell–based therapies for retinal degeneration

No.	Study title	Sponsor/ collaborators	Study design	Intervention	Age	Ph	No. of subject	Period	Status	Study ID
1	A study of transplantation of autologous-induced pluripotent stem cell (iPSC)-derived retinal pigment epithelium (RPE) cell sheet in subjects with exudative age-related macular degeneration	The Laboratory for Retinal Regeneration, RIKEN Center for Developmental Biology	Intervention model: single group assignment; masking: none (open label); primary purpose: safety	Autologous human iPSC (hiPSC)-derived RPE cell sheet	50 yr and older	P1	1	Oct. 2013/ Sept. 2018	Completed	UMIN000011929
2	Autologous transplantation of iPSC-derived RPE for geographic atrophy associated with age-related macular degeneration	National Institutes of Health Clinical Center, Bethesda, Maryland, USA	Intervention model: single group assignment; masking: none (open label); primary purpose: treatment	Combination product: hiPSC-derived RPE/ polylactic-co-glycolic acid (PLGA) scaffold	55 yr and older	P1/II	20	July 2020/ Mar. 2029	Recruiting	NCT04339764

Continued

Table 1. *Continued*

No.	Study title	Sponsor/ collaborators	Study design	Intervention	Age	Ph	No. of subject	Period	Status	Study ID
3	A study of transplantation of allogeneic iPSC-derived RPE cell suspension in subjects with neovascular age-related macular degeneration	The Laboratory for Retinal Regeneration, RIKEN Center for Developmental Biology, Kobe, Japan/Kobe City Medical Center General Hospital, Kobe, Japan	Intervention model: single group assignment; masking: none (open label); primary purpose: safety	Subretinal transplantation of allogeneic hiPSC-derived RPE cells	50 yr to 85 yr	P1	5	Feb. 2017/ Oct. 2021	Active, not recruiting	UMIN000026003
4	Clinical research of allogeneic iPSC-RPE cell strips transplantation for RPE impaired disease	Kobe Eye Hospital	Intervention model: single group assignment; masking: none (open label); primary purpose: treatment	Allogeneic iPSC-RPE cell strips	20 yr and older	P1/2	50	Feb. 2022/ Feb. 2032	Recruiting	jRCTa050210178

Referenced clinical trials are either registered with clinicaltrials.gov or jrct.niph.go.jp.

Cite this article as *Cold Spring Harb Perspect Med* doi: 10.1101/cshperspect.a041308

tion are needed to maintain or restore visual function (Fig. 1). Research on RPE cell transplantation began to attract attention in the late 1980s. Transplanting human RPE cells into the subretinal space of monkeys showed engraftment on Bruch's membrane (Gouras et al. 1985). Since then, several reports have been published on the protective effect of RPE cell transplantation on neural retinas in animal models (Singh et al. 2020). These studies demonstrated the proof-of-concept (POC) of cell therapy with RPE for diseases of the outer retinal layer.

Peyman et al. (1991) first reported RPE transplantation in humans with AMD in 1991. In the first case, autologous cell transplantation was performed after removing proliferative tissue under the macula. The nearby RPE was transplanted into the macula to improve visual acuity. In the second case, the RPE was exfoliated from the donor's eye as a sheet and transplanted, but no visual acuity improvement was observed. In another study, the CNV of AMD was removed and a cell sheet obtained by culturing fetal-derived RPE was transplanted into a sheet (Algvere et al. 1994, 1997); however, immune rejection occurred after the operation. Weisz et al. also reported that when fetal RPE was injected as a cell suspension, no improvement in visual acuity or graft fibrosis was observed (Weisz et al. 1999). Del Priore et al. (2001) transplanted a donor RPE sheet after CNV removal, but engraftment was poor and visual acuity did not improve. In this way, almost all transplants using allografts in eyes that have destroyed the blood–retinal barrier by CNV removal showed rejection and deterioration in visual acuity.

Autologous transplantation is ideal to avoid rejection and RPE collected from the peripheral area is frequently transplanted (Joussen et al. 2006; Maaijwee et al. 2007; MacLaren et al. 2007). Reports suggest that although some patients had improved visual acuity, it is difficult to collect sufficient autologous RPE cells with stable quality, and serious adverse events frequently occur due to surgical intervention. Furthermore, when peripheral RPE patches with choroid were transplanted, some of the patients obtained good visual acuity. However, surgery had a higher risk of cutting out patches and the choroid could act as a fibrous tissue if it was not connected to the host choroidal vessels.

As a countermeasure against these problems, we reviewed the cell source of the transplant and suggested that RPE cells derived from ES-RPE and iPSC-RPE are promising candidates as graft cells (Haruta et al. 2004; Hirami et al. 2009; Osakada et al. 2009). It has been observed that both ES-RPE and iPSC-RPE have the same functions as those derived from living organisms, such as the formation of cell sheets with a collection of hexagonal cells with tight junctions. These cells, which can be prepared more easily than primary cultured RPE cells, have led to dramatic developments in cell therapy for AMD. Recent advances in RPE cell transplantation research among various pluripotent stem cells can be attributed to the fact that ES-RPE/iPSC-RPE have all the following conditions suitable for their clinical application: (1) they have the required cell functions (quality), (2) the retina requires a small number of cells so that enough cells can be manufactured for transplantation (amount), (3) cells with certified quality for clinical use can always be obtained (reproducibility), and (4) their purity is satisfactory (safety). Furthermore, subretinal surgeries such as CNV removal has already been performed. Thus, the field of ophthalmology, as described above, has contributed significantly to the area of clinical application of iPSCs.

Autologous iPSC-RPE Cell Sheet Transplantation

In August 2013, we initiated clinical research on autologous iPSC-RPE cell sheet transplantation through joint research with RIKEN, the Institute of Biomedical Research and Innovation Hospital, and Kobe City Medical Center General Hospital (UMIN000011929). The skin of the patient was collected in November 2013, and CNV removal and RPE sheet transplant surgery were performed in September 2014. In September 2015, 12 mo after transplant surgery, safety and effectiveness were evaluated as the primary and secondary end points, respectively (Mandai et al. 2017). The 4-yr report has already been pub-

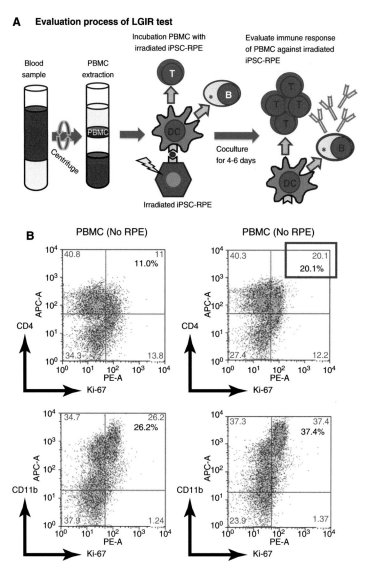

Figure 4. Monitoring immune rejection against allogeneic-induced pluripotent stem cell retinal pigment epithelial (iPSC-RPE) after transplantation. A lymphocyte graft immune reaction (LGIR) test was developed and used to detect the immune response of the transplanted RPE cells (*A*). Peripheral blood mononuclear cells (PBMCs) were collected and incubated with irradiated iPSC-RPE cells. The immune response of PBMCs against irradiated iPSC-RPE cells was monitored by flow cytometry. The LGIR results and findings of the fundus and optical coherence tomography (OCT) images of a patient with wet-type age-related macular degeneration in clinical research on allogeneic iPSC-RPE cell suspension transplantation are shown after transplantation. Mild immune rejection was suspected 5 wk after transplantation according to an increase in the activated PBMC population (red frame in *B*), and exudative changes in fundus images (white arrows in *C* and *D*), and OCT images (yellow arrow in *E*). (*Legend continues on following page.*)

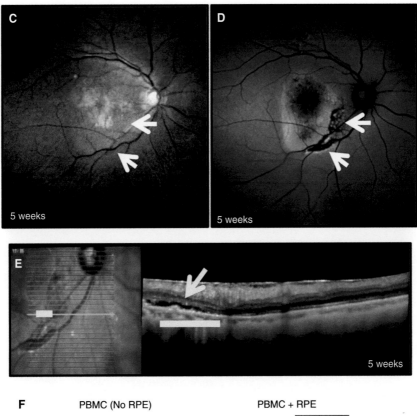

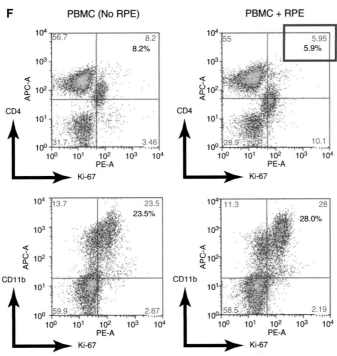

Figure 4. (*Continued*.) Immune rejection was ameliorated at 8 wk after transplantation due to a decrease in the activated PBMC population (*F*, red frame), and attenuated exudative changes in fundus images (white arrows in *G* and *H*), and OCT images (yellow arrow in *I*) by treatment with subcapsular injection of triamcinolone. (T) T cell, (B) B cell, (DC) dendritic cell. (Panels *B–E* reprinted from Maeda et al. 2021 because original article was published under an open access Creative Common CC BY license.)

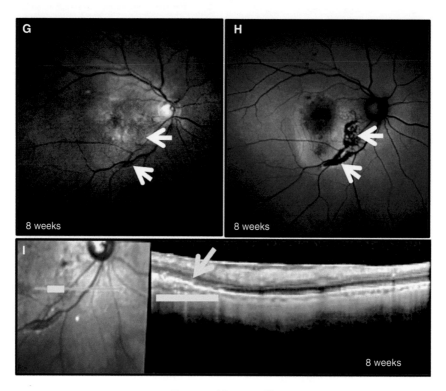

Figure 4. (*Continued.*)

lished (Takagi et al. 2019), and the 5-yr follow-up has been completed (Fig. 2). No intraoperative complications, tumorigenesis, engraftment failure, rejection, or other serious complications of transplanted cells, which were the primary end points, were observed 5 yr after surgery. No recurrence of CNV was observed in patients in the absence of additional anti-VEGF antibody treatment. Corrected visual acuity was maintained at 0.09 preoperatively. When comparing the preoperative and final observations, the foveal retinal thickness decreased from 0.298 mm before transplantation to 0.170 mm 1 yr after transplantation. However, it increased to 0.569 mm, 5 yr after transplantation due to the development of macular edema, although macular edema was dramatically decreased by topical steroid treatment (Fig. 2B). Regarding the graft, the major axis, minor axis, and thickness observed were 2.667 mm, 0.623 mm, and 0.33 mm, respectively, 3 d after transplantation. Six months later, the major and minor axis increased to 3.261 mm and 1.635 mm, respectively, and a further increase to 3.366 mm and 2.232 mm, respectively, was observed 5 yr later. The area of the graft was 1.521 mm^2 3 d after transplantation and a threefold increase to 5.471 mm^2 was seen 1 yr after transplantation. The size of the RPE sheet was relatively stable, with an area of 6.532 mm^2 at 3 yr and 5.769 mm^2 at 5 yr after transplantation. The choroidal volume was relatively stable from 0.56 mm^3 before transplantation to 0.43 mm^3 5 yr after transplantation immediately below the transplantation site but decreased from 2.31 mm^3 to 1.40 mm^3 around the transplantation site. In addition, according to the National Eye Institute (NEI), evaluation of the safety and feasibility of subretinal transplantation of iPSC-RPE that is grown as a monolayer on a biodegradable polylactic-co-glycolic acid (PLGA) scaffold, as a potential autologous cell-based therapy for GA preparations associated with AMD, is underway.

Allogeneic iPSC-RPE Cell Suspension Transplantation

The world's first autologous iPSC-RPE cell transplantation was carefully studied, and the results suggested that autologous iPSC-RPE transplantation is safe and effective (Mandai et al. 2017). Our next aim was to study allogeneic transplantation. First, we established a test system that can evaluate and manage immune rejection for allogeneic RPE transplantation, called the lymphocyte graft immune reaction (LGIR) test (Fig. 4). We also established a test to detect grafted RPE-specific antibodies (donor-specific antibodies [DSAs]) (Sugita et al. 2020).

In our preclinical studies (Sugita et al. 2016a, b; Fujii et al. 2020), we confirmed the reliability of the LGIR test in determining immune rejection after RPE cell transplantation. Thereafter, a local steroid administration protocol, a clinical study of allogeneic iPSC-RPE suspension transplantation (UMIN000026003), was conducted in collaboration with RIKEN, Center for iPS Cell Research and Application, Kyoto University (CiRA), Osaka University, and Kobe City Medical Center General Hospital in Japan. This study aimed to investigate the safety of six HLA loci-matched allogeneic cell transplantations under local steroids only, to develop/establish future standard cell therapy with iPSC-RPE (Sugita et al. 2020).

In the period of March to September 2017, transplantation was performed on five patients with exudative AMD who had the same HLA haplotype as allogeneic iPSC-RPE. Twelve months after transplantation surgery, safety and efficacy were evaluated as primary and secondary end points, respectively. The following are the notable points taken from that study: (1) The raw material was established from an HLA 6-locus homozygote donor manufactured by CiRA, Kyoto University; (2) Dosage of a cell suspension that is easy to store and transport and is considered less invasive by transplantation was selected; (3) A frozen stock of RPE cells was created as an intermediate, which was thawed as per requirement on the date of transplantation. Recovery culture was performed for 2 weeks, and the cell suspension was prepared using a dedicated transplant medium; (4) At the time of transplantation, the procedure for removal of neovascularization was not performed in autologous RPE transplantation, and a commercially available ophthalmic cannula (PolyTip cannula 25 g/38 g; MedOne, Sarasota, FL) was used as a dedicated transplantation device for the cell suspension; and (5) Immune rejection after transplantation was evaluated using a test system (LGIR and DSA) that assessed the immune response of the participant's peripheral lymphocytes to the transplanted cells in vitro, RPE-specific antibody, and OCT imaging to detect any exudative findings at the RPE-transplanted lesion.

There were no intraoperative complications, and the RPE cell suspension was implanted in the subretinal space as planned in all five cases. According to the protocol, anti-VEGF antibodies and topical ocular steroids were administered at the time of transplantation to treat the underlying disease and suppress rejection. In a follow-up examination after transplantation, only one out of five cases were suspected of having mild immune rejection from OCT findings. LGIR was found to be slightly positive, indicating subtle immune rejection. In this case, administration of additional sub-Tenon topical steroids resulted in successful management. However, no noticeable rejection of transplanted cells was observed during the observation period. In case of any occurrence of rejection, it can be managed with topical ocular steroids. Among the three cases in which a positive reaction was observed in LGIR, only one case showed clinical findings suggestive of rejection of transplanted cells, whereas none of the cases showed damage to photoreceptor cells directly above the transplanted cells. The epiretinal membrane was observed in all cases, whereas macular edema resistant to anti-VEGF antibody treatment was observed only in one case and vitreous surgery was performed for its removal. The study concluded that grafted RPE cells survived in all five cases for more than 2 yr and further suggests that the instances of immune rejection and complications that occurred during this study could be managed appropriately (Fig. 5; Sugita et al. 2020).

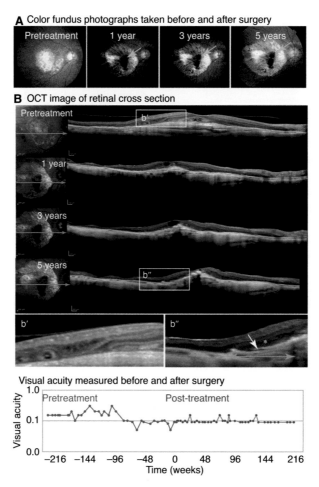

A Color fundus photographs taken before and after surgery

Pretreatment | 1 year | 3 years | 5 years

B OCT image of retinal cross section

Pretreatment

1 year

3 years

5 years

b′ | b″

Visual acuity measured before and after surgery

Pretreatment | Post-treatment

Figure 5. Clinical findings of induced pluripotent stem cell retinal pigment epithelial (iPSC-RPE) transplantation to wet-type age-related macular degeneration (AMD) patients. Survival of the autologous iPSC-RPE sheet was observed stably for 5 yr in subretinal transplanted lesions while maintaining pigmentation and a slight increase in graft size (*A*, green arrows). Changes in the retinal structure before and after surgery were monitored using optical coherence tomography (OCT) (*B*). The outer nuclear layer (*) and inner and outer segment (IS/OS) junction lines were recognized at the RPE sheet-transplanted lesion (above the orange arrow), whereas the retinal structure was disrupted before surgery (b′). The corrected visual acuity of the patient was stably maintained for 5 yr without significant changes, and anti-VEGF antibody treatment was completely discontinued after surgery (*C*). Quantitative assessment of transplanted iPSC-RPE cells in a representative case of the clinical research on iPSC-RPE cell suspension transplantation. Color fundus photographs and early-phase fluorescein angiography (FA) images were obtained during pretreatment (*C*) and 1 yr after treatment (*D*). (*E*) Window defect (WD) shown by binary image processing of the FA images at pretreatment. The FA image was processed using binary imaging (*E*, *left* panel), and the vessel images were manually removed (*E*, *right* panel). Overlays of WD binary images for pretreatment FA (*F*) and FA at 1 yr after treatment (*G*). The WD area is displayed in pixels. (*H*) Automated measurement of the WD area with soft tissue was performed using deep learning. The decrease in the WD area due to RPE engraftment is indicated by the score (pixel). Polarization-sensitive OCT showed that the presence of pigmented RPE cells indicated that the high-entropy area was above the RPE basement membrane and that there was a time-dependent decrease in the low-entropy area within the fovea-centered 3-mm-diameter circle. The low-entropy areas at 1, 7, and 12 mo after transplantation are shown in black on the entropy map for each time point with the percentage of the black area within the red circle. Low-entropy areas for each time point were aligned with the retinal vessels and are shown in the *right* panel to demonstrate consistency in the pattern (*H*). Time course of a representative section view at the white line on the *left* color fundus image, which shows the continuity of the presumably melanin-containing RPE cells covering the surface of the fibrous tissue 12 mo after transplantation. (Panels *A* and *B* reprinted from Maeda et al. 2021 because original article was published under an open access Creative Common CC BY license.)

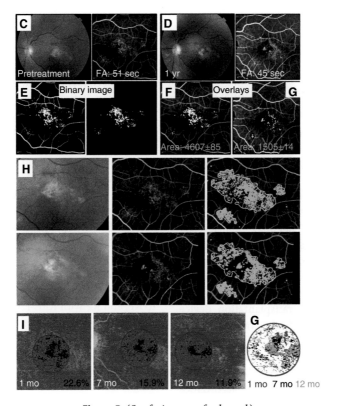

Figure 5. (*See facing page for legend.*)

REGENERATIVE MEDICINE-RELATED LAWS: TOWARD THE REALIZATION OF SAFE AND HIGH-QUALITY MEDICAL CARE

The Regenerative Medicine Promotion Act was enacted in April 2014 to quickly and safely promote the practical applications of regenerative medicine. The basic philosophy of the Act includes comprehensive efforts aimed at the realization of safe research development, and the spread of treatments based on the consideration of bioethics associated with treatments using human cells. Therefore, it is permitted to outsource the cultivation and processing of cells and tissues, used for regenerative medicine, to a certified corporate factory outside the medical institution to promote industrialization and commercialization. Furthermore, apart from its promotion, it is stipulated that the basic policy should be reviewed at least every 3 years if required.

In connection with this law, the Act on the Safety of Regenerative Medicine was enacted in 2014, which sets regulations for all clinical studies and treatments led by hospitals using cells or genes. According to this law, depending on the cell type applied to humans, first-, second-, and third-class tiers of regenerative medicine were defined. The first class is for pluripotent stem cells and other allogeneic cell therapies. The criteria for determining which category each medical technology falls into will be reviewed in accordance with technological progress and changes over time. Of note, in the United States, the 21st Century Cures Act was enacted at the end of 2016 and progress is being made toward the establishment of a system similar to the conditional and time-limited approval system in Japan. In particular, the same section defines a new category of "regenerative medicine advanced therapy" (RMAT) and stipulates that the above-mentioned accelerated approval system can be applied to products that meet its requirements (www.fda.gov/regulatory-information/selected-amendments-fdc-act/21st-century-cures-act#:~

:text=The%2021st%20Century%20Cures%20Act,
them%20faster%20and%20more%20efficiently).

DEVELOPMENT OF REGENERATIVE MEDICINE: FROM MANUFACTURING TO CLINICAL APPLICATIONS

Unlike small molecule compounds, regenerative medicines should use cells that are heterogeneous and changeable at any time. They undergo a quality control test and a highly controlled manufacturing process (induction of differentiation if derived from iPSCs); however, cells are not yet homogeneous. They may change characteristics even after transplantation according to the host environment. Furthermore, when the final product forms a tissue, transplantation to a diseased site is a prerequisite, and it may be necessary to prepare a transplantation device for this purpose and study the transplantation techniques. The safety and efficacy of regenerative medicine products in these developmental stages are verified through nonclinical animal tests, and after being evaluated in accordance with the criteria described later, clinical studies and trials are conducted. For those cells that exist in the body, the clinical efficacy will be determined by surgical techniques and the retaining ability of the host tissue. However, it is difficult to speculate on the treatment effect only by randomized controlled trials (RCTs), or in other words, RCT results cannot be applied to every surgery. Therefore, suitable regulations are required for such new fields of medicine.

FUTURE PROSPECTS AND CHALLENGES IN RETINAL REGENERATIVE MEDICINE

New Category of Disease Group and Medication for Retinal Degeneration

While RPE is responsible for maintaining retinal homeostasis (Boulton and Dayhaw-Barker 2001; Sparrow et al. 2010; Palczewski 2014), it has been suggested that functional deterioration of RPE may be a major cause of some hereditary and nonhereditary retinal degenerative diseases, such as AMD (Hageman et al. 2001; Sparrow et al. 2010; Ach et al. 2014). RPE is a layer of

pigment epithelial cells that exists in the outer layer of the retina and plays an important role in maintaining homeostasis of the retina such as stress relief in the photo response of retinal photoreceptor cells and maintenance of photoreceptor function. Retinal disease, which is included in the hereditary disease group, is caused by age-related pathological changes such as genetic abnormalities expressed in RPE, oxidative stress associated with aging, and abnormal accumulation of waste products. It has been suggested that it can be a major cause of RP and AMD, which have been the target diseases of clinical studies using RPE transplantation. There are several other retinal degenerative diseases mainly caused by RPE deficiency and are grouped into one disease group called RPE-impaired diseases. These rare diseases include RP, diseases related to RP, and RP with RPE-related gene abnormalities (those with abnormalities in genes such as *RPE65*, *RDH5*, and *MERTK*). This group also includes AMD, which is a common cause of blindness in the elderly, and is recognized as one of the intractable diseases of the eye. Although the pathogenesis of these diseases is different, RPE cell dysfunction and degeneration are common, and a standard treatment for RPE cell dysfunction and degeneration has not been established to date. Cell transplantation may be effective, but this requires further research. Therefore, retinal degenerative disease, a common pathological condition for which this treatment method has not been established yet, was targeted as a disease group called RPE-impaired disease. Clinical research is being conducted on corneal epithelial stem cell exhaustion as a target disease for regenerative medicine of the corneal epithelium, which has been proposed under the same concept as RPE-impaired disease.

Objective Evaluation of RPE Transplantation for Retinal Degeneration

Because of the variation in disease types in RPE-impaired diseases, setting a primary end point that can be objectively evaluated among these multiple diseases and incorporating various visual function tests as secondary end points is indispensable for performing clinical studies efficiently. This evalu-

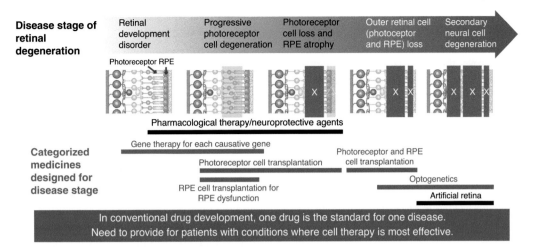

Figure 6. Treatment strategy with categorized medicine for retinal degeneration. Categorized medicine is a therapeutic strategy based on the pathology of the retina, rather than on a disease-by-disease basis. In the early stage of retinal degeneration, the photoreceptor cells and retinal pigment epithelial cells to be treated are intact; therefore, gene therapy or drug therapy with neuroprotective factors for these cells is indicated. Gene therapy or cell transplantation is indicated at the stage of severe dysfunction or degeneration of the retinal cells. Cell transplantation is indicated when retinal degeneration progresses and photoreceptor cells and retinal pigment epithelial cells disappear. Optogenetic or artificial retinas are indicated in the final stages of damage to the inner retina. (Figure based on data in Scholl et al. 2016.)

ation will enable the identification of diseases for which RPE cell transplantation can be effective. To address issues related to RPE-impaired diseases, evaluation methods using a window defect (WD) and clinical findings of fluorescein angiography (FA), which is an imaging test used in general ophthalmic practice, were designed. Since the WD shows an RPE abnormal region in the FA as a lesion with hyperfluorescence, measurement of the decrease in WD after RPE transplantation is suggested to represent engraftment of transplanted cells. This method was successfully used to quantify the engrafted area in a previous study (Sugita et al. 2020) and the quality of analyses was improved using automated measurement software driven by deep learning (Motozawa et al. 2022). It is possible to develop a treatment method for rare diseases by collectively evaluating the efficacy using this concept. In fact, as in a past case, it is indicated for patients with severe myopia who have decreased visual acuity due to CNV, as well as in exudative AMD, even though an anti-VEGF drug was likely to be effective. Since it took 7 years to be approved, it may be useful to conduct clinical trials on a group of diseases to examine the

safety and efficacy of diseases with common pathological conditions. From these observations, proper treatments can be provided according to the stage of the disease in retinal degeneration with categorized medicines in combination with other types of treatments (Fig. 6).

Improvement of Formulation for Better Efficacy

In the allogeneic iPSC-RPE cell suspension transplantation performed so far for wet-type AMD, the formation of an anterior retinal membrane, which is thought to be caused by cell leakage from the transplantation site, is frequently observed (Sugita et al. 2020). This has also been reported in clinical trials of RPE cell suspensions derived from ES cells by another group (Maeda et al. 2021). No direct adverse events have occurred due to anterior retinal membrane formation itself, and it can be dealt with by vitreous surgery performed in general medical care. However, the effects of cell transplantation treatment are the reconstruction and functional recovery of the RPE layer on the premise of engraftment of transplanted cells, the effect on visual function due to anterior retinal membrane formation, and the risk of vitreous surgery as a countermeasure. Based on the above, it is desirable to improve the transplantation technique for prompt engraftment of transplanted cells at the subretinal transplantation site, thereby suppressing the leakage of nonadherent cells. Several nonclinical studies have confirmed that transplanting cells with a simple aggregated strip provides shape, facilitates observation of the transplanted cells, and suppresses the risk of postoperative leakage (Nishida et al. 2021). Preparations for clinical research using this technique are currently in progress (Table 1).

Other Technical Improvements in Retinal Regenerative Medicine

A strategy to consistently establish manufacturing and treatment methods is important for the practical application of retinal regenerative medicine. For example, cost reduction can be expected by reviewing the cells used as raw materials and the manufacturing method in a timely manner. In fact, for research purposes, the Kyoto iPS Cell Research Institute, Japan has started to provide iPSCs that are partially KO HLA. Since these cells are less likely to be rejected even by recipients with different HLA haplotypes, there is a possibility that the cost of cell raw materials can be reduced if they are put into practical use. Furthermore, in currently planned retinal cell transplantations, the number of transplanted cells and the transplantation site are limited; thus, significant improvements in visual acuity and visual field cannot be expected. Therefore, it is important to evaluate the anatomical recovery and normalization of the retinal structure at the transplantation site. Polarization-sensitive OCT (PS-OCT) and AO are new diagnostic imaging techniques for this problem (Fig. 5). Since PS-OCT can visualize melanin pigment that is abundant in healthy RPE cells, it is possible to distinguish normal RPE sites from abnormal ones where RPE is deficient or dysfunctional. In addition, AO enables retinal observations at the cellular level (Fig. 5). Using these techniques, a more precise evaluation can be attained if cells are engrafted at

an abnormal RPE site and normalization of the retinal structure is seen.

CONCLUDING REMARKS

Cell therapies with iPSC-RPE have significant potential as curative treatments for retinal degeneration because of the distinct advantages of retinal characteristics, and such diseases are an attractive target for applications/implementations of regenerative medicine. However, several important issues remain yet to be addressed, and the relevant basic research areas must continue to solve these practical problems. It is expected that advances in the clinical applications of stem cell–derived retinal cells will be made with the help of various technologies from several/diverse/disparate fields, and cooperation with regulatory systems to design more suitable clinical studies for regenerative medicine. In the future, comprehensive therapeutic strategies should be developed and made available for the pharmacological treatment of retinal degeneration, along/together with other therapies/remedial treatments (e.g., gene therapy).

ACKNOWLEDGMENTS

We would like to thank Dr. Yasuo Kurimoto, Dr. Michiko Mandai, Dr. Sunao Sugita, Dr. Yasuhiko Hirami, and Dr. Akiko Maeda (Kobe Eye Center Hospital) for their valuable comments and support.

REFERENCES

Ach T, Huisingh C, McGwin G, Messinger JD, Zhang T, Bentley MJ, Gutierrez DB, Ablonczy Z, Smith RT, Sloan KR, et al. 2014. Quantitative autofluorescence and cell density maps of the human retinal pigment epithelium. *Invest Ophthalmol Vis Sci* 55: 4832–4841. doi:10.1167/iovs.14-14802

Algvere PV, Berglin L, Gouras P, Sheng Y. 1994. Transplantation of fetal retinal pigment epithelium in age-related macular degeneration with subfoveal neovascularization. *Graefes Arch Clin Exp Ophthalmol* 232: 707–716. doi:10.1007/BF00184273

Algvere PV, Berglin L, Gouras P, Sheng Y, Kopp ED. 1997. Transplantation of RPE in age-related macular degeneration: observations in disciform lesions and dry RPE atrophy. *Graefes Arch Clin Exp Ophthalmol* 235: 149–158. doi:10.1007/BF00941722

Al-Merjan JI, Pandova MG, Al-Ghanim M, Al-Wayel A, Al-Mutairi S. 2005. Registered blindness and low vision in Kuwait. *Ophthalmic Epidemiol* 12: 251–257. doi:10.1080/09286580591005813

Boulton M, Dayhaw-Barker P. 2001. The role of the retinal pigment epithelium: topographical variation and ageing changes. *Eye* 15: 384–389. doi:10.1038/eye.2001.141

Buch H, Vinding T, Nielsen NV. 2001. Prevalence and causes of visual impairment according to World Health Organization and United States criteria in an aged, urban Scandinavian population: the Copenhagen city eye study. *Ophthalmology* 108: 2347–2357. doi:10.1016/S0161-6420(01)00823-5

da Cruz L, Fynes K, Georgiadis O, Kerby J, Luo YH, Ahmado A, Vernon A, Daniels JT, Nommiste B, Hasan SM, et al. 2018. Phase 1 clinical study of an embryonic stem cell-derived retinal pigment epithelium patch in age-related macular degeneration. *Nat Biotechnol* 36: 328–337. doi:10.1038/nbt.4114

Daniel E, Maguire MG, Grunwald JE, Toth CA, Jaffe GJ, Martin DF, Ying GS, Comparison of Age-Related Macular Degeneration Treatments Trials Research Group. 2020. Incidence and progression of nongeographic atrophy in the comparison of age-related macular degeneration treatments trials (CATT) clinical trial. *JAMA Ophthalmol* 138: 510–518. doi:10.1001/jamaophthalmol.2020.0437

Del Priore LV, Kaplan HJ, Tezel TH, Hayashi N, Berger AS, Green WR. 2001. Retinal pigment epithelial cell transplantation after subfoveal membranectomy in age-related macular degeneration: clinicopathologic correlation. *Am J Ophthalmol* 131: 472–480. doi:10.1016/S0002-9394(00)00850-3

Fleckenstein M, Mitchell P, Freund KB, Sadda S, Holz FG, Brittain C, Henry EC, Ferrara D. 2018. The progression of geographic atrophy secondary to age-related macular degeneration. *Ophthalmology* 125: 369–390. doi:10.1016/j.ophtha.2017.08.038

Fujii S, Sugita S, Futatsugi Y, Ishida M, Edo A, Makabe K, Kamao H, Iwasaki Y, Sakaguchi H, Hirami Y, et al. 2020. A strategy for personalized treatment of iPS-retinal immune rejections assessed in cynomolgus monkey models. *Int J Mol Sci* 21: 3077. doi:10.3390/ijms21093077

GBD 2019 Blindness and Vision Impairment Collaborators. 2021. Trends in prevalence of blindness and distance and near vision impairment over 30 years: an analysis for the Global Burden of Disease Study. *Lancet Glob Health* 9: e130–e143.

Gouras P, Flood MT, Kjedbye H, Bilek MK, Eggers H. 1985. Transplantation of cultured human retinal epithelium to Bruch's membrane of the owl monkey's eye. *Curr Eye Res* 4: 253–265. doi:10.3109/02713688509000857

Hageman GS, Luthert PJ, Victor Chong NH, Johnson LV, Anderson DH, Mullins RF. 2001. An integrated hypothesis that considers drusen as biomarkers of immune-mediated processes at the RPE-Bruch's membrane interface in aging and age-related macular degeneration. *Prog Retin Eye Res* 20: 705–732. doi:10.1016/S1350-9462(01)00010-6

Haruta M, Sasai Y, Kawasaki H, Amemiya K, Ooto S, Kitada M, Suemori H, Nakatsuji N, Ide C, Honda Y, et al. 2004. In vitro and in vivo characterization of pigment epithelial

cells differentiated from primate embryonic stem cells. *Invest Ophthalmol Vis Sci* 45: 1020–1025. doi:10.1167/iovs.03-1034

Hirami Y, Osakada F, Takahashi K, Okita K, Yamanaka S, Ikeda H, Yoshimura N, Takahashi M. 2009. Generation of retinal cells from mouse and human induced pluripotent stem cells. *Neurosci Lett* 458: 126–131. doi:10.1016/j.neulet.2009.04.035

Joussen AM, Heussen FM, Joeres S, Llacer H, Prinz B, Rohrschneider K, Maaijwee KJ, van Meurs J, Kirchhof B. 2006. Autologous translocation of the choroid and retinal pigment epithelium in age-related macular degeneration. *Am J Ophthalmol* 142: 17–30.e8. doi:10.1016/j.ajo.2006.01.090

Kashani AH, Lebkowski JS, Rahhal FM, Avery RL, Salehi-Had H, Dang W, Lin CM, Mitra D, Zhu D, Thomas BB, et al. 2018. A bioengineered retinal pigment epithelial monolayer for advanced, dry age-related macular degeneration. *Sci Transl Med* 10: eaao4097. doi:10.1126/scitranslmed.aao4097

Kashani AH, Lebkowski JS, Rahhal FM, Avery RL, Salehi-Had H, Chen S, Chan C, Palejwala N, Ingram A, Dang W, et al. 2021. One-year follow-up in a phase 1/2a clinical trial of an allogeneic RPE cell bioengineered implant for advanced dry age-related macular degeneration. *Transl Vis Sci Technol* 10: 13. doi:10.1167/tvst.10.10.13

Kuroda Y, Yamashiro K, Miyake M, Yoshikawa M, Nakanishi H, Oishi A, Tamura H, Ooto S, Tsujikawa A, Yoshimura N. 2015. Factors associated with recurrence of age-related macular degeneration after anti-vascular endothelial growth factor treatment: a retrospective cohort study. *Ophthalmology* 122: 2303–2310. doi:10.1016/j.ophtha.2015.06.053

Kuroda Y, Yamashiro K, Tsujikawa A, Ooto S, Tamura H, Oishi A, Nakanishi H, Miyake M, Yoshikawa M, Yoshimura N. 2016. Retinal pigment epithelial atrophy in neovascular age-related macular degeneration after ranibizumab treatment. *Am J Ophthalmol* 161: 94–103.e1. doi:10.1016/j.ajo.2015.09.032

Maaijwee K, Heimann H, Missotten T, Mulder P, Joussen A, van Meurs J. 2007. Retinal pigment epithelium and choroid translocation in patients with exudative age-related macular degeneration: long-term results. *Graefes Arch Clin Exp Ophthalmol* 245: 1681–1689. doi:10.1007/s00417-007-0607-4

MacLaren RE, Uppal GS, Balaggan KS, Tufail A, Munro PM, Milliken AB, Ali RR, Rubin GS, Aylward GW, da Cruz L. 2007. Autologous transplantation of the retinal pigment epithelium and choroid in the treatment of neovascular age-related macular degeneration. *Ophthalmology* 114: 561–570.e2. doi:10.1016/j.ophtha.2006.06.049

Maeda A, Mandai M, Takahashi M. 2019. Gene and induced pluripotent stem cell therapy for retinal diseases. *Annu Rev Genomics Hum Genet* 20: 201–216. doi:10.1146/annurev-genom-083118-015043

Maeda T, Sugita S, Kurimoto Y, Takahashi M. 2021. Trends of stem cell therapies in age-related macular degeneration. *J Clin Med* 10: 1785. doi:10.3390/jcm10081785

Mandai M, Watanabe A, Kurimoto Y, Hirami Y, Morinaga C, Daimon T, Fujihara M, Akimaru H, Sakai N, Shibata Y, et al. 2017. Autologous induced stem-cell-derived retinal cells for macular degeneration. *N Engl J Med* **376:** 1038–1046. doi:10.1056/NEJMoa1608368

Mehat MS, Sundaram V, Ripamonti C, Robson AG, Smith AJ, Borooah S, Robinson M, Rosenthal AN, Innes W, Weleber RG, et al. 2018. Transplantation of human embryonic stem cell-derived retinal pigment epithelial cells in macular degeneration. *Ophthalmology* **125:** 1765–1775. doi:10.1016/j.ophtha.2018.04.037

Morizane Y, Morimoto N, Fujiwara A, Kawasaki R, Yamashita H, Ogura Y, Shiraga F. 2019. Incidence and causes of visual impairment in Japan: the first nation-wide complete enumeration survey of newly certified visually impaired individuals. *Jpn J Ophthalmol* **63:** 26–33. doi:10.1007/s10384-018-0623-4

Motozawa N, Miura T, Ochiai K, Yamamoto M, Horinouchi T, Tsuzuki T, Kanda GN, Ozawa Y, Tsujikawa A, Takahashi K, et al. 2022. Automated evaluation of retinal pigment epithelium disease area in eyes with age-related macular degeneration. *Sci Rep* **12:** 892. doi:10.1038/s41598-022-05006-3

Nagiel A, Freund KB, Spaide RF, Munch IC, Larsen M, Sarraf D. 2013. Mechanism of retinal pigment epithelium tear formation following intravitreal anti-vascular endothelial growth factor therapy revealed by spectral-domain optical coherence tomography. *Am J Ophthalmol* **156:** 981–988.e2. doi:10.1016/j.ajo.2013.06.024

Nishida M, Tanaka Y, Tanaka Y, Amaya S, Tanaka N, Uyama H, Masuda T, Onishi A, Sho J, Yokota S, et al. 2021. Human iPS cell derived RPE strips for secure delivery of graft cells at a target place with minimal surgical invasion. *Sci Rep* **11:** 21421. doi:10.1038/s41598-021-00703-x

Osakada F, Ikeda H, Sasai Y, Takahashi M. 2009. Stepwise differentiation of pluripotent stem cells into retinal cells. *Nat Protoc* **4:** 811–824. doi:10.1038/nprot.2009.51

Palczewski K. 2014. Chemistry and biology of the initial steps in vision: the Friedenwald lecture. *Invest Ophthalmol Vis Sci* **55:** 6651–6672. doi:10.1167/iovs.14-15502

Peyman GA, Blinder KJ, Paris CL, Alturki W, Nelson NC Jr, Desai U. 1991. A technique for retinal pigment epithelium transplantation for age-related macular degeneration secondary to extensive subfoveal scarring. *Ophthalmic Surg* **22:** 102–108. doi:10.3928/1542-8877-19910201-12

Scholl HP, Strauss RW, Singh MS, Dalkara D, Roska B, Picaud S, Sahel JA. 2016. Emerging therapies for inherited retinal degeneration. *Sci Transl Med* **8:** 368rv366. doi:10.1126/scitranslmed.aaf2838

Schwartz SD, Regillo CD, Lam BL, Eliott D, Rosenfeld PJ, Gregori NZ, Hubschman JP, Davis JL, Heilwell G, Spirn M, et al. 2015. Human embryonic stem cell-derived retinal pigment epithelium in patients with age-related macular degeneration and Stargardt's macular dystrophy: follow-up of two open-label phase 1/2 studies. *Lancet* **385:** 509–516. doi:10.1016/S0140-6736(14)61376-3

Singh MS, Park SS, Albini TA, Canto-Soler MV, Klassen H, MacLaren RE, Takahashi M, Nagiel A, Schwartz SD, Bharti K. 2020. Retinal stem cell transplantation: balancing safety and potential. *Prog Retin Eye Res* **75:** 100779. doi:10.1016/j.preteyeres.2019.100779

Song WK, Park KM, Kim HJ, Lee JH, Choi J, Chong SY, Shim SH, Del Priore LV, Lanza R. 2015. Treatment of macular degeneration using embryonic stem cell-derived retinal pigment epithelium: preliminary results in Asian patients. *Stem Cell Reports* **4:** 860–872. doi:10.1016/j.stemcr.2015.04.005

Sparrow JR, Hicks D, Hamel CP. 2010. The retinal pigment epithelium in health and disease. *Curr Mol Med* **10:** 802–823. doi:10.2174/156652410793937813

Sugita S, Iwasaki Y, Makabe K, Kamao H, Mandai M, Shiina T, Ogasawara K, Hirami Y, Kurimoto Y, Takahashi M. 2016a. Successful transplantation of retinal pigment epithelial cells from MHC homozygote iPSCs in MHC-matched models. *Stem Cell Reports* **7:** 635–648. doi:10.1016/j.stemcr.2016.08.010

Sugita S, Iwasaki Y, Makabe K, Kimura T, Futagami T, Suegami S, Takahashi M. 2016b. Lack of T cell response to iPSC-derived retinal pigment epithelial cells from HLA homozygous donors. *Stem Cell Reports* **7:** 619–634. doi:10.1016/j.stemcr.2016.08.011

Sugita S, Mandai M, Hirami Y, Takagi S, Maeda T, Fujihara M, Matsuzaki M, Yamamoto M, Iseki K, Hayashi N, et al. 2020. HLA-matched allogeneic iPS cells-derived RPE transplantation for macular degeneration. *J Clin Med* **9:** 2217. doi:10.3390/jcm9072217

Takagi S, Mandai M, Gocho K, Hirami Y, Yamamoto M, Fujihara M, Sugita S, Kurimoto Y, Takahashi M. 2019. Evaluation of transplanted autologous induced pluripotent stem cell-derived retinal pigment epithelium in exudative age-related macular degeneration. *Ophthalmol Retina* **3:** 850–859. doi:10.1016/j.oret.2019.04.021

Weisz JM, Humayun MS, De Juan E Jr, Del Cerro M, Sunness JS, Dagnelie G, Soylu M, Rizzo L, Nussenblatt RB. 1999. Allogenic fetal retinal pigment epithelial cell transplant in a patient with geographic atrophy. *Retina* **19:** 540–545. doi:10.1097/00006982-199911000-00011

Wong WL, Su X, Li X, Cheung CM, Klein R, Cheng CY, Wong TY. 2014. Global prevalence of age-related macular degeneration and disease burden projection for 2020 and 2040: a systematic review and meta-analysis. *Lancet Glob Health* **2:** e106–e116. doi:10.1016/S2214-109X(13)70145-1

Xu H, Wang B, Ono M, Kagita A, Fujii K, Sasakawa N, Ueda T, Gee P, Nishikawa M, Nomura M, et al. 2019. Targeted disruption of HLA genes via CRISPR-Cas9 generates iPSCs with enhanced immune compatibility. *Cell Stem Cell* **24:** 566–578.e7. doi:10.1016/j.stem.2019.02.005

Young M, Chui L, Fallah N, Or C, Merkur AB, Kirker AW, Albiani DA, Forooghian F. 2014. Exacerbation of choroidal and retinal pigment epithelial atrophy after anti-vascular endothelial growth factor treatment in neovascular age-related macular degeneration. *Retina* **34:** 1308–1315. doi:10.1097/IAE.0000000000000081

Considerations for Developing an Autologous Induced Pluripotent Stem Cell (iPSC)-Derived Retinal Pigment Epithelium (RPE) Replacement Therapy

Devika Bose, Davide Ortolan, Mitra Farnoodian, Ruchi Sharma, and Kapil Bharti

Ocular and Stem Cell Translational Research, National Eye Institute, National Institutes of Health, Bethesda, Maryland 20892, USA

Correspondence: Kapil.bharti@nih.gov

Cell-replacement therapies are a new class of treatments, which include induced pluripotent stem cell (iPSC)-derived tissues that aim to replace degenerated cells. iPSCs can potentially be used to generate any cell type of the body, making them a powerful tool for treating degenerative diseases. Cell replacement for retinal degenerative diseases is at the forefront of cell therapies, given the accessibility of the eye for surgical procedures and a huge unmet medical need for retinal degenerative diseases with no current treatment options. Clinical trials are ongoing in different parts of the world using stem cell–derived retinal pigment epithelium (RPE). This review focuses on scientific and regulatory considerations when developing an iPSC-derived RPE cell therapy from the development of a robust and efficient differentiation protocol to critical quality control assays for cell validation, the choice of an appropriate animal model for preclinical testing, and the regulatory aspects that dictate the final approval for proceeding to a first-in-human clinical trial.

The recent use of the induced pluripotent stem cell (iPSC) technology to generate different cell types has revolutionized the field of regenerative medicine (Takahashi et al. 2007; Yu et al. 2007; Hirschi et al. 2014). The problems associated with immune rejection, insufficient availability of replacement tissues, and how well the body can integrate a new allogeneic cell/tissue can be circumvented by using the patient's own iPSCs to generate new and healthy autologous tissues and, potentially, organs (Vonk et al. 2015; Madrid et al. 2021). Stem cell–based therapy is being used to treat retinal degenerative diseases like age-related macular degeneration (AMD) (Schwartz et al. 2012, 2015; Song et al. 2015; Da Cruz et al. 2018; Kashani et al. 2018), retinitis pigmentosa (RP) (Uy et al. 2013; Tuekprakhon et al. 2021), diabetic retinopathy, and Stargardt's retinal degeneration (Schwartz et al. 2015). Retinal pigment epithelium (RPE)-based cell therapy is one of the most advanced treatments for some of these diseases (Bharti et al. 2011; Monsarrat et al. 2016; Deinsberger et al. 2020).

RPE is a polarized monolayer present at the back of the eye, which performs many functions critical for healthy vision; some of these include nourishing the overlying photoreceptors and removing waste products of the visual cycle (Bharti et al. 2006). Healthy RPE cells are therefore responsible for good vision and retinal homeostasis. A patient's fibroblasts or peripheral blood mononuclear cells (PBMCs) can be isolated and reprogrammed into iPSCs. These cells are then differentiated to form RPE by different protocols, including spontaneous or directed differentiation (Osakada et al. 2009b; Bharti et al. 2011; Pennington et al. 2015; Ben M'barek et al. 2017; Sharma et al. 2019). Studying the developmental pathways of the RPE in vivo underlies which signaling pathways and associated growth factors are important for RPE differentiation in vitro. Differentiation of iPSCs toward RPE requires activation and inhibition of different pathways at different phases of the differentiation cycle (Song et al. 2015; Da Cruz et al. 2018; Sharma et al. 2022). Our laboratory has developed a triphasic differentiation protocol to generate RPE from iPSCs, in which media with different growth factors are used in all three phases (Sharma et al. 2022).

As per regulatory guidelines and for patient safety, the quality control (QC) criteria are to be stringent for RPE cells that are planned to be transplanted into a patient. As the differentiation process is very long and there are many factors influencing differentiation, it is necessary to monitor this process at every step. As part of good manufacturing practices (GMPs) and Food and Drug Administration (FDA) guidelines, a variety of tests must be performed at every stage of the differentiation process starting with the source material—the iPSCs—and ending with the final product—the RPE (Rao and Malik 2012; Baghbaderani et al. 2015; Jha et al. 2021). In addition to regularly monitoring sterility of cultures (these tests are not discussed in this review), QC tests include testing for iPSC and RPE purity and maturity markers by flow cytometry, measuring the *trans*-epithelial resistance of RPE tissue after they mature, and performing microscopic evaluation to further confirm RPE maturity (Schwartz et al. 2015; Mandai

et al. 2017; Kashani et al. 2018; Sharma et al. 2019; Nishida et al. 2021). There are many regulatory guidelines that need to be followed when using an iPSC-RPE product as an investigational new drug (IND) (Jha et al. 2021). These are discussed in detail later in this review. Under Title 21 Code of Federal Regulations (CFR) guidelines, the iPSC-RPE has to be tested in animals to determine its safety and efficacy (Jha and Bharti 2015). It is vital to see whether, in preclinical studies, transplanted RPE cells are effective at mitigating the retinal degeneration in an efficacy model, and whether they have the potential to cause a tumor or any other adverse effect in a safety model (Jha et al. 2021).

RPE DEVELOPMENT AND DIFFERENTIATION

RPE has a central role in maintaining the health of the outer blood–retina barrier (oBRB) and its dysfunction and degeneration are associated with retinal degenerations (Bharti et al. 2014). This property makes RPE a key target for cell therapies—RPE replacement could halt or slow down retinal degenerations. To develop cell therapies for retinal diseases, RPE cells derived from iPSCs need to closely resemble the native cells, phenotypically and functionally. To this end, it is essential to know which signaling pathways act during the development of the human RPE to reproduce them in vitro during stem cell differentiation.

The vertebrate eye develops from an evagination of the eye field in the ventral forebrain to form the optic vesicle. The proximal region of the optic vesicle will become the optic stalk, the distal region will become neural retina, while the dorsal region will become the RPE. Once the evagination of the optic vesicle reaches the surface ectoderm, its distal part invaginates forming the optic cup. The tissues surrounding the optic cup influence specification of cell types. Four signaling pathways are particularly important: the transforming growth factor β (TGF-β) superfamily, WNT, the hedgehog (HH) family, and fibroblast growth factors (FGFs) (Amato et al. 2004; Yang 2004; Bharti et al. 2006). The mesenchyme surrounding the eye directly influences RPE development. After removal of the mesenchyme, the chick optic vesicle shows down-regulation of RPE markers and up-regulation of neuroretinal markers. ACTIVIN A, a member of the TGF-β superfamily, activates the TGF-β pathway and was shown to compensate for the missing mesenchyme ex vivo (Fuhrmann et al. 2000). A different branch of the TGF-β super-family, the bone morphogenetic protein (BMP) pathway, also proved to be essential for RPE development (Müller et al. 2007). *Bmp4* and *Bmp7* are expressed in the surface ectoderm, the mes-enchyme surrounding the optic vesicle and the presumptive RPE. Inhibiting BMP signaling, with the protein NOGGIN, prevents RPE devel-opment and induces expression of neuroretinal genes (Steinfeld et al. 2017). On the other hand, stimulating BMP signaling in the optic vesicle induces RPE development in the presumptive optic stalk and neuroretina (Müller et al. 2007). WNT activation is essential for RPE specifica-tion, since RPE commitment was blocked upon β-CATENIN genetic inactivation (Hägglund et al. 2013). The HH pathway is also thought to play a role in RPE development since proteins of this pathway have been detected in RPE (Neu-mann and Nuesslein-Volhard 2000; Stenkamp et al. 2000). Interestingly, inhibiting HH signal-ing in *Xenopus* leads to a reduction or loss of RPE markers (Perron et al. 2003). FGFs are negative regulators of early RPE development (Bharti et al. 2012). The surface ectoderm is the main source of FGFs for the eye primordium, specifi-cally FGF1 and FGF2 (De Iongh and McAvoy 1993; Pittack et al. 1997). Removal of the surface ectoderm induces the transition of the presump-tive neuroretina into RPE-like cells, while expo-sure of the presumptive RPE to FGF alters its development to neuroretina (Pittack et al. 1997; Hyer et al. 1998; Nguyen and Arnheiter 2000).

Several groups attempted in vitro RPE dif-ferentiation using spontaneous differentiation or developmentally guided protocols (Schwartz et al. 2012, 2015; Sharma et al. 2022). Sponta-neous differentiation requires replacing iPSC culture medium with one that does not contain any specific growth factor. This process is inef-ficient since it requires 20–25 wk of culture for RPE differentiation and the yield of RPE cells is <10%. Developmentally guided or directed dif-ferentiation uses the knowledge from work done on embryonic RPE development by supple-menting culture media with specific growth fac-tors at the right time point (Osakada et al. 2009a; Sharma et al. 2022). This system improves effi-ciency, shortens differentiation time from 25 wk to 10 wk, and reduces iPSC line to line variabil-ity. The first step for RPE production is the in-duction of the anterior neuroepithelium and the eye field. The role of insulin-like growth factor (IGF) in directing differentiation toward the anterior neuroepithelium was first described in *Xenopus*, where ectopic expression of IGF mRNA led to the induction of ectopic eyes and head-like structures containing brain tissue (Pera et al. 2001). Efficient neural induction from stem cells can be achieved with dual inhi-bition of SMAD signaling (Chambers et al. 2009). In addition, WNT/β-CATENIN and BMP inhibitors were shown to be up-regulated during eye field specification (Meyer et al. 2009). To recreate this process in vitro, we supply IGF-1 in combination with dual SMAD inhibition (TGF-β, SB431452; BMP, LDN193189) and WNT inhibitor, CK1-7 (Fig. 1; Sharma et al. 2022). The second step is the induction of the RPE from the anterior neuroepithelium. We add an FGF inhibitor, PD0325901, to the neuroecto-derm-induction media (Fig. 1; Sharma et al. 2022), since FGF removal is sufficient to convert the presumptive neuroretina to RPE (Pittack et al. 1997). The third step is the appearance of RPE from the eye field. At this point, activation of BMP, TGF-β, WNT, and HH pathways ap-pear to be important in determining RPE fate, as described above. We found that supplying a medium containing ACTIVIN A that triggers TGF-β/SMAD pathway activation is sufficient to generate cells with a committed RPE pheno-type (Sharma et al. 2022). Other studies enhance RPE derivation by adding a WNT agonist to the ACTIVIN A–containing medium (Nadar et al. 2015). Because the differentiation process alone may not yield a pure population of RPE cells, an enrichment process is often needed. Several lab-oratories manually select and expand pigmented colonies (Pennington et al. 2015; Ben M'barek et al. 2017; Da Cruz et al. 2018). Instead, our laboratory enriches RPE cultures by negative se-

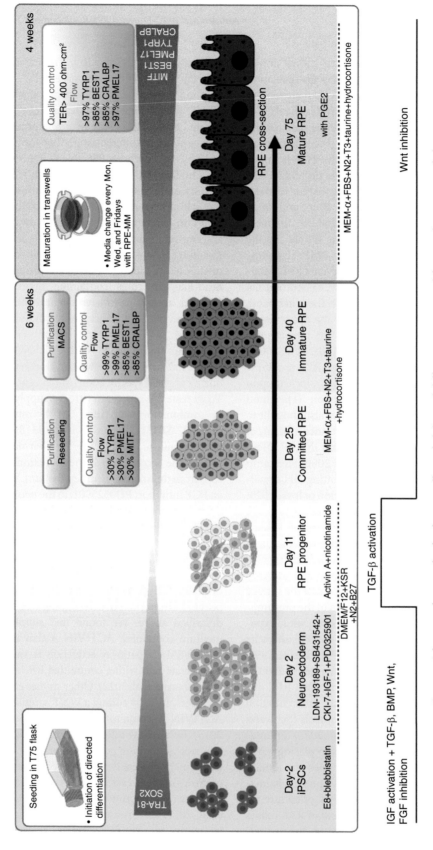

Figure 1. Schematic showing the developmentally guided directed differentiation protocol for retinal pigment epithelium (RPE) generation. (Figure adapted from Sharma et al. 2022, with permission from Elsevier © 2022.)

lection of cells expressing neuronal surface markers with CD24 and CD56 antibodies (Sharma et al. 2019, 2022). Finally, to obtain a fully mature RPE culture ready to be used as a clinical product, WNT inhibition through primary cilium stimulation with PGE2 was shown to enhance iPSC-RPE maturation (May-Simera et al. 2018; Sharma et al. 2022).

iPSC-RPE CELL-BASED THERAPY: IN-PROCESS AND CLINICAL PRODUCT VALIDATION

When using tissue differentiated from iPSCs for developing a replacement therapy, stringent QC assays to characterize every step of the manufacturing process and the final product have become imperative. There are FDA guidelines available to check safety when using cells as a source of treatment (Mendicino et al. 2019). However, iPSC-based technologies are still in their infancy as far as the FDA roadmap is concerned. iPSC-based treatments are broadly categorized into autologous or allogeneic approaches. Autologous or patient-specific cell therapies use the patients' own cells to make iPSC cells and the iPSC-derived product is transplanted back into the patient, whereas allogeneic therapies use iPSCs generated from one specific healthy donor and the derived tissue is used to treat larger populations. For the autologous approach, the process is the product; since every individual gets their iPSC-derived tissue transplanted, validating the process is as critical as the product. But for allogeneic transplants, hypothetically, one master iPSC bank can be used to treat the entire population; hence, the validation steps are focused more on the final product. The therapeutic and interventional clinical trial space is using both the allogeneic and autologous approaches. The iPSC-RPE field is currently using both these strategies; two groups are using the autologous approach to target neovascular wet AMD and dry AMD, while two other groups are exploiting the allogeneic approach for developing therapies for geography atrophy (dry AMD) (Mandai et al. 2017; Sharma et al. 2019) (ClinicalTrials.gov identifiers: NCT04339764, NCT02463344, NCT01344993). Here, we will primarily focus on the autologous-based cell-therapy approach for dry AMD and will discuss the critical steps of the manufacturing pipeline, QC of the product, and validation of the process. We have categorized this section into iPSC validation and iPSC-derived RPE validation.

iPSC Validation

1. Somatic cell donor screening,

2. Quality of iPSC, and

3. Sterility: endotoxin, mycoplasma, bacteria, fungus testing.

Somatic Cell Donor Screening

For making iPSCs, somatic cells such as blood cells and fibroblasts are often used. The Centers for Disease Control and Prevention (CDC) and the American Association of Blood Banks (AABB) have a list of assays to conduct for screening patients for pathogenic diseases (Mendicino et al. 2019; Jha et al. 2021). For autologous cell therapy, the donor screening (www.cdc.gov/transplantsafety/protecting-patient/screening-testing.html) is done mainly to protect GMP operators and there is no strict regulatory requirement to do so. Hence, once donors are screened for disease pathogens (hepatitis B, HIV, Nile virus, etc.), it is not critical to screen the source material before starting the process of iPSC induction (Creasey et al. 2019).

iPSC Quality Assessment

Reprogramming of somatic cells to iPSC is a time-extensive process. The process of generating iPSCs has been refined since its discovery (González et al. 2011). Previously, integrating viral vectors (e.g., retroviral, lentiviral, and inducible lentiviral) were the only options, but now nonintegrating transgene expressing technologies (e.g., Sendai, adenoviral, plasmid DNA transfer, loxp lentivirus, piggyBac, polyarginine-tagged polypeptide, RNA-modified synthetic mRNA) are also available (Yu et al. 2011; Rao and Malik 2012). There is a wide range of somatic cell types that can be used and, depending upon the type, the reprogramming efficiency varies (Rao and Malik 2012). At the National Eye Institute (NEI) phase I/IIa clinical trial (ClinicalTrials.gov identifier: NCT04339764) we are using episomal vectors (Sharma et al. 2019). As far as iPSC-based RPE clinical trials, the choice has been skin fibroblasts or peripheral blood CD34[+] cells (Mandai et al. 2017; Sharma et al. 2019). The limiting factor and a point for consideration is whether there are GMP protocols for generating iPSCs for a specific cell type; for example, CD34[+] cells have protocols established for GMP of iPSC lines (Mack et al. 2011). Figure 2 highlights the streamlined autologous GMP of iPSC-RPE for the NEI phase I/IIa clinical trial to treat dry AMD (Sharma et al. 2019).

Regardless of the method used for iPSC generation, clinical-grade iPSC quality is validated by checking for the expression of iPSC markers, either by qRT-PCR, flow cytometry or immunofluorescence of surface (SSEA4, TRA-1-81) and nuclear (OCT-4, SOX-2) markers (Rao and Malik 2012; Baghbaderani et al. 2015). Stringent QC thresholds for iPSC quality in terms of percentage-positive iPSC markers are usually preferred. In iPSC-derived RPE cell therapy, the Japanese group led by Dr. Takahashi used immunostaining and teratoma assay to assess the pluripotency of the iPSC lines (Mandai et al. 2017). The iPSCs also need to be characterized for sterility (endotoxin, mycoplasma, fungus, bacteria), donor matching (short-tandem repeat assay or HLA-matching), and zero footprints—absence of the reprograming vectors (plasmid loss determination by copy number) (Rao and Malik 2012; Baghbaderani et al. 2015; Steichen et al. 2019).

To ensure the genomic integrity of iPSCs, different assays can be carried out. For example, conventional G-banding determines the potential karyotypic abnormalities, whole genome or exome sequencing can determine the status of oncogenic and disease-inducing alterations, copy number variations (CNVs), or insertion or deletion mutations (INDELs) (Sharma et al. 2020). The very first autologous iPSC-derived RPE transplantation clinical study in Japan was halted because of potential oncogenic mutations discovered in iPSCs of the second patient enrolled in their trial (Mandai et al. 2017).

RPE Validation during Differentiation and Maturation

1. Molecular validation,

2. Structural validation,

3. Functional validation,

4. Junctional integrity validation, and

5. Tumorigenicity, dose toxicity, and distribution.

The quality of the final product depends on the differentiation protocol; details of the NEI protocol have been covered in the previous section and published extensively (May-Simera et al. 2018; Sharma et al. 2020, 2021, 2022). Here we focus on the assays that validate RPE purity, maturity, and functionality. Several of the other RPE differentiation protocols have assays that focus on the final product (Ben M'barek et al. 2017; Mandai et al. 2017; Kashani et al. 2018). However, our differentiation protocol has three stages of RPE development: RPE progenitors (day 25), immature RPE (intermediate, day 40), and mature RPE (day 75, final product)—this has allowed us to develop "go/no go" assays for the clinical manufacturing process (Sharma et al. 2019, 2022).

The final RPE product has been transplanted either in cell suspension or as a monolayer patch (Schwartz et al. 2015; Mandai et al. 2017; Kashani et al. 2018). There are various kinds of natural, synthetic materials like parylene or biodegradable materials like poly(lactic-co-glycolic acid) (PLGA), and polyester that have been used to seed RPE cells and transplant the tissue as a sheet (Kashani et al. 2018; Sharma et al. 2019). Poly(glycerol sebacate) (PGS) scaffolds are biodegradable scaffolds used in the transplantation of other retinal cells like photoreceptors (Lee et al. 2021). Biodegradable scaffolds like PLGA or PGS are beneficial because they provide a support to secrete extracellular matrix proteins, an essential factor in cellular interactions and cell signaling (Sharma et al. 2020). Moreover, they enable cells to build native niches like

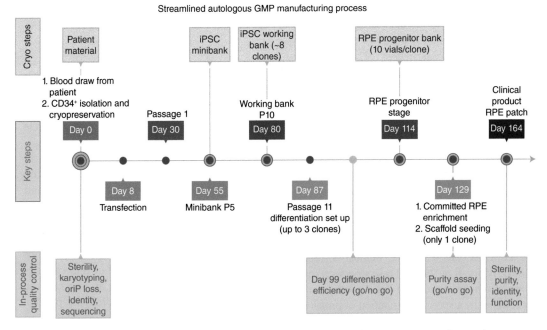

Figure 2. Schematic of clinical manufacturing process of the induced pluripotent stem cell-retinal pigment epithelium (iPSC-RPE) patch at the National Eye Institute (NEI) for phase I/IIa autologous cell-based replacement therapy for dry age-related macular degeneration (AMD). (oriP) Minimal replicator of Epstein–Barr virus.

the Bruch's membrane underneath iPSC-RPE (Sharma et al. 2019). This allows generation of a mature functional iPSC-RPE monolayer with basal infoldings, which are otherwise missing on a plastic surface (Sharma et al. 2020). A significant and obvious benefit of using a biodegradable matrix is that, following transplantation and degradation of the scaffold, there will be no hindrance to the exchange of nutrients and metabolites. At the same time, another important point to consider is that the substrate, even though it is biodegradable, should have enough physical strength to be easily manipulated during the transplantation procedure.

RPE sheets have also been grown on a collagen substrate without scaffold support, and later the collagen was dissolved using collagenase enzyme to obtain only the cell sheet that was transplanted in one patient (Mandai et al. 2017). A recent report from Nishida et al. showed transplantation in animals of iPSC-derived RPE sheets grown in a polydimethylsiloxane (PDMS)-based device, which is 19.5 mm in length, 1 mm in width, and 1.6 mm in depth

(Nishida et al. 2021). Authors transplanted albino nude rats and rabbits and showed RPE transplant integration in the back of the eye.

In the next section, we highlight the QC steps at the intermediate and the end-stage product. The process of characterization and validation of the differentiating tissue can be designed during various manufacturing stages. It helps in benchmarking the quality of the product.

Molecular Validation

The developing RPE has a specific gene-expression pattern in its early and late stages of maturity. These signature genes, discovered or established by various laboratories, can be used to study the molecular maturity of differentiating RPE by assays such as qRT-PCR, flow cytometry, western blot (WB), or immunofluorescence (IF) staining. For instance, the early signs of RPE commitment fate are determined by MITF and PAX6 coexpression (Bharti et al. 2012). As the cells mature, TYRP1 and CRALBP start to appear, while BEST1, RPE65, and ALDHA3 markers decide the final stage of maturity (Sharma et al. 2019). Our group uses the flow cytometry assay to determine the purity of differentiating cells. Other groups have used qRT-PCR and immunostaining-based assays to confirm the maturity of the end product (Mandai et al. 2017).

Structural Validation

RPE has a unique cellular architecture that can be observed by high-resolution scanning and transmission electron microscopic (SEM, TEM) techniques. The apically located melanosomes, the apical mesh of microvilli, basally located nucleus, and basal infoldings confirm the polarity and structural maturity of the iPSC-RPE monolayer (Strauss 2005; Bharti et al. 2011). These structures can be validated by SEM and TEM (Fig. 3). RPE polarity is preserved by a specific distribution of proteins on its apical and basal sides. For example, EZRIN and Na/K ATPase are expressed on the apical membrane, while COLLAGEN IV is the marker for the basal side of RPE cells (Miyagishima et al. 2016). RPE monolayer secretes pigment epithelium-derived factor (PEDF) predominantly on the apical side for photoreceptor health and vascular endothelial-derived growth factor (VEGF) predominantly on the basal side for choriocapillaris (Strauss 2005; Maminishkis et al. 2006; Miyagishima et al. 2016). ELISA assay is typically used to detect these cytokine levels and can be used to confirm the polarity of RPE tissue in vitro. Several groups use VEGF and PEDF secretion assays to confirm the maturity of RPE tissue (Osakada

et al. 2009a; Ben M'barek et al. 2017; Mandai et al. 2017; Da Cruz et al. 2018; Kashani et al. 2018).

Functional Validation

Inside the eye, RPE remains in direct contact with the outer segments (OS) of photoreceptors to complete the replenishment of visual cycle pigments and uptake shed OS through phagocytosis (Lakkaraju et al. 2020). Established in vitro assays can assess RPE phagocytic ability via WB, IF, or flow cytometry for uptake and digestion of OS and rhodopsin WB—a key OS protein (Lakkaraju et al. 2020). In the laboratory, RPE cells are "fed" with bovine OS, and, after 4 h of "feeding," cells are tested for the presence of rhodopsin either by WB, IF, or flow cytometry. For example, Mandai et al. checked the phagocytosis capacity by feeding the porcine photoreceptor outer segment (POS) labeled with FITC (Osakada et al. 2009a; Mandai et al. 2017). For flow cytometry-based assays, OS are labeled with pH-sensitive or any other fluorescent dye. The phagocytic ability can be directly correlated with the fluorescent intensity, which can be quantified by flow cytometry-based assay. Our data show that iPSC-RPE are comparable to primary human RPE in their ability to phagocytose OS (Miyagishima et al. 2016).

Morphometric Validation

RPE is a monolayer of hexagonal cells and its hexagonality is thought to correlate with RPE

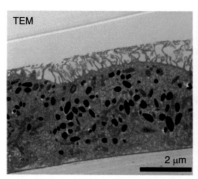
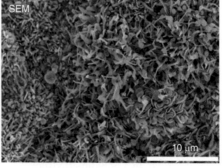

Figure 3. Transmission and scanning electron microscopic (TEM and SEM) images of induced pluripotent stem cell-retinal pigment epithelium (iPSC-RPE) validates maturity at the structural level.

health and maturity (Schaub et al. 2020; Ortolan et al. 2022). Thus, morphometric analysis can indicate this tissue's health. Our group has developed an artificial intelligence (AI)-based software that can determine shape metrics, such as cell hexagonality and number of neighbors of each RPE cell (Schaub et al. 2020; Ortolan et al. 2022). The cells are first stained for border markers, using anti-ZO-1 antibodies or phalloidin (stains for F-ACTIN), and subsequently imaged with a fluorescence microscope (Fig. 4). Images are then segmented with our machine-learning-based software—RESHAPE. This morphometric assay is used for QC of the iPSC-RPE patch (Sharma et al. 2019, 2020). Others have used anti-ZO-1 and phalloidin staining to qualitatively assess RPE shape (Schwartz et al. 2015; Song et al. 2015).

Junctional Integrity

Another important RPE maturity feature is related to the tight junctions that the cells express in the monolayer (Strauss 2005; Maminishkis et al. 2006). As RPE cells mature into a monolayer, these junctional complexes get stronger by addition of more proteins onto them, leading to fully sealed paracellular spaces between cells (Rizzolo 2007). The junctional integrity of an RPE monolayer is measured by passing an electric current from the apical toward the basal side of the monolayer. The resistance to the flow of current defines the tightness of RPE junctions. There are several ways to study this—with EVOM or ENDOM or using a modified Ussing chamber (Maminishkis et al. 2006). Our clinical study is the only clinical study to date that uses this functional readout of RPE monolayer maturity as several hundred ohm·cm^2 of TER.

The in vitro validation of the end product is followed by safety and efficacy testing in animal models. The choice of animal model is based on the target disease and the mode of transplantation.

ANIMAL MODELS FOR PRECLINICAL STUDIES

Preclinical efficacy and toxicity studies are required for regulatory approval before the transplant can be tested in humans (Chader 2002). For a first-in-human trial, toxicity studies are required to be performed as per good laboratory practice (GLP) standards and are discussed in our regulatory section. Here, we focus on efficacy studies that are typically performed in a retinal degeneration animal model for an RPE-based transplant. Immune rejection of a xeno transplant by the animal is a major cause of failure of human transplants in such preclinical studies; hence, a strong immune-suppression regimen is required to allow survival of the human cells over the duration of the study. Important factors that contribute to the success of cellular therapy are the mode of injection, how cells integrate into the eye, and whether the transplanted cells survive (Frey-Vasconcells et al. 2012; Sharma et al. 2020; Arzi et al. 2021). Some of the earliest RPE transplantations were done in monkeys and

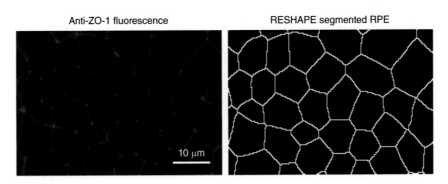

Anti-ZO-1 fluorescence | RESHAPE segmented RPE

10 μm

Figure 4. Example of induced pluripotent stem cell-retinal pigment epithelium (iPSC-RPE) stained with a ZO-1 antibody and its corresponding cell border segmentation performed by RESHAPE, a machine-learning software for morphometric analysis.

in Royal College of Surgeon Rats (RCS) (Binder et al. 2007). The RCS rat model is a well-established animal model used for RPE patch transplantation (Binder et al. 2007). In this rat model, a homozygous mutation in the MERTK gene renders the host RPE cells incapable of phagocytosing shed POS, causing retinal degeneration and secondary photoreceptor loss (Binder et al. 2007). Researchers have tested the ability of human RPE cells injected as a suspension or a patch to rescue retinal degeneration seen in this model (Wang et al. 2008). However, rescue effects also observed in some cases following sham surgery have confounded some of the results obtained from this model (Wang et al. 2008). Our group has tested their RPE transplants in pigs. The pig is a useful model to study human RPE transplants because the pig eye contains a cone photoreceptor-rich area, called the visual streak, which is reminiscent of the human macula that degenerates in AMD (Hafezi et al. 2000). Furthermore, the size and anatomy of the pig eye are very similar to the human eye, making it practical to test surgical approaches meant for the human eye (Choi et al. 2021). For these reasons, we tested our iPSC-derived RPE patch in a pig eye with laser-damaged RPE, such that the human RPE patch could rescue the pig retina from degenerating (Sharma et al. 2019). Our work shows the feasibility of delivering a patch of the size intended for a human eye, into a pig eye. Follow-up of the RPE patch with clinically relevant techniques such as fundus imaging, optical coherence tomography, and electroretinograms of the pig retina confirmed RPE-transplant integration and its ability to rescue the pig retina from degenerating (Sharma et al. 2019). Our experience suggests that testing of an RPE patch in an animal model that better recapitulates the human eye and human disease condition helps build confidence in the clinical product to be delivered to patients.

REGULATORY CHALLENGES FOR DEVELOPING AN iPSC-BASED CELL THERAPY

Many regulatory challenges need to be overcome to develop a pluripotent stem cell–based therapy. Here, we focus on an iPSC-based product for clinical testing. These challenges may significantly impact the final product and must be adequately addressed at the outset of product development. Among these challenges are the establishment of a reliable and consistent manufacturing process, the validation of analytical in-process controls—including the specificity, sensitivity, accuracy, and reproducibility of each assay—and the execution of the necessary preclinical studies to validate the product's safety and efficacy prior to use in humans.

The FDA's Center for Biologics Evaluation and Research (CBER) governs cell-based therapies in the United States. Several sections of the CFR offer general guidelines for the development of an iPSC-derived product (Mendicino et al. 2019).

The development process for cell therapy products differs depending on the chosen strategy between autologous and allogeneic. Because each strategy has its own requirements and challenges, it is essential to identify these limitations early to implement strategies that improve the safety and efficacy of the product for a particular clinical intervention. See Jha et al. (2021) and Creasey et al. (2019) for additional information on the latest regulatory considerations for developing autologous cell therapy and the approval pathway for the cell therapy biologics license application (BLA).

Overall, the regulatory consideration for developing a phase I IND application for cell-based therapies requires three major sections: chemistry, manufacturing, and control (CMC), preclinical studies, and clinical studies (Fig. 5; FDA 2008a,b).

CMC information is a detailed description of the clinical product that includes the cell source, the collection method, and any associated handling, culturing, processing, storage, shipping, and testing. It is one of the most essential components of a phase I IND application for cell therapy (FDA 2008a). To ensure product safety, characterization, quality, purity, stability, and strength (including potency) (details in 21 CFR 312.22(a) for the U.S. FDA), FDA requires sufficient CMC information (Fig. 6).

Critical quality attributes (CQAs) are the properties of cell therapy products that provide

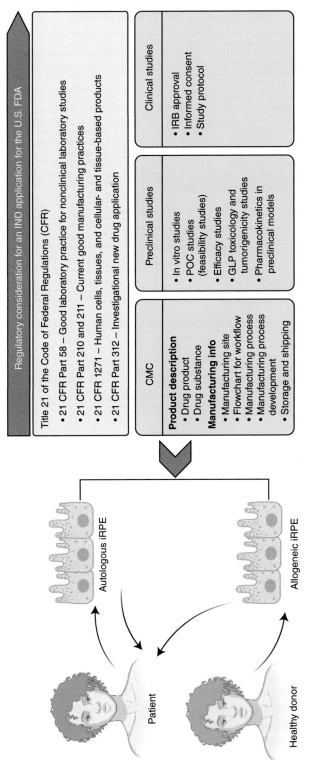

Figure 5. General requirements for an investigational new drug (IND) application for the U.S. Food and Drug Administration (FDA). In the Code of Federal Regulations (CFR), the FDA has issued guidelines for the development of regulated products. Several sections of Title 21 of the CFR provide general guidelines for developing an induced pluripotent stem cell (iPSC)-derived product. (CMC) Chemistry, manufacturing, and control, (POC) proof-of-concept, (GLP) good laboratory practice, (IRB) institutional review board, (iRPE) iPSC-derived retinal pigment epithelium.

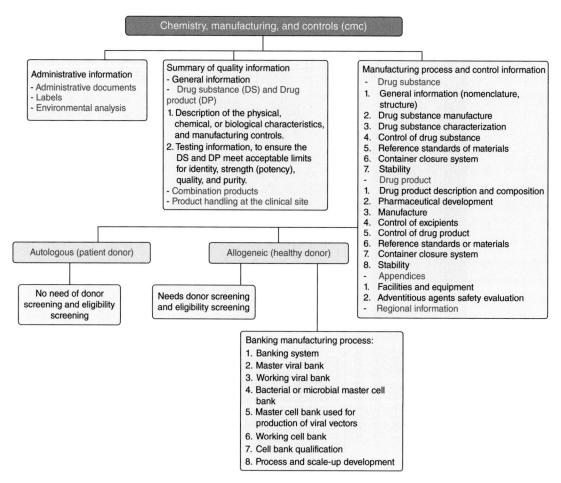

Figure 6. Chemistry manufacturing and controls requirements for a phase I investigational new drug (IND) application for autologous and allogeneic induced pluripotent stem cell (iPSC) product.

a mechanistic understanding of product characterization and ensure manufacturing consistency and stability. CQAs are particularly advantageous for the development of autologous products because they assist in identifying variability and its source during the manufacturing process (Jha et al. 2021). The FDA mandates preclinical studies that need to be GLP-compliant (details available in 21 CFR Part 58 of the FDA) to evaluate the safety of iPSC-derived cell therapy products intended for clinical use (Mendicino et al. 2019). These studies evaluate the tumorigenic, toxic, and migratory properties of iPSC-derived cell therapy products. The functionality of a cell therapy product is another critical quality issue that preclinical studies should

address. The functionality will likely determine the success of integration of the transplanted cells in the target tissue and the ability to become part of a functional unit. To ensure that transplanted human cells survive long enough in animals to reveal their tumorigenic potential, preclinical studies employ a variety of animal models, including both immunocompetent (with immune suppression) and immunocompromised animals (Harding and Mirochnitchenko 2014; Jha et al. 2021).

In addition to FDA approval of the IND application, an institutional review board (IRB) and a data safety monitoring board help ensure patient safety. Establishing the product's safety in a patient cohort is the foundation for all subsequent trials. Because a phase I study is intended to be a safety trial, the first patient cohort should be selected so that if the product fails to meet its safety profile, it will cause minimal or no harm to patients. The identification and comprehension of a patient's prognosis are crucial to effective risk management. Patients must be made aware of the potential dangers associated with a first-in-human procedure.

CLINICAL DEVELOPMENT OF AUTOLOGOUS iPSC-RPE PATCH TRANSPLANT

Our laboratory at the NEI is conducting a phase I/IIa trial for testing the safety of autologous iPSC-RPE patches for treating dry AMD patients. The protocol plans to enroll up to 16 patients with a primary end point of 1 yr and secondary end point follow-up of 5 yr. The first autologous transplantation of an iPSC-RPE scaffold in the eye of a patient with dry AMD was completed in August 2022 at the NEI (www.nei.nih.gov/about/news-and-events/news/first-us-patient-receives-autologous-stem-cell-therapy-treat-dry-amd).

The estimated completion date of Clinical Trial NCT04339764 is 2026–2028. With the current timeline, if successful, this technology would likely be avaiable for FDA approval 8–10 yr from now.

The time taken at NEI to manufacture an iPSC-RPE patch is 164 d (Fig. 2). Once the iPSC culture is ready, it takes 40 d of differentiation to obtain pure RPE cells. Our RPE cells grow on PLGA scaffolds for an additional 5 wk before the cell therapy product is ready to be transplanted.

Previously, it was suggested that the costs incurred in manufacturing clinical grade iPSCs are close to $800,000 (Huang et al. 2019). Our manufacturing cost (reagents, supplies, and assays) is well below $50,000. Because of the academic nature of this trial, the cost of GMP facility operation and management is not feasible to calculate at this stage. It is anticipated that GMP facility operation costs will drop significantly as this project reaches phase III when products for multiple patients are being manufactured simultaneously.

The success rate of iPSC reprograming is quite high in our manufacturing process; on average, we have been able to pick 20–30 clones from every donor. The major advantage of our autologous approach is that the therapy does not require systemic immunosuppression. Given the typical age of dry AMD patients, they are predisposed to multiple life-threatening diseases. Having a healthy immune system greatly increases the chances of success. The main disadvantages of the autologous approach are the large costs of manufacture and the fact that the technology of generating personalized iPSC-RPE patches is logistically cumbersome. To alleviate this issue, we have set up several freezing points along the manufacturing process that allow us to keep backups of the product intermediates. With ongoing technological innovation in microfluidics and AI-based image analysis, it is anticipated that, in the coming decade, manufacturing of autologous cell therapies will be streamlined and the cost will drop by several orders of magnitude.

CONCLUDING REMARKS

The current decade has witnessed an increasing demand for the use of stem cell–based therapy for the treatment of several diseases, including retinal degenerative diseases (Bharti et al. 2014). Visual health is an important area of research—eye diseases if left untreated can progressively lead to blindness (Flaxman et al. 2021). There are many hurdles for developing iPSC-derived products for clinic care. Herein we have covered the essential steps that led to the development of iPSC-RPE clinical-grade tissue and led to a first-in-human study for the treatment of dry AMD. Our data suggest that it is critical to develop a tissue that faithfully resembles the native tissue by using the knowledge accumulated by studies on tissue development; proper QC assays to assess the quality and functionality of the product; testing its safety and efficacy by transplanting it in relevant animal models; and, finally, following the guidelines set by the FDA to ensure timely reach to the patients.

In vivo, the RPE interacts with other cell types in the retina-like photoreceptors, endothelial cells, pericytes, and fibroblasts (Sharma et al. 2020; Song et al. 2022). So, the next step of cell-replacement therapy would be going from a two-dimensional culture to three-dimensional culture to increase the success of integration of the new tissue and to treat late-stage diseases. Our group has recently developed an in vitro system that recapitulates the oBRB, by embedding endothelial cells, pericytes, and fibroblasts in a bio-ink, which is then bioprinted on the basal side of a biodegradable scaffold on which RPE cells were seeded (Song et al. 2022).

The RPE is primarily responsible for the health of the photoreceptors and can support preservation of vision only when photoreceptors are still present. In cases in which photoreceptors have already been lost, RPE transplantation alone will not suffice. As such, other groups have aimed at the generation of photoreceptors from iPSC as a viable option for cell-replacement therapy (Lee et al. 2021). Transplantation of iPSC photoreceptors is still at the proof-of-concept stage, and safety and efficacy studies of iPSC photoreceptor scaffolds is being tested in animals (Lee et al. 2021). Currently, researchers are looking into ways to develop the technology that would enable transplantation of RPE photoreceptors as a dual patch for cell-replacement therapy. Hopefully, more clinical trials can be developed in the near future by leveraging our experience to cure currently untreatable diseases.

REFERENCES

Amato MA, Boy S, Perron M. 2004. Hedgehog signaling in vertebrate eye development: a growing puzzle. *Cell Mol Life Sci* **61**: 899–910. doi:10.1007/s00018-003-3370-7

Arzi B, Webb TL, Koch TG, Volk SW, Betts DH, Watts A, Goodrich L, Kallos MS, Kol A. 2021. Cell therapy in veterinary medicine as a proof-of-concept for human therapies: perspectives from the North American Veterinary Regenerative Medicine Association. *Front Vet Sci* **8**: 779109. doi:10.3389/fvets.2021.779109

Baghbaderani BA, Tian X, Neo BH, Burkall A, Dimezzo T, Sierra G, Zeng X, Warren K, Kovarcik DP, Fellner T, et al. 2015. cGMP-manufactured human induced pluripotent stem cells are available for pre-clinical and clinical applications. *Stem Cell Reports* **5**: 647–659. doi:10.1016/j.stemcr.2015.08.015

Ben M'barek K, Habeler W, Plancheron A, Jarraya M, Regent F, Terray A, Yang Y, Chatrousse L, Domingues S, Masson Y, et al. 2017. Human ESC-derived retinal epithelial cell sheets potentiate rescue of photoreceptor cell loss in rats with retinal degeneration. *Sci Transl Med* **9**: 7471. doi:10.1126/scitranslmed.aai7471

Bharti K, Nguyen M-TTT, Skuntz S, Bertuzzi S, Arnheiter H. 2006. The other pigment cell: specification and development of the pigmented epithelium of the vertebrate eye. *Pigment Cell Res* **19**: 380–394.

Bharti K, Miller SS, Arnheiter H. 2011. The new paradigm: retinal pigment epithelium cells generated from embryonic or induced pluripotent stem cells. *Pigment Cell Melanoma Res* **24**: 21–34. doi:10.1111/j.1755-148X.2010.00772.x

Bharti K, Gasper M, Ou J, Brucato M, Clore-Gronenborn K, Pickel J, Arnheiter H. 2012. A regulatory loop involving PAX6, MITF, and WNT signaling controls retinal pigment epithelium development. *PLoS Genet* **8**: e1002757. doi:10.1371/journal.pgen.1002757

Bharti K, Rao M, Hull SC, Stroncek D, Brooks BP, Feigal E, van Meurs JC, Huang CA, Miller SS. 2014. Developing cellular therapies for retinal degenerative diseases. *Invest Ophthalmol Vis Sci* **55**: 1191–1201. doi:10.1167/iovs.13-13481

Binder S, Stanzel BV, Krebs I, Glittenberg C. 2007. Transplantation of the RPE in AMD. *Prog Retin Eye Res* **26**: 516–554. doi:10.1016/j.preteyeres.2007.02.002

Chader GJ. 2002. Animal models in research on retinal degenerations: past progress and future hope. *Vision Res* **42**: 393–399. doi:10.1016/S0042-6989(01)00212-7

Chambers SM, Fasano CA, Papapetrou EP, Tomishima M, Sadelain M, Studer L. 2009. Highly efficient neural conversion of human ES and iPS cells by dual inhibition of SMAD signaling. *Nat Biotechnol* **27**: 275–280. doi:10.1038/nbt.1529

Choi KE, Anh VTQ, Oh JH, Yun C, Kim SW. 2021. Normative data of axial length, retinal thickness measurements, visual evoked potentials, and full-field electroretinography in female, wild-type minipigs. *Transl Vis Sci Technol* **10**: 3–3. doi:10.1167/tvst.10.12.3

Creasey AA, Stacey G, Bharti K, Sato Y, Lubiniecki A. 2019. A strategic road map to filing a biologics license application for a pluripotent stem cell derived therapeutic product. *Biologicals* **59**: 68–71. doi:10.1016/j.biologicals.2019.03.007

Da Cruz L, Fynes K, Georgiadis O, Kerby J, Luo YH, Ahmado A, Vernon A, Daniels JT, Nommiste B, Hasan SM, et al. 2018. Phase 1 clinical study of an embryonic stem cell–derived retinal pigment epithelium patch in age-related macular degeneration. *Nat Biotechnol* **36**: 328–337. doi:10.1038/nbt.4114

Deinsberger J, Reisinger D, Weber B. 2020. Global trends in clinical trials involving pluripotent stem cells: a systematic multi-database analysis. *NPJ Regen Med* **5**: 1–13. doi:10.1038/s41536-020-00100-4

De Iongh R, McAvoy JW. 1993. Spatio-temporal distribution of acidic and basic FGF indicates a role for FGF in rat lens morphogenesis. *Dev Dyn* **198**: 190–202. doi:10.1002/aja.1001980305

FDA. 2008a. Guidance for FDA Reviewers and Sponsors: Content and Review of Chemistry, Manufacturing, and

Control (CMC) Information for Human Somatic Cell Therapy Investigational New Drug Applications (INDs). https://www.regulations.gov/docket/FDA-2008-D-0206/document

FDA. 2008b. Guidance for Industry CGMP for Phase 1 Investigational Drugs. https://www.regulations.gov/document/FDA-2005-D-0157-0005

Flaxman AD, Wittenborn JS, Robalik T, Gulia R, Gerzoff RB, Lundeen EA, Saaddine J, Rein DB; Vision and Eye Health Surveillance System Study Group. 2021. Prevalence of visual acuity loss or blindness in the US: a Bayesian meta-analysis. *JAMA Ophthalmol* **139**: 717–723. doi:10.1001/jamaophthalmol.2021.0527

Frey-Vasconcells J, Whittlesey KJ, Baum E, Feigal EG. 2012. Translation of stem cell research: points to consider in designing preclinical animal studies. *Stem Cells Transl Med* **1**: 353–358. doi:10.5966/sctm.2012-0018

Fuhrmann S, Levine EM, Reh TA. 2000. Extraocular mesenchyme patterns the optic vesicle during early eye development in the embryonic chick. *Development* **127**: 4599–4609. doi:10.1242/dev.127.21.4599

González F, Boué S, Belmonte JCI. 2011. Methods for making induced pluripotent stem cells: reprogramming à la carte. *Nat Rev Genet* **12**: 231–242. doi:10.1038/nrg2937

Hafezi F, Grimm C, Simmen BC, Wenzel A, Remé CE. 2000. Molecular ophthalmology: an update on animal models for retinal degenerations and dystrophies. *Br J Ophthalmol* **84**: 922–927. doi:10.1136/bjo.84.8.922

Hägglund AC, Berghard A, Carlsson L. 2013. Canonical Wnt/β-catenin signalling is essential for optic cup formation. *PLoS ONE* **8**: e81158. doi:10.1371/journal.pone.0081158

Harding J, Mirochnitchenko O. 2014. Preclinical studies for induced pluripotent stem cell-based therapeutics. *J Biol Chem* **289**: 4585–4593. doi:10.1074/jbc.R113.463737

Hirschi KK, Li S, Roy K. 2014. Induced pluripotent stem cells for regenerative medicine. *Annu Rev Biomed Eng* **16**: 277–294. doi:10.1146/annurev-bioeng-071813-105108

Huang CY, Liu CL, Ting CY, Chiu YT, Cheng YC, Nicholson MW, Hsieh PCH. 2019. Human iPSC banking: barriers and opportunities. *J Biomed Sci* **26**: 87. doi:10.1186/s12929-019-0578-x

Hyer J, Mima T, Mikawa T. 1998. FGF1 patterns the optic vesicle by directing the placement of the neural retina domain. *Development* **125**: 869–877. doi:10.1242/dev.125.5.869

Jha BS, Bharti K. 2015. Regenerating retinal pigment epithelial cells to cure blindness: a road towards personalized artificial tissue. *Curr Stem Cell Rep* **1**: 79–91. doi:10.1007/s40778-015-0014-4

Jha BS, Farnoodian M, Bharti K. 2021. Regulatory considerations for developing a phase I investigational new drug application for autologous induced pluripotent stem cells-based therapy product. *Stem Cells Transl Med* **10**: 198–208. doi:10.1002/sctm.20-0242

Kashani AH, Lebkowski JS, Rahhal FM, Avery RL, Salehi-Had H, Dang W, Lin CM, Mitra D, Zhu D, Thomas BB, et al. 2018. A bioengineered retinal pigment epithelial monolayer for advanced, dry age-related macular degeneration. *Sci Transl Med* **10**: eaao4097. doi:10.1126/scitranslmed.aao4097

Lakkaraju A, Umapathy A, Tan L, Daniele L, Philp N, Boesze-Battaglia K, Williams D. 2020. The cell biology of the retinal pigment epithelium. *Prog Retin Eye Res* **78**: 100846. doi:10.1016/j.preteyeres.2020.100846

Lee IK, Ludwig AL, Phillips MJ, Lee J, Xie R, Sajdak BS, Jager LD, Gong S, Gamm DM, Ma Z. 2021. Ultrathin micromolded 3D scaffolds for high-density photoreceptor layer reconstruction. *Sci Adv* **7**. doi:10.1126/sciadv.abf0344

Mack AA, Kroboth S, Rajesh D, Wang WB. 2011. Generation of induced pluripotent stem cells from CD34⁺ cells across blood drawn from multiple donors with non-integrating episomal vectors. *PLoS ONE* **6**: e27956. doi:10.1371/journal.pone.0027956

Madrid M, Sumen C, Aivio S, Saklayen N. 2021. Autologous induced pluripotent stem cell–based cell therapies: promise, progress, and challenges. *Curr Protoc* **1**: e88. doi:10.1002/cpz1.88

Maminishkis A, Chen S, Jalickee S, Banzon T, Shi G, Wang FE, Ehalt T, Hammer JA, Miller SS. 2006. Confluent monolayers of cultured human fetal retinal pigment epithelium exhibit morphology and physiology of native tissue. *Invest Ophthalmol Vis Sci* **47**: 3612–3624. doi:10.1167/iovs.05-1622

Mandai M, Watanabe A, Kurimoto Y, Hirami Y, Morinaga C, Daimon T, Fujihara M, Akimaru H, Sakai N, Shibata Y, et al. 2017. Autologous induced stem-cell-derived retinal cells for macular degeneration. *N Engl J Med* **376**: 1038–1046. doi:10.1056/NEJMoa1608368

May-Simera HL, Wan Q, Jha BS, Hartford J, Khristov V, Dejene R, Chang J, Patnaik S, Lu Q, Banerjee P, et al. 2018. Primary cilium-mediated retinal pigment epithelium maturation is disrupted in ciliopathy patient cells. *Cell Rep* **22**: 189–205. doi:10.1016/j.celrep.2017.12.038

Mendicino M, Fan Y, Griffin D, Gunter KC, Nichols K. 2019. Current state of U.S. Food and Drug Administration regulation for cellular and gene therapy products: potential cures on the horizon. *Cytotherapy* **21**: 699–724. doi:10.1016/j.jcyt.2019.04.002

Meyer JS, Shearer RL, Capowski EE, Wright LS, Wallace KA, McMillan EL, Zhang SC, Gamm DM. 2009. Modeling early retinal development with human embryonic and induced pluripotent stem cells. *Proc Natl Acad Sci* **106**: 16698–16703. doi:10.1073/pnas.0905245106

Miyagishima KJ, Wan Q, Corneo B, Sharma R, Lotfi MR, Boles NC, Hua F, Maminishkis A, Zhang C, Blenkinsop T, et al. 2016. In pursuit of authenticity: induced pluripotent stem cell–derived retinal pigment epithelium for clinical applications. *Stem Cell Transl Med* **5**: 1562–1574.

Monsarrat P, Vergnes JN, Planat-Bénard V, Ravaud P, Kémoun P, Sensebé L, Casteilla L. 2016. An innovative, comprehensive mapping and multiscale analysis of registered trials for stem cell-based regenerative medicine. *Stem Cells Transl Med* **5**: 826–835. doi:10.5966/sctm.2015-0329

Müller F, Rohrer H, Vogel-Höpker A. 2007. Bone morphogenetic proteins specify the retinal pigment epithelium in the chick embryo. *Development* **134**: 3483–3493. doi:10.1242/dev.02884

Nadar VP, Buchholz DE, Lowenstein SE, Clegg DO, Clegg DO. 2015. Canonical/β-catenin Wnt pathway activation improves retinal pigmented epithelium derivation from human embryonic stem cells. *Invest Ophthalmol Vis Sci* **56:** 1002–1013. doi:10.1167/iovs.14-15835

Neumann CJ, Nuesslein-Volhard C. 2000. Patterning of the zebrafish retina by a wave of sonic hedgehog activity. *Science* **289:** 2137–2139. doi:10.1126/science.289.5487.2137

Nguyen M, Arnheiter H. 2000. Signaling and transcriptional regulation in early mammalian eye development: a link between FGF and MITF. *Development* **127:** 3581–3591. doi:10.1242/dev.127.16.3581

Nishida M, Tanaka Y, Tanaka Y, Amaya S, Tanaka N, Uyama H, Masuda T, Onishi A, Sho J, Yokota S, et al. 2021. Human iPS cell derived RPE strips for secure delivery of graft cells at a target place with minimal surgical invasion. *Sci Rep* **11:** 1–14. doi:10.1038/s41598-021-00703-x

Ortolan D, Sharma R, Volkov A, Maminishkis A, Hotaling NA, Huryn LA, Cukras C, Di Marco S, Bisti S, Bharti K. 2022. Single-cell-resolution map of human retinal pigment epithelium helps discover subpopulations with differential disease sensitivity. *Proc Natl Acad Sci* **119:** e2117553119. doi:10.1073/pnas.2117553119

Osakada F, Ikeda H, Sasai Y, Takahashi M. 2009a. Stepwise differentiation of pluripotent stem cells into retinal cells. *Nat Protoc* **4:** 811–824. doi:10.1038/nprot.2009.51

Osakada F, Jin ZB, Hirami Y, Ikeda H, Danjyo T, Watanabe K, Sasai Y, Takahashi M. 2009b. In vitro differentiation of retinal cells from human pluripotent stem cells by small-molecule induction. *J Cell Sci* **122:** 3169–3179. doi:10.1242/jcs.050393

Pennington BO, Clegg DO, Melkoumian ZK, Hikita ST. 2015. Defined culture of human embryonic stem cells and xeno-free derivation of retinal pigmented epithelial cells on a novel, synthetic substrate. *Stem Cells Transl Med* **4:** 165–177. doi:10.5966/sctm.2014-0179

Pera EM, Wessely O, Li SY, De Robertis EM. 2001. Neural and head induction by insulin-like growth factor signals. *Dev Cell* **1:** 655–665. doi:10.1016/S1534-5807(01)00069-7

Perron M, Boy S, Amato MA, Viczian A, Koebernick K, Pieler T, Harris WA. 2003. A novel function for *Hedgehog* signalling in retinal pigment epithelium differentiation. *Development* **130:** 1565–1577. doi:10.1242/dev.00391

Pittack C, Grunwald GB, Reh TA. 1997. Fibroblast growth factors are necessary for neural retina but not pigmented epithelium differentiation in chick embryos. *Development* **124:** 805–816. doi:10.1242/dev.124.4.805

Rao MS, Malik N. 2012. Assessing iPSC reprogramming methods for their suitability in translational medicine. *J Cell Biochem* **113:** 3061–3068. doi:10.1002/jcb.24183

Rizzolo LJ. 2007. Development and role of tight junctions in the retinal pigment epithelium. *Int Rev Cytol* **258:** 195–234. doi:10.1016/S0074-7696(07)58004-6

Schaub NJ, Hotaling NA, Manescu P, Padi S, Wan Q, Sharma R, George A, Chalfoun J, Simon M, Ouladi M, et al. 2020. Deep learning predicts function of live retinal pigment epithelium from quantitative microscopy. *J Clin Invest* **130:** 1010–1023. doi:10.1172/JCI131187

Schwartz SD, Hubschman JP, Heilwell G, Franco-Cardenas V, Pan CK, Ostrick RM, Mickunas E, Gay R, Klimanskaya I, Lanza R. 2012. Embryonic stem cell trials for macular degeneration: a preliminary report. *Lancet* **379:** 713–720. doi:10.1016/S0140-6736(12)60028-2

Schwartz SD, Regillo CD, Lam BL, Eliott D, Rosenfeld PJ, Gregori NZ, Hubschman JP, Davis JL, Heilwell G, Spirn M, et al. 2015. Human embryonic stem cell-derived retinal pigment epithelium in patients with age-related macular degeneration and Stargardt's macular dystrophy: follow-up of two open-label phase 1/2 studies. *Lancet* **385:** 509–516. doi:10.1016/S0140-6736(14)61376-3

Sharma R, Khristov V, Rising A, Jha BS, Dejene R, Hotaling N, Li Y, Stoddard J, Stankewicz C, Wan Q, et al. 2019. Clinical-grade stem cell-derived retinal pigment epithelium patch rescues retinal degeneration in rodents and pigs. *Sci Transl Med* **11:** eaat5580. doi:10.1126/scitranslmed.aat5580

Sharma R, Bose D, Maminishkis A, Bharti K. 2020. Retinal pigment epithelium replacement therapy for age-related macular degeneration: are we there yet? *Annu Rev Pharmacol Toxicol* **60:** 553–572.

Sharma R, George A, Nimmagadda M, Ortolan D, Karla BS, Qureshy Z, Bose D, Dejene R, Liang G, Wan Q, et al. 2021. Epithelial phenotype restoring drugs suppress macular degeneration phenotypes in an iPSC model. *Nat Commun* **12:** 7293. doi:10.1038/s41467-021-27488-x

Sharma R, Bose D, Montford J, Ortolan D, Bharti K. 2022. Triphasic developmentally guided protocol to generate retinal pigment epithelium from induced pluripotent stem cells. *STAR Protoc* **3:** 101582. doi:10.1016/j.xpro.2022.101582

Song WK, Park KM, Kim HJ, Lee JH, Choi J, Chong SY, Shim SH, Del Priore LV, Lanza R. 2015. Treatment of macular degeneration using embryonic stem cell-derived retinal pigment epithelium: preliminary results in Asian patients. *Stem Cell Reports* **4:** 860–872. doi:10.1016/j.stemcr.2015.04.005

Song MJ, Quinn R, Nguyen E, Hampton C, Sharma R, Park TS, Koster C, Voss T, Tristan C, Weber C et al. 2022. Bioprinted 3D outer retina barrier uncovers RPE-dependent choroidal phenotype in advanced macular degeneration. *Nat Methods* **20:** 149–161. doi:10.1038/s41592-022-01701-1

Steichen C, Hannoun Z, Luce E, Hauet T, Dubart-Kupperschmitt A. 2019. Genomic integrity of human induced pluripotent stem cells: reprogramming, differentiation and applications. *World J Stem Cells* **11:** 729–747. doi:10.4252/wjsc.v11.i10.729

Steinfeld J, Steinfeld I, Bausch A, Coronato N, Hampel ML, Depner H, Layer PG, Vogel-Höpker A. 2017. BMP-induced reprogramming of the neural retina into retinal pigment epithelium requires Wnt signalling. *Biol Open* **6:** 979–992.

Stenkamp DL, Frey RA, Prabhudesai SN, Raymond PA. 2000. Function for Hedgehog genes in zebrafish retinal development. *Dev Biol* **220:** 238–252. doi:10.1006/dbio.2000.9629

Strauss O. 2005. The retinal pigment epithelium in visual function. *Physiol Rev* **85:** 845–881. doi:10.1152/physrev.00021.2004

Takahashi K, Tanabe K, Ohnuki M, Narita M, Ichisaka T, Tomoda K, Yamanaka S. 2007. Induction of pluripotent stem cells from adult human fibroblasts by defined factors. *Cell* **131:** 861–872. doi:10.1016/j.cell.2007.11.019

Tuekprakhon A, Sangkitporn S, Trinavarat A, Pawestri AR, Vamvanij V, Ruangchainikom M, Luksanapruksa P, Pongpaksupasin P, Khorchai A, Dambua A, et al. 2021. Intravitreal autologous mesenchymal stem cell transplantation: a non-randomized phase I clinical trial in patients with retinitis pigmentosa. *Stem Cell Res Ther* **12:** 1–15. doi:10.1186/s13287-020-02122-7

Uy H, Pik M, Chan S, Franz M, Cruz M. 2013. Stem cell therapy: a novel approach for vision restoration in retinitis pigmentosa. *Med Hypothesis Discov Innov Ophthalmol* **2:** 52.

Vonk LA, De Windt TS, Slaper-Cortenbach ICM, Saris DBF. 2015. Autologous, allogeneic, induced pluripotent stem cell or a combination stem cell therapy? Where are we headed in cartilage repair and why: a concise review.

Stem Cell Res Ther **6:** 1–11. doi:10.1186/s13287-015-0086-1

Wang S, Lu B, Girman S, Holmes T, Bischoff N, Lund RD. 2008. Morphological and functional rescue in RCS rats after RPE cell line transplantation at a later stage of degeneration. *Invest Ophthalmol Vis Sci* **49:** 416–421. doi:10.1167/iovs.07-0992

Yang X-J. 2004. Roles of cell-extrinsic growth factors in vertebrate eye pattern formation and retinogenesis. *Semin Cell Dev Biol* **15:** 91–103. doi:10.1016/j.semcdb.2003.09.004

Yu J, Vodyanik MA, Smuga-Otto K, Antosiewicz-Bourget J, Frane JL, Tian S, Nie J, Jonsdottir GA, Ruotti V, Stewart R, et al. 2007. Induced pluripotent stem cell lines derived from human somatic cells. *Science* **318:** 1917–1920. doi:10.1126/science.1151526

Yu J, Chau KF, Vodyanik MA, Jiang J, Jiang Y. 2011. Efficient feeder-free episomal reprogramming with small molecules. *PLoS ONE* **6:** e17557. doi:10.1371/journal.pone.0017557

Photoreceptor Cell Replacement Using Pluripotent Stem Cells: Current Knowledge and Remaining Questions

Christelle Monville,[1,2] Olivier Goureau,[3] and Karim Ben M'Barek[1,2,4]

[1]INSERM U861, I-Stem, AFM, Institute for Stem Cell Therapy and Exploration of Monogenic Diseases, 91100 Corbeil-Essonnes, France

[2]Université Paris-Saclay, Université d'Evry, U861, 91100 Corbeil-Essonnes, France

[3]Sorbonne Université, Institut de la Vision, INSERM, CNRS, 75012 Paris, France

[4]Centre d'Etude des Cellules Souches, 91100 Corbeil-Essonnes, France

Correspondence: cmonville@istem.fr; olivier.goureau@inserm.fr; kbenmbarek@istem.fr

Retinal degeneration is an increasing global burden without cure for the majority of patients. Once retinal cells have degenerated, vision is permanently lost. Different strategies have been developed in recent years to prevent retinal degeneration or to restore sight (e.g., gene therapy, cell therapy, and electronic implants). Herein, we present current treatment strategies with a focus on cell therapy for photoreceptor replacement using human pluripotent stem cells. We will describe the state of the art and discuss obstacles and limitations observed in preclinical animal models as well as future directions to improve graft integration and functionality.

Vision is an essential sense used in almost every aspect of everyday life and, in particular, in our modern societies with the increasing number of screens (smartphones, computers, TVs, etc.) and information transmitted through them. Thus, loss of vision has dramatic impacts in daily life and is a major economic burden for society (Wittenborn et al. 2013; GBD 2019 Blindness and Vision Impairment Collaborators; Vision Loss Expert Group of the Global Burden of Disease Study 2021a,b). In 2020, an estimated 596 million people had distance vision impairment worldwide, of whom 43 million were blind (Burton et al. 2021). Major causes of vision impairment are uncorrected refractive errors and cataracts for which effective treatments are available (Flaxman et al. 2017). On the other hand, retinal degenerative diseases are the leading cause of untreatable sight loss in the industrialized world.

The retina is composed of several cell types including photoreceptors, which are a specialized type of neurons that convert light inputs into electrical signals. This signal is further processed and integrated by different other cell types of the retina until axons of ganglion cells (forming the optic nerve). On contact with photoreceptors, retinal pigment epithelial (RPE) cells form a specialized epithelium that provides a critical trophic support to these photoreceptors and maintain their homeostasis. As terminally differentiated cells without regenerative capabilities in humans, damage and loss of photoreceptors result in diseases leading to permanent visual impairment, such as age-related macular degeneration (AMD) and retinitis pigmentosa (RP).

RETINAL DEGENERATIVE DISEASES

Age-Related Macular Degeneration

AMD is the main cause of central vision loss in patients older than 55 years (Flaxman et al. 2017; Burton et al. 2021) and is caused by the degeneration of RPE cells. The main risk factor is aging. Mechanisms causing RPE cell loss may involve at least in part inflammation, oxidative stress, and complement system that alter surrounding cells and the supportive Bruch's membrane to which RPE cells are attached (Brown et al. 2018; Handa et al. 2019; Zarbin et al. 2019; Hussain et al. 2020).

Initially asymptomatic, the disease evolves to central vision distortion and finally central scotomas (Mitchell et al. 2018). At late stages, two forms are described: wet AMD, which is defined by the presence of macular choroidal neovascularization (CNV; 10%–20% of cases), and dry AMD characterized by macular atrophy (corresponding to 80%–90% of cases) (Mitchell et al. 2018; Al-Khersan et al. 2019). No treatment is available for the dry form of AMD. An anti-VEGF therapy is usually delivered to wet AMD patients to slow or prevent vision degradation. CNVs can also be removed by surgery.

Retinitis Pigmentosa

RP forms a heterogeneous group of inherited retinal dystrophies that affects 1.5 million patients worldwide (Hartong et al. 2006; Verbakel et al. 2018; Pfeiffer et al. 2020). Symptoms are night blindness at early stages; later during disease progression, the visual field becomes more and more reduced starting from the periphery (tunnel vision) (Hartong et al. 2006). To date, more than 90 genes involved in RP have been described (sph.uth.edu/retnet/sum-dis.htm). Mutations affect photoreceptor functions and, for about 5% of cases, RPE cell functions (Ben M'Barek et al. 2018). The other cell layers are initially well preserved but, after decades of degeneration, rewiring, glial hypertrophy, and global cell death may occur (Pfeiffer et al. 2020). Only one approved treatment is available for patients with *RPE65* gene mutations (2% of RP cases). It consists of a gene therapy (Luxturna [voretigene neparvovecrzyl]) that improves navigational abilities and light sensitivity (Maguire et al. 2019, 2021). Forty to fifty percent of RP patients may develop cataracts that can be removed by surgery (Auffarth et al. 1997; Bayyoud et al. 2013).

Current Strategies under Development

Current treatment strategies under development involve gene and cell therapies or electronic implants (Roska and Sahel 2018). These strategies address two challenges: preventing retinal degeneration before complete cell loss and restoring sight in late disease stages (Fig. 1).

Gene therapy can be applied to RP patients, either by replacing the mutant gene with a healthy copy or by correcting the underlying mutations, prior to complete photoreceptor cell degeneration to achieve preservation of the remaining cells. However, a specific gene therapy should be developed to address each of the known RP-inducing genes. Such a gene therapy approach is expensive as very few RP patients are affected by one specific gene (e.g., $425,000 per eye for LUXTURNA [Pennesi and Schlecther 2020]). Of note, gene mutations causing RP are not known in 30% of nonsyndromic and 50% of autosomal-dominant RP patients (Hartong et al. 2006; Verbakel et al. 2018). Nevertheless, several gene therapies are in the pipeline of clinical development (Sahel et al. 2019). In the meantime, scientists are looking for alternative mutation-independent approaches. The discovery of the rod-derived cone viability factor (RdCVF) and its ability to convey neuroprotection and delay photoreceptor degeneration is an example of a neuroprotective strategy (Léveillard and Sahel 2010). Gene therapy with RdCVF is envisioned as a potential strategy

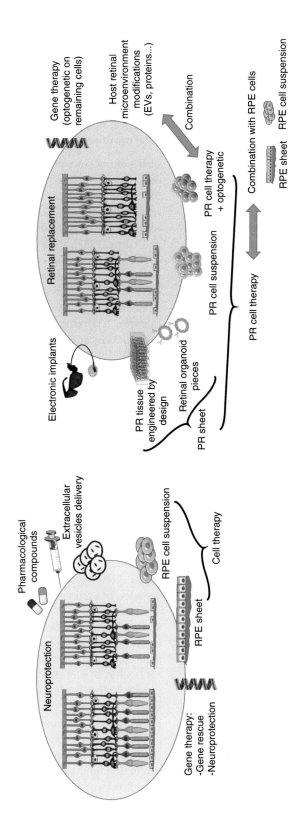

Figure 1. Scheme describing different therapeutic options envisioned to prevent degeneration or restore vision of patients with retinal degenerative disorders. (PR) Photoreceptors, (EVs) extracellular vesicles.

to prevent oxidative stress and provide neuroprotection (Clérin et al. 2020).

The replacement of RPE cells that are not functional or degenerating in AMD and some forms of RP is also considered as a cell therapy strategy to protect photoreceptors. Our group has developed protocols to generate RPE cells, identified the formulation that conveys the most potent therapeutic effects, and elaborated strategies to deliver the engineered retinal tissue in rodent and primates (Ben M'Barek et al. 2017, 2020; Ben M'Barek and Monville 2019). This work led in 2019 to an ongoing phase I/II clinical trial for RP patients (with known mutations affecting RPE cells) based on these technologies. Other groups developed similar approaches for AMD with already published results (Mandai et al. 2017b; da Cruz et al. 2018; Kashani et al. 2018; Qiu 2019).

Electronic implants aim to replace the function of dead photoreceptors through the conversion of images collected by camera into electrical signals that are transmitted to the retinal circuitry downstream photoreceptors. Current implants showed recently promising results but the technology is still in its infancy due to the very low-resolution vision (low number and density of electrodes) (Roska and Sahel 2018; Cehajic-Kapetanovic et al. 2022). Another approach of gene therapy is based on optogenetics. The overall strategy is to convert surviving retinal neurons (ganglion cells, bipolar cells, and dormant cones) into light-sensitive cells through transfer of gene coding for different microbial opsins. These modified retinal cells acquire the potential to convert light into electrical signals (artificial photoreceptors) (Busskamp et al. 2010; Klapper et al. 2016; Garita-Hernandez et al. 2018; Khabou et al. 2018). The first proof-of-concept of this strategy was recently obtained with the partial visual recovery in a late-stage blind RP patient (Sahel et al. 2021). However, two main hurdles are associated with this strategy: the choice of the light sensitivity of the selected protein (as it does not have the sensitivity and complexity of the different photoreceptor subtypes) and the loss of the sophisticated signal integration mediated by the different retinal cell subtypes when photoreceptors are bypassed. Finally, the replacement of dead photoreceptors by new exogenous photoreceptors through cell therapy will be specifically discussed in the following sections.

PHOTORECEPTOR CELL REPLACEMENT

Historical Perspective: Transplantation Using Fetal or Adult Retinas

First grafting experiments of triturated rat embryonic or neonatal retinas into rat retinal lesion eyes in the late 1980s demonstrated the potential of a retinal graft to survive and continue its development into a host eye (Turner and Blair 1986; Blair and Turner 1987). Since then, a number of studies explored the potential of embryonic or neonatal retinal cells to engraft into host retinas leading to the first clinical trials (for review, see Seiler and Aramant 2012; Ludwig and Gamm 2021). For example, fetal embryonic sheets composed of neural retinas and RPE cells were used for transplantation in clinical trials involving patients with late-stage RP and AMD (Radtke et al. 2002, 2008). While the first study did not report visual improvements, the latter one showed positive visual outcomes measured using the ETDRS scale (early treatment of diabetic retinopathy study scale that quantifies visual acuity) in seven of the 10 patients transplanted (Radtke et al. 2008). This improvement lasted for at least 6 yr in one patient but it remains difficult to determine whether the graft was integrated into the retinal circuitry or whether it provided a trophic effect preserving remaining photoreceptors. No immunosuppression was used to prevent rejection. Nevertheless, this study suggested overall the safety of a retinal transplantation. Such retinal sheet transplantation has also been performed in sighted RP patients (Berger et al. 2003). Indeed, in a clinical trial, eight patients were transplanted with photoreceptor sheets obtained from cadavers (within 24 h of death) without immunosuppression. Mean reading speed or visual acuity did not change during the 1-yr follow-up (no improvements or degradation).

These transplantation studies shed light onto several limitations associated with the graft origin that limit reproducibility of experiments, as well as large-scale clinical trials and potential future use in clinical practice. Fetal human cells obtained from abortion are surrounded with ethical and legal constraints that are different from one country to another. The availability of this material is scarce and the age of fetuses may be variable. Adult retinas from cadavers may not be able to integrate and their procurement is also difficult. The emergence of human pluripotent stem cells (hPSCs) discovered in 1998 stimulated this research field through the promise of easier access to human embryonic retinal cells. hPSCs including hESCs (human embryonic stem cells [Thomson et al. 1998]) and hiPSC (human-induced pluripotent stem cells [Takahashi et al. 2007]) are characterized by a self-renewal potential and the ability to differentiate into any cell type of the adult body, including retinal cells. Thus, providing the development of efficient protocols to differentiate hPSCs into photoreceptors, retinal cell material suitable for transplantation will no longer be a limiting factor.

Photoreceptor Differentiation from Pluripotent Stem Cells

Differentiation of hPSCs into the various retinal cell types follows a sequence of events and cellular intermediate similar to what is observed in vivo (Ben M'Barek and Monville 2019; Gagliardi et al. 2019; O'Hara-Wright and Gonzalez-Cordero 2020). These steps are reproduced in vitro using a combination of chemical factors and cytokines added to the culture medium. The best results in producing photoreceptors are obtained through the generation of self-organized three-dimensional tissue cultures as retinal organoids, which can be compared to optic vesicles or optic cups observed in vivo (Nakano et al. 2012; Reichman et al. 2014, 2017; Zhong et al. 2014; Kuwahara et al. 2015; Ohlemacher et al. 2015; Parfitt et al. 2016; Capowski et al. 2019). These organoids are laminated by a superposition of different retinal cell types similar to in vivo retina: photoreceptors located at the surface of organoids and, at the opposite, ganglion cells located deep inside retinal organoids. Some degree of photoreceptor maturation is observed after long culture duration (several months) with a timeline similar to human in vivo development (Cowan et al. 2020).

Recently, Saha and colleagues (2022) observed light-evoked electrical responses in cones (35% of measured cones) from long-term retinal organoid cultures (240–270 d of differentiation). Thus, these retinal organoids represent a source of functional photoreceptors suitable for transplantation. However, photoreceptors may need to be isolated from other cells inside retinal organoids before transplantation. Different methods of cell isolation based on surface antigens were developed to either exclude contaminating cells or to specifically isolate photoreceptors (Lakowski et al. 2015, 2018; Santos-Ferreira et al. 2016b; Welby et al. 2017; Gagliardi et al. 2018). Finally, efforts were made to standardize organoid differentiation protocols across various hPSCs through the definition of three morphological stages of differentiation (Capowski et al. 2019).

Cell Therapy Formulation

Cell Suspension

Once photoreceptors are produced, different strategies were developed to formulate the final cell therapy product that will be transplanted. Initial studies grafted cells as suspension or small clumps of cells (when obtained from fetuses). Such formulation has the advantage of an easy manipulation and does not require sophisticated implantation tools.

When implanted as a cell suspension, the majority of photoreceptor precursors fail to properly integrate and complete their maturation. Visual outcomes following grafting in rodents with retinal degeneration were evaluated through electrophysiology (retinal electrical response to light) and/or visual behaviors (pupil light response or optokinetic reflex), and were usually moderately or not improved (Pearson et al. 2012; Barber et al. 2013; Singh et al. 2013; Gagliardi et al. 2018). In addition, these observed functional visual outcomes were mainly elicited by a phenomenon of cytoplasmic material transfer (Pearson et al. 2012, 2016; Santos-Ferreira et al. 2016a; Singh et al. 2016). This material transfer allows the exchange of cytoplasmic proteins and/or mRNAs (including those used to label donor photoreceptors) that are missing in the degenerated host retina. Host photoreceptors become functional and can elicit moderate visual functionality in rodents, thanks to the formation of a nanotube-like process between donor and host photoreceptors, facilitating the transfer of this material (Kalargyrou et al. 2021; Ortin-Martinez et al. 2021).

Some recent studies suggested that long-term follow-up in rodent models following implantation are required to observe an improved maturation. Degenerative context might also play a role: most studies focused on end-stage retinal degeneration models—where integration might be less favorable than conditions where photoreceptors, susceptible to provide support to the grafted cells, remain. Gasparini and collaborators recently evaluated this hypothesis. Indeed, this group used as grafting material cones isolated by cell sorting from Day 200 (D200) retinal organoids, thanks to a specific fluorescent reporter (Gasparini et al. 2022). These photoreceptors were injected into Cpfl1 (cone photoreceptor function loss 1) deficient mice in which cones degenerate but rods remain preserved. After a follow-up of 6 mo under local immune suppression, the authors observed an improved integration and maturation of donor photoreceptors with the presence of inner and outer segments. However, no proof of functionality in vivo was shown (only ex vivo electrophysiology). Ribeiro and collaborators also suggested increasing the number of grafted cells to improve integration/maturation in long-term studies (Ribeiro et al. 2021). To facilitate survival of transplanted human cells, they used the immunocompromised $rd1/Foxn1^{nu}$ mice model that presents a complete loss of rods and central cones at 3 mo of age. Cones were isolated by cell sorting from D120 retinal organoids previously transduced with AAV vector carrying green fluorescent protein (GFP) under the control of a cone promoter. Three months after subretinal injection of 500,000 cones, they observed modest maturation improvements (presence of nascent segment-like protrusions) in 20% of grafted cones and positive visual outcomes. More interestingly, they confirmed that the functionality observed was due to functional grafted cones as the grafting of nonfunctional cones (from mutant hiPSCs) did not elicit the same response (strongly suggesting that

there was no material transfer or trophic effect involvements). Photoreceptors derived from D74–D106 organoids were also subretinally delivered to photoreceptor-ablated retina in nonhuman primates, using vitrectomy as for human surgery (Aboualizadeh et al. 2020). Follow-up analysis showed that the transplanted photoreceptors did not reach full morphological maturity (presence of outer segments) even 41 wk after transplantation. Of note, they reported that injected cells could reflux from the retinotomy or concentrate in the inferior area of the bleb due presumably to gravity. Thus, the authors suggested keeping the monkeys horizontal for 3–4 h after the surgery. These are important points to consider for future clinical trials.

Tissue Formulation

Similar to RPE cell therapy, scientists evaluated other formulations for photoreceptor transplantation. Early studies indicated that neonatal retinal cells organized as aggregates had a better survival and organization than cell suspension (for review, see Seiler and Aramant 2012). Thus, sheet formulation was explored mainly through the direct use of pieces of retinal organoids for transplantation (Assawachananont et al. 2014; Shirai et al. 2016; Mandai et al. 2017a; Iraha et al. 2018; McLelland et al. 2018; Tu et al. 2019). Shirai and collaborators used as grafting material small pieces of 0.5 mm obtained from retinal organoids derived from hPSCs (Shirai et al. 2016). Different stages of organoid maturation (from D50 to D100) were evaluated following transplantation in an immunodeficient rat model of photoreceptor degeneration ($RhoS344^{ter}/Foxn1^{nu}$). The authors did not report any major differences in the thickness of the graft that reflects the number of photoreceptor nuclei, ~250 d post-transplantation. To reduce culture duration at minimum (and reduce associated manufacturing costs), D50–D60 was selected as graft age for following experiments. These grafts developed after transplantation and formed outer and inner nuclear layer–like structures. These donor inner nuclear layers are susceptible to limit donor photoreceptor integration with host bipolar cells. In addition, donor photoreceptors formed rosettes that prevent interactions with host RPE cells. Outer segments are indeed located inside the lumen of these rosettes (Shirai et al. 2016; Mandai et al. 2017a; Iraha et al. 2018). The same approach was performed with hPSC-derived retinal organoids at D64–D66 grafted in the immunocompromised $rd1/Foxn1^{nu}$ mice model at 2 mo of age (Iraha et al. 2018). Immunohistological analyses revealed a long-term survival of the graft (almost 6 mo post-surgery) and some in vivo maturation of the grafted organoid sheet with the detection of both rods and cones presenting inner/outer segment-like structures (Iraha et al. 2018). Multielectrode array (MEA) recordings measuring light responses of ex vivo transplanted retinas indicated that some of them (three out of eight retinas) were responsive to light. However, in vivo full-field electroretinogram (ERG) recordings in response to light stimuli remained flat (no response). The number of integrated photoreceptors was suggested to be too low to elicit consistent responses (below 150,000 cells) (Iraha et al. 2018). When implanted in nonhuman primates, sheets of D59–D63 retinal organoids also formed rosettes (Tu et al. 2019). Visual function (behavioral test) was modestly improved at 1.5 yr in one monkey in the grafted laser-lesioned area compared to control retinal area, but no improvement was recorded by focal ERG. A recent study in dogs reported that cell clusters of photoreceptor precursor cells obtained from D104–D151 organoids survived up to 3–5 mo in the subretinal space of normal dogs and can extend axons beyond the outer limiting membrane when transplanted in dogs with retinal degeneration ($rcd1/PDE6B$ mutations) (Ripolles-Garcia et al. 2022).

Thus, all these experiments demonstrated that retinal organoids are able to continue their development following grafting into host retinas (even degenerated retinas) and to form de novo organized outer nuclear layers. However, a number of challenges still need to be overcome to improve integration and functionality of grafts: (1) limit the presence of other retinal cell types into the graft, (2) limit the formation of rosettes that prevent the interaction with RPE cells, and (3) increase the proportion of cones to improve visual outcomes in humans.

Optimization of Cell Integration and Functionality

To optimize functionality of grafted photoreceptors, different strategies are under investigation. These include refining the formulation of cell therapy products, combining with optogenetics or modifying the local microenvironment of the degenerative host retina to improve cell integration.

Selection of the Cell Types to Be Grafted

To improve survival and functional visual preservation, one recently proposed approach was to transplant, at the same time, both RPE cells and retinal progenitor cells (RPCs) that could give rise to photoreceptors. Injections of RPE cells or RPCs alone (D45–D50 of differentiation in culture prior implantation)—both derived from hPSCs and labeled with GFP—were compared to injections of a combination of both cell types in RCS rats (presenting an RPE dysfunction) before photoreceptor degeneration (Salas et al. 2021). A combination of RPE cells and RPCs triggered a better graft survival at 12 wk postsurgery as monitored by fluorescence fundus imaging to detect GFP in immunosuppressed animals. This survival was associated with a better preservation of host photoreceptors allowing a better restoration of visual functions (scotopic ERGs) compared to the same cell types injected alone (Salas et al. 2021). However, the integration was not formally evaluated and the immunosuppression strategy chosen was not optimal for long-term morphological and functional evaluation (i.e., difficulty of controlling the uptake of the immunosuppressive drug cyclosporine by the rodents). The visual outcomes observed in these experiments could be due to neuroprotective effects. Experiments with genetically immunocompromised models of retinal degeneration (Thomas et al. 2018) will better address the long-term integration of different cell types.

Instead of combining RPE and RPCs in cell suspension, another approach is to combine pieces of retinal organoids with a preformed RPE sheet. Thomas and collaborators assembled RPE sheets on parylene with retinal organoid pieces using either gelatin, alginate, or Matrigel (Thomas et al. 2021). Alginate provided better performance as a bio-adhesive and was selected to assemble the co-graft. These co-grafts were implanted into immunodeficient RCS rats (*RCS-p+/Foxn1^{nu}* rats) at a stage of advanced retinal degeneration and graft survival was observed up to 7.7 mo (maximum follow-up time). Optokinetic tests suggested a neuroprotective effect rather than functionality of co-grafted photoreceptors. Unfortunately, the co-graft was not compared to either RPE cells or retinal organoid sheets grafted alone. This multilayer strategy did not prevent the formation of rosettes when implanted in vivo due to the structure of the organoid and the RPE sheet was not entirely covered with the organoid (Thomas et al. 2021).

Finally, the last strategy is to genetically modify cells inside organoids to trigger selective depletion of cell populations not required for future transplantation. In this context, Yamasaki and collaborators generated hPSCs with the deletion of the *ISLET-1* (*ISL1*) gene (Yamasaki et al. 2022). Differentiation of these *ISL1^{-/-}* hPSCs into retinal organoids leads to a reduction of bipolar cells while preserving photoreceptors, Müller glia, and horizontal cells. Both wild-type and *ISL1^{-/-}* retinal organoids (stage D60) were cut into pieces and grafted into immunodeficient rat model of end-stage photoreceptor degeneration. Six months post-transplantation, multiples rosettes presenting photoreceptor inner and outer segments in their lumen were observed with both grafts. Interestingly, better host-graft contacts between host bipolar cells and grafted photoreceptors were reported in *ISL1^{-/-}* grafts compared to wild-type grafts. At 8–10 mo post-surgery, MEA recordings revealed a significant restoration of light responsiveness in host ganglion cells (Yamasaki et al. 2022). This response was improved with *ISL1^{-/-}* retinal organoids compared to wild-type grafts, suggesting that the selective depletion of bipolar cells inside organoids favors the contacts between grafted photoreceptors and host bipolar cells, leading to the formation of functional synapses even into this xenogeneic context.

Tissue Engineering by Design

To organize photoreceptors prior to implantation, different approaches were envisioned such as decellularized retinas in which RPE cells and ocular progenitors differentiated from hPSCs can be seeded (Maqueda et al. 2021) or polymers (or mixtures of polymers) that are not structured by design (Lavik et al. 2005; Tucker et al. 2010; Singh et al. 2018). Besides such scaffolds, probably one of the most promising strategies is to design a specific 3D microstructuration to guide the organization of photoreceptor precursors and to prevent the formation of rosettes. Indeed, different attempts were published using a variety of polymers (biodegradable or not) that can support this microstructuration such as poly(dimethylsiloxane) (PDMS), poly(lactic-co-glycolic acid) (PLGA), poly (glycerol-sebacate) (PGS), or acrylated poly(caprolactone) (PCL) (Neeley et al. 2008; McUsic et al. 2012; Jung et al. 2018; Thompson et al. 2019). The 3D microstructuration design of the scaffold is critical to achieve both a sufficient density and a relevant polarized maturation. Thus, different micropore designs were proposed (Neeley et al. 2008; McUsic et al. 2012; Worthington et al. 2017; Jung et al. 2018; Lee et al. 2021).

Worthington and collaborators directly created microstructured scaffolds with two-photon lithography printing. This approach allowed the designing of highly complex 3D structures, composed of vertical micropores, which can theoretically be loaded with photoreceptors and horizontal micropores to favor exchange between cells (Worthington et al. 2017). This technical choice induced long writing steps to produce only one scaffold at a time despite their efforts to optimize printing steps. RPCs derived from retinal organoids at D30 plated into these scaffolds for 2 d survived and formed neuronal processes inside micropores. In addition, this group developed PCL biodegradable polymers (Thompson et al. 2019) as well as extracellular matrix–based polymers (mixture of gelatin and hyaluronic acid) (Shrestha et al. 2020) for scaffolding. In vivo toxicity studies revealed that the PCL polymer was well tolerated, biocompatible, and safe (Thompson et al. 2019). PCL scaffolds

Cite this article as *Cold Spring Harb Perspect Med* doi: 10.1101/cshperspect.a041309

were loaded with RPCs derived from retinal organoids at D70 and transplanted into the eye of nude rats to evaluate the tolerance of the product (Han et al. 2022). The PCL scaffold loaded with cells was demonstrated to be safe but no functionality studies were conducted.

Another technical choice was based on the creation of a negative mold that will be reused a number of times to create numerous scaffolds (micromolding). Using this approach, Neeley and collaborators proposed a cylindrical micropore where retinal cells can grow and differentiate (Neeley et al. 2008; Redenti et al. 2009). 3D microstructured PLGA scaffolds using a similar cylindrical design containing retinal cells can also be cocultured with RPE cells at least for 14 d (McUsic et al. 2012). However, this cylindrical design does not prevent cells from crossing the scaffold. Therefore, Jung and collaborators proposed an alternative "wine glass" design to retain cells on a reservoir. Thus, this design is composed of a cut shape reservoir where one to three photoreceptors can be loaded and a microchannel in which photoreceptors can grow extensions that can mature into inner/outer segment–like structures (Jung et al. 2018). Polymers used for this scaffold included PDMS or PGS, the last being biodegradable in vivo. Photoreceptor precursors isolated from retinal organoids at D80 continue to mature after 3 mo in vitro by developing basal axon extensions on microchannels and expressing rod-specific markers. Optimization of the scaffold by the same team led to creation of an "ice cube tray" design (Lee et al. 2021). This evolution allowed to increase photoreceptor density and reduced the amount of synthetic biomaterial used to generate the scaffold (increase of the ratio cells vs. polymer). This design is composed of a reservoir layer that receives a mean load of 18 photoreceptors and a base layer with pores (Lee et al. 2021). Interestingly, photoreceptors isolated from D120 retinal organoids seeded into these scaffolds seemed polarized after 5 d in cell culture, even though immunofluorescence staining did not clearly show a well-defined orientation of maturing photoreceptors.

Collectively, these studies started to explore a tissue engineering by design strategy that may improve outcomes following retinal implantation in vivo. Optimization of micropore designs as well as functionality of photoreceptors into these scaffolds is still required, as well as in vivo proof-of-concept.

Combination of Optogenetic and Cell Transplantation

Functional integration of photoreceptors entails connecting to the inner host retina but also development of light-sensitive outer segments, requiring interaction with the underlying RPE. An alternative strategy to tissue engineering is to combine stem cell–based therapy and optogenetics, thereby conferring light sensitivity to donor cells (immature photoreceptors). This strategy allows overcoming the issue of maturation with formation of inner/outer segments into the host retina and the lack of contacts with endogenous RPE cells, by the production of functional photoreceptors thanks to the microbial opsin activity. Using specific AAV vectors, Garita-Hernandez and collaborators have been able to deliver a hyperpolarizing microbial opsin into photoreceptor precursors from D42 retinal organoids (Garita-Hernandez et al. 2019). Patch clamp recording on cell suspension from D70 retinal organoids demonstrated robust optogenetic light responses in these optogenetically transformed photoreceptors lacking light-sensitive outer segments. Furthermore, in vivo studies demonstrated that light-driven responses at the ganglion cell level can be observed in blind mice, after transplantation of these photoreceptors equipped with a microbial opsin but not recorded after transplantation of "control" photoreceptors (organoids transfected only with GFP). However, it remains unclear whether microbial opsin may elicit adverse immune responses in humans (Cehajic-Kapetanovic et al. 2022). Long-term follow-up using immunodeficient blind rodent models are also required to evaluate visual recovery after a longer period of maturation.

Modification of the Microenvironment

An aspect yet underestimated in the context of photoreceptor transplantation is related to the retinal microenvironment. Indeed, most research groups focused on improving the transplant to ameliorate visual outcomes but few considered the retinal degenerative environment. Indeed, during the process of retinal degeneration, a number of signaling pathways deregulating gene expression are involved (inflammation, endoplasmic reticulum stress, oxidative stress, aberrant autophagy, calcium homeostasis dysfunctions) (Gorbatyuk et al. 2020). Therefore, a "reconfiguration" of this host microenvironment might improve integration and functionality of donor photoreceptors.

Several studies showed that injection of purified solutions of extracellular vesicles (EVs; secreted by almost all cells and containing a cargo composed of DNA, RNA, proteins, and lipids) are susceptible to limit inflammation (Mead and Tomarev 2020; Jarrige et al. 2021). For example, following subretinal injection in an RP rat model, EVs derived from neural progenitor cells were mostly internalized by microglia, which was therefore inhibited and induced the down-regulation of proinflammatory cytokines (Peng et al. 2014; Bian et al. 2020). We could envision a strategy of injecting EVs prior or concomitantly to cell transplantation to modulate inflammation and favor integration/maturation of grafted cells (Jarrige et al. 2021). Other groups suggested a role of inhibitory extracellular matrix such as CD44 and neurocan, which accumulate due to glial hypertrophy during retinal degeneration (Tucker et al. 2010; Yao et al. 2011). Matrix metalloproteinase 2 (MMP2) incorporated into PLGA beads were proposed as cotransplants with RPCs to favor integration of donor cells (Yao et al. 2011).

CONCLUDING REMARKS

The field has made significant progress these last years to improve our knowledge related to photoreceptor cell grafting, in particular understanding material transfer mechanisms and developing more complex cell therapies. There is still a long way to go to develop efficient cell therapy for photoreceptor replacement perhaps structured as engineered tissues. Nevertheless, first patients with advanced RP were already implanted with hPSC-derived neuroretinal sheets (RIKEN, JRCT ID jRCTa050200027) (Maeda et al. 2022). We

hope this first-in-man study will pave the way for clinical trials exploring other types of photoreceptor cell therapy products.

ACKNOWLEDGMENTS

This work was supported by grants from the ANR (RebuildingRETINA: ANR-19-CE18-0004) and the Fondation pour la Recherche Medicale (Transplantation and Cell Therapy - PME201906008797) to K.B.M. I-Stem is part of the Biotherapies Institute for Rare Diseases supported by the Association Française contre les Myopathies-Téléthon. The figure was created using Servier Medical Art (smart.servier.com).

REFERENCES

Aboualizadeh E, Phillips MJ, McGregor JE, DiLoreto DA, Strazzeri JM, Dhakal KR, Bateman B, Jager LD, Nilles KL, Stuedemann SA, et al. 2020. Imaging transplanted photoreceptors in living nonhuman primates with single-cell resolution. *Stem Cell Reports* 15: 482–497. doi:10.1016/j.stemcr.2020.06.019

Al-Khersan H, Hussain RM, Ciulla TA, Dugel PU. 2019. Innovative therapies for neovascular age-related macular degeneration. *Exp Opin Pharmacother* 20: 1879–1891. doi:10.1080/14656566.2019.1636031

Assawachananont J, Mandai M, Okamoto S, Yamada C, Eiraku M, Yonemura S, Sasai Y, Takahashi M. 2014. Transplantation of embryonic and induced pluripotent stem cell-derived 3D retinal sheets into retinal degenerative mice. *Stem Cell Reports* 2: 662–674. doi:10.1016/j.stemcr.2014.03.011

Auffarth GU, Tetz MR, Krastel H, Blankenagel A, Völcker HE. 1997. Complicated cataracts in various forms of retinitis pigmentosa. Type and incidence. *Ophthalmologe* 94: 642–646. doi:10.1007/s003470050175

Barber AC, Hippert C, Duran Y, West EL, Bainbridge JW, Warre-Cornish K, Luhmann UF, Lakowski J, Sowden JC, Ali RR, et al. 2013. Repair of the degenerate retina by photoreceptor transplantation. *Proc Natl Acad Sci* 110: 354–359. doi:10.1073/pnas.1212677110

Bayyoud T, Bartz-Schmidt KU, Yoeruek E. 2013. Long-term clinical results after cataract surgery with and without capsular tension ring in patients with retinitis pigmentosa: a retrospective study. *BMJ Open* 3: e002616. doi:10.1136/bmjopen-2013-002616

Ben M'Barek K, Monville C. 2019. Cell therapy for retinal dystrophies: from cell suspension formulation to complex retinal tissue bioengineering. *Stem Cells Int* 2019: 4568979. doi:10.1155/2019/4568979

Ben M'Barek K, Habeler W, Plancheron A, Jarraya M, Regent F, Terray A, Yang Y, Chatrousse L, Domingues S, Masson Y, et al. 2017. Human ESC-derived retinal epithelial cell sheets potentiate rescue of photoreceptor cell loss in rats with retinal degeneration. *Sci Transl Med* **9**: eaai7471. doi:10.1126/scitranslmed.aai7471

Ben M'Barek K, Habeler W, Monville C. 2018. Stem cell-based RPE therapy for retinal diseases: engineering 3D tissues amenable for regenerative medicine. *Adv Exp Med Biol* **1074**: 625–632. doi:10.1007/978-3-319-75402-4_76

Ben M'Barek K, Bertin S, Brazhnikova E, Jaillard C, Habeler W, Plancheron A, Fovet CM, Demilly J, Jarraya M, Bejanariu A, et al. 2020. Clinical-grade production and safe delivery of human ESC derived RPE sheets in primates and rodents. *Biomaterials* **230**: 119603. doi:10.1016/j.biomaterials.2019.119603

Berger AS, Tezel TH, Del Priore LV, Kaplan HJ. 2003. Photoreceptor transplantation in retinitis pigmentosa: short-term follow-up. *Ophthalmology* **110**: 383–391. doi:10.1016/S0161-6420(02)01738-4

Bian B, Zhao C, He X, Gong Y, Ren C, Ge L, Zeng Y, Li Q, Chen M, Weng C, et al. 2020. Exosomes derived from neural progenitor cells preserve photoreceptors during retinal degeneration by inactivating microglia. *J Extracell Vesicles* **9**: 1748931. doi:10.1080/20013078.2020.1748931

Blair JR, Turner JE. 1987. Optimum conditions for successful transplantation of immature rat retina to the lesioned adult retina. *Brain Res* **433**: 257–270. doi:10.1016/0165-3806(87)90029-0

Brown CN, Green BD, Thompson RB, den Hollander AI, Lengyel I, and on behalf of the EYE-RISK consortium. 2018. Metabolomics and age-related macular degeneration. *Metabolites* **9**: 4. doi:10.3390/metabo9010004

Burton MJ, Ramke J, Marques AP, Bourne RRA, Congdon N, Jones I, Ah Tong BAM, Arunga S, Bachani D, Bascaran C, et al. 2021. The Lancet Global Health Commission on Global Eye Health: vision beyond 2020. *Lancet Glob Health* **9**: e489–e551. doi:10.1016/S2214-109X(20)30488-5

Busskamp V, Duebel J, Balya D, Fradot M, Viney TJ, Siegert S, Groner AC, Cabuy E, Forster V, Seeliger M, et al. 2010. Genetic reactivation of cone photoreceptors restores visual responses in retinitis pigmentosa. *Science* **329**: 413–417. doi:10.1126/science.1190897

Capowski EE, Samimi K, Mayerl SJ, Phillips MJ, Pinilla I, Howden SE, Saha J, Jansen AD, Edwards KL, Jager LD, et al. 2019. Reproducibility and staging of 3D human retinal organoids across multiple pluripotent stem cell lines. *Development* **146**: dev171686. doi:10.1242/dev.171686

Cehajic-Kapetanovic J, Singh MS, Zrenner E, MacLaren RE. 2022. Bioengineering strategies for restoring vision. *Nat Biomed Eng* doi:10.1038/s41551-021-00836-4

Clérin E, Marussig M, Sahel JA, Léveillard T. 2020. Metabolic and redox signaling of the nucleoredoxin-like-1 gene for the treatment of genetic retinal diseases. *Int J Mol Sci* **21**: 1625. doi:10.3390/ijms21051625

Cowan CS, Renner M, De Gennaro M, Gross-Scherf B, Goldblum D, Hou Y, Munz M, Rodrigues TM, Krol J, Szikra T, et al. 2020. Cell types of the human retina and its organoids at single-cell resolution. *Cell* **182**: 1623–1640.e34. doi:10.1016/j.cell.2020.08.013

da Cruz L, Fynes K, Georgiadis O, Kerby J, Luo YH, Ahmado A, Vernon A, Daniels JT, Nommiste B, Hasan SM, et al. 2018. Phase 1 clinical study of an embryonic stem cell-derived retinal pigment epithelium patch in age-related macular degeneration. *Nat Biotechnol* **36**: 328–337. doi:10.1038/nbt.4114

Flaxman SR, Bourne RRA, Resnikoff S, Ackland P, Braithwaite T, Cicinelli MV, Das A, Jonas JB, Keeffe J, Kempen JH, et al. 2017. Global causes of blindness and distance vision impairment 1990-2020: a systematic review and meta-analysis. *Lancet Glob Health* **5**: e1221–e1234. doi:10.1016/S2214-109X(17)30393-5

Gagliardi G, Ben M'Barek K, Chaffiol A, Slembrouck-Brec A, Conart JB, Nanteau C, Rabesandratana O, Sahel JA, Duebel J, Orieux G, et al. 2018. Characterization and transplantation of CD73-positive photoreceptors isolated from human iPSC-derived retinal organoids. *Stem Cell Reports* **11**: 665–680. doi:10.1016/j.stemcr.2018.07.005

Gagliardi G, Ben M'Barek K, Goureau O. 2019. Photoreceptor cell replacement in macular degeneration and retinitis pigmentosa: a pluripotent stem cell-based approach. *Prog Retin Eye Res* **71**: 1–25. doi:10.1016/j.preteyeres.2019.03.001

Garita-Hernandez M, Guibbal L, Toualbi L, Routet F, Chaffiol A, Winckler C, Harinquet M, Robert C, Fouquet S, Bellow S, et al. 2018. Optogenetic light sensors in human retinal organoids. *Front Neurosci* **12**: 789. doi:10.3389/fnins.2018.00789

Garita-Hernandez M, Lampič M, Chaffiol A, Guibbal L, Routet F, Santos-Ferreira T, Gasparini S, Borsch O, Gagliardi G, Reichman S, et al. 2019. Restoration of visual function by transplantation of optogenetically engineered photoreceptors. *Nat Commun* **10**: 4524. doi:10.1038/s41467-019-12330-2

Gasparini SJ, Tessmer K, Reh M, Wieneke S, Carido M, Völkner M, Borsch O, Swiersy A, Zuzic M, Goureau O, et al. 2022. Transplanted human cones incorporate and function in a murine cone degeneration model. *J Clin Invest* **132**: e154619. doi:10.1172/JCI154619

GBD 2019 Blindness and Vision Impairment Collaborators; Vision Loss Expert Group of the Global Burden of Disease Study. 2021a. Causes of blindness and vision impairment in 2020 and trends over 30 years, and prevalence of avoidable blindness in relation to VISION 2020: the Right to Sight: an analysis for the Global Burden of Disease Study. *Lancet Glob Health* **9**: e144–e160. doi:10.1016/S2214-109X(20)30489-7

GBD 2019 Blindness and Vision Impairment Collaborators; Vision Loss Expert Group of the Global Burden of Disease Study. 2021b. Trends in prevalence of blindness and distance and near vision impairment over 30 years: an analysis for the Global Burden of Disease Study. *Lancet Glob Health* **9**: e130–e143. doi:10.1016/S2214-109X(20)30425-3

Gorbatyuk MS, Starr CR, Gorbatyuk OS. 2020. Endoplasmic reticulum stress: new insights into the pathogenesis and treatment of retinal degenerative diseases. *Prog Retin Eye Res* **79**: 100860. doi:10.1016/j.preteyeres.2020.100860

Han IC, Bohrer LR, Gibson-Corley KN, Wiley LA, Shrestha A, Harman BE, Jiao C, Sohn EH, Wendland R, Allen BN, et al. 2022. Biocompatibility of human induced pluripotent stem cell-derived retinal progenitor cell grafts in immunocompromised rats. *Cell Transplant* **31**: 9636897221104451. doi:10.1177/09636897221104451

Handa JT, Bowes Rickman C, Dick AD, Gorin MB, Miller JW, Toth CA, Ueffing M, Zarbin M, Farrer LA. 2019. A systems biology approach towards understanding and treating non-neovascular age-related macular degeneration. *Nat Commun* **10:** 3347. doi:10.1038/s41467-019-11262-1

Hartong DT, Berson EL, Dryja TP. 2006. Retinitis pigmentosa. *Lancet* **368:** 1795–1809. doi:10.1016/S0140-6736(06)69740-7

Hussain AA, Lee Y, Marshall J. 2020. Understanding the complexity of the matrix metalloproteinase system and its relevance to age-related diseases: age-related macular degeneration and Alzheimer's disease. *Prog Retin Eye Res* **74:** 100775. doi:10.1016/j.preteyeres.2019.100775

Iraha S, Tu HY, Yamasaki S, Kagawa T, Goto M, Takahashi R, Watanabe T, Sugita S, Yonemura S, Sunagawa GA, et al. 2018. Establishment of immunodeficient retinal degeneration model mice and functional maturation of human ESC-derived retinal sheets after transplantation. *Stem Cell Reports* **10:** 1059–1074. doi:10.1016/j.stemcr.2018.01.032

Jarrige M, Frank E, Herardot E, Martineau S, Darle A, Benabides M, Domingues S, Chose O, Habeler W, Lorant J, et al. 2021. The future of regenerative medicine: cell therapy using pluripotent stem cells and acellular therapies based on extracellular vesicles. *Cells* **10:** 240. doi:10.3390/cells10020240

Jung YH, Phillips MJ, Lee J, Xie R, Ludwig AL, Chen G, Zheng Q, Kim TJ, Zhang H, Barney P, et al. 2018. 3D microstructured scaffolds to support photoreceptor polarization and maturation. *Adv Mater* **30:** e1803550. doi:10.1002/adma.201803550

Kalargyrou AA, Basche M, Hare A, West EL, Smith AJ, Ali RR, Pearson RA. 2021. Nanotube-like processes facilitate material transfer between photoreceptors. *EMBO Rep* **22:** e53732. doi:10.15252/embr.202153732

Kashani AH, Lebkowski JS, Rahhal FM, Avery RL, Salehi-Had H, Dang W, Lin CM, Mitra D, Zhu D, Thomas BB, et al. 2018. A bioengineered retinal pigment epithelial monolayer for advanced, dry age-related macular degeneration. *Sci Transl Med* **10:** eaao4097. doi:10.1126/scitranslmed.aao4097

Khabou H, Garita-Hernandez M, Chaffiol A, Reichman S, Jaillard C, Brazhnikova E, Bertin S, Forster V, Desrosiers M, Winckler C, et al. 2018. Noninvasive gene delivery to foveal cones for vision restoration. *JCI Insight* **3:** e96029. doi:10.1172/jci.insight.96029

Klapper SD, Swiersy A, Bamberg E, Busskamp V. 2016. Biophysical properties of optogenetic tools and their application for vision restoration approaches. *Front Syst Neurosci* **10:** 74. doi:10.3389/fnsys.2016.00074

Kuwahara A, Ozone C, Nakano T, Saito K, Eiraku M, Sasai Y. 2015. Generation of a ciliary margin-like stem cell niche from self-organizing human retinal tissue. *Nat Commun* **6:** 6286. doi:10.1038/ncomms7286

Lakowski J, Gonzalez-Cordero A, West EL, Han YT, Welby E, Naeem A, Blackford SJ, Bainbridge JW, Pearson RA, Ali RR, et al. 2015. Transplantation of photoreceptor precursors isolated via a cell surface biomarker panel from embryonic stem cell-derived self-forming retina. *Stem Cells* **33:** 2469–2482. doi:10.1002/stem.2051

Lakowski J, Welby E, Budinger D, Di Marco F, Di Foggia V, Bainbridge JWB, Wallace K, Gamm DM, Ali RR, Sowden JC. 2018. Isolation of human photoreceptor precursors via a cell surface marker panel from stem cell-derived

retinal organoids and fetal retinae. *Stem Cells* **36:** 709–722. doi:10.1002/stem.2775

Lavik EB, Klassen H, Warfvinge K, Langer R, Young MJ. 2005. Fabrication of degradable polymer scaffolds to direct the integration and differentiation of retinal progenitors. *Biomaterials* **26:** 3187–3196. doi:10.1016/j.biomaterials.2004.08.022

Lee IK, Ludwig AL, Phillips MJ, Lee J, Xie R, Sajdak BS, Jager LD, Gong S, Gamm DM, Ma Z. 2021. Ultrathin micromolded 3D scaffolds for high-density photoreceptor layer reconstruction. *Sci Adv* **7:** eabf0344. doi:10.1126/sciadv.abf0344

Léveillard T, Sahel JA. 2010. Rod-derived cone viability factor for treating blinding diseases: from clinic to redox signaling. *Sci Transl Med* **2:** 26ps16. doi:10.1126/scitranslmed.3000866

Ludwig AL, Gamm DM. 2021. Outer retinal cell replacement: putting the pieces together. *Transl Vis Sci Technol* **10:** 15. doi:10.1167/tvst.10.10.15

Maeda T, Mandai M, Sugita S, Kime C, Takahashi M. 2022. Strategies of pluripotent stem cell-based therapy for retinal degeneration: update and challenges. *Trends Mol Med* **28:** 388–404. doi:10.1016/j.molmed.2022.03.001

Maguire AM, Russell S, Wellman JA, Chung DC, Yu ZF, Tillman A, Wittes J, Pappas J, Elci O, Marshall KA, et al. 2019. Efficacy, safety, and durability of voretigene neparvovec-rzyl in RPE65 mutation-associated inherited retinal dystrophy: results of phase 1 and 3 trials. *Ophthalmology* **126:** 1273–1285. doi:10.1016/j.ophtha.2019.06.017

Maguire AM, Russell S, Chung DC, Yu ZF, Tillman A, Drack AV, Simonelli F, Leroy BP, Reape KZ, High KA, et al. 2021. Durability of voretigene neparvovec for biallelic RPE65-mediated inherited retinal disease: phase 3 results at 3 and 4 years. *Ophthalmology* **128:** 1460–1468. doi:10.1016/j.ophtha.2021.03.031

Mandai M, Fujii M, Hashiguchi T, Sunagawa GA, Ito SI, Sun J, Kaneko J, Sho J, Yamada C, Takahashi M. 2017a. iPSC-derived retina transplants improve vision in rd1 end-stage retinal-degeneration mice. *Stem Cell Reports* **8:** 1112–1113. doi:10.1016/j.stemcr.2017.03.024

Mandai M, Watanabe A, Kurimoto Y, Hirami Y, Morinaga C, Daimon T, Fujihara M, Akimaru H, Sakai N, Shibata Y, et al. 2017b. Autologous induced stem-cell-derived retinal cells for macular degeneration. *N Engl J Med* **376:** 1038–1046. doi:10.1056/NEJMoa1608368

Maqueda M, Mosquera JL, García-Arumí J, Veiga A, Duarri A. 2021. Repopulation of decellularized retinas with hiPSC-derived retinal pigment epithelial and ocular progenitor cells shows cell engraftment, organization and differentiation. *Biomaterials* **276:** 121049. doi:10.1016/j.biomaterials.2021.121049

McLelland BT, Lin B, Mathur A, Aramant RB, Thomas BB, Nistor G, Keirstead HS, Seiler MJ. 2018. Transplanted hESC-derived retina organoid sheets differentiate, integrate, and improve visual function in retinal degenerate rats. *Invest Ophthalmol Vis Sci* **59:** 2586–2603. doi:10.1167/iovs.17-23646

McUsic AC, Lamba DA, Reh TA. 2012. Guiding the morphogenesis of dissociated newborn mouse retinal cells and hES cell-derived retinal cells by soft lithography-patterned microchannel PLGA scaffolds. *Biomaterials* **33:** 1396–1405. doi:10.1016/j.biomaterials.2011.10.083

Cite this article as *Cold Spring Harb Perspect Med* doi: 10.1101/cshperspect.a041309

Mead B, Tomarev S. 2020. Extracellular vesicle therapy for retinal diseases. *Prog Retin Eye Res* **79:** 100849. doi:10.1016/j.preteyeres.2020.100849

Mitchell P, Liew G, Gopinath B, Wong TY. 2018. Age-related macular degeneration. *Lancet* **392:** 1147–1159. doi:10.1016/S0140-6736(18)31550-2

Nakano T, Ando S, Takata N, Kawada M, Muguruma K, Sekiguchi K, Saito K, Yonemura S, Eiraku M, Sasai Y. 2012. Self-formation of optic cups and storable stratified neural retina from human ESCs. *Cell Stem Cell* **10:** 771–785. doi:10.1016/j.stem.2012.05.009

Neeley WL, Redenti S, Klassen H, Tao S, Desai T, Young MJ, Langer R. 2008. A microfabricated scaffold for retinal progenitor cell grafting. *Biomaterials* **29:** 418–426. doi:10.1016/j.biomaterials.2007.10.007

O'Hara-Wright M, Gonzalez-Cordero A. 2020. Retinal organoids: A window into human retinal development. *Development* **147:** dev189746. doi:10.1242/dev.189746

Ohlemacher SK, Iglesias CL, Sridhar A, Gamm DM, Meyer JS. 2015. Generation of highly enriched populations of optic vesicle-like retinal cells from human pluripotent stem cells. *Curr Protoc Stem Cell Biol* **32:** 1H.8.1–1H.8.20. doi:10.1002/9780470151808.sc01h08s32

Ortin-Martinez A, Yan NE, Tsai ELS, Comanita L, Gurdita A, Tachibana N, Liu ZC, Lu S, Dolati P, Pokrajac NT, et al. 2021. Photoreceptor nanotubes mediate the in vivo exchange of intracellular material. *EMBO J* **40:** e107264. doi:10.15252/embj.2020107264

Parfitt DA, Lane A, Ramsden CM, Carr AJ, Munro PM, Jovanovic K, Schwarz N, Kanuga N, Muthiah MN, Hull S, et al. 2016. Identification and correction of mechanisms underlying inherited blindness in human iPSC-derived optic cups. *Cell Stem Cell* **18:** 769–781. doi:10.1016/j.stem.2016.03.021

Pearson RA, Barber AC, Rizzi M, Hippert C, Xue T, West EL, Duran Y, Smith AJ, Chuang JZ, Azam SA, et al. 2012. Restoration of vision after transplantation of photoreceptors. *Nature* **485:** 99–103. doi:10.1038/nature10997

Pearson RA, Gonzalez-Cordero A, West EL, Ribeiro JR, Aghaizu N, Goh D, Sampson RD, Georgiadis A, Waldron PV, Duran Y, et al. 2016. Donor and host photoreceptors engage in material transfer following transplantation of post-mitotic photoreceptor precursors. *Nat Commun* **7:** 13029. doi:10.1038/ncomms13029

Peng B, Xiao J, Wang K, So KF, Tipoe GL, Lin B. 2014. Suppression of microglial activation is neuroprotective in a mouse model of human retinitis pigmentosa. *J Neurosci* **34:** 8139–8150. doi:10.1523/JNEUROSCI.5200-13.2014

Pennesi ME, Schlechter CL. 2020. The evolution of retinal gene therapy: from clinical trials to clinical practice. *Ophthalmology* **127:** 148–150. doi:10.1016/j.ophtha.2019.12.003

Pfeiffer RL, Marc RE, Jones BW. 2020. Persistent remodeling and neurodegeneration in late-stage retinal degeneration. *Prog Retin Eye Res* **74:** 100771. doi:10.1016/j.preteyeres.2019.07.004

Qiu TG. 2019. Transplantation of human embryonic stem cell-derived retinal pigment epithelial cells (MA09-hRPE) in macular degeneration. *NPJ Regen Med* **4:** 19. doi:10.1038/s41536-019-0081-8

Radtke ND, Seiler MJ, Aramant RB, Petry HM, Pidwell DJ. 2002. Transplantation of intact sheets of fetal neural retina with its retinal pigment epithelium in retinitis pigmentosa patients. *Am J Ophthalmol* **133:** 544–550. doi:10.1016/S0002-9394(02)01322-3

Radtke ND, Aramant RB, Petry HM, Green PT, Pidwell DJ, Seiler MJ. 2008. Vision improvement in retinal degeneration patients by implantation of retina together with retinal pigment epithelium. *Am J Ophthalmol* **146:** 172–182.e1. doi:10.1016/j.ajo.2008.04.009

Redenti S, Neeley WL, Rompani S, Saigal S, Yang J, Klassen H, Langer R, Young MJ. 2009. Engineering retinal progenitor cell and scrollable poly(glycerol-sebacate) composites for expansion and subretinal transplantation. *Biomaterials* **30:** 3405–3414. doi:10.1016/j.biomaterials.2009.02.046

Reichman S, Terray A, Slembrouck A, Nanteau C, Orieux G, Habeler W, Nandrot EF, Sahel JA, Monville C, Goureau O. 2014. From confluent human iPS cells to self-forming neural retina and retinal pigmented epithelium. *Proc Natl Acad Sci* **111:** 8518–8523. doi:10.1073/pnas.1324212111

Reichman S, Slembrouck A, Gagliardi G, Chaffiol A, Terray A, Nanteau C, Potey A, Belle M, Rabesandratana O, Duebel J, et al. 2017. Generation of storable retinal organoids and retinal pigmented epithelium from adherent human iPS cells in xeno-free and feeder-free conditions. *Stem Cells* **35:** 1176–1188. doi:10.1002/stem.2586

Ribeiro J, Procyk CA, West EL, O'Hara-Wright M, Martins MF, Khorasani MM, Hare A, Basche M, Fernando M, Goh D, et al. 2021. Restoration of visual function in advanced disease after transplantation of purified human pluripotent stem cell-derived cone photoreceptors. *Cell Rep* **35:** 109022. doi:10.1016/j.celrep.2021.109022

Ripolles-Garcia A, Dolgova N, Phillips MJ, Savina S, Ludwig AL, Stuedemann SA, Nlebedum U, Wolfe JH, Garden OA, Maminishkis A, et al. 2022. Systemic immunosuppression promotes survival and integration of subretinally implanted human ESC-derived photoreceptor precursors in dogs. *Stem Cell Reports* **17:** 1824–1841. doi:10.1016/j.stemcr.2022.06.009

Roska B, Sahel JA. 2018. Restoring vision. *Nature* **557:** 359–367. doi:10.1038/s41586-018-0076-4

Saha A, Capowski E, Fernandez Zepeda MA, Nelson EC, Gamm DM, Sinha R. 2022. Cone photoreceptors in human stem cell-derived retinal organoids demonstrate intrinsic light responses that mimic those of primate fovea. *Cell Stem Cell* **29:** 460–471.e463. doi:10.1016/j.stem.2022.01.002

Sahel JA, Bennett J, Roska B. 2019. Depicting brighter possibilities for treating blindness. *Sci Transl Med* **11:** eaax2324. doi:10.1126/scitranslmed.aax2324

Sahel JA, Boulanger-Scemama E, Pagot C, Arleo A, Galluppi F, Martel JN, Esposti SD, Delaux A, de Saint Aubert JB, de Montleau C, et al. 2021. Partial recovery of visual function in a blind patient after optogenetic therapy. *Nat Med* **27:** 1223–1229. doi:10.1038/s41591-021-01351-4

Salas A, Duarri A, Fontrodona L, Ramírez DM, Badia A, Isla-Magrané H, Ferreira-de-Souza B, Zapata MA, Raya A, Veiga A, et al. 2021. Cell therapy with hiPSC-derived RPE cells and RPCs prevents visual function loss in a rat model of retinal degeneration. *Mol Ther Methods Clin Dev* **20:** 688–702. doi:10.1016/j.omtm.2021.02.006

Santos-Ferreira T, Llonch S, Borsch O, Postel K, Haas J, Ader M. 2016a. Retinal transplantation of photoreceptors results in donor-host cytoplasmic exchange. *Nat Commun* **7:** 13028. doi:10.1038/ncomms13028

Santos-Ferreira T, Völkner M, Borsch O, Haas J, Cimalla P, Vasudevan P, Carmeliet P, Corbeil D, Michalakis S, Koch E, et al. 2016b. Stem cell-derived photoreceptor transplants differentially integrate into mouse models of cone-rod dystrophy. *Invest Ophthalmol Vis Sci* **57**: 3509–3520. doi:10.1167/iovs.16-19087

Seiler MJ, Aramant RB. 2012. Cell replacement and visual restoration by retinal sheet transplants. *Prog Retin Eye Res* **31**: 661–687. doi:10.1016/j.preteyes.2012.06.003

Shirai H, Mandai M, Matsushita K, Kuwahara A, Yonemura S, Nakano T, Assawachananont J, Kimura T, Saito K, Terasaki H, et al. 2016. Transplantation of human embryonic stem cell-derived retinal tissue in two primate models of retinal degeneration. *Proc Natl Acad Sci* **113**: E81–E90. doi:10.1073/pnas.1512590113

Shrestha A, Allen BN, Wiley LA, Tucker BA, Worthington KS. 2020. Development of high-resolution three-dimensional-printed extracellular matrix scaffolds and their compatibility with pluripotent stem cells and early retinal cells. *J Ocul Pharmacol Ther* **36**: 42–55. doi:10.1089/jop.2018.0146

Singh MS, Charbel Issa P, Butler R, Martin C, Lipinski DM, Sekaran S, Barnard AR, MacLaren RE. 2013. Reversal of end-stage retinal degeneration and restoration of visual function by photoreceptor transplantation. *Proc Natl Acad Sci* **110**: 1101–1106. doi:10.1073/pnas.1119416110

Singh MS, Balmer J, Barnard AR, Aslam SA, Moralli D, Green CM, Barnea-Cramer A, Duncan I, MacLaren RE. 2016. Transplanted photoreceptor precursors transfer proteins to host photoreceptors by a mechanism of cytoplasmic fusion. *Nat Commun* **7**: 13537. doi:10.1038/ncomms13537

Singh D, Wang SB, Xia T, Tainsh L, Ghiassi-Nejad M, Xu T, Peng S, Adelman RA, Rizzolo LJ. 2018. A biodegradable scaffold enhances differentiation of embryonic stem cells into a thick sheet of retinal cells. *Biomaterials* **154**: 158–168. doi:10.1016/j.biomaterials.2017.10.052

Takahashi K, Tanabe K, Ohnuki M, Narita M, Ichisaka T, Tomoda K, Yamanaka S. 2007. Induction of pluripotent stem cells from adult human fibroblasts by defined factors. *Cell* **131**: 861–872. doi:10.1016/j.cell.2007.11.019

Thomas BB, Zhu D, Lin TC, Kim YC, Seiler MJ, Martinez-Camarillo JC, Lin B, Shad Y, Hinton DR, Humayun MS. 2018. A new immunodeficient retinal dystrophic rat model for transplantation studies using human-derived cells. *Graefes Arch Clin Exp Ophthalmol* **256**: 2113–2125. doi:10.1007/s00417-018-4134-2

Thomas BB, Lin B, Martinez-Camarillo JC, Zhu D, McLelland BT, Nistor G, Keirstead HS, Humayun MS, Seiler MJ. 2021. Co-grafts of human embryonic stem cell derived retina organoids and retinal pigment epithelium for retinal reconstruction in immunodeficient retinal degenerate Royal College of Surgeons rats. *Front Neurosci* **15**: 752958. doi:10.3389/fnins.2021.752958

Thompson JR, Worthington KS, Green BJ, Mullin NK, Jiao C, Kaalberg EE, Wiley LA, Han IC, Russell SR, Sohn EH, et al. 2019. Two-photon polymerized poly(caprolactone) retinal cell delivery scaffolds and their systemic and retinal biocompatibility. *Acta Biomater* **94**: 204–218. doi:10.1016/j.actbio.2019.04.057

Thomson JA, Itskovitz-Eldor J, Shapiro SS, Waknitz MA, Swiergiel JJ, Marshall VS, Jones JM. 1998. Embryonic stem cell lines derived from human blastocysts. *Science* **282**: 1145–1147. doi:10.1126/science.282.5391.1145

Tu HY, Watanabe T, Shirai H, Yamasaki S, Kinoshita M, Matsushita K, Hashiguchi T, Onoe H, Matsuyama T, Kuwahara A, et al. 2019. Medium- to long-term survival and functional examination of human iPSC-derived retinas in rat and primate models of retinal degeneration. *EBioMed* **39**: 562–574. doi:10.1016/j.ebiom.2018.11.028

Tucker BA, Redenti SM, Jiang C, Swift JS, Klassen HJ, Smith ME, Wnek GE, Young MJ. 2010. The use of progenitor cell/biodegradable MMP2-PLGA polymer constructs to enhance cellular integration and retinal repopulation. *Biomaterials* **31**: 9–19. doi:10.1016/j.biomaterials.2009.09.015

Turner JE, Blair JR. 1986. Newborn rat retinal cells transplanted into a retinal lesion site in adult host eyes. *Brain Res* **391**: 91–104. doi:10.1016/0165-3806(86)90011-8

Verbakel SK, van Huet RAC, Boon CJF, den Hollander AI, Collin RWJ, Klaver CCW, Hoyng CB, Roepman R, Klevering BJ. 2018. Non-syndromic retinitis pigmentosa. *Prog Retin Eye Res* **66**: 157–186. doi:10.1016/j.preteyes.2018.03.005

Welby E, Lakowski J, Di Foggia V, Budinger D, Gonzalez-Cordero A, Lun ATL, Epstein M, Patel A, Cuevas E, Kruczek K, et al. 2017. Isolation and comparative transcriptome analysis of human fetal and iPSC-derived cone photoreceptor cells. *Stem Cell Reports* **9**: 1898–1915. doi:10.1016/j.stemcr.2017.10.018

Wittenborn JS, Zhang X, Feagan CW, Crouse WL, Shrestha S, Kemper AR, Hoerger TJ, Saaddine JB; Vision Cost-Effectiveness Study Group. 2013. The economic burden of vision loss and eye disorders among the United States population younger than 40 years. *Ophthalmology* **120**: 1728–1735. doi:10.1016/j.ophtha.2013.01.068

Worthington KS, Wiley LA, Kaalberg EE, Collins MM, Mullins RF, Stone EM, Tucker BA. 2017. Two-photon polymerization for production of human iPSC-derived retinal cell grafts. *Acta Biomater* **55**: 385–395. doi:10.1016/j.actbio.2017.03.039

Yamasaki S, Tu HY, Matsuyama T, Horiuchi M, Hashiguchi T, Sho J, Kuwahara A, Kishino A, Kimura T, Takahashi M, et al. 2022. A genetic modification that reduces ON-bipolar cells in hESC-derived retinas enhances functional integration after transplantation. *iScience* **25**: 103657. doi:10.1016/j.isci.2021.103657

Yao J, Tucker BA, Zhang X, Checa-Casalengua P, Herrero-Vanrell R, Young MJ. 2011. Robust cell integration from co-transplantation of biodegradable MMP2-PLGA microspheres with retinal progenitor cells. *Biomaterials* **32**: 1041–1050. doi:10.1016/j.biomaterials.2010.09.063

Zarbin M, Sugino I, Townes-Anderson E. 2019. Concise review: update on retinal pigment epithelium transplantation for age-related macular degeneration. *Stem Cells Transl Med* **8**: 466–477. doi:10.1002/sctm.18-0282

Zhong X, Gutierrez C, Xue T, Hampton C, Vergara MN, Cao LH, Peters A, Park TS, Zambidis ET, Meyer JS, et al. 2014. Generation of three-dimensional retinal tissue with functional photoreceptors from human iPSCs. *Nat Commun* **5**: 4047. doi:10.1038/ncomms5047

Cell-Based Therapies: Strategies for Regeneration

Marina Pavlou and Thomas A. Reh

Department of Biological Structure, University of Washington School of Medicine, Institute of Stem Cells and Regenerative Medicine, Seattle, Washington 98195, USA

Correspondence: tomreh@uw.edu

The neural retina of mammals, like most of the rest of the central nervous system, does not regenerate new neurons after they are lost through damage or disease. The ability of non-mammalian vertebrates, like fish and amphibians, is remarkable, and lessons learned over the last 20 years have revealed some of the mechanisms underlying this potential. This knowledge has recently been applied to mammals to develop methods that can stimulate regeneration in mice. In this review, we highlight the progress in this area, and propose a "wish list" of how the clinical implementation of regenerative strategies could be applicable to various human retinal diseases.

The retina of mammals, including humans, like most of the central nervous system (CNS), lacks the capacity to regenerate new neurons when they are lost to injury or disease. This has inspired the development and testing of various therapeutic strategies aimed at replenishing the missing neurons. The most popular strategy has been cell replacement, primarily focused on generating neurons in vitro, starting with pluripotent stem cells or retinal progenitors, and then transplanting these cells to the site of neuronal loss (see Monville et al. 2022). While good progress is being made with this approach and clinical trials are underway, there are many technical difficulties with transplantation and replacement cell sourcing that still need to be addressed. In our review, we focus on a very different approach for cell replacement: to stimulate regeneration of new retinal neurons from "intrinsic" sources to replace those neurons that have de-

generated from disease. This strategy would not require transplantation and subsequent integration of the cells from either the subretinal space or the vitreous, since the new neurons are generated from within the retina. Moreover, no cell manufacturing would be required, thereby avoiding the complexity inherent with this process.

Endogenous regeneration strategies are based on biology: several nonmammalian species readily regenerate their retinas after injury (for review, see Todd and Reh 2022). In these species, retinal injury or cell loss causes one or more types of nonneuronal cell to "dedifferentiate" into a cell resembling a retinal progenitor, reenter the cell cycle, and generate new retinal neurons much like the retinal progenitors that make retinal neurons during development. The progenitors generate the neurons while going through multiple rounds of cell division, and can replace any type of retinal neuron, and in extreme cases can replace the entire laminated retina in a few weeks. The main sources of retinal regeneration are (1) retinal stem/progenitor cells at the margin of the retina, (2) the retinal pigment epithelium (RPE), and (3) the Müller glia (MG). Depending on the species and the type of injury, any of these three cellular sources for regeneration can be employed; however, in this review, we will focus on MG, since these are likely to be engaged for vision restoration in humans.

Although it had been known particularly from the pioneering work of Pamela Raymond and her colleagues that teleost fish were able to regenerate retinal neurons from a source intrinsic to the retina (Lenkowski and Raymond 2014), the focus on MG as a source for retinal regeneration came from studies in bird retina by Fischer and Reh (2001). Subsequently, Dan Goldman and colleagues (Fausett and Goldman 2006) lineage-traced regenerated neurons from MG in adult zebrafish, and a large number of studies have confirmed and extended these initial findings (Goldman 2014). In fish, MG respond to injury by reentering the cell cycle and dedifferentiating into multipotent progenitors (Konar et al. 2021). The mobilization of these cells involves a transient expression of inflammation-related genes and cytoskeletal remodeling (Lahne et al. 2015; Nagashima and Hitchcock 2021). These progenitors help repopulate the injured retina by giving rise to new neurons that integrate in the existing network and restore tissue function, albeit not to the original levels (Sherpa et al. 2014; D'Orazi et al. 2016; Hammer et al. 2022).

In mice, where most research on retinal regeneration in mammals has been focused, the MG response to injury is very different. Although the initial response of MG to neuron loss is dominated by an up-regulation in inflammation-associated genes, the MG of fish (and to a lesser extent birds) rapidly activate a program of neurogenesis, whereas this does not occur in mice (Hoang et al. 2020). In mice, there is no evidence for reexpression of developmental genes related to neurogenesis and little evidence of damage-induced mitotic proliferation of the MG (Karl et al. 2008). Thus, there appears to be a bifurcation in the transcriptional response to injury in the MG depending on the species; in mammals, the inflammatory response is sustained and may prevent the expression of a regenerative program, whereas in fish, the inflammatory response is more transient and is required to initiate regeneration (White et al. 2017). Therefore, stimulating a more fish-like program of regeneration in mammalian MG will need to stimulate both the proliferation of the MG and the acquisition of a neurogenic potential, both of which occur spontaneously after injury in fish, but are lacking in mammals.

DEVELOPMENT OF A RETINAL REGENERATION APPROACH TO VISION RESTORATION

The process of regeneration typically involves both cell proliferation and changes in gene expression to acquire a progenitor state; these processes appear to be somewhat separable, and both may need to be addressed in the development of a regeneration therapy. During normal eye development, eye-field-committed progenitor cells in the forebrain give rise to the eyecup (Hägglund et al. 2011), where multipotent retinal progenitors will divide repeatedly and give rise to neurons. These new neurons differentiate into the six main neuron classes (ganglion cells, cones, horizontal cells, amacrines, bipolar cells, rods) in the retina in a sequential manner, and at the end of neurogenesis, the remaining progenitors differentiate into MG. The MG do not normally reenter the cell cycle, and several studies have attempted to define what controls their terminal differentiation, looking at both intrinsic and extrinsic factors.

With regard to intrinsic factors, cell-cycle regulators play a central role. For example, cyclin D1 is essential for cell proliferation of retinal progenitors (Sicinski et al. 1995), and deletion of the cyclin-dependent kinase inhibitor, p57 (Dyer and Cepko 2000) or p27kip (Levine et al. 2000), leads to sustained MG proliferation after the normal period of histogenesis, although the cells typically proliferate one or two more rounds of division. Furthermore, p53 knockout (KO) leads to an increase in MG proliferation in vitro

(Ueki et al. 2012), suggesting that DNA damage may limit MG cell-cycle reentry. This is consistent with other observations (Nomura-Komoike et al. 2016) where MG cell-cycle reentry was accompanied by increase in DNA damage markers, like H2X, in mice, but not zebrafish. The NFI transcription factors (TFs) were also shown to control cell-cycle exit and generation of late-born cell types in the retina, including MG (G1/S phase markers [e.g., *Pcna*, *Ccne2*] and G2/M phase [e.g., *Ccnbl*, *Ube2c*]) (Clark et al. 2019). To manipulate these intrinsic pathways, the overexpression of certain TFs may also increase cell proliferation in MG, such as overexpression of Ascl1 and Lin28 in fish and mice (Elsaeidi et al. 2018). In fish, preventing Ascl1 up-regulation after injury prevents cell-cycle reentry of MG (Fausett et al. 2008; Gorsuch et al.

2017), and the same was true when down-regulating proliferating cell nuclear antigen (PCNA) during light damage, which lead to loss of Pax6 expression and inhibition of MG division (Thummel et al. 2008). Indeed, overexpression of Ascl1 in mouse MG leads to their reentry into the cell cycle, and this is accentuated by coadministration of extrinsic mitogens like epidermal growth factor (EGF) (Table 1; Jorstad et al. 2017).

These intrinsic regulators of MG proliferation are also influenced by signaling molecules. The most well-studied mitogenic factor for MG is EGF. EGF has been shown to stimulate MG proliferation in fish, birds, mice (Close et al. 2006; Karl et al. 2008; Ueki et al. 2012), rats (Close et al. 2005), rabbits (Scherer and Schnitzer 1994), guinea pig (Milenkovic et al. 2003), and human (Hollborn et al.

Table 1. Factors that affect Müller glial proliferation and neurogenesis

Factor	Species	References
Intrinsic		
Cyclin D1	Mouse	Sicinski et al. 1995
P57	Mouse	Dyer and Cepko 2000
P27kip	Mouse	Levine et al. 2000
P53	Mouse	Ueki et al. 2012
NFI	Mouse	Clark et al. 2019
Ascl1	Fish, mouse	Fausett et al. 2008; Gorsuch et al. 2017; Jorstad et al. 2017; Elsaeidi et al. 2018
Ascl1/Atoh1	Mouse	Todd et al. 2021
Lin28	Fish, mouse	Elsaeidi et al. 2018
PCNA/Pax6	Fish	Thummel et al. 2008
Extrinsic		
EGF	Fish, chicken, mouse, rat, rabbit, guinea pig, human	Scherer and Schnitzer 1994; Close et al. 2005, 2006; Hollborn et al. 2005; Karl et al. 2008; Ueki et al. 2012
HB-EGF	Fish, chicken	Wan et al. 2012; Todd et al. 2015
CNTF	Fish	Kassen et al. 2009
BMP	Mouse	Ueki and Reh 2013
IGF, insulin	Chicken	Fischer et al. 2002
FGF	Chicken	Fischer et al. 2002
P2Y-receptor activation	Guinea pig	Milenkovic et al. 2003
PDGF	Guinea pig	Milenkovic et al. 2003
TGF-β	Mouse	Close et al. 2005
STAT pathway	Mouse	Jorstad et al. 2020
Microglia depletion	Mouse	Todd et al. 2020
YAP/TAZ pathway	Mouse	Hamon et al. 2019; Rueda et al. 2019
mTORC-1	Mouse	Lim et al. 2021
Notch pathway	Mouse	Hojo et al. 2000; Nelson et al. 2007
MMP2	Chicken	Campbell et al. 2019
MMP9	Fish	Silva et al. 2020

2005). EGF stimulates proliferation of progenitors in the developing CNS as well as astrocytes and unregulated activation of epidermal growth factor receptor (EGFR) is frequently associated with gliomas (Su Huang et al. 1997; Halatsch et al. 2006). EGF signaling leading to MG proliferation engages PI3K and MEK/ERK1/2, as well as other signaling pathways such as ciliary neurotrophic factor (CNTF)/leukemia inhibitory factor (LIF) and bone morphogenetic protein (BMP), in fish (Kassen et al. 2009), birds (Todd et al. 2015), and mice (Ueki and Reh 2013), and up-regulates cyclin D1 expression. In addition to EGF, insulin-like growth factor (IGF), insulin, fibroblast growth factor (FGF), P2Y-receptor activation, heparin-binding (HB)-EGF, and platelet-derived growth factor (PDGF) stimulate MG proliferation after intravitreal injection in birds (Ikeda and Puro 1995; Fischer et al. 2002; Todd et al. 2015), mice (Karl et al. 2008; Todd et al. 2015), and fish (Wan et al. 2012). In fish, retinal injury induces expression of many of these mitogens and their receptors in MG (Goldman 2014), suggesting that a coordinated up-regulation of multiple parallel signaling molecules supports the robust proliferation observed during regeneration.

In addition to positive regulators of MG proliferation, the MG also are under negative regulation by signaling factors. TGF-β is one of the regulators of progenitor proliferation as inhibiting the TGF-β pathway leads to an increase in MG proliferation in vivo and in vitro in postnatal rat, while EGF stimulates MG proliferation (Close et al. 2005). These factors were shown to affect the level of cyclin-dependent kinase inhibitor p27, thus providing a potential link between the extrinsic and intrinsic regulators of cell proliferation. However, in mice heterozygous deletion of the inhibitory Smad protein, Smad7, causes an increase in progenitor proliferation in postnatal animals (Kugler et al. 2017), potentially leading to an increase in MG. These somewhat contradictory findings may be partly explained by the fact that Smad7 inhibits both BMP and TGF-β signaling, and BMP signaling also promotes MG differentiation (Ueki and Reh 2013; Ueki et al. 2015). Gain-of-function

via up-regulation of the YAP/TAZ pathway (intravitreal injection of adeno-associated virus [AAV]/CMV-YAP5SA) leads to MG exit from quiescence state and cell-cycle reentry in mouse retina by functional interaction with EGFR signaling (Hamon et al. 2019), thereby overcoming the Hippo pathway blockade on MG proliferation following injury in the retina (Rueda et al. 2019). Also, hyperactivation of mTORC-1 leads to mammalian MG proliferation; however, this accelerates the aging process and leads to premature cell death in an Hif1a-dependent manner (Lim et al. 2021). Interestingly, different mouse strains can undergo varying levels of MG proliferation following injury (Suga et al. 2014), suggesting a major contextual impact on MG response during degeneration.

This begs the question, why do fish, amphibian, and bird MG reenter the mitotic cell cycle after injury and mammalian MG do not (Fig. 1)? Many of the initial events in the response of MG to retinal injury are the same in fish and other vertebrates, including mammals. The initial response to up-regulate inflammatory signaling is conserved across species; however, after these early changes, the fish glia reenter the cell cycle while mouse glia do not. There are some key differences: Ascl1 is spontaneously increased in fish MG after injury and as noted above, KO of Ascl1 prevents the MG from cell-cycle reentry (Fausett et al. 2008). In fish, dedifferentiated MG divide asymmetrically to produce a proliferating retinal progenitor and an MG (Nagashima et al. 2013; Nagashima and Hitchcock 2021), while this may not occur in mammals, even after mitotic stimulation. Another key difference seems to be in the Notch pathway. In fish, the Notch3 receptor and DeltaB maintain MG quiescence and negatively regulate regeneration following light damage (Campbell et al. 2020; Sahu et al. 2021). By contrast, in mice, the Notch pathway activation promotes MG differentiation and inhibition of Notch signaling in mice in mature retina has not been reported to induce proliferation in these cells (Hojo et al. 2000). Furthermore, during mouse retina development it is clear that Notch inhibition leads to cell-cycle exit of the progenitors (Nelson et al. 2007). Further studies on the differences in Notch-responsive

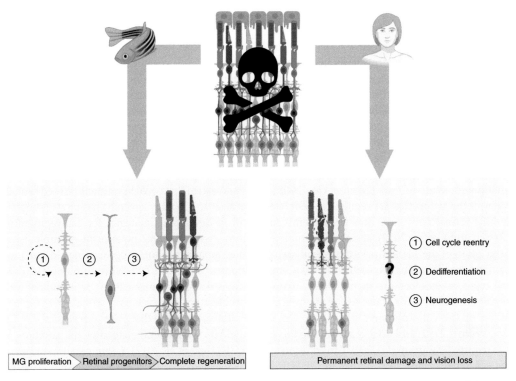

Figure 1. Schematic representation of different cellular responses to retinal injury between zebrafish, as an example of a regenerating organism, and human. Following damage, Müller glia (MG) in zebrafish respond in a stepwise manner by (1) reentering the cell cycle, (2) dedifferentiating into retinal progenitors, and (3) giving rise to new neurons to repopulate the damaged tissue. These responses are absent in the human retina leading to permanent retinal damage after injury, which creates an impetus for asking how we can stimulate a regenerative response from human MG.

genes may lead to a better understanding of this key difference.

Other environmental variables may also be distinct across species and influence mammalian MG response to injury. For example, the cell–ECM interaction in the mammalian retina may influence interkinetic nuclear migration of MG, which is necessary for their proliferation during development and regeneration (Lahne and Hyde 2016). Gelatinase activity can also modulate MG proliferation, with evidence from the avian retina that injury decreases gelatinase activity and MMP2 inhibition shifts MG to a progenitor fate (Campbell et al. 2019). Furthermore, evidence from the zebrafish also implicates the role of MMP9 in regeneration (Silva et al. 2020), although this has not been studied in the mammalian retina. Inflammation may

also induce the activation of cell-cycle genes in fish, but not in mice (Nagashima and Hitchcock 2021). As noted above, CNTF and STAT signaling are important in the MG response to injury in fish, mice, and birds. Some of the activation of this pathway may come from local inflammatory signals released by immune cells. Recent studies have shown that manipulating microglia following injury can affect the MG response in all these species (White et al. 2017; Mitchell et al. 2019; Todd et al. 2020; Nagashima and Hitchcock 2021) and further studies into how the immune response shapes the local environment for MG proliferation are warranted.

The process of making the diversity of neurons during development requires many specific TFs that control genesis of different types and subtypes. The process of specification begins prior to neurogenesis, when a specific set of TFs, called eye-field TFs, collaborate to specify a region of the anterior neural tube to become the neural retinas. Once neurogenesis begins after optic cup formation, the eye-field TFs, along with additional factors, are required for both progenitor proliferation, and the competence of the progenitors to generate specific fates. Pax6, for example, is required early in retinal development as an eye-field determining factor and, later, required in retinal progenitors to maintain their multipotent state (Oron-Karni et al. 2008). Many of the factors that are required to generate specific retinal fates have now been identified (Bassett and Wallace 2012), although a complete description of the TF networks that specify retinal fates is still lacking. Nevertheless, for some cell types, photoreceptors in particular, many key TFs are known; for example, for the specification of the cone photoreceptor fates, Otx2, Crx, Prdm1, Trβ2, and RXR-γ are among those TFs required (Swaroop et al. 2010). In addition to the cell-type-specific TFs, studies in the retina and elsewhere in the CNS have identified "proneural" TFs that promote neurogenesis in nonneural cells (e.g., fibroblasts or glia) (Bocchi et al. 2022). These include Ascl1, Neurogenin2, and Neurod1. These TFs provide neurogenic potential, but do not necessarily restrict cells to a specific type of neuron (Imayoshi and Kageyama 2014).

STIMULATION OF RETINAL REGENERATION IN MICE

The work in retinal development highlights the enormous complexity that would theoretically need to be engaged in MG to initiate retinal repair. While this might seem a daunting task, happily studies that have compared gene expression in retinal progenitors and MG have found that many of the eye-field TFs are expressed in MG at similar levels to the retinal progenitors (Nelson et al. 2008). In addition, many of the networks of TFs present in progenitors persist in the MG (Karl et al. 2008; Nelson et al. 2008; Hoang et al. 2020). This has led to attempts to replace some of the missing factors in MG, either in vitro or in vivo, and determine whether some

critical factors could stimulate neurogenesis from these cells.

Although some of the early attempts to reprogram MG to progenitors were not successful at demonstrating convincing neurogenesis, in the past 10 years the situation changed with improvement in the methods for in vitro cultures of MG from mice and transgenic methods for manipulating TF expression. A first step toward identifying potential reprogramming factors for stimulating neurogenesis from MG was to establish an in vitro system that could be used as a test bed (Pollak et al. 2013). In vitro screening has proven successful in developing strategies for cell reprogramming, with the most noteworthy example being the Yamanaka factors for generating induced pluripotent stem cells (iPSCs) from fibroblasts (Takahashi and Yamanaka 2006). In a study of MG proliferation in developing retina using explant cultures, we found that prior to postnatal day 12, the MG would proliferate after the addition of EGF (Ueki et al. 2012). Using parallel studies of dissociated retinal cultures, we determined that by postnatal day 10 there were no longer progenitors in the mouse retina, but MG could still proliferate in dissociated retinal cells from postnatal day P11–P12, with a consistent enrichment of MG markers after passaging (Ueki et al. 2012). We subsequently found that MG from adult mice (>10 wk), can be maintained in dissociated cell cultures, although these do not expand much and do best when cultured on a "feeder layer" of P12 MG (Wohl and Reh 2016).

Once methods were in hand to maintain MG in dissociated cell cultures, these were used to test TF candidates (e.g., those expressed by developing retinal progenitors, but not expressed in MG). Of the initial factors that we tested, the proneural TF Ascl1 was the most effective in reprogramming the MG to neurogenic progenitors (Pollak et al. 2013). The MG-derived progenitors express many genes associated with neurogenesis, including Notch, Dll1/3, Hes1/5/6, and others. The MG-derived progenitors undergo mitotic cell divisions at a higher rate than the MG in the cultures, and generate new neurons, defined by morphology, lineage tracing with coexpression of immunofluorescence markers of neurons, single-cell transcriptomic data, and electrophysiology (Pollak et al. 2013). Multiple genes have now been tested in this system and we find that it can be predictive of TFs that have similar neurogenic potential in vivo (see below).

Following the discovery of pioneer factor Ascl1 and its capacity to reprogram mammalian MG into neurons in vitro, we developed mouse models where proneural TFs were expressed in a tamoxifen-inducible manner only in MG (Fig. 2A′; Ueki et al. 2015). The model had a glial-specific Cre-recombinase ER-T2, a floxed tTA (tetracycline activator protein) and a TRE-Ascl1-GFP; in this mouse, injection of tamoxifen induces Cre-mediated recombination of the tTA, which then activates the TRE and drives Ascl1 expression specifically in MG. We initially tested this mouse line in neonatal mice and found that overexpression of Ascl1 with this system induced neurogenesis from MG, up to postnatal day 14, but not in older mice (Ueki et al. 2015). However, by administering the histone deacetylase inhibitor Trichostatin A (TSA) with an intravitreal injection, we found that neurogenesis could be induced from the MG following retinal injury in adult mice (Jorstad et al. 2017).

The paradigm for inducing regeneration in adult mice MG is as follows (Fig. 2A″). First the animal receives tamoxifen to induce the Ascl1 expression in the MG, and then the mice receive an intravitreal injection of *N*-methyl-D-aspartate (NMDA) to induce retina injury, followed by an injection of TSA. In the days following the injury, we find that many of the same progenitor markers that are spontaneously expressed after injury in fish are now induced in the mouse Ascl1-expressing MG. Cells with neuron morphology can be lineage traced from the MG within a few weeks of the injury, and these resembled bipolar cells and amacrine cells. The MG-derived neurons make synapses with existing neurons and responded to light activation of photoreceptors. Single-cell RNA-seq showed the MG-derived neurons had a transcriptomic profile of bipolar neurons, primarily, though small numbers of amacrine cells were also observed (Fig. 2A–F; Jorstad et al. 2017).

Since the initial study, we have found several additional features of Ascl1-mediated MG reprogramming that are important for future

translation. The STAT pathway is more highly activated in a subset of MG after injury, and this appears to interfere with the neurogenic competence of the MG. We found that neurogenesis was significantly improved by inhibiting the STAT pathway (Jorstad et al. 2020). The increase in neurogenesis observed with STAT pathway inhibition allowed us to also see that MG undergo proliferation after Ascl1 expression in vivo and many of the new neurons are derived from mitotic divisions of the MG-derived progenitors. Another finding relevant to the role of inflammation in MG reprogramming was the observation that microglia become highly active after retinal injury and closely associated with MG after Ascl1 overexpression. We found that ablating microglia from the retina also results in a large increase in neurogenic competence of Ascl1 expressing MG (Todd et al. 2020).

Additional TFs can further expand the types of neurons regenerated from MG by expanding the reprogramming cocktail to include, for example, TFs relevant to retinal ganglion cell (RGC) development. Atoh7 is critical for RGC development, and we have found that overexpression of the related Atonal family member Atoh1 significantly increases neurogenesis and does so without any injury or TSA (Fig. 2G). The types of neurons generated by the MG now more closely resemble RGCs, although other neuronal types are observed as well (Todd et al. 2021). In addition to positive factors that can promote neurogenesis from MG, studies have also identified factors that repress neurogenesis in MG, and when deleted enable the MG to acquire some potential for generating new neurons. An example of neurogenic repressors are NFI factors, Nfia/b/x (Clark et al. 2019); manipulation of nuclear factor I (NFI) factors in combination with a neurogenic cocktail may more effectively promote neurogenesis from MG.

While the studies with transgenic mice have shown robust and reproducible induction of neurogenesis in MG, ultimately it will be necessary to use a viral strategy to overexpress these factors in a clinical setting. Some studies have also attempted to reprogram MG with AAV-based strategies, but these studies have led to considerable controversy, and have generally not been reproduced. For ex-

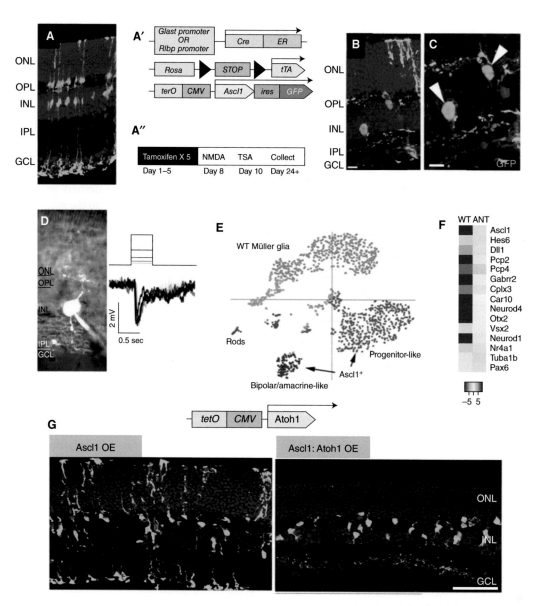

Figure 2. Summary of in vivo data demonstrating the potential of mammalian Müller glia (MG) to be reprogrammed into new neurons (adapted from Jorstad et al. 2017; Todd et al. 2021). (A) Immunohistochemistry image of lineage-traced mouse retinal section, showing MG in green and nuclei in blue as a result of a transgenic line (A') that can trigger Ascl1-GFP overexpression in MG in a tamoxifen-inducible manner (A"). Following injury, these MG can give rise to new neurons in the inner nuclear layer (INL) (B) that resemble bipolar morphology shown in green with white arrowheads (C). These MG-derived neurons show bipolar-like electrophysiological properties (D) and their transcriptomic signature resembles that of bipolar cells or retinal progenitors (F). (E) UMAP representation of clusters obtained following scRNAseq analysis, demonstrating the classes of cells obtained after Ascl1-mediated reprogramming of MG. The combined overexpression of Atoh1 together with Ascl1 in mouse MG led to a significant increase in reprogramming efficiency (G). Scale bars, 10 μm (B, C); 50 μm (G). (Panels A, A', A", B, D, E, F reprinted from Jorstad et al. 2017 with permission from the authors. Panels in G are reprinted from Todd et al. 2021 under Creative Commons CC BY-NC-ND 4.0 license.)

ample, investigators reported that AAV delivered Ptbp1 can stimulate MG to generate RGCs and photoreceptors (Fu et al. 2020; Zhou et al. 2020). Revisiting these results, with more stringent controls, showed that Ptbp1 knockdown had no effect on neurogenesis in the mouse retina (Hoang et al. 2022); these and other reports have highlighted the pitfalls associated with tracing cell fate with cell-type-specific promoters delivered with AAVs (Blackshaw and Sanes 2021). Claims of vision restoration following AAV-mediated reprogramming of MG to photoreceptors (Yao et al. 2018) or cell-fusion-mediated photoreceptor regeneration in vivo (Sanges et al. 2016) have further fueled the field with questions about appropriate controls when using AAV-delivered TFs. Similar claims of viral vector-mediated reprogramming of brain astrocytes to neurons (Guo et al. 2014; Brulet et al. 2017) have not been substantiated; more recent evidence indicates the putative glial-derived neurons were in fact endogenous neurons (Wang et al. 2021). As such, results based on transgenic animal models have merited more trust due to a favorable reproducibility record.

The ability of MG to serve as a source for new neurons in the adult mammalian retina now provides potential opportunities for retinal repair, like what the fish accomplishes naturally. It is remarkable that the newly generated neurons connect with the existing retina neurons and can respond to light in a similar manner as existing neurons (though not as robustly). The ability to potentially control the types of neurons generated from the Ascl1-reprogrammed MG also offers the possibility of tailoring the TF combination to the specific disease, to more precisely replace only those neuronal types lost in the patient. However, there are still many outstanding questions that will need to be addressed to better define the applicability of this approach for vision restoration. Some of these are detailed below.

Does the type of injury affect the types of new neurons that get regenerated? Most of the studies on MG reprogramming in mice have used a neurotoxic injury (NMDA). In fish, there is evidence that the type of neuronal injury may affect the response, and potentially bias the MG-

derived progenitors to regenerate those neurons that have been lost in the damage (D'Orazi et al. 2020; Lahne et al. 2020). Additional studies of other types of retinal injury will be needed to determine whether a similar cell-type-specific regeneration will occur in MG-derived progenitors after Ascl1 expression. Along the same lines, no study has yet looked at the response of Ascl1-expressing MG to the type of slow, progressive retinal injury that occurs in many human degenerative diseases. We do not know whether MG can be reprogrammed to a neurogenic state with Ascl1 in very old mice. Will the age limit the potential for regeneration? We have found that Ascl1 expression in MG induces a progenitor program, and we find that many of the MG now reenter the mitotic cell cycle (Fig. 2E–F). So far, this has been confined to a limited period after the Ascl1 expression, and it does not appear that the cells undergo multiple rounds of mitotic division. However, retinal progenitors proliferate extensively during development and so this is something that will need careful monitoring. In addition, the studies in mice also suggest that at least some of the MG directly "transdifferentiate" into neurons. Depending on the ratio of the transdifferentiation versus proliferative neurogenesis, there could be a problem with depletion of the MG. There are also indications that foveal MG have features not present in other MG; will they respond to reprogramming differently? Last, while we have found that the MG-derived neurons can function at the cellular level, no group has yet demonstrated vision recovery in a relevant disease model.

WHAT DISEASES MIGHT BE AMENABLE TO THIS APPROACH?

The ideal scenario is that we develop a regeneration regime that can be applied to all contexts, irrespective of the underlying disease, but it is more likely that different TF combinations will be needed to target replacement of specific cell types and tailored to disease type, stage, and severity of neuronal loss.

One potential target would be cone replacement in age-related macular degeneration (AMD). This multifactorial disease results in the death of RPE cells and disruption of the RPE/choroid and Bruch's membrane interface leading to drusen formation (Ambati and Fowler 2012; Mitchell et al. 2018). Vision loss is caused by the degeneration of photoreceptors, specifically cone photoreceptors primarily in central retina (Mitchell et al. 2018). AMD patients would therefore benefit from a regenerative regimen that would trigger the genesis of new cone photoreceptors.

Diabetic retinopathy, with the loss multiple types of retinal neurons, is another potential target for regeneration therapy (Lechner et al. 2017; Forrester et al. 2020). It is important to note that in addition to the hostile inflammatory environment, the disruption of retinal vasculature poses an additional barrier to neurogenesis, as pH and oxygen/nutrient levels are abnormal (Lechner et al. 2017). Thus, before therapeutic intervention it would be crucial to first stage the disease progression and allow for vasculature restoration before neurogenesis is triggered, to help the survival of new cells.

In retinopathy of prematurity (ROP), inner retinal neurons are lost as a consequence of transient vasculature overgrowth in preterm infants (Hellström et al. 2013). Bipolar cells in the inner retina are most susceptible to this pathology in animal models (Smith et al. 1994; Hartnett and Penn 2012), leading to an interruption of signal relay between photoreceptor and RGCs. Since Ascl1 overexpression in MG leads to Otx2$^+$ bipolar cell regeneration (Jorstad et al. 2017), particularly effective in young mice, this disease would be a promising target for an existing reprogramming strategy. In contrast to diabetic retinopathy, the abnormal vasculature of ROP retinas eventually reverts back to normal (Hellström et al. 2013), which suggests that regeneration of inner nuclear layer (INL) neurons would be more successful in these patients after disease staging.

Patients with glaucoma suffer from abnormalities in the anterior structures of the eye, important for the drainage of incoming aqueous humor, which leads to an increased intraocular pressure. This in turn leads to the death of RGCs as the innermost neuron layer and severs the connection that relays electrochemical signals from our eyes to the brain (Jonas et al. 2017).

RGCs are a large and diverse subtype of neurons, with >40 types annotated in mammals (Rheaume et al. 2018; Shekhar et al. 2022), and it is not known which or how many of these subtypes will be most impactful to replace for vision restoration, but developing the appropriate combinations of TFs might allow control in directing MG-derived progenitors to "generic" RGCs that may mature to the required subtypes in a context-dependent manner based on environmental cues.

WHAT WOULD A REGENERATIVE THERAPY LOOK LIKE?

In most of the diseases described above, a considerable percentage of one or more types of retinal neurons have been lost. Therefore, an ideal therapy would both stimulate (1) the production of more cells, and (2) specifically targeting the differentiation of the new cells to the appropriate neuronal type. Thus, methods for controlling both the regulation of cell proliferation and the regulation of neurogenesis will ideally need to be developed.

The first step of a therapeutic intervention would be to stage the disease progression with regard to cell types that have degenerated and the fidelity of the tissue in terms of vasculature leakiness and fibrosis/gliosis. This staging could then inform on a semi-tailor-made regenerative therapy to match the patient. To implement a regenerative therapy in vivo, we must consider the existing toolbox available. For ocular diseases, AAV vectors have become the gold standard, with both natural and synthetic serotypes used to target the CNS and retina. Using AAVs, an appropriate cocktail of proneural TFs would be delivered intraocularly in the form of a vector injection with the aim of targeting MG. Intravitreal or subretinal injections could be performed to transduce MG either through their vitreal end-feet at the inner limiting membrane or their processes forming the outer limiting membrane, respectively.

MG must be targeted specifically to avoid off-target effects of expressing proneural TFs in existing neurons. To this end, two aspects of AAV vector design are important to consider:

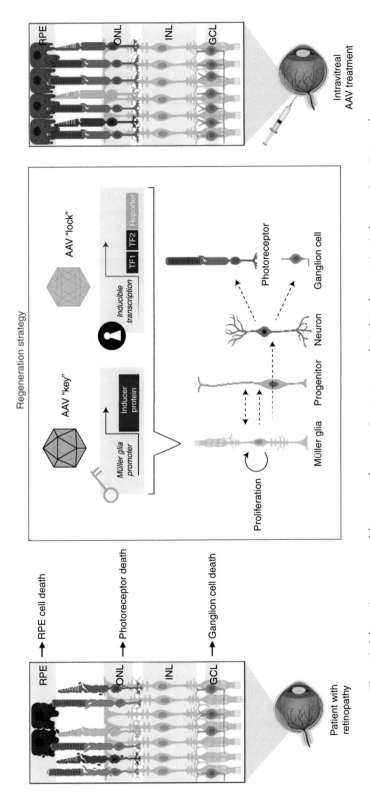

Figure 3. Schematic summary of the proposed regeneration strategy as clinical implementation in human. In patients with various forms of retinopathy, neuron classes such as photoreceptors and ganglion cells will degenerate leading to permanent blindness. Using the most popular viral vectors, namely adeno-associated virus (AAV), a regeneration strategy could be implemented where a transcription factor (TF) cocktail is introduced to Müller glia (MG) specifically to trigger their proliferation, dedifferentiation, and subsequent neurogenesis to replenish the missing neuron classes. This vector-mediated strategy could be injected intraocularly in patients, which is an intervention well established in the field of ophthalmology.

capsid and promoter specificity. AAV capsids have been shown to transduce different retinal cell types depending on the injection orientation and the cell groups proximal to the injection site (Castle et al. 2016). It is plausible that specificity may improve in degenerating retinas, as the absence of some neuron classes could limit the number of unspecific targets. So far, only the engineered capsid AAV.SHH10 has been described to have MG-specific tropism (Klimczak et al. 2009; Pellissier et al. 2014) although the potency of the vector may vary in humans and in pathological contexts. A strong MG-specific promoter, such as Rlbp1, could drive sufficient levels of a TF cocktail (Vázquez-Chona et al. 2009; Pellissier et al. 2014), although it would be crucial to confirm specificity in the specific regimen as promoter specificity was shown to differ depending on the downstream coding sequence (e.g., glial fibrillary acidic protein [GFAP] promoter activity in neurons) (Wang et al. 2021). In addition, once the MG are reprogrammed to neural progenitors/neurons, they will no longer activate the MG-specific promoter, and this may prevent a stable adoption of the neuron fate.

How can we improve existing technologies? We can deliver the components of a regenerative therapy in multiple pieces that can only be effective when all are present. By splitting the transgene cassette into two AAVs it is possible to create a lock-and-key configuration, where the "lock" AAV delivers an inducible cassette encoding the proneural TF(s) and the "key" AAV delivers a cassette with a cell-specific promoter driving the inducer protein (Fig. 3). Most conditional gene expression systems, such as the tetracycline (tet) inducible system and the site-directed recombination systems Cre-Lox and Flp-FRT, come from bacteria or yeast and have been used successfully in mammalian cells both in vitro and in vivo (Sternberg and Hamilton 1981; Gossen and Bujard 1992; Gossen et al. 1995; Jensen et al. 2020). The efficiency however of inducible systems has been shown to vary depending on the context, whether in cell lines or animal models (Song and Palmiter 2018), which has led to considerable efforts to validate their potential in therapies and counteract leakiness using molecular techniques

such as crossover-insensitive ATG-out vectors (Fischer et al. 2019).

CONCLUDING REMARKS

The possibility that we may someday stimulate retinal repair from within, by an MG-based regeneration approach, is becoming a reality. While still some ways off from implementing this in a clinical setting, it is clear from work done in the last 10 years, that regeneration of new neurons from MG is possible in the mouse retina, using TF reprogramming of their fate. The new neurons that are regenerated in the mature mouse retina differentiate into recognized types, by electrophysiological, morphological, and transcriptomic criteria. The regenerated neurons "wire" into the existing circuits and can respond to light through synapses with photoreceptors. A more thorough understanding of the TF networks that specify cell identities should allow more precise control of the types and numbers of neurons regenerated to best suit a particular disease. Moreover, it is critical to validate these promising results from mice in primate and human retina, and to develop best practices for ensuring accurate targeting of MG with AAVs. Together, these new developments will provide further impetus to this emerging field of cell fate engineering for retinal disease.

ACKNOWLEDGMENTS

Everyone in the Reh and Bermingham-McDonogh laboratories for useful feedback and discussion. We particularly thank Dr. Levi Todd for comments on the manuscript. The authors also thank the Foundation Fighting Blindness and the National Eye Institute (NEI) for their support over many years in developing this approach. M.P. acknowledges Institute for Stem Cell and Regenerative Medicine (ISCRM) for support.

REFERENCES

*Reference is also in this subject collection.

Ambati J, Fowler BJ. 2012. Mechanisms of age-related macular degeneration. *Neuron* 75: 26–39. doi:10.1016/J .NEURON.2012.06.018

Bassett EA, Wallace VA. 2012. Cell fate determination in the vertebrate retina. *Trends Neurosci* **35**: 565–573. doi:10 .1016/j.tins.2012.05.004

Blackshaw S, Sanes JR. 2021. Turning lead into gold: reprogramming retinal cells to cure blindness. *J Clin Invest* **131**: e146134. doi:10.1172/jci146134

Bocchi R, Masserdotti G, Götz M. 2022. Direct neuronal reprogramming: fast forward from new concepts toward therapeutic approaches. *Neuron* **110**: 366–393. doi:10 .1016/J.NEURON.2021.11.02

Brulet R, Matsuda T, Zhang L, Miranda C, Giacca M, Kaspar BK, Nakashima K, Hsieh J. 2017. NEUROD1 instructs neuronal conversion in non-reactive astrocytes. *Stem Cell Rep* **8**: 1506–1515. doi:10.1016/J.STEMCR.2017.04 .013

Campbell WA, Deshmukh A, Blum S, Todd L, Mendonca N, Weist J, Zent J, Hoang TV, Blackshaw S, Leight J, et al. 2019. Matrix-metalloproteinase expression and gelatinase activity in the avian retina and their influence on Müller glia proliferation. *Exp Neurol* **320**: 112984. doi:10.1016/J .EXPNEUROL.2019.112984

Campbell LJ, Hobgood JS, Jia M, Boyd P, Hipp RI, Hyde DR. 2021. Notch3 and DeltaB maintain Müller glia quiescence and act as negative regulators of regeneration in the light-damaged zebrafish retina. *Glia* **69**: 546–566. doi:10.1002/ glia.23912

Castle MJ, Turunen HT, Vandenberghe LH, Wolfe JH. 2016. Controlling AAV tropism in the nervous system with natural and engineered capsids. *Methods Mol Biol* **1382**: 133–149. doi:10.1007/978-1-4939-3271-9_10

Clark BS, Stein-O'Brien GL, Shiau F, Cannon GH, Davis-Marcisak E, Sherman T, Santiago CP, Hoang TV, Rajaii F, James-Esposito RE, et al. 2019. Single-cell RNA-seq analysis of retinal development identifies NFI factors as regulating mitotic exit and late-born cell specification. *Neuron* **102**: 1111–1126.e5. doi:10.1016/J.NEURON.2019.04 .010

Close JL, Gumuscu B, Reh TA. 2005. Retinal neurons regulate proliferation of postnatal progenitors and Müller glia in the rat retina via TGFβ signaling. *Development* **132**: 3015–3026. doi:10.1242/DEV.01882

Close JL, Liu J, Gumuscu B, Reh TA. 2006. Epidermal growth factor receptor expression regulates proliferation in the postnatal rat retina. *Glia* **54**: 94–104. doi:10.1002/GLIA .20361

D'Orazi FD, Zhao WF, Wong RO, Yoshimatsu T. 2016. Mismatch of synaptic patterns between neurons produced in regeneration and during development of the vertebrate retina. *Curr Biol* **26**: 2268–2279. doi:10.1016/j.cub.2016 .06.063

D'Orazi FD, Suzuki SC, Darling N, Wong RO, Yoshimatsu T. 2020. Conditional and biased regeneration of cone photoreceptor types in the zebrafish retina. *J Comp Neurol* **528**: 2816–2830. doi:10.1002/CNE.24933

Dyer MA, Cepko CL. 2000. P57(Kip2) regulates progenitor cell proliferation and amacrine interneuron development in the mouse retina. *Development* **127**: 3593–3605. doi:10 .1242/DEV.127.16.3593

Elsaeidi F, Macpherson P, Mills EA, Jui J, Flannery JG, Goldman D. 2018. Notch suppression collaborates with Ascl1 and Lin28 to unleash a regenerative response in fish ret-

ina, but not in mice. *J Neurosci* **38**: 2246–2261. doi:10 .1523/JNEUROSCI.2126-17.2018

Fausett BV, Goldman D. 2006. A role for A1 tubulin-expressing Müller glia in regeneration of the injured zebrafish retina. *J Neurosci* **26**: 6303–6313. doi:10.1523/JNEUR OSCI.0332-06.2006

Fausett BV, Gumerson JD, Goldman D. 2008. The proneural basic helix-loop-helix gene Ascl1a is required for retina regeneration. *J Neurosci* **28**: 1109–1117. doi:10.1523/ JNEUROSCI.4853-07.2008

Fischer AJ, Reh TA. 2001. Müller glia are a potential source of neural regeneration in the postnatal chicken retina. *Nat Neurosci* **4**: 247–252. doi:10.1038/85090

Fischer KB, Collins HK, Callaway EM. 2019. Sources of off-target expression from recombinase dependent AAV vectors and mitigation with cross-over insensitive ATG-out vectors. *Proc Natl Acad Sci* **116**: 27001–27010. doi:10 .1073/PNAS.1915974116/-/DCSUPPLEMENTAL

Fischer AJ, McGuire CR, Dierks BD, Reh TA. 2002. Insulin and fibroblast growth factor 2 activate a neurogenic program in Müller glia of the chicken retina. *J Neurosci* **22**: 9387–9398. doi:10.1523/JNEUROSCI.22-21-09387.2002

Forrester JV, Kuffova L, Delibegovic M. 2020. The role of inflammation in diabetic retinopathy. *Front Immunol* **11**: 583687. doi:10.3389/FIMMU.2020.583687

Fu X, Zhu J, Duan Y, Li G, Cai H, Zheng L, Qian H, Zhang C, Jin Z, Fu XD, et al. 2020. Visual function restoration in genetically blind mice via endogenous cellular reprogramming. BioRxiv doi:10.1101/2020.04.08.030981

Goldman D. 2014. Müller glial cell reprogramming and retina regeneration. *Nat Rev Neurosci* **15**: 431–442. doi:10 .1038/nrn3723

Gorsuch RA, Lahne M, Yarka CE, Petravick ME, Li J, Hyde DR. 2017. Sox2 regulates Müller glia reprogramming and proliferation in the regenerating zebrafish retina via Lin28 and Ascl1a. *Exp Eye Res* **161**: 174–192. doi:10.1016/j.exer .2017.05.012

Gossen M, Bujard H. 1992. Tight control of gene expression in mammalian cells by tetracycline-responsive promoters. *Proc Natl Acad Sci* **89**: 5547–5551. doi:10.1073/PNAS .89.12.5547

Gossen M, Freundlieb S, Bender G, Müller G, Hillen W, Bujard H. 1995. Transcriptional activation by tetracyclines in mammalian cells. *Science* **268**: 1766–1769. doi:10.1126/science.7792603

Guo Z, Zhang L, Wu Z, Chen Y, Wang F, Chen G. 2014. In vivo direct reprogramming of reactive glial cells into functional neurons after brain injury and in an Alzheimer's disease model. *Cell Stem Cell* **14**: 188–202. doi:10.1016/j .stem.2013.12.001

Hägglund AC, Dahl L, Carlsson L. 2011. Lhx2 is required for patterning and expansion of a distinct progenitor cell population committed to eye development. *PloS ONE* **6**: e23387. doi:10.1371/JOURNAL.PONE.0023387

Halatsch ME, Schmidt U, Behnke-Mursch J, Unterberg A, Wirtz CR. 2006. Epidermal growth factor receptor inhibition for the treatment of glioblastoma multiforme and other malignant brain tumours. *Cancer Treat Rev* **32**: 74–89. doi:10.1016/J.CTRV.2006.01.003

Hammer J, Röppenack P, Yousuf S, Schnabel C, Weber A, Zöller D, Koch E, Hans S, Brand M. 2022. Visual function is gradually restored during retina regeneration in adult zebrafish. *Front Cell Dev Biol* **9**: 3952. doi:10.3389/FCELL .2021.831322/BIBTEX

Hamon A, García-García D, Ail D, Bitard J, Chesneau A, Dalkara D, Locker M, Roger JE, Perron M. 2019. Linking YAP to Müller glia quiescence exit in the degenerative retina. *Cell Rep* **27**: 1712–1725.e6. doi:10.1016/j.celrep .2019.04.045

Hartnett ME, Penn JS. 2012. Mechanisms and management of retinopathy of prematurity. *N Engl J Med* **367**: 2515–2526. doi:10.1056/NEJMRA1208129

Hellström A, Smith LEH, Dammann O. 2013. Retinopathy of prematurity. *Lancet* **382**: 1445–1457. doi:10.1016/S0140-6736(13)60178-6

Hoang T, Wang J, Boyd P, Wang F, Santiago C, Jiang L, Yoo S, Lahne M, Todd LJ, Jia M, et al. 2020. Gene regulatory networks controlling vertebrate retinal regeneration. *Science* **370**: eabb8598. doi:10.1126/SCIENCE.ABB8598

Hoang T, Kim DW, Appel H, Pannullo NA, Leavey P, Ozawa M, Zheng S, Yu M, Peachey NS, Blackshaw S. 2022. Genetic loss of function of Ptbp1 does not induce glia-to-neuron conversion in retina. *Cell Rep* **39**: 110849. doi:10 .1016/J.CELREP.2022.110849

Hojo M, Ohtsuka T, Hashimoto N, Gradwohl G, Guillemot F, Kageyama R. 2000. Glial cell fate specification modulated by the BHLH gene Hes5 in mouse retina. *Development* **127**: 2515–2522. doi:10.1242/DEV.127.12.2515

Hollborn M, Tenckhoff S, Jahn K, Iandiev I, Biedermann B, Schnurrbusch UEK, Limb GA, Reichenbach A, Wolf S, Wiedemann P, et al. 2005. Changes in retinal gene expression in proliferative vitreoretinopathy: glial cell expression of HB-EGF. *Mol Vis* **11**: 397–413. https:// pubmed.ncbi.nlm.nih.gov/15988409

Ikeda T, Puro DG. 1995. Regulation of retinal glial cell proliferation by antiproliferative molecules. *Exp Eye Res* **60**: 435–443. doi:10.1016/S0014-4835(05)80100-9

Imayoshi I, Kageyama R. 2014. BHLH factors in self-renewal, multipotency, and fate choice of neural progenitor cells. *Neuron* **82**: 9–23. doi:10.1016/J.NEURON.2014.03 .018

Jensen O, Ansari S, Gebauer L, Müller SF, Lowjaga KAAT, Geyer J, Tzvetkov MV, Brockmöller J. 2020. A double-Flp-in method for stable overexpression of two genes. *Sci Rep* **10**: 1–14. doi:10.1038/s41598-020-71051-5

Jonas JB, Aung T, Bourne RR, Bron AM, Ritch R, Panda-Jonas S. 2017. Glaucoma. *Lancet* **390**: 2183–2193. doi:10 .1016/S0140-6736(17)31469-1

Jorstad NL, Wilken MS, Grimes WN, Wohl SG, Vandenbosch LS, Yoshimatsu T, Wong RO, Rieke F, Reh TA. 2017. Stimulation of functional neuronal regeneration from Müller glia in adult mice. *Nature* **548**: 103–107. doi:10.1038/nature23283

Jorstad NL, Wilken MS, Todd L, Finkbeiner C, Nakamura P, Radulovich N, Hooper MJ, Chitsazan A, Wilkerson BA, Rieke F, et al. 2020. STAT signaling modifies Ascl1 chromatin binding and limits neural regeneration from Müller glia in adult mouse retina. *Cell Rep* **30**: 2195–2208.e5 doi:10.1016/J.CELREP.2020.01.075

Karl MO, Hayes S, Nelson BR, Tan K, Buckingham B, Reh TA. 2008. Stimulation of neural regeneration in the mouse retina. *Proc Natl Acad Sci* **105**: 19508–19513. doi:10.1073/PNAS.0807453105

Kassen SC, Thummel R, Campochiaro LA, Harding MJ, Bennett NA, Hyde DR. 2009. CNTF induces photoreceptor neuroprotection and Müller glial cell proliferation through two different signaling pathways in the adult zebrafish retina. *Exp Eye Res* **88**: 1051–1064. doi:10 .1016/J.EXER.2009.01.007

Klimczak RR, Koerber JT, Dalkara D, Flannery JG, Schaffer DV. 2009. A novel adeno-associated viral variant for efficient and selective intravitreal transduction of rat Müller cells. *PLoS ONE* **4**: e7467. doi:10.1371/journal.pone .0007467

Konar GJ, Ferguson C, Flickinger Z, Kent MR, Patton JG. 2021. MiRNAs and Müller glia reprogramming during retina regeneration. *Front Cell Dev Biol* **8**: 632632. doi:10.3389/FCELL.2020.632632

Kugler M, Schlecht A, Fuchshofer R, Schmitt SI, Kleiter I, Aigner L, Tamm ER, Braunger BM. 2017. SMAD7 deficiency stimulates Müller progenitor cell proliferation during the development of the mammalian retina. *Histochem Cell Biol* **148**: 21–32. doi:10.1007/S00418-017-1549-5

Lahne M, Hyde DR. 2016. Interkinetic nuclear migration in the regenerating retina. *Adv Exp Med Biol* **854**: 587–593. doi:10.1007/978-3-319-17121-0_78

Lahne M, Li J, Marton RM, Hyde DR. 2015. Actin-cytoskeleton- and rock-mediated INM are required for photoreceptor regeneration in the adult zebrafish retina. *J Neurosci* **35**: 15612–15634. doi:10.1523/JNEUROSCI.5005-14 .2015

Lahne M, Nagashima M, Hyde DR, Hitchcock PF. 2020. Reprogramming Müller glia to regenerate retinal neurons. *Annu Rev Vis Sci* **6**: 171–193. doi:10.1146/ANNUREV-VISION-121219-081808

Lechner J, O'Leary OE, Stitt AW. 2017. The pathology associated with diabetic retinopathy. *Vision Res* **139**: 7–14. doi:10.1016/J.VISRES.2017.04.003

Lenkowski JR, Raymond PA. 2014. Müller glia: stem cells for generation and regeneration of retinal neurons in teleost fish. *Prog Retin Eye Res* **40**: 94–123. doi:10.1016/J .PRETEYERES.2013.12.007

Levine EM, Close J, Fero M, Ostrovsky A, Reh TA. 2000. P27Kip1 regulates cell cycle withdrawal of late multipotent progenitor cells in the mammalian retina. *Dev Biol* **219**: 299–314. doi:10.1006/DBIO.2000.9622

Lim S, Kim YJ, Park S, Choi JH, Sung Y, Nishimori K, Kozmik Z, Lee HW, Kim JW. 2021. MTORC1-induced retinal progenitor cell overproliferation leads to accelerated mitotic aging and degeneration of descendent Müller glia. *eLife* **10**: e70079. doi:10.7554/eLife.70079

Milenkovic I, Weick M, Wiedemann P, Reichenbach A, Bringmann A. 2003. P2Y receptor-mediated stimulation of Müller glial cell DNA synthesis: dependence on EGF and PDGF receptor transactivation. *Invest Ophthalmol Vis Sci* **44**: 1211–1220. doi:10.1167/IOVS.02-0260

Mitchell P, Liew G, Gopinath B, Wong TY. 2018. Age-related macular degeneration. *Lancet* **392**: 1147–1159. doi:10 .1016/S0140-6736(18)31550-2

Mitchell DM, Sun C, Hunter SS, New DD, Stenkamp DL. 2019. Regeneration associated transcriptional signature of retinal microglia and macrophages. *Sci Rep* **9**: 4768. doi:10 .1038/s41598-019-41298-8

* Monville C, Goureau O, M'Barek K. 2022. Photoreceptor cell replacement using pluripotent stem cells: current knowl-

edge and remaining questions. *Cold Spring Harb Perspect Med* doi:10.1101/cshperspect.a0413009

Nagashima M, Hitchcock PF. 2021. Inflammation regulates the multi-step process of retinal regeneration in zebrafish. *Cells* 10: 783. doi:10.3390/CELLS10040783

Nagashima M, Barthel LK, Raymond PA. 2013. A self-renewing division of zebrafish Müller glial cells generates neuronal progenitors that require N-cadherin to regenerate retinal neurons. *Development* 140: 4510–4521. doi:10.1242/DEV.090738

Nelson BR, Hartman BH, Georgi SA, Lan MS, Reh TA. 2007. Transient inactivation of notch signaling synchronizes differentiation of neural progenitor cells. *Dev Biol* 304: 479–498. doi:10.1016/J.YDBIO.2007.01.001

Nelson AD, Suzuki M, Svendsen CN. 2008. A high concentration of epidermal growth factor increases the growth and survival of neurogenic radial glial cells within human neurosphere cultures. *Stem Cells* 26: 348–355. doi:10.1634/stemcells.2007-0299

Nomura-Komoike K, Saitoh F, Komoike Y, Fujieda H. 2016. DNA damage response in proliferating Müller glia in the mammalian retina. *Invest Ophthalmol Vis Sci* 57: 1169–1182. doi:10.1167/IOVS.15-18101

Oron-Karni V, Farhy C, Elgart M, Marquardt T, Remizova L, Yaron O, Xie Q, Cvekl A, Ashery-Padan R. 2008. Dual requirement for Pax6 in retinal progenitor cells. *Development* 135: 4037–4047. doi:10.1242/DEV.028308

Pellissier LP, Hoek RM, Vos RM, Aartsen WM, Klimczak RR, Hoyng SA, Flannery JG, Wijnholds J. 2014. Specific tools for targeting and expression in Müller glial cells. *Mol Ther Methods Clin Dev* 1: 14009. doi:10.1038/mtm.2014.9

Pollak J, Wilken MS, Ueki Y, Cox KE, Sullivan JM, Taylor RJ, Levine EM, Reh TA. 2013. ASCL1 reprograms mouse Müller glia into neurogenic retinal progenitors. *Development* 140: 2619–2631. doi:10.1242/dev.091355

Rheaume BA, Jereen A, Bolisetty M, Sajid MS, Yang Y, Renna K, Sun L, Robson P, Trakhtenberg EF. 2018. Single cell transcriptome profiling of retinal ganglion cells identifies cellular subtypes. *Nat Commun* 9: 1–17. doi:10.1038/s41467-018-05134-3

Rueda EM, Hall BM, Hill MC, Swinton PG, Tong X, Martin JF, Poché RA. 2019. The hippo pathway blocks mammalian retinal Müller glial cell reprogramming. *Cell Rep* 27: 1637–1649.e6. doi:10.1016/J.CELREP.2019.04.047

Sahu A, Devi S, Jui J, Goldman D. 2021. Notch signaling via Hey1 and Id2b regulates Müller glia's regenerative response to retinal injury. *Glia* 69: 2882–2898. doi:10.1002/GLIA.24075

Sanges D, Simonte G, Di Vicino U, Romo N, Pinilla I, Nicolás M, Cosma MP. 2016. Reprogramming Müller glia via in vivo cell fusion regenerates murine photoreceptors. *J Clin Invest* 126: 3104–3116. doi:10.1172/JCI85193

Scherer J, Schnitzer J. 1994. Growth factor effects on the proliferation of different retinal glial cells in vitro. *Brain Res Dev Brain Res* 80: 209–221. doi:10.1016/0165-3806(94)90106-6

Shekhar K, Whitney IE, Butrus S, Peng YR, Sanes JR. 2022. Diversification of multipotential postmitotic mouse retinal ganglion cell precursors into discrete types. *eLife* 11: e73809. doi:10.7554/ELIFE.73809

Sherpa T, Lankford T, McGinn TE, Hunter SS, Frey RA, Sun C, Ryan M, Robison BD, Stenkamp DL. 2014. Retinal regeneration is facilitated by the presence of surviving neurons. *Dev Neurobiol* 74: 851–876. doi:10.1002/DNEU.22167

Sicinski P, Donaher JL, Parker SB, Li T, Fazeli A, Gardner H, Haslam SZ, Bronson RT, Elledge SJ, Weinberg RA. 1995. Cyclin D1 provides a link between development and oncogenesis in the retina and breast. *Cell* 82: 621–630. doi:10.1016/0092-8674(95)90034-9

Silva NJ, Nagashima M, Li J, Kakuk-Atkins L, Ashrafzadeh M, Hyde DR, Hitchcock PF. 2020. Inflammation and matrix metalloproteinase 9 (Mmp-9) regulate photoreceptor regeneration in adult zebrafish. *Glia* 68: 1445–1465. doi:10.1002/GLIA.23792

Smith LEH, Wesoloiuski E, Mclellan A, Kostyk SK, D'amato XR, Sullivan R, D'amore PA. 1994. Oxygen-induced retinopathy in the mouse. *Invest Ophthalmol Vis Sci* 35: 101–111.

Song AJ, Palmiter RD. 2018. Detecting and avoiding problems when using the Cre–Lox system. *Trends Genet* 34: 333–340. doi:10.1016/j.tig.2017.12.008

Sternberg N, Hamilton D. 1981. Bacteriophage P1 site-specific recombination. I: Recombination between LoxP sites. *J Mol Biol* 150: 467–486. doi:10.1016/0022-2836(81)90375-2

Suga A, Sadamoto K, Fujii M, Mandai M, Takahashi M. 2014. Proliferation potential of Müller glia after retinal damage varies between mouse strains. *PLoS ONE* 9: e94556. doi:10.1371/JOURNAL.PONE.0094556

Su Huang HJ, Nagane M, Klingbeil CK, Lin H, Nishikawa R, Ji XD, Huang CM, Gill GN, Wiley HS, Cavenee WK. 1997. The enhanced tumorigenic activity of a mutant epidermal growth factor receptor common in human cancers is mediated by threshold levels of constitutive tyrosine phosphorylation and unattenuated signaling. *J Biol Chem* 272: 2927–2935. doi:10.1074/JBC.272.5.2927

Swaroop A, Kim D, Forrest D. 2010. Transcriptional regulation of photoreceptor development and homeostasis in the mammalian retina. *Nat Rev Neurosci* 11: 563–576. doi:10.1038/NRN2880

Takahashi K, Yamanaka S. 2006. Induction of pluripotent stem cells from mouse embryonic and adult fibroblast cultures by defined factors. *Cell* 126: 663–676. doi:10.1016/j.cell.2006.07.024

Thummel R, Kassen SC, Montgomery JE, Enright JM, Hyde DR. 2008. Inhibition of Müller glial cell division blocks regeneration of the light-damaged zebrafish retina. *Dev Neurobiol* 68: 392–408. doi:10.1002/DNEU.20596

Todd L, Reh TA. 2022. Comparative biology of vertebrate retinal regeneration: restoration of vision through cellular reprogramming. *Cold Spring Harb Perspect Biol* 14: a040816. doi:10.1101/CSHPERSPECT.A040816

Todd L, Volkov LI, Zelinka C, Squires N, Fischer AJ. 2015. Heparin-binding EGF-like growth factor (HB-EGF) stimulates the proliferation of Müller glia-derived progenitor cells in avian and murine retinas. *Mol Cell Neurosci* 69: 54–64. doi:10.1016/J.MCN.2015.10.004

Todd L, Finkbeiner C, Wong CK, Hooper MJ, Reh TA. 2020. Microglia suppress Ascl1-induced retinal regeneration in mice. *Cell Rep* 33: 108507. doi:10.1016/j.celrep.2020.108507

Todd L, Hooper MJ, Haugan AK, Finkbeiner C, Jorstad N, Radulovich N, Wong CK, Donaldson PC, Jenkins W, Chen Q, et al. 2021. Efficient stimulation of retinal regeneration from Müller glia in adult mice using combinations of proneural BHLH transcription factors. *Cell Rep* **37:** 109857. doi:10.1016/J.CELREP.2021.109857

Ueki Y, Reh TA. 2013. EGF stimulates Müller glial proliferation via a BMP dependent mechanism. *Glia* **61:** 778–789. doi:10.1002/GLIA.22472

Ueki Y, Karl MO, Sudar S, Pollak J, Taylor RJ, Loeffler K, Wilken MS, Reardon S, Reh TA. 2012. P53 is required for the developmental restriction in Müller glial proliferation in mouse retina. *Glia* **60:** 1579–1589. doi:10.1002/GLIA.22377

Ueki Y, Wilken MS, Cox KE, Chipman L, Jorstad N, Sternhagen K, Simic M, Ullom K, Nakafuku M, Reh TA. 2015. Transgenic expression of the proneural transcription factor Ascl1 in Müller glia stimulates retinal regeneration in young mice. *Proc Natl Acad Sci* **112:** 13717–13722. doi:10.1073/pnas.1510595112

Vázquez-Chona F, Clark AM, Levine EM. 2009. Rlbp1 promoter drives robust Müller glial GFP expression in transgenic mice. *Invest Ophthalmol Vis Sci* **50:** 3996–4003. doi:10.1167/IOVS.08-3189

Wan J, Ramachandran R, Goldman D. 2012. HB-EGF is necessary and sufficient for Müller glia dedifferentiation and retina regeneration. *Dev Cell* **22:** 334–347. doi:10.1016/J.DEVCEL.2011.11.020

Wang LL, Serrano C, Zhong X, Ma S, Zou Y, Zhang CL. 2021. Revisiting astrocyte to neuron conversion with lineage tracing in vivo. *Cell* **184:** 5465–5481.e16. doi:10.1016/J.CELL.2021.09.005

White DT, Sengupta S, Saxena MT, Xu Q, Hanes J, Ding D, Ji H, Mumm JS. 2017. Immunomodulation-accelerated neuronal regeneration following selective rod photoreceptor cell ablation in the zebrafish retina. *Proc Natl Acad Sci* **114:** E3719–E3728. doi:10.1073/PNAS.1617721114/SUPPL_FILE/PNAS.1617721114.SM08.AVI

Wohl SG, Reh TA. 2016. MiR-124-9-9* potentiates Ascl1-induced reprogramming of cultured Müller glia. *Glia* **64:** 743–762. doi:10.1002/glia.22958

Yao K, Qiu S, Wang YV, Park SJH, Mohns EJ, Mehta B, Liu X, Chang B, Zenisek D, Crair MC, et al. 2018. Restoration of vision after de novo genesis of rod photoreceptors in mammalian retinas. *Nature* **560:** 484–488. doi:10.1038/S41586-018-0425-3

Zhou H, Su J, Hu X, Zhou C, Li H, Chen Z, Xiao Q, Wang B, Wu W, Sun Y, et al. 2020. Glia-to-neuron conversion by CRISPR-CasRx alleviates symptoms of neurological disease in mice. *Cell* **181:** 590–603.e16. doi:10.1016/J.CELL.2020.03.024

Cite this article as *Cold Spring Harb Perspect Med* doi: 10.1101/cshperspect.a041306

The Importance of Natural History Studies in Inherited Retinal Diseases

Allison Ayala,[1] Janet Cheetham,[2] Todd Durham,[2] and Maureen Maguire[1]

[1]Jaeb Center for Health Research, Tampa, Florida 33647, USA

[2]Foundation Fighting Blindness, Columbia, Maryland 21045, USA

Correspondence: aayala@jaeb.org

Natural history studies of inherited retinal diseases (IRDs) play a critical role in the design and implementation of treatment trials. Study objectives ideally encompass (1) understanding the time course and pattern of disease progression, (2) within genotypic and phenotypic subtypes of patient populations, and (3) characterizing a range of measures of vision function, retinal structure, and functional vision that may serve as endpoints. In rare disease, data quality standards are paramount to optimizing smaller sample sizes, including a prospective, standardized, and longitudinal approach to data collection. Multicenter studies additionally facilitate strength in numbers and generalizability, and multidisciplinary collaboration ensures a holistic approach to study design and knowledge-building. Dissemination of natural history study results, data sets, and lessons learned will stimulate further innovation and progress in IRD therapeutic research, including setting up future trial designs for their best chance of success.

Inherited retinal diseases (IRDs) represent a genetically heterogeneous group of progressive retinal disorders caused by variants in at least 280 genes confirmed to date (sph.uth .edu/retnet). Despite progress in therapy development (Sahel et al. 2019), and a growing number of interventional trials for IRDs (Thompson et al. 2020; www.clinicaltrials.gov), there remain significant hurdles to designing trials and advancing therapies. Recent papers have reviewed the unmet needs and identified top priorities to move the promise of treatment forward among a complex landscape of IRD research (Csaky et al. 2017; Duncan et al. 2018; Thompson et al. 2020). A common theme is the vital need for natural history studies, the foundation for trial design and therapy development.

ROLE OF NATURAL HISTORY STUDIES IN THERAPY DEVELOPMENT

A natural history study is an observational data collection that summarizes the course of a disease in the absence of intervention. This may also include tracking the course of disease in the presence of a standard care therapy (e.g., arginine-restricted dietary regimens to reduce ornithine levels in patients with gyrate atrophy) and is recognized by the Food and Drug Administration (FDA) as a potential part of understanding natural history (Food and Drug Administration 2019b). Natural history study design options include prospective versus retrospective and longitudinal versus cross-sectional, which are described in detail in the FDA guidance. This manuscript is primarily focused on considerations of prospective, longitudinal natural history studies, which allow for higher data quality and more comprehensive data collection. However, it is worth noting that retrospective or cross-sectional natural history studies may be necessary to consider due to cost, time, or other logistics.

Incorporating knowledge of a disease's natural history is an essential part of the drug development process, as it informs clinical trial design. In particular, the FDA defines "adequate and well controlled" investigations according to seven key design elements: clear research objectives, valid comparison with a control, appropriate selection of subjects, method of assignment to treatment, methods to minimize bias, well-defined and reliable methods to assess response, and adequate analysis of results (Food and Drug Administration 2010). Figure 1 summarizes how natural history studies inform many of these and is also well described in FDA guidance (Food and Drug Administration 2019a,b). One important objective of a natural history study is to evaluate the rate of disease progression, which will reveal how quickly changes beyond day-to-day variation occur in the absence of treatment. This informs trial duration and frequency of data collection in the form of

visit and testing schedules and must be coupled with selection of outcome measures as potential trial endpoints. Identifying the best candidate endpoint for measuring effect of treatment on disease progression in a trial requires consideration of many properties (Fig. 2), including sensitivity to changes in disease stage, subject/tester/grader reproducibility, correlation with other measures of disease stage, how much within-person change is beyond measurement variability, and whether within-person change is clinically meaningful. Biomarkers (defined as objective measures of biological or pathological process that can predict a clinically meaningful benefit, such as the area of the ellipsoid zone [EZ] as measured from spectral-domain optical coherence tomography [SD-OCT]) may also be developed or validated as surrogate endpoints as part of exploring candidates. Understanding and describing the patient population may also influence the selection of outcome measures. Factors that could impact disease progression may include demographic, genetic, environmental, and other disease characteristics. Identifying characteristics of patients with faster progression rates identifies who may benefit most from treatment and ultimately inform trial inclusion criteria. Collectively, addressing these objectives can yield estimates of variability around rates of progression within target patient populations and on endpoints of interest, which can then be used for sample size calculations and scenario planning for a future trial.

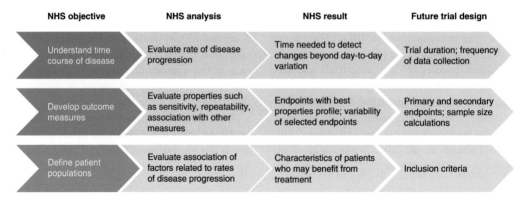

Figure 1. How natural history studies (NHS) inform clinical trial design: A summary of the flow from each NHS objective, to the analyses and results those objectives yield, and ultimately how those results are used in designing future trials.

Properties of assessment procedure	
Accurate	Measures the intended quantity
Reproducible	Test–retest, intersession, intergrader, intragrader
Range	Floor or ceiling effects within the range of interest
Objectively measured	Regulatory preference over subjective measures, reduces bias
Association with the disease	
Clinically meaningful	Directly measures (or is predictive of) how a person feels, functions, or survives
Correlation	Correlates with other measures of disease stage, duration, or rate of progression
Sensitive	Ability to detect changes early, and high "signal-to-noise" ratio (mean change is large relative to standard deviation)
Ability to detect "real" changes	For discrete events, change is greater than measurement error
Feasibility	
Low cost	Equipment, training, independent expert assessments
Availability	Equipment available at clinical sites
Ease of test administration	Level of study personnel training needed
Ability to perform	Study population considerations (e.g., very young age, poor ocular media clarity)
Goals of future trial	
Phase of trial	Early (exploratory) or late (must demonstrate clinically significant change)
Expected benefit of treatment	Reverse (improve) or stop/slow disease progression
Biological considerations	Mechanism or site of action

Figure 2. Desirable properties of candidate endpoints to be considered when identifying the best candidate endpoint for a future trial.

Another potential objective of natural history data may include its use as an external control group for a trial. Although the introduction of bias is a major concern (e.g., differences in enrollment criteria, outcome measurement methods), the FDA allows this in special circumstances when concurrent controls are impractical or unethical. Acceptance of an external control requires discussion with regulatory agencies and careful planning, including data collection under conditions where external control participants are similar to trial participants in all respects of disease severity and risk factors, as detailed in FDA guidance (Food and Drug Administration 2019a,b). Beyond its use as a formal external control group, a well-designed natural history study will also generally provide a good historical basis for expected changes in a trial's concurrent control group, which may aid in interpretation of missing data in the clinical trial, albeit with the same noted limitations.

Outside of these scientific objectives, there are countless intangible insights and practical groundwork to be gained from natural history studies that can be applied to future trials. Natural history studies should be designed with sufficient duration to observe clinically meaningful changes, frequent enough measures to establish timing of those changes, and from a variety of measures based on features of disease and what is currently known. Testing and data-collection methods should be standardized to reduce variability (including testing equipment, staff training, and procedures manuals) and include methods to improve accuracy and reduce bias of measurements, such as independent expert grading of images. Development of these many standards requires input from a variety of subject matter experts, the experience of real-world implementation (especially on a multicenter scale), iterations of refinement based on lessons learned, and validation of methods (such as test–retest assessments or inter-/intragrader reproducibility). This important journey of ironing out details early provides a foundation for high-quality and efficient future trials, and establishes communication pathways, identifies disease-specific centers of excellence, brings clinicians and patient communities together, and improves the understanding of standard of care practices.

SPECIAL CONSIDERATIONS IN RARE DISEASE

FDA guidance states "the natural history of rare diseases is often poorly understood … the need for prospectively designed, protocol-driven natural history studies initiated in the earliest drug development planning stages cannot be overemphasized" but acknowledges that traditional knowledge gaps are "more difficult to address in rare disease" (Food and Drug Administration 2019a). Lack of specialized clinical centers, methods for diagnosis, or knowledge about potential endpoints are hallmark challenges of rare disease research (Food and Drug Administration 2012, 2014; Ogorka and Chanchu 2017). More directly, small sample sizes inherent in rare disease impact the precision of estimates of progression rates, the cornerstone of understanding natural history. Disease heterogeneity (in terms of both genotypes and phenotypes in IRDs) further exacerbates small sample size issues, as disease subtypes may have different manifestations of progression rate or severity. This means that objectives for understanding risk factors for progression and correlation of outcomes may be exploratory or inconclusive.

To address these challenges, natural history studies in rare disease should give special emphasis to the following:

Data quality. Standardization of testing procedures and data collection are important to reduce variability. Training and certification of study staff coupled with careful monitoring of protocol adherence and data validations by a central coordinating center will also enforce implementation of standardized procedures and improve precision of data collected. Independent and standardized expert grading of key outcomes, such as reading center evaluation of the SD-OCT EZ area, can provide more accurate measures, which may result in endpoints that are more sensitive to detecting changes in disease. Centralized ex-

 Cite this article as *Cold Spring Harb Perspect Med* doi: 10.1101/cshperspect.a041297

pert review of eligibility criteria will ensure the study cohort is limited precisely to the disease under study. An example of this in IRDs would be confirmation by a centralized genetic expert that the laboratory-reported variants of the gene under study are likely pathogenic and the cause of each participant's retinal disease. Efforts to minimize missing data is also critical. Engaging patient communities early in the protocol development process may help to understand the potential burden of study procedures and motivate protocol adjustments to maximize compliance and retention.

Statistical approaches to maximize value of data collected. Longitudinal data with multiple time points improves precision within a limited sample size. Testing and analyzing data from both eyes when evaluating ocular outcome measures will also increase the effective sample size, although high correlation between the eyes will reduce this impact. Determining the degree of symmetry between the eyes may be an objective of the natural history study. Change over time may not be linear, so efforts should be made to identify the pattern of change. For example, loss may be a constant percentage of the current value (exponential decay), or not be detectable until a specific threshold of duration of disease. Statistical objectives and methods to evaluate outcome measures should focus on exploration rather than testing prespecified hypotheses. This includes descriptive statistics and graphical displays of distributions, correlations, and estimates of variability. Visual plots of individual patient trajectories can also be helpful in understanding progression in a smaller study.

Multicenter approach: strength in numbers. A multicenter approach to rare disease is essential to achieving feasible sample sizes, especially for evaluating subgroups. The Foundation Fighting Blindness (FFB) Consortium 2021 IRD Gene Poll found, in the 48 most common genes with a total consortium-wide patient count greater than 100, the median within-center count was less than 20 for all except three genes, and the consortium-wide total for each gene is, on average, 5 times greater than the

maximum single center count (source: FFB Consortium, unpubl.). In addition to the absolute numbers, the efforts for achieving data quality noted above require significant logistical and budgetary considerations to carry out, and a multicenter approach to research can facilitate efficiencies, economy of scale, and knowledge-building that is not possible in small single-center studies.

SPECIFIC KNOWLEDGE GAPS IN IRDs THAT NATURAL HISTORY STUDIES CAN ADDRESS

The specific knowledge gaps in IRDs have been extensively described in recent publications (Csaky et al. 2017; Duncan et al. 2018; Thompson et al. 2020). Each of these reports point to natural history studies to address two major gaps most urgently: the identification of optimal IRD patient populations for target therapies and the development and validation of outcome measures for IRDs.

Define IRD Patient Populations

The challenge in defining IRD patient populations for target therapies is the genetic heterogeneity of hundreds of IRDs, which manifest in vastly different phenotypes. This creates the need to identify genetic factors impacting disease severity and progression, including the impact of mutation-specific variations within a given gene. Natural history studies are thereby needed within each gene-specific population and should ideally aim to understand progression in subgroups at the finest level possible to more specifically target treatments. This includes the need to evaluate a variety of genetic subfactors (within variants or types of variants) and a range of phenotypes (including duration and severity of disease). This becomes even more challenging in ultrarare genes and highlights the desirability to develop methods to pool genes based on similar disease mechanisms. Verbakel et al. (2018) described principal pathways affected in retinitis pigmentosa (RP), including phototransduction cascade (10 RP genes), the visual cycle (7 RP genes), and ciliary structure and transport (35 RP genes). Natural history study data are needed to determine whether these or other classifications of genes may allow pooling of patients to better explore other factors related to disease progression and refined criteria for candidates for therapies.

Develop Endpoints for IRDs

Specifically in the context of gene therapy for retinal disorders, the FDA "encourages sponsors to explore a wide spectrum of potential clinical endpoints" and "to develop and propose novel endpoints to measure clinically meaningful effects" (Food and Drug Administration 2020). The concept of "clinically meaningful" is critical to evaluating endpoints. The FDA-NIH Biomarker Working Group BEST (Biomarkers, Endpoints, and other Tools) Resource (2016) defines clinical benefit as "a positive clinically meaningful effect of an intervention (i.e., a positive effect on how an individual feels, functions, or survives)" and defines a clinical outcome as a measure of this benefit, which can be assessed as (1) clinician-reported outcomes (which we refer to as "visual function measures" in the context of IRDs), or as (2) patient/observer-reported outcomes or performance outcomes (which we categorize collectively as "functional vision measures"). Regulatory agencies also support development of surrogate endpoints, which are measures that are reasonably likely to predict a clinical benefit (which we use to categorize "structural measures" of IRDs).

Other characteristics of endpoints that are acceptable to regulatory bodies to demonstrate efficacy include those that are validated, reliable, and sensitive to change, among other properties noted previously and in Figure 2 (Csaky et al. 2017; Food and Drug Administration 2020; Thompson et al. 2020). The list of IRD endpoints is large and growing, and many are nicely summarized in other recent reports (Csaky et al. 2017; Cideciyan et al. 2021; Sahel et al. 2021). Some key IRD endpoints discussed or accepted by the FDA are summarized in Figure 3, grouped by the type of outcome measure. It is important to note that, although an endpoint may have established FDA acceptance, it may not be ap-

propriate for a specific IRD, so natural history studies are still needed to validate endpoint properties within a given genotype. An overview of the types of IRD measures and gaps to be addressed by natural history studies are as follows.

Visual function measures. Visual function measures are intended to capture performance of the various components of the visual system within the clinical environment. Traditionally, the FDA has accepted definitions for clinically meaningful changes in visual function measures based on within-person thresholds. There has been some evolution over time from emphasis on a clinically meaningful change within a person to a clinically meaningful difference in means (Beck et al. 2007). In general, smaller sample sizes are required to detect a difference between treatment groups in mean change than to detect a difference in proportions of patients achieving a specific amount of change. More work is needed to build the case for defining clinical meaningfulness of visual function measures in terms of mean changes, when applicable. Of the visual function tests available, visual acuity has gained the most widespread acceptance because of its proven simplicity and reliability. However, visual acuity testing does not provide insight into aspects of visual functioning across the entire retina. Light sensitivity captured by perimetry measures such as static perimetry and microperimetry provide more spatial information across the visual field. Improvement in microperimetry of ≥ 7 decibels at ≥ 5 prespecified points has been discussed as an endpoint acceptable to regulators and presumably has the potential to be considered clinically meaningful (Weinreb and Kaufman 2009; Yang and Dunbar 2021). Hill of vision changes have also been discussed with the FDA but require more specific criteria for clinically meaningful changes, and evidence to support any criteria developed (Csaky et al. 2017). Other potential visual function measures such as full-field stimulus threshold, low luminance visual acuity, contrast sensitivity, and color vision have been listed by the FDA as worthy of consideration and many are being used as endpoints in current IRD trials (Csaky et al. 2017; Duncan et al.

Type of measure	Test	Key endpoints measured	Prior FDA acceptance or discussion on criteria for clinically meaningful	Sources
Visual function measures				
	Best corrected visual acuity	Early Treatment of Diabetic Retinopathy Study letter score	FDA has historically accepted 15-letter changes in retina therapy trials.	FDA Guidance (Food and Drug Administration 2020)
	Static perimetry	Hill of vision	FDA has discussed using changes in hill of vision as a reasonable candidate measure in IRDs but would require evidence supporting criteria for clinically meaningful changes.	Csaky et al. 2017
	Microperimetry	Retinal sensitivity at specific loci	FDA has discussed using number of points demonstrating change on an established threshold sensitivity, specifically considering 5 or more points showing changes in 7 or more decibels as reasonable criteria in the context of glaucoma.	Weinreb and Kaufman 2009; Yang and Dunbar 2021
	Contrast sensitivity	Contrast sensitivity	FDA has discussed using significant changes at 2 or more frequencies as a reasonable candidate measure in IRDs but would require evidence supporting criteria clinically meaningful changes.	Csaky et. al. 2017
Functional vision measures				
	Multiluminance Mobility Test	Speed and accuracy to navigate mobility course	FDA has accepted changes in light level required to pass the course, with change of 2 lux considered clinically meaningful.	Csaky et al. 2017; Food and Drug Administration 2020
Structural measures				
	Fundus autofluorescence	Hyper- or hypofluorescent lesion size	FDA has discussed changes in lesion area in Stargardt disease with no clear guidance other than correlation with functional measures will be important to demonstrate that changes are clinically meaningful.	Csaky et al. 2017
	Optical coherence tomography	Ellipsoid zone area	FDA has noted changes in mean area of intact photoreceptors on at least 2 images with intervals of 6 months or more, evaluated using best curve fit analysis to exceed measurement uncertainty would be considered clinically meaningful. FDA has also discussed clinically meaningful based on extent and location of change, and that changes outside the "fuzzy border" edge of the EZ are likely to be acceptable.	Csaky et al. 2017; Food and Drug Administration 2020

Figure 3. A summary of (inherited retinal disease [IRD]) endpoints historically discussed or accepted by the Food and Drug Administration (FDA).

2018; Food and Drug Administration 2020; Thompson et al. 2020). However, there is still little to go by in defining the extent of change that is clinically significant and establishing evidence that may be accepted by regulatory agencies.

Functional vision measures. Functional vision measures are intended to capture how well patients perform vision-related activities of daily living. Mobility course performance tests assess this in a physical environment. One multiluminance mobility test has been used to establish efficacy for FDA approval of gene therapy for mutations in RPE65 (Russell et al. 2017) and is recognized in FDA guidance (Food and Drug Administration 2020) as an endpoint that was used to support marketing approval. Newer technology has allowed for development of virtual mobility course platforms to simulate urban environments or test object detection while reducing logistics to implement (Lombardi et al. 2018; Aleman et al. 2021). Patient-reported outcomes (PROs) are also useful tools for evaluating real-life challenges faced by patients. Although a wide range of vision function and health-related quality of life instruments for retinal diseases exist (Prem Senthil et al. 2017) and more recent instruments have been developed specifically targeted to IRD patients (Lacy et al. 2021), there is an urgent need to validate these instruments for specific IRDs, based on rod versus cone dysfunction, central or peripheral visual field progression, and other disease-specific manifestations. Continued development and validation efforts within IRD natural history studies will increase the ability of therapies to demonstrate efficacy based directly on these outcomes or the association of structure and function endpoints with these measures of impact on daily living.

Structural measures. Structural measures are intended as surrogate endpoints that are reasonably likely to predict a clinically meaningful benefit and may have the benefit to detect disease progression earlier than visual function measures. The FDA highlights the rate of photoreceptor loss as an established efficacy endpoint that can be used to evaluate clinical benefit for

treatment of retinal disorders (Food and Drug Administration 2020). The EZ area captures the extent of intact photoreceptors on SD-OCT imaging and has been shown to correlate with visual field loss in RP patients (Birch et al. 2015). However, the extent and location of EZ area changes acceptable to the FDA as clinically meaningful is less clear and requires additional evidence (Csaky et al. 2017). Fundus autofluorescence allows quantification of atrophic lesion growth in Stargardt disease (Ervin et al. 2019; Strauss et al. 2019) and in geographic atrophy (Schmitz-Valckenberg et al. 2011). Further development of these and other structural outcome measures (including adaptive optics scanning laser ophthalmoscopy) (Csaky et al. 2017) is an expanding area in IRDs as newer technology, better retinal imaging acquisition, and interpretation techniques may improve sensitivity, accuracy, and objectivity. IRD research may also benefit from a photographic-based disease severity scale, in much the same way the diabetic retinopathy grading scale developed by the Early Treatment Diabetic Retinopathy Study Research Group (1991) advanced treatment assessment methods in the field. Natural history studies are needed to further define these measures, provide evidence of association with functional endpoints to support clinically meaningful criteria, and to evaluate other properties of these endpoints like reproducibility and feasibility of implementation.

EXAMPLES OF NATURAL HISTORY STUDIES IN IRDs AND LESSONS LEARNED

The history of studies of the course of disease for specific IRDs has provided the groundwork for understanding aspects of disease progression and potential endpoints, but largely includes studies from single centers using protocols that may not generalize to other centers, retrospective studies that may be biased toward individuals whose disease is progressing more rapidly and are therefore seeking care, or studies using outdated methods or technology (Berson et al. 1985; Roesch et al. 1998; Birch et al. 1999; Sandberg et al. 2008). As a recent example, three natural history studies in Usher syndrome type

1B provide in combination an overall impression of this IRD-specific disease course (Jacobson et al. 2011; Lenassi et al. 2014; Testa et al. 2017). All three were longitudinal with variable follow-up duration of as much as 10 to 15 years in some patients, and sample sizes ranging from 10 to 33. In combination, these studies suggest visual field loss in Usher 1B patients occurs at a rate of 8% to 14% per year, visual acuity loss averages 2% to 4% per year, and legal blindness occurs in half of individuals by approximately age 40. The strength of these studies is the duration of data, which provide a good sense of long-term prognosis, including a zoomed-out view of visual field progression that suggests it is not linear. Understanding where on the progression curve a particular patient is may provide insights into the therapeutic window. The limitations of small sample sizes, single centers, and lack of standardized data collection, however, leave other trial design questions unanswered. Longitudinal data collected on a larger multicenter scale with standardized methods are needed to provide more precise estimates of annual rates of change, variability, and correlation of structure and function, to better define endpoints to be used for future trials. More recent multicenter studies initiated by the FFB have begun to address many of these limitations and allow for a larger scale assessment of challenges faced and insights gained for future trial development.

Stargardt Disease and ProgStar Studies

The Progression of Atrophy Secondary to Stargardt Disease (ProgStar) studies were designed to measure progression of Stargardt disease on fundus autofluorescence imaging, OCT, and microperimetry as possible efficacy measures for clinical trials (NCT01977846). These multicenter, longitudinal natural history studies included both a retrospective ($N = 251$ participants) and prospective ($N = 259$ participants) component. The measurable impact of the ProgStar studies is extensive and includes 20 publications to date (PubMed search April 2022), the vast majority of which are from the prospective study, reflecting the inability to glean much from insufficient quality retrospective data. Deidentified data sets have been made available free of charge to 26 requestors (17 industry and nine academic) to date (source: Jaeb Center for Health Research, host of ProgStar public data set). A workshop organized by the study sponsor, FFB, was held to review key findings and lessons learned, and are summarized in Figure 4 (Ervin et al. 2019). Discussion of the most promising endpoints for treatment trials included the EZ area on OCT, area of definitely decreased autofluorescence, and sensitivity around scotoma on microperimetry, all of which were found to be sensitive to change at 2 years. The study also affirmed that visual acuity was not a sensitive outcome measure for a trial. Moreover, the lessons learned include ideas for cost and time efficiencies (e.g., OCT manual segmentation is time consuming to grade and reducing the number of boundaries for segmentation may help) as well as improving properties of candidate outcome measures (e.g., changes in transition zones may be more sensitive to disease progression and new technology for frequency tracking and autocalibrating may help with fixation issues and reliability of microperimetry measures). These shared experiences offer insights for future trial designers to fine-tune endpoints while saving valuable resources.

FFB Consortium Natural History Studies

Building on the success of the ProgStar studies, FFB sought to establish a standing infrastructure from which to launch natural history studies more efficiently (Durham et al. 2021). In 2016, FFB initiated an international consortium of clinical centers to conduct IRD research, with the goal to accelerate development of treatments for IRDs. The vision for the consortium mission includes (1) investigators collaborating on ideas for hypotheses, study designs, and publications, (2) highly standardized studies providing long-term data to evaluate disease onset, progression, and sensitive structural and functional outcome measures, and (3) an open central repository of completed data sets to stimulate further hypothesis generation and innovation (public.jaeb.org/ffb). The organizational structure of the consor-

	Optical coherence tomography (OCT)	Fundus autofluorescence (FAF)	Microperimetry (MP)	Visual acuity (VA)
Outcomes	• Total retinal thickness • Ellipsoid zone (EZ) area	• Area of definitely decreased AF (DDAF) • Area of questionably decreased AF (QDAF)	• Mean macular sensitivity • Deep scotoma count • Sensitivity at lesion edges	• Best corrected VA by ETDRS (Early Treatment Diabetic Retinopathy Study)
Advantages	• Sensitive to change 2 years	• Sensitive to change 2 years • Software assists w/grading	• Sensitive measure of central vision beyond the fovea, correlates with OCT	• Easy • Important to patients
Disadvantages	• Time/difficult to grade • Not all retinal layers identifiable		• Changes in fixation (not appropriate late-stage)	• Insensitive
Lessons learned	• Reduce the number of boundaries for segmentation, to manage time and cost • Consider how to account for disruptions in intact boundaries due to abnormal retinal structures and other pathologies • Incorporate reproducibility studies into grading protocols	• Poorly demarcated lesions of QDAF should be integrated into the grading scheme, as these may represent earlier disease stages in which photoreceptors and retinal pigment epithelium might be still amenable to rescue • Complexities of interpreting FAF lesions in Stargardt disease participants may be even more difficult with color fundus photos; FAF turned out to be helpful in distinguishing several characteristics	• Changes in transition zones may be more sensitive to disease progression • Evolving technology may enhance the reliability of MP (frequency tracking and autocalibrating) • Scotopic MP subject to additional confounding factors such as the degree of light shielding within the test room and length of dark adaptation, that must be carefully controlled	
Most promising outcomes	• EZ area	• DDAF lesion area	• Mean macular sensitivity • Deep scotoma count • Sensitivity around scotoma	• Not a suitable outcome measure except for distinct subgroups

Figure 4. Summarizes key findings and lessons learned of the ProgStar study, as discussed at a workshop organized by the study sponsor, and shared through publication (Ervin et al. 2019).

Cite this article as *Cold Spring Harb Perspect Med* doi: 10.1101/cshperspect.a041297

tium is comprised of an executive committee, operations committee, coordinating center, genetics committee, study chairs, reading centers, subject matter experts, investigators, coordinators, technicians, and patients and families. Figure 5 provides an example overview of a multidisciplinary approach to design and conduct of natural history studies in IRDs, similar to that of the consortium. The consortium's established infrastructure allows for a more efficient study startup, including master agreements for clinical centers and vendors, reusable database and case report form templates, and procedure manuals and technician certifications for standard testing modalities, which are applicable across consortium studies. An international network of IRD centers also gathers a larger pool of IRD patients together for common research goals and encourages experts across centers to share ideas, improve methods, establish standards, and more easily build upon knowledge gained along the way.

Three prospective, longitudinal natural history studies have been launched by the

FFB Consortium to date: Rate of Progression in USH2A-Related Retinal Degeneration (RUSH2A; NCT03146078), Rate of Progression in EYS-Related Retinal Degeneration (Pro-EYS; NCT04127006), and Rate of Progression in PCDH15-Related Retinal Degeneration in Usher Syndrome 1F (RUSH1F; NCT04765345). As of this publication, RUSH2A was nearing completion of the final 4-year visits, which will provide the data to evaluate annual rates of change on various outcome measures and to evaluate correlations between structure and function as well as risk factors related to change on those measures. In preparation for these analyses, the consortium leadership has developed a template to summarize and compare properties of endpoint candidates provided in Figure 6 as an example of the general type of tool that may be used in evaluating multiple outcome measures as future trial endpoints.

More recently, the FFB Consortium has considered the special challenge of studying ultra-rare IRD genes, which represent a significant portion of IRD genes. Three hundred and twen-

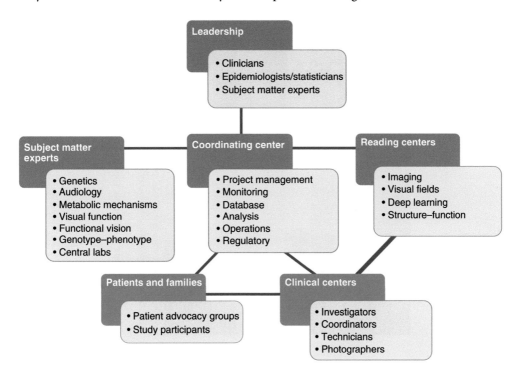

Figure 5. An example organizational chart featuring a multidisciplinary approach for conducting natural history studies in inherited retinal diseases (IRDs).

	Static perimetry V$_{TOT}$ (hill of vision, total volume)	Static perimetry V$_{30}$ (hill of vision, 30 degrees)	Static perimetry V$_{PERIPH}$ (peripheral = total minus 30 degrees)	Static perimetry mean sensitivity	Micro-perimetry mean sensitivity	Micro-perimetry pointwise sensitivity	Best corrected visual acuity	Full-field stimulus threshold	OCT ellipsoid zone area	OCT central subfield thickness
Coefficient of repeatability										
Sensitivity*										
Correlation with duration										
Floor or ceiling effects										
Relative patient burden†										
Degree of subjectivity (patient or examiner)†										
Clinically meaningful†										

* Measured as "signal-to-noise ratio" (mean change / standard deviation of change)
† Qualitative assessment of low/medium/high, by committee of subject matter experts

Figure 6. Example tool that may be used to evaluate and compare multiple candidate endpoints for a future trial.

Cite this article as *Cold Spring Harb Perspect Med* doi: 10.1101/cshperspect.a041297

ty-six (326) genes out of 374 potential IRD genes listed in the FFB Consortium 2021 Gene Poll had less than 100 total patients counted consortium-wide as having IRD linked to that causal gene, across 32 sites reporting in the poll (unpubl.). Individual natural history studies for each rare IRD gene are not feasible. Many centers have as few as one or two patients for a particular IRD gene and may not be able to devote resources needed to implement each study. Individual studies also require considerable startup time (e.g., contracts, ethics committee approvals) and study management expenses regardless of the number of patients. A single, universal protocol under which all rare IRD genes may be enrolled would address these challenges. The FFB consortium is launching a Universal Rare Gene Study (Uni-Rare), featuring a registry open to all rare RD genes, to cross-sectionally characterize (genotype, structure, and function) patients so they are ready to be enrolled into the universal longitudinal natural history study, which will open up to targeted genes (full protocol available on public website public.jaeb.org/ffb/stdy). This two-phase study will eliminate repetitive processes like certification, training, regulatory approval, contract agreements, and ultimately reduce costs and accelerate timelines for the natural history studies. The longitudinal natural history objectives for each gene are to (1) characterize the natural history of retinal degeneration on various measures of structure, function, and PROs, (2) explore whether structural outcome measures can be validated as surrogates for visual function outcomes, and (3) explore possible risk factors for progression of outcome measures. For a given gene, the sample size will impact the precision around the point estimates for changes in the outcome measures of interest (objective 1) and the correlation between the outcome measures of interest (objective 2), and will also affect the power to detect differences among subgroups (objective 3). The statistical chapter of the Uni-Rare protocol provides tables showing the impact of sample size and varying assumptions on these objectives. Even with collective enrollment across consortium centers, some very rare IRD genes will have very small sample sizes and

therefore limited ability to evaluate all the noted objectives. As an exploratory objective, the Uni-Rare platform will also leverage the collective sample size and standardized data collection across all IRD genes to explore the extent to which genes with common mechanisms of disease have similar clinical manifestations, with the goal to determine whether and how some genes may be pooled in some analyses.

CONCLUSION

The success of IRD treatment trials depends on natural history data. Patient populations should be evaluated based on the finest level of genetic, phenotypic, and environmental factors possible to identify who may benefit from treatment and more carefully target therapy trials. Endpoint candidates should include a wide spectrum of vision function, structure, and functional vision measures. The heterogeneity of disease manifestation across IRDs also means that accepted endpoints for one gene may need to be validated within another. Numerous endpoint properties must be considered, including accuracy and reproducibility of the measure itself, sensitivity and clinical meaningfulness, feasibility, and goals of a future trial.

Well-designed natural history studies should emphasize data quality standards, such as prospective and standardized testing procedures and independent expert grading of outcomes. Longitudinal data with multiple time points can improve precision of estimates. Multicenter studies facilitate larger sample sizes and cultivate standards with broader applicability. Input from multidisciplinary teams fosters knowledge-building and sharing of ideas for a more holistic approach to study design, data collection, and data analysis. Natural history studies are also an opportunity to iron out details, work out kinks, and uncover unknowns. Publications on lessons learned can help future trial designers fine-tune study design, endpoints, and procedures, which may expedite timelines and ensure greater chances of success of future treatment trials.

The FFB Consortium's Uni-Rare study is a unique approach to IRD natural history studies and provides the opportunity to efficiently characterize disease progression of most IRD genes in a multicenter, prospective, standardized data collection. The consortium envisions Uni-Rare will result in mutually beneficial partnerships between IRD researchers and companies, including early access to study data sets and joint development of novel outcome measures. Results from the Uni-Rare studies will be widely disseminated as deidentified public data sets and publications to stimulate further innovation and progress in IRD therapeutic research.

REFERENCES

Aleman TS, Miller AJ, Maguire KH, Aleman EM, Serrano LW, O'Connor KB, Bedoukian EC, Leroy BP, Maguire AM, Bennett J. 2021. A virtual reality orientation and mobility test for inherited retinal degenerations: testing a proof-of-concept after gene therapy. *Clin Ophthalmol* **15**: 939–952. doi:10.2147/OPTH.S292527

Beck RW, Maguire MG, Bressler NM, Glassman AR, Lindblad AS, Ferris FL. 2007. Visual acuity as an outcome measure in clinical trials of retinal diseases. *Ophthalmology* **114**: 1804–1809. doi:10.1016/j.ophtha.2007.06.047

Berson EL, Sandberg MA, Rosner B, Birch DG, Hanson AH. 1985. Natural course of retinitis pigmentosa over a three-year interval. *Am J Ophthalmol* **99**: 240–251. doi:10.1016/0002-9394(85)90351-4

Birch DG, Anderson JL, Fish GE. 1999. Yearly rates of rod and cone functional loss in retinitis pigmentosa and cone-rod dystrophy. *Ophthalmology* **106**: 258–268. doi:10.1016/S0161-6420(99)90064-7

Birch DG, Locke KG, Felius J, Klein M, Wheaton DK, Hoffman DR, Hood DC. 2015. Rates of decline in regions of the visual field defined by frequency-domain optical coherence tomography in patients with RPGR-mediated X-linked retinitis pigmentosa. *Ophthalmology* **122**: 833–839. doi:10.1016/j.ophtha.2014.11.005

Cideciyan AV, Krishnan AK, Roman AJ, Sumaroka A, Swider M, Jacobson SG. 2021. Measures of function and structure to determine phenotypic features, natural history, and treatment outcomes in inherited retinal diseases. *Annu Rev Vis Sci* **7**: 747–772. doi:10.1146/annurev-vision-032321-091738

Csaky K, Ferris F III, Chew EY, Nair P, Cheetham JK, Duncan JL. 2017. Report from the NEI/FDA Endpoints Workshop on age-related macular degeneration and inherited retinal diseases. *Invest Ophthalmol Vis Sci* **58**: 3456–3463. doi:10.1167/iovs.17-22339

Duncan JL, Pierce EA, Laster AM, Daiger SP, Birch DG, Ash JD, Iannaccone A, Flannery JG, Sahel JA, Zack DJ, et al. 2018. Inherited retinal degenerations: current landscape and knowledge gaps. *Transl Vis Sci Technol* **7**: 6. doi:10.1167/tvst.7.4.6

Durham TA, Duncan JL, Ayala AR, Birch DG, Cheetham JK, Ferris FL, Hoyng CB, Pennesi ME, Sahel JA; Foundation Fighting Blindness Consortium Investigator Group. 2021. Tackling the challenges of product development through a collaborative rare disease network: the Foundation Fighting Blindness Consortium. *Transl Vis Sci Technol* **10**: 23–23. doi:10.1167/tvst.10.4.23

Early Treatment Diabetic Retinopathy Study Research Group. 1991. Grading diabetic retinopathy from stereoscopic color fundus photographs—an extension of the modified Airlie House classification. ETDRS report number 10. *Ophthalmology* **98**: 786–806. doi:10.1016/S0161-6420(13)38012-9

Ervin AM, Strauss RW, Ahmed MI, Birch D, Cheetham J, Ferris FL III, Ip MS, Jaffe GJ, Maguire MG, Schönbach EM, et al. 2019. A workshop on measuring the progression of atrophy secondary to Stargardt disease in the ProgStar studies: findings and lessons learned. *Transl Vis Sci Technol* **8**: 16–16. doi:10.1167/tvst.8.2.16

Food and Drug Administration. 2010. 21 CFR 314.126—adequate and well-controlled studies. FDA, Silver Spring, Maryland.

Food and Drug Administration. 2012. *Workshop on natural history studies of rare diseases: meeting the needs of drug development and research workshop summary*, pp. 1–41. FDA, Silver Spring, Maryland.

Food and Drug Administration. 2014. Report: complex issues in developing drugs and biological products for rare diseases and accelerating the development of therapies for pediatric rare diseases including strategic plan: accelerating the development of therapies for pediatric rare diseases, pp. 1–86. FDA, Silver Spring, Maryland.

Food and Drug Administration. 2019a. Rare diseases: common issues in drug development guidance for industry, pp. 1–24. FDA, Silver Spring, Maryland.

Food and Drug Administration. 2019b. Rare diseases: natural history studies for drug development guidance for industry, pp. 1–19. FDA, Silver Spring, Maryland.

Food and Drug Administration. 2020. Human gene therapy for retinal disorders guidance for industry, pp. 1–12. FDA, Silver Spring, Maryland.

Food and Drug Administration National Institute of Health Working Group. 2016. BEST (Biomarkers, Endpoints, and other Tools) Resource. FDA, Silver Spring, Maryland.

Jacobson SG, Cideciyan AV, Gibbs D, Sumaroka A, Roman AJ, Aleman TS, Schwartz SB, Olivares MB, Russell RC, Steinberg JD, et al. 2011. Retinal disease course in Usher syndrome 1B due to *MYO7A* mutations. *Invest Ophthalmol Vis Sci* **52**: 7924–7936. doi:10.1167/iovs.11-8313

Lacy GD, Abalem MF, Andrews CA, Abuzaitoun R, Popova LT, Santos EP, Yu G, Rakine HY, Baig N, Ehrlich JR, et al. 2021. The Michigan Vision-Related Anxiety Questionnaire: a psychosocial outcomes measure for inherited retinal degenerations. *Am J Ophthalmol* **225**: 137–146. doi:10.1016/j.ajo.2020.12.001

Lenassi E, Saihan Z, Cipriani V, Le Quesne Stabej P, Moore AT, Luxon LM, Bitner-Glindzicz M, Webster AR. 2014. Natural history and retinal structure in patients with Usher syndrome type 1 owing to MYO7A mutation. *Ophthalmology* **121**: 580–587. doi:10.1016/j.ophtha.2013.09.017

Lombardi M, Zenouda A, Azoulay-Sebban L, Lebrisse M, Gutman E, Brasnu E, Hamard P, Sahel JA, Baudouin C, Labbé A. 2018. Correlation between visual function and performance of simulated daily living activities in glaucomatous patients. *J Glaucoma* **27:** 1017–1024. doi:10 .1097/IJG.0000000000001066

Ogorka T, Chanchu G. 2017. Researchers conduct NH studies for rare diseases and drug development. *Applied Clinical Trials*, October 16. https://www.appliedclini caltrialsonline.com/view/researchers-conduct-nh-studies-rare-diseases-and-drug-development

Prem Senthil M, Khadka J, Pesudovs K. 2017. Assessment of patient-reported outcomes in retinal diseases: a systematic review. *Surv Ophthalmol* **62:** 546–582. doi:10.1016/j .survophthal.2016.12.011

Roesch MT, Ewing CC, Gibson AE, Weber BH. 1998. The natural history of X-linked retinoschisis. *Can J Ophthalmol* **33:** 149–158.

Russell S, Bennett J, Wellman JA, Chung DC, Yu ZF, Tillman A, Wittes J, Pappas J, Elci O, McCague S, et al. 2017. Efficacy and safety of voretigene neparvovec (AAV2-hRPE65v2) in patients with RPE65-mediated inherited retinal dystrophy: a randomised, controlled, open-label, phase 3 trial. *Lancet* **390:** 849–860. doi:10.1016/S0140-6736(17)31868-8

Sahel JA, Bennett J, Roska B. 2019. Depicting brighter possibilities for treating blindness. *Sci Transl Med* **11:** eaax2324. doi:10.1126/scitranslmed.aax2324

Sahel JA, Grieve K, Pagot C, Authié C, Mohand-Said S, Paques M, Audo I, Becker K, Chaumet-Riffaud AE, Azoulay L, et al. 2021. Assessing photoreceptor status in retinal dystrophies: from high-resolution imaging to functional vision. *Am J Ophthalmol* **230:** 12–47. doi:10.1016/j.ajo .2021.04.013

Sandberg MA, Rosner B, Weigel-DiFranco C, McGee TL, Dryja TP, Berson EL. 2008. Disease course in patients with autosomal recessive retinitis pigmentosa due to the USH2A gene. *Invest Ophthalmol Vis Sci* **49:** 5532–5539. doi:10.1167/iovs.08-2009

Schmitz-Valckenberg S, Fleckenstein M, Göbel AP, Hohman TC, Holz FG. 2011. Optical coherence tomography and autofluorescence findings in areas with geographic atrophy due to age-related macular degeneration. *Invest Ophthalmol Vis Sci* **52:** 1–6. doi:10.1167/iovs.10-5619

Strauss RW, Kong X, Ho A, Jha A, West S, Ip M, Bernstein PS, Birch DG, Cideciyan AV, Michaelides M, et al. 2019. Progression of Stargardt disease as determined by fundus autofluorescence over a 12-month period: ProgStar Report No. 11. *JAMA Ophthalmol* **137:** 1134–1145. doi:10 .1001/jamaophthalmol.2019.2885

Testa F, Melillo P, Bonnet C, Marcelli V, de Benedictis A, Colucci R, Gallo B, Kurtenbach A, Rossi S, Marciano E, et al. 2017. Clinical presentation and disease course of Usher syndrome because of mutations in MYO7A or USH2A. *Retina* **37:** 1581–1590. doi:10.1097/IAE.000000000000 1389

Thompson DA, Iannaccone A, Ali RR, Arshavsky VY, Audo I, Bainbridge JWB, Besirli CG, Birch DG, Branham KE, Cideciyan AV, et al. 2020. Advancing clinical trials for inherited retinal diseases: recommendations from the Second Monaciano Symposium. *Transl Vis Sci Technol* **9:** 2. doi:10.1167/tvst.9.7.2

Verbakel SK, van Huet RAC, Boon CJF, den Hollander AI, Collin RWJ, Klaver CCW, Hoyng CB, Roepman R, Klevering BJ. 2018. Non-syndromic retinitis pigmentosa. *Prog Retin Eye Res* **66:** 157–186. doi:10.1016/j.preteyeres.2018 .03.005

Weinreb RN, Kaufman PL. 2009. The glaucoma research community and FDA look to the future: a report from the NEI/FDA CDER Glaucoma Clinical Trial Design and Endpoints Symposium. *Invest Ophthalmol Vis Sci* **50:** 1497–1505. doi:10.1167/iovs.08-2843

Yang Y, Dunbar H. 2021. Clinical perspectives and trends: microperimetry as a trial endpoint in retinal disease. *Ophthalmologica* **244:** 418–450. doi:10.1159/000 515148

Adaptive Optics Imaging of Inherited Retinal Disease

Jacque L. Duncan[1] and Joseph Carroll[2]

[1]Department of Ophthalmology, University of California, San Francisco, California 94143-4081, USA

[2]Department of Ophthalmology & Visual Sciences, Medical College of Wisconsin Eye Institute, Milwaukee, Wisconsin 53226, USA

Correspondence: jcarroll@mcw.edu

The human retina is amenable to direct, noninvasive visualization using a wide array of imaging modalities. In the ~140 years since the publication of the first image of the living human retina, there has been a continued evolution of retinal imaging technology. Advances in image acquisition and processing speed now allow real-time visualization of retinal structure, which has revolutionized the diagnosis and management of eye disease. Enormous advances have come in image resolution, with adaptive optics (AO)-based systems capable of imaging the retina with single-cell resolution. In addition, newer functional imaging techniques provide the ability to assess function with exquisite spatial and temporal resolution. These imaging advances have had an especially profound impact on the field of inherited retinal disease research. Here we will review some of the advances and applications of AO retinal imaging in patients with inherited retinal disease.

Our focus on adaptive optics (AO)-based imaging methods is not intended to convey that other imaging approaches have not been valuable in the study of inherited retinal disease; however, the field of noninvasive retinal imaging is so expansive it is simply not possible to comprehensively review the entirety of retinal imaging approaches in the space provided. We refer the reader to some excellent reviews on scanning laser ophthalmoscopy (SLO), optical coherence tomography (OCT), OCT-angiography, and fundus autofluorescence, as well as newer techniques like photothermal OCT and fluorescence lifetime imaging (Van Velthoven et al. 2007; Schmitz-Valckenberg et al. 2008; Abràmoff et al. 2010; Kashani et al. 2017; Lapierre-Landry et al. 2018; Spaide et al. 2018; Sauer et al. 2021).

AO is not an imaging method per se, but rather is an "add-on" that can be integrated into the full gamut of conventional retinal imaging platforms. An excellent review of AO from a technical perspective can be found in Burns et al. (2019), so we cover only the basics here. Generically, AO refers to a technology that dynamically compensates for wavefront aberrations in an imaging system, including microscopes, telescopes, and ophthalmoscopes. Within the retinal imaging domain there are three classes of AO systems: AO-fundus imaging, adaptive optics optical coherence tomography (AOOCT), and adaptive optics scanning laser ophthalmoscopy (AOSLO). Most operate in a similar fashion, which is to measure the eye's monochromatic aberrations using a wavefront sensor (typically a Shack–Hartmann design) and then correct these aberrations using a deformable mirror or other active optical element. While wavefront-sensorless approaches have been explored (Hofer et al. 2011; Wong et al. 2015), they have yet to become mainstream in the AO community. AO retinal imaging systems achieve nearly diffraction-limited resolution of the living retina in humans, allowing resolution of individual rods (Dubra et al. 2011), cones (Williams 2011), ganglion cells (Liu et al. 2017; Rossi et al. 2017), retinal pigmented epithelium (RPE) cells (Liu et al. 2018; Bower et al. 2021), and macrophages and hyalocytes (Hammer et al. 2020a,b; Migacz et al. 2022). Within inherited retinal degenerations, the focus has largely been on the rod and cone photoreceptors, given the relative ease with which they can be resolved. While dozens of retinal diseases have been examined using AO imaging, we highlight here a few conditions where AO imaging has provided key insights into understanding pathophysiology of the disease. In addition, we briefly examine efforts to elucidate structure–function relationships of the cone mosaic and discuss development of photoreceptor-based biomarkers and their relevance for advancing clinical trials.

IMAGING TO IMPROVE UNDERSTANDING OF PATHOPHYSIOLOGY IN DISEASE

Red-Green Color Vision Deficiency

Normal human color vision is trichromatic, with the cone mosaic being comprised of three types of cone, termed long (L), middle (M), and short-wavelength-sensitive (S) based on the region of the visible spectrum in which they show maximum sensitivity (Neitz and Neitz 2011). In fact, an AO-fundus camera was used to conduct single-cell retinal densitometry to provide direct visualization of the number and arrangement of the three cone types in small patches of retina (Roorda and Williams 1999; Hofer et al. 2005a). Subsequent AOSLO and phase-sensitive AOOCT-based methods have been developed that allow more rapid classification of cone type (Sabesan et al. 2015; Zhang et al. 2019).

This capability is now being leveraged to better understand how the cone mosaic underlies our perception of colors (Hofer et al. 2005b; Sabesan et al. 2016; Schmidt et al. 2018).

Interestingly, one of the first "clinical" applications of AO imaging was also related to color vision, namely, red-green color vision deficiency. Inherited color vision deficiency is quite common (affecting about 8% of males) and can present with a wide spectrum of clinical manifestations and severity. These defects arise due to mutations in the *OPN1LW* and *OPN1MW* opsin gene array on the X chromosome (Neitz and Neitz 2011). The milder types of red-green deficiency arise when the first two genes in the array encode spectrally distinct opsins of the same general type (i.e., L or M), resulting in a retina that contains either two types of L cone (deuteranomalous trichromacy) or two types of M cone (protanomalous trichromacy). The more severe forms of red-green deficiency arise when there is only a single functional gene in the array, which can be due to mutations within the other gene(s) in the array or a deletion of all but one of the genes in the array. The result is either deuteranopia (a single functional *OPN1LW* gene) or protanopia (a single functional *OPN1MW* gene).

The structure of the cone mosaic in individuals with red-green color vision deficiency has been extensively examined using multiple AO imaging tools. Using an AO fundus camera, it was shown that single-gene dichromats had contiguous cone mosaics of normal density (Carroll et al. 2004, 2009; Wagner-Schuman et al. 2010) —consistent with known mechanisms of gene expression within the gene array. In contrast, more recent work with phase-sensitive AOOCT reported normal cone density in individuals harboring a single *OPN1LW* or *OPN1MW* gene but altered cone mosaic geometry and frequent dark gaps in the mosaic (Zhang et al. 2021). Individuals with the Cys203Arg missense mutation in their opsin gene(s) showed reduced cone density but normal mosaic geometry, consistent with early degeneration of cones expressing Cys203Arg (Carroll et al. 2009). While AOOCT work found no difference in cone density, there was altered mosaic geometry as indicated by a reduced proportion of cones having

Cite this article as *Cold Spring Harb Perspect Med* doi: 10.1101/cshperspect.a041285

hexagonal Voronoi domains (Zhang et al. 2021). These differences between studies could be due to differences in AO imaging modality or real differences in disease mechanism between patients—regardless, this demonstrates the utility of AO imaging to explore genotype–phenotype correlations with unprecedented resolution.

Other opsin gene variants result in exon skipping (and, as a result, no functional photopigment) (Neitz et al. 2019). Imaging of these individuals reveals a Swiss cheese–like cone mosaic (Fig. 1), with dark gaps interspersed among normally appearing cones (Carroll et al. 2004). Subsequent imaging with nonconfocal (split detection) AOSLO revealed remnant cone inner segments occupying these gaps (Patterson et al. 2018). The proportion of non-waveguiding cones in the mosaic was highly variable across individuals, mirroring the normal variation in L:M cone ratio. Even brothers with the same opsin gene array showed discrepant amounts of mosaic disruption, suggesting either variable effects of cone migration accompanying foveal pit development, or a role for genetic elements outside the opsin gene array in regulating the relative expression of these genes (Patterson et al. 2018).

Achromatopsia

Achromatopsia (ACHM) is a condition in which cone function is absent or severely reduced. There can be a number of genetic causes for the disease; most involve components of the phototransduction cascade (e.g., cyclic nucleotide gated ion channel, transducin, or phosphodiesterase) but mutations in *ATF6* have also been linked to ACHM and other cone dystrophies. AO imaging revealed a common phenotype among patients with the *CNGA3* or *CNGB3* forms of ACHM—minimal photoreceptor structure at the fovea with large cone-sized gaps with interleaved rods in the parafovea (Genead et al. 2011; Merino et al. 2011). The gaps were hypothesized to represent non-waveguiding but surviving cones, which was of critical importance as gene replacement therapy was being advanced in preclinical animal models at the time. Follow-up imaging with nonconfocal (split-detection) AOSLO revealed inner segment structures occupying these gaps, all but confirming their identity as remnant cone cells (Langlo et al. 2016; Georgiou et al. 2019a). Interestingly, imaging at the fovea showed highly variable numbers of remnant cone cells across individuals (Fig. 2), which could certainly impact the potential

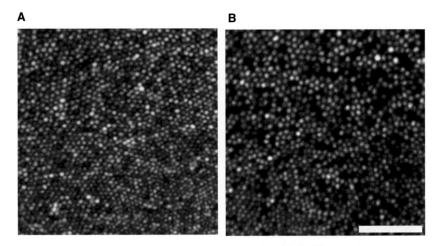

A

B

Figure 1. Disrupted cone mosaic appearance in red-green color vision deficiency. Panel *A* shows a confocal adaptive optics scanning laser ophthalmoscopy (AOSLO) image of the parafoveal cone mosaic from an individual with two *OPN1MW* genes in their opsin gene array. Panel *B* shows a confocal AOSLO image of the parafoveal cone mosaic from an individual with both an *OPN1LW* and an *OPN1MW* gene in the opsin gene array, though the *OPN1MW* gene encodes an exon-skipping haplotype. Scale bar, 50 μm.

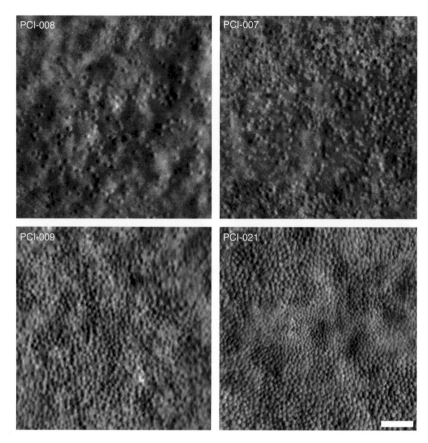

Figure 2. Variable foveal cone inner segment structure in achromatopsia (ACHM). Shown are split-detection AOSLO images from the central fovea in four individuals with *CNGB3*-associated ACHM. The number and distribution of remnant inner segments is highly variable within and between individuals (see text). Scale bar, 50 μm. (Figure reprinted from Langlo et al. 2016 under a Creative Commons Attribution-NonCommercial-NoDerivatives 4.0 International License.)

response to therapeutic intervention. Further AOSLO studies have shown relatively stable cone structure over time (Langlo et al. 2017), and a high degree of interocular symmetry of remnant cone structure within individuals (Litts et al. 2020)—both representing important findings as it relates to treatment potential in ACHM.

While individuals with the other genetic forms of ACHM generally present with similar clinical phenotypes, AOSLO has revealed marked differences in the underlying cone mosaic in these cases. For example, patients with *GNAT2*-associated ACHM have surprisingly well-preserved cone structure (Georgiou et al. 2020), which seems to correlate with residual cone function (Stockman et al. 2007). Conversely, there is

near absence of cone structure in all patients with *ATF6*-associated ACHM (Mastey et al. 2019). Finally, individuals with *PDE6C*-associated ACHM show a slowly progressive maculopathy and little residual macular cone structure into adulthood (Georgiou et al. 2019b). The ability to map high-resolution genotype–phenotype correlations within ACHM not only advances understanding of mechanism but suggests variable therapeutic potential across individuals.

Albinism

While it occupies a small portion of the retinal area, the various anatomical specializations of the fovea support high acuity vision. Elucidating the developmental origins of the primate fovea has been challenging, as primates are the only mammals with a fovea. However, studying foveal structure and function in patients with altered foveal development could provide some insights into normal foveal development. One such disorder is albinism—an inherited disorder that disrupts melanin biosynthesis and presents with hypopigmentation of the skin, hair, and/or eyes. Regardless of the genetic type, all forms of albinism are associated with foveal hypoplasia and other structural abnormalities of the visual system (e.g., iris transillumination, macular translucency, and aberrant decussation at the optic chiasm). In addition, patients with albinism often have moderate to severe nystagmus and reductions in visual acuity. Visual acuity can range from as good as 20/25 down to 20/200 (Summers 1996). Of particular interest has been examining how disruptions in foveal structure correlate with visual function. Many studies have shown that the severity of foveal hypoplasia does scale with the reduction in acuity, though there can be significant overlap in acuity for individuals with very similar foveal morphology (Thomas et al. 2011). Moreover, many individuals with poorly defined foveal pits can have relatively preserved visual acuity (Harvey et al. 2006). This motivated studies with AOSLO to map the cone mosaic topography in individuals with albinism. Surprisingly, a strong link between peak cone density and visual acuity has not been observed (Wilk et al. 2014), which suggests that post-receptoral defects in foveal cone pathways may be disrupted. Future work using AO-based acuity methods could be used to evaluate the integrity of the 1:1 midget connectivity in the albinotic fovea (Rossi and Roorda 2010).

IMAGING STRUCTURE–FUNCTION CORRELATIONS OF THE CONE MOSAIC

Retinitis Pigmentosa

Primary photoreceptor degenerations cause progressive dysfunction and death of photoreceptors; when rods are affected primarily, the condition is called rod-cone degeneration or retinitis pigmentosa (RP), while cone dystrophy or cone-rod dystrophy describes photoreceptor degenerations that affect cones to a greater extent than rods. To date mutations in over 300 genes have been associated with photoreceptor degeneration (sph.uth.edu/retnet/sum-dis.htm, accessed April 24, 2022). Many genes associated with photoreceptor degeneration encode proteins that are expressed in both rods and cones at the photoreceptor connecting cilium, a region that is critical for transport of proteins from the nucleus to the outer segment where phototransduction occurs (Shamseldin et al. 2020, 2022; Chandra et al. 2022). Other genes associated with RP encode proteins that are essential for phototransduction and are expressed exclusively in rods, such as *RHO* (OMIM Gene/Locus MIM number: 180380), which encodes rhodopsin; in *RHO*-related RP, cones eventually degenerate even though they do not express the mutated gene (Narayan et al. 2016). A number of studies have used AO imaging to examine photoreceptor structure in patients with RP, revealing abnormalities of the foveal cone mosaic despite normal central function and normal OCT appearance in many eyes (Gale et al. 2016; Sun et al. 2016; Kortuem et al. 2022). Nonconfocal techniques, like split-detection AOSLO, permits disambiguation of cone from rod photoreceptors in parafoveal images, which is especially important in RP as degenerating cells can have absent or abnormal reflectivity profiles (Kortuem et al. 2022). Of great importance for emerging trials in RP and other disorders is advancing robust biomarkers of photoreceptor structure and function, although there can often be disconnects between structural and functional measures (Sahel et al. 2021). AOSLO has been used to compare cone structure and function in eyes with RP associated with *RHO*, a primary phototransduction gene expressed only in rods, with eyes that have mutations in *RPGR* (OMIM Gene/Locus MIM number: 312620), a gene expressed at the connecting cilium of both rods and cones (Foote et al. 2020). AO microperimetry was used to probe visual sensitivity of cones in patients with *RHO*- and *RPGR*-related RP and revealed reduced sensitivity per cone in the eyes with *RPGR*-related RP (Fig. 3). The results demonstrated differences in cone sensitiv-

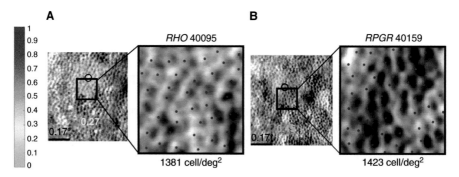

Figure 3. Similar cone density in retinal regions with different adaptive optics microperimetry (AOMP)-derived sensitivity threshold. Shown are adaptive optics scanning laser ophthalmoscopy (AOSLO) split-detection images from two different patients with the threshold values superimposed as color-coded circle (color scale bar provided to the *left*). The open black circle indicates the actual stimulus size, and individual cones are marked in red within the *inset* images. The image in panel *A* is from a patient with an *RHO* mutation (AOSLO image from 3.6° eccentricity), while the image in panel *B* is from a patient with an *RPGR* mutation (AOSLO image from 1.1° eccentricity). Retinal sensitivity-threshold values in color-coded circles are shaded from green (normal) to red (stimulus not seen) based on the thresholds measured at each location. Scale bar, 0.17°. (Figure reprinted from Foote et al. 2020 under a Creative Commons Attribution-NonCommercial-NoDerivatives 4.0 International License.)

ity among different mechanisms of rod-cone degeneration and provide evidence that cone function may be more affected than can be predicted by structural measures alone. Treatments for RP associated with genes expressed at the connecting cilium (and expressed by both rods and cones) may be more likely to not only delay progressive degeneration and vision loss, but may improve visual function if partially degenerated photoreceptors can be treated successfully.

Choroideremia

Choroideremia is an X-linked retinal degeneration that causes progressive loss of night vision, followed by loss of peripheral vision, with eventual loss of central vision and visual acuity. Despite being described in the late 1800s, the mechanism of retinal degeneration in choroideremia is not fully understood (Barnard et al. 2014). The *CHM* gene (OMIM Gene/Locus MIM number: 300390) encodes rab escort protein 1 (REP1), which is involved in intracellular vesicle trafficking and is expressed in all cells (Barnard et al. 2014). However, genetic mutations in the *CHM* gene cause choroideremia without causing adverse effects in any non-ocu-

lar cells, perhaps because there is a similar protein, REP2, which can compensate for the lack of REP1 in cells outside the eye (Barnard et al. 2014). Since REP1 is expressed in all cells, the primary cell affected by mutations in the *CHM* gene is unclear. The earliest symptoms are night blindness; some reports have shown rod dysfunction as the earliest manifestation (Jacobson et al. 2006), while other reports have shown loss of RPE cells or reduced choriocapillaris perfusion as the earliest findings visible using structural imaging (Morgan et al. 2014; Foote et al. 2019b). As shown in Figure 4, AOSLO images have demonstrated persistence of cone structure beyond the margins of preserved RPE cells (Foote et al. 2019b). AOSLO microperimetry has demonstrated visual loss in outer retinal tubulations that retained outer nuclear layer and inner segment structures but with RPE cell and photoreceptor outer segment loss (Tuten et al. 2019). These reports are not incompatible, and likely reflect early functional loss of rod sensitivity followed by sequential RPE cell, then photoreceptor outer segment, and finally inner segment, loss. AOSLO studies in choroideremia have demonstrated cone mosaic integrity in 8/9 eyes 1 mo after subretinal injection of AAV-mediated gene replacement, although foveal cone loss occurred

R1 = 4.12%   R4 = 14.6%   R1 = 3.79%   R4 = 18.5%

R2 = 5.12%   R5 = 25.7%   R2 = 4.77%   R5 = 28.2%

R3 = 9.05%   R6 = 34.8%   R3 =12.3%   R6 = 34.4%

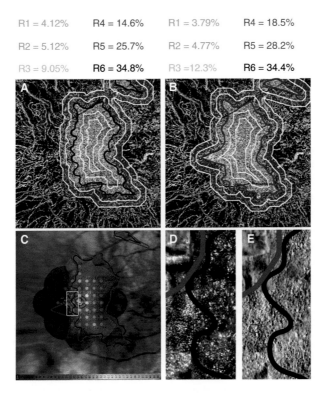

Figure 4. Assessing structure and function in a patient with choroideremia. Panel *A* shows a swept source optical coherence tomography angiography (SS-OCTA) slab extracted at the level of the choriocapillaris and demarcates the flow void (shown as colored pixels and expressed as %) in regions 1–6 (R1–R6). The area of retained retinal pigment epithelium (RPE) (assessed from short-wavelength autofluorescence images) is outlined in black. Panel *B* shows an SS-OCTA slab extracted at the level of the choriocapillaris and demarcates the flow void (expressed as %) in regions R1–R6. The area of preserved RPE (assessed from SS-OCT images) autofluorescence is outlined in blue. Panel *C* shows a map of retinal sensitivity from fundus-guided microperimetry, with the boundaries of retained RPE shown in black (short-wavelength autofluorescence [SW-AF]) and blue (SS-OCT). Panels *D* and *E* show adaptive optics scanning laser ophthalmoscopy (AOSLO) images from the region in *C* marked by the white rectangle. Panel *D* was acquired using confocal AOSLO, while panel *E* was acquired using split-detector AOSLO. For *D* and *E*, red boxes indicate select regions where cone spacing was measured. (Figure reprinted from Foote et al. 2019b under a Creative Commons Attribution-NonCommercial-NoDerivatives 4.0 International License.)

in 1/9 treated eyes (Morgan et al. 2022). The cellular-level resolution afforded by AOSLO images demonstrated that subfoveal delivery of gene therapy can be performed without accelerating foveal cone loss in choroideremia.

However, even high-resolution, multimodal imaging approaches are not able to identify the earliest changes caused by *CHM* mutations that result in measurable reductions in visual function or cellular structures. This lack of mechanistic understanding on a cellular level has complicated efforts to develop treatments for choroideremia. Advances in RPE structural

imaging using AO are a step toward this goal (Bower et al. 2021), but to date have not demonstrated RPE cellular function. Future work to develop methods that can provide measures of cellular metabolism would be invaluable to improve understanding of mechanisms that lead to photoreceptor dysfunction and degeneration. Visualizing cellular dysfunction in living eyes could identify targets for therapeutic intervention, characterize outcome measures of their safety and efficacy, and accelerate development of treatment for these blinding diseases.

CURRENT AND EMERGING PHOTORECEPTOR-BASED BIOMARKERS

Structural

The single-cell resolution provided by AOSLO and other AO-based imaging tools lends itself to a myriad of quantitative metrics to describe cellular phenotypes. Metrics used to describe the cone mosaic generally include density, spacing, and regularity (Rodieck 1991; Martin et al. 2000; Li and Roorda 2007; Chui et al. 2008; Kram et al. 2010; Li et al. 2010; Dees et al. 2011; Lombardo et al. 2014; Cooper et al. 2016b; Wells-Gray et al. 2016; Keeley et al. 2020). Just as variable are the methods used to extract these metrics—for example, cone-spacing methods include use of the direct Fourier transform of an image of a contiguous mosaic to extract modal spacing (Cooper et al. 2013), direct calculation of cone spacing from a list of cone coordinates (Cooper et al. 2016b), or use of the density recovery profile (Rodieck 1991; Foote et al. 2019a). Even with density, there can be differences in the size/shape of the area used to integrate. There is a great need to specify precise methods and details regarding mosaic quantification to assist comparison of results across different studies. In addition, there have been numerous studies examining the reliability, reproducibility, and repeatability of various cone metrics, which may not be the same for different imaging modalities or measurement techniques.

The first example of using a quantitative cone mosaic metric in a clinical trial was a sub-study of a multicenter trial of ciliary neurotrophic factor (CNTF), a neurotrophic factor that could potentially slow retinal degeneration progression (LaVail et al. 1992; MacDonald et al. 2007). In this trial, each patient had one eye randomly assigned to receive sustained-release CNTF, with the fellow eye receiving sham treatment. While no changes in standard clinical outcome measures were observed over 24 mo (e.g., visual acuity, visual field sensitivity, or ERG response), the sham-treated eyes showed a significantly larger decrease in cone density over time compared to the CNTF-treated eyes (Talcott et al. 2011). This was the first demonstration of the potential use of AOSLO imaging as a valuable measure for assessing treatment response. This study provided strong rationale for use of photoreceptor-based biomarkers in treatment trials, and the number of studies including AO imaging as an ancillary outcome measure has increased over time. For example, a group of academic institutions with AOSLO capability will support AOSLO imaging as an ancillary study to an NIH-sponsored randomized controlled trial of N-acetylcysteine in patients with RP (UG1EY033262) (Kong et al. 2021). To control for differences between AOSLO systems, the investigators collaborated with researchers at the U.S. Food and Drug Administration who created a phantom to calibrate the scale of images acquired using different systems (Kedia et al. 2019; Lamont et al. 2020). Certified, trained personnel at each site will image the phantom eye before each patient-imaging session, acquire images, assemble them into montages, and submit them to a cloud-based portal for review and grading by trained graders at the AOSLO Reading Center. The project should provide proof-of-concept and validation of the infrastructure and methods needed to accelerate the adoption of AOSLO-based measures of retinal structure as outcome measures of safety and/or efficacy for randomized clinical trials.

As mentioned above, there are many metrics that can be used to describe the cone mosaic. It has been shown that not all metrics are equally sensitive in detecting changes in the mosaic (Cooper et al. 2016b). For example, spacing measures (e.g., nearest neighbor distance or intercone distance) are very robust metrics—meaning that they do not change in response to small changes in cell numbers. This can be a strength if the method used to identify cells has a known level of uncertainty, but it comes with the cost of being insensitive to real loss of small numbers of cells. Conversely, regularity-based metrics can be hyper-sensitive to small changes in the mosaic and may flag cell identification errors as bona fide changes in cell structure. In addition, it is important to be aware of how distortions in AOSLO images can impact metrics (Cooper et al. 2016a), though higher-speed AO devices can mitigate this (Rha et al. 2006; Lu et al. 2017, 2018; Pandiyan et al. 2020a). The above are important factors to consider when choosing a metric for a

Cite this article as *Cold Spring Harb Perspect Med* doi: 10.1101/cshperspect.a041285

trial and should be balanced against the rate of cell loss in the pathology being studied, as well as the degree and type of changes in the mosaic expected from the treatment/intervention.

Functional

While assessing the number and distribution of photoreceptors in an AO image is the most obvious approach to assessing the health of the cone mosaic, additional information can be gleaned from examining the intensity of the cones in the image. Both rod and cone photoreceptors vary in their reflectivity over space and time (Zhang et al. 2006; Rossi and Roorda 2010; Cooper et al. 2011). Cones also show reduced intensity in AO images with eccentric pupil illumination (Roorda and Williams 2002; Gao et al. 2008), which is due to the Stiles–Crawford effect and known waveguiding mechanisms of the cells. However, it is the changes in reflectivity due to disease that can be most informative. For example, as discussed above, some forms of red–green color vision deficiency can have a subset of cones that appear dark on AO fundus or AOSLO images. These gaps were shown to be nonfunctional using AO-microperimetry (Makous et al. 2006) and suggested a link between cone reflectivity and cone function. Such a link is further supported by findings in ACHM, where patients with *CNGB3*- and *CNGA3*-associated ACHM have no cone function, and universally reduced or absent reflectivity of their remaining cones on AO imaging (Langlo et al. 2016, 2017). Conversely, individuals with *GNAT2*-associated ACHM show greater cone reflectivity together with measurable residual cone function (Dubis et al. 2014; Georgiou et al. 2020). However, it is important to recall the cases of dark cones in many retinas that show normal function, termed "dysflective" cones (Tu et al. 2017; Duncan and Roorda 2019; Bensinger et al. 2022). As such, cone reflectivity cannot be taken as a universal biomarker for cone function—although continued efforts to map structure–function correlations in other retinal diseases are needed.

The above examples all relate to static assessment of cone reflectivity. More recent studies have explored the temporal variability of cone reflectance as another measure of cone function. For example, variability in cone reflectance over time has been linked to shedding and regeneration of cone outer segments (Jonnal et al. 2010; Pircher et al. 2010; Kocaoglu et al. 2016). Perhaps most exciting are the changes in reflectivity that occur after exposure to visual stimuli. These optical responses are believed to be caused by changes induced by phototransduction processes (Hillmann et al. 2016; Cooper et al. 2017; Zhang et al. 2017). With membrane potential changes and osmosis that accompany phototransduction, there is an initial rapid contraction of the outer segment followed by a slower expansion. These cellular changes are detectable as a change in the optical phase of the OCT signal between the cone inner segments and tips of the outer segments (Pandiyan et al. 2020a). This response is conceptually analogous to the electroretinogram (a classical clinical measure of photoreceptor function) and has thus been referred to as the optoretinogram (Azimipour et al. 2020; Pandiyan et al. 2020a,b). This technique enables direct comparison of photoreceptor structure and function on a single-cell scale. While this would be especially valuable in assessing photoreceptor function in response to treatment, it would also be highly valuable in mapping disease progression in patients with retinal degeneration. This latter possibility was recently demonstrated using phase-sensitive AOOCT in patients with RP (Lassoued et al. 2021). They found that the optoretinographic responses decreased with increasing RP severity, but also that in regions where cones were present and apparently normal in number, their function was compromised. This is consistent with the known sequence of cone degeneration in RP (Milam et al. 1998), and illustrates the advantages over relying solely on structural AO assessments.

CONCLUDING REMARKS

While AO-based imaging devices currently exist primarily as academic research tools, as clinical trials focused on treatments for inherited retinal degenerations become more frequent, concurrent incorporation of AO imaging is necessary to support development and advancement of novel therapies. One of the main challenges to widespread use of AO imaging techniques is the relative absence of standardized hardware. While a commercial AO fundus camera is available, it lacks the ability to resolve rods and foveal cones, though its high speed is a benefit when imaging patients with nystagmus and/or unstable fixation. There is also a large data processing and analysis burden associated with a technique that allows visualization of tens of thousands of cells. Advances in automated image processing pipelines show great promise in reducing this burden (Huang et al. 2012; Chen et al. 2016; Salmon et al. 2017, 2021; Davidson et al. 2018b). In addition, automated image analysis tools (including machine learning approaches) can help reduce the level of expertise needed to accurately analyze large volumes of AO images (Cunefare et al. 2016, 2018, 2019; Bergeles et al. 2017; Davidson et al. 2018a). Continued efforts in this regard will help make AO imaging technology more accessible, and thus easier to integrate into future clinical trials.

ACKNOWLEDGMENTS

The authors thank Dr. Niamh Wynne and Owen Bowie for helpful comments on an earlier version of this manuscript.

REFERENCES

Abràmoff MD, Garvin MK, Sonka M. 2010. Retinal imaging and image analysis. *IEEE Rev Biomed Eng* **3:** 169–208. doi:10.1109/RBME.2010.2084567

Azimipour M, Valente D, Vienola KV, Werner JS, Zawadzki RJ, Jonnal RS. 2020. Optoretinogram: optical measurement of human cone and rod photoreceptor responses to light. *Opt Lett* **45:** 4658–4661. doi:10.1364/OL.398868

Barnard AR, Groppe M, MacLaren RE. 2014. Gene therapy for choroideremia using an adeno-associated viral (AAV) vector. *Cold Spring Harb Perspect Med* **5:** a017293. doi:10.1101/cshperspect.a017293

Bensinger E, Wang Y, Roorda A. 2022. Patches of dysflective cones in eyes with no known disease. *Invest Ophthalmol Vis Sci* **63:** 29. doi:10.1167/iovs.63.1.29

Bergeles C, Dubis AM, Davidson B, Kasilian M, Kalitzeos A, Carroll J, Dubra A, Michaelides M, Ourselin S. 2017. Unsupervised identification of cone photoreceptors in non-confocal adaptive optics scanning light ophthalmoscope images. *Biomed Opt Express* **8:** 3081–3094. doi:10.1364/BOE.8.003081

Bower AJ, Liu T, Aguilera N, Li J, Liu J, Lu R, Giannini JP, Huryn LA, Dubra A, Liu Z, et al. 2021. Integrating adaptive optics-SLO and OCT for multimodal visualization of the human retinal pigment epithelial mosaic. *Biomed Opt Express* **12:** 1449–1466. doi:10.1364/BOE.413438

Burns SA, Elsner AE, Sapoznik KA, Warner RL, Gast TJ. 2019. Adaptive optics imaging of the human retina. *Prog Retin Eye Res* **68:** 1–30. doi:10.1016/j.preteyeres.2018.08.002

Carroll J, Neitz M, Hofer H, Neitz J, Williams DR. 2004. Functional photoreceptor loss revealed with adaptive optics: an alternate cause of color blindness. *Proc Natl Acad Sci* **101:** 8461–8466. doi:10.1073/pnas.0401440101

Carroll J, Baraas RC, Wagner-Schuman M, Rha J, Siebe CA, Sloan C, Tait DM, Thompson S, Morgan JI, Neitz J, et al. 2009. Cone photoreceptor mosaic disruption associated with Cys203Arg mutation in the M-cone opsin. *Proc Natl Acad Sci* **106:** 20948–20953. doi:10.1073/pnas.0910128106

Chandra B, Tung ML, Hsu YN, Scheetz T, Sheffield VC. 2022. Retinal ciliopathies through the lens of Bardet-Biedl syndrome: past, present and future. *Prog Retin Eye Res* **89:** 101035. doi:10.1016/j.preteyeres.2021.101035

Chen M, Cooper RF, Han GK, Gee J, Brainard DH, Morgan JI. 2016. Multi-modal automatic montaging of adaptive optics retinal images. *Biomed Opt Express* **7:** 4899–4918. doi:10.1364/BOE.7.004899

Chui TYP, Song HX, Burns SA. 2008. Adaptive-optics imaging of human cone photoreceptor distribution. *J Opt Soc Am A Opt Image Sci Vis* **25:** 3021–3029. doi:10.1364/JOSAA.25.003021

Cooper RF, Dubis AM, Pavaskar A, Rha J, Dubra A, Carroll J. 2011. Spatial and temporal variation of rod photoreceptor reflectance in the human retina. *Biomed Opt Express* **2:** 2577–2589. doi:10.1364/BOE.2.002577

Cooper RF, Langlo CS, Dubra A, Carroll J. 2013. Automatic detection of modal spacing (Yellott's ring) in adaptive optics scanning light ophthalmoscope images. *Ophthalmic Physiol Opt* **33:** 540–549. doi:10.1111/opo.12070

Cooper RF, Sulai YN, Dubis AM, Chui TY, Rosen RB, Michaelides M, Dubra A, Carroll J. 2016a. Effects of intraframe distortion on measures of cone mosaic geometry from adaptive optics scanning light ophthalmoscopy. *Transl Vis Sci Technol* **5:** 10. doi:10.1167/tvst.5.1.10

Cooper RF, Wilk MA, Tarima S, Carroll J. 2016b. Evaluating descriptive metrics of the human cone mosaic. *Invest Ophthalmol Vis Sci* **57:** 2992–3001. doi:10.1167/iovs.16-19072

Cooper RF, Tuten WS, Dubra A, Brainard DH, Morgan JIW. 2017. Non-invasive assessment of human cone photoreceptor function. *Biomed Opt Express* **8:** 5098–5112. doi:10.1364/BOE.8.005098

Cunefare D, Cooper RF, Higgins B, Katz DF, Dubra A, Carroll J, Farsiu S. 2016. Automatic detection of cone photoreceptors in split detector adaptive optics scanning light ophthalmoscope images. *Biomed Opt Express* **7:** 2036–2050. doi:10.1364/BOE.7.002036

Cunefare D, Langlo CS, Patterson EJ, Blau S, Dubra A, Carroll J, Farsiu S. 2018. Deep learning based detection of cone photoreceptors with multimodal adaptive optics scanning light ophthalmoscope images of achromatopsia.

Cite this article as *Cold Spring Harb Perspect Med* doi: 10.1101/cshperspect.a041285

Biomed Opt Express **9:** 3740–3756. doi:10.1364/BOE.9
.003740

Cunefare D, Huckenpahler AL, Patterson EJ, Dubra A, Carroll J, Farsiu S. 2019. RAC-CNN: multimodal deep learning based automatic detection and classification of rod and cone photoreceptors in adaptive optics scanning light ophthalmoscope images. *Biomed Opt Express* **10:** 3815–3832. doi:10.1364/BOE.10.003815

Davidson B, Kalitzeos A, Carroll J, Dubra A, Ourselin S, Michaelides M, Bergeles C. 2018a. Automatic cone photoreceptor localisation in healthy and Stargardt afflicted retinas using deep learning. *Sci Rep* **8:** 7911. doi:10.1038/s41598-018-26350-3

Davidson B, Kalitzeos A, Carroll J, Dubra A, Ourselin S, Michaelides M, Bergeles C. 2018b. Fast adaptive optics scanning light ophthalmoscope retinal montaging. *Biomed Opt Express* **9:** 4317–4328. doi:10.1364/BOE.9
.004317

Dees EW, Dubra A, Baraas RC. 2011. Variability in parafoveal cone mosaic in normal trichromatic individuals. *Biomed Opt Express* **2:** 1351–1358. doi:10.1364/BOE.2
.001351

Dubis AM, Cooper RF, Aboshiha J, Langlo CS, Sundaram V, Liu B, Collison F, Fishman GA, Moore AT, Webster AR, et al. 2014. Genotype-dependent variability in residual cone structure in achromatopsia: towards developing metrics for assessing cone health. *Invest Ophthalmol Vis Sci* **55:** 7303–7311. doi:10.1167/iovs.14-14225

Dubra A, Sulai Y, Norris JL, Cooper RF, Dubis AM, Williams DR, Carroll J. 2011. Noninvasive imaging of the human rod photoreceptor mosaic using a confocal adaptive optics scanning ophthalmoscope. *Biomed Opt Express* **2:** 1864–1876. doi:10.1364/BOE.2.001864

Duncan JL, Roorda A. 2019. Dysflective cones. *Adv Exp Med Biol* **1185:** 133–137. doi:10.1007/978-3-030-27378-1_22

Foote KG, De la Huerta I, Gustafson K, Baldwin A, Zayit-Soudry S, Rinella N, Porco TC, Roorda A, Duncan JL. 2019a. Cone spacing correlates with retinal thickness and microperimetry in patients with inherited retinal degenerations. *Invest Ophthalmol Vis Sci* **60:** 1234–1243. doi:10.1167/iovs.18-25688

Foote KG, Rinella N, Tang J, Bensaid N, Zhou H, Zhang Q, Wang RK, Porco TC, Roorda A, Duncan JL. 2019b. Cone structure persists beyond margins of short-wavelength autofluorescence in choroideremia. *Invest Ophthalmol Vis Sci* **60:** 4931–4942. doi:10.1167/iovs.19-27979

Foote KG, Wong JJ, Boehm AE, Bensinger E, Porco TC, Roorda A, Duncan JL. 2020. Comparing cone structure and function in *RHO*- and *RPGR*- associated retinitis pigmentosa. *Invest Ophthalmol Vis Sci* **61:** 42. doi:10
.1167/iovs.61.4.42

Gale MJ, Feng S, Titus HE, Smith TB, Pennesi ME. 2016. Interpretation of flood-illuminated adaptive optics images in subjects with retinitis pigmentosa. *Adv Exp Med Biol* **854:** 291–297. doi:10.1007/978-3-319-17121-0_39

Gao W, Cense B, Zhang Y, Jonnal RS, Miller DT. 2008. Measuring retinal contributions to the optical Stiles-Crawford effect with optical coherence tomography. *Opt Express* **16:** 6486–6501. doi:10.1364/OE.16.006486

Genead MA, Fishman GA, Rha J, Dubis AM, Bonci DM, Dubra A, Stone EM, Neitz M, Carroll J. 2011. Photoreceptor structure and function in patients with congenital

achromatopsia. *Invest Ophthalmol Vis Sci* **52:** 7298–7308.
doi:10.1167/iovs.11-7762

Georgiou M, Litts KM, Kalitzeos A, Langlo CS, Kane T, Singh N, Kassilian M, Hirji N, Kumaran N, Dubra A, et al. 2019a. Adaptive optics retinal imaging in *CNGA3*-associated achromatopsia: retinal characterization, interocular symmetry, and intrafamilial variability. *Invest Ophthalmol Vis Sci* **60:** 383–396. doi:10.1167/iovs.18-25880

Georgiou M, Robson AG, Singh N, Pontikos N, Kane T, Hirji N, Ripamonti C, Rotsos T, Dubra A, Kalitzeos A, et al. 2019b. Deep phenotyping of *PDE6C*-associated achromatopsia. *Invest Ophthalmol Vis Sci* **60:** 5112–5123. doi:10
.1167/iovs.19-27761

Georgiou M, Singh N, Kane T, Robson AG, Kalitzeos A, Hirji N, Webster A, Dubra A, Carroll J, Michaelides M. 2020. Photoreceptor structure in *GNAT2*-associated achromatopsia. *Invest Ophthalmol Vis Sci* **61:** 40. doi:10.1167/iovs
.61.3.40

Hammer DX, Agrawal A, Villanueva R, Saeedi O, Liu Z. 2020a. Label-free adaptive optics imaging of human retinal macrophage distribution and dynamics. *Proc Natl Acad Sci* **117:** 30661–30669. doi:10.1073/pnas.201
0943117

Hammer DX, Liu Z, Cava J, Carroll J, Saeedi O. 2020b. On the axial location of Gunn's dots. *Am J Ophthalmol Case Rep* **19:** 100757. doi:10.1016/j.ajoc.2020.100757

Harvey PS, King RA, Summers CG. 2006. Spectrum of foveal development in albinism detected with optical coherence tomography. *J AAPOS* **10:** 237–242. doi:10.1016/j.jaapos
.2006.01.008

Hillmann D, Spahr H, Pfäffle C, Sudkamp H, Franke G, Hüttmann G. 2016. In vivo optical imaging of physiological responses to photostimulation in human photoreceptors. *Proc Natl Acad Sci* **113:** 13138–13143. doi:10.1073/pnas.1606428113

Hofer H, Carroll J, Neitz J, Neitz M, Williams DR. 2005a. Organization of the human trichromatic cone mosaic. *J Neurosci* **25:** 9669–9679. doi:10.1523/JNEUROSCI.2414-05.2005

Hofer H, Singer B, Williams DR. 2005b. Different sensations from cones with the same photopigment. *J Vis* **5:** 444–454. doi:10.1167/5.5.5

Hofer H, Sredar N, Queener H, Li C, Porter J. 2011. Wavefront sensorless adaptive optics ophthalmoscopy in the human eye. *Opt Express* **19:** 14160–14171. doi:10.1364/OE.19.014160

Huang G, Qi X, Chui TY, Zhong Z, Burns SA. 2012. A clinical planning module for adaptive optics SLO imaging. *Optom Vis Sci* **89:** 593–601. doi:10.1097/OPX
.0b013e318253e081

Jacobson SG, Cideciyan AV, Sumaroka A, Aleman TS, Schwartz SB, Windsor EA, Roman AJ, Stone EM, MacDonald IM. 2006. Remodeling of the human retina in choroideremia: rab escort protein 1 (*REP-1*) mutations. *Invest Ophthalmol Vis Sci* **47:** 4113–4120. doi:10.1167/iovs.06-0424

Jonnal RS, Besecker JR, Derby JC, Kocaoglu OP, Cense B, Gao W, Wang Q, Miller DT. 2010. Imaging outer segment renewal in living human cone photoreceptors. *Opt Express* **18:** 5257–5270. doi:10.1364/OE.18.005257

Kashani AH, Chen CL, Gahm JK, Zheng F, Richter GM, Rosenfeld PJ, Shi Y, Wang RK. 2017. Optical coherence tomography angiography: a comprehensive review of current methods and clinical applications. *Prog Retin Eye Res* **60**: 66–100. doi:10.1016/j.preteyeres.2017.07.002

Kedia N, Liu Z, Sochol RD, Tam J, Hammer DX, Agrawal A. 2019. 3-D printed photoreceptor phantoms for evaluating lateral resolution of adaptive optics systems. *Opt Lett* **44**: 1825–1828. doi:10.1364/OL.44.001825

Keeley PW, Eglen SJ, Reese BE. 2020. From random to regular: variation in the patterning of retinal mosaics. *J Comp Neurol* **528**: 2135–2160. doi:10.1002/cne.24880

Kocaoglu OP, Liu Z, Zhang F, Kurokawa K, Jonnal RS, Miller DT. 2016. Photoreceptor disc shedding in the living human eye. *Biomed Opt Express* **7**: 4554–4568. doi:10.1364/BOE.7.004554

Kong X, Trotochaud S, Naufal F, Campochiaro PA. 2021. The design and patient acceptability of NAC attack a phase-3 clinical trial for retinitis pigmentosa (RP). *Invest Ophthalmol Vis Sci* **62**: 9. doi:10.1167/iovs.62.15.9

Kortuem F, Kempf M, Kuehlewein L, Nasser F, Kortuem C, Paques M, Kohl S, Ueffing M, Wissinger B, Zrenner E, et al. 2022. Adaptive optics ophthalmoscopy in retinitis pigmentosa (RP): typical patterns. *Acta Ophthalmol* doi:10.1111/aos.15183

Kram YA, Mantey S, Corbo JC. 2010. Avian cone photoreceptors tile the retina as five independent, self-organizing mosaics. *PLoS ONE* **5**: e8992. doi:10.1371/journal.pone.0008992

Lamont AC, Restaino MA, Alsharhan AT, Liu Z, Hammer DX, Sochol RD, Agrawal A. 2020. Direct laser writing of a titanium dioxide-laden retinal cone phantom for adaptive optics-optical coherence tomography. *Opt Express* **10**: 2757–2767. doi:10.1364/OME.400450

Langlo CS, Patterson EJ, Higgins BP, Summerfelt P, Razeen MM, Erker LR, Parker M, Collison FT, Fishman GA, Kay CN, et al. 2016. Residual foveal cone structure in *CNGB3*-associated achromatopsia. *Invest Ophthalmol Vis Sci* **57**: 3984–3995. doi:10.1167/iovs.16-19313

Langlo CS, Erker LR, Parker M, Patterson EJ, Higgins BP, Summerfelt P, Razeen MM, Collison FT, Fishman GA, Kay CN, et al. 2017. Repeatability and longitudinal assessment of foveal cone structure in *CNGB3*-associated achromatopsia. *Retina* **37**: 1956–1966. doi:10.1097/IAE.0000000000001434

Lapierre-Landry M, Carroll J, Skala MC. 2018. Imaging retinal melanin: a review of current technologies. *J Biol Eng* **12**: 1–13. doi:10.1186/s13036-018-0124-5

Lassoued A, Zhang F, Kurokawa K, Liu Y, Bernucci MT, Crowell JA, Miller DT. 2021. Cone photoreceptor dysfunction in retinitis pigmentosa revealed by optoretinography. *Proc Natl Acad Sci* **118**: e2107444118. doi:10.1073/pnas.2107444118

LaVail MM, Unoki K, Yasumura D, Matthes MT, Yancopoulos GD, Steinberg RH. 1992. Multiple growth factors, cytokines, and neurotrophins rescue photoreceptors from the damaging effects of constant light. *Proc Natl Acad Sci* **89**: 11249–11253. doi:10.1073/pnas.89.23.11249

Li KY, Roorda A. 2007. Automated identification of cone photoreceptors in adaptive optics retinal images. *J Opt Soc Am A Opt Image Sci Vis* **24**: 1358–1363. doi:10.1364/JOSAA.24.001358

Li KY, Tiruveedhula P, Roorda A. 2010. Intersubject variability of foveal cone photoreceptor density in relation to eye length. *Invest Ophthalmol Vis Sci* **51**: 6858–6867. doi:10.1167/iovs.10-5499

Litts KM, Georgiou M, Langlo CS, Patterson EJ, Mastey RR, Kalitzeos A, Linderman RE, Lam BL, Fishman GA, Pennesi ME, et al. 2020. Interocular symmetry of foveal cone topography in congenital achromatopsia. *Curr Eye Res* **45**: 1257–1264. doi:10.1080/02713683.2020.1737138

Liu Z, Kurokawa K, Zhang F, Lee JJ, Miller DT. 2017. Imaging and quantifying ganglion cells and other transparent neurons in the living human retina. *Proc Natl Acad Sci* **114**: 12803–12808. doi:10.1073/pnas.1711734114

Liu Z, Tam J, Saeedi O, Hammer DX. 2018. Trans-retinal cellular imaging with multimodal adaptive optics. *Biomed Opt Express* **9**: 4246–4262. doi:10.1364/BOE.9.004246

Lombardo M, Serrao S, Lombardo G. 2014. Technical factors influencing cone packing density estimates in adaptive optics flood illuminated retinal images. *PLoS ONE* **9**: e107402. doi:10.1371/journal.pone.0107402

Lu J, Gu B, Wang X, Zhang Y. 2017. High-speed adaptive optics line scan confocal retinal imaging for human eye. *PLoS ONE* **12**: e0169358. doi:10.1371/journal.pone.0169358

Lu J, Gu B, Wang X, Zhang Y. 2018. High speed adaptive optics ophthalmoscopy with an anamorphic point spread function. *Opt Express* **26**: 14356–14374. doi:10.1364/OE.26.014356

MacDonald IM, Sauvé Y, Sieving PA. 2007. Preventing blindness in retinal disease: ciliary neurotrophic factor intraocular implants. *Can J Ophthalmol* **42**: 399–402. doi:10.3129/i07-039

Makous W, Carroll J, Wolfing JI, Lin J, Christie N, Williams DR. 2006. Retinal microscotomas revealed with adaptive-optics microflashes. *Invest Ophthalmol Vis Sci* **47**: 4160–4167. doi:10.1167/iovs.05-1195

Martin PR, Grünert U, Chan TL, Bumsted K. 2000. Spatial order in short-wavelength-sensitive cone photoreceptors: a comparative study of the primate retina. *J Opt Soc Am A Opt Image Sci Vis* **17**: 557–579. doi:10.1364/JOSAA.17.000557

Mastey RR, Georgiou M, Langlo CS, Kalitzeos A, Patterson EJ, Kane T, Singh N, Vincent A, Moore AT, Tsang SH, et al. 2019. Characterization of retinal structure in *ATF6*-associated achromatopsia. *Invest Ophthalmol Vis Sci* **60**: 2631–2640. doi:10.1167/iovs.19-27047

Merino D, Duncan JL, Tiruveedhula P, Roorda A. 2011. Observation of cone and rod photoreceptors in normal subjects and patients using a new generation adaptive optics scanning laser ophthalmoscope. *Biomed Opt Express* **2**: 2189–2201. doi:10.1364/BOE.2.002189

Migacz JV, Otero-Marquez O, Zhou R, Rickford K, Murillo B, Zhou DB, Castanos MV, Sredar N, Dubra A, Rosen RB, et al. 2022. Imaging of vitreous cortex hyalocyte dynamics using non-confocal quadrant-detection adaptive optics scanning light ophthalmoscopy in human subjects. *Biomed Opt Express* **13**: 1755–1773. doi:10.1364/BOE.449417

Milam AH, Li ZY, Fariss RN. 1998. Histopathology of the human retina in retinitis pigmentosa. *Prog Retin Eye Res* **17**: 175–205. doi:10.1016/S1350-9462(97)00012-8

Morgan JIW, Han G, Klinman E, Maguire WM, Chung DC, Maguire AM, Bennett J. 2014. High-resolution adaptive optics retinal imaging of cellular structure in choroideremia. *Invest Ophthalmol Vis Sci* **55:** 6381–6397. doi:10.1167/iovs.13-13454

Morgan JIW, Jiang YY, Vergilio GK, Serrano LW, Pearson DJ, Bennett J, Maguire AM, Aleman TS. 2022. Short-term assessment of subfoveal injection of adeno-associated virus-mediated *hCHM* gene augmentation in choroideremia using adaptive optics ophthalmoscopy. *JAMA Ophthalmol* **140:** 411–420. doi:10.1001/jamaophthalmol.2022.0158

Narayan DS, Wood JPM, Chidlow G, Casson RJ. 2016. A review of the mechanisms of cone degeneration in retinitis pigmentosa. *Acta Ophthalmol* **94:** 748–754.

Neitz J, Neitz M. 2011. The genetics of normal and defective color vision. *Vision Res* **51:** 633–651. doi:10.1016/j.visres.2010.12.002

Neitz M, Patterson SS, Neitz J. 2019. Photopigment genes, cones, and color update: disrupting the splicing code causes a diverse array of vision disorders. *Curr Opin Behav Sci* **30:** 60–66. doi:10.1016/j.cobeha.2019.05.004

Pandiyan VP, Jiang XT, Maloney-Bertelli A, Kuchenbecker JA, Sharma U, Sabesan R. 2020a. High-speed adaptive optics line-scan OCT for cellular-resolution optoretinography. *Biomed Opt Express* **11:** 5274–5296. doi:10.1364/BOE.399034

Pandiyan VP, Maloney-Bertelli A, Kuchenbecker JA, Boyle KC, Ling T, Chen ZC, Park BH, Roorda A, Palanker D, Sabesan R. 2020b. The optoretinogram reveals the primary steps of phototransduction in the living human eye. *Sci Adv* **6:** eabc1124. doi:10.1126/sciadv.abc1124

Patterson EJ, Kalitzeos A, Kasilian M, Gardner JC, Neitz J, Hardcastle AJ, Neitz M, Carroll J, Michaelides M. 2018. Residual cone structure in patients with X-linked cone opsin mutations. *Invest Ophthalmol Vis Sci* **59:** 4238–4248. doi:10.1167/iovs.18-24699

Pircher M, Kroisamer JS, Felberer F, Sattmann H, Götzinger E, Hitzenberger CK. 2010. Temporal changes of human cone photoreceptors observed in vivo with SLO/OCT. *Biomed Opt Express* **2:** 100–112. doi:10.1364/BOE.2.000100

Rha J, Jonnal RS, Thorn KE, Qu J, Zhang Y, Miller DT. 2006. Adaptive optics flood-illumination camera for high speed retinal imaging. *Opt Express* **14:** 4552–4569. doi:10.1364/OE.14.004552

Rodieck RW. 1991. The density recovery profile: a method for the analysis of points in the plane applicable to retinal studies. *Vis Neurosci* **6:** 95–111. doi:10.1017/S0952523800001049X

Roorda A, Williams DR. 1999. The arrangement of the three cone classes in the living human eye. *Nature* **397:** 520–522. doi:10.1038/17383

Roorda A, Williams DR. 2002. Optical fiber properties of individual human cones. *J Vis* **2:** 404–412. doi:10.1167/2.5.4

Rossi EA, Roorda A. 2010. The relationship between visual resolution and cone spacing in the human fovea. *Nat Neurosci* **13:** 156–157. doi:10.1038/nn.2465

Rossi EA, Granger CE, Sharma R, Yang Q, Saito K, Schwarz C, Walters S, Nozato K, Zhang J, Kawakami T, et al. 2017. Imaging individual neurons in the retinal ganglion cell layer of the living eye. *Proc Natl Acad Sci* **114:** 586–591. doi:10.1073/pnas.1613445114

Sabesan R, Hofer H, Roorda A. 2015. Characterizing the human cone photoreceptor mosaic via dynamic photopigment densitometry. *PLoS ONE* **10:** e0144891. doi:10.1371/journal.pone.0144891

Sabesan R, Schmidt BP, Tuten WS, Roorda A. 2016. The elementary representation of spatial and color vision in the human retina. *Sci Adv* **2:** e1600797. doi:10.1126/sciadv.1600797

Sahel JA, Grieve K, Pagot C, Authié C, Mohand-Said S, Paques M, Audo I, Becker K, Chaumet-Riffaud A-E, Azoulay L, et al. 2021. Assessing photoreceptor status in retinal dystrophies: from high-resolution imaging to functional vision. *Am J Ophthalmol* **230:** 12–47. doi:10.1016/j.ajo.2021.04.013

Salmon AE, Cooper RF, Langlo CS, Baghaie A, Dubra A, Carroll J. 2017. An automated reference frame selection (ARFS) algorithm for cone imaging with adaptive optics scanning light ophthalmoscopy. *Transl Vis Sci Technol* **6:** 9. doi:10.1167/tvst.6.2.9

Salmon AE, Cooper RF, Chen M, Higgins B, Cava JA, Chen N, Follett HM, Gaffney M, Heitkotter H, Heffernan E, et al. 2021. Automated image processing pipeline for adaptive optics scanning light ophthalmoscopy. *Biomed Opt Express* **12:** 3142–3168. doi:10.1364/BOE.418079

Sauer L, Vitale AS, Modersitzki NK, Bernstein PS. 2021. Fluorescence lifetime imaging ophthalmoscopy: autofluorescence imaging and beyond. *Eye* **35:** 93–109. doi:10.1038/s41433-020-01287-y

Schmidt BP, Sabesan R, Tuten WS, Neitz J, Roorda A. 2018. Sensations from a single M-cone depend on the activity of surrounding S-cones. *Sci Rep* **8:** 8561. doi:10.1038/s41598-018-26754-1

Schmitz-Valckenberg S, Holz FG, Bird AC, Spaide RF. 2008. Fundus autofluorescence imaging: review and perspectives. *Retina* **28:** 385–409. doi:10.1097/IAE.0b013e31816a4907

Shamseldin HE, Shaheen R, Ewida N, Bubshait DK, Alkuraya H, Almardawi E, Howaidi A, Sabr Y, Abdalla EM, Alfaifi AY, et al. 2020. The morbid genome of ciliopathies: an update. *Genet Med* **22:** 1051–1060. doi:10.1038/s41436-020-0761-1

Shamseldin HE, Shaheen R, Ewida N, Bubshait DK, Alkuraya H, Almardawi E, Howaidi A, Sabr Y, Abdalla EM, Alfaifi AY, et al. 2022. The morbid genome of ciliopathies: an update. *Genet Med* **24:** 966. doi:10.1016/j.gim.2022.01.019

Spaide RF, Fujimoto JG, Waheed NK, Sadda SR, Staurenghi G. 2018. Optical coherence tomography angiography. *Prog Retin Eye Res* **64:** 1–55. doi:10.1016/j.preteyeres.2017.11.003

Stockman A, Smithson HE, Michaelides M, Moore AT, Webster AR, Sharpe LT. 2007. Residual cone vision without α-transducin. *J Vis* **7:** 8. doi:10.1167/7.4.8

Summers CG. 1996. Vision in albinism. *Trans Am Ophthalmol Soc* **94:** 1095–1155.

Sun LW, Johnson RD, Langlo CS, Cooper RF, Razeen MM, Russillo MC, Dubra A, Connor TB Jr, Han D, Pennesi ME, et al. 2016. Assessing photoreceptor structure in retinitis pigmentosa and Usher syndrome. *Invest Ophthalmol Vis Sci* **57:** 2428–2442. doi:10.1167/iovs.15-18246

Talcott KE, Ratnam K, Sundquist S, Lucero AS, Lujan BJ, Tao W, Porco TC, Roorda A, Duncan JL. 2011. Longitudinal study of cone photoreceptors during retinal degeneration and in response to ciliary neurotrophic factor treatment. *Invest Ophthalmol Vis Sci* **52:** 2219–2226. doi:10.1167/iovs.10-6479

Thomas MG, Kumar A, Mohammad S, Proudlock FA, Engle EC, Andrews C, Chan WM, Thomas S, Gottlob I. 2011. Structural grading of foveal hypoplasia using spectral-domain optical coherence tomography: a predictor of visual acuity? *Ophthalmology* **118:** 1653–1660. doi:10.1016/j.ophtha.2011.01.028

Tu JH, Foote KG, Lujan BJ, Ratnam K, Qin J, Gorin MB, Cunningham ET Jr, Tuten WS, Duncan JL, Roorda A. 2017. Dysflective cones: visual function and cone reflectivity in long-term follow-up of acute bilateral foveolitis. *Am J Ophthalmol Case Rep* **7:** 14–19. doi:10.1016/j.ajoc.2017.04.001

Tuten WS, Vergilio GK, Young GJ, Bennett J, Maguire AM, Aleman TS, Brainard DH, Morgan JIW. 2019. Visual function at the atrophic border in choroideremia assessed with adaptive optics microperimetry. *Ophthalmol Retina* **3:** 888–899. doi:10.1016/j.oret.2019.05.002

Van Velthoven MEJ, Faber DJ, Verbraak FD, Van Leeuwen TG, De Smet MD. 2007. Recent developments in optical coherence tomography for imaging the retina. *Prog Retin Eye Res* **26:** 57–77. doi:10.1016/j.preteyeres.2006.10.002

Wagner-Schuman M, Neitz J, Rha J, Williams DR, Neitz M, Carroll J. 2010. Color-deficient cone mosaics associated with Xq28 opsin mutations: a stop codon versus gene deletions. *Vision Res* **50:** 2396–2402. doi:10.1016/j.visres.2010.09.015

Wells-Gray EM, Choi SS, Bries A, Doble N. 2016. Variation in rod and cone density from the fovea to the mid-periphery in healthy human retinas using adaptive optics scanning laser ophthalmoscopy. *Eye* **30:** 1135–1143. doi:10.1038/eye.2016.107

Wilk MA, McAllister JT, Cooper RF, Dubis AM, Patitucci TN, Summerfelt P, Anderson JL, Stepien KE, Costakos DM, Connor TB Jr, et al. 2014. Relationship between foveal cone specialization and pit morphology in albinism. *Invest Ophthalmol Vis Sci* **55:** 4186–4198. doi:10.1167/iovs.13-13217

Williams DR. 2011. Imaging single cells in the living retina. *Vision Res* **51:** 1379–1396. doi:10.1016/j.visres.2011.05.002

Wong KS, Jian Y, Cua M, Bonora S, Zawadzki RJ, Sarunic MV. 2015. In vivo imaging of human photoreceptor mosaic with wavefront sensorless adaptive optics optical coherence tomography. *Biomed Opt Express* **6:** 580–590. doi:10.1364/BOE.6.000580

Zhang Y, Cense B, Rha J, Jonnal RS, Gao H, Zawadzki RJ, Werner JS, Jones S, Olivier S, Miller DT. 2006. High-speed volumetric imaging of cone photoreceptors with adaptive optics spectral-domain optical coherence tomography. *Opt Express* **14:** 4380–4394. doi:10.1364/OE.14.004380

Zhang P, Zawadzki RJ, Goswami M, Nguyen PT, Yarov-Yarovoy Y, Burns ME, Pugh EN Jr. 2017. In vivo optophysiology reveals that G-protein activation triggers osmotic swelling and increased light scattering of rod photoreceptors. *Proc Natl Acad Sci* **114:** E2937–E2946.

Zhang F, Kurokawa K, Lassoued A, Crowell JA, Miller DT. 2019. Cone photoreceptor classification in the living human eye from photostimulation-induced phase dynamics. *Proc Natl Acad Sci* **116:** 7951–7956. doi:10.1073/pnas.1816360116

Zhang F, Kurokawa K, Bernucci MT, Jung HW, Lassoued A, Crowell JA, Neitz J, Neitz M, Miller DT. 2021. Revealing how color vision phenotype and genotype manifest in individual cone cells. *Invest Ophthalmol Vis Sci* **62:** 8. doi:10.1167/iovs.62.2.8

Beyond the NEI-VFQ: Recent Experience in the Development and Utilization of Patient-Reported Outcomes for Inherited Retinal Diseases

Todd Durham,[1] Judit Banhazi,[2] Francesco Patalano,[2] and Thiran Jayasundera[3]

[1]Foundation Fighting Blindness, Columbia, Maryland 21045, USA

[2]Novartis, Basel-Stadt 4056, Switzerland

[3]University of Michigan Kellogg Eye Center, Department of Ophthalmology and Visual Sciences, Ann Arbor, Michigan 48105, USA

Correspondence: tdurham@fightingblindness.org

Patient-reported outcome measures (PROMs) are tools designed to capture how a patient feels or functions, without the input or interpretation of anyone else. The earliest PROMs used in studies of inherited retinal diseases (IRDs) lack the validity required for therapy development today. The NEI-VFQ was one of the earliest PROMs developed using concept elicitation and cognitive debriefing of patients, but it lacks items that are common to patients with IRDs and it has poor measurement properties. Recent advances in PROM development include the Michigan Retinal Degeneration Questionnaire (MRDQ) and the ViSIO-PRO for nonsyndromic retinitis pigmentosa (RP), both of which have been qualitatively and quantitatively validated. As these new tools are used in clinical studies, they will generate additional evidence about their measurement characteristics. With the latest advances in PROM development for IRDs, it is now possible to move beyond the NEI-VFQ to measure what is truly important to patients.

In 1998, the National Eye Institute (NEI) first reported their development of the 51-item NEI Visual Function Questionnaire (NEI-VFQ), which was designed to understand the impacts of vision loss in 246 patients with glaucoma, diabetic retinopathy, age-related macular degeneration (AMD), cataract, cytomegalovirus retinitis, and low vision from all causes (Mangione et al. 1998a). The NEI-VFQ is an example of many patient-reported outcome measures (PROMs) that are designed to capture the "status of a patient's health condition that comes directly from the patient, without interpretation of the patient's response by a clinician or anyone else" (U.S. Department of Health and Human Services Food and Drug Administration et al. 2009). PROMs may be used to demonstrate the beneficial or harmful effects of a treatment in a clinical trial and they play an increasingly important role in health technology assessments of products (Whittal et al. 2021; Jayasundera et al. 2022). When a condition has a single concept of interest (e.g., pain intensity), a PROM may be developed to measure that single concept.

However, as suggested by the scope of the initial research for the NEI-VFQ, patients with blinding conditions have a diversity of subjective experiences. As a result, instrument developers often design PROMs to measure multiple concepts (e.g., severity of visual symptoms, difficulty performing activities of daily living) that are identified as and, thus, important to, patients. Once a PROM has been developed, researchers must consider the extent to which the content (i.e., the statements or questions about their status to which the patient responds) of the existing instrument is valid for a particular clinical study or trial population. In the case of inherited retinal diseases (IRDs), this assessment will lead to the recognition that there is no one-size-fits-all because phenotypic heterogeneity is more often the rule than the exception.

IRDs are a group of rare and blinding conditions such as syndromic and nonsyndromic retinitis pigmentosa (RP), Stargardt disease, achromatopsia, and choroideremia, which have an estimated prevalence of 1 in 3100 (Daiger et al. 2007), 1 in 10,000 (Michaelides et al. 2003), 1 in 30,000 (Sharpe et al. 1999), and 1 in 50,000 (Khan et al. 2016), respectively. Each of the IRDs is caused by pathogenic variants in 1 of 280 genes (RetNet: sph.uth.edu/retnet) and their clinical manifestations are highly variable. Photoreceptors (rods and cones) may degenerate at different rates and in different locations of the retina and these cellular changes impact vision in different ways. For example, RP is characterized by the initial loss of rods in the mid-peripheral retina followed by cones in the central retina (Fahim et al. 2000). The progressive pattern of photoreceptor loss in RP can explain the typical course of visual symptoms: the earliest is often night blindness, followed by progressive loss of peripheral vision, with central visual acuity (VA) preserved well into the advanced stages of disease. In contrast to RP, Stargardt disease initially affects the central retina with a resulting loss of VA that often progresses, at varying rates, to legal blindness (Tanna et al. 2017). Despite having typical patterns of progression, both Stargardt disease and RP have forms with early (childhood) and late (adulthood) onset. In fact, early childhood onset retinal degeneration (or Leber congenital amaurosis [LCA]) results in severe vision loss that is evident in the first few months of a child's life (Kumaran et al. 2017). The phenotypic variability within and across various IRDs, particularly with respect to ages of onset, poses a challenge for the selection of a valid PROM. The urgency of this challenge is highlighted by the product pipeline in May 2022 that has more than 35 investigational products under development for IRDs (www.fightingblindness.org/clinical-trial-pipeline).

The objectives of this narrative review are as follows: to provide a foundation of knowledge by summarizing relevant guidance and best practices on the use of PROMs in clinical trials, particularly for rare diseases; to summarize literature describing the use of existing PROMs in studies of IRDs; to highlight recent advances in the development of new PROMs; and to provide practical guidance on the selection or development of PROMs to be used in clinical trials of interventions being tested for individuals with IRDs.

REGULATORY CONSIDERATIONS FOR PROMs IN PRODUCT DEVELOPMENT

Regulatory guidance and perspectives from the U.S. Food and Drug Administration (U.S. FDA) and the European Medicines Authority (EMA) underscore the need to establish and document the content validity of a selected PROM relative to the intended clinical trial population (i.e., to establish that the instrument is "fit for purpose"). In its guidance of 2009, the FDA provided comprehensive information on how its reviewers evaluate the appropriateness of PROMs when claims generated from them are to be included in product labels (U.S. Department of Health and Human Services Food and Drug Administration et al. 2009). A recent series of workshops and guidance documents (U.S. Department of Health and Human Services Food and Drug Administration et al. 2020, 2022) on patient-focused drug development from the FDA further detail the regulatory expectations for PROMs. When included in the prescribing information, the FDA will review documentation on the target study population, the statistical role of the

PROM in the clinical trial (i.e., its relationship to other end points), the conceptual framework of the PROM (i.e., how items relate to each other, to domains, and concepts), and measurement characteristics of the selected PROM. The latter includes the content validity (e.g., how the items were generated or validated using qualitative research and whether the items are understood), the reliability and responsiveness of the instrument, and any modifications to the instrument over time.

When PROMs are to be developed de novo, the FDA guidance describes the steps required to document the instrument's characteristics starting with drafting a conceptual framework, to concept elicitation to generate relevant items (based on qualitative research among patients in the population of interest), cognitive debriefing of the draft instrument to ensure it is understood by patients, scoring algorithms, and language and cultural translation (Fig. 1). Successful PROM development requires detailed knowledge of advanced statistical and psychometric methods (Frost et al. 2007), as well as use of qualitative methods for item generation and instrument modification (Lasch et al. 2010). Whether a PROM is being developed de novo, modified from an existing instrument, or applied as is, a PROM should be shown to have four characteristics in the following priority: (1) content or qualitative validity (i.e., it measures the concepts of interest in the target population); (2) quantitative validity, defined as "concurrent validity" (the ability to differentiate known groups, like severity) and "convergent validity" (evidence of anticipated associations with other clinical measures); (3) reliability (consistency under similar conditions); and (4) sensitivity (ability to detect change). Like the FDA, the EMA emphasizes the importance of establishing the construct validity (i.e., both qualitative and quantitative validity) of a PROM prior to confirmatory studies and clarifies the distinction between health-related quality of life (HRQOL)—a broad multidimensional concept—and other PROMs that are more limited in scope (e.g., those focusing on activities of daily living, or the severity of symptoms) (European Medicines Agency 2005).

RECOMMENDATIONS TO OVERCOME CHALLENGES OF PROM SELECTION IN RARE DISEASE AND PEDIATRIC POPULATIONS

As the regulatory perspectives make clear, establishing and documenting the construct validity and measurement characteristics of PROMs require a thorough understanding of natural history of progression and numerous studies in the population of interest. It may not be easy for researchers to meet these evidence requirements for IRDs because they are rare conditions, clinically heterogeneous, often poorly understood, and affect individuals from early childhood to adulthood.

Two expert consensus documents by the International Society for Pharmacoeconomics and Outcomes Research (ISPOR) address the special challenges and practical recommendations for PROM selection in rare diseases and pediatric populations. The 2017, ISPOR report identified four main challenges of PROM selection in rare diseases, all of which apply to the IRDs: phenotypic heterogeneity within and across diseases, incomplete knowledge of the natural history of disease, large proportions of children in the population of interest, and association with progressive and disabling conditions (Benjamin et al. 2017). The consequences of these challenges are quite substantial. There is unlikely to be an appropriate existing PROM for every IRD. Further, the inability to recruit sufficient numbers of participants may call into question whether content validity can be established: achieving concept saturation—when no new information is likely to be learned with new interviews—may require at least 25 interviews (Turner-Bowker et al. 2018).

Considering the difficulty in meeting typical evidence standards for PROMs, the ISPOR task force offers several practical solutions in the context of rare diseases, including the following: use all sources of data in natural history (published and unpublished); involve patient advocacy organizations to understand natural history and design clinical studies; focus on the most common symptoms and impacts of disease, given the therapy's effects and the population of interest;

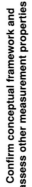
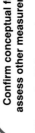

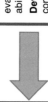
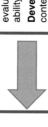
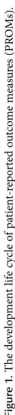

Draft instrument with validated content

Research: (1) Concept elicitation through patient interviews; (2) patient cognitive interviews on draft items to ensure the items are understood

Develop: (1) Draft items; (2) recall period, response options, and format; (3) mode/method of data collection; (4) pilot test draft instrument and compare to the hypothesized framework to establish content validity

Methods: Qualitative interviews; coding of interviews

Preliminary instrument development with a conceptual framework

Research: (1) Determine hypothesized concepts and what needs to be measured (the construct); (2) determine the intended population; (3) conduct literature and expert reviews on concepts relevant to patients

Develop: (1) Hypothesized conceptual framework (how concepts relate to each other); (2) end point model to show how the new instrument will relate to other end points in the trial

Methods: Literature search

Confirm conceptual framework and assess other measurement properties

Research: (1) Prospective study that enables evaluation of reliability, construct validity, and ability to detect change

Develop: (1) Scoring rules; (2) final instrument content, scoring, formats, and training materials

Methods: Psychometric methods to establish reliability; factor analyses to examine item discrimination; measures of association to characterize construct

Modify instrument

Develop: Modified instrument (wording, response options, mode/method of data collection); translation and cultural adaption; other modifications

Methods: Qualitative interviews

Evaluate PROM data collected from a clinical trial

Research: Clinical trial data collection and analysis to include evaluation of treatment response

Develop: Interpretation of treatment benefit in relation to the intended label claim

Methods: Use of distribution- or anchor-based methods to define a minimally important difference

Figure 1. The development life cycle of patient-reported outcome measures (PROMs).

Cite this article as *Cold Spring Harb Perspect Med* doi: 10.1101/cshperspect.a041298

seek to understand regional variations through a variety of data sources; use multiple types of measures to span diverse age groups (e.g., PROMs and observer-reported outcomes [ObsROs]); consider using item banks to match the concepts of interest and study population; use individual items or subscales of existing instruments if these can be shown to have valid content for the population; use a generic (non-disease-specific) PROM, while recognizing their lack of specificity may make them insensitive to change; and recruit a broad representation of patients (Benjamin et al. 2017).

When the target study population includes children, the measurement strategy needs to consider developmental differences and the ability of the child to reliably report the status of their health. For this situation, the proposed good research practices by another ISPOR consensus task force are invaluable (Matza et al. 2013). In general, the task force proposes that children 12–18 years of age can and should self-report their health status. To establish the content validity of a new or existing instrument in this age group, children should be involved (when necessary) in concept elicitation and cognitive debriefing. For children less than 12, it may be necessary to develop or implement a proxy report (ideally on observable impacts) or ObsRO. In both cases, the validity of the content would be developed or confirmed using a qualitative study and other aspects of instrument validity and measurement characteristics would be evaluated using quantitative studies.

IRD PROMs DEVELOPED PRIOR TO THE 2009 FDA GUIDANCE

Numerous PROMs have been developed for and applied to studies of participants with IRDs. Some of these instruments have been developed for a specific IRD while others have been more general in their scope—either developed to apply to multiple IRDs or more generally across blinding diseases. We identified and screened relevant publications in Medline/PubMed using the following search strategy: ("inherited" OR "genetic") AND ("retina" OR "retinal") AND ("patient-reported outcome" OR "PROM" OR "quality of

life" OR "QOL"). We also reviewed any individual references included in review papers and ARVO abstracts identified using a similar search strategy. What follows is a brief review of the instruments identified through this search, primarily focused on the criteria to establish content validity, namely, generation of items from qualitative research followed by cognitive debriefing.

Prem Senthil and colleagues (2017a) conducted a systematic review and quality evaluation of PROMs for retinal diseases that includes publications up to 2014. The authors identified one ophthalmic, non-disease-specific PROM, the NEI-VFQ, and 11 IRD-specific PROMs (nine for RP, one for Stargardt disease, and one for congenital stationary night blindness), including the following: MDQ (Geruschat et al. 1998), the IMQ (Turano et al. 1999), FEQ (Kennedy et al. 1977), PVFQ (Lodha et al. 2003), EDTQ (Lowe and Drasado 1992), V-ADL (Somani et al. 2006), ADVQ (Szlyk et al. 1998), DTPQ (Szlyk et al. 2001), NVQ-39 (Bijveld et al. 2013), VDQ (Sumi et al. 2000), and SMDVQ (Miedziak et al. 2000). These disease-specific instruments cover only one or two domains across mobility, health concerns, and activity limitations, while the NEI-VFQ (Mangione et al. 1998a) covers activity limitations, emotional well-being, social participation, and ocular comfort (Table 1). Of the PROMs evaluated in this review, the authors concluded that the IMQ (Turano et al. 1999), despite only measuring a single domain of mobility, was the highest quality instrument because of its use of Rasch analysis, measurement precision, item fit, and concurrent validity. As Lacy and colleagues (2020a) describe in their review paper, the existing IRD-specific PROMs were not developed from content elicited from patients, were not cognitively debriefed to ensure understanding, and were often lacking in detailed documentation. Consequently, the earliest IRD-specific instruments cannot be recommended for use in clinical trials.

Another early PROM was developed by Misajon and colleagues (2005) to perform economic evaluations of eye care programs. The resulting six-item QOL instrument (VisQOL) was devel-

Table 1. Patient-reported outcome measures (PROMs) for inherited retinal diseases (IRDs): Content generation

Instrument/objective	Methods used for item generation	Composition of sample for item generation	Cognitive debriefing	Number of items	References
Field Expander Questionnaire (FEQ)/evaluate experience with a field expander device for retinitis pigmentosa (RP) patients	Items were developed by the investigators based on clinical experience and literature review	Not applicable	None reported	25	Kennedy et al. 1977
EDTQ/assess own abilities at everyday tasks	Not available	Not available	None reported	16	Lowe and Drasdo 1992
MDQ/assess perceptions of difficulties with mobility	Items were written by the investigators based on experience	Not applicable	None reported	4	Geruschat et al. 1998
ADVQ/assess RP patients perceived functioning on selected everyday tasks	Modified from Activities of Daily Vision Scale (for individuals with cataracts), Functional Assessment Self-Report Inventory, and new items developed to target difficult activities involving peripheral vision or dim light	Not applicable	None reported	33	Szlyk et al. 1998
National Eye Institute Visual Function Questionnaire (NEI-VFQ) (51-item)/measure vision-targeted health-related quality of life (HRQOL)	Condition-specific focus groups with structured interview; coded transcriptions	Glaucoma ($N = 82$); diabetic retinopathy ($N = 58$); cataract ($N = 42$); age-related macular degeneration (AMD) ($N = 35$); cytomegalovirus (CMV) retinitis ($N = 17$); low vision (visual acuity [VA] in better eye 20/200 or worse OR < 10° field) ($N = 12$)	Yes	51	Mangione et al. 1998a
Independent Mobility Questionnaire (IMQ)/assess perceived difficulty with independent mobility	Items were developed by the investigators based on clinical experience and literature review	Not applicable	None reported	35	Turano et al. 1999
SMDVQ/assess symptoms and impacts on activities of daily living in Stargardt	Not available	Not available	Not available	35	Miedziak et al. 2000
VDQ/evaluate visual disability in daily life	Not available	Not available	Not available	35	Sumi et al. 2000

Cite this article as *Cold Spring Harb Perspect Med* doi: 10.1101/cshperspect.a041298

Instrument/purpose	Development	Population	Responsiveness	No.	Reference
NEI-VFQ (25 item)/create a short form of the 51-item NEI-VFQ	The 51-item NEI-VFQ was reduced in size to 25 items after eliminating all three items in the "expectations for future vision" subscale (based on cognitive interviews), redundant items in each subscale (as indicated by the amount of variance explained by a smaller set of items) or suggested by floor or ceiling effects	Glaucoma ($N = 77$); diabetic retinopathy ($N = 123$); cataract ($N = 93$); AMD ($N = 108$); CMV retinitis ($N = 37$); low vision (VA in better eye 20/200 or worse OR $< 10°$ field) ($N = 90$); normal reference ($N = 122$)	Yes	25	Mangione et al. 2001
DTPQ/assess daily task performance in individuals with RP	Included 33 items from the ADVQ and an additional 20 items developed by investigators to capture activities potentially problematic for individuals with RP	Not applicable	None reported	53	Szlyk et al. 2001
PVFQ/assess subjective near and global visual functioning	Not available	Not available	Not available		Lodha et al. 2003
Vision-related quality of life (VisQOL)/evaluate economic costs and benefits of programs using a multi-attribute utility measure of VisQOL	Semi-structured interviews with focus group participants	Adults with vision impairment (VA in better eye worse than 20/20; $N = 70$) due to AMD, glaucoma, Stevens–Johnson syndrome, macular dystrophy, among others; and adults with normal vision (VA in better eye of 20/20; $N = 86$)	Not reported	6	Misajon et al. 2005
Vision-related activities of daily living (V-ADL)/assess distance, intermediate, near, and peripheral tasks to evaluate spectacle-mounted prisms for patients with RP	Modified from an existing instrument, the Belfast Activities of Daily Living questionnaire for low vision	Not applicable	None reported	23	Somani et al. 2006
Night Vision Questionnaire (NVQ)-39/to assess how often patients experience night vision in various situations	Modifications of two existing instruments: 35-item instrument (IMQ by Turano et al. 1999) and an instrument to assess vision problems under low luminance in AMD	Not applicable	None reported	39	Bijveld et al. 2013

Continued

Table 1. *Continued*

Instrument/objective	Methods used for item generation	Composition of sample for item generation	Cognitive debriefing	Number of items	References
IRD item bank for QOL/explore impact of IRD across all aspects of QOL	Qualitative research	23 RP patients; 32 patients (23 RP, two cone dystrophy, seven macular dystrophy)	Yes	Total not reported	Prem Senthil et al. 2017b,c
Visual Function Scale (VFS)-Plus/evaluate vision-related activity in patients with RP	Adopt all 15 items from the VFS of the NEI-VFQ plus an additional four driving items from the NEI-VFQ to improve targeting	Not applicable; the expanded instrument was psychometrically evaluated in a retrospective analysis of 594 individuals with RP (109 dominant, 95 recessive, 39 X-linked, 190 isolated, 161 unknown or simplex)	Yes—as part of NEI-VFQ	19	Costela et al. 2020
Michigan Retinal Degeneration Questionnaire (MRDQ)/evaluate patient-reported benefits of gene therapies that correspond to measures of visual function	Semi-structured in-depth interviews guided by 86 open-ended questions in the following topic areas: symptoms prior to diagnosis, night vision problems, day vision problems, glare, photosensitivity, light/dark adaptation, photopsia, peripheral vision, mid-peripheral vision, central vision, contrast sensitivity, floaters, distance vision, color vision, headaches and eye pain, driving, and other vision problems; recorded transcripts were coded and codes were mapped to themes	26 IRD patients with a variety of IRD diagnoses—Stargardt, RP/rod-cone dystrophy [RCD], Usher syndrome/RCD, Best macular dystrophy, cone-rod dystrophy [CRD], achromatopsia, choroideremia), best corrected VA (ranging in the better seeing eye from no light perception [NLP] to 20/20), Goldmann visual field area (ranging in the better seeing eye from 0 to 20,897 mm^2), and age (ranging from 21 to 71 years)	Yes	59	Lacy et al. 2021a
Michigan Vision-Related Anxiety Questionnaire (MVAQ)/	Semi-structured in-depth interviews	26 IRD patients with a variety of IRD diagnoses (Stargardt, RP/RCD, Usher syndrome/RCD, CRD, achromatopsia, choroideremia), best corrected VA (ranging in the better seeing eye from NLP to 20/20), Goldmann visual field area (ranging in the better seeing eye from 0 to 20,897 mm^2), and age (ranging from 21 to 71 years)	Yes	14	Lacy et al. 2021b

Cite this article as *Cold Spring Harb Perspect Med* doi: 10.1101/cshperspect.a041298

Continued

Attitudes to Gene Therapy for the Eye (AGT-Eye)/"to investigate the knowledge and perceived value of gene therapy interventions that have been approved for patients with IRDs or will be approved in the future"	Generation of themes by expert clinicians that could be evaluated by patients using a Likert scale ranging from "strongly disagree" to "strongly agree"; review of proposed items by seven affected IRD patients and two parents of affected minors; revision for clarity and readability by researchers	Expert clinicians, seven affected IRD patients, and two parents of affected minors	Yes	22	Mack et al. 2021; McGuinness et al. 2022
ViSIO-PRO/evaluate RP/Leber congenital amaurosis (LCA)-specific visual impairments and impacts on vision-dependent activities of daily living (ADL)	Semi-structured qualitative interviews with thematic analysis of interview transcripts	In the USA: 16 adults, one adolescent and one child–caregiver pair with clinical and genetic diagnoses of RP with the following disease-causing genes: RPGR (*N* = 7); EYS (*N* = 3); PRPF31 (*N* = 2); USH2A (*N* = 2); RHO (*N* = 2); RPE65 (*N* = 2); In the USA, Germany, and France: seven adults, one adolescent, three children 6–11 years, five caregivers of children 3–11 years all of whom had clinical and genetic diagnoses of RPE65-associated RP/LCA; In Germany and France: nine adults, five adolescents, five children, and 11 caregivers with clinical and genetic diagnoses of RP with the following disease-causing genes: RPE65 (*N* = 11); RPGR (*N* = 5); CEP290 (*N* = 3); AIPL1 (*N* = 2); LRAT (*N* = 1); PDE6B (*N* = 1); RDH12 (*N* = 1); RP2 (*N* = 1)	Yes	49	Kay et al. 2020, 2021, 2022; Audo et al. 2021, 2022

Table 1. *Continued*

Instrument/objective	Domain/part	Items	References
Field Expander Questionnaire (FEQ)/evaluate experience with a field expander device for RP patients	Not applicable	Examples: "field expander made walking more difficult," "things to the side could be seen more easily through the device," "the device made objects appear to be farther away," "the device is cosmetically acceptable"	Kennedy et al. 1977
EDTQ/assess own abilities at everyday tasks	Visual search and mobility	Degree of difficulty: locating small article at table level; locating small article at floor level; purchasing an item alone in a small shop; purchasing an item alone in a large shop; ascending and descending unfamiliar stairs alone; crossing a road with relatively little traffic; crossing a road with frequent traffic	Lowe and Drasdo 1992
MDQ/assess perceptions of difficulties with mobility	Not applicable	"Do you primarily walk alone or with others?"; "do you use any mobility aids or devices?"; "are you satisfied with your present level of travel?"; "when walking around, do you have difficulties with avoiding obstacles in your path; identifying drop-offs; negotiating stairs; getting around office buildings, hospitals, or schools; maintaining orientation during travel; reestablishing orientation if lost?"	Geruschat et al. 1998
ADVQ/assess RP patients perceived functioning on selected everyday tasks	Activities involving central vision (10 items)	Threading a needle; reading street signs at night; reading directions on medicine bottles; reading ingredients on cans of food; reading street signs during the day; seeing faces across a street; reading ordinary newspaper print; playing cards; reading numbers on television screen; finding destination in unfamiliar buildings	Szlyk et al. 1998
	Miscellaneous (12 items)	Writing checks; engaging in physical exercise; watching a movie at a theater; using a ruler; walking outdoors during the day; preparing meals; grooming; using a screwdriver; using escalators; watching television; grocery shopping; using public transportation	

Continued

	Mobility (five items)	Finding a seat in a movie theater; finding particular items in a store; walking outdoors at night; participating in social gatherings; walking through shopping malls	Mangione et al. 1998a
	Driving (three items)	Driving at night; driving during the day; driving in unfamiliar areas	
	Negotiating steps (two items)	Walking down steps in dim light; walking down steps during daylight	
NEI-VFQ (51-item)/measure vision-targeted HRQOL	Eating meals (one item)	Eating meals	
	General health (two items)	5-level rating; 0–10 health rating	
	General vision (two items)	6-level rating; 0–10 vision rating	
	Ocular pain (two items)	Amount pain; amount time: pain	
	Near vision (seven items)	Difficulty with following: reading normal newsprint; reading small print; seeing well up close; seeing for games/cards; finding objects on crowded shelf; reading mail/bills for accuracy; shaving/styling hair/makeup	
	Distance vision (seven items)	Difficulty with following: reading street signs; going downstairs in daylight; going downstairs at night; recognizing faces from across room; seeing television programs; participating in sports or outdoor activities; going out to movies/plays/sporting events	
	Vision-specific social functioning (four items)	Difficulty with following: seeing how people react; with normal social activities; entertaining at home; visiting others	
	Vision-specific mental health (eight items)	Amount of time for following: worrying about eyesight; thinking about eyesight; frustrated due to eyesight; often irritable	
		Amount true for following: worry eyesight will cause embarrassment to self/others; irritable toward others; feel frustrated a lot of time; much less control over things	

Table 1. *Continued*

Instrument/objective	Domain/part	Items	References
	Expectations for visual function (three items)	Amount true for following: expect worse eyesight; expect better eyesight; better/worse: expectations for the next year	
	Vision-specific role functioning (five items)	Amount of time for following: accomplish less; have more help; let others do more work; limited in things I can do; limited in endurance	
	Dependency due to vision (five items)	Amount true for following: stay at home most of time; others know personal business; do not leave home alone; rely too much on others' word; need much help from others	
	Driving (four items)	Difficulty driving during daytime: in familiar places; in unfamiliar places; difficulty driving: at night; in difficult conditions	
	Peripheral vision (one item)	Difficulty noticing objects off to side	
	Color vision (one item)	Difficulty picking/matching clothes	
Independent Mobility Questionnaire (IMQ)/assess perceived difficulty with independent mobility	Not applicable	Level of difficulty you feel in the situation without any assistance: walking in familiar areas; walking in unfamiliar areas; moving about in home, work, classroom, stores, outdoors; moving about in crowded situations; walking at night; using public transportation; detecting ascending stairwells; detecting descending stairwells; walking up steps; walking down steps; stepping onto curbs; stepping off curbs; walking through doorways; walking in high-glare areas; adjusting to lighting changes during the day: indoor to outdoor, outdoor to indoor; adjusting to lighting changes at night: indoor to streetlights, streetlights to indoor; walking in dimly lit indoor areas; being aware of another person's presence; avoiding bumping into people, walls, head-height objects, shoulder-height objects, waist-height objects, knee-height objects, low-lying objects; avoiding tripping over uneven travel surfaces; moving around in social gatherings; finding restrooms in public places; seeing cars at intersection	Turano et al. 1999

Cite this article as *Cold Spring Harb Perspect Med* doi: 10.1101/cshperspect.a041298

Instrument/purpose	Domain (items)	Description/response	Reference
SMDVQ/assess symptoms and impacts on activities of daily living in Stargardt	Not available		Miedziak et al. 2000
VDQ/evaluate visual disability in daily life	Not available		Sumi et al. 2000
NEI-VFQ (25-item)/create a short form of the 51-item NEI-VFQ	General health (one item)	5-level rating	Mangione et al. 2001
	General vision (one item)	6-level rating	
	Ocular pain (two items)	Amount pain; amount time: pain	
	Near vision (three items)	Difficulty with following: reading normal newsprint; seeing well up close; finding objects on crowded shelf	
	Distance vision (three items)	Difficulty with following: reading street signs; going downstairs at night; going out to movies/plays/sporting events	
	Distance vision (three items)	Difficulty with following: reading street signs; going downstairs at night; going out to movies/plays/sporting events	
	Vision-specific social functioning (two items)	Difficulty with following: seeing how people react; visiting others	
	Vision-specific mental health (four items)	Amount of time for following: worrying about eyesight Amount true for following: worry eyesight will cause embarrassment to self/others; feel frustrated a lot of time; much less control over things	
	Vision-specific role functioning (two items)	Amount of time for following: accomplish less; limited in endurance	
	Dependency due to vision (three items)	Amount true for following: stay at home most of time; rely too much on others' word; need much help from others	
	Driving (three items)	Difficulty driving during daytime in familiar places; difficulty driving at night; in difficult conditions	
	Peripheral vision (one item)	Difficulty noticing objects off to side	
	Color vision (one item)	Difficulty picking/matching clothes	

Continued

Table 1. *Continued*

Instrument/objective	Domain/part	Items	References
DTPQ/assess daily task performance in individuals with RP	Reading; mobility; peripheral detection (a complete categorization of all items was not reported)	Ranked difficulty with the following: adjusting to daylight; carrying out activities requiring visual concentration; changing lanes in traffic; driving at night; driving during the day; driving in unfamiliar areas; eating meals; engaging in physical exercise; finding a seat in a movie theater; finding destination in unfamiliar buildings; finding particular items in a store; getting acquainted with new places; grocery shopping; grooming; judging distances; judging level of liquid; locating house or store with address number; locating items on dinner table; looking for an item in crowded drawer; noticing things to the side; participating in social gatherings; playing cards; preparing meals; reading directions on medicine bottles; reading fast-food restaurant menus; reading ingredients on canned food labels; reading numbers on a television; reading street signs at night; reading street signs during the day; reading the newspaper; recognizing faces across a street; responding to things popping into field of view; seeing moving objects when driving at night; seeing oncoming headlights or street lights when driving at night; selecting items from refrigerator; slicing food; threading a needle; tracking birds or airplanes; tracking traffic at intersection; using a ruler; using a screwdriver; using directory at shopping mall; using escalators; using public transportation; using vending machines; walking down steps during daylight; walking down steps in dim light; walking outdoors at night; walking outdoors during the day; walking through shopping malls; watching a movie at a theater; watching television; writing checks	Szlyk et al. 2001

Cite this article as *Cold Spring Harb Perspect Med* doi: 10.1101/cshperspect.a041298

Measure/purpose	Domains	Items	Reference
PVFQ/assess subjective near and global visual functioning	Near visual function, global visual function	Not available	Lodha et al. 2003
VisQOL/evaluate economic costs and benefits of programs using a multi-attribute utility measure of vision-related quality of life	Single domain: QOL	"Does my vision make it likely I will injure myself (i.e., when moving around the house, yard, neighborhood, or workplace)?"; "does my vision make it difficult to cope with the demands in my life?"; "does my vision affect my ability to have friendships?"; "do I have difficulty organizing any assistance I may need?"; "does my vision make it difficult to fulfill the roles I would like to fulfill in life (e.g., family roles, work roles, community roles, etc.)?"; "does my vision affect my confidence to join in everyday activities?"	Misajon et al. 2005
Vision-related activities of daily living (V-ADL)/assess distance, intermediate, near, and peripheral tasks to evaluate spectacle-mounted prisms for patients with RP	Distance vision-related activities (eight items)	Difficulty with the following: "read street signs," "recognize faces outside," "enjoy scenery when out for a drive," "recognize seasonal changes in the garden," "walk alone in the neighborhood," "walk alone outside your neighborhood," "adjust to dark coming from light," "adjust to light coming from dark"	Somani et al. 2006
	Intermediate vision-related activities (eight items)	Difficulty with the following: "watching television," "distinguish a person's features in the room," "distinguish objects in the room," "notice steps and use them," "prepare food in the kitchen," "handle food on your plate," "pour yourself a drink," "cut your fingernails"	

Continued

Table 1. *Continued*

Instrument/objective	Domain/part	Items	References
	Near vision related activities (four items)	Difficulty with the following: "read newspaper headlines," "read regular print material," "write and sign documents," "can you identify money"	
	Peripheral vision-related activities (three items)	Difficulty with the following: "notice stationary or moving targets with your side vision," "navigate your way among stationary or moving targets," "locate a target from among other targets crowding the field"	
Night Vision Questionnaire (NVQ)-39/to assess how often patients experience night vision in various situations	Lighting in home environment and how often go out alone	Lighting in "living environment"; how often go out alone in winter; how often go out alone in summer	Bijveld et al. 2013
	Activity restrictions at night	Open-ended	
	Modes of transportation used in various situations	Transportation by foot, bike, moped, "scoot-mobile/disabled vehicle," car, or other in the following situations: "daytime," "in twilight or more than sufficient streetlight," "in the dark (but with a flashlight/bicycle light/headlight," "I do not use this means of transportation in twilight or in the dark because of your vision at night," "I do not use this means of transportation because of other reasons"	
	Strategies used when walking outside in the dark	How frequently you use the following strategies when walking outside in the dark: "I use a cane," "I make sure someone goes with me," "I go from lamppost to lamppost," "I take a flashlight with me," "I use a different kind of aid, namely," "I take a different kind of action, namely …"	
	How often specific outdoor situations cause problems in the dark without the use of an aid	When it is dark, how often the following situations arise: "I have difficulty getting an overview," "I experience problems moving around in a familiar environment," "I have difficulty finding my way in a familiar environment," "I experience problems moving about in an unfamiliar environment," "I have difficulty finding my way in an unfamiliar environment," "I have difficulty noticing traffic at intersections," "I find it hard to use public transportation," "I experience	

 Cite this article as *Cold Spring Harb Perspect Med* doi: 10.1101/cshperspect.a041298

Continued

			Prem Senthil et al. 2017b,c
	problems stepping up and down the sidewalk," "I find it hard to walk across uneven travel surfaces," "I have difficulty not to fall or stumble," "I have difficulty going out to, for instance, sporting events, cinema, friends, church, restaurants, places of entertainment, etc.," "I go out less often than I would want because of my vision at night"		
How often specific indoor situations cause problems when there is "poor or insufficient lighting" and without the use of an aid	"I have difficulty noticing the furniture in a room," "I have difficulty noticing the furniture in a room," "I have difficulty finding small objects," "I have difficulty reading the paper or a book," "in restaurants, I have difficulty reading the menu," "I have difficulty avoiding bumping into obstacles or persons," "I have difficulty recognizing faces"		
How often general situations cause problems	"I experience problems going from light to dark," "If it is dark, I experience problems moving about in crowded situations," "I feel blind at night," "at a social event when there is dim light, I feel insecure," "I feel restricted because of my vision at night," "when it is dark, I feel dependent on others to help me because of my vision at night"		
IRD item bank for QOL/explore impact of IRD across all aspects of QOL	Activity limitation/activity limitation (47 items); activity limitation/reading (15 items); activity limitation/driving (eight items); activity limitation/lighting (11 items); health concerns/general health concerns (32 items); health concerns/concerns about the disease progression (seven items); emotional (53 items); economic (17 items); convenience (16 items); social (28 items); visual symptoms; (20 items); mobility (23 items)	Not yet reported	

Table 1. *Continued*

Instrument/objective	Domain/part	Items	References
Visual Function Scale (VFS)-Plus/evaluate vision-related activity in patients with retinitis pigmentosa	Visual function scale (15 items)	Eyesight; read ordinary print in newspapers; see well up close; find something on a crowded shelf; read street signs or the names of stores; going down steps, stairs, or curbs in dim light or at night; notice objects off to the side while walking; pick and match own clothes; go out to see movies, plays, or sports events; read small print in a telephone book, on a medicine bottle, or on legal forms; figure out whether bills received are accurate; doing things like shaving, styling hair, or putting on makeup; recognize people across a room; take part in active sports or other outdoor activities; see and enjoy programs on TV; driving in familiar places; driving during daytime; driving at night; driving in difficult situations	Costela et al. 2020
	Driving (four items)	Driving in familiar places; driving during daytime; driving at night; driving in difficult situations	
Michigan Retinal Degeneration Questionnaire (MRDQ)/evaluate patient-reported benefits of gene therapies that correspond to measures of visual function	Central/difficulty	Reading books, magazines, or mail?; reading on a computer or tablet?; reading on cell phone screens?; reading the newspaper, food labels, price tags, or medication labels?; reading direction signs?; reading store names?	Lacy et al.2021a
	Central/accommodations	Scan a page or line of text to find the "right spot" to read?; adjust the amount of room light to read?; move closer to objects to read?; use vision aids for close reading (i.e., magnifying glasses, zoom function)?; use vision aids for distance reading (i.e., telescopes or bioptics)?	
	Color/difficulty	"Distinguishing between colors of similar shades (i.e., blues and blacks, blues and blues, or tones of pastel)?; distinguishing bright colors (i.e., stop lights or crosswalk signs)?"	
	Color/accommodations	"Ask for help to distinguish colors?; adjust the light/ brightness to help distinguish colors?"	

Cite this article as *Cold Spring Harb Perspect Med* doi: 10.1101/cshperspect.a041298

Continued

Contrast/difficulty	"Recognizing faces?; finding a white object on a white table?; chopping an onion on a light-colored board?; eating rice and chicken on a white plate?; seeing doorways?; seeing curbs, sidewalks, or uneven ground?"
Contrast/accommodations	Ask for help to find a white object on a white table?
Scotopic/difficulty	Adapting to the dark (i.e., moving from a well-lit room to a darker room)?; finding a seat in a poorly lit restaurant?; finding a seat in a movie theatre?; peripheral vision during the night?; seeing children or pets outside of your central vision during the night?; seeing stairs or steps during the night?; taking the garbage outside during the night?; crossing the street during the night?; walking in crowded areas during the night?
Scotopic/accommodations	Ask for help with finding objects outside of your visual field during the night?; touch things around you to move during the night?; use someone's arm to walk during the night?
Mesopic peripheral/difficulty	Peripheral vision in poorly lit areas?; seeing children or pets outside of your central vision in poorly lit areas?; seeing stairs or steps in poorly lit areas?; taking the garbage outside in poorly lit areas?; crossing the street in poorly lit areas?; walking in crowded areas in poorly lit areas?
Mesopic peripheral/accommodations	Ask for help with finding objects outside of your visual field in poorly lit areas?; touch things around you to move in poorly lit areas?; use someone's arm to walk in poorly lit areas?
Photopic peripheral/difficulty	"Peripheral vision during the day?; seeing children or pets outside of your central vision during the day?; seeing stairs or steps during the day?; taking the garbage outside during the day?; crossing the street during the day?; walking in crowded areas during the day?"

Table 1. *Continued*

Instrument/objective	Domain/part	Items	References
	Photopic peripheral/accommodations	Ask for help with finding objects outside of your visual field during the day?; touch things around you to move during the day?; use someone's arm to walk during the day?	
	Photosensitivity/difficulty	Sensitivity to bright lights?; sensitivity to fluorescent lights in a store or office?; sensitivity to oncoming headlights?; sensitivity to bright sunlight?	
	Photosensitivity/accommodations	Use tinted/transition lenses, sunglasses or hats when outdoors because you are bothered by bright light?; squint your eyes when not using sunglasses because you are bothered by bright light?; worry about seeing in places with bright fluorescent lights when you are alone?	Lacy et al. 2021b
Michigan Vision-Related Anxiety Questionnaire (MVAQ)	Rod function-related anxiety	Worry bumping into people/objects during the night; worry bumping into people/objects in poorly lit areas; worry about seeing during the night; worry about seeing in poorly lit areas; worry about uneven ground during the night; worry about uneven ground in poorly lit areas	
	Cone function-related anxiety	Worry when reading up close; worry when reading at a distance; worry when distinguishing colors; worry when seeing against similar backdrops; worry about recognizing faces; worry when going to unfamiliar places during the day; worry about bright fluorescent lights; worry about going out on bright sunny days	
Attitudes to Gene Therapy for the Eye (AGT-Eye)/ "To investigate the knowledge and perceived value of gene therapy interventions that have been approved for patients with IRDs or will be approved in the future"	Awareness of treatment (one item)	"I have good knowledge about gene therapy for inherited retinal disease"	Mack et al. 2021; McGuinness et al. 2022
	Sources of information (one item)	"I have obtained information about gene therapy treatment from: my ophthalmologist; other medical or health professional; registry, for example, Australian Inherited Retinal Disease Register; disease register; research group; newspapers; internet; social media; patient support group; family/friends"	

Continued

Knowledge of clinical trials vs. approved treatment (one item)	"I understand the difference between an experimental treatment provided by a clinical trial and a treatment that has already been approved by the Australian government"
Timing and method of treatment (four items)	"Gene therapy for the eye is suitable at any stage of a person's life"; "generally, gene therapy for inherited retinal disease is delivered to both eyes"; "gene therapy for the eye is injected into the bloodstream through the arm"; "gene therapy and stem cell therapy are the same treatment"
Understanding of outcomes (eight items)	"Gene therapy for the eye can restore vision back to normal"; "gene therapy for the eye is a treatment that may slow down the disease"; "treatment complications to my eyes, such as permanent blindness, are possible with an approved gene therapy"; "gene therapy in my eye may have side effects elsewhere in my body"; "having gene therapy for their eye condition means a person will not pass on an eye condition to any children they may have in the future"; "I may not be eligible for financial or other government benefits if my gene therapy for my eye condition is unsuccessful"; "gene therapy for inherited retinal diseases will require many years of follow-up with my eyecare practitioner"; "receiving gene therapy for my inherited retinal disease means I won't be eligible for future genetic treatments"
Awareness of treatment (two items)	"I will lose my privacy if I undergo gene therapy, and my data will be in the public domain," "if I undergo gene therapy, it will affect my eligibility or terms of conditions in life, disability or health insurance in the future"

Table 1. *Continued*

Instrument/objective	Domain/part	Items	References
	Understanding the cost and opportunity cost of treatment (five items)	"The government should pay all costs of my gene therapy," "government subsidy of my treatment would be an effective use of taxpayer money," "if gene therapy for my condition was not available in my state I would consider travelling interstate to access it"; "my private health insurance should pay all out of pocket costs for my gene therapy," "I would consider a payment plan for my gene therapy"	Audo et al. 2021, 2022; Kay et al. 2021, 2022
ViSIO-PRO/evaluate RP/LCA-specific visual impairments and impacts on vision-dependent ADLs	Not yet reported	Not yet reported	

Cite this article as *Cold Spring Harb Perspect Med* doi: 10.1101/cshperspect.a041298

oped based on focus group interviews in 70 adults with vision impairment, defined as visual acuity (VA) in the better eye of worse than 20/20 (Table 1). The affected participants had a variety of conditions, but were primarily AMD, glaucoma, Stevens–Johnson syndrome, macular dystrophy, and others. An initial set of 33 items across six domains (physical well-being, independence, social well-being, emotional well-being, self-actualization, and planning and organization) was reduced based on psychometric analyses of dimensionality and statistical redundancy. Methodology to convert the responses to the six-item VisQOL into health utility scores has been published (Peacock et al. 2008).

Unlike the earliest IRD-specific PROMs, the 51-item NEI-VFQ was developed using methodologies that are recognizable in the 2009 FDA guidance. To generate the items for the instrument, investigators at the NEI conducted condition-specific focus groups with structured interviews and coded the transcripts to identify the salient content (Mangione et al. 1998a). The conditions included glaucoma (82 participants), diabetic retinopathy (58 participants), cataract (42 participants), AMD (35 participants), cytomegalovirus (CMV) retinitis (17 participants), and low vision from any cause (VA in better eye of 20/200 or worse or <10° field; 12 participants). The authors did not indicate whether any of the low vision participants had an IRD. Based on the qualitative research, the investigators developed 51 items across 13 domains (Table 1). After developing the item content, the items were evaluated through cognitive debriefing to ensure individuals understood each item (Mangione et al. 1998b). In a subsequent study, the 51-item instrument was reduced to a shorter form with 25 items after eliminating items based on cognitive interviews, statistical redundancy, and the presence of ceiling or floor effects (Mangione et al. 2001). The 25-item NEI-VFQ has been translated into numerous languages (eprovide .mapi-trust.org), making it an attractive PROM for use in global clinical trials.

Before adopting the NEI-VFQ for a clinical trial, researchers should be aware that Pesudovs and colleagues (2010) reported that the NEI-VFQ had serious flaws in terms of multidimensionality (meaning it measured more than a single construct of vision-related quality of life) and targeting of items to person ability. As demonstrated in this study, Rasch methods can appropriately scale the scores, diagnose incorrect assumptions, and rectify mistargeting of items through calibration of scores to person ability. These advantages demonstrate how Rasch analysis, a specific application of item response theory, may be preferred over scoring applications using classical test theory (Cappelleri et al. 2014; Petrillo et al. 2015).

In several studies of IRD cohorts, there is documented support for convergent validity of the NEI-VFQ, particularly related to peripheral vision in RP. For example, in 108 RP patients, 95% of whom were classified as severely low vision or worse, the NEI-VFQ was highly correlated with a combination of BCVA from both eyes ($r = 0.60$; $P < 0.001$) and a combination of Goldmann perimetry III4e fields from both eyes ($r = 0.44$; $P < 0.001$; Seo et al. 2009). The association with peripheral vision, but not BCVA, was reported in another study of 40 RP patients by Sugawara and colleagues. In their study, there was a significant association ($r = -0.519$; $P < 0.001$) between NEI-VFQ and graded (seven levels) monocular visual fields, which were measured using a Goldmann perimetry V4e target, but the correlation with BCVA was small ($r = 0.016$; $P = 0.922$) (Sugawara et al. 2010). Another study of 33 RP patients with central VF < 20° reported a strong correlation ($r = 0.802$; $P < 0.001$) between NEI-VFQ and the extent of the central visual field (Altinbay and Taskin 2021). In another study of 30 RP patients with decimal BCVA ≥ 0.6, NEI-VFQ scores were significantly associated with mean sensitivity in the central 10° measured by the Nidek MP1 ($r = 0.67$; $P < 0.001$), but not VA ($r = -0.17$; $P = 0.36$) (Sugawara et al. 2011). A strong association between NEI-VFQ scores and mean sensitivity ($r = 0.72$) was also reported in a study of 16 Stargardt patients (Murro et al. 2017).

IRD PROMs DEVELOPED SINCE THE 2009 FDA GUIDANCE

Among the recent innovations for IRD-specific PROMs is the Michigan Retinal Degeneration

Questionnaire (MRDQ), which was developed by Lacy and colleagues (2020b) to translate the effects of gene therapy on measures of visual function into the patient experience. To develop the items for this instrument, researchers interviewed 26 IRD patients with a range of IRD diagnoses (Stargardt, RP/rod-cone dystrophy [RCD], Usher syndrome/RCD, Best macular dystrophy, cone-rod dystrophy [CRD], achromatopsia, choroideremia), best corrected VA (ranging in the better seeing eye from no light perception [NLP] to 20/20), Goldmann visual field area (ranging in the better seeing eye from 0 to 20,897 mm²), and age (ranging from 21 to 71 years). The interviews were guided by open-ended questions around the following topic areas: symptoms prior to diagnosis, night vision problems, day vision problems, glare, photosensitivity, light/dark adaptation, photopsia, peripheral vision, mid-peripheral vision, central vision, contrast sensitivity, floaters, distance vision, color vision, headaches and eye pain, driving, and other vision problems. The in-depth interviews were subsequently coded using software for qualitative analyses. The initial items were drafted and grouped into domains. The items were refined further based on cognitive interviews and pilot interviews in 16 and 13 IRD patients, respectively. After reducing the number of items based on psychometric analyses, the final MRDQ instrument is comprised of 59 items across seven domains, including central vision, color vision, contrast sensitivity, scotopic vision, photopic peripheral vision, mesopic peripheral vision, and photosensitivity (Table 1).

Lacy and colleagues documented the quantitative characteristics of the MRDQ through psychometric analysis of completed instruments in a sample of 128 IRD patients, 25 of whom completed the instrument a second time for purposes of evaluating reliability (Lacy et al. 2021a). In this study, the domains appeared to measure the intended constructs. For example, the greatest proportion of variance for the central, color, contrast, and photopic peripheral domain scores were attributed to corrected VA scores (a measure of cone function), whereas the variance in scotopic, mesopic peripheral, and photosensitiv-

ity domain scores were mostly attributable to IRD phenotype (measuring the involvement of primarily rods or cones; rod-cone vs. cone/cone-rod vs. macular). Upon re-testing of 25 participants within ≈2 weeks, the domain scores were highly correlated (r values ranging across domains from 0.84 to 0.95) and their between-visit means were close to zero. Since its initial development, the MRDQ has been translated and adapted for Portuguese speakers (Marques et al. 2022).

Lacy and colleagues also developed a new instrument, the Michigan Vision-Related Anxiety Questionnaire (MVAQ) to evaluate the therapeutic effects of vision-related anxiety in patients with IRDs (Lacy et al. 2021b). From in-depth interviews with 128 IRD patients, 26 items related to "anxiety" or "worry" were identified and formed the preliminary instrument. Individual items were refined through an iterative process of patient feedback and item revision. The final instrument has 14 items in two domains, rod- and cone-related anxiety (Table 1). Psychometric analyses demonstrated that the MVAQ has high intervisit reliability (correlations of 0.81–0.83 in the two domains) and significant associations with participant characteristics. IRD phenotype accounts for most of the variance of the rod function-related anxiety while VA in the better eye accounted for a majority of the variance of the cone function-related anxiety. Like the MRDQ, the MVAQ has been translated and adapted for Portuguese-speaking IRD patients (Marques et al. 2022).

As a potentially time-saving alternative to fixed-length instruments like the MRDQ, item banks enable researchers to select a subset of appropriate domains for use in their research. Item banks can be administered adaptively via computer and, thus, may require less time to complete than fixed length instruments. Prem Senthil and colleagues developed item banks from two qualitative studies, one in 23 RP patients (Prem Senthil et al. 2017b) and the other in 32 patients (23 RP, two cone dystrophy, seven macular dystrophy; Prem Senthil et al. 2017c) and reviewing existing instruments (Prem Senthil et al. 2017a). The item banks comprised 10 domains from those closely related to vision (e.g., visual symptoms, mobility, activity limitations) to others more distal to vision (e.g., economic, general health concerns) (Prem Senthil et al. 2019). The item banks were tested in 233 participants with IRDs to evaluate their psychometric properties. Across the domains, the number of items ranged from 8 to 53 in the driving and emotional domains (Table 1), but computer-assisted administration achieved high measurement precision using only 8–11 items from the full domain-specific item banks. Quantitative validation of the item banks has not yet been reported.

Costela and colleagues (2020) showed that it is possible to modify an existing PROM to improve its measurement characteristics. Using retrospective analyses from several studies of 594 patients with RP, they showed that a customized instrument, represented by a subset of items from the NEI-VFQ, could capture vision-related ability, was correlated with traditional measures of vision, and was responsive to change over 4 years of follow-up (Costela et al. 2020). The instrument, termed "VFS-plus" by the authors, was made up of items from the NEI-VFQ, namely 15 items related to visual function and four items from the driving scale. The addition of the latter increased the average difficulty, and thus improved the targeting, of the overall scale. The Rasch analyses of the VFS-plus demonstrated unidimensionality (consistent with a single scale), excellent fit, high reliability coefficients, and little evidence of differential item functioning (i.e., items performing differently for evaluated groups of participants). The convergent validity of the VS-plus score was demonstrated by highly positive correlations with Goldmann visual field area, 30 Hz ERG amplitude, and better VA. Importantly, the overall scores decreased significantly over time, indicative of an instrument that is responsive to change.

Researchers from Novartis and their partners Adelphi Values have been developing a new PRO (and ObsRO) for individuals with RP or LCA after concluding that the NEI-VFQ did not have adequate coverage or relevance in individuals with *RLBP1*-associated RP (Green et al. 2020). The content for the new PRO was informed by semi-structured interviews of 19 in-dividuals in the United States with RP or LCA from various genetic causes (Kay et al. 2020), of 16 participants across the United States, France, and Germany with *RPE65*-associated RP/LCA (Kay et al. 2021), and 19 RP-affected individuals and 11 caregivers in Germany and France (Audo et al. 2021). Across these studies (Table 1), common visual symptoms included night blindness, restricted peripheral vision, dark–light adaptation, and color vision. The severity of these RP-related impacts depended on lighting conditions and the familiarity of surroundings, two mediating factors that were incorporated into the instrument. The draft instrument, termed "ViSIO-PRO," was found to have qualitative validity (i.e., valid content and well-understood items) in a study of 66 participants (including RP-affected adults and adolescents, and caregivers) (Kay et al. 2022). Subsequently, psychometric properties of the instrument were evaluated in a study of 83 adults and adolescents with RP of various causes (Audo et al. 2022). The instrument was found to have convergent validity through correlations with other visual function measures, moderate-to-high test–retest reliability (intraclass coefficients 0.66–0.98) and could be divided and scored separately for visual function symptoms, mobility, vision-related ADL, and broader health-related quality of life. Manuscripts for this work are in progress as of this writing.

Not all PROMs are designed to evaluate the effect of a treatment. As an example, Mack and colleagues developed a novel instrument, the AGT-Eye, to measure the knowledge and attitudes of IRD patients about gene therapy (Mack et al. 2021). The items for this instrument were drafted by expert clinicians, reviewed by IRD patients or caregivers for clarity and appropriateness, and finalized by expert researchers. The instrument contains 22 items in six unique domains: "awareness of treatment," "sources of information," "knowledge of clinical trials vs. approved treatment," "timing and method of treatment," "understanding of outcomes," and "understanding the cost and opportunity cost of treatment." To describe the measurement properties of the AGT-Eye, McGuiness and colleagues analyzed the responses of 681 IRD patients. The researchers found that the instrument could not separate individuals into different levels of knowledge about gene therapy because the most common response was "neither agree nor disagree." On this basis, the authors concluded that the lack of discrimination limits the utility of the instrument in its current form.

INSIGHTS FROM QUALITATIVE RESEARCH IN PATIENTS WITH IRDs

Qualitative studies play an essential role in the development, modification, and adoption of PROMs for a particular study because they can identify the most common visual symptoms, major impacts on daily living, and the most important impacts of IRDs. We identified qualitative studies in IRDs using a PubMed search with the following search strategy: (qualitative OR interview OR focus group) AND (retinitis pigmentosa OR Leber congenital amaurosis OR Stargardt OR retinoschisis OR Usher syndrome OR cone-rod OR cone rod). Six of the qualitative studies identified most common symptoms and impacts on daily living associated with an IRD (Table 2). In multiple studies of RP and Usher syndrome, commonly reported symptoms included night blindness, loss of peripheral vision, and poor light adaptation (Prem Senthil et al. 2017b; Green et al. 2020; Lange et al. 2021). Activity limitations or other impacts included reading, driving, navigation in unfamiliar places, sports, and emotional well-being. While Stargardt patients identified these same activity limitations, their most common symptoms (photosensitivity and loss of central vision) differed quite a bit from RP (Roborel de Climens et al. 2021). Last, limitations with sports and driving were common concerns of parents whose boys have X-linked retinoschisis (Turriff et al. 2020). Five qualitative studies (Table 3) examined other aspects of living with IRDs like coping and views on work (Hayeems et al. 2005; Bittner et al. 2010; Ehn et al. 2019, 2020; Zelihić et al. 2020).

DISCUSSION AND RECOMMENDATIONS

This brief narrative summary has highlighted that the earliest PROMs used in studies of IRDs do not meet a minimum contemporary standard for documented qualitative validity (i.e., that item content is supported by a conceptual framework and that it is generated from and understood by patients). In terms of qualitative validity, the development and refinement of the NEI-VFQ represented a step in the right direction. However, the item generation for the NEI-VFQ did not include any documented patients with IRDs and thus it is likely to exclude concepts that are important to patients with IRDs. In fact, one study in this review documented the existence of this gap for *RLBP1*-associated RP. Nonetheless, the NEI-VFQ offers some appeal to investigators today since it has been translated into many languages. However, its lack of specificity for IRDs, owing to IRD patients being excluded from content generation, and suboptimal psychometric properties merit careful consideration by researchers before adopting the NEI-VFQ as the sole PROM for their clinical trials.

Several recent advances in PROM development offer promising alternatives to the NEI-VFQ. The MRDQ is a qualitatively and quantitatively validated instrument that was designed following FDA and other contemporary guidance to translate standard clinical measures of vision for IRDs in general into patient-centered symptomatic benefits for patients. Utilization of this instrument in future studies (including clinical trials) will contribute to its development and refinement. These new studies will help to establish the instrument's sensitivity, estimate the minimally important difference, and confirm that the instrument's items include all the relevant concepts for a particular IRD. Another alternative is the ViSIO-PRO, which has been shown to be qualitatively and quantitatively valid and reliable. This instrument was developed following contemporary guidance by eliciting content from patients with a diversity of genetic causes of their RP. Compared to the MRDQ, the ViSIO-PRO has a wider range of domains including visual function symptoms (the single domain in the MRDQ), vision-dependent daily activities, mobility, and distal HRQOL. Like the MRDQ, the ViSIO-PRO will benefit from additional studies and refinement. Last, item banks, which are still early in development, offer a

Table 2. Qualitative studies of symptoms or other impacts on daily activities in patients with inherited retinal diseases (IRDs)

IRDs studied	Location	Sample size	Methodology	Most common symptoms	Limitations or other impacts	References
Retinitis pigmentosa (RP)	Australia	23 adult patients	Semi-structured interview with transcripts coded using software and an inductive approach	Night blindness; restricted visual field; progressive visual loss; defective color vision; poor light adaptation; poor contrast vision	Reading; seeing in changing light conditions; shopping; driving; navigation in unfamiliar places; playing sports; walking outdoors; using computers; engage in leisure activities	Prem Senthil et al. 2017b
RP associated with *RLBP1* gene	Canada and Sweden	21 patients	Open-ended concept elicitation	Night blindness; difficulty adapting to changes in lighting; difficulties seeing in bright lighting	Reading; driving; navigation; sports/physical activity; frustration; sadness; having to rely on others; shopping	Green et al. 2020
RP with restricted peripheral vision (≤20° using III4e target from Goldmann visual field)	USA	19 adult patients	Semi-structured interview with coded transcripts	Not reported	Activity limitations (e.g., unfamiliar places, concerts); driving; emotional well-being; reading; mobility; social function	Lange et al. 2021
Stargardt disease	USA and France	21 patients and seven parents	Semi-structured interview with coded transcripts	Photosensitivity; loss of central vision	Difficulty with sports/physical activities; frustration and worry; reduced ability to concentrate; problems with face recognition; impacts on driving and reading; difficulties at school/work	Roborel de Climens et al. 2021
Usher syndrome type 1	USA and France	18 patients and nine parents	Semi-structured interview with coded transcripts	Night blindness; loss of peripheral vision	Difficulty moving; fear of falling; difficulties at school/work	Roborel de Climens et al. 2020
X-linked retinoschisis (XLRS)	USA	19 parents of boys with XLRS	Semi-structured interview with coded transcripts	Not reported	Fear of unknown; limitations with sports; limitations with driving	Turriff et al. 2020

Table 3. Qualitative studies of other impacts in patients with inherited retinal diseases (IRDs)

IRDs studied	Location	Sample size	Methodology	Primary themes reported	References
Bardet–Biedl syndrome	Norway	Five parents with children 0–16 years of age	Semi-structured in-depth interviews with transcripts coded inductively	Experiences of parents: distress about the initial diagnosis; difficulty communicating their child's condition to others; not being informed of benefits available to them; maintaining positive interactions through work; being open about their child as a coping strategy	Zelihić et al. 2020
RP	USA	43 adult patients	Focus groups and semi-structured interviews; qualitative coding of transcripts	After diagnosis, patients seek to understand the meaning in their lives; to make functional changes as a result of RP required a shift in personal identity to a visually impaired person	Hayeems et al. 2005
RP (legally blind)	USA	Eight adult patients	Focus groups	Related to vision loss: loss of independence; usefulness of assistive devices; helpful to keep hope for a treatment or cure; high degree of resilience about vision; coping strategies: humor; communicating with others	Bittner et al. 2010
Usher syndrome type 2A	Sweden	14 adult patients	Focus group interviews with transcripts coded inductively	Life strategies to manage: remaining active; using devices; using support; sharing knowledge; appreciating the present; maintaining a positive image; alleviating emotional pain	Ehn et al. 2019
Usher syndrome type 2A	Sweden	Seven adult patients	Semi-structured interviews analyzed by interpretative phenomenological analysis	Experiences with work: feeling of satisfaction; commitment that needs balancing; facing limitations (e.g, feeling exhausted or insufficient); feelings of uncertainty	Ehn et al. 2020

Cite this article as *Cold Spring Harb Perspect Med* doi: 10.1101/cshperspect.a041298

different concept altogether. Using these, researchers may combine individual items to construct any number of disease-specific PROMs.

While these latest advances in PROMs are promising, they may not address all the challenges represented by therapy development for rare diseases like IRDs. The ISPOR guidance on PROMs for rare disease leads us to the following recommendations when developing a PROM strategy for a clinical trial: start with a thorough understanding of the natural history of disease and the likely benefits of the new therapy; if not documented, conduct qualitative research to determine the most common or important symptoms or disease impacts (e.g., navigating unfamiliar environments in dim lighting); determine which common disease impacts are potentially modifiable by the new therapy, given its mechanism of action; identify whether any PROM or set of items from a PROM could address the anticipated therapeutic benefits. Armed with this fundamental information, therapy developers have the beginning of a PROM strategy that may, as the ISPOR guidance suggests, require creativity and collaboration with regulators and payors. Development of PROMs is a multidisciplinary effort requiring clinical experience and expertise in a variety of research methodologies. Perhaps most important of these is the ability to design qualitative studies that capture the richness of patient experience. Incorporating these insights into an appropriate PROM will make the trial data more reflective of benefits to patients. With the latest advances in PROM development, it is now possible to move beyond the NEI-VFQ to show how treatments can affect what is truly important to patients with IRDs.

REFERENCES

Altinbay D, Taskin I. 2021. Evaluation of vision-related quality of life in retinitis pigmentosa patients with low vision. *Jpn J Ophthalmol* **65:** 777–785. doi:10.1007/s10384-021-00875-z

Audo I, Williamson N, Bradley H, Barclay M, Sims J, Arbuckle R, Patalano F, Spera C, Naujoks C, Afroz N, et al. 2021. Qualitative exploration of patient and caregiver experiences of visual function impairments and impacts on vision-dependent activities of daily living and health-related quality of life associated with retinitis pigmentosa

and Leber congenital amaurosis in Germany and France. *Invest Ophthalmol Vis Sci* **62:** 3585.

Audo I, Williamson N, Barclay M, Sims J, Boparai K, Bradley H, Patalano F, Naujoks C, Spera C, Banhazi J, et al. 2022. Abstract 3711269. In *ARVO 2022*. May 1–4, Denver.

Benjamin K, Vernon MK, Patrick DL, Perfetto E, Nestler-Parr S, Burke L. 2017. Patient-reported outcome and observer-reported outcome assessment in rare disease clinical trials: an ISPOR COA emerging good practices task force report. *Value Health* **20:** 838–855. doi:10.1016/j.jval.2017.05.015

Bijveld M, van Genderen M, Hoeben F, Katzin A, van Nispen R, Riemslag F, Kappers A. 2013. Assessment of night vision problems in patients with congenital stationary night blindness. *PLoS ONE* **8:** e62927. doi:10.1371/journal.pone.0062927

Bittner A, Edwards L, George M. 2010. Coping strategies to manage stress related to vision loss and fluctuations in retinitis pigmentosa. *Optometry* **81:** 461–468. doi:10.1016/j.optm.2010.03.006

Cappelleri J, Lundy J, Hays R. 2014. Overview of classical test theory and item response theory for the quantitative assessment of items in developing patient-reported outcomes measures. *Clin Ther* **36:** 648–662. doi:10.1016/j.clinthera.2014.04.006

Costela F, Pesudovs K, Sandberg M, Weigel-DiFranco C, Woods R. 2020. Validation of a vision-related activity scale for patients with retinitis pigmentosa. *Health Qual Life Outcomes* **18:** 196. doi:10.1186/s12955-020-01427-8

Daiger S, Bowne S, Sullivan L. 2007. Perspective on genes and mutations causing retinitis pigmentosa. *Arch Ophthalmol* **125:** 151–158. doi:10.1001/archopht.125.2.151

Ehn M, Anderzén-Carlsson A, Möller C, Wahlqvist M. 2019. Life strategies of people with deafblindness due to Usher syndrome type 2a—a qualitative study. *Int J Qual Stud Health Well-being* **14:** 1656790. doi:10.1080/17482631.2019.1656790

Ehn M, Wahlqvist M, Möller C, Anderzén-Carlsson A. 2020. The lived experiences of work and health of people living with deaf-blindness due to Usher syndrome type 2. *Int J Qual Stud Health Well-being* **15:** 1846671. doi:10.1080/17482631.2020.1846671

European Medicines Agency. 2005. Reflection paper on the regulatory guidance for the use of health-related quality of life (HRQL) measures in the evaluation of medicinal products. Committee for Medicinal Products for Human Use (CHMP). Amsterdam.

Fahim A, Daiger S, Weleber R. 2000. Nonsyndromic retinitis pigmentosa overview. In *GeneReviews* (ed. Adam MP, Ardinger HH, Pagon RA), pp. 1993–2019. University of Washington, Seattle.

Frost M, Reeve B, Liepa A, Stauffer J, Hays R. 2007. What is sufficient evidence for the reliability and validity of patient-reported outcome measures? *Value Health* **10:** S94–S105. doi:10.1111/j.1524-4733.2007.00272.x

Geruschat D, Turano K, Stahl J. 1998. Traditional measures of mobility performance and retinitis pigmentosa. *Optom Vis Sci* **75:** 525–537. doi:10.1097/00006324-199807000-00022

Green J, Tolley C, Bentley S, Arbuckle R, Burstedt M, Whelan J, Holopigian K, Stasi K, Sloesen B, Spera C, et al. 2020. Qualitative interviews to better understand the patient experience and evaluate patient-reported outcomes (PRO) in RLBP1 retinitis pigmentosa (RLBP1 RP). *Adv Ther* 37: 2884–2901. doi:10.1007/s12325-020-01275-4

Hayeems R, Geller G, Finkelstein D, Faden R. 2005. How patients experience progressive loss of visual function: a model of adjustment using qualitative methods. *Br J Ophthalmol* 89: 615–620. doi:10.1136/bjo.2003.036046

Jayasundera KT, Abuzaitoun RO, Lacy GD, Abalem MF, Saltzman GM., Ciulla TA, Johnson MW. 2022. Challenges of cost-effectiveness analyses of novel therapeutics for inherited retinal diseases. *Am J Ophthalmol* 235: 90–97. doi:10.1016/j.ajo.2021.08.009

Kay C, Banhazi J, Williamson N, Arbuckle R, Tolley C, Spera C, Green J, Fischer M, Audo I, Patalano F, et al. 2020. Patient and caregiver experiences of functional vision impairment and health-related quality of life limitations associated with hereditary retinitis pigmentosa. *Invest Ophthalmol Vis Sci* 61: 1562.

Kay C, Williamson N, Bradley H, Barclay M, Sims J, Arbuckle R, Spera C, Naujoks C, Afroz N, Fischer M, et al. 2021. Qualitative interviews with patients and caregivers regarding visual function impairments and impacts on vision-dependent activities of daily living and health-related quality of life in RPE65-related retinitis pigmentosa and Leber congenital amaurosis. *Invest Ophthalmol Vis Sci* 62: 3589.

Kay C. et al. 2022. Abstract 3712801. In *ARVO 2022*. May 1–4, Denver.

Kennedy W, Rosten J, Young L, Ciuffreda K, Levin M. 1977. A field expander for patients with retinitis pigmentosa: a clinical study. *Am J Optom Physiol Opt* 54: 744–755. doi:10.1097/00006324-197711000-00002

Khan K, Islam F, Moore A, Michaelides M. 2016. Clinical and genetic features of choroideremia in childhood. *Ophthalmology* 123: 2158–2165. doi:10.1016/j.ophtha.2016.06.051

Kumaran N, Moore AT, Weleber RG, Michaelides M. 2017. Leber congenital amaurosis/early-onset severe retinal dystrophy: clinical features, molecular genetics and therapeutic interventions. *Br J Ophthalmol* 101: 1147–1154. doi:10.1136/bjophthalmol-2016-309975

Lacy G, Abalem M, Musch D, Jayasundera K. 2020a. Patient-reported outcome measures in inherited retinal degeneration gene therapy trials. *Ophthalmic Genet* 41: 1–6. doi:10.1080/13816810.2020.1731836

Lacy G, Abalem M, Popova L, Santos E, Yu G, Rakine H, Rosenthal J, Ehrlich J, Musch D, Jayasundera K. 2020b. Content generation for patient-reported outcome measures for retinal degeneration therapeutic trials. *Ophthalmic Genet* 41: 315–324. doi:10.1080/13816810.2020.1776337

Lacy G, Abalem M, Andrews C, Popova L, Santos E, Yu G, Rakine H, Baig N, Ehrlich J, Fahim A, et al. 2021a. The Michigan Retinal Degeneration Questionnaire: a patient-reported outcomes instrument for inherited retinal degenerations. *Am J Ophthalmol* 222: 60–68. doi:10.1016/j.ajo.2020.08.032

Lacy G, Abalem M, Andrews C, Abuzaitoun R, Popova L, Santos E, Yu G, Rakine H, Baig N, Ehrlich J, et al. 2021b. The Michigan Vision-Related Anxiety Questionnaire: a psychosocial outcomes measure for inherited retinal de-

generations. *Am J Ophthalmol* 225: 137–146. doi:10.1016/j.ajo.2020.12.001

Lange R, Kumagai A, Weiss S, Zaffke K, Day S, Wicker D, Howson A, Jayasundera K, Smolinski L, Hedlich C, et al. 2021. Vision-related quality of life in adults with severe peripheral vision loss: a qualitative interview study. *J Patient Rep Outcomes* 5: 7. doi:10.1186/s41687-020-00281-y

Lasch K, Marquis P, Vigneux M, Abetz L, Arnould B, Bayliss M, Crawford B, Rosa K. 2010. PRO development: rigorous qualitative research as the crucial foundation. *Qual Life Res* 19: 1087–1096. doi:10.1007/s11136-010-9677-6

Lodha N, Westall C, Brent M, Abdolell M, Héon E. 2003. A modified protocol for the assessment of visual function in patients with retinitis pigmentosa. *Adv Exp Med Biol* 533: 49–57. doi:10.1007/978-1-4615-0067-4_7

Lowe J, Drasdo N. 1992. Patients' responses to retinitis pigmentosa. *Optom Vis Sci* 69: 182–185. doi:10.1097/00006324-199203000-00003

Mack H, Chen F, Grigg J, Jamieson R, De Roach J, O'Hare F, Britten-Jones A, McGuiness M, Tindill N, Ayton L, et al. 2021. Perspectives of people with inherited retinal diseases on ocular gene therapy in Australia: protocol for a national survey. *BMJ Open* 11: e048361. doi:10.1136/bmjopen-2020-048361

Mangione C, Berry S, Spritzer K, Janz N, Klein R, Owsley C, Lee P. 1998a. Identifying the content area for the 51-item national eye institute visual function questionnaire: results from focus groups with visually impaired persons. *Arch Ophthalmol* 116: 227–233.

Mangione C, Lee P, Pitts J, Gutierrez M, Berry S, Hays R. 1998b. Psychometric properties of the national eye institute visual function questionnaire (NEI-VFQ). NEI-VFQ field test investigators. *Arch Ophthalmol* 116: 1496–1504. doi:10.1001/archopht.116.11.1496

Mangione C, Lee P, Gutierrez P, Spritzer K, Berry S, Hays R. 2001. Development of the 25-item national eye institute visual function questionnaire. *Arch Ophthalmol* 119: 1050–1058. doi:10.1001/archopht.119.7.1050

Marques J, Bernardes L, Oliveira C, Fonseca G, Gil J, Sotero L, Relvas A, Murta J, Silva R, Lacy G, et al. 2022. Portuguese translation and linguistic validation of the Michigan retinal degeneration questionnaire and the Michigan vision-related anxiety questionnaire in a cohort with inherited retinal degenerations. *Ophthalmic Genet* 43: 137–139. doi:10.1080/13816810.2022.2025609

Matza L, Patrick D, Riley A, Alexander J, Rajmil L, Pleil A, Bullinger M. 2013. Pediatric patient-reported outcome instruments for research to support medical product labeling: report of the ISPOR PRO good research practices for the assessment of children and adolescents task force. *Value Health* 16: 461–479. doi:10.1016/j.jval.2013.04.004

McGuinness M, Britten-Jones A, Ayton L, Finger R, Chen F, Grigg J, Mack H. 2022. Measurement properties of the attitudes to gene therapy for the eye (AGT-Eye) instrument for people with inherited retinal diseases. *Transl Vis Sci Technol* 11: 14. doi:10.1167/tvst.11.2.14

Michaelides M, Hunt D, Moore A. 2003. The genetics of inherited macular dystrophies. *J Med Genet* 40: 641–650. doi:10.1136/jmg.40.9.641

Miedziak A, Perski T, Andrews P, Donoso L. 2000. Stargardt's macular dystrophy—a patient's perspective. *Optometry* **71:** 165–176.

Misajon R, Hawthorne G, Richardson J, Barton J, Peacock S, Iezzi A, Keeffe J. 2005. Vision and quality of life: the development of a utility measure. *Invest Ophthalmol Vis Sci* **46:** 4007–4015. doi:10.1167/iovs.04-1389

Murro V, Sodi A, Giacomelli G, Mucciolo D, Pennino M, Virgili G, Rizzo S. 2017. Reading ability and quality of life in Stargardt disease. *Eur J Ophthalmol* **27:** 740–745. doi:10.5301/ejo.5000972

Peacock S, Misajon R, Iezzi A, Richardson J, Hawthorne G, Keeffe J. 2008. Vision and quality of life: development of methods for the VisQoL vision-related utility instrument. *Ophthalmic Epidemiol* **15:** 218–223. doi:10.1080/09286580801979417

Pesudovs K, Gothwal V, Wright T, Lamoureux E. 2010. Remediating serious flaws in the national eye institute visual function questionnaire. *J Cataract Refract Surg* **36:** 718–732. doi:10.1016/j.jcrs.2009.11.019

Petrillo J, Cano S, McLeod L, Coon C. 2015. Using classical test theory, item response theory, and Rasch measurement theory to evaluate patient-reported outcome measures: a comparison of worked examples. *Value Health* **18:** 25–34. doi:10.1016/j.jval.2014.10.005

Prem Senthil M, Khadka J, Pesudovs K. 2017a. Assessment of patient-reported outcomes in retinal diseases: a systematic review. *Surv Ophthalmol* **62:** 546–582. doi:10.1016/j.survophthal.2016.12.011

Prem Senthil M, Khadka J, Pesudovs K. 2017b. Seeing through their eyes: lived experiences of people with retinitis pigmentosa. *Eye (Lond)* **31:** 741–748. doi:10.1038/eye.2016.315

Prem Senthil M, Khadka J, Gilhotra J, Simon S, Pesudovs K. 2017c. Exploring the quality of life issues in people with retinal diseases: a qualitative study. *J Patient Rep Outcomes* **1:** 15. doi:10.1186/s41687-017-0023-4

Prem Senthil M, Khadka J, De Roach J, Lamey T, McLaren T, Campbell I, Fenwick E, Lamoureux E, Pesudovs K. 2019. Development and psychometric assessment of novel item banks for hereditary retinal diseases. *Optom Vis Sci* **96:** 27–34. doi:10.1097/OPX.0000000000001317

Roborel de Climens A, Tugaut B, Piscopo A, Arnould B, Buggage R, Brun-Strang C. 2020. Living with type I Usher syndrome: insights from patients and their parents. *Ophthalmic Genet* **41:** 240–251. doi:10.1080/13816810.2020.1737947

Roborel de Climens A, Tugaut B, Dias Barbosa C, Buggage R, Brun-Strang C. 2021. Living with Stargardt disease: insights from patients and their parents. *Ophthalmic Genet* **42:** 150–160. doi:10.1080/13816810.2020.1855663

Seo J, Yu H, Lee B. 2009. Assessment of functional vision score and vision-specific quality of life in individuals with retinitis pigmentosa. *Korean J Ophthalmol* **23:** 164–168. doi:10.3341/kjo.2009.23.3.164

Sharpe L, Stockman A, Jagle H, Nathans J. 1999. Opsin genes, cone photopigments, color vision, and color blindness. In *Color vision: from genes to perception* (ed. Gegenfurtner K, Sharpe LT), pp. 3–52. Cambridge University Press, Cambridge, UK.

Somani S, Brent M, Markowitz S. 2006. Visual field expansion in patients with retinitis pigmentosa. *Can J Ophthalmol* **41:** 27–33. doi:10.1016/S0008-4182(06)80062-1

Sugawara T, Hagiwara A, Hiramatsu A, Ogata K, Mitamura Y, Yamamoto S. 2010. Relationship between peripheral visual field loss and vision-related quality of life in patients with retinitis pigmentosa. *Eye (Lond)* **24:** 535–539. doi:10.1038/eye.2009.176

Sugawara T, Sato E, Baba T, Hagiwara A, Tawada A, Yamamoto S. 2011. Relationship between vision-related quality of life and microperimetry-determined macular sensitivity in patients with retinitis pigmentosa. *Jpn J Ophthalmol* **55:** 643–646. doi:10.1007/s10384-011-0080-9

Sumi I, Matsumoto S, Okajima O, Shirato S. 2000. The relationship between visual disability and visual scores in patients with retinitis pigmentosa. *Jpn J Ophthalmol* **44:** 82–87. doi:10.1016/S0021-5155(99)00171-9

Szlyk J, Fishman G, Grover S, Revelins B, Derlacki D. 1998. Difficulty in performing everyday activities in patients with juvenile macular dystrophies: comparison with patients with retinitis pigmentosa. *Br J Ophthalmol* **82:** 1372–1376. doi:10.1136/bjo.82.12.1372

Szlyk J, Seiple W, Fishman G, Alexander K, Grover S, Mahler C. 2001. Perceived and actual performance of daily tasks: relationship to visual function tests in individuals with retinitis pigmentosa. *Ophthalmology* **108:** 65–75. doi:10.1016/S0161-6420(00)00413-9

Tanna P, Strauss R, Fujinami K, Michaelides M. 2017. Stargardt disease: clinical features, molecular genetics, animal models and therapeutic options. *Br J Ophthalmol* **101:** 25–30. doi:10.1136/bjophthalmol-2016-308823

Turano K, Geruschat D, Stahl J, Massof R. 1999. Perceived visual ability for independent mobility in persons with retinitis pigmentosa. *Invest Ophthalmol Vis Sci* **40:** 865–877.

Turner-Bowker D, Lamoureux R, Stokes J, Litcher-Kelly L, Galipeau N, Yaworsky A, Solomon J, Shields A. 2018. Informing a priori sample size estimation in qualitative concept elicitation interview studies for clinical outcome assessment instrument development. *Value Health* **21:** 839–842. doi:10.1016/j.jval.2017.11.014

Turriff A, Nolen R, D'Amanda C, Biesecker B, Cukras C, Sieving PA. 2020. "There are hills and valleys": experiences of parenting a son with X-linked retinoschisis. *Am J Ophthalmol* **212:** 98–104. doi:10.1016/j.ajo.2019.11.023

U.S. Department of Health and Human Services Food and Drug Administration; Center for Drug Evaluation and Research (CDER); Center for Biologics Evaluation and Research (CBER); Center for Devices and Radiological Health (CDRH). 2009. Guidance for industry—patient-reported outcome measures: use in medical product development to support labeling claims. FDA, Rockville, MD.

U.S. Department of Health and Human Services Food and Drug Administration; Center for Drug Evaluation and Research (CDER); Center for Biologics Evaluation and Research (CBER). 2020. Guidance for industry—patient-focused drug development: collecting comprehensive and representative input. FDA, Rockville, MD.

U.S. Department of Health and Human Services Food and Drug Administration; Center for Drug Evaluation and Research (CDER); Center for Biologics Evaluation and Research (CBER). 2022. Guidance for industry—patient-focused drug development: methods to identify what is important to patient. FDA, Rockville, MD.

Whittal A, Meregaglia M, Nicod E. 2021. The use of patient-reported outcome measures in rare diseases and implica-tions for health technology assessment. *Patient* **14:** 485–503. doi:10.1007/s40271-020-00493-w

Zelihić D, Hjardemaal F, Lippe C. 2020. Caring for a child with Bardet–Biedl syndrome: a qualitative study of the parental experiences of daily coping and support. *Eur J Med Genet* **63:** 103856. doi:10.1016/j.ejmg.2020.103856

Cite this article as *Cold Spring Harb Perspect Med* doi: 10.1101/cshperspect.a041298

Mobility Testing and Other Performance-Based Assessments of Functional Vision in Patients with Inherited Retinal Disease

Daniel Chung,[1] Colas Authié,[2] and Laure Blouin[3]

[1]SparingVision, Philadelphia, Pennsylvania 19103, USA

[2]StreetLab, Institut de la Vision, UMR 7210 CNRS - UPMC - INSERM - CHNO, 75012 Paris, France

[3]SparingVision, 75008 Paris, France

Correspondence: daniel.chung@sparingvision.com

In the field of clinical ophthalmology, many of the common visual function study end points do not effectively reflect the significant morbidity of inherited retinal diseases (IRDs) and its effect on the patient's quality of life. In the last decade, emphasis has been placed on the development and implementation of patient-performance or task-focused end points, that may have greater ability to demonstrate the improvement or preservation of the patient's quality of life provided by therapeutic interventions. This article reviews performance-based tools developed to assess functional vision, such as the multi-luminance mobility test (MLMT) or the functional low-vision observer-rated assessment (FLORA), and highlights some of the recent advancements used in clinical development for IRD or ocular interventional therapies.

In the last few decades, significant advances have been made in the area of gene-based medicine to address inherited retinal diseases (IRDs). This was exemplified by the 2017 regulatory approval for voretigene neparvovec, the first gene therapy to address an IRD, in this case caused by biallelic variants in the *RPE65* gene. Our understanding of the functional and structural changes caused by IRDs and their resultant impact on vision has greatly aided the development of gene-based therapeutic strategies for these diseases, which continue to have a high unmet need. IRDs consist of a heterogeneous group of diseases commonly caused by variants in a single gene. They include cone-

rod, cone and rod-cone dystrophies such as retinitis pigmentosa (RP) or choroideremia, as well as many other clinical classifications such as Leber congenital amaurosis (LCA), Stargardt disease, Best disease, or blue cone monochromacy. They are all characterized by a dysfunction of the photoreceptors and/or retinal pigment epithelium of the retina. Worldwide, these pathologies cause vision deficits in millions of patients.

Since the success of the first gene therapy approved for an IRD, the number of clinical development programs for IRDs has significantly expanded. They typically use gene-based strategies—the most common being gene augmentation therapy—but more recently, gene editing and antisense oligonucleotide strategies are also being investigated.

Advances in technology have allowed the development of different methods to deliver genetic material to the retina using viral and nonviral vectors, with the aim of reversing, stopping, or slowing down the progression of these diseases. Additional focus has been placed on vector optimization and safety, immunomodulation, and the identification of more relevant clinical study end points.

By nature, IRDs are considered a rare disease, although in aggregate they affect millions of patients worldwide. Their etiology is also highly disparate, with over 300 different genes responsible for syndromic and nonsyndromic forms of the disease. Therefore, the development of therapies for IRDs is faced with the common challenges of clinical development for rare diseases: low patient numbers, limited natural history studies, and difficult market access and commercialization. In addition, the slow progression of most IRDs and the lack of significant biomarkers to monitor this progression have been major challenges in the clinical development of effective therapies. Appropriate clinical end points will need to effectively document the changes in visual performance, regardless of the therapeutic aim of reversing, stopping, or slowing down disease progression. Currently, many of the common visual function study end points do not effectively reflect the significant morbidity of the individual diseases, with its effect on the patient's quality of life.

In response to some of these challenges, emphasis has been placed on the development and implementation of patient-performance or task-focused end points, that may have greater ability to demonstrate the improvement or preservation of the patient's quality of life provided by therapeutic interventions. These performance end points are often referred to as functional vision, versus visual function, which is typically assessed by ophthalmic measures (Bennett et al. 2019). Functional vision is the ability to conduct visually dependent activities, which is critical for an individual's autonomy to perform tasks of daily living, and consequently

maintain their overall quality of life and a degree of independence. A such, the maintenance of functional vision may delay a patient's dependency on a caregiver due to their visual deficit.

These functional end points have gained further validity and interest, considering that the primary end point in the pivotal phase 3 trial of voretigene neparvovec was a novel functional-vision mobility end point called the multi-luminance mobility test (MLMT). This review will look at some of the functional end points such as MLMT, functional low-vision observer-rated assessment (FLORA), and some of the recent advancements used in clinical development for IRD or ocular interventional therapies.

MULTI-LUMINANCE MOBILITY TEST (MLMT)

The MLMT was designed to evaluate a patient's ability for visually based performance on a defined mobility course, at various standardized lights levels. It was originally developed to evaluate subjects in the clinical development of voretigene neparvovec, a gene therapy for patients with biallelic variants in the *RPE65* gene (Russell et al. 2017). Subjects with *RPE65*-associated IRDs usually experience a rapid and early onset of retinal degeneration, starting with rod photoreceptors responsible for dim-light vision, gradually leading to loss-of-light sensitivity. The MLMT was designed to integrate visual function parameters—such as visual acuity, visual field, and light sensitivity—into a quantifiable measure that could be used to show gains in mobility at lower light intensities. This end point marked one of the first quantifiable performance-based assessments of vision. Its success was due to its high reproducibility, a robust and refined testing rubric, completion of a content and construct validation study, and its use in several published clinical studies (Russell et al. 2017; Chung et al. 2018).

In brief, the test was administered at baseline and then at set intervals of follow-up, for up to 5 years after subretinal administration of voretigene neparvovec (Bennett et al. 2021). At enrollment, subjects were introduced to a training course: they were instructed to follow arrows

 Cite this article as *Cold Spring Harb Perspect Med* doi: 10.1101/cshperspect.a041299

on the MLMT course while avoiding obstacles in or adjacent to their path, to step on every arrowed tile, and to avoid off-course movement. The test was scored in metrics of time to complete the course and the accuracy in completing them. At the first testing visit, prior to intervention, the lowest light level was determined at which they could successfully navigate the course. At testing light levels, and following dark adaptation, subjects were tested for each eye separately (the contralateral eye was patched) in random sequence, and then with both eyes unpatched, as the primary measure. All course attempts were video- and audio-recorded, coded, and sent to independent Orientation and Mobility (O&M)-trained graders who evaluated the test performance based on a predetermined grading rubric, which scored speed of travel and number of obstacles hit (i.e., accuracy). This allowed for quantification of the performance score, which compared baseline measures with post-intervention performance. Passing scores required reaching two preset time and accuracy thresholds.

In 2017 and 2018, respectively, the U.S. and European Union regulatory authorities accepted the MLMT test results as a successful primary end point of functional vision in a pivotal trial. The success of this novel end point can be attributed to its straightforward design, but also to a separate study demonstrating the construct and content validity of the test.

The mobility course was printed on large canvases, which allowed easy course changes while maintaining the consistent layout of each course. The pathway consisted of a sequence of adjacent squares with arrows used to create 12 different courses. All courses included the same number of arrows, squares, turns, and obstacles. The obstacles included objects of various heights placed both next to and on the arrowed path, that the subject would have to navigate around or step over. During testing, the sequence of courses presented to the patient were randomly selected, and all 12 courses were verified to be of equal difficulty. The light levels ranged from 1 lux—similar to a moonless summer night—to 400 lux, which is equal to a brightly lit office. In total, seven light levels were chosen to mimic light intensities commonly encountered in scenarios of daily living. Scoring was based on the lowest light level at which the subject could successfully traverse the mobility test, with a comparison before and after intervention. Following gene therapy administration, the vast majority of the subjects showed improved mobility scores, meaning they could navigate the mobility test successfully at lower light levels after intervention, compared to untreated control subjects who did not show significant improvement (Russell et al. 2017).

Furthermore, a separate study was carried out to test the content and construct validity of the MLMT (Chung et al. 2018). Its results showed (1) construct validity (i.e., the test's ability to differentiate between subjects with nonimpaired vision from those with impaired vision); (2) reliability, demonstrated by high inter-, intra-, and test–retest grader reproducibility; (3) content validity, as speed and accuracy at the seven light levels correlated to a visual function test, the full-field light stimulation threshold (FST) test, with passing thresholds reported for visual acuity, visual field, and patient questionnaires; and (4) its ability to detect changes in functional vision over time in IRD subjects.

Although the MLMT constitutes the first functional vision test successfully used to assess patients with IRD in a successful pivotal trial for gene therapy, different mobility courses have been developed for other ocular indications.

ORIENTATION AND MOBILITY ASSESSMENT FOR A RETINAL PROSTHESIS

In the mid-2000s, Optobionics Corporation developed an artificial silicon retina (ASR) comprised of 5000 passive microphotodiodes powered purely from ambient light. In a safety and feasibility trial, six legally blind patients affected by RP were implanted with the 2-mm-wide array in their right eye. All patients reported improvements in visual function over several weeks, even though it could not be attributed solely to the implant (Chow and Chow 2007).

In preparation for a commercialization of their implant, the company—that was liquidated before reaching that stage—developed a controlled mobility course to assess O&M in eight patients with ultralow vision defined as a visual acuity below 20/1600 (Geruschat et al. 2012). The mobility course consisted in an 18-m-long narrow corridor painted and carpeted in light colors, and evenly illuminated. Every 1.5 m, an obstacle was placed in the patient's way: either a tube of dark foam was suspended from the ceiling, or a dark rug was placed on the floor. By varying the type and location of the obstacles, 96 different configurations were possible for this obstacle course.

Patients had to walk the mobility course and back, trying to avoid a total of 24 obstacles distributed over 36 m. Patients performed this test three times: once using only their treated eye, once using only their untreated eye, and once using their binocular vision. Each run was scored using the time it took the patient to walk the obstacle course and the number of obstacles they accidentally touched.

O&M assessment did not detect improvements in patients implanted with the ASR, and therefore did not corroborate the vision improvement that patients reported. The low sensitivity of this controlled mobility course was thought to be partially due to its lack of complexity. It is also worth noting that visual acuity did not constitute a good predictor of mobility in this study, and authors reckoned that stronger predictors such as contrast sensibility or visual field probably could have been better correlates.

FUNCTIONAL LOW-VISION OBSERVER-RATED ASSESSMENT (FLORA)

Although mobility testing has been used in recent gene therapy trials, patient-performance testing has also been developed not based on mobility. In 2011, Second Sight developed a tool to objectively assess mobility in patients with low vision. Following a recommendation from the FDA, the FLORA was designed to assess real-world functional vision and well-being in subjects participating in a phase I clinical trial of the Argus II retinal prosthesis.

The Argus II prosthesis was a retinal implant used to electrically stimulate cells of the inner retina that remain partially functional in patients with late-stage RP. In a first-in-man study opened in 2007, 30 subjects with ultralow vision (VA < 20/1600) were treated with the Argus II (Ahuja et al. 2011). Twenty-nine subjects had RP, and one suffered from choroideremia. All subjects had bare light perception for a mean of 16 years prior to enrolling in the trial.

The FLORA assessments were administered to 26 participants. Half of them had been implanted with the retinal prosthesis for over 3 years on average, and the other half for around 1.7 years (this difference in follow-up was due to the temporary interruption of patient recruitment) (Geruschat et al. 2015). The FLORA assessments typically took 3–4 hours to complete with the help of an evaluator. It was structured as a three-part approach: self-report, observation of performance, and case summary.

The self-report consisted of 14 open-ended questions assessing the impact of the retinal prosthesis on the well-being of the treated patient, from their point of view. The large majority of the questions were answered, and no question was passed up more than twice.

The observation part of the FLORA instrument included activities of daily living (ADLs) and tasks of O&M that the subject performed with the retinal prosthesis turned on and turned off, under the assessment of an external evaluator. For their observation, the evaluator selected tasks ranging from assignments that could likely be performed only with light perception or projection (i.e., locate a light source, find an open doorway, or determine whether the lights are on or off) to assignments that required some extent of visual acuity and more elaborate oculomotor abilities (i.e., recognize shapes, estimate the size of an object). However, tasks requiring a level of vision beyond what the prosthesis could afford were excluded from the FLORA (i.e., reading 12-point print, identifying faces or colors).

The tasks were organized in five categories: body awareness and orientation (only performed when the Argus II was turned off), visual orientation (e.g., using light contrasts to detect windows or doors), vision for mobility (e.g., following crosswalks, or avoiding obstacles), daily living tasks (e.g., sort out dark from light-colored laundry), and social interactions (e.g., detect people in room or walking by). Evaluators selected which tasks to observe, depending on the subject's self-reported abilities and goals. Ease of performance was graded impossible, difficult, moderate, or easy. The amount of vision required for task accomplishment was also rated from no vision involved, to vision only.

All 35 tasks available for assessment were selected at least once by an observer, with on average 20 subjects performing a given task (range: 5–26). The tasks selected by observers were evenly distributed in terms of level of difficulty.

The third part of FLORA was a narrative case report summarizing the findings and observations, considering both the subject's and the evaluator's point of view: the effects of treatment on functional vision were reported by the observer, and well-being and satisfaction were reported by the subject. The results of these highly individualized reports written by different evaluators were not discussed by Geruschat et al. (2015).

In March of 2020, a clinical trial was opened to validate the FLORA-20 instrument—comprising 20 functional vision tasks commonly performed around the house—in profoundly blind individuals. The FLORA-20 was designed as the primary end point of the pivotal clinical trial of the Orion Visual Cortical Prosthesis System, a brain implant intended to provide useful artificial vision to blind patients. However, the validation trial of the FLORA-20 instrument was suspended due to the covid-19 pandemic and plans to review and restart the study are currently being evaluated.

VISION-GUIDED MOBILITY ASSESSMENT

In 2016, a vision-guided mobility assessment was developed by the University College of London to assess mobility in patients with RPE65-associated retinal dystrophy (*RPE65-RD*). This test was also used in a phase I–II clinical trial of AAV2/5-OPTIRPE65 gene therapy (NCT02781480). The tool was later optimized as a research platform named Pedestrian Accessibility Movement Environment Labora-

tory (PAMELA) and validated in 2020 (Kumaran et al. 2020).

This mobility assessment instrument was comprised of three sections: a 10-m straight line, a 13-m simple maze with moveable barriers, and a second 10-m straight line including two obstacles that simulate sidewalk curbs. A series of tests were performed at decreasing illumination levels (from 246 down to 1 lux), following a period of light adaptation. That was specifically designed to assess vision mobility with progressive difficulty, in this population of patients suffering from nyctalopia.

For each trial, the following measures were collected: time to complete the course, walking speed, and number of errors made (disorientation or contact with obstacle). Walking speed and course time were the most accurate measures to discriminate between affected and non-affected patients.

Test–retest did not indicate any learning effect, despite a rather large coefficient of repeatability. The vision-guided mobility assessment showed both convergent and discriminant (divergent) validity, respectively, as mean retinal sensitivity and total hill of vision could predict walking speed, when visual acuity and contrast sensitivity did not.

Furthermore, it appeared that faster walking speed was correlated with higher retinal sensitivity. Finally, walking speed was associated with the difficulties in mobility reported in quality-of-life questionnaires.

StreetLab AND THE MOBILITY STANDARDIZED TEST (MOST)

In 2013, clinicians and researchers at the Institut de la Vision (Paris, France) designed a research facility dedicated to the development of new methods to evaluate and train patients with low vision. The StreetLab center is committed to assess therapeutic benefits and innovative solutions for mobility in real-life conditions, and support the comprehensive investigation of behavioral and adaptive mechanisms in visually impaired patients.

This facility includes four evaluation platforms: an artificial street, a test apartment, a virtual reality platform, and a driving simulator. The artificial street recreates a wide-street environment (9 × 7 m) with controlled light levels (0–2000 lux), color temperature (2700–6500 K), and 3D sound system. The fully controlled conditions can be tailored to accommodate a broad array of experimental conditions in terms of light, sound, and adjustable scenery (decor, furniture, etc.). Besides, mobility assessment can be combined with objective eye tracking and full-body motion-capture systems.

The virtual reality platform allows patients to be immersed in standardized tasks inspired by daily life. The advantages of virtual reality include the ability to assess patient's behavior in conditions that are difficult to evaluate in real life, and to reproduce these experimental constraints in multiple investigation centers.

StreetLab platforms have been used to assess O&M in several clinical studies. For example, simulated tasks of daily living were evaluated in 32 patients with glaucoma: "mobility" and obstacle avoidance using the artificial street environment, "reaching and grasping" large and small objects on a kitchen work surface, "localization of people," and "face orientation recognition" (Lombardi et al. 2018). In this pilot study, visual performance was not analyzed based on subjective quality-of-life questionnaires, but on the objective evaluation of a patient's abilities to perform tasks of daily living. Results of the daily-living tasks significantly correlated with parameters of binocular visual field and mean deviation in the best-seeing eye. Moreover, mobility performance was significantly impacted by glare disability observed in patients with moderate and severe glaucoma (Bertaud et al. 2021). However, no correlation was found between results of the daily-living tasks and results of the NEI VFQ-25 quality-of-life questionnaire (Azoulay-Sebban et al. 2020).

Mobility performance was also assessed in IRDs. In patients with RP, visual field was the most significant predictor of mobility performance under low light (1 lux), while contrast sensitivity best correlated with the number of collisions and segments in the trajectory (Sahel et al. 2021a). Moreover, compensatory adapta-

tions in gaze/eye movements were identified during locomotion in RP patients with peripheral visual field loss (Authié et al. 2017). In two patients (one adult, one child) with LCA due to a mutation in the *RPE65* gene, positive effects were observed on travel speed and number of collisions, especially at low luminance, 6 months after gene therapy with voretigene neparvovec (Luxturna) (Sahel et al. 2021a). The StreetLab platforms were also used to detect the first partial functional recovery after optogenetic therapy in a patient with severe vision loss due to RP (Sahel et al. 2021b).

Finally, the driving simulator at StreetLab was used to safely assess the driving performance of individuals with normal vision and visually impaired patients. This platform helped reveal that, during simulated car racing, driving performance and safety were better when visual acuity was artificially reduced in the dominant eye compared to purely monocular vision (Adrian et al. 2019); and that glaucoma patients exhibited unsafe driving behaviors despite the driving and eye-scanning compensatory mechanisms they put in place to counterbalance their visual impairment (Adrian et al. 2022).

Recently, a new mobility test called "mobility standardized test" (MOST) was developed and validated by the researchers at StreetLab, to monitor the progression of retinal disease and assess the efficacy of new treatments (Authié et al. 2022). This test can be performed either in real-life or virtual conditions (MOST-IRL or MOST-VR), and demonstrated excellent reproducibility, sensitivity, and high agreement between both conditions. Moreover, the virtual test MOST-VR has two advantages over its real-life version MOST-IRL: it is easily exported and implemented in multicentric studies, and it allows the assessment of patient performance without the intervention of a human observer.

DISCUSSION

Quantitative patient performance testing has been a challenge to develop for the assessment of visual impairment in patients with IRD. Mobility testing scenarios in real-world conditions are difficult to standardize, and can potentially be unsafe for the subjects in clinical trials. Therefore, patient-performance testing in controlled study settings was developed as a surrogate for real-world testing. The field of ophthalmology has seen a rise in the clinical development of therapies for rare IRDs—with the advent of voretigene neparvovec, the first gene therapy to receive global regulatory approval for IRDs associated with biallelic variants in the *RPE65* gene—and this has revealed the need for additional outcome measures. There are currently no well-accepted systemic biomarkers of ophthalmological function, so clinical development relies heavily on visual function tests to measure therapeutic benefits. Unfortunately, the threshold of 0.3 LogMAR or 15-letter change in visual acuity measured by the Early Treatment Diabetic Retinopathy Study (ETDRS) chart, commonly used to assess treatments for macular edema, is not as relevant when it comes to rare IRDs.

The MLMT was the first quantifiable functional vision test to be successfully used in a pivotal clinical trial for an IRD, which has led almost all clinical development programs for rare ocular diseases to incorporate mobility testing in their protocols. It should be noted, however, that a given mobility test may not be suited for all diseases. For example, MLMT is able to measure performance at various levels of illumination and is designed to detect improvement in mobility due to an increase in light sensitivity. This should be appropriate for most rod-cone dystrophies, but cone and cone-rod dystrophies may not be properly assessed with this test, at least in its current design.

Each type of mobility test needs to be evaluated for what it is designed to measure. The question of what to measure should ideally start with patient community input, to identify the most prominent deficit in visual function that causes impairment and degradation of their quality of life. Performance-based testing is primarily used to show the impact of a therapeutic benefit on the individual's quality of life. Investigation and development of these end points have gained more interest and acceptance as a valid and pertinent method for demonstrating a positive therapeutic effect after treatment intervention. As there is a great need to develop and refine ocular outcome measures, performance-based testing will remain one of the major objectives for the clinical development of ocular therapeutics.

REFERENCES

Adrian J, Le Brun J, Miller N, Sahel JA, Saillant G, Bodaghi B. 2019. Implications of monocular vision for racing drivers. *PLoS ONE* **14**: e0226308. doi:10.1371/journal.pone.0226308

Adrian J, Authié C, Lebrun J, Lombardi M, Zenouda A, Gutman E, Brasnu E, Hamard P, Sahel JA, Baudouin C, et al. 2022. Driving behaviour and visual compensation in glaucoma patients: evaluation on a driving simulator. *Clin Exp Ophthalmol* **50**: 420–428. doi:10.1111/ceo.14062

Ahuja AK, Dorn JD, Caspi A, McMahon MJ, Dagnelie G, Dacruz L, Stanga P, Humayun MS, Greenberg RJ; Argus II Study Group. 2011. Blind subjects implanted with the Argus II retinal prosthesis are able to improve performance in a spatial-motor task. *Br J Ophthalmol* **95**: 539–543. doi:10.1136/bjo.2010.179622

Authié C, Berthoz A, Sahel JA, Safran A. 2017. Adaptive gaze strategies for locomotion with constricted visual field. *Front Hum Neurosci* **11**: 38. doi:10.3389/fnhum.2017.00387

Authié CN, Poujade M, Talebi A, Defer A, Zenouda A, Coen C, Zhang Y, Sahel JA, Mohand-Said S, Chaumet-Riffaud P, et al. 2022. Development and validation of a mobility test for inherited retinal disease in real and virtual conditions—preliminary results. *Invest Ophthalmol Vis Sci* **63**: 715–F0443.

Azoulay-Sebban L, Zhao Z, Zenouda A, Lombardi M, Gutman E, Brasnu E, Hamard P, Sahel JA, Baudouin C, Labbé A. 2020. Correlations between subjective evaluation of quality of life, visual field loss, and performance in simulated activities of daily living in glaucoma patients. *J Glaucoma* **29**: 970–974. doi:10.1097/IJG.0000000000001597

Bennett CR, Bex PJ, Bauer CM, Merabet LB. 2019. The assessment of visual function and functional vision. *Semin Pediatr Neurol* **31**: 30–40. doi:10.1016/j.spen.2019.05.006

Bennett J, Russell SR, High KA, Drack AV, Yu ZF, Chung DC, Reape K, Maguire AM. 2021. Five-year post-injection results of the phase 3 trial of voretigene neparvovec-rzyl in biallelic RPE65 mutation-associated inherited retinal disease. *Invest Ophthalmol Vis Sci* **62**: 3540.

Bertaud S, Zenouda A, Lombardi M, Authié C, Brasnu E, Hamard P, Sahel JA, Baudouin C, Labbé A. 2021. Glare and mobility performance in glaucoma: a pilot study. *J Glaucoma* **30**: 963–970. doi:10.1097/IJG.0000000000001936

Chow AY, Chow VY. 2007. Subretinal artificial silicon retina microchip implantation in retinitis pigmentosa. In *Ophthalmology research. Visual prosthesis and ophthalmic devices*. Humana Press, Totowa, NJ.

Chung DC, McCague S, Yu ZF, Thill S, DiStefano-Pappas J, Bennett J, Cross D, Marshall K, Wellman J, High KA. 2018. Novel mobility test to assess functional vision in patients with inherited retinal dystrophies. *Clin Exp Ophthalmol* **46:** 247–259. doi:10.1111/ceo.13022

Geruschat DR, Bittner AK, Dagnelie G. 2012. Orientation and mobility assessment in retinal prosthetic clinical trials. *Optom Vis Sci* **89:** 1308–1315. doi:10.1097/OPX.0b013e3182686251

Geruschat DR, Flax M, Tanna N, Bianchi M, Fisher A, Goldschmidt M, Fisher L, Dagnelie G, Deremeik J, Smith A, et al. 2015. FLORA™: phase I development of a functional vision assessment for prosthetic vision users. *Clin Exp Optom* **98:** 342–347. doi:10.1111/cxo.12242

Kumaran N, Ali RR, Tyler NA, Bainbridge JWB, Michaelides M, Rubin GS. 2020. Validation of a vision-guided mobility assessment for *RPE65*-associated retinal dystrophy. *Transl Vis Sci Technol* **9:** 5. doi:10.1167/tvst.9.10.5

Lombardi M, Zenouda A, Azoulay-Sebban L, Lebrisse M, Gutmann E, Brasnu E, Hamard P, Sahel JA, Baudouin C, Labbé A. 2018. Correlation between visual function and performance of simulated daily living activities in glaucomatous patients. *J Glaucoma* **27:** 1017–1024. doi:10.1097/IJG.0000000000001066

Russell S, Bennett J, Wellman JA, Chung DC, Yu ZF, Tillman A, Wittes J, Pappas J, Elci O, McCague S, et al. 2017. Efficacy and safety of voretigene neparvovec (AAV2-hRPE65v2) in patients with RPE65-mediated inherited retinal dystrophy: a randomised, controlled open-label, phase 3 trial. *Lancet* **390:** 849–860. doi:10.1016/S0140-6736(17)31868-8

Sahel JA, Grieve K, Pagot C, Authié C, Mohand-Said S, Paques M, Audo I, Becker K, Chaumet-Riffaud AE, Azoulay L, et al. 2021a. Assessing photoreceptor status in retinal dystrophies: from high-resolution imaging to functional vision. *Am J Ophthalmol* **230:** 12–47. doi:10.1016/j.ajo.2021.04.013

Sahel JA, Boulanger-Scemama E, Pagot C, Arleo A, Galluppi F, Martel J, Degli Esposti S, Delaux A, de Saint Aubert JB, de Montleau C, et al. 2021b. Partial recovery of visual function in a blind patient after optogenetic therapy. *Nat Med* **27:** 1223–1229. doi:10.1038/s41591-021-01351-4

Current Status of Clinical Trials Design and Outcomes in Retinal Gene Therapy

Boris Rosin,[1] Eyal Banin,[2] and José-Alain Sahel[1,2,3]

[1]The UPMC Vision Institute, University of Pittsburgh, Pittsburgh, Pennsylvania 15219, USA

[2]Division of Ophthalmology, Hadassah-Hebrew University Medical Center, Jerusalem 91120, Israel

[3]Institut Hospitalo-Universitaire FOReSIGHT, Paris 75012, France

Correspondence: brosin@pitt.edu

With the rapid expansion of methods encompassed by the term gene therapy, new trials exploring the safety and efficacy of these methods are initiated more frequently. As a result, important questions arise pertaining the design of these trials and patient participation. One of the most important aspects of any clinical trial is the ability to measure the trial's outcome in a manner that will reflect the effect of the treatment and allow its quantification, whether the trial is aimed at preservation or restoration of retinal cells (photoreceptors and others), vision, or both. Here we will review the existing methods for quantification of trial outcomes, stressing the importance of assessing the participant's visual function and not just visual acuity. We will also describe the key considerations in trial design. Finally, as patient safety remains the primary concern in any trial participation, we will outline the key principles in that regard.

The FDA approval of voretigene neparvovec rzyl (AAV2-hRPE65v2), a subretinal injection of a viral vector for the treatment of Leber's congenital amaurosis (LCA) consecutive to mutations in the *RPE65* gene (LCA2; NCT00999609), ushered in a new era of gene therapy trials and, more broadly, vision/visual function restoration trials. With well over 250 known genes causing inherited retinal dystrophies (IRDs) (Pontikos et al. 2020), the potential for novel treatments using gene therapy opened a very large perspective. Gene-replacement techniques continue to evolve and improve. Adjustments to existing technique include methods to enhance mitochondrial function (Chadderton et al. 2023), employed in mitochondrial DNA

mutations such as Leber's hereditary optic neuropathy (LHON) (Newman et al. 2021). Interestingly, such approaches need not be limited to gene therapy, as much simpler interventions (e.g., increasing the intraocular pressure as a means of induction of ocular stress) were shown to enhance the transfer of gene therapy for LHON (McGrady et al. 2023). However, gene therapy is by no means limited to the classic gene-replacement approach, exemplified by voretigene neparvovec rzyl, as the term encompasses many different techniques.

Gene-editing techniques, such as CRISPR-Cas9, have shown great initial promise in in vitro studies (Zhang et al. 2021) and are now being tested in clinical trials in human patients affected by IRDs (NCT03872479). In a subtype of IRDs characterized by a gain-of-function mutation, gene replacement needs to be paired with gene-silencing techniques, some of which act at the RNA level and are designed to control/interfere with the expression of an aberrant protein causing the disorder (Orlans et al. 2021). Gene augmentation, the change of function of existing cells and genes to achieve a therapeutic goal, is another novel approach to gene therapy (Xi et al. 2022). While the approaches described above require surviving target cells, either photoreceptors or ganglion cells, for success, optogenetics, a novel gene therapy approach to the treatment of IRDs, can be used even in cases of widespread photoreceptor loss. The introduction of opsins into the surviving inner retinal cells by means of gene therapy in essence converts them into photoreceptors, with initial safety studies showing great promise (Sahel et al. 2021a) and clinical trials continuing (NCT03326336). Finally, employing gene therapy for introduction of trophic factors known to increase the survival of photoreceptors (e.g., rod-derived cone viability factor [RdCVF]) was shown to promote protection of photoreceptors in murine models of cone-rod dystrophy (Byrne et al. 2015), leading to ongoing phase Ib-IIa trials in patients (NCT05748873).

Unfortunately, far from all gene therapy trials culminate in success, as was the case with the first X-linked *RPGR* gene therapy trial (NCT03116113), despite showing promise in safety trials and some post hoc analyses (von Krusenstiern et al. 2023). Similarly, an RNA-based approach for the treatment of LCA10, while initially showing promise in safety trials (Russell et al. 2022), failed to reach the predefined end points in the subsequent phase 3 trial (NCT03913143). However, such "failures" may reflect flaws in the design of trials. Thus, the need for improving trial design as well as the methods for estimation of outcomes, such as vision/visual function and retinal structure, is self-evident.

The above is not meant to represent a comprehensive review of gene therapy approaches and trials, but rather to impress upon the reader the current scope of the field. This includes in particular the marked differences between the approaches encompassed by the term "gene

therapy," as well as the variability of outcomes, even in treatments initially showing great promise. We have not even mentioned nongene therapy approaches, such as cell therapy and retinal prostheses, for instance.

METHODS FOR OUTCOME ESTIMATION

Visual Acuity and Contrast Sensitivity

While visual acuity is the main method for estimation of visual system function in the clinical setting, and it remains a main component of every attempt to estimate the outcomes of a therapeutic intervention, its usefulness in clinical trials for the treatment of IRDs is somewhat limited. In many of the patients considered for IRD treatment trials, visual acuity is rudimentary. Such is the case in LCA, where poor vision from birth is one of the defining features of the disorder described by Leber in 1869 (Leber 1869). In many cases, ascertaining poor visual acuity is an important parameter for patient inclusion in the study, as patients with preserved visual acuity could potentially lose some of that acuity in an unsuccessful trial. With gene-replacement attempts aimed toward preservation of remaining cells and not their restoration, one does not expect visual acuity to change significantly in a case of a successful intervention. Nevertheless, in trials targeting macular dystrophies and optic nerve disorders, visual acuity may provide compelling data.

Estimation of visual acuity could be performed by the classic ETDRS (Ferris et al. 1982) or the Bailey–Lovie letter charts (Bailey and Lovie 1976). Contrast sensitivity, classically measured by the Pelli–Robson charts (Pelli et al. 1988), could also be estimated by more novel technological approaches (Pelli and Bex 2013). Interestingly, studies have shown that contrast sensitivity (along with visual field) affects functional vision, as estimated by mobility performance, more significantly than visual acuity (Marron and Bailey 1982). In children and nonverbal adults, both visual acuity and contrast sensitivity could be estimated by objective measures employing vision-dependent reflexes, such as the optokinetic nystagmus (OKN) (Hyon et al. 2010), albeit the relationship between these

Cite this article as *Cold Spring Harb Perspect Med* doi: 10.1101/cshperspect.a041301

parameters is complex (Çetinkaya et al. 2008). Of note, OKN responses are the main method for estimation of visual acuity in laboratory animals, and many commercial systems employing the OKN exist (Prusky et al. 2004).

In patients with low vision, the measurement of vison off-chart is less accurate and various attempts to provide reliable quantitative measurements have been put forth (see collections.lib.utah.edu/ark:/87278/s6768n5w) (Schulze-Bonsel et al. 2006; Karanjia et al. 2016).

An alternative approach used in estimation of functional vision in low-vision patients is the use of self-reporting questionnaires, which incorporate the patient's self-assessment of their performance of tasks of daily living. These include the Veterans Affairs Low-Vision Visual Functioning Questionnaire (Stelmack et al. 2004) and the National Eye Institute Visual Function Questionnaire (Mangione et al. 2001), among others. Patient-reported outcomes are becoming increasingly important in this respect (Lacy et al. 2021).

Advanced Psychophysics

Electrophysiology

Since its original description by Ragnar Granit in 1933 (Granit 1933), the full-field electroretinogram (FFERG) has been the mainstay of electrophysiological testing of retinal function in generalized retinal dystrophies. In a similar manner, since the almost simultaneous description of Adrian and Matthews in 1934 (Adrian and Matthews 1934), the visual-evoked potentials (VEPs) test has been used largely for the estimation of function of the visual pathways and during the pre–magnetic resonance imaging (MRI) era was in fact considered to be an important testing modality for the diagnosis of multiple sclerosis presenting with optic neuritis (Halliday et al. 1972). Notably, the VEP response is predominated by macular function and can thus serve as a measure of interventions aimed at the macula (Holder 2004). Multifocal ERG (MFERG) is another useful tool to estimate macular function and offer localization of retinal defects (Hoffmann et al. 2021). In pattern VEP, stimuli are used to corre-

late optic pathways function to visual acuity and checkered pattern VEP has been used to that aim for many years (Harter and White 1968; Regan 1973). Pattern ERG is another method (Riggs et al. 1964) employed for estimation of both retina and optic pathways function (Berninger et al. 1988). The International Society for Clinical Electrophysiology of Vision (ISCEV) defines standards for the reporting of electrophysiological recordings and their analysis (Hamilton et al. 2021; Robson et al. 2022).

Color Vision

Farnsworth hue testing (Kinnear and Sahraie 2002) and the Ishihara plates (Ishihara 1972) have been the mainstay of color vision testing and provide a good estimation of macular function and by extension of the optic nerve (Ménage et al. 1993), where the macular fibers have a much more prominent representation than the fibers originating in the peripheral retina (Holder 2004). Of these, the Farnsworth–Munsell D-15 is perhaps the most useful in the setting of IRDs, where it has been successfully used to estimate cone function (Okajima et al. 1982; Wissinger et al. 2008). This is especially true since the Ishihara and other color vision tests require significantly preserved levels of visual acuity, as opposed to the hue recognition–based tests (Ng and Shih 2017).

Dark Adaptation

Dark adaptation testing is another useful modality for the estimation of retinal function. In particular, the longer latency rod dark adaptation curve is useful in quantifying rod photoreceptor function (Roman et al. 2005), whereas the absence of the rod-cone break is a useful tool in the estimation of cone dysfunction in achromatopsia (Aboshiha et al. 2014), which has recently emerged as the target for gene therapy in several trials (NCT02935517, NCT02599922).

Visual Fields

Visual fields are progressively constricted in many of the IRDs, causing significant dysfunction and impacting the patients' quality of life (Sugawara et al. 2009). The use of the static Humphrey visual fields, the mainstay of clinical practice in the management of glaucoma, is limited in the evaluation and management of IRDs. However, the 10-2 field has been used in more advanced disease with only a central island of viable photoreceptors remaining (Sayo et al. 2017). Nevertheless, kinetic perimetry has traditionally been the modality of choice for the evaluation of visual fields in IRD patients (Berson et al. 1985). In the past two decades, the classic Goldmann kinetic visual field test has been gradually replaced by the Octopus semiautomatic kinetic visual field, and studies have found the two testing modalities to be comparable (Barnes et al. 2019). Recently, the static GATE (German adaptive threshold estimation) protocol has been used more frequently in the evaluation of visual fields of patients participating in clinical trials (Schiefer et al. 2009; Buckley et al. 2022). In addition, microperimetry, somewhat better termed fundus-controlled perimetry, is slowly gaining a very central role in the management of patients of IRDs. In this testing modality, the stimuli are projected directly onto the retina with retinal image registration, allowing to control for patients' eye movements, and the test provides a localized measure of retinal sensitivity mapping (Bagdonaite-Bejarano et al. 2019). As such, this approach allows to map out the preferential retinal locus (PRL) of each individual patient (Schönbach et al. 2022), which is of utmost importance for clinical trials aimed at preservation of the remaining photoreceptors (Yang and Dunbar 2021) as well as the planning of interventions better served by avoiding the PRL, such as in retinal prostheses implantation (Palanker et al. 2022).

Imaging in Relation to Psychophysics

Fundus autofluorecense (FAF) has been demonstrated to be a useful adjunct in the estimation of retinal function, as an abnormal fluorescence area in FAF negatively correlates with the extent of the patients' visual field (Oishi et al. 2013). With the considerable advancements of ocular coherence tomography

(OCT) technologies, the OCT analysis of IRD patients has taken the leap beyond the mere volumetric changes, which still provide significant amounts of useful information (Oh et al. 2020). OCT angiography is used to demonstrate angiographic changes in IRD patients (Cabral et al. 2020) and even monitor progression (Jauregui et al. 2018). Furthermore, due to the high resolution of imaging achieved by OCT, techniques to image the substructures of the photoreceptors have proven to be useful in ascertaining their viability. Thus, in an ongoing study, a specialized algorithm looking at OCTs of patients with generalized IRDs demonstrated a substantial subpopulation of such patients with a measurable volume of alive but dormant cone photoreceptors, making them perhaps amenable to gene therapy and other preservation therapy approaches (Janeschitz-Kriegl et al. 2022). In addition, capitalizing on the ability of the newer OCT devices to demonstrate changes on the micrometer scale, such changes were demonstrated to occur in the initial phase of phototransduction and were found to be repeatable and quantifiable. This, in essence, introduced a new discipline bridging imaging and psychophysics, termed optoretinography (Pandiyan et al. 2020). Potential implications are profound, as one can envision incorporating functional testing into the standard OCT testing performed for many of the patients seen in a retinal clinic. Adaptive optics, an imaging technique allowing in essence resolution on the level of a single cell, in itself an important imaging modality in assessing photoreceptor health (Salmon et al. 2017), further adds to the capability of optoretinography (Cooper et al. 2020).

Visual Function versus Functional Vision

Introduction

The difference between visual acuity, defined as the ability to discern optotypes at a given distance, and visual function, defined as the ability to perform a vision-dependent task, is well established. For instance, it has long been known that visual acuity in patients with advanced age-related macular degeneration does not predict the ability to recognize certain objects and faces, given the same contrast sensitivity levels (Alexander et al. 1988). In the recent preliminary results of IRD treatment by means of optogenetics, an algae-derived opsin, ChrimsonR, was introduced into the surviving cells of the inner retina of a subject with advanced retinitis pigmentosa (RP) and light perception (LP) vision. Following treatment, he was able to detect objects when using the specialized goggles required for the activation of ChrimsonR, while his visual acuity remained LP, in a clear separation between visual acuity and function (Sahel et al. 2021a). On the other hand, patients with RP and visual field constriction, reported a significant functional impairment using the vision-related quality of life questionnaire, despite having relatively preserved visual acuity (Lange et al. 2021). Thus, the importance of developing methods to estimate visual function independently of visual acuity is paramount. To that means, the FDA has put forth guidelines, the Investigational Device Exemption (IDE) Guidance for Retinal Prostheses, describing the essential requirements for any test aimed toward quantifying visual function in trials evaluating retinal prosthetic devices (www.fda.gov/regulatory-information/search-fda-guidance-documents/investigational-device-exemption-ide-guidance-retinal-prostheses).

Object Recognition

As described above, object recognition has recently been shown as a useful method of visual function estimation (Sahel et al. 2021a). Similar approaches include picture discrimination tests (Gulati et al. 2011) and tools designed to assess instrumental activities of daily living in low vision patients (Finger et al. 2014). While these may seem as rudimentary levels of visual function, especially compared to these of patients with measureable visual acuity, the impact on patient's lives can be dramatic. Furthermore, while IRDs are relatively rare, these disorders represent a frequent cause of blindness in both children and young adults, whereas blindness in these age groups is considered to be one of the major socioeconomic burdens on medical-relat-

ed expenditures in the developed world (Frick et al. 2007, 2010).

Navigation Tasks

Introduction

When examining the components of disability of patients with retinal dystrophies, one of the most frequently reported issues is the inability to navigate in unfamiliar environments (Prem Senthil et al. 2017). Thus, navigation tasks have quickly become the preferred method for estimation of visual function in IRD patients.

The MLMT

The multiluminance mobility test (MLMT) (see Chung et al. 2023) was the functional test used during the trials leading to the FDA approval of voretigene neparvovec rzyl (Chung et al. 2018). In this test, the subject performs a navigational task upon a relatively small (7×12 feet) canvas divided into squares. The desired path is denoted by arrows of sufficient size to allow visualization by an individual with a visual acuity of 20/200. Obstacles are introduced in squares both within and outside of the desired path, either conceptually (e.g., black squares representing holes) or physically (e.g., elevated squares within the path). A randomized path is created before each trial. The speed of completion as well as accuracy are scored and combined into a single score.

The importance of the MLMT is undoubtedly in the introduction of a standardized method to assess patient mobility. However, its design had some significant drawbacks. First and foremost, the limited navigation space required patients to adjust their navigation speed to the constricted environment. Furthermore, the composition of the score, reliant only on speed and accuracy of completion and offering strict discretization (lowest score of −1 to highest score of 6), did not adequately reflect the intrinsic complexities of the mobility challenges experienced by patients with IRDs. Finally, the use of conceptual rather than real obstacles created an unrealistic environment poorly representative of day-to-day navigational tasks.

The Streetlab

The Streetlab is an indoor simulation environment designed to mimic the complexities of a real urban street. Its large size (30 × 23 feet) is further enhanced by images projected on the walls of the setup (Fig. 1). Real-time obstacles (e.g., plants, garbage bins, stepladder) are introduced. A sound system is used to introduce real street sounds into the environment.

Multiple parameters are recorded and analyzed. In addition to the accuracy and time to completion, as measured by the MLMT, time to motion initiation after the "go" signal, time to walk 12 feet in a straight line without obstacles, and other similar parameters are recorded. Furthermore, the subjects' motion is recorded by a closed-loop video system and their gait is analyzed to include, in addition to their trajectory, the number of turns and collisions. The tasks are performed under different illumination conditions (Sahel et al. 2021b).

In addition to providing the means to create a controlled environment for visual function testing, the Streetlab offers several advantages over the MLMT. First, it creates a realistic environment of a real-life situation, such as navigating an unfamiliar street, a situation which IRD patients consistently report as one of the most challenging aspects of their visual disability (Sugawara et al. 2009). Furthermore, it offers a multitude of parameters for the quantification of the changes in visual function, adequately representing the intricacies of all the aspects of a successful navigational task. Finally, the use of highly flexible and adaptable environment, allows the utilization of the individual patient's "coping mechanisms" (i.e., the strategies they adapt to improve their visual function) (Authié et al. 2017; Sahel et al. 2021b).

Virtual Reality Constructs

With the use of augmented and virtual reality gaining a more central place in our lives, the use of virtual reality constructs is an intuitive approach to creation of custom navigational tasks for visual function estimation. To date, no uniform approach to the design of such tasks exists

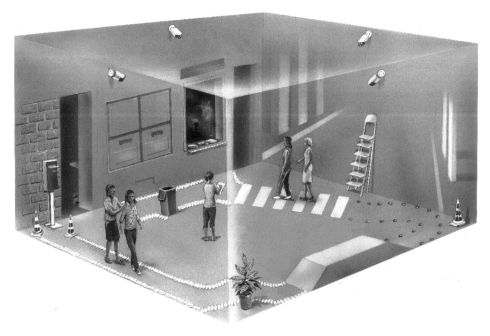

Figure 1. A schematic representation of the Streetlab. Each patient is accompanied by a mobility specialist. A central coordinator is monitoring their performance and taking notes. Video recording is stored for offline analysis of gait and movement initiation. (Illustration provided by Tuvia Kurtz.)

and standardization is required to incorporate such tests as acceptable outcome measures in both observational and interventional trials (Authié et al. 2023; Pur et al. 2023).

Considerations in the Design of Clinical Trials

Introduction

With IRDs presenting a significant cause of visual disability worldwide (Cross et al. 2022), standardization of performing clinical trials is of the utmost importance. The Second Monaciano Symposium for the Advancement of Clinical Trials for IRFDs set forth recommendations for the performance of such trials (Thompson et al. 2020). While a comprehensive discussion regarding such strategies is beyond the scope of this review, we will mention here what we believe to be the most pivotal points when designing a study aimed at furthering the understanding and developing treatments of IRDs.

Observational Studies

These should ideally be performed prior to the interventional study, with the aim to adequately describe the natural history of a genetic condition. Naturally, for any study aimed at furthering the understanding of or developing a new treatment modality for IRDs, a precise genetic diagnosis of the condition is crucial. This will not only exclude nongenetic cases, but could also provide information about the significance of different mutations in disease phenotype. Notably, phenotypes tend to express variation even for the same mutation in different patients.

Ideally, an observational study should collect as much clinical information as possible regarding the IRD in question. Practically, and as shown in this review, the large amount of different testing modalities makes it impossible to perform all for each study. Out of the modalities listed above, visual acuity, contrast sensitivity, color vision, visual fields, basic imaging (fundus photos, FAF, and OCT) and a baseline FFERG are essential. The latter is also useful as an end point test, provided the baseline ERG is recordable. Additional testing modalities should be adapted to fit the disease in question (e.g., MFERG for maculopathies vs. dark adaptation for achromatopsia). Visual function tests are very useful to quantify the resultant disability.

Interventional Studies

Perhaps the most important aspect of an interventional study is the selection of an appropriate outcome measure. Many times, no single appropriate testing modality will exist, and multiple modalities or even custom-developed testing modalities will have to be used as the outcome measures. Custom modalities will need to be standardized and validated. As shown above, functional tests are of the utmost importance for any interventional study, as they cannot only ensure benefit but also guard against possible harm.

Among the key questions to address while designing a trial are the following

- Is the expected outcome vision restoration or solely preservation? What are the patient's expectations?

- Are solid, reliable natural history data available to refine outcome measures?

- What are ways to cope with the natural variability of structural and functional parameters?

- Is efficacy better demonstrated using structural versus functional changes, or both, and over what time period?

Ethical considerations are of utmost importance for any interventional trial. We need to ensure that the patient receives all the information about the intended treatment in accessible language and is allowed enough time to reach an informed decision about participation. *Primum non nocere* should continue to be the main guiding principle for all interventions. We should strive to ensure that patients of any socioeconomic status would be able to benefit from a novel treatment in an equal manner. Finally, with a multitude of information available online, we should be prepared to provide guidance to patients seeking our advice regarding a planned trial offering them participation.

SUMMARY

As we enter a new and exciting era of a multitude of therapies and approaches being either developed or, in some cases, already available for IRDs, we should strive to continue to improve all aspects of clinical trials. Where possible, standardization of outcome measures should be employed. Testing modalities should be tailored to the individual patient, aiming to not only to allow better quantification of interventional outcomes, but also to ease the patient's clinical burden associated with trial participation.

REFERENCES

*Reference is also in this subject collection.

Aboshiha J, Luong V, Cowing J, Dubis AM, Bainbridge JW, Ali RR, Webster AR, Moore AT, Fitzke FW, Michaelides M. 2014. Dark-adaptation functions in molecularly confirmed achromatopsia and the implications for assessment in retinal therapy trials. *Invest Ophthalmol Vis Sci* **55:** 6340. doi:10.1167/iovs.14-14910

Adrian ED, Matthews BHC. 1934. The Berger rhythm: potential changes from the occipital lobes in man. *Brain* **57:** 355–385. doi:10.1093/brain/57.4.355

Alexander MF, Maguire MG, Lietman TM, Snyder JR, Elman MJ, Fine SL. 1988. Assessment of visual function in patients with age-related macular degeneration and low visual acuity. *Arch Ophthalmol* **106:** 1543–1547. doi:10.1001/archopht.1988.01060140711040

Authié CN, Berthoz A, Sahel JA, Safran A. 2017. Adaptive gaze strategies for locomotion with constricted visual field. *Front Hum Neurosci* **11:** 387. doi:10.3389/fnhum.2017.00387

Authié CN, Poujade M, Talebi A, Defer A, Zenouda A, Coen C, Mohand-Said S, Chaumet-Riffaud P, Audo I, Sahel JA. 2023. Development and validation of a novel mobility test for rod-cone dystrophies, from reality to virtual reality. *Am J Ophthalmol* doi:10.1016/j.ajo.2023.06.028

Bagdonaite-Bejarano L, Hansen RM, Fulton AB. 2019. Microperimetry in three inherited retinal disorders. *Semin Ophthalmol* **34:** 334–339. doi:10.1080/08820538.2019.1622025

Bailey IL, Lovie JE. 1976. New design principles for visual acuity letter charts. *Am J Optom Physiol Opt* **53:** 740–745. doi:10.1097/00006324-197611000-00006

Barnes CS, Schuchard RA, Birch DG, Dagnelie G, Wood L, Koenekoop RK, Bittner AK. 2019. Reliability of semiautomated kinetic perimetry (SKP) and Goldmann kinetic perimetry in children and adults with retinal dystrophies. *Transl Vis Sci Technol* **8:** 36–36. doi:10.1167/tvst.8.3.36

Berninger TA, Arden GB, Arden GB. 1988. The pattern electroretinogram. *Eye* **2:** S257–S283. doi:10.1038/eye.1988.149

Berson EL, Sandberg MA, Rosner B, Birch DG, Hanson AH. 1985. Natural course of retinitis pigmentosa over a three-year interval. *Am J Ophthalmol* **99:** 240–251. doi:10.1016/0002-9394(85)90351-4

Buckley TMW, Josan AS, Taylor LJ, Jolly JK, Cehajic-Kapetanovic J, MacLaren RE. 2022. Characterizing visual fields in *RPGR* related retinitis pigmentosa using octopus static-automated perimetry. *Transl Vis Sci Technol* **11:** 15. doi:10.1167/tvst.11.5.15

Byrne LC, Dalkara D, Luna G, Fisher SK, Clérin E, Sahel JA, Léveillard T, Flannery JG. 2015. Viral-mediated RdCVF and RdCVFL expression protects cone and rod photoreceptors in retinal degeneration. *J Clin Invest* **125:** 105–116. doi:10.1172/JCI65654

Cabral D, Coscas F, Pereira T, Français C, Geraldes C, Laiginhas R, Rodrigues C, Kashi AK, Nogueira V, Falcão M, et al. 2020. Quantitative optical coherence tomography angiography biomarkers in a treat-and-extend dosing regimen in neovascular age-related macular degeneration. *Transl Vis Sci Technol* **9:** 18. doi:10.1167/tvst.9.3.18

Çetinkaya A, Oto S, Akman A, Akova YA. 2008. Relationship between optokinetic nystagmus response and recognition visual acuity. *Eye (Lond)* **22:** 77–81. doi:10.1038/sj.eye.6702529

Chadderton N, Palfi A, Maloney DM, Carrigan M, Finnegan LK, Hanlon KS, Shortall C, O'Reilly M, Humphries P, Cassidy L, et al. 2023. Optimisation of AAV-NDI1 significantly enhances its therapeutic value for correcting retinal mitochondrial dysfunction. *Pharmaceutics* **15:** 322. doi:10.3390/pharmaceutics15020322

Chung DC, McCague S, Yu ZF, Thill S, DiStefano-Pappas J, Bennett J, Cross D, Marshall K, Wellman J, High KA. 2018. Novel mobility test to assess functional vision in patients with inherited retinal dystrophies. *Clin Exp Ophthalmol* **46:** 247–259. doi:10.1111/ceo.13022

* Chung D, Authié C, Blouin L. 2023. Mobility testing and other performance-based assessments of functional vision in patients with inherited retinal disease. *Cold Spring Harb Perspect Med* doi: 10.1101/cshperspect.a041299

Cooper RF, Brainard DH, Morgan JIW. 2020. Optoretinography of individual human cone photoreceptors. *Opt Express* **28:** 39326. doi:10.1364/OE.409193

Cross N, van Steen C, Zegaoui Y, Satherley A, Angellillo L. 2022. Retinitis pigmentosa: burden of disease and current unmet needs. *Clin Ophthalmol* **16:** 1993–2010. doi:10.2147/OPTH.S365486

Ferris FL, Kassoff A, Bresnick GH, Bailey I. 1982. New visual acuity charts for clinical research. *Am J Ophthalmol* **94:** 91–96. doi:10.1016/0002-9394(82)90197-0

Finger RP, McSweeney SC, Deverell L, O'Hare F, Bentley SA, Luu CD, Guymer RH, Ayton LN. 2014. Developing an instrumental activities of daily living tool as part of the low vision assessment of daily activities protocol. *Invest Ophthalmol Vis Sci* **55:** 8458–8466. doi:10.1167/iovs.14-14732

Frick KD, Gower EW, Kempen JH, Wolff JL. 2007. Economic impact of visual impairment and blindness in the United States. *Arch Ophthalmol* **125:** 544. doi:10.1001/archopht.125.4.544

Frick KD, Kymes SM, Lee PP, Matchar DB, Pezzullo ML, Rein DB, Taylor HR; Vancouver Economic Burden of Vision Loss Group. 2010. The cost of visual impairment: purposes, perspectives, and guidance. *Invest Ophthalmol Vis Sci* **51:** 1801–1805. doi:10.1167/iovs.09-4469

Cite this article as *Cold Spring Harb Perspect Med* doi: 10.1101/cshperspect.a041301

Granit R. 1933. The components of the retinal action potential in mammals and their relation to the discharge in the optic nerve. *J Physiol* **77:** 207–239. doi:10.1113/jphysiol.1933.sp002964

Gulati R, Roche H, Thayaparan K, Hornig R, Rubin GS. 2011. The development of a picture discrimination test for people with very poor vision. *Invest Ophthalmol Vis Sci* **52:** 1197–1197

Halliday AM, Mcdonald WI, Mushin J. 1972. Delayed visual evoked response in optic neuritis. *Lancet* **1:** 982–985. doi:10.1016/S0140-6736(72)91155-5

Hamilton R, Bach M, Heinrich SP, Hoffmann MB, Odom JV, McCulloch DL, Thompson DA. 2021. ISCEV extended protocol for VEP methods of estimation of visual acuity. *Doc Ophthalmol* **142:** 17–24. doi:10.1007/s10633-020-09780-1

Harter MR, White CT. 1968. Effects of contour sharpness and check-size on visually evoked cortical potentials. *Vision Res* **8:** 701–711. doi:10.1016/0042-6989(68)90044-8

Hoffmann MB, Bach M, Kondo M, Li S, Walker S, Holopigian K, Viswanathan S, Robson AG. 2021. ISCEV standard for clinical multifocal electroretinography (mfERG) (2021 update). *Doc Ophthalmol* **142:** 5–16. doi:10.1007/s10633-020-09812-w

Holder GE. 2004. Electrophysiological assessment of optic nerve disease. *Eye* **18:** 1133–1143. doi:10.1038/sj.eye.6701573

Hyon JY, Yeo HE, Seo JM, Lee IB, Lee JH, Hwang JM. 2010. Objective measurement of distance visual acuity determined by computerized optokinetic nystagmus test. *Investig Ophthalmol Vis Sci* **51:** 752–757. doi:10.1167/iovs.09-4362

Ishihara S. 1972. *Tests for colour-blindness.* Kanehara Shuppan, Tokyo.

Janeschitz-Kriegl L, Calzetti G, Michaelides M, Sahel JA, Nagy Z, Stringl K, Zi-Bing J, Duncan JL, Banin E, Lam BL, et al. 2022. Worldwide multicenter ocular imaging study (EyeConic) to identify patients eligible for cone-based optogenetics therapy. *Invest Ophthalmol Vis Sci* **63:** 455–455

Jauregui R, Park KS, Duong JK, Mahajan VB, Tsang SH. 2018. Quantitative progression of retinitis pigmentosa by optical coherence tomography angiography. *Sci Rep* **8:** 1–7. doi:10.1038/s41598-018-31488-1

Karanjia R, Hwang TJ, Chen AF, Pouw A, Tian JJ, Chu ER, Wang MY, Tran JS, Sadun AA. 2016. Correcting finger counting to Snellen acuity. *Neuroophthalmology* **40:** 219–221. doi:10.1080/01658107.2016.1209221

Kinnear PR, Sahraie A. 2002. New Farnsworth-Munsell 100 hue test norms of normal observers for each year of age 5–22 and for age decades 30–70. *Br J Ophthalmol* **86:** 1408–1411. doi:10.1136/bjo.86.12.1408

Lacy GD, Abalem MF, Andrews CA, Popova LT, Santos EP, Yu G, Rakine HY, Baig N, Ehrlich JR, Fahim AT, et al. 2021. The Michigan Retinal Degeneration Questionnaire: a patient-reported outcome instrument for inherited retinal degenerations. *Am J Ophthalmol* **222:** 60–68. doi:10.1016/j.ajo.2020.08.032

Lange R, Kumagai A, Weiss S, Zaffke KB, Day S, Wicker D, Howson A, Jayasundera KT, Smolinski L, Hedlich C, et al. 2021. Vision-related quality of life in adults with severe peripheral vision loss: a qualitative interview study. *J Patient Rep Outcomes* **5:** 7. doi:10.1186/s41687-020-00281-y

Leber T. 1869. Ueber retinitis pigmentosa und angeborene amaurose. *Arch für Opthalmologie* **15:** 1–25. doi:10.1007/BF02721213

Mangione CM, Lee PP, Gutierrez PR, Spritzer K, Berry S, Hays RD; National Eye Institute Visual Function Questionnaire Field Test Investigators. 2001. Development of the 25-item National Eye Institute Visual Function Questionnaire. *Arch Ophthalmol* **119:** 1050–1058. doi:10.1001/archopht.119.7.1050

Marron JA, Bailey IL. 1982. Visual factors and orientation-mobility performance. *Optom Vis Sci* **59:** 413–426. doi:10.1097/00006324-198205000-00009

McGrady NR, Boal AM, Risner ML, Taiel M, Sahel JA, Calkins DJ. 2023. Ocular stress enhances contralateral transfer of lenadogene nolparvovec gene therapy through astrocyte networks. *Mol Ther* **31:** 2005–2013. doi:10.1016/J.YMTHE.2023.03.035

Ménage MJ, Papakostopoulos D, Dean Hart JC, Papakostopoulos S, Gogolitsyn Y. 1993. The Farnsworth-Munsell 100 hue test in the first episode of demyelinating optic neuritis. *Br J Ophthalmol* **77:** 68–74. doi:10.1136/bjo.77.2.68

Newman NJ, Yu-Wai-Man P, Carelli V, Moster ML, Biousse V, Vignal-Clermont C, Sergott RC, Klopstock T, Sadun AA, Barboni P, et al. 2021. Efficacy and safety of intravitreal gene therapy for Leber hereditary optic neuropathy treated within 6 months of disease onset. *Ophthalmology* **128:** 649–660. doi:10.1016/j.ophtha.2020.12.012

Ng JS, Shih B. 2017. Level of visual acuity necessary to avoid false-positives on the HRR and Ishihara color vision tests. *Eur J Ophthalmol* **27:** 363–366. doi:10.5301/ejo.5000855

Oh JK, Nuzbrokh Y, Lima de Carvalho JR, Ryu J, Tsang SH. 2020. Optical coherence tomography in the evaluation of retinitis pigmentosa. *Ophthalmic Genet* **41:** 413–419. doi:10.1080/13816810.2020.1780619

Oishi A, Ogino K, Makiyama Y, Nakagawa S, Kurimoto M, Yoshimura N. 2013. Wide-field fundus autofluorescence imaging of retinitis pigmentosa. *Ophthalmology* **120:** 1827–1834. doi:10.1016/j.ophtha.2013.01.050

Okajima O, Tanino T, Okamoto M. 1982. Color vision defects in pigmentary retinal dystrophy. *Jpn J Ophthalmol* **26:** 292–301.

Orlans HO, McClements ME, Barnard AR, Martinez-Fernandez de la Camara C, MacLaren RE. 2021. Mirtron-mediated RNA knockdown/replacement therapy for the treatment of dominant retinitis pigmentosa. *Nat Commun* **12:** 4934. doi:10.1038/s41467-021-25204-3

Palanker D, Le Mer Y, Mohand-Said S, Sahel JA. 2022. Simultaneous perception of prosthetic and natural vision in AMD patients. *Nat Commun* **13:** 1–6. doi:10.1038/s41467-022-28125-x

Pandiyan VP, Maloney-Bertelli A, Kuchenbecker JA, Boyle KC, Ling T, Chen ZC, Park BH, Roorda A, Palanker D, Sabesan R. 2020. The optoretinogram reveals the primary steps of phototransduction in the living human eye. *Sci Adv* **6:** eabc1124. doi:10.1126/sciadv.abc1124

Pelli DG, Bex P. 2013. Measuring contrast sensitivity. *Vision Res* **90:** 10–14. doi:10.1016/j.visres.2013.04.015

Pelli DG, Robson JG, Wilkins AJ. 1988. The design of a new letter chart for measuring contrast sensitivity. *Clin Vis Sci* **2:** 187–199.

Pontikos N, Arno G, Jurkute N, Schiff E, Ba-Abbad R, Malka S, Gimenez A, Georgiou M, Wright G, Armengol M, et al. 2020. Genetic basis of inherited retinal disease in a molecularly characterized cohort of more than 3000 families from the United Kingdom. *Ophthalmology* **127:** 1384–1394. doi:10.1016/j.ophtha.2020.04.008

Prem Senthil M, Khadka J, Pesudovs K. 2017. Seeing through their eyes: lived experiences of people with retinitis pigmentosa. *Eye* **31:** 741–748. doi:10.1038/eye.2016.315

Prusky GT, Alam NM, Beekman S, Douglas RM. 2004. Rapid quantification of adult and developing mouse spatial vision using a virtual optomotor system. *Invest Ophthalmol Vis Sci* **45:** 4611–4616. doi:10.1167/iovs.04-0541

Pur DR, Lee-Wing N, Bona MD. 2023. The use of augmented reality and virtual reality for visual field expansion and visual acuity improvement in low vision rehabilitation: a systematic review. *Graefes Arch Clin Exp Ophthalmol* **261:** 1743–1755. doi:10.1007/s00417-022-05972-4

Regan D. 1973. Rapid objective refraction using evoked brain potentials. *Invest Ophthalmol* **12:** 669–679.

Riggs LA, Parker Johnson E, Schick AML. 1964. Electrical responses of the human eye to moving stimulus patterns. *Science* **144:** 567–567. doi:10.1126/science.144.3618.567

Robson AG, Frishman LJ, Grigg J, Hamilton R, Jeffrey BG, Kondo M, Li S, McCulloch DL. 2022. ISCEV standard for full-field clinical electroretinography (2022 update). *Doc Ophthalmol* **144:** 165–177. doi:10.1007/s10633-022-098 72-0

Roman AJ, Schwartz SB, Aleman TS, Cideciyan AV, Chico JD, Windsor EA, Gardner LM, Ying GS, Smilko EE, Maguire MG, et al. 2005. Quantifying rod photoreceptor-mediated vision in retinal degenerations: dark-adapted thresholds as outcome measures. *Exp Eye Res* **80:** 259–272. doi:10.1016/j.exer.2004.09.008

Russell SR, Drack AV, Cideciyan AV, Jacobson SG, Leroy BP, Van Cauwenbergh C, Ho AC, Dumitrescu AV, Han IC, Martin M, et al. 2022. Intravitreal antisense oligonucleotide sepofarsen in Leber congenital amaurosis type 10: a phase 1b/2 trial. *Nat Med* **28:** 1014–1021. doi:10.1038/s41591-022-01755-w

Sahel JA, Boulanger-Scemama E, Pagot C, Arleo A, Galluppi F, Martel JN, Esposti SD, Delaux A, de Saint Aubert JB, de Montleau C, et al. 2021a. Partial recovery of visual function in a blind patient after optogenetic therapy. *Nat Med* **27:** 1223–1229. doi:10.1038/s41591-021-01351-4

Sahel JA, Grieve K, Pagot C, Authié C, Mohand-Said S, Paques M, Audo I, Becker K, Chaumet-Riffaud AE, Azoulay L, et al. 2021b. Assessing photoreceptor status in retinal dystrophies: from high-resolution imaging to functional vision. *Am J Ophthalmol* **230:** 12–47. doi:10.1016/j.ajo.2021.04.013

Salmon AE, Cooper RF, Langlo CS, Baghaie A, Dubra A, Carroll J. 2017. An automated reference frame selection (ARFS) algorithm for cone imaging with adaptive optics scanning light ophthalmoscopy. *Transl Vis Sci Technol* **6:** 9. doi:10.1167/tvst.6.2.9

Sayo A, Ueno S, Kominami T, Nishida K, Inooka D, Nakanishi A, Yasuda S, Okado S, Takahashi K, Matsui S, et al. 2017. Longitudinal study of visual field changes determined by Humphrey field analyzer 10-2 in patients with retinitis pigmentosa. *Sci Rep* **7:** 16383. doi:10.1038/s41598-017-16640-7

Schiefer U, Pascual JP, Edmunds B, Feudner E, Hoffmann EM, Johnson CA, Lagrèze WA, Pfeiffer N, Sample PA, Staubach F, et al. 2009. Comparison of the new perimetric GATE strategy with conventional full-threshold and SITA standard strategies. *Invest Ophthalmol Vis Sci* **50:** 488. doi:10.1167/iovs.08-2229

Schönbach EM, Strauss RW, Cattaneo MEGV, Fujinami K, Birch DG, Cideciyan AV, Sunness JS, Zrenner E, Sadda SR, Scholl HPN, et al. 2022. Longitudinal changes of fixation stability and location within 24 months in Stargardt disease: ProgStar Report No. 16. *Am J Ophthalmol* **233:** 78–89. doi:10.1016/j.ajo.2021.07.013

Schulze-Bonsel K, Feltgen N, Burau H, Hansen L, Bach M. 2006. Visual acuities "hand motion" and "counting fingers" can be quantified with the Freiburg visual acuity test. *Invest Ophthalmol Vis Sci* **47:** 1236–1240. doi:10 .1167/iovs.05-0981

Stelmack JA, Szlyk JP, Stelmack TR, Demers-Turco P, Williams RT, Moran D, Massof RW. 2004. Psychometric properties of the Veterans Affairs Low-Vision Visual Functioning Questionnaire. *Invest Ophthalmol Vis Sci* **45:** 3919–3928. doi:10.1167/iovs.04-0208

Sugawara T, Hagiwara A, Hiramatsu A, Ogata K, Mitamura Y, Yamamoto S. 2009. Relationship between peripheral visual field loss and vision-related quality of life in patients with retinitis pigmentosa. *Eye* **24:** 535–539. doi:10 .1038/eye.2009.176

Thompson DA, Iannaccone A, Ali RR, Arshavsky VY, Audo I, Bainbridge JWB, Besirli CG, Birch DG, Branham KE, Cideciyan AV, et al. 2020. Advancing clinical trials for inherited retinal diseases: recommendations from the Second Monaciano Symposium. *Transl Vis Sci Technol* **9:** 2. doi:10.1167/tvst.9.7.2

von Krusenstiern L, Liu J, Liao E, Gow JA, Chen G, Ong T, Lotery AJ, Jalil A, Lam BL, MacLaren RE, et al. 2023. Changes in retinal sensitivity associated with cotoretigene toliparvovec in X-linked retinitis pigmentosa with RPGR gene variations. *JAMA Ophthalmol* **141:** 275–283. doi:10 .1001/jamaophthalmol.2022.6254

Wissinger B, Dangel S, Jägle H, Hansen L, Baumann B, Rudolph G, Wolf C, Bonin M, Koeppen K, Ladewig T, et al. 2008. Cone dystrophy with supernormal rod response is strictly associated with mutations in KCNV2. *Invest Ophthalmol Vis Sci* **49:** 751–757. doi:10.1167/iovs .07-0471

Xi Z, Vats A, Sahel JA, Chen Y, Byrne LC. 2022. Gene augmentation prevents retinal degeneration in a CRISPR/Cas9-based mouse model of PRPF31 retinitis pigmentosa. *Nat Commun* **13.** doi:10.1038/s41467-022-35361-8

Yang Y, Dunbar H. 2021. Clinical perspectives and trends: microperimetry as a trial endpoint in retinal disease. *Ophthalmol Int J Ophthalmol* **244:** 418–450. doi:10.1159/000515148

Zhang X, Zhang D, Thompson JA, Chen SC, Huang Z, Jennings L, McLaren TL, Lamey TM, De Roach JN, Chen FK, et al. 2021. Gene correction of the *CLN3* c.175G > A variant in patient-derived induced pluripotent stem cells prevents pathological changes in retinal organoids. *Mol Genet Genomic Med* **9:** 1601. doi:10.1002/mgg3.1601

Index

A

AAV. *See* Adeno-associated virus (AAV) gene therapy vectors
ABCA4
    retinitis pigmentosa, 4
    splice site mutations, 328
    Stargardt disease mutations, 4, 26, 29, 30
Achromatopsia
    cone dysfunction, 3
    genetic mutations, 6
    imaging for pathophysiology, 495–496
    models
        BEST1-related dystrophies, 80–83
        CNGA3, 79–80
        CNGB3, 80
        overview, 79
    prevalence, 28
Adaptive immune system, 180–181, 190
Adaptive optics (AO), 493–494
Adeno-associated virus (AAV) gene therapy vectors
    approaches to AAV engineering
        ancestral screening, 170–171
        biomining, 167–170
        high-throughput approaches, 171
        next-generation AAVs, 172
        promoters and *cis*-regulatory elements, 172–173
        rational mutagenesis, 170
        scAAVenger, 171
        in silico design, 171–172
    assessing full vs. empty capsids, 138–139
    choroideremia, 202
    gene editing strategies, 311
    humoral antiAAV2 neutralizing antibodies, 141–143
    immune response, 96–97
    innate immune response, 188–191
    obstacles within
        immune response, 166–167
        inner limiting membrane penetration, 165–166
        limited tropism, 165
        small packaging capacity, 166
    optogenetics, 285–286
    outcome measures, 143–144
    overview, 163–164
    rationale for, 164–165
    retinal regeneration, 472
    retinal transduction, 302
    RHO mutations, 233–234
    role in gene editing, 309–310
    RPE65 delivery, 130–131, 136–137
    safety of delivery device, 138

standard in ocular disease, 470
structure of AAV, 164
XLRS, 251–255
ADVQ, 512, 516
Afferent pupillary defect (APD), 143
Age-related macular degeneration (AMD)
    choroidal neovascularization, 38
    clinical features, 412
    clinical research on iPSC-RPE transplantation
        allogenic cell suspension, 421–423
        autologous cell sheet, 417–420
        overview, 414–417
    etiology, 42
    genetic models, 41–43
    geographic atrophy, 390
    overlap with Stargardt disease, 12
    overview, 448
    photoreceptor cell death, 38
    retinal replacement for treatment of, 469–470
    stem cell therapies in, 410–414
Albinism, 496–497
Alternative RNA splicing
    high throughput sequencing
        isoform identification and RNA-seq, 329–330
        long-read sequencing (LRS), 330
        single-cell resolution of isoforms, 330–331
    mutations in splicing factors
        RNA-binding proteins, 329
        spliceosome, 329
    overview, 325–326
    retinal organoid models, 331
    therapies for modulation of splicing
        antisense oligonucleotides (ASOs), 334–335
        CRISPR-based splicing, 332–334
        mature mRNAs and proteins, 335–336
        overview, 331–332
        spliceosome machinery therapeutics, 334
        trans-splicing-mediated therapies, 335
    types of
        alternative splice sites, 326–327
        cassette exon inclusion or skipping, 326
        intron retention, 327–329
        mutually exclusive exons, 329
        overview, 326
AMD. *See* Age-related macular degeneration
Antisense oligonucleotides (ASOs), 235, 312–314, 334–335
AO. *See* Adaptive optics
APD. *See* Afferent pupillary defect
Apoptosis, 263, 343–344
Argus II epiretinal prosthesis, 400–401

Index

ASOs. *See* Antisense oligonucleotides
Attitudes to Gene Therapy for the Eye (AGT-Eye), 515,
    526–528
Autophagy, 345–346, 350

B

Bardet–Biedl syndrome (BBS)
    clinical features, 2
    dog models, 63
    emblematic ciliopathy, 52
    gene mutations, 55
    human cell models, 64
    mouse models, 59–63
    nonhuman primate models, 63
    qualitative studies on, 534
    zebrafish models, 58–59
Base editing, 311–312
Batten disease, CLN3 variant, 5
BBS. *See* Bardet–Biedl syndrome
BBSome complex module, 54–55
BDNF. *See* Brain-derived neurotrophic factor
Best vitelliformmacular dystrophy, 4
BEST1
    gene-augmentation therapy, 82
    models, 80–81, 83
Blood–retinal barrier (BRB), 181–182, 184
Brain-derived neurotrophic factor (BDNF), 36, 277, 358

C

C3, age-related macular degeneration, 42
CABP4, congenital stationary night blindness mutations,
    81, 83
Cas12, 310–312
Cas13 and ADAR, 312, 315
Cas14, 312
Cas9, 310, 314
Cassette exon inclusion or skipping, 326–327
CCR2, 184
Cell death pathways, 183, 343–344, 347–348, 351
Cell therapy
    cell suspension, 451–452
    early studies, 417, 421
    organoids in, 113
    overview, 112
    retinal pigment epithelium (RPE) in, 429, 434, 438–441,
    449
    tissue formulation, 452–453
CEP290
    cat model, 74
    gene therapy, 128, 130, 315–317
    intronic mutations, 335
    LCA, 6, 73, 311, 314, 326, 331
    mouse model, 60
    splice site mutations in, 328
CFH, age-related macular degeneration susceptibility
    studies, 42–43

cGMP-signaling, 343, 344–345, 348, 350–351
Channelrhodopsin-2 (ChR2)
    gene therapy, 130
    optogenetics, 289–291, 300–304
Chemokine fractalkine (CX3CL1), 182, 184
CHM
    choroideremia imaging, 498–499
    choroideremia mutations, 201–202, 205
        clinical genetics of, 209–210
        female carriers, 208–209
    disease mechanism of in choroideremia, 210–211
Choroidal neovascularization (CNV), age-related macular
        degeneration, 38, 411–414, 417, 448
Choroideremia
    clinical genetics, 209–210
    clinical phenotype
        differential diagnosis, 206–207
        female carriers, 208–209
        images, 206–207
        overview, 202–206
    clinical trials
        inclusion of patients with late choroideremia, 212–213
        overview, 212
        RPE disfunction in late disease, 213–214
        short duration of, 212
        summary of, 203–204
        surgical detachment of fovea, 213
    disease mechanism, 210–211
    imaging structure-function correlations of cone mosaic,
        498–499
    near-infrared fluorescence imaging, 215
    overview, 201–202
    regulatory approval of gene therapy
        modification of process, 215–216
        novel end points, 214–215
    retinal appearance in, 205
ChrimsonR, 293–294, 303
Cilia
    overview, 52
    proteins, 53–55
    schematic, 53
Ciliary neurotrophic factor (CNTF), 358–360
Ciliopathy
    nonvertebrate models, 57–58
    phenotypes and genotypes, 52–57
    RPGR-associated, 223–225
    vertebrate models
        dog models, 63
        human cell models, 64
        mouse models, 59–63
        nonhuman primate models, 63
        zebrafish models, 58–59
CNGB1, 74–76
CNGC, 344–345, 347, 351
CNTF. *See* ciliary neurotrophic factor
CNV. *See* choroidal neovascularization
Cone mosaic, imaging structure-function correlations
    choroideremia, 498–499
    retinitis pigmentosa, 497–498

Cone-rod degenerations/dystrophies (CORDs)
    genetics, 6
    RPGR, 221–223
Congenital stationary night blindness (CSNB)
    gene mutations, 3, 6
    models, 81, 83
    phenotypes, 29–30
    photoreceptor to bipolar cell connectivity mutations, 83
    prevalence, 28
Contrast sensitivity, 548–549
CORDs. *See* Cone-rod degenerations/dystrophies
CRB1, 6, 40, 43, 326
cre-lox gene targeting, 43–44
CRISPR/Cas9, 310, 311, 332–334
CRX
    cat model, 72–74
    in LCA, 6
CSNB. *See* congenital stationary night blindness

D

Damage-associated molecular patterns (DAMPs), 181–183, 189–191
DAMPs. *See* Damage-associated molecular patterns
Diabetic retinopathy
    genetic manipulations, 98
    immune system in retinal transplants, 95–97
    molecular manipulations, 98
    overview, 94–95
    retinal gene editing, 99–100
    retinal gene therapy, 100–102
    transgenic models, 98–99
Diabetic retinopathy, retinal regeneration as treatment, 470
Digenic disease, 12, 18
DNA editing
    antisense oligonucleotides (ASOs), 313–314
    base editing, 312–313
    Cas 12, 310–312
    Cas 13 and ADARs, 315
    Cas 14, 312
    CRISPR/Cas9, 310
    prime editing, 313
    RNA editing, 313
    short-hairpin RNAs (shRNAs), 314–315
Docosahexaenoic acid, 226
DTPQ, 511, 513, 520

E

EDTQ, 511–512, 516
Electrical stimulation of neurons, 391–392
Electronic retinal prostheses
    approaches to
        anatomical position
            epiretinal implants, 392–393
            subretinal implants, 393–394
        delivery of power and data, 394–395
        electrical stimulation of neurons, 391–392
        overview, 389–391

clinical evaluation
    Argus II epiretinal prosthesis, 400–401
    criteria for, 400
    other clinical results, 402–403
    overview, 400
    photovoltaic subretinal implant PRIMA, 401–402
    subretinal implant Alpha IMS/AMS, 401
    suprachoroidal systems, 402
outlook, 403
    electric field shaping for high resolution in subretinal approach, 403–404
    flexible implants for wide visual field, 404
    image processing, 404–405
    selective stimulation of RGCs, 404
preclinical evaluation
    in vivo characterization
        contrast sensitivity, 399–400
        frequency dependence, 400
        lateral resolution, 399
        overview, 398–399
    retinal response to stimulation
        contrast sensitivity, 397–398
        electric receptive fields, 395–396
        lateral resolution, 396–397
Embryoid bodies, 113–114, 116, 332
Energy metabolism in photoreceptor cells, 347–348, 350
ERAD and autophagy, 346–347
Eye size
    dosing, 137–138
    pig eyes, 92–93

F

ff-ERG. *See* Full-field electroretinogram
FGF. *See* Fibroblast growth factor
Fibroblast growth factor (FGF), 37, 358–359, 431–432, 463
Field Expander Questionnaire, 512, 516
FLORA. *See* Functional low-vision observer-rated assessment
Full-field electroretinogram (ff-ERG), 2
Functional low-vision observer-rated assessment (FLORA), 542–543

G

GDNF. *See* Glial-derived neurotrophic factor
Gene editing. *See also* Adeno-associated virus (AAV) gene therapy vectors; CRISPR/Cas9; DNA editing
    adeno-associated virus (AAV), 309–310
    CRISPR/Cas9, 277, 310
    lentiviruses, 310
    overview, 232–233, 311–312
    pig models in retinal disease, 99–100
    RHO, 234
Gene expression control, 301–302
Gene therapy
    assessing full vs. empty capsids, 138–139
    choroideremia, 210
    clinical trials, 144–145
        choroideremia, 212–214
        color vision, 549

Gene therapy (*Continued*)
    dark adaptation, 549
    design and outcomes
        design considerations, 553
        electrophysiology, 549
        navigation tasks, 551–553
        overview, 547–548
        psychophysics, 549–550
        visual acuity and contrast sensitivity, 548–549
        visual fields, 549–50
        visual function vs. functional vision, 550–551
    cone survival in RP
        alterations in rod metabolism, 384–385
        gluconeogenesis, 384
        mTOR, 384
        rdCVF, 384
        Txnip, 384
    current clinical targets, 127–128
    development, 139–143
    dosing and model differences, 137–138
    immune response to viral vector, 187–191
    Leber hereditary optic neuropathy (LHON)
        overview, 263–265
        phase I and II clinical trials, 267–274
        phase III clinical trials, 274–276
        preclinical studies, 265–267
    microRNA, 239
    model systems for testing in RHO mutations, 232–233
    neuroprotection in, 449
    outcome measures, 143–144
    overview, 111, 125–126
    questions and challenges
        gain-of-function mutations, 129–130
        gene-agnostic approaches, 130
        route of administration, 128–129
        vector design, 129
    retinal organiods, 112–113
    RPE65, 130–131
    RPGR, 226–227
    safety of delivery devices, 138
    vector development, 292
    vectors, 126–127
    vertical transmission, 143
Glaucoma
    glutamate excitotoxicity, 39
    intraocular pressure, 38
    model for, 41
    retinal regeneration treatment, 470
Glial-derived neurotrophic factor (GDNF), 182, 190, 237, 358–359
Glucose metabolism
    insufficient glucose in cones, 382–384
    overview in retinitis pigmentosa, 381–382
GPCR, 231, 284, 301, 303
GUCY2D, 344–345

H

HGP. *See* Human Genome Project
Human embryonic stem cells, 451

Human Genome Project (HGP), 13–14
Human pluripotent stem cells, 451
Human-induced pluripotent stem cells, 451

I

Immune system
    adaptive in retinitis pigmentosa, 180–181
    innate in retinitis pigmentosa, 181–182
Immunomodulation, 186–187
Immunosuppression, 186–187
Independent Mobility Questionnaire, 512, 518
Induced pluripotent stem cells
    organoid regeneration, 116
    overview, 409
    regenerative medicine resource, 410, 429
    retinal pigment epithelial transplantation
        allogeneic cell suspension, 421–422
        animal models for preclinical studies, 437–438
        autologous cell sheet, 417–420
        autologous iPSC-RPE patch transplant, 441
        clinical development overview, 433
        clinical development validation
            differentiation and maturation, 434–435
            functional validation, 436
            iPSC quality assessment, 433–434
            junctional validation, 437
            molecular validation, 435–436
            morphometric validation, 436–437
            somatic cell donor screening, 433
            structural validation, 436
        overview, 411, 413–417
        regulatory challenges, 438–441
Inflammation, 179–180
Inherited retinal diseases (IRDs)
    adaptive optics imaging
        imaging structure-function correlations of cone mosaic, 497–499
        overview, 493–494, 501–502
        pathophysiology, 494–497
    canine and feline models, 71–72
    choroideremia, 201
    chromosomal assignment, 13
    clinical trials, 7–8
    disease prevalence
        versus genetic prevalence, 24–30
        overview, 23–24
    early research, 12–13
    epigenetics, 7
    future clinical development, 350–352
    gene discovery, 11
    history of terms and concept changes, 11–12
    Human Genome Project (HGP), 13–14
    inflammation in, 179–180
    knowledge gaps addressed by natural history studies
        defining patient populations, 481–482
        developing clinical endpoints, 482–484
    massive parallel sequencing applied to, 5–7

mobility testing
  functional low-vision observer-rated assessment (FLORA), 542–543
  multi-luminance mobility test (MLMT), 540–541, 545
  orientation and mobility assessment for retinal prostheses, 541–542
  overview, 539–540
  StreetLab and mobility standardized test (MOST), 543–5444
  vision-guided mobility assessment, 543
modern clinical science
  definition of IRD gene, 15
  expanding human genetics, 17–18
  mutation databases, 16–17
  population-based genetic screening, 15–16
  research trends, 14–15
modern era of genetics, 14
natural history studies in therapy development, 477–480
overview, 1–2, 477
overview of neurotrophic factors, 357–358
pathomechanisms for, 343–344
patient-reported outcomes, 507–508
phenotypic delineation, 7–8
phenotypic variability, 2–5
present and future research, 18–19
qualitative research, 532
research support, 12
therapeutic gene editing (*See* DNA editing; gene editing)
therapy development
  improving energy metabolism, 350
  rebalancing photoreceptor proteostasis, 348–350
  targeting CNGC and PKG, 348
Inherited retinal dystrophy, 51–52
Innate intercellular signaling, 182
Intraocular pressure, 38
Intron retention, 327–329
Isoform identification/quantification with short-read RNA sequencing (RNA-seq), 329–330

J

Joubert syndrome, 52, 57

L

Laser-induced subretinal inflammation, 38
LCA. *See* Leber congenital amaurosis
Leber congenital amaurosis (LCA)
  assessment with NEI-VFQ, 531
  gene therapy, 125
  genetic causes, 6, 12, 29
  models
    CEP290, 74, 315–317, 327
    CRX, 72–74
    NPHP5, 72
    RD3, 74
    RPE65, 72, 139, 315

patient outcomes, 515
prevalence, 26–28
Leber hereditary optic neuropathy (LHON)
  clinical features, 260–261
  future research, 276–277
  gene therapy, 41
  ophthalmological images, 261
  other approaches, 277–278
  overview, 259–260, 263–265
  pathogenetic mechanisms, 261–263
  phase I and II clinical trials, 267–274
  phase III clinical trials, 274–276
  preclinical studies, 265–267
Lentiviruses, 310–311
LHON. *See* Leber hereditary optic neuropathy
Light damage, 38
Long-read sequencing, 330
LRIT3, congenital stationary night blindness mutations, 6, 81, 83

M

Macrophages
  peripherally derived, 183–184
  phenotypes, 185–186
Mainzer–Saldino syndrome, 57
Massive parallel sequencing, 5–7
MDQ, 511–512, 516
MERTK
  LCA, 6
  microglia and macrophage phenotypes, 185
  retinal degeneration, 40, 328
  retinitis pigmentosa, 41, 196, 424
MG. *See* Müller glia
Michigan Retinal Degeneration Questionnaire (MRDQ), 514, 524–526, 529–530, 532
Michigan Vision-Related Anxiety Questionnaire (MVAQ), 514, 526, 530
Microglia phenotypes, 185–186
microRNA, 239
Mitochondria, 262
MLMT. *See* Multi-luminance mobility test
Mobility standardized test (MOST), 543–544
Mobility testing
  functional low-vision observer-rated assessment (FLORA), 542–543
  multi-luminance mobility test (MLMT), 540–541, 545
  orientation and mobility assessments for retinal prostheses, 541–542
  overview, 539–540
  StreetLab and Mobility Standardized Test (MOST), 543–544
  vision-guided mobility assessment, 543
Molecular manipulations, pig models, 98
Monogenic disease, 12, 179, 358
MOST. *See* Mobility standardized test
MRDQ. *See* Michigan Retinal Degeneration Questionnaire
MVAQ. *See* Michigan Vision-Related Anxiety Questionnaire
mRNAs and protein therapies, 335–336

mtDNA, 261–263
Müller glia (MG)
    factors affecting proliferation of, 463–465
    in regenerative therapy, 470–472
    as source of retinal regeneration, 462
    stimulation of regeneration in mice, 466–469
Multi-luminance mobility test (MLMT), 144, 153, 540–541,
    545, 551
Mutation databases, 16–17

N

National Eye Institute Visual Function Questionnaire (NEI-
    VFQ), 512–513, 517, 519, 529, 531–532
Natural history studies
    examples of in IRDs
        FFB Consortium, 485–489
        overview, 484–485
        Stargardt disease and ProgStar, 485
    informing clinical trial design, 478
    overview, 477
    rare diseases, 480–481
    role of in therapy development, 477–480
    utility in knowledge gaps
        defining patient populations, 481–482
        developing clinical endpoints, 482–484
        overview, 481
NEI-VFQ. *See* National Eye Institute Visual Function
    Questionnaire
Nephronophthisis (NPHP), 52, 54, 57
Neurotrophic factors, 232, 237
    CNTF, 359–360
    FGF, 359
    GDNF, 359
    overview, 357–358, 361–362
    RdCVF, 360–361
Next-generation-sequencing, 5, 7, 330
Night Vision Questionnaire, 513, 522
NPHP5
    dog model, 72, 73
    mouse model, 63
NXNL, 372–374
NXNL1
    characterization, 367–368
    metabolic and redox signaling, 370–372
    therapeutic development, 375
    thioredoxin RdCVFL, 368–370
NXNL2, 374–375

O

ON bipolar cells, 283, 290, 304
Opsin genes, 239
Opsins, 284–285
Optical coherence tomography, 146
Optogenetic vision restoration
    activation of ON bipolar cells, 304
    activation of RGCs, 302–304
    administration, 286–287
    animal model studies, 289–291
    clinical trials, 294
    expression control, 301–302
    gene transfer, 302
    new methods, 294
    new optogenetic proteins
        ChrimsonR, 293–294
        overview, 292–293
    new promoters, 288–292
    opsins, 284–285
    overview, 283–284
    promoters, 287–288
    reactivating dormant cone photoreceptors, 304–305
    tools, 300–301
    vector development, 292
    vectors, 285–286
    visual acuity measures, 294–295
Oxidative phosphorylation, 262
Oxygen-induced retinopathy, 39

P

PAMPs. *See* Pathogen-associated molecular patterns
Pathogen-associated molecular patterns (PAMPs), 181, 191
Pathophysiology, imaging for
    achromatopsia, 495–496
    albinism, 496–497
    red-green color vision deficiency, 494–495
Patient-reported outcome measures
    discussion and recommendations, 532–535
    overview, 507–508
    prior to 2009 FDA guidance
        discussion, 511, 529
        table of instruments, 512–528
    in rare diseases and pediatric populations, 509–511
    regulatory considerations for product development,
        508–509
    since 2009 FDA guidance, 529–532
Pattern recognition receptors, 181
PDE6A, dog model, 74–75
PDE6B, dog model, 75–76
Peripherally derived macrophages, 183–184
Photoreceptors
    bipolar cell connectivity disorders, 83
    cGMP-signaling in physiology and pathophysiology,
        344–345
    energy metabolism in cell death and survival, 347–348
    functional biomarkers in imaging, 501
    historical perspectives of cell replacement
        cell therapy formulation, 451–453
        differentiation from pluripotent stem cells, 451
        optimization of cell integration and functionality,
            453–456
        of transplantation with fetal or adult retinas,
            450–451
    preserving viability of
        microRNA gene therapy, 239
        modulation of retinal bioenergetics, 237–238
        neurotrophic factors, 237

suppression of unfolded protein response (UPR), 237
rebalancing proteostasis, 350–352
structural biomarkers in imaging, 500–501
Photovoltaic subretinal implant PRIMA, 401–402
Pig models
    diabetic retinopathy
        genetic manipulations, 98
        immune systems in retinal transplants, 95–97
        molecular manipulations, 98
        overview, 94–95
        retinal gene editing, 99–100
        retinal gene therapy, 100–102
        transgenic models, 98–99
    eye size and retinal morphology, 92–93
    overview, 91–92
    physical characteristics, 92
    retinal development, 93–94
Pluripotent stem cells, 113–114
    organoid generation, 109
Population-based genetic screening, 15–16
Primary retinal ischemia, 39
Prime editing, 311, 313
ProgStar studies, 485–486
Prosthetic vision. *See* Electronic retinal prostheses
Proteasomal degradation, 345–346
Protein kinase G (PKG), 345, 348, 351
Proteostasis, 345–346, 348–350
PRPF31, 18
PRPH2, 40
Psychophysics, 549–550
PVFQ, 513, 521

Q

Quality of Life (QOL), 514, 523

R

RD3, 74
RDH5, 81, 83–85
Red-green color vision deficiency, 494–495
Regenerative medicine
    development of, 424
    future prospects and challenges
        improved efficacy, 425–426
        new categories of disease groups and medications, 424
        objective evaluation, 424–425
        technical improvements, 426
    human eyes, 412
    induced pluripotent stem cells (iPSCs) as resource in, 410
    laws for, 423–424
    overview, 409–410
Resident microglia, 183–184
Retina
    anatomy overview, 299–300
    cell type composition, 447–448
Retinal bioenergetics, 237–238
Retinal degeneration. *See also* Retinitis pigmentosa

degenerative mechanisms in, 351
development of treatment strategies, 448–450
inflammation, 179–180
overview, 300
pharmacological models, 39
retinitis pigmentosa, 448
stem cell–based therapies, 410–416, 429
Retinal development, pig models, 93–94
Retinal explant cultures, 37
Retinal function, ex vivo study
    cre-lox gene targeting, 43–44
    increased intraocular pressure, 38
    induced genetic models, 41–43
    laser-induced subretinal inflammation, 38
    light damage, 38
    naturally occurring models, 39–41
    overview, 37–38
    oxygen-induced retinopathy, 39
    pharmacological models, 39
Retinal ganglion cells
    loss of, 35
    optogenetic activation, 302–305
    in optogenetics, 287–288
    overview, 299–300
    in vitro culture, 36
Retinal gene editing, 99–100. *See also* Gene editing
Retinal gene therapy, 100–102. *See also* Gene therapy
Retinal morphology of pig eyes, 92–93
Retinal organoids
    analysis methods, 119
    high-throughput culture
        culture time, 115
        functional assays, 118–119
        imaging, 115, 119
        live imaging, 115–117
        molecular assays, 117–119
        organoid morphology, 114–115
        organoid analysis, 115
        overview, 112–114
    human as model systems
        comparison to human retina, 110–111
        mimicking retinal development, 110
        splicing-related retinal disease, 331
    overview, 109–110
    scaling up, 112
    therapy development, 111–112
Retinal pigment epithelium
    allogeneic cell suspension transplantation, 420–422
    autologous cell sheet transplantation, 417–419
    autologous patch transplantation, 435, 441
    clinical research on transplantation AMD, 414–417
    degeneration of in AMD, 448
    degeneration of in choroideremia, 201–202, 205, 211
    development and differentiation, 430–433
    efficacy of transplantation, 425–426
    evaluation of transplantation, 424–425

Retinal pigment epithelium (*Continued*)
  glucose transport in, 383
  in immune function, 182
  juctional integrity in transplants, 437
  metabolism of, 381–382
  molecular validation in transplants, 435–436
  morphometric validation in transplants, 436–437
  organoid culture, 116
  photoreceptor function, 2
  retinal degeneration, 424, 429
  role of in vision, 430
  RPE65 expressed in, 153
  structural validation in transplants, 436
  validation in transplants, 434–435
  in vitro culture of, 36
Retinal prostheses, 541–542
Retinal regeneration
  cone replacement in AMD, 469–470
  development of approaches to, 462–466
  overview, 461–462
  stimulation of in mice, 466–469
  therapy, 470–472
  treatment of diabetic retinopathy, 470
Retinal replacement, 449, 450–456, 461–462
Retinal transplants
  developing alternatives, 461–462
  historical perspectives, 450–451
  immune systems in viral-mediated gene therapy, 95–97
Retinitis pigmentosa (RP)
  adaptive immune system in, 180–181
  assessment with ADVQ, 516
  assessment with DTPQ, 520
  assessment with NEI-VFQ, 531
  assessment with V-ADL, 521
  clinical features, 2–4, 390–391, 412
  damage-associated molecular patterns, 182–183
  digenic diseases, 12
  disease versus genetic prevalence, 24–26
  gene therapy for cone survival
    alterations in rod metabolism, 384–385
    gluconeogenesis, 384
    mTOR, 384
    rdCVF, 384
    Txnip, 384
  genetic variability in, 300
  genetics of, 3–6
  history of, 13
  history of inflammation in, 179–180
  imaging structure-function correlations of cone mosaic, 497–498
  immune response to viral vector-associated gene therapy, 187–191
  immunosuppression and immunomodulation, 186–187
  incidence, 2
  inflammation, 179–180
  innate immune system, 181–182
  innate intercellular signaling, 182
  insufficient glucose in cones, 382–384

metabolism overview, 381–382
mobility standardized test (MOST), 544
models
  CNGB1, 74
  in dogs, 78–79
  PDE6A, 74–76
  PDE6B, 76
  RHO, 76–78
  RPGR, 78
neurotrophic factors, 358
overview, 1, 448
photoreceptor cell death, 38
progression of, 365–366
qualitative studies of, 533–534
resident microglia vs. peripherally derived macrophages, 183–184
RHO, 231–232, 317–18
spectrum of microglia/macrophage phenotypes, 185–186
Retinopathy of prematurity, 39, 470
RGR, 206–207
RHO. *See* Rhodopsin
Rhodopsin (RHO)
  in choroideremia, 206
  dog model, 75
  gene editing
    antisense oligonucleotides (ASOs), 235
    overview, 234
    RNA replacement, 235–236
    transcriptional repression, 235
  gene therapy
    adRP, 317–318
    model systems, 232–233
    other delivery methods, 234
    targeting overview, 234
    viral vectors for, 233–234
  overview of mutations, 231–232
  preserving viability of photoreceptors
    microRNA gene therapy, 238
    modulation of retinal bioenergetics, 237–238
    neurotrophic factors, 237
    overview, 236
    suppression of unfolded protein response (UPR), 237
  retinitis pigmentosa imaging, 497
  retinitis pigmentosa mutations, 2–5, 76–78
RNA interference (RNAi), 335
RNA replacement, 235–236
RNA splicing. *See* alternative RNA splicing
Rod-cone cellular interactions, evolution of, 372–376
Rod-derived cone viability factor (RdCVF), 360–362, 366–368, 371, 374, 382
Rod-derived cone viability factor long (RdCVFL), 368–371, 374
RP. *See* Retinitis pigmentosa
RP1, 13–14
RP2, 221
RPE65
  choroideremia, 206
  clinical trials, 139–140, 144–145

development, 139–141
discovery of, 13–14
extrapolation to inherited retinal degenerations, 146–147
gene therapy, 1, 35, 85, 130–131, 136–137
LCA dog model, 72
Luxturna, 315, 361
role of in visual cycle, 155
variations and predictions of efficacy, 141
RPGR
animal models, 40, 75, 78, 225
COD and CORD phenotypes, 222–223
female carriers, 223
gene-replacement therapy, 226–227
molecular genetics, 224
overview, 221
phenotypes and clinical features, 222
rod-cone dystrophy, 222
structure and function, 224–225
syndromic ciliopathy, 223–224
treatment principles, 225–226
RPGRIP1, 6, 75, 78, 224
RS1, 249–251

S

Senior–Loken syndrome, 57
Short-hairpin RNAs (shRNAs), 312, 314–315, 381
shRNAs. *See* short-hairpin RNAs
SMDVQ, 512, 519
Spinocerebellar ataxia, 319
Splice-complex proteins, 18
Spliceosome, 329, 334
Stargardt disease
genetics, 26–27, 29
overlap with age-related macular degeneration, 12
overview, 26
prevalence, 25, 27
ProgStar studies, 485
Stem cell therapies overview, 410–414
StreetLab, 543–544, 552
Subretinal implant Alpha IMS/AMS, 401
Suprachoroidal implant systems, 402

T

Thioredoxin, 372
Thioredoxin RdCVFL, 368–370
Trans-splicing-mediated therapeutics, 335
Transcription factors, 410, 463, 472
Transcriptional repression, 235
Transgenic pig models, 98–99
Tumor necrosis factor-α, retinal ganglion cells, 36

U

Unfolded protein response (UPR), 237
UPR. *See* Unfolded protein response
USH2A, 318–319
Usher syndrome

gene mutations, 18
gene therapy, 41–42
overview, 27–28
prevalence, 25, 27–28
qualitative studies of, 533–534
USH2A, 4, 18, 318–319

V

V-ADL. *See* Vision-related activities of daily living
Vascular endothelial growth factor, 36
VDQ, 512, 519
VFS. *See* Vision Function Scale
Viral-mediated gene therapy, 95–97
Virtual reality, 552–553
ViSIO-PRO, 515, 528
Vision Function Scale (VFS), 524
Vision-guided mobility assessment, 543
Vision-related activities of daily living (V-ADL), 513, 521
Vision-related Quality of Life (VisQOL), 513, 521
VisQOL. *See* Vision-related Quality of Life
Visual acuity, 548–549, 550–551
Visual Function Scale (VFS), 514
Voretigene neparvovec-rzyl (Luxturna)
age and effectiveness, 144–145
assessing safety, 141–143
clinical trials, 139–141
clinical development process, 152
FDA advisory committee, 159–160
natural history studies, 160–161
novel primary end point, 156–158
overview, 151–152
secondary and exploratory endpoints, 158–159
trial design, 152–156
development and approval, 135–136
LCA treatment, 315
limits of application, 357
route of administration, 136–137

W

Warburg effect, 381
Whole-exome sequencing, 5
Whole-genome sequencing, 5

X

X-linked retinitis pigmentosa (XLRP), 222
X-linked retinoschisis (XLRS)
clinical disease overview, 247–249
diagnostics, 249–250
gene therapy, 251–255
images, 248
inheritance, gene and cell biology, 249
medical management, 250–251
mouse models, 251
qualitative studies, 533
XLRP. *See* X-linked retinitis pigmentosa
XLRS. *See* X-linked retinoschisis